Pharmacotherapy Handbook

NOTICE

Medicine is an ever-changing science. As new research and clinical experience broaden our knowledge, changes in treatment and drug therapy are required. The authors and the publisher of this work have checked with sources believed to be reliable in their efforts to provide information that is complete and generally in accord with the standards accepted at the time of publication. However, in view of the possibility of human error or changes in medical sciences, neither the authors nor the publisher nor any other party who has been involved in the preparation or publication of this work warrants that the information contained herein is in every respect accurate or complete, and they disclaim all responsibility for any errors or omissions or for the results obtained from use of the information contained in this work. Readers are encouraged to confirm the information contained herein with other sources. For example and in particular, readers are advised to check the product information sheet included in the package of each drug they plan to administer to be certain that the information contained in this work is accurate and that changes have not been made in the recommended dose or in the contraindications for administration. This recommendation is of particular importance in connection with new or infrequently used drugs.

Pharmacotherapy Handbook

Eighth Edition

Barbara G. Wells, PharmD, FASHP, FCCP, BCPP

Dean and Professor
Executive Director, Research Institute of Pharmaceutical Sciences
School of Pharmacy, The University of Mississippi
Oxford, Mississippi

Joseph T. DiPiro, PharmD, FCCP

Professor and Executive Dean
South Carolina College of Pharmacy
Medical University of South Carolina, Charleston,
and University of South Carolina, Columbia

Terry L. Schwinghammer, PharmD, FCCP, FASHP, FAPhA, BCPS

Professor and Chair, Department of Clinical Pharmacy
School of Pharmacy, West Virginia University
Morgantown, West Virginia

Cecily V. DiPiro, PharmD

Consultant Pharmacist
Mount Pleasant, South Carolina

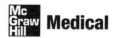

New York   Chicago   San Francisco   Lisbon   London   Madrid   Mexico City
Milan   New Delhi   Paris   San Juan   Seoul   Singapore   Sydney   Toronto

Pharmacotherapy Handbook, Eighth Edition

Copyright © 2012 by The McGraw-Hill Companies, Inc. All rights reserved. Printed in United States of America. Except as permitted under the United States Copyright Act of 1976, no part of this publication may be reproduced or distributed in any form or by any means, or stored in a database or retrieval system, without the prior written permission of the publisher.

Previous edition copyright © 2009, 2006, 2003, 2000, by The McGraw-Hill Companies, Inc.; copyright © 1998 by Appleton & Lange.

3 4 5 6 7 8 9 0   DOC/DOC   15 14 13

ISBN 978-0-07-174834-6
MHID 0-07-174834-2

This book was set in Minion Pro by Thomson Digital.
The editors were Michael Weitz and Karen G. Edmonson.
The Production Supervisor was Sherri Souffrance.
Project management was provided by Aakriti Kathuria, Thomson Digital.
The designer was Alan Barnett; the cover photo by David Mack/PhotoResearchers, Inc.
RR Donnelley was the printer and binder.

Library of Congress Cataloging-in-Publication Data
Pharmacotherapy handbook / [edited by] Barbara G. Wells ... [et al.]. — 8th ed.
   p. ; cm.
 Includes bibliographical references and index.
 ISBN-13: 978-0-07-174834-6 (soft cover : alk. paper)
 ISBN-10: 0-07-174834-2 (soft cover : alk. paper)
 1. Drugs—Handbooks, manuals, etc. 2. Chemotherapy—Handbooks, manuals, etc. I. Wells, Barbara G.
 [DNLM: 1. Drug Therapy—Handbooks. WB 39]
 RM301.12.P46 2011
 615.5'8—dc23

                                                               2011024912

INTERNATIONAL EDITION ISBN 978-0-07-178846-5; MHID 0-07-178846-8
Copyright © 2012. Exclusive rights by The McGraw-Hill Companies, Inc., for manufacture and export. This book cannot be re-exported from the country to which it is consigned by McGraw-Hill. The International Edition is not available in North America.

Contents

SECTION 1: BONE AND JOINT DISORDERS

Edited by Terry L. Schwinghammer

SECTION 2: CARDIOVASCULAR DISORDERS

Edited by Terry L. Schwinghammer

SECTION 3: DERMATOLOGIC DISORDERS

Edited by Terry L. Schwinghammer

SECTION 4: ENDOCRINOLOGIC DISORDERS

Edited by Terry L. Schwinghammer

Contents

SECTION 9: NEUROLOGIC DISORDERS

Edited by Barbara G. Wells

SECTION 10: NUTRITIONAL DISORDERS

Edited by Cecily V. DiPiro

SECTION 11: ONCOLOGIC DISORDERS

Edited by Cecily V. DiPiro

SECTION 12: OPHTHALMIC DISORDERS

Edited by Cecily V. DiPiro

Contents

Preface

This pocket companion to *Pharmacotherapy: A Pathophysiologic Approach*, eighth edition, is designed to provide practitioners and students with critical information that can be easily used to guide drug therapy decision making in the clinical setting. To ensure brevity and portability, the bulleted format provides the user with essential textual information, key tables and figures, and treatment algorithms.

Corresponding to the major sections in the main text, disorders are alphabetized within the following sections: Bone and Joint Disorders, Cardiovascular Disorders, Dermatologic Disorders, Endocrinologic Disorders, Gastrointestinal Disorders, Gynecologic and Obstetric Disorders, Hematologic Disorders, Infectious Diseases, Neurologic Disorders, Nutritional Disorders, Oncologic Disorders, Ophthalmic Disorders, Psychiatric Disorders, Renal Disorders, Respiratory Disorders, and Urologic Disorders. Drug-induced conditions associated with allergic and pseudoallergic reactions, hematologic disorders, liver disease, pulmonary disorders, and kidney disease appear in five tabular appendices. Information on the management of pharmacotherapy in the elderly is also included as an appendix. Also in the eighth edition, a chapter has been added on renal cell carcinoma.

Carrying over a popular feature from *Pharmacotherapy: A Pathophysiologic Approach*, each chapter is organized in a consistent format:

- Disease state definition
- Pathophysiology
- Clinical presentation
- Diagnosis
- Desired outcome
- Treatment
- Monitoring

The treatment section may include nonpharmacologic therapy, drug selection guidelines, dosing recommendations, adverse effects, pharmacokinetic considerations, and important drug–drug interactions. When more in-depth information is required, the reader is encouraged to refer to the primary text, *Pharmacotherapy: A Pathophysiologic Approach*, eighth edition.

It is our sincere hope that students and practitioners find this book helpful as they continuously strive to deliver highest quality patient-centered care. We invite your comments on how we may improve subsequent editions of this work.

Barbara G. Wells
Joseph T. DiPiro
Terry L. Schwinghammer
Cecily V. DiPiro

Please provide your comments about this book—Wells et al., *Pharmacotherapy Handbook,* eighth edition—to its authors and publisher by writing to *pharmacotherapy@mcgraw-hill.com*. Please indicate the author and title of this handbook in the subject line of your e-mail.

Acknowledgments

The editors wish to express their sincere appreciation to the authors whose chapters in the eighth edition of *Pharmacotherapy: A Pathophysiologic Approach* served as the basis for this book. The dedication and professionalism of these outstanding practitioners, teachers, and clinical scientists are evident on every page of this work. The authors of the chapters from the eighth edition are acknowledged at the end of each respective *Handbook* chapter.

To the Reader

Basic and clinical research provides a continuous flow of biomedical information that enables practitioners to use medications more effectively and safely. The editors, authors, and publisher of this book have made every effort to ensure accuracy of information provided. However, it is the responsibility of all practitioners to assess the appropriateness of published drug therapy information, especially in light of the specific clinical situation and new developments in the field. The editors and authors have taken care to recommend dosages that are consistent with current published guidelines and other responsible literature. However, when dealing with new and unfamiliar drug therapies, students and practitioners should consult several appropriate information sources.

CHAPTER 1

Gout and Hyperuricemia

DEFINITIONS

- The term *gout* describes a disease spectrum including hyperuricemia, recurrent attacks of acute arthritis associated with monosodium urate crystals in leukocytes found in synovial fluid leukocytes, deposits of monosodium urate crystals in tissues in and around joints (tophi), interstitial renal disease, and uric acid nephrolithiasis.

- The underlying metabolic disorder of gout is hyperuricemia (serum urate concentration >7 mg/dL [416 μmol/L] in men or >6 mg/dL [357 μmol/L] in women), but hyperuricemia may be an asymptomatic condition.

PATHOPHYSIOLOGY

- In humans, uric acid is the end product of purine degradation. It is a waste product that serves no known physiologic purpose. The size of the urate pool is increased severalfold in individuals with gout. This excess accumulation may result from either overproduction or underexcretion.

- The purines from which uric acid is produced originate from three sources: dietary purine, conversion of tissue nucleic acid to purine nucleotides, and de novo synthesis of purine bases.

- Abnormalities in the enzyme systems that regulate purine metabolism may result in overproduction of uric acid. Increased activity of phosphoribosyl pyrophosphate (PRPP) synthetase leads to increased concentration of PRPP, a key determinant of purine synthesis and uric acid production. A deficiency of hypoxanthine–guanine phosphoribosyl transferase (HGPRT) may also result in overproduction of uric acid. HGPRT converts guanine to guanylic acid and hypoxanthine to inosinic acid. These two conversions require PRPP as the cosubstrate and are important reutilization reactions involved in nucleic acid synthesis. A deficiency in the HGPRT enzyme leads to increased metabolism of guanine and hypoxanthine to uric acid and more PRPP to interact with glutamine in the first step of the purine pathway.

- Uric acid may be overproduced as a consequence of increased breakdown of tissue nucleic acids, as with myeloproliferative and lymphoproliferative disorders. Cytotoxic drugs used to treat these disorders can also result in overproduction of uric acid due to lysis and the breakdown of cellular matter.

- Dietary purines play an unimportant role in the generation of hyperuricemia in the absence of some derangement in purine metabolism or elimination.

1

- About two thirds of the uric acid produced each day is excreted in the urine. The remainder is eliminated through the GI tract after enzymatic degradation by colonic bacteria. A decline in the urinary excretion of uric acid to a level below the rate of production leads to hyperuricemia and an increased miscible pool of sodium urate.
- Drugs that decrease renal clearance of uric acid through modification of filtered load or one of the tubular transport processes include diuretics, nicotinic acid, salicylates (<2 g/day), ethanol, pyrazinamide, levodopa, ethambutol, cyclosporine, and cytotoxic drugs.
- The average person produces 600 to 800 mg of uric acid daily and excretes <600 mg in urine. Individuals who excrete >600 mg after being on a purine-free diet for 3 to 5 days are considered overproducers. Hyperuricemic individuals who excrete <600 mg of uric acid per 24 hours on a purine-free diet are defined as underexcretors of uric acid. On a regular diet, excretion >1,000 mg per 24 hours reflects overproduction; less than this is probably normal.
- Deposition of urate crystals in synovial fluid results in an inflammatory process involving chemical mediators that causes vasodilation, increased vascular permeability, complement activation, and chemotactic activity for polymorphonuclear leukocytes. Phagocytosis of urate crystals by leukocytes results in rapid lysis of cells and a discharge of proteolytic enzymes into the cytoplasm. The ensuing inflammatory reaction is associated with intense joint pain, erythema, warmth, and swelling.
- Uric acid nephrolithiasis occurs in 10% to 25% of patients with gout. Predisposing factors include excessive urinary excretion of uric acid, acidic urine, and highly concentrated urine.
- In acute uric acid nephropathy, acute renal failure occurs as a result of blockage of urine flow secondary to massive precipitation of uric acid crystals in the collecting ducts and ureters. This syndrome is a well-recognized complication in patients with myeloproliferative or lymphoproliferative disorders and results from massive malignant cell turnover, particularly after initiation of chemotherapy. Chronic urate nephropathy is caused by the long-term deposition of urate crystals in the renal parenchyma.
- Tophi (urate deposits) are uncommon in gouty subjects and are a late complication of hyperuricemia. The most common sites of tophaceous deposits in patients with recurrent acute gouty arthritis are the base of the great toe, helix of the ear, olecranon bursae, Achilles tendon, knees, wrists, and hands.

CLINICAL PRESENTATION

- Acute attacks of gouty arthritis are characterized by rapid onset of excruciating pain, swelling, and inflammation. The attack is typically mono-articular at first, most often affecting the first metatarsophalangeal joint (podagra), and then, in order of frequency, the insteps, ankles, heels, knees, wrists, fingers, and elbows. Attacks commonly begin at night, with the patient awakening from sleep with excruciating pain. The affected joints are erythematous, warm, and swollen. Fever and leukocytosis are common. Untreated attacks may last from 3 to 14 days before spontaneous recovery.

- Although acute attacks of gouty arthritis may occur without apparent provocation, attacks may be precipitated by stress, trauma, alcohol ingestion, infection, surgery, rapid lowering of serum uric acid by ingestion of uric acid–lowering agents, and ingestion of certain drugs known to elevate serum uric acid concentrations.

DIAGNOSIS

- A definitive diagnosis requires aspiration of synovial fluid from the affected joint and identification of intracellular crystals of monosodium urate monohydrate in synovial fluid leukocytes.
- When joint aspiration is not a viable option, a presumptive diagnosis of acute gouty arthritis is based on the presence of the characteristic signs and symptoms, as well as the response to treatment.

DESIRED OUTCOME

- The treatment goals for gout are to terminate the acute attack, prevent recurrent attacks of gouty arthritis, and prevent complications associated with chronic deposition of urate crystals in tissues.

TREATMENT

ACUTE GOUTY ARTHRITIS

See Fig. 1–1 for a treatment algorithm for acute gouty arthritis.

Nonpharmacologic Therapy

- Patients should be advised to reduce their dietary intake of saturated fats and meats high in purines (e.g., organ meats), avoid alcohol, increase fluid intake, and lose weight if obese.
- Joint rest for 1 to 2 days should be encouraged, and local application of ice may be beneficial.

Nonsteroidal Antiinflammatory Drugs

- Nonsteroidal antiinflammatory drugs (NSAIDs) are the mainstay of therapy because of their excellent efficacy and minimal toxicity with short-term use. There is little evidence to support one NSAID as more efficacious than another, and three drugs—indomethacin, naproxen, and sulindac—have FDA approval for this indication (Table 1–1).
- Therapy should be initiated with maximum recommended doses for gout at the onset of symptoms and continued for 24 hours after complete resolution of an acute attack, then tapered quickly over 2 to 3 days. Acute attacks generally resolve within 5 to 8 days after initiating therapy.
- The most common adverse effects involve the GI system (gastritis, bleeding, and perforation), kidneys (renal papillary necrosis and reduced creatinine clearance [CL_{cr}]), cardiovascular system (increased blood pressure and sodium and fluid retention), and CNS (impaired cognitive function, headache, and dizziness).

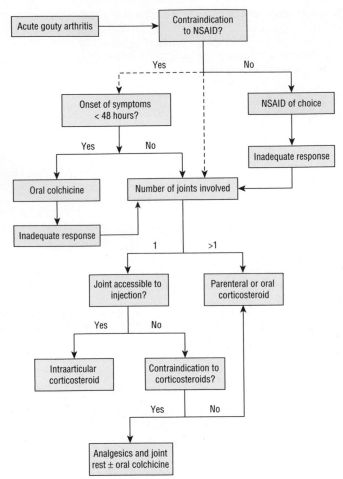

FIGURE 1–1. Treatment algorithm for acute gouty arthritis. (NSAID, nonsteroidal antiinflammatory drug.)

- Although the risk of GI complications is relatively small with short-term therapy, coadministration with a proton pump inhibitor should be considered in elderly patients and others at increased GI risk. NSAIDs should be used with caution in individuals with a history of peptic ulcer disease, heart failure, uncontrolled hypertension, renal insufficiency, or coronary artery disease or if they are receiving anticoagulants concurrently.
- The efficacy and safety of cyclooxygenase-2 (COX-2) selective inhibitors (e.g., celecoxib) have not been fully assessed in gouty arthritis, but they are more costly than conventional NSAIDs and are unlikely to result in fewer GI complications because of the short duration of therapy.

TABLE 1–1	Dosage Regimens of Oral Nonsteroidal Antiinflammatory Drugs for Treatment of Acute Gouty Arthritis
Generic Name	**Dosage and Frequency**
Etodolac	300 mg twice daily
Fenoprofen	300–600 mg three or four times daily
Ibuprofen	800 mg four times daily
Indomethacin	25–50 mg four times daily for 3 days, then taper to twice daily for 4 to 7 days
Ketoprofen	75 mg four times daily
Naproxen	500 mg twice daily for 3 days, then 250–500 mg daily for 4 to 7 days
Piroxicam	20 mg once daily or 10 mg twice daily
Sulindac	200 mg twice daily for 7 to 10 days

Corticosteroids

- Recent evidence indicates that corticosteroids are equivalent to NSAIDs for treatment of acute gout flares. They can be used either systemically or by intraarticular injection.
- The recommended dose is **prednisone** 30 to 60 mg (or an equivalent dose of another corticosteroid) orally once daily for 3 to 5 days. Because rebound attacks may occur upon corticosteroid withdrawal, the dose should be gradually tapered in 5 mg increments over 10 to 14 days and discontinued.
- A single intramuscular injection of a long-acting corticosteroid (e.g., **triamcinolone acetonide** 60 mg) can be used as an alternative to the oral route if patients are unable to take oral therapy. If not contraindicated, low-dose colchicine can be used as adjunctive therapy to injectable corticosteroids to prevent rebound flare-ups.
- Intraarticular administration of **triamcinolone acetonide** 5 to 20 mg for small joints or 10 to 40 mg for large joints may be useful for acute gout limited to one or two joints.
- **Adrenocorticotropic hormone (ACTH)** gel, 40 to 80 USP units, may be given intramuscularly every 6 to 8 hours for 2 or 3 days and then discontinued. Studies with ACTH are limited, and it should be reserved for patients with contraindications to first-line therapies (e.g., heart failure, chronic renal failure, or history of GI bleeding).

Colchicine

- **Colchicine** is an antimitotic drug that is highly effective in relieving acute gout attacks but has a low benefit-to-toxicity ratio. For this reason, it is used less often than NSAIDs in the United States and is generally reserved as a second-line therapy when NSAIDs or corticosteroids are contraindicated or ineffective.
- When colchicine is started within the first 24 hours of an acute attack, about two thirds of patients respond within several hours. The likelihood of success decreases substantially if treatment is delayed longer than 48 hours after symptom onset.

- **Colcrys** is an FDA-approved form of colchicine available in 0.6 mg tablets for oral use. The recommended dose is 1.2 mg (two tablets) initially, followed by 0.6 mg (one tablet) 1 hour later. In patients with renal impairment, the dose should not be repeated more often than once every 2 weeks.
- Oral colchicine causes dose-dependent GI adverse effects (nausea, vomiting, and diarrhea). Non-GI adverse effects include neutropenia and axonal neuromyopathy, which may be worsened in patients taking other myopathic drugs (e.g., statins) or in those with renal insufficiency. Colchicine should not be used concurrently with P-glycoprotein or strong CYP450 3A4 inhibitors (e.g., clarithromycin) because reduced biliary excretion may lead to increased plasma colchicine levels and toxicity.
- IV colchicine has resulted in fatalities and is no longer available.

PROPHYLACTIC THERAPY OF INTERCRITICAL GOUT

General Approach

- Prophylactic treatment can be withheld if the first episode of acute gouty arthritis was mild and responded promptly to treatment, the patient's serum urate concentration was only minimally elevated, and the 24-hour urinary uric acid excretion was not excessive (<1,000 mg/24 hours on a regular diet).
- If the patient had a severe attack of gouty arthritis, a complicated course of uric acid nephrolithiasis, a substantially elevated serum uric acid (>10 mg/dL [595 μmol/L]), or a 24-hour urinary excretion of uric acid > 1,000 mg, then prophylactic treatment should be instituted immediately after resolution of the acute episode.
- Prophylactic therapy is cost-effective for patients who have two or more attacks per year, even if the serum uric acid concentration is normal or only minimally elevated.

Colchicine

- **Colchicine** given in low oral doses (0.6 mg once daily) may be effective in preventing recurrent arthritis in patients with no evidence of visible tophi and a normal or slightly elevated serum urate concentration. Treated patients who sense the onset of an acute attack should increase the dose to 1.2 mg, followed by one repeat dose of 0.6 mg in 1 hour. Discontinuation of prophylaxis may be attempted if the serum urate concentration remains normal and the patient remains symptom free for 1 year. However, treatment discontinuation may be followed by an exacerbation of acute gouty arthritis.

Uric Acid–lowering Therapy

- Patients with a history of recurrent acute gouty arthritis and a significantly elevated serum uric acid concentration are probably best managed with uric acid–lowering therapy. Urate-lowering therapy should not begin during an acute attack but 6 to 8 weeks after resolution.
- The goal of urate-lowering therapy is to achieve and maintain a serum uric acid concentration <6 mg/dL (357 μmol/L) and preferably <5 mg/dL (297 μmol/L).

- Reduction of the serum urate concentration can be accomplished by decreasing uric acid synthesis (xanthine oxidase inhibitors) or by increasing the renal excretion of uric acid (uricosurics).
- Colchicine 0.6 mg once daily should be administered for at least the first 8 weeks of antihyperuricemic therapy to minimize the risk of acute attacks that may occur during initiation of uric acid–lowering therapy.

XANTHINE OXIDASE INHIBITORS

- Xanthine oxidase inhibitors reduce uric acid by impairing the conversion of hypoxanthine to xanthine and xanthine to uric acid. Because they are effective in both overproducers and underexcretors of uric acid, they are the most widely prescribed agents for long-term prevention of recurrent gout attacks.
- **Allopurinol** lowers uric acid levels in a dose-dependent manner. Because of the long half-life of its metabolite (oxypurinol), allopurinol can be given once daily. It is typically initiated at a dose of 100 mg daily and increased by 100 mg daily at 1-week intervals to achieve a serum uric acid level ≤6 mg/dL (357 μmol/L). Serum uric acid levels can be checked about 1 week after starting therapy or modifying the dose. Although typical doses are 100 to 300 mg daily, occasionally doses of 600 to 800 mg daily are necessary. The dose should be reduced in patients with renal insufficiency (≤200 mg/day for CL_{cr} 60 mL/min and ≤100 mg/day for CL_{cr} 30 mL/min).
- Mild adverse effects of allopurinol include skin rash, leukopenia, GI problems, headache, and urticaria. More severe adverse reactions include severe rash (toxic epidermal necrolysis, erythema multiforme, or exfoliative dermatitis) and an allopurinol hypersensitivity syndrome characterized by fever, eosinophilia, dermatitis, vasculitis, and renal and hepatic dysfunction that occurs rarely but is associated with a 20% mortality rate.
- **Febuxostat** (Uloric) also lowers serum uric acid in a dose-dependent manner. The recommended starting dose is 40 mg once daily. The dose should be increased to 80 mg once daily for patients who do not achieve target serum uric acid concentrations after 2 weeks of therapy. It is well tolerated, with adverse events mostly limited to nausea, arthralgias, and minor hepatic transaminase elevations. Febuxostat does not require dose adjustment in mild to moderate hepatic or renal dysfunction. Due to rapid mobilization of urate deposits with initiation of therapy, concomitant therapy with colchicine or an NSAID should be given for at least the first 8 weeks of therapy to prevent acute gout flare-ups.

URICOSURIC DRUGS

- **Probenecid** and **sulfinpyrazone** (not currently available in the United States) increase the renal clearance of uric acid by inhibiting the postsecretory renal proximal tubular reabsorption of uric acid. They should only be used in patients with documented underexcretion of uric acid (<800 mg/24 hours on a regular diet or 600 mg/24 hours on a purine-restricted diet). Therapy with uricosuric drugs should be started at a low dose to avoid marked uricosuria and possible stone formation. Maintenance of adequate urine flow and alkalinization of the urine during the first several days of uricosuric therapy further decrease the likelihood of uric acid stone formation.

- Probenecid is given initially at a dose of 250 mg twice daily for 1 to 2 weeks, then 500 mg twice daily for 2 weeks. Thereafter, the daily dose is increased by 500 mg increments every 1 to 2 weeks until satisfactory control is achieved or a maximum dose of 2 g/day is reached.
- The initial dose of sulfinpyrazone is 50 mg twice daily for 3 or 4 days, then 100 mg twice daily, increasing the daily dose by 100 mg increments each week up to 800 mg/day.
- The major side effects associated with uricosuric therapy are GI irritation, rash and hypersensitivity, precipitation of acute gouty arthritis, and stone formation. These drugs are contraindicated in patients with impaired renal function (CL_{cr} < 50 mL/min) or a history of renal calculi, as well as in patients who are overproducers of uric acid.

EVALUATION OF THERAPEUTIC OUTCOMES

- A serum uric acid level should be checked in patients suspected of having an acute gout attack, particularly if it is not the first attack and a decision is to be made about starting prophylactic therapy. However, acute gout can occur in the presence of normal serum uric acid concentrations. Repeat serum uric acid measurements do not need to be monitored routinely except during the titration phase of allopurinol or febuxostat to achieve a goal serum urate <6 mg/dL (357 μmol/L).
- Patients with acute gout should be monitored for symptomatic relief of joint pain, as well as potential adverse effects and drug interactions related to drug therapy. The acute pain of an initial attack of gouty arthritis should begin to ease within about 8 hours of treatment initiation. Complete resolution of pain, erythema, and inflammation usually occurs within 48 to 72 hours.
- Patients receiving hypouricemic medications should have baseline assessment of renal function, hepatic enzymes, complete blood count, and electrolytes. The tests should be rechecked every 6 to 12 months in patients receiving long-term prophylaxis.
- Because of comorbidity with diabetes, dyslipidemia, hypertension, and stroke, the presence of increased serum uric acid levels or gout should prompt evaluation for cardiovascular disease and the need for appropriate risk reduction measures. Clinicians should also look for possible correctable causes of hyperuricemia (e.g., medications, obesity, and alcohol abuse).

See Chapter 102, Gout and Hyperuricemia, authored by Michael E. Ernst and Elizabeth C. Clark, for a more detailed discussion of this topic.

2 Osteoarthritis

DEFINITION

- Osteoarthritis (OA) is a common, slowly progressive disorder affecting primarily the weight-bearing diarthrodial joints of the peripheral and axial skeleton. It is characterized by progressive deterioration and loss of articular cartilage, resulting in osteophyte formation, pain, limitation of motion, deformity, and progressive disability. Inflammation may or may not be present in the affected joints.

PATHOPHYSIOLOGY

- *Primary (idiopathic) OA,* the most common type, has no known cause. Subclasses of primary OA are *localized OA* (involving one or two sites) and *generalized OA* (affecting three or more sites). The term *erosive OA* indicates the presence of erosion and marked proliferation in the proximal and distal interphalangeal (PIP and DIP) hand joints.
- *Secondary OA* is associated with a known cause, such as rheumatoid arthritis or another inflammatory arthritis, trauma, metabolic or endocrine disorders, and congenital factors.
- OA usually begins with damage to articular cartilage through injury, excess joint loading from obesity or other reasons, or joint instability or injury that causes abnormal loading. Damage to cartilage increases the metabolic activity of chondrocytes in an attempt to repair the damage; this leads to increased synthesis of matrix constituents with cartilage swelling. The normal balance between cartilage breakdown and resynthesis can be lost, with a shift toward increasing destruction and cartilage loss.
- Destruction of aggrecans (long molecules of proteoglycans linked with hyaluronic acid) by the proteolytic enzyme ADAMTS-5 is thought to play a key role. A collagen receptor called DRR-2 on the chondrocyte cell surface may also be involved. In healthy cartilage, DRR-2 is inactive, shielded from contact with collagen by aggrecans. Damage to cartilage triggers aggrecan destruction, thereby exposing DRR-2 to collagen. The active DRR-2 then increases activity of matrix metalloproteinase (MMP) 13, which destroys collagen. Collagen breakdown products stimulate further DRR-2 activation, resulting in more cartilage destruction.
- Subchondral bone adjacent to articular cartilage also undergoes pathologic changes that allow progression of damage to articular cartilage. In OA, subchondral bone releases vasoactive peptides and MMPs. Neovascularization and subsequent increased permeability of the adjacent cartilage occur, which contribute further to cartilage loss.
- Substantial loss of cartilage causes joint space narrowing and leads to painful, deformed joints. The remaining cartilage softens and develops fibrillations, and there is splitting, further cartilage loss, and exposure of underlying bone. Cartilage is eventually eroded completely, leaving denuded subchondral bone that becomes dense, smooth, and glistening (eburnation).

A more brittle, stiffer bone results, with decreased weight-bearing ability and development of sclerosis and microfractures. New bone formations (osteophytes) appear at joint margins distant from cartilage destruction; evidence indicates that osteophytes help to stabilize OA joints.

- Local inflammatory changes occur in the joint capsule and synovium. The synovium becomes infiltrated with T cells, and immune complexes appear. Crystals or cartilage shards in synovial fluid may contribute to inflammation. There are also increased levels of interleukin-1, prostaglandin E_2, tumor necrosis factor, and nitric oxide in synovial fluid. Inflammatory changes result in effusions and synovial thickening.
- The pain of OA arises from activation of nociceptive nerve endings within joints by mechanical and chemical irritants. OA pain may result from distention of the synovial capsule by increased joint fluid; microfracture; periosteal irritation; or damage to ligaments, synovium, or the meniscus.

CLINICAL PRESENTATION

- The prevalence and severity of OA increase with age. Potential risk factors include obesity, repetitive use through work or leisure activities, joint trauma, and heredity.
- The clinical presentation depends on the duration and severity of disease and the number of joints affected. The predominant symptom is a localized deep, aching pain associated with the affected joint. Early in OA, pain accompanies joint activity and decreases with rest. With progression, pain occurs with minimal activity or at rest.
- Joints most commonly affected are the DIP and PIP joints of the hand, the first carpometacarpal joint, knees, hips, cervical and lumbar spine, and the first metatarsophalangeal joint of the toe.
- In addition to pain, limitation of motion, stiffness, crepitus, and deformities may occur. Patients with lower extremity involvement may report a sense of weakness or instability.
- Upon arising, joint stiffness typically lasts <30 minutes and resolves with motion. Joint enlargement is related to bony proliferation or to thickening of the synovium and joint capsule. The presence of a warm, red, and tender joint may suggest an inflammatory synovitis.
- Joint deformity may be present in the later stages as a result of subluxation, collapse of subchondral bone, formation of bone cysts, or bony overgrowths.
- Physical examination of the affected joints reveals tenderness, crepitus, and possibly joint enlargement. Heberden and Bouchard nodes are bony enlargements (osteophytes) of the DIP and PIP joints, respectively.

DIAGNOSIS

- The diagnosis of OA is dependent on patient history, clinical examination of the affected joint(s), radiologic findings, and laboratory testing.
- Criteria for the classification of OA of the hips, knees, and hands were developed by the American College of Rheumatology (ACR). The criteria

include the presence of pain, bony changes on examination, a normal erythrocyte sedimentation rate (ESR), and radiographs showing characteristic osteophytes or joint space narrowing.

- For hip OA, a patient must have hip pain and two of the following: (1) an ESR <20 mm/hour, (2) radiographic femoral or acetabular osteophytes, and/or (3) radiographic joint space narrowing.
- For knee OA, a patient must have knee pain and radiographic osteophytes in addition to one or more of the following: (1) age >50 years, (2) morning stiffness of 30 minutes' or less duration, (3) crepitus on motion, (4) bony enlargement, (6) bony tenderness, and/or (7) palpable joint warmth.
- No specific clinical laboratory abnormalities occur in primary OA. The ESR may be slightly elevated in patients with generalized or erosive inflammatory OA. The rheumatoid factor test is negative. Analysis of the synovial fluid reveals fluid with high viscosity. This fluid demonstrates a mild leukocytosis (<2,000 white blood cells/mm^3[<2 × 10^9/L]) with predominantly mononuclear cells.

DESIRED OUTCOME

- The major goals for the management of OA are to (1) educate the patient, family members, and caregivers; (2) relieve pain and stiffness; (3) maintain or improve joint mobility; (4) limit functional impairment; and (5) maintain or improve quality of life.

TREATMENT

NONPHARMACOLOGIC THERAPY

- The first step is to educate the patient about the extent of the disease, prognosis, and management approach. Dietary counseling and a structured weight loss program are recommended for overweight OA patients.
- Physical therapy—with heat or cold treatments and an exercise program—helps to maintain and restore joint range of motion and reduce pain and muscle spasms. Exercise programs using isometric techniques can strengthen muscles, improve joint function and motion, and decrease disability, pain, and the need for analgesic use.
- Assistive and orthotic devices such as canes, walkers, braces, heel cups, and insoles can be used during exercise or daily activities.
- Surgical procedures (e.g., osteotomy, partial or total arthroplasty, and joint fusion) are indicated for patients with functional disability and/or severe pain unresponsive to conservative therapy.

PHARMACOLOGIC THERAPY

General Approach

- Drug therapy in OA is targeted at relief of pain. Because OA often occurs in older individuals who have other medical conditions, a conservative approach to drug treatment is warranted.

- An individualized approach to treatment is necessary (**Fig. 2-1**). For mild or moderate pain, topical analgesics or acetaminophen can be used. If these measures fail or if there is inflammation, nonsteroidal antiinflammatory drugs (NSAIDs) may be useful. Appropriate nondrug therapies should be continued when drug therapy is initiated.

Acetaminophen

- **Acetaminophen** is recommended by the ACR as first-line drug therapy for pain management of OA. The dose is 325 to 650 mg every 4 to 6 hours on a scheduled basis (maximum dose 4 g/day; maximum 2 g/day if there is chronic alcohol intake or underlying liver disease). Comparable relief of mild to moderate OA pain has been demonstrated for acetaminophen (2.6–4 g/day) compared with aspirin (650 mg four times daily), ibuprofen (1,200 or 2,400 mg daily), and naproxen (750 mg daily). However, some patients respond better to NSAIDs.

- Acetaminophen is usually well tolerated, but potentially fatal hepatotoxicity with overdose is well documented. It should be used with caution in patients with liver disease and those who chronically abuse alcohol; when used in this setting, the duration should be limited, and the dose should not exceed 2 g daily. Chronic alcohol users (three or more drinks daily) should be warned about an increased risk of liver damage or GI bleeding with acetaminophen. Other individuals do not appear to be at increased risk for GI bleeding. Renal toxicity is also possible with long-term use; use of nonprescription combination products containing acetaminophen and NSAIDs is discouraged because of an increased risk of renal failure.

Nonsteroidal Antiinflammatory Drugs

- NSAIDs at prescription strength are often prescribed for OA patients after treatment with acetaminophen proves ineffective or for patients with inflammatory OA. Analgesic effects begin within 1 to 2 hours, whereas antiinflammatory benefits may require 2 to 3 weeks of continuous therapy.

- Nonselective NSAIDs and cyclooxygenase-2 (COX-2) selective NSAIDs are superior to acetaminophen for improving symptoms and functional limitations in OA. All NSAIDs have similar efficacy in reducing pain and inflammation in OA (**Table 2-1**), although individual patient response differs among NSAIDs.

- Selection of an NSAID depends on prescriber experience, medication cost, patient preference, toxicities, and adherence issues. An individual patient should be given a trial of one drug that is adequate in time (2–3 wk) and dose. If the first NSAID fails, another agent in the same or another chemical class can be tried; this process may be repeated until an effective drug is found. Combining two NSAIDs increases adverse effects without providing additional benefit.

- COX-2 selective inhibitors (e.g., celecoxib) demonstrate analgesic benefits that are similar to traditional nonselective NSAIDs. Although COX-2 selective inhibition was designed to reduce NSAID-induced gastropathy (e.g., ulcers, bleeding, and/or perforation), concerns about

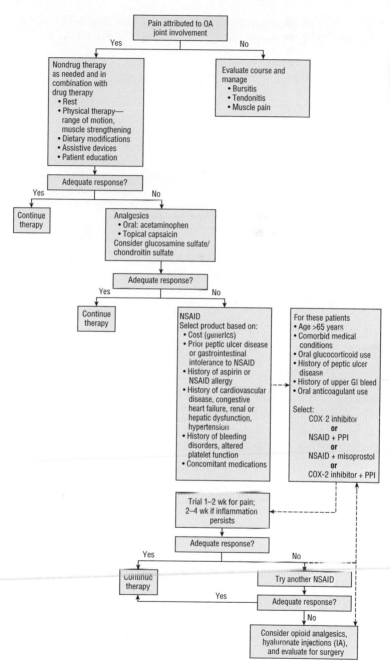

FIGURE 2–1. Treatment for osteoarthritis. (COX, cyclooxygenase; IA, intraarticular; NSAID, nonsteroidal antiinflammatory drug; OA, osteoarthritis; PPI, proton pump inhibitor.)

TABLE 2–1 Medications Commonly Used in the Treatment of Osteoarthritis

Medication	Dosage and Frequency	Maximum Dosage (mg/day)
Oral analgesics		
Acetaminophen	325–650 mg every 4 to 6 hours or 1 g three or four times daily	4,000
Tramadol	50–100 mg every 4 to 6 hours	400
Acetaminophen/codeine	300–1,000 mg/15–60 mg every 4 hours as needed	4,000/360
Acetaminophen/ oxycodone	325–650 mg/2.5–10 mg every 6 hours as needed	4,000/40
Topical analgesics		
Capsaicin 0.025% or 0.075%	Apply to affected joint three or four times daily	–
Nutritional supplements		
Glucosamine sulfate/ chondroitin sulfate	500 mg/400 mg three times daily	1,500/1,200
Nonsteroidal antiinflammatory drugs (NSAIDs)		
Carboxylic acids		
Acetylated salicylates		
Aspirin, plain, buffered, or enteric-coated[d]	325–650 mg every 4 to 6 hours for pain; antiinflammatory doses start at 3,600 mg/day in divided doses	3,600[a]
Nonacetylated salicylates		
Salsalate	500–1,000 mg two or three times daily	3,000[a]
Diflunisal	500–1,000 mg two times daily	1,500
Choline salicylate[b]	500–1,000 mg two or three times daily	3,000[a]
Choline magnesium salicylate	500–1,000 mg two or three times daily	3,000[a]
Acetic acids		
Etodolac	800–1,200 mg/day in divided doses	1,200
Diclofenac	100–150 mg/day in divided doses	200
Indomethacin	25 mg two or three times daily; 75 mg SR once daily	200/150
Ketorolac[c]	10 mg every 4 to 6 hours	40
Nabumetone[d]	500–1,000 mg once or twice daily	2,000
Propionic acids		
Fenoprofen	300–600 mg three or four times daily	3,200
Flurbiprofen	200–300 mg/day in 2 to 4 divided doses	300
Ibuprofen	1,200–3,200 mg/day in 3 or 4 divided doses	3,200
Ketoprofen	150–300 mg/day in 3 or 4 divided doses	300
Naproxen	250–500 mg twice daily	1,500
Naproxen sodium	275–550 mg twice daily	1,375
Oxaprozin	600–1,200 mg daily	1,800

(continued)

TABLE 2–1	Medications Commonly Used in the Treatment of Osteoarthritis *(Continued)*	
Medication	**Dosage and Frequency**	**Maximum Dosage (mg/day)**
Nonsteroidal antiinflammatory drugs (NSAIDs)		
Fenamates		
Meclofenamate	200–400 mg/day in 3 or 4 divided doses	400
Mefenamic acid[e]	250 mg every 6 hours	1,000
Oxicams		
Piroxicam	10–20 mg daily	20
Meloxicam	7.5 mg daily	15
Coxibs		
Celecoxib	100 mg twice daily or 200 mg once daily	200 (400 for RA)

RA, rheumatoid arthritis; SR, sustained-release
[a]Monitor serum salicylate levels over 3–3.6 g/day.
[b]Only available as a liquid; 870 mg salicylate/5 mL.
[c]Not approved for treatment of OA for more than 5 days.
[d]Nonorganic acid, but metabolite is an acetic acid.
[e]Not approved for treatment of OA.

adverse cardiovascular events (e.g., myocardial infarction and stroke) have led authorities to recommend their use only in patients who are at high risk for NSAID-related GI effects and low risk for cardiovascular toxicity.

- GI complaints are the most common adverse effects of NSAIDs. Minor complaints such as nausea, dyspepsia, anorexia, abdominal pain, flatulence, and diarrhea occur in 10% to 60% of patients. NSAIDs should be taken with food or milk, except for enteric-coated products (milk or antacids may destroy the enteric coating and cause increased GI symptoms in some patients).
- All NSAIDs have the potential to cause gastric and duodenal ulcers and bleeding through direct (topical) or indirect (systemic) mechanisms. Risk factors for NSAID-associated ulcers and ulcer complications (perforation, gastric outlet obstruction, and GI bleeding) include increased age, comorbid medical conditions (e.g., cardiovascular disease), concomitant corticosteroid or anticoagulant therapy, and history of peptic ulcer disease or upper GI bleeding.
- For OA patients who need an NSAID but are at high risk for GI complications, the ACR recommendations include either a COX-2 selective inhibitor or a nonselective NSAID in combination with either a proton pump inhibitor or misoprostol.
- NSAIDs may also cause kidney diseases, hepatitis, hypersensitivity reactions, rash, and CNS complaints of drowsiness, dizziness, headaches, depression, confusion, and tinnitus. All nonselective NSAIDs inhibit COX-1-dependent thromboxane production in platelets, thereby increasing

bleeding risk. NSAIDs should be avoided in late pregnancy because of the risk of premature closure of the ductus arteriosus.

- The most potentially serious drug interactions include the concomitant use of NSAIDs with lithium, warfarin, oral hypoglycemics, methotrexate, antihypertensives, angiotensin-converting enzyme inhibitors, β-blockers, and diuretics.

Topical Therapies

- **Capsaicin,** an extract of red peppers that causes release and ultimately depletion of substance P from nerve fibers, has been beneficial in providing pain relief in OA when applied topically over affected joints. It may be used alone or in combination with oral analgesics or NSAIDs. To be effective, capsaicin must be used regularly, and it may require up to 2 weeks to take effect. It is well tolerated, but one third of patients experience burning and/or stinging at the site of application that usually subsides with repeated application. Patients should be warned not to get the cream in their eyes or mouth and to wash their hands after application. Application of the cream, gel, or lotion is recommended four times daily, but tapering to twice-daily application may enhance long-term adherence with adequate pain relief.
- **Topical NSAIDs** can provide effective OA treatment while avoiding the serious adverse effects of systemic therapy. They may be considered when first-line agents fail, are contraindicated, or are poorly tolerated. The mechanism of action is thought to be related to local inhibition of COX-2 enzymes. Common adverse effects include pruritus, burning, pain, and rash at the site of application. Patients using topical products should avoid oral NSAIDs to minimize the potential for additive side effects. Topical **diclofenac 1.5% solution** (Pennsaid) and **diclofenac 1% gel** (Voltaren Gel) are applied four times daily according to labeling instructions.
- Topical rubefacients containing **methyl salicylate, trolamine salicylate,** and other salicylates may have modest, short-term efficacy for treating acute pain associated with OA. Local skin reactions occur rarely.

Glucosamine and Chondroitin

- **Glucosamine** and **chondroitin** are dietary supplements that were shown to stimulate proteoglycan synthesis from articular cartilage in vitro. Although their excellent safety profile makes them appealing for patients at high risk of adverse drug events, results of a large, well-controlled clinical trial sponsored by the National Institutes of Health demonstrated no significant clinical response to glucosamine alone, chondroitin alone, or combination therapy when compared with placebo across all patients. In subgroup analyses, patients with moderate to severe knee pain showed a response to combination glucosamine–chondroitin therapy superior to placebo, but this finding did not reach the predetermined threshold for pain reduction.
- Because of their relative safety, a trial of glucosamine–chondroitin may be reasonable in patients with moderate to severe knee OA considering alternatives to traditional OA treatment. However, two recent

evidence-based guidelines recommend against their use. Dosing should be at least glucosamine sulfate 1,500 mg/day and chondroitin sulfate 1,200 mg/day in divided doses.

- Glucosamine adverse effects are mild and include GI gas, bloating, and cramps; it should not be used in patients with shellfish allergies. The most common adverse effect of chondroitin is nausea.

Corticosteroids

- Systemic corticosteroid therapy is not recommended in OA, given the lack of proven benefit and the well-known adverse effects with long-term use.

- Intraarticular corticosteroid injections can provide excellent pain relief, particularly when a joint effusion is present. Average doses for injection of large joints in adults are **methylprednisolone acetate** 20 to 40 mg or **triamcinolone hexacetonide** 10 to 20 mg. After aseptic aspiration of the effusion and corticosteroid injection, initial pain relief may occur within 24 to 72 hours, with peak relief occurring after 7 to 10 days and lasting for 4 to 8 weeks. The patient should minimize joint activity and stress on the joint for several days after the injection. Therapy is generally limited to three or four injections per year because of potential systemic effects and because the need for more frequent injections indicates poor response to therapy.

Hyaluronate Injections

- High-molecular-weight hyaluronic acid is a constituent of synovial fluid that provides lubrication with motion and shock absorbency during rapid movements. Because the concentration and molecular size of endogenous hyaluronic acid decrease in OA, exogenous administration has been studied in an attempt to reconstitute synovial fluid and reduce symptoms.

- Hyaluronic acid injections temporarily and modestly increase synovial fluid viscosity and were reported to decrease pain, but many studies were short term and poorly controlled with high placebo response rates.

- Six intraarticular preparations and regimens are available for treating knee pain associated with OA:
  - ✓ **Sodium hyaluronate 20 mg/2 mL** (Hyalgan) once weekly for five injections
  - ✓ **Sodium hyaluronate 20 mg/2 mL** (Euflexxa) once weekly for three injections
  - ✓ **Sodium hyaluronate 25 mg/2.5 mL** (Supartz) once weekly for five injections
  - ✓ **Hylan polymers 16 mg/2 mL** (Synvisc) once weekly for three injections
  - ✓ **Hylan polymers 48 mg/6 mL** (Synvisc-One) single injection (with efficacy for up to 26 weeks)
  - ✓ **Hyaluronan 30 mg/2 mL** (Orthovisc) once weekly for three injections

- Injections are well tolerated, but acute joint swelling, effusion, and stiffness, as well as local skin reactions (e.g., rash, ecchymoses, or pruritus), have been reported.

- These products may be beneficial for knee OA that is unresponsive to other therapies, but they are expensive because treatment includes both drug and administration costs.

Opioid Analgesics

- Low-dose opioid analgesics (e.g., **oxycodone**) may be useful for patients who experience no relief with acetaminophen, NSAIDs, intraarticular injections, or topical therapy.
- They are particularly useful in patients who cannot take NSAIDs because of renal failure or cardiovascular disease, or for patients in whom all other treatment options have failed and who are at high surgical risk, precluding joint arthroplasty.
- A low-dose opioid should be used initially, allowing a sufficient duration between dose increases to permit an assessment of efficacy and safety. Sustained-release compounds usually offer better pain control throughout the day and are used when immediate-release opioids do not provide a sufficient duration of pain control.

Tramadol

- Tramadol with or without acetaminophen has modest analgesic effects in patients with OA. It may also be effective as add-on therapy in patients taking concomitant NSAIDs or COX-2 selective inhibitors. As with opioids, tramadol may be helpful for patients who cannot take NSAIDs or COX-2 selective inhibitors.
- Tramadol should be initiated at a lower dose (100 mg/day in divided doses) and titrated as needed for pain control to a dose of 200 mg/day. It is available in a combination tablet with acetaminophen and as a sustained-release tablet.
- Opioid-like adverse effects such as nausea, vomiting, dizziness, constipation, headache, and somnolence are common.

EVALUATION OF THERAPEUTIC OUTCOMES

- To monitor efficacy, the patient's baseline pain can be assessed with a visual analog scale, and range of motion for affected joints can be assessed with flexion, extension, abduction, or adduction.
- Depending on the joint affected, measurement of grip strength and 50-feet walking time can help assess hand and hip/knee OA, respectively.
- Baseline radiographs can document the extent of joint involvement and follow disease progression with therapy.
- Other measures include the clinician's global assessment based on the patient's history of activities and limitations caused by OA, the Western Ontario and McMaster Universities Arthrosis Index, Stanford Health Assessment Questionnaire, and documentation of analgesic or NSAID use.
- Patients should be asked if they are having adverse effects from their medications. They should also be monitored for any signs of drug-related effects, such as skin rash, headaches, drowsiness, weight gain, or hypertension from NSAIDs.

- Baseline serum creatinine, hematology profiles, and serum transaminases with repeat levels at 6- to 12-month intervals are useful in identifying specific toxicities to the kidney, liver, GI tract, or bone marrow.

See Chapter 101, Osteoarthritis, authored by Lucinda M. Buys and Mary Elizabeth Elliott, for a more detailed discussion of this topic.

Osteoporosis

DEFINITION

- Osteoporosis is a bone disorder characterized by low bone density, impaired bone architecture, and compromised bone strength predisposing a person to increased fracture risk.
- Categories of osteoporosis include (1) postmenopausal osteoporosis, (2) age-related osteoporosis, and (3) secondary osteoporosis.

PATHOPHYSIOLOGY

- Bone loss occurs when bone resorption exceeds bone formation, usually from high bone turnover when the number and/or depth of bone resorption sites greatly exceed the rate and ability of osteoblasts to form new bone.
- In addition to reduced bone mineral density (BMD), bone quality and structural integrity are impaired because of the increased quantity of immature bone that is not yet adequately mineralized.
- Men and women begin to lose a small amount of bone mass starting in the third or fourth decade as a consequence of reduced bone formation. Estrogen deficiency during menopause increases proliferation, differentiation, and activation of new osteoclasts and prolongs survival of mature osteoclasts; this increases bone resorption more than formation. Men do not undergo a period of accelerated bone resorption similar to menopause. The etiology of male osteoporosis is multifactorial; secondary causes and aging are the most common contributing factors.
- Age-related osteoporosis occurs mainly because of hormone, calcium, and vitamin D deficiencies leading to accelerated bone turnover and reduced osteoblast formation.
- Drug-induced osteoporosis may result from systemic corticosteroids (prednisone doses greater than >7.5 mg/day), thyroid hormone replacement, some antiepileptic drugs (e.g., phenytoin and phenobarbital), depot medroxyprogesterone acetate, and other agents.

CLINICAL PRESENTATION

- Many patients are unaware that they have osteoporosis and only present after fracture. Fractures can occur after bending, lifting, or falling or independent of any activity.
- The most common osteoporosis-related fractures involve the vertebrae, proximal femur, and distal radius (wrist or Colles fracture). Two thirds of patients with vertebral fractures are asymptomatic; the remainder present with moderate to severe back pain that radiates down a leg after a new vertebral fracture. The pain usually subsides significantly after 2 to 4 weeks, but residual, chronic, low-back pain may persist. Multiple vertebral fractures

decrease height and sometimes curve the spine (kyphosis or lordosis) with or without significant back pain.
- Patients with a nonvertebral fracture frequently present with severe pain, swelling, and reduced function and mobility at the fracture site.

DIAGNOSIS

- Risk factors for osteoporosis and osteoporotic fractures included in the World Health Organization (WHO) Fracture Risk Assessment Tool (FRAX) include low BMD, female gender, race/ethnicity, history of a previous low-trauma (fragility) fracture as an adult, osteoporotic fracture in a first-degree relative (especially parental hip fracture), low body weight or body mass index, premature menopause (before 45 years old), rheumatoid arthritis, systemic corticosteroid therapy, current cigarette smoking, and alcohol intake of three or more drinks per day.
- Physical examination findings include bone pain, postural changes (i.e., kyphosis), and loss of height (>1.5 in [3.8 cm]).
- Laboratory testing may include complete blood count, creatinine, blood urea nitrogen, calcium, phosphorus, alkaline phosphatase, albumin, thyroid-stimulating hormone, free testosterone, 25-hydroxyvitamin D, and 24-hour urine concentrations of calcium and phosphorus. Urine or serum biomarkers (e.g., osteocalcin and cross-linked N-telopeptides of type I collagen) are sometimes used.
- Measurement of central (hip and spine) BMD with dual-energy x-ray absorptiometry (DXA) is the gold standard for osteoporosis diagnosis. Measurement at peripheral sites (forearm, heel, and phalanges) with ultrasound or DXA is used only for screening purposes and to determine the need for further testing.
- A T-score is a comparison of the patient's measured BMD to the mean BMD of a healthy, young (20- to 29-year-old), gender-matched, white reference population. The T-score is the number of standard deviations from the mean of the reference population.
- The diagnosis of osteoporosis based on a low-trauma fracture or central hip and/or spine DXA using WHO T-score thresholds. Normal bone mass is a T-score >−1, osteopenia is a T-score of −1 to −2.4, and osteoporosis is a T-score ≤−2.5.

DESIRED OUTCOME

- The primary goal of osteoporosis management is prevention. Optimizing skeletal development and peak bone mass accrual in childhood, adolescence, and early adulthood will reduce the future incidence of osteoporosis.
- Once osteopenia or osteoporosis develops, the objective is to stabilize or improve bone mass and strength and prevent fractures.
- Goals in patients who have already suffered osteoporotic fractures include reducing pain and deformity, improving functional capacity, reducing future falls and fractures, and improving quality of life.

PREVENTION AND TREATMENT

Fig. 3–1 provides an osteoporosis management algorithm for postmenopausal women and men 50 years and older that incorporates both nonpharmacologic and pharmacologic approaches.

NONPHARMACOLOGIC THERAPY

- All individuals should have a balanced diet with adequate intake of **calcium** and **vitamin D** (Table 3–1). Achieving daily calcium requirements from calcium-containing foods (which also contain other essential nutrients) is preferred.
  - ✓ Consumers can calculate the amount of calcium in a food serving by adding a zero to the percentage of the daily value listed on food labels. For example, one serving of milk (8 oz or 240 mL) has 30% of the daily value of calcium; this converts to 300 mg of calcium per serving.
  - ✓ To calculate the amount of vitamin D in a food serving, multiply the percent daily value of vitamin D listed on the food label by 4. For example, 20% vitamin D = 80 units.
- Excessive alcohol intake increases osteoporosis risk because of poor nutrition, impaired calcium and vitamin D metabolism, and an increased risk for falls. Alcohol consumption should not exceed one drink per day for women and two drinks per day for men.
- Excessive caffeine consumption may increase calcium excretion, increase the rate of bone loss, and perhaps increase fracture risk. Ideally, caffeine intake should be limited to two or fewer servings per day. Moderate caffeine intake (two to four servings per day) is not of concern if adequate calcium intake is achieved.
- Consumption of cola beverages, even without caffeine, may be associated with decreased BMD and increased fracture risk, perhaps because phosphoric acid content alters calcium balance.
- Smoking cessation can help to optimize peak bone mass, minimize bone loss, and ultimately reduce fracture risk.
- Weight-bearing aerobic and strengthening exercises can decrease the risk of falls and fractures by improving muscle strength, coordination, balance, and mobility.
- Because of the link between falls and fractures, individuals at risk for falls should undergo a falls assessment and potentially a multidisciplinary falls prevention program.

PHARMACOLOGIC THERAPY

ANTIRESORPTIVE THERAPY

Calcium Supplementation

- **Calcium** should be ingested in adequate amounts to prevent secondary hyperparathyroidism and bone destruction. Although calcium increases

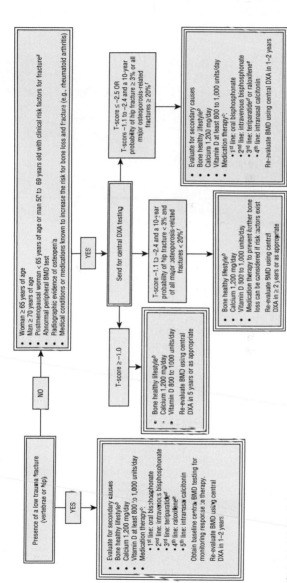

FIGURE 3–1. Algorithm for the management of osteoporosis in postmenopausal women and men ages 50 and older.

Presence of a low trauma fracture (vertebrae or hip)

YES

- Evaluate for secondary causes
- Bone healthy lifestyle[b]
- Calcium 1,200 mg/day
- Vitamin D at least 800 to 1,000 units/day
- Medication therapy[c]:
  - 1st line: oral bisphosphonate
  - 2nd line: intravenous bisphosphonate
  - 3rd line: teriparatide[d]
  - 4th line: raloxifene[e]
  - 5th line: intranasal calcitonin

Obtain baseline central BMD testing for monitoring response to therapy.

Re-evaluate BMD using central DXA in 1–2 years

NO

- Woman ≥ 65 years of age
- Men ≥ 70 years of age
- Postmenopausal woman < 65 years of age or man 50 to 69 years old with clinical risk factors for fracture[a]
- Abnormal peripheral BMD test
- Radiographic evidence of osteopenia
- Medical conditions or medications known to increase the risk for bone loss and fracture (e.g., rheumatoid arthritis)

YES

Send for central DXA testing

T-score ≥ –1.0

- Bone healthy lifestyle[b]
- Calcium 1,200 mg/day
- Vitamin D 800 to 1000 units/day
- Re-evaluate BMD using central DXA in 5 years or as appropriate

T-score –1.1 to –2.4 and a 10-year probability of hip fracture < 3% and of all major osteoporosis-related fractures < 20%[f]

- Bone healthy lifestyle[b]
- Calcium 1,200 mg/day
- Vitamin D 300 to 1,000 units/day
- Medication therapy to prevent further bone loss can be considered if risk factors exist
- Re-evaluate BMD using central DXA in ≥ 2 years or as appropriate

T-score ≤ –2.5 OR T-score –1.1 to –2.4 and a 10-year probability of hip fracture ≥ 3% or all major osteoporosis-related fractures ≥ 20%[f]

- Evaluate for secondary causes
- Bone healthy lifestyle[b]
- Calcium 1,200 mg/day
- Vitamin D at least 800 to 1,000 units/day
- Medication therapy[c]:
  - 1st line: oral bisphosphonate
  - 2nd line: intravenous bisphosphonate
  - 3rd line: teriparatide[d] or raloxifene[e]
  - 4th line: intranasal calcitonin
- Re-evaluate BMD using central DXA in 1–2 years

[a]Major clinical risk factors for fracture: current smoker, low body weight or body mass index, history of osteoporosis/ low trauma fracture in a first-degree relative, personal history of fracture as an adult (after age 50 years), excessive alcohol intake

[b]Bone-healthy lifestyle includes smoking cessation, limit alcohol intake, well-balanced diet with adequate calcium and vitamin D intakes, weight-bearing/resistance exercises, and fall prevention

[c]Men with hypogonadism might also receive testosterone replacement; women with menopausal symptoms might receive low dose hormone therapy for a short time

[d]Teriparatide can be considered a 1st line option in patients with a T-score < –3.5 or if multiple low trauma fractures

[e]Raloxifene might be a good option in women at high risk for breast cancer

[f]WHO absolute fracture risk assessment tool (FRAX) for osteoporotic fracture risk estimations

(BMD, bone mineral density; DXA, dual-energy x-ray absorptiometry)

TABLE 3–1	Calcium and Vitamin D Recommended Dietary Allowances[a]	
Group and Ages	**Elemental Calcium (mg)**	**Vitamin D (units)**
Infants		
Birth to 6 months	200	400
6–12 months	260	400
Children/adolescents		
1–3 years	700	600
4–8 years	1,000	600
9–18 years	1,300	600
Adults		
19–50 years	1,000	600
51–70 years (men)	1,000	600
51–70 years (women)	1,200	600
>70 years	1,200	800
14–18 years, pregnant/lactating	1,300	600
19–50 years, pregnant/lactating	1,000	600

[a]2010 Recommendations from the U.S. Institute of Medicine of the National Academy of Sciences (http://www.iom.edu/calcium).

BMD, fracture prevention is minimal. It should be combined with vitamin D and osteoporosis medications when needed. Because the fraction of calcium absorbed decreases with increasing dose, maximum single doses ≤600 mg of elemental calcium are recommended.

- **Calcium carbonate** is the salt of choice because it contains the highest concentration of elemental calcium (40%) and is the least expensive. It should be ingested with meals to enhance absorption from increased acid secretion.
- **Calcium citrate** absorption is acid independent and need not be taken with meals. It may have fewer GI side effects (e.g., flatulence) than calcium carbonate.
- **Tricalcium phosphate** contains 38% calcium, but calcium-phosphate complexes could limit overall calcium absorption. It might be helpful in patients with hypophosphatemia that cannot be resolved with increased dietary intake.
- Constipation is the most common adverse reaction; it can be treated with increased water intake, dietary fiber (given separately from calcium), and exercise. Calcium carbonate can create gas, sometimes causing flatulence or upset stomach. Calcium causes kidney stones rarely.

Vitamin D Supplementation

- **Vitamin D** deficiency results from insufficient intake, decreased sun exposure, decreased skin production, decreased liver and renal metabolism, and winter residence in northern climates. Supplemental vitamin D maximizes intestinal calcium absorption and has been shown to increase BMD; it may also reduce fractures.

- Supplementation is usually provided with daily nonprescription cholecalciferol (vitamin D_3) products. Higher dose prescription ergocalciferol (vitamin D_2) regimens given weekly, monthly, or quarterly may be used for replacement and maintenance therapy.
- Seniors and patients being treated for osteoporosis should ingest the recommended dietary allowances in **Table 3–1** through food and supplementation with a goal to maintain their 25 (OH) vitamin D concentration at 30 ng/mL (75 nmol/L) or higher. Intake of 100 units of cholecalciferol (vitamin D_3) will raise the vitamin D concentration by ~1 ng/mL (2.5 nmol/L). Because the half-life of vitamin D is about 1 month, a repeat vitamin D concentration should be obtained after about 3 months of therapy to allow a new steady state to be achieved.

Bisphosphonates

- Bisphosphonates (**Table 3–2**) mimic pyrophosphate, an endogenous bone resorption inhibitor, resulting in decreased osteoclast maturation, number, recruitment, bone adhesion, and life span. Bisphosphonates become incorporated into bone, giving them long biologic half-lives of up to 10 years.
- Of the antiresorptive agents available, bisphosphonates provide the greatest BMD increases and fracture risk reductions. Fracture reductions are demonstrated as early as 6 months, with the greatest fracture reduction seen in patients with lower initial BMD and in those with the greatest BMD changes with therapy.
- BMD increases are dose dependent and greatest in the first 6 to 12 months of therapy. Small increases continue over time at the lumbar spine but plateau after 2 to 5 years at the hip. After discontinuation, the increased BMD is sustained for a prolonged period that varies depending on the bisphosphonate used.
- **Alendronate, risedronate,** and **oral ibandronate** are approved by the FDA for prevention and treatment of postmenopausal osteoporosis. **IV ibandronate** and **zoledronic acid** are indicated only for treatment of postmenopausal women. Risedronate and alendronate are also approved for male and glucocorticoid-induced osteoporosis.
- Bisphosphonates must be administered carefully to optimize the clinical benefit and minimize the risk of adverse GI effects. All bisphosphonates are poorly absorbed (bioavailability 1–5%) even under optimal conditions. Each oral tablet should be taken in the morning with at least 6 oz of plain tap water (not coffee, juice, mineral water, or milk) at least 30 minutes (60 minutes for oral ibandronate) before consuming any food, supplement, or medication. The patient should remain upright (sitting or standing) for at least 30 minutes after alendronate and risedronate and 1 hour after ibandronate administration to prevent esophageal irritation and ulceration.
- Most patients prefer once-weekly or once-monthly bisphosphonate administration over daily therapy. If a patient misses a weekly dose, it can be taken the next day. If more than 1 day has elapsed, that dose is skipped until the next scheduled ingestion. If a patient misses a monthly dose, it can be taken up to 7 days before the next scheduled dose.
- The most common bisphosphonate adverse effects are nausea, abdominal pain, and dyspepsia. Esophageal, gastric, or duodenal irritation, perforation,

Medications Used to Prevent and Treat Osteoporosis

Drug	Adult Dosages	Pharmacokinetics	Adverse Effects	Drug Interactions
Calcium	Adequate intake (Table 3–1) in divided doses	Absorption—predominantly active transport with some passive diffusion, fractional absorption 10–60%, fecal elimination for the unabsorbed and renal elimination for the absorbed calcium	Constipation, gas, upset stomach, rare kidney stones	Carbonate products–decreased absorption with proton pump inhibitors Decreased absorption of iron, tetracycline, quinolones, bisphosphonates, phenytoin, and fluoride when given concomitantly Antagonist of verapamil May induce hypercalcemia with thiazide diuretics Fiber laxatives, oxalates, phytates, and sulfates can decrease calcium absorption if given concomitantly
Vitamin D₃ (cholecalciferol)	Adequate intake (Table 3–1); if malabsorption or multiple anticonvulsants, might require higher doses	Hepatic metabolism to 25(OH) vitamin D and then renal metabolism to active compound 1,25(OH)₂ vitamin D, other active and inactive metabolites	Hypercalcemia, (weakness, headache, somnolence, nausea, and/or cardiac rhythm disturbance), hypercalciuria	Phenytoin, barbiturates, carbamazepine, and rifampin increase vitamin D metabolism
Vitamin D₂ (ergocalciferol)	For vitamin D deficiency, 50,000 units once or twice weekly for 8 to 12 weeks; repeat as needed until therapeutic concentrations; occasionally, 50,000 units monthly for maintenance			Cholestyramine, colestipol, orlistat, and mineral oil decrease vitamin D absorption

Drug	Dose	Pharmacokinetics	Adverse Effects	Comments
1,25(OH)₂ vitamin D (calcitriol, Rocaltrol po, Calcijex IV)	0.25–0.5 mcg orally or 1–2 mcg/mL IV daily for renal osteodystrophy, hypoparathyroidism, or refractory rickets			Might induce hypercalcemia with thiazide diuretics in hypoparathyroid patients
Bisphosphonates				
Alendronate (Fosamax, Fosamax plus D, generic)	5 mg daily, 35 mg weekly (prevention) 10 mg daily, 70 mg tablet, 70 mg tablet with vitamin D 2,800 or 5,600 units, or 75 mL liquid weekly (treatment)	Poorly absorbed—<1% decreasing to zero with food or beverage intake—long $T_{1/2}$ (<10 years); renal elimination (of absorbed) and fecal elimination (unabsorbed)	Common: nausea, dyspepsia (oral), transient flu-like illness (injectables) Rare: GI perforation, ulceration, and/or bleeding (oral); musculoskeletal pain, ONJ, atypical fractures	Do not coadminster with any other medication or supplements (including calcium and vitamin D)
Risedronate (Actonel)	5 mg daily, 35 mg weekly, 75 mg on 2 consecutive days once monthly, 150 mg monthly			
Ibandronate (Boniva)	2.5 mg daily, 150 mg once monthly; 3 mg IV every 3 months			
Zoledronic acid (Reclast)	5 mg IV infusion; yearly (treatment) 5 mg IV infusion every 2 years (prevention)			
Estrogen agonist/antagonist				
Raloxifene (Evista)	60 mg daily	Hepatic metabolism	Hot flushes, leg cramps, venous thromboembolism, peripheral edema, rare cataracts and gallbladder disease; black box warning for fatal stroke	None

(continued)

TABLE 3–2 Medications Used to Prevent and Treat Osteoporosis (*Continued*)

Drug	Adult Dosages	Pharmacokinetics	Adverse Effects	Drug Interactions
Calcitonin (Miacalcin)	200 units intranasally daily, alternating nares every other day	Renal elimination; 3% nasal availability	Rhinitis, epistaxis	None
Denosumab (Prolia)	60 mcg subcutaneously every 6 months	T_{max} 10 days, $T_{1/2}$ 25.4 days	Back, extremity, and musculoskeletal pain; hypercholesterolemia; cystitis; serious infections; ONJ	
Teriparatide (PTH 1–34 units, Forteo)	20 mcg subcutaneously daily for up to 2 years	95% bioavailability T_{max} ~30 minutes $T_{1/2}$ ~60 minutes Hepatic metabolism	Pain at injection site, nausea, headache, dizziness, leg cramps, rare increase in uric acid, slightly increased calcium	None

GI, gastrointestinal; IM, intramuscular; ONJ, osteonecrosis of the jaw; T_{max}, time to maximum concentration; $T_{1/2}$, half-life.

ulceration, or bleeding may occur when administration directions are not followed or when bisphosphonates are prescribed for patients with contraindications. The most common adverse effects of IV bisphosphonates include fever, flu-like symptoms, and local injection-site reactions.

- Rare adverse effects include osteonecrosis of the jaw (ONJ) and subtrochanteric femoral (atypical) fractures. ONJ occurs more commonly in patients with cancer, chemotherapy, radiation, and glucocorticoid therapy receiving higher-dose IV bisphosphonate therapy.

Mixed Estrogen Agonists/Antagonists

- **Raloxifene** is an estrogen agonist on bone but an antagonist on the breast and uterus. It is approved for prevention and treatment of postmenopausal osteoporosis. Other estrogen agonists/antagonists are under development (e.g., bazedoxifene and lasofoxifene).
- Raloxifene decreases vertebral fractures and increases spine and hip BMD, but to a lesser extent than bisphosphonates. After discontinuation, the beneficial effect is lost, and bone loss returns to age- or disease-related rates.
- Raloxifene (like tamoxifen) is associated with decreased breast cancer risk. Raloxifene is associated with decreases in total and low-density lipoprotein cholesterol, neutral effects on high-density lipoprotein cholesterol, but slight increases in triglycerides; no beneficial cardiovascular effects have yet been demonstrated.
- Raloxifene is well tolerated overall. Hot flushes occur more frequently in women recently finishing menopause or discontinuing estrogen therapy. Endometrial bleeding occurs rarely. Raloxifene is contraindicated in women with an active or past history of venous thromboembolism. Therapy should be stopped if a patient anticipates extended immobility. Because a slight increase in fatal stroke was documented in a large clinical trial, the prescribing information contains a black box warning urging caution in women at risk for stroke.

Calcitonin

- **Calcitonin** is an endogenous hormone released from the thyroid gland when serum calcium is elevated. Salmon calcitonin is used clinically because it is more potent and longer lasting than the mammalian form. Calcitonin is reserved as a third-line agent because efficacy is less robust than with the other antiresorptive therapies.
- Calcitonin is indicated for osteoporosis treatment for women at least 5 years past menopause. Although limited data suggest beneficial effects in men and concomitantly with glucocorticoids, these indications are not FDA approved.
- Only vertebral fractures have been documented to decrease with intranasal calcitonin therapy. Calcitonin does not consistently affect hip BMD and does not decrease hip fracture risk.
- Calcitonin may provide pain relief to some patients with acute vertebral fractures. If used, it should be prescribed for short-term treatment (4 weeks) and should not be used in place of other more effective and less expensive analgesics, nor should it preclude the use of more appropriate osteoporosis therapy.

- The intranasal dose is 200 units daily, alternating nares every other day. Subcutaneous administration of 100 units daily is available but rarely used because of adverse effects and cost.

Denosumab

- **Denosumab** (Prolia) is a fully human monoclonal antibody that binds to RANKL, blocking its ability to bind to its receptor activator of nuclear factor kappa B (RANK) on the surface of osteoclasts. Denosumab inhibits osteoclast formation, function, and survival.
- It is indicated for treatment of women with postmenopausal osteoporosis who are at high risk for fracture (i.e., history of osteoporotic fracture or multiple risk factors for fracture) or patients who have failed or cannot tolerate other therapies. It has been shown to reduce the incidence of vertebral, nonvertebral, and hip fractures.
- Denosumab is administered as a 60 mg subcutaneous injection in the upper arm, upper thigh, or abdomen once every 6 months.
- The most common adverse events in clinical trials were back or musculoskeletal pain, pain in the extremities, hypercholesterolemia, cystitis, decreased serum calcium, and skin reactions. The drug is contraindicated in patients with hypocalcemia until the condition iscorrected. Serious but rare adverse effects include serious infections, ONJ, and suppression of bone turnover. A medication guide must be given to patients with each filled prescription.

Estrogen Therapy

- Estrogens are approved by the FDA for prevention of osteoporosis, but they should only be used short-term in women who need estrogen therapy (ET) for the management of menopausal symptoms such as hot flushes. The risks of long-term ET outweigh the potential bone benefits.
- ET with or without a progestogen significantly reduces fracture risk. Increases in BMD are less than with bisphosphonates, denosumab, or teriparatide but greater than with raloxifene or calcitonin. Oral and transdermal estrogens at equivalent doses and continuous or cyclic regimens have similar BMD effects. Effect on BMD is dose dependent, with some benefit seen with lower estrogen doses. When ET is discontinued, bone loss accelerates, and fracture protection is lost.
- The lowest effective dose that prevents and controls menopausal symptoms should be used, with use discontinued as soon as possible. Many contraindications to ET and hormone replacement therapy exist and must be identified before starting therapy.

Testosterone

- A few studies of testosterone or **methyltestosterone** replacement in men and women, respectively, have demonstrated increases in BMD, but no data on fracture prevention exist. Testosterone replacement should not be used solely for prevention or treatment of osteoporosis, but it might be beneficial to reduce bone loss in patients needing therapy for hypogonadal symptoms or for women with low libido.

ANABOLIC THERAPIES

Teriparatide

- **Teriparatide** (Forteo) is a recombinant product representing the first 34 amino acids in human parathyroid hormone (PTH). Teriparatide increases bone formation, the bone remodeling rate, and osteoblast number and activity. Both bone mass and architecture are improved.

- Teriparatide is FDA approved for postmenopausal women, men, and patients taking corticosteroids who are at high risk for fracture. Examples of candidates for therapy include patients with a history of osteoporotic fracture, multiple risk factors for fracture, very low bone density (e.g., T-score <−3.5), or those who have failed or are intolerant of previous bisphosphonate therapy.

- The drug reduces fracture risk in postmenopausal women, but no fracture data are available in men or for patients taking corticosteroids. Lumbar spine BMD increases are higher than with other osteoporosis medications. Although wrist BMD is decreased, wrist fractures are not increased.

- Discontinuation of therapy results in a decrease in BMD, which can be alleviated with subsequent antiresorptive therapy. Use of a second course of teriparatide is controversial.

- The teriparatide dose is 20 mcg subcutaneously once daily in the thigh or abdominal area for up to 2 years (see **Table 3–2**). The initial dose should be given with the patient either lying or sitting, in case orthostatic hypotension occurs. Each prefilled 3 mL pen device delivers a 20 mcg dose each day for up to 28 days; the pen device should be kept refrigerated.

- Transient hypercalcemia rarely occurs. A trough serum calcium concentration is recommended 1 month after initiation of therapy.

- Teriparatide is contraindicated in patients at baseline increased risk for osteosarcoma (e.g., Paget bone disease, unexplained alkaline phosphatase elevations, pediatric patients, young adults with open epiphyses, or patients with prior radiation therapy involving the skeleton).

GLUCOCORTICOID-INDUCED OSTEOPOROSIS

- Glucocorticoids decrease bone formation through decreased proliferation and differentiation, as well as enhanced apoptosis of osteoblasts. They also increase bone resorption, decrease calcium absorption, and increase renal calcium excretion.

- Bone losses are rapid, with the greatest decrease occurring during the first 6 to 12 months of therapy. Low to medium doses of inhaled glucocorticoids have no appreciable effect on BMD or fracture risk. Patients using high-dose, inhaled glucocorticoids should be evaluated for osteopenia or osteoporosis.

- Guidelines for managing corticosteroid-induced osteoporosis recommend measuring baseline BMD using central DXA for all patients starting on prednisone 5 mg or more daily (or equivalent) for at least 6 months. BMD testing should also be considered at baseline in patients being started on shorter durations of systemic glucocorticoids if they are at high risk for low bone mass and fractures. Because bone loss can occur rapidly, central DXA can be repeated every 6 to 12 months if needed.

- All patients starting or receiving long-term systemic glucocorticoid therapy should receive at least 1,500 mg of elemental calcium and 800 to 1,200 units of vitamin D daily and practice a bone-healthy lifestyle.
- Oral alendronate and risedronate and IV zoledronic acid have documented efficacy and are FDA approved for glucocorticoid-induced osteoporosis. The American College of Rheumatology guidelines recommend that all patients newly starting on systemic glucocorticoids (≥5 mg/day of prednisone equivalent) for an anticipated duration of at least 3 months should receive preventive bisphosphonate therapy.
- Zoledronic acid is approved for patients with an anticipated steroid duration of at least 1 year. A more conservative approach might be considered in premenopausal women of childbearing potential.
- Bisphosphonate therapy is also recommended for patients starting or receiving long-term glucocorticoid therapy with documented low bone density (T-score <−1) or evidence of a low-trauma fracture.
- Teriparatide can be used if bisphosphonates are not tolerated or contraindicated. Testosterone replacement therapy may be considered in men, and high-dose hormonal oral contraceptives can be considered for premenopausal women with documented hypogonadism.

EVALUATION OF THERAPEUTIC OUTCOMES

- Patients receiving pharmacotherapy for low bone mass should be examined at least annually.
- Patients should be asked about possible fracture symptoms (e.g., bone pain or disability) at each visit.
- Medication adherence and tolerance should be evaluated at each visit.
- Central DXA BMD measurements can be obtained every 1 to 2 years for monitoring bone loss and every 2 years for assessing treatment response. More frequent monitoring may be warranted in patients with conditions associated with higher rates of bone loss (e.g., glucocorticoid use).

See Chapter 99, Osteoporosis and Other Metabolic Bone Diseases, authored by Mary Beth O'Connell and Sheryl F. Vondracek, for a more detailed discussion of this topic.

4   Rheumatoid Arthritis

DEFINITION

- Rheumatoid arthritis (RA) is a chronic and usually progressive inflammatory disorder of unknown etiology characterized by polyarticular symmetric joint involvement and systemic manifestations.

PATHOPHYSIOLOGY

- RA results from a dysregulation of the humoral and cell-mediated components of the immune system. Most patients produce antibodies called rheumatoid factors; these seropositive patients tend to have a more aggressive course than patients who are seronegative.
- Immunoglobulins (Igs) can activate the complement system, which amplifies the immune response by enhancing chemotaxis, phagocytosis, and release of lymphokines by mononuclear cells that are then presented to T lymphocytes. The processed antigen is recognized by the major histocompatibility complex proteins on the lymphocyte surface, resulting in activation of T and B cells.
- Tumor necrosis factor (TNF), interleukin-1 (IL-1), and IL-6 are proinflammatory cytokines important in the initiation and continuance of inflammation.
- Activated T cells produce cytotoxins, which are directly toxic to tissues, and cytokines, which stimulate further activation of inflammatory processes and attract cells to areas of inflammation. Macrophages are stimulated to release prostaglandins and cytotoxins.
- Activated B cells produce plasma cells, which form antibodies that, in combination with complement, result in the accumulation of polymorphonuclear leukocytes. These leukocytes release cytotoxins, oxygen free radicals, and hydroxyl radicals that promote cellular damage to synovium and bone.
- Vasoactive substances (histamine, kinins, and prostaglandins) are released at sites of inflammation, increasing blood flow and vascular permeability. This causes edema, warmth, erythema, and pain and makes it easier for granulocytes to pass from blood vessels to sites of inflammation.
- Chronic inflammation of the synovial tissue lining the joint capsule results in tissue proliferation (pannus formation). Pannus invades cartilage and eventually the bone surface, producing erosions of bone and cartilage and leading to joint destruction. The end results may be loss of joint space, loss of joint motion, bony fusion (ankylosis), joint subluxation, tendon contractures, and chronic deformity.

CLINICAL PRESENTATION

- Nonspecific prodromal symptoms that develop insidiously over weeks to months may include fatigue, weakness, low-grade fever, loss of appetite, and joint pain. Stiffness and myalgias may precede development of synovitis.

- Joint involvement tends to be symmetric and affect the small joints of the hands, wrists, and feet; the elbows, shoulders, hips, knees, and ankles may also be affected.
- Joint stiffness typically is worse in the morning, usually exceeds 30 minutes, and may persist all day.
- On examination, joint swelling may be visible or may be apparent only by palpation. The tissue feels soft, spongy, and warm and may appear erythematous, especially early in the disease course. Chronic joint deformities may involve subluxations of the wrists, metacarpophalangeal joints, and proximal interphalangeal joints (swan neck deformity, boutonnière deformity, and ulnar deviation).
- Extra-articular involvement may include rheumatoid nodules, vasculitis, pleural effusions, pulmonary fibrosis, ocular manifestations, pericarditis, cardiac conduction abnormalities, bone marrow suppression, and lymphadenopathy.

DIAGNOSIS

- A working group of the American College of Rheumatology (ACR) and the European League Against Rheumatism (EULAR) developed the 2010 Rheumatoid Arthritis Classification Criteria (*Arthritis Rheum* 2010;62:2569–2581). The six new criteria are intended to diagnose the disease earlier so patients can be started on disease-modifying treatments sooner to prevent erosive damage and improve outcomes. Two criteria are considered essential by the panel: at least one joint with definite clinical synovitis (swelling) and absence of another disease that would better explain the synovitis. The remaining four criteria are evaluated on a scoring system, with a combined score of 6 or more indicating that the patient has definite RA: joint involvement, serology, acute phase reactants, and duration of symptoms. These criteria differ substantially from the previous 1987 criteria; symmetric joint involvement and the presence of structural joint damage or rheumatoid nodules are not required, and the new criteria set a lower threshold for the number of involved joints.
- Laboratory abnormalities that may be seen include normocytic, normochromic anemia; thrombocytosis or thrombocytopenia; leukopenia; elevated erythrocyte sedimentation rate and C-reactive protein; positive rheumatoid factor (60–70% of patients); positive anticyclic citrullinated peptide antibody (50–85% of patients); and positive antinuclear antibodies (25% of patients).
- Examination of aspirated synovial fluid may reveal turbidity, leukocytosis, reduced viscosity, and normal or low glucose relative to serum concentrations.
- Radiologic findings early in the disease course may include soft tissue swelling and osteoporosis near the joint (periarticular osteoporosis). Erosions occurring later in the disease course are usually seen first in the metacarpophalangeal and proximal interphalangeal joints of the hands and metatarsophalangeal joints of the feet.

DESIRED OUTCOME

- The ultimate goal of RA treatment is to induce a complete remission, although this may be difficult to achieve.
- The primary objectives are to reduce joint swelling, stiffness, and pain; preserve range of motion and joint function; improve quality of life; prevent systemic complications; and slow destructive joint changes.

TREATMENT

NONPHARMACOLOGIC THERAPY

- Adequate rest, weight reduction if obese, occupational therapy, physical therapy, and use of assistive devices may improve symptoms and help maintain joint function.
- Patients with severe disease may benefit from surgical procedures such as tenosynovectomy, tendon repair, and joint replacements.
- Patient education about the disease and the benefits and limitations of drug therapy is important.

PHARMACOLOGIC THERAPY

General Approach

- A disease-modifying antirheumatic drug (DMARD) should be started within the first 3 months of symptom onset. DMARDs should be used in all patients except those with limited disease. Early use of DMARDs results in a more favorable outcome and can reduce mortality.
- First-line nonbiologic DMARDs include **methotrexate (MTX), hydroxychloroquine, sulfasalazine, and leflunomide** (Fig. 4–1). The order of agent selection is not clearly defined, but MTX is often chosen initially because long-term data suggest superior outcomes compared with other DMARDs and lower cost than biologic agents. Leflunomide appears to have long-term efficacy similar to MTX.
- Combination therapy with two or more nonbiologic DMARDs may be effective when single-DMARD treatment is unsuccessful. Recommended

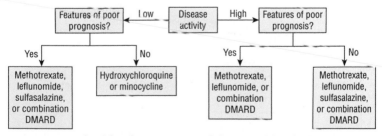

FIGURE 4–1. Algorithm for treatment of rheumatoid arthritis using non-biologic disease-modifying antirheumatic drugs (DMARDs). (MTX, methotrexate; NSAID, nonsteroidal antiinflammatory drug.)

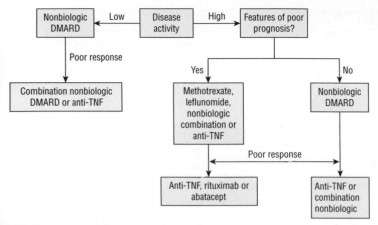

FIGURE 4–2. Algorithm for treatment of rheumatoid arthritis using biologic DMARDs. (TNF, tumor necrosis factor.)

combinations include (1) MTX plus hydroxychloroquine, (2) MTX plus leflunomide, and (2) MTX plus sulfasalazine.

- Biologic agents with disease-modifying activity include the anti-TNF agents **etanercept, infliximab, adalimumab, certolizumab,** and **golimumab**; the costimulation modulator **abatacept**; the IL-6 receptor antagonist **tocilizumab**; and **rituximab**, which depletes peripheral B cells. Biologic DMARDs are effective for patients who fail treatment with other DMARDs (**Fig. 4–2**).

- DMARDs that are less frequently used include **anakinra** (an IL-1 receptor antagonist), **azathioprine, penicillamine, gold salts** (including **auranofin**), **minocycline, cyclosporine,** and **cyclophosphamide**. These agents have either less efficacy or higher toxicity, or both.

- Nonsteroidal antiinflammatory drugs (NSAIDs) and/or corticosteroids may be used for symptomatic relief if needed. They provide relatively rapid improvement compared with DMARDs, which may take weeks to months before benefit is seen. However, NSAIDs have no impact on disease progression, and corticosteroids have the potential for long-term complications.

- See **Tables 4–1** and **4–2** for usual dosages and monitoring parameters for DMARDs and NSAIDs used in RA.

Nonsteroidal Antiinflammatory Drugs

- NSAIDs act primarily by inhibiting prostaglandin synthesis, which is only a small portion of the inflammatory cascade. They possess both analgesic and antiinflammatory properties and reduce stiffness, but they do not slow disease progression or prevent bony erosions or joint deformity. NSAIDs should seldom be used as monotherapy for RA; instead, they should be viewed as adjuncts to DMARD treatment. Common NSAID dosage regimens are shown in **Table 4–3**.

TABLE 4–1 Usual Doses and Monitoring Parameters for Antirheumatic Drugs.

Drug	Usual Dose	Initial Monitoring Tests	Maintenance Monitoring Tests
NSAIDs	See Table 4–3	S_c or BUN, CBC every 2 to 4 weeks after starting therapy for 1 to 2 months; salicylates: serum salicylate levels if therapeutic dose and no response	Same as initial plus stool guaiac every 6 to 12 months
Corticosteroids	Oral, IV, IM, IA, and soft-tissue injections, variable	Glucose; blood pressure every 3 to 6 months	Same as initial
Methotrexate	Oral or IM: 7.5 to 15 mg/wk	Baseline: AST, ALT, ALK-P, albumin, total bilirubin, hepatitis B and C studies, CBC with platelets, S_c	CBC with platelets, AST, albumin every 1 to 2 months
Leflunomide	Oral: 100 mg daily for 3 days, then 10 to 20 mg daily, or 10 to 20 mg daily without loading dose	Baseline: ALT, CBC with platelets	CBC with platelets and ALT monthly initially, then every 6 to 8 weeks
Hydroxychloroquine	Oral: 200 to 300 mg twice daily; after 1 to 2 months may decrease to 200 mg once or twice daily	Baseline: color fundus photography and automated central perimetric analysis	Ophthalmoscopy every 9 to 12 months and Amsler grid at home every 2 weeks
Sulfasalazine	Oral: 500 mg twice daily, then increase to 1 g twice daily max	Baseline: CBC with platelets, then every week for 1 month	Same as initial every 1 to 2 months
Etanercept	50 mg SC once weekly	Tuberculin skin test	None
Infliximab	3 mg/kg IV at 0, 2, and 6 weeks, then every 8 weeks	Tuberculin skin test	None
Adalimumab	40 mg SC every 2 weeks	Tuberculin skin test	None
Certolizumab	400 mg (2 doses of 200 mg) SC at weeks 0, 2, and 4, followed by 200 mg every 2 weeks	Tuberculin skin test	None
Golimumab	50 mg SC once monthly	Tuberculin skin test	None
Abatacept	30-minute IV weight-based infusion: <60 kg = 500 mg; 60–100 kg = 750 mg; >100 kg = 1,000 mg	None	None

(continued)

TABLE 4–1 Usual Doses and Monitoring Parameters for Antirheumatic Drugs. *(Continued)*

Drug	Usual Dose	Initial Monitoring Tests	Maintenance Monitoring Tests
Rituximab	Two 1,000 mg IV infusions separated by 2 weeks	None	None
Tocilizumab	4–8 mg/kg every 4 weeks	AST/ALT, CBC with platelets, lipids	AST/ALT, CBC with platelets, lipids every 4 to 8 weeks
Anakinra	100 mg SC daily	Neutrophil count	Neutrophil count monthly for 3 months, then quarterly for up to 1 year
Auranofin	Oral: 3 mg once or twice daily	Baseline: UA, CBC with platelets	Same as initial every 1 to 2 months
Gold thiomalate	IM: 10 mg test dose, then weekly dosing 25–50 mg; after response may increase dosing interval	Baseline and until stable: UA, CBC with platelets preinjection	Same as initial every other dose
Azathioprine	Oral: 50–150 mg daily	CBC with platelets, AST every 2 weeks for 1 to 2 months	Same as initial every 1 to 2 months
Cyclophosphamide	Oral: 1–2 mg/kg/day	UA, CBC with platelets every week for 1 month	Same tests as initial but every 2 to 4 weeks
Cyclosporine	Oral: 2.5 mg/kg/day	S_{cr}, blood pressure every month	Same as initial
Minocycline	Oral: 100–200 mg daily	None	None
Penicillamine	Oral: 125–250 mg daily, may increase by 125–250 mg every 1 to 2 months; max 750 mg/day	Baseline: UA, CBC with platelets, then every week for 1 month	Same as initial every 1 to 2 months, but every 2 weeks if dose changes

ALK-P, alkaline phosphatase; ALT, alanine aminotransferase; AST, aspartate aminotransferase; BUN, blood urea nitrogen; CBC, complete blood cell count; IA, intraarticular; IM, intramuscular; NSAIDs, nonsteroidal antiinflammatory drugs; SC, subcutaneous; Scr, serum creatinine; UA, urinalysis.

TABLE 4–2	Clinical Monitoring of Drug Therapy in Rheumatoid Arthritis	
Drug	**Toxicities Requiring Monitoring**	**Symptoms to Inquire About[a]**
NSAIDs and salicylates	GI ulceration and bleeding, renal damage	Blood in stool, black stool, dyspepsia, nausea/vomiting, weakness, dizziness, abdominal pain, edema, weight gain, shortness of breath
Corticosteroids	Hypertension, hyperglycemia, osteoporosis[b]	Blood pressure if available, polyuria, polydipsia, edema, shortness of breath, visual changes, weight gain, headaches, broken bones or bone pain
Methotrexate	Myelosuppression, hepatic fibrosis, cirrhosis, pulmonary infiltrates or fibrosis, stomatitis, rash	Symptoms of myelosuppression, shortness of breath, nausea/vomiting, lymph node swelling, coughing, mouth sores, diarrhea, jaundice
Leflunomide	Hepatitis, GI distress, alopecia	Nausea/vomiting, gastritis, diarrhea, hair loss, jaundice
Hydroxychloroquine	Macular damage, rash, diarrhea	Visual changes, including a decrease in night or peripheral vision, rash, diarrhea
Sulfasalazine	Myelosuppression, rash	Symptoms of myelosuppression, photosensitivity, rash, nausea/vomiting
Etanercept, adalimumab, certolizumab, golimumab, tocilizumab, anakinra	Local injection site reactions, infection	Symptoms of infection
Infliximab, rituximab, abatacept	Immune reactions, infection	Postinfusion reactions, symptoms of infection
Azathioprine	Myelosuppression, hepatotoxicity, lymphoproliferative disorders	Symptoms of myelosuppression (extreme fatigue, easy bleeding or bruising, infection), jaundice
Gold (intramuscular or oral)	Myelosuppression, proteinuria, rash, stomatitis	Symptoms of myelosuppression, edema, rash, oral ulcers, diarrhea
Penicillamine	Myelosuppression, proteinuria, stomatitis, rash, dysgeusia	Symptoms of myelosuppression, edema, rash, diarrhea, altered taste perception, oral ulcers

NSAIDs, nonsteroidal antiinflammatory drugs.

[a]Altered immune function increases infection, which should be considered, particularly in patients taking azathioprine, methotrexate, corticosteroids, or other drugs that may produce myelosuppression.

[b]Osteoporosis is not likely to manifest early in treatment, but all patients should be taking appropriate steps to prevent bone loss.

TABLE 4–3	Dosage Regimens for Nonsteroidal Antiinflammatory Drugs		
	Recommended Total Daily Antiinflammatory Dosage		
Drug	**Adult**	**Children**	**Dosing Schedule**
Aspirin	2.6–5.2 g	60–100 mg/kg	Four times daily
Celecoxib	200–400 mg	–	Once or twice daily
Diclofenac	150–200 mg	–	Three or four times daily; extended release: twice daily
Diflunisal	0.5–1.5 g	–	Twice daily
Etodolac	0.2–1.2 g (max 20 mg/kg)	–	Two to four times daily
Fenoprofen	0.9–3 g	–	Four times daily
Flurbiprofen	200–300 mg	–	Two to four times daily
Ibuprofen	1.2–3.2 g	20–40 mg/kg	Three or four times daily
Indomethacin	50–200 mg	2–4 mg/kg (max 200 mg)	Two to four times daily; extended release: once daily
Meclofenamate	200–400 mg	–	Three to four times daily
Meloxicam	7.5–15 mg	–	Once daily
Nabumetone	1–2 g	–	Once or twice daily
Naproxen	0.5–1 g	10 mg/kg	Twice daily; extended release: once daily
Naproxen sodium	0.55–1.1 g	–	Twice daily
Nonacetylated salicylates	1.2–4.8 g	–	Two to six times daily
Oxaprozin	0.6–1.8 g (max 26 mg/kg)	–	One to three times daily
Piroxicam	10–20 mg	–	Once daily
Sulindac	300–400 mg	–	Twice daily
Tolmetin	0.6–1.8 g	15–30 mg/kg	Two to four times daily

Nonbiologic DMARDs

METHOTREXATE

- **MTX** inhibits cytokine production and purine biosynthesis, which may be responsible for its antiinflammatory properties. Its onset is relatively rapid (as early as 2–3 wk), and 45% to 67% of patients remained on it in studies ranging from 5 to 7 years.
- Toxicities are GI (stomatitis, diarrhea, nausea, and vomiting), hematologic (thrombocytopenia and leukopenia), pulmonary (fibrosis and pneumonitis), and hepatic (elevated enzymes and rarely cirrhosis). Concomitant folic acid may reduce some adverse effects without loss of efficacy. Liver injury tests (aspartate aminotransferase [AST] or alanine aminotransferase [ALT]) should be monitored periodically, but a liver biopsy is recommended during therapy only in patients with persistently

elevated hepatic enzymes. MTX is teratogenic, and patients should use contraception and discontinue the drug if conception is planned.

- MTX is contraindicated in pregnant and nursing women, chronic liver disease, immunodeficiency, pleural or peritoneal effusions, leukopenia, thrombocytopenia, preexisting blood disorders, and creatinine clearance <40 mL/min.

LEFLUNOMIDE

- **Leflunomide** (Arava) inhibits pyrimidine synthesis, which reduces lymphocyte proliferation and modulation of inflammation. Its efficacy for RA is similar to that of MTX.
- A loading dose of 100 mg/day for the first 3 days may result in a therapeutic response within the first month. The usual maintenance dose of 20 mg/day may be lowered to 10 mg/day in cases of GI intolerance, complaints of hair loss, or other dose-related toxicity.
- The drug may cause liver toxicity and is contraindicated in patients with preexisting liver disease. The ALT should be monitored monthly initially and periodically thereafter. Leflunomide may cause bone marrow toxicity; a complete blood cell count with platelets is recommended monthly for 6 months, then every 6 to 8 weeks thereafter. It is teratogenic and should be avoided during pregnancy.

HYDROXYCHLOROQUINE

- **Hydroxychloroquine** lacks the myelosuppressive, hepatic, and renal toxicities seen with some other DMARDs, which simplifies monitoring. Its onset may be delayed for up to 6 weeks, but the drug should not be considered a therapeutic failure until after 6 months of therapy with no response.
- Short-term toxicities include GI (nausea, vomiting, and diarrhea), ocular (accommodation defects, benign corneal deposits, blurred vision, scotomas, night blindness, and preretinopathy), dermatologic (rash, alopecia, and skin pigmentation), and neurologic (headache, vertigo, and insomnia) effects. Periodic ophthalmologic examinations are necessary for early detection of reversible retinal toxicity.

SULFASALAZINE

- **Sulfasalazine** use is often limited by adverse effects. Antirheumatic effects should be seen in 2 months.
- Adverse effects include GI (anorexia, nausea, vomiting, and diarrhea), dermatologic (rash and urticaria), hematologic (leukopenia and rarely agranulocytosis), and hepatic (elevated enzymes) effects. GI symptoms may be minimized by starting with low doses, dividing the dose more evenly throughout the day, and taking the drug with food.

OTHER NONBIOLOGIC DMARDS

- **Gold salts, azathioprine, penicillamine, cyclosporine,** and **cyclophosphamide** can be effective and may be of value in certain clinical settings. However, they are used less frequently today because of toxicity, lack of long-term benefits, or both. Tables 4–2 and 4–3 provide information on dosing and monitoring.

Biologic DMARDs

TNF-α INHIBITORS

- Inhibitors of the inflammatory cytokine TNF-α are generally the first biologic DMARDs used for RA treatment. About 30% of patients eventually discontinue their use due to inadequate efficacy or adverse effects. In such situations, addition of a nonbiologic DMARD may be beneficial if the patient is not already taking one. Choosing an alternative TNF inhibitor may benefit some patients; treatment with rituximab or abatacept may also be effective in patients failing TNF inhibitors. Combination biologic DMARD therapy is not recommended because of the increased risk for infection.

- Congestive heart failure (HF) is a relative contraindication for anti-TNF agents due to reports of increased cardiac mortality and HF exacerbations with several agents. Patients with a history of uncompensated HF or recent hospital admissions for HF should not use anti-TNF therapy. The drugs should be discontinued in patients whose HF worsens during treatment.

- Anti-TNF therapy has been reported to induce a multiple sclerosis (MS)–like illness or exacerbate MS in patients with the disease. Patients with neurologic symptoms suggestive of MS should discontinue therapy.

- TNF inhibitors are associated with increased risk of cancer, especially lymphoproliferative cancers. The drugs contain a black box warning about increased risk of lymphoproliferative and other cancers in children and adolescents treated with these drugs.

- These drugs (and other biologic DMARDs) carry a small increased risk for infection. Tuberculin skin testing is recommended prior to treatment so that latent tuberculosis can be detected. These agents should be avoided in patients with preexisting infection and in those at high risk for developing infection. Treatment should be discontinued temporarily if an infection develops during therapy. No laboratory monitoring is required with anti-TNF agents.

  - ✓ **Etanercept** (Enbrel) is a fusion protein consisting of two p75-soluble TNF receptors linked to an Fc fragment of human IgG_1. It binds to and inactivates TNF, preventing it from interacting with the cell-surface TNF receptors and thereby activating cells. Clinical trials used etanercept in patients who failed DMARDs, and responses were seen in 60% to 75% of patients. It has been shown to slow erosive disease progression to a greater degree than oral MTX in patients with inadequate response to MTX monotherapy. Adverse effects include local injection site reactions, and there have been case reports of pancytopenia and neurologic demyelinating syndromes.

  - ✓ **Infliximab** (Remicade) is a chimeric anti-TNF antibody fused to a human constant-region IgG_1. It binds to TNF and prevents its interaction with TNF receptors on inflammatory cells. To prevent formation of antibodies to this foreign protein, MTX should be given orally in doses used to treat RA for as long as the patient continues on infliximab. In clinical trials, the combination of infliximab and MTX halted progression of joint damage and was superior to MTX monotherapy.

Infliximab may increase the risk of infection. An acute infusion reaction with fever, chills, pruritus, and rash may occur within 1 to 2 hours after administration. Autoantibodies and lupus-like syndrome have also been reported.

✓ **Adalimumab** (Humira) is a human IgG$_1$ antibody to TNF that is less antigenic than infliximab. It has response rates similar to other TNF inhibitors. Local injection site reactions were the most common adverse event reported in clinical trials.

✓ **Certolizumab** (Cimzia) is a humanized antibody specific for TNF-α.

✓ **Golimumab** (Simponi) is another human antibody to TNF-α (see Tables 4–1 and 4–2 for dosing and monitoring information).

ABATACEPT

- **Abatacept** (Orencia) is a costimulation modulator approved for patients with moderate to severe disease who fail to achieve an adequate response from one or more DMARDs. By binding to CD80/CD86 receptors on antigen-presenting cells, abatacept inhibits interactions between the antigen-presenting cells and T cells, preventing T cells from activating to promote the inflammatory process. The drug is well tolerated, with infusion reactions, headache, nasopharyngitis, dizziness, cough, back pain, hypertension, dyspepsia, urinary tract infection, rash, and extremity pain reported more frequently in clinical trials.

RITUXIMAB

- **Rituximab** (Rituxan) is a monoclonal chimeric antibody consisting of mostly human protein with the antigen-binding region derived from a mouse antibody to CD20 protein found on the cell surface of mature B lymphocytes. Binding of rituximab to B cells results in nearly complete depletion of peripheral B cells, with a gradual recovery over several months. Rituximab is useful in patients failing MTX or TNF inhibitors. Methylprednisolone 100 mg should be given 30 minutes prior to rituximab to reduce the incidence and severity of infusion reactions. Acetaminophen and antihistamines may also benefit patients who have a history of reactions. MTX should be given concurrently in the usual doses for RA to achieve the best therapeutic outcomes.

TOCILIZUMAB

- **Tocilizumab** (Actemra) attaches to IL 6 receptors, which prevents the cytokine from interacting with cells. It has been used as monotherapy or in combination with MTX. Infusion reactions, increased plasma lipids, and increased infections have been reported.

ANAKINRA

- **Anakinra** (Kineret) is an IL-1 receptor antagonist; it is considered to be less effective than other biologic DMARDs and is not included in the current ACR treatment recommendations. It can be used alone or in combination with any of the other DMARDs except for TNF-blocking agents.

Corticosteroids

- **Corticosteroids** have antiinflammatory and immunosuppressive properties. They interfere with antigen presentation to T lymphocytes, inhibit prostaglandin and leukotriene synthesis, and inhibit neutrophil and monocyte superoxide radical generation.
- Oral corticosteroids (e.g., **prednisone** and **methylprednisolone**) can be used to control pain and synovitis while DMARDs are taking effect ("bridging therapy"). This is often used in patients with debilitating symptoms when DMARD therapy is initiated.
- Low-dose, long-term corticosteroid therapy may be used to control symptoms in patients with difficult-to-control disease. Prednisone doses below 7.5 mg/day (or equivalent) are well tolerated but are not devoid of the long-term corticosteroid adverse effects. The lowest dose that controls symptoms should be used. Alternate-day dosing of low-dose oral corticosteroids is usually ineffective in RA.
- High-dose oral or IV bursts may be used for several days to suppress disease flares. After symptoms are controlled, the drug should be tapered to the lowest effective dose.
- The intramuscular route is preferable in nonadherent patients. Depot forms (**triamcinolone acetonide, triamcinolone hexacetonide,** and **methylprednisolone acetate**) provide 2 to 6 weeks of symptomatic control. The onset of effect may be delayed for several days. The depot effect provides a physiologic taper, avoiding hypothalamic-pituitary axis suppression.
- Intraarticular injections of depot forms may be useful when only a few joints are involved. If effective, injections may be repeated every 3 months. No one joint should be injected more than two or three times per year.
- Adverse effects of systemic glucocorticoids limit their long-term use. Dosage tapering and eventual discontinuation should be considered at some point in patients receiving chronic therapy.

EVALUATION OF THERAPEUTIC OUTCOMES

- Clinical signs of improvement include reduction in joint swelling, decreased warmth over actively involved joints, and decreased tenderness to joint palpation.
- Symptom improvement includes reduction in joint pain and morning stiffness, longer time to onset of afternoon fatigue, and improvement in ability to perform daily activities.
- Periodic joint radiographs may be useful in assessing disease progression.
- Laboratory monitoring is of little value in monitoring response to therapy but is essential for detecting and preventing adverse drug effects (see **Table 4–2**).
- Patients should be questioned about the presence of symptoms that may be related to adverse drug effects (see **Table 4–3**).

See Chapter 100, Rheumatoid Arthritis, authored by Arthur A. Schuna, for a detailed discussion of this topic.

5 Acute Coronary Syndromes

DEFINITIONS

- Acute coronary syndromes (ACSs) include all clinical syndromes compatible with acute myocardial ischemia resulting from an imbalance between myocardial oxygen demand and supply.
- In contrast to stable angina, an ACS results primarily from diminished myocardial blood flow secondary to an occlusive or partially occlusive coronary artery thrombus.
- ACSs are classified according to electrocardiographic (ECG) changes into (1) ST-segment-elevation (STE) ACS or STE MI and (2) non–ST-segment-elevation (NSTE) ACS, which includes non–ST-segment-elevation myocardial infarction (NSTE MI) and unstable angina (UA).
- After an STE MI, pathologic Q waves are seen frequently on the ECG and usually indicate transmural MI. Non–Q-wave MI, which is seen predominantly in NSTE MI, is limited to the subendocardial myocardium.
- NSTE MI differs from UA in that ischemia is severe enough to produce myocardial necrosis, resulting in release of detectable amounts of biochemical markers, primarily troponin I or T and creatine kinase myocardial band (CK-MB) from the necrotic myocytes into the bloodstream.

PATHOPHYSIOLOGY

- The formation of atherosclerotic plaques is the underlying cause of coronary artery disease (CAD) and ACS in most patients. Endothelial dysfunction leads to formation of fatty streaks in the coronary arteries and eventually to atherosclerotic plaques. Factors responsible for development of atherosclerosis include hypertension, age, male gender, tobacco use, diabetes mellitus, obesity, and dyslipidemia.
- The cause of ACS in >90% of patients is rupture, fissuring, or erosion of an unstable atheromatous plaque. Plaques most susceptible to rupture have an eccentric shape; thin, fibrous cap; large, fatty core; high content of inflammatory cells, such as macrophages and lymphocytes; limited amounts of smooth muscle; and significant compensatory enlargement.
- A partially or completely occlusive clot forms on top of the ruptured plaque. Exposure of collagen and tissue factor induces platelet adhesion and activation, which promote release of adenosine diphosphate and thromboxane A_2 from platelets. These produce vasoconstriction and potentiate platelet activation. A change in the conformation of the glycoprotein (GP) IIb/IIIa surface receptors of platelets occurs that cross-links platelets to each

45

other through fibrinogen bridges (the final common pathway of platelet aggregation).

- Simultaneously, activation of the extrinsic coagulation cascade occurs as a result of exposure of blood to the thrombogenic lipid core and endothelium, which are rich in tissue factor. This pathway ultimately leads to the formation of a fibrin clot composed of fibrin strands, cross-linked platelets, and trapped red blood cells.

- Ventricular remodeling occurs after an MI and is characterized by changes in the size, shape, and function of the left ventricle that may lead to cardiac failure. Factors contributing to ventricular remodeling include neurohormonal factors (e.g., activation of the renin–angiotensin–aldosterone and sympathetic nervous systems), hemodynamic factors, mechanical factors, changes in gene expression, and modifications in myocardial matrix metalloproteinase activity and their inhibitors. This process may lead to cardiomyocyte hypertrophy, loss of cardiomyocytes, and increased interstitial fibrosis, which promote both systolic and diastolic dysfunction.

- Complications of MI include cardiogenic shock, heart failure (HF), valvular dysfunction, various arrhythmias, pericarditis, stroke secondary to left ventricular (LV) thrombus embolization, venous thromboembolism, and LV free-wall rupture.

CLINICAL PRESENTATION

- The predominant symptom of ACS is midline anterior chest discomfort (usually occurring at rest), severe new-onset angina, or increasing angina that lasts at least 20 minutes. The discomfort may radiate to the shoulder, down the left arm, to the back, or to the jaw. Accompanying symptoms may include nausea, vomiting, diaphoresis, and shortness of breath. Elderly patients, patients with diabetes, and women are less likely to present with classic symptoms.

- There are no specific features indicative of ACS on physical examination. However, patients with ACS may present with signs of acute HF or arrhythmias.

DIAGNOSIS

- A 12-lead ECG should be obtained within 10 minutes of patient presentation. Key findings indicating myocardial ischemia or MI are ST-segment elevation, ST-segment depression, and T-wave inversion (Fig. 5–1). These changes in certain groupings of leads help to identify the location of the involved coronary artery. The appearance of a new left bundle-branch block accompanied by chest discomfort is highly specific for acute MI. Some patients with myocardial ischemia have no ECG changes, so biochemical markers and other risk factors for CAD should be assessed to determine the patient's risk for experiencing a new MI or other complications.

- Biochemical markers of myocardial cell death are important for confirming the diagnosis of MI. An evolving MI is defined as a typical rise and

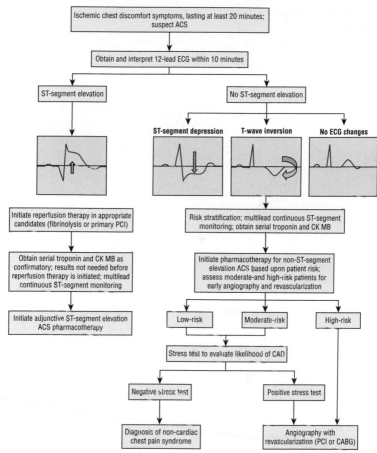

FIGURE 5–1. Evaluation of the acute coronary syndrome (ACS) patient.
(CABG, coronary artery bypass graft surgery; CAD, coronary artery disease; CK-MB, creatine kinase myocardial band; ECG, electrocardiogram; PCI, percutaneous coronary intervention.) *(Reprinted with permission from the American College of Clinical Pharmacy. Spinler SA. Acute coronary syndromes. In: Dunsworth TS, Richardson MM, Cheng JWM, et al., eds. Pharmacotherapy Self-Assessment Program, 7th ed. Cardiology II module. Kansas City: American College of Clinical Pharmacy, 2010:99.)*

gradual fall in troponin I or T or a more rapid rise and fall of CK-MB (**Fig. 5–2**). Typically, blood is obtained at least two times, once in the emergency department and again in 6 to 9 hours. An MI is identified if at least one troponin value is greater than the MI decision limit set by the hospital laboratory with a typical rise or fall. If a troponin test is not available, an increased CK-MB may be used to make the diagnosis. Both troponins and CK-MB are detectable within 6 hours of MI. Troponins remain elevated for 7 to 14 days, whereas CK-MB returns to normal within 48 hours.

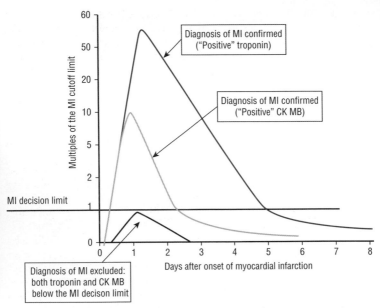

FIGURE 5–2. Biochemical markers in suspected acute coronary syndrome.

- Patient symptoms, past medical history, ECG, and troponin or CK-MB determinations are used to stratify patients into low, medium, or high risk of death, initial MI, reinfarction, or likelihood of failing pharmacotherapy and needing urgent coronary angiography and percutaneous coronary intervention (PCI).

DESIRED OUTCOME

- Short-term goals of therapy include (1) early restoration of blood flow to the infarct-related artery to prevent infarct expansion (in the case of MI) or prevent complete occlusion and MI (in UA), (2) prevention of complications and death, (3) prevention of coronary artery reocclusion, (4) relief of ischemic chest discomfort, and (5) resolution of ST-segment and T-wave changes on ECG.

TREATMENT

GENERAL APPROACH

- General treatment measures include hospital admission, oxygen administration if saturation is <90%, continuous multilead ST-segment monitoring for arrhythmias and ischemia, glycemic control, frequent measurement of vital signs, bedrest for 12 hours in hemodynamically stable patients, use of stool softeners to avoid Valsalva maneuver, and pain relief.

- Blood chemistry tests that should be performed include potassium and magnesium, glucose, serum creatinine, baseline complete blood cell count (CBC) and coagulation tests, and fasting lipid panel. The fasting lipid panel should be drawn within the first 24 hours of hospitalization because values for cholesterol (an acute phase reactant) may be falsely low after that period.
- It is important to triage and treat patients according to their risk category (see **Fig. 5–1**).
- Patients with STE MI are at high risk of death, and efforts to reestablish coronary perfusion should be initiated immediately (without evaluation of biochemical markers).
- Patients with NSTE ACS who are considered to be at low risk (based on thrombolysis in myocardial infarction [TIMI] risk score) should have serial biochemical markers obtained. If they are negative, the patient may be admitted to a general medical floor with ECG telemetry monitoring, undergo a noninvasive stress test, or be discharged.
- High-risk NSTE ACS patients should undergo early coronary angiography (within 12–24 h) and revascularization if a significant coronary artery stenosis is found. Moderate-risk patients with positive biochemical markers typically also undergo angiography and revascularization, if indicated.
- Moderate-risk patients with negative biochemical markers may also undergo angiography and revascularization or may initially undergo a noninvasive stress test, with only select patients with positive tests proceeding to angiography.

NONPHARMACOLOGIC THERAPY

- For patients with STE ACS, either fibrinolysis or immediate primary PCI (with either balloon angioplasty or stent placement) is the treatment of choice for reestablishing coronary artery blood flow when the patient presents within 3 hours of symptom onset. Primary PCI may be associated with a lower mortality rate than fibrinolysis, possibly because PCI opens >90% of coronary arteries compared with <60% opened with fibrinolytics. The risks of intracranial hemorrhage (ICH) and major bleeding are also lower with PCI than with fibrinolysis. Primary PCI is generally preferred if institutions have skilled interventional cardiologists and other necessary facilities, in patients with cardiogenic shock, patients with contraindications to fibrinolytics, and patients presenting with symptom onset more than 3 hours prior.
- For patients with NSTE ACS, clinical practice guidelines recommend either PCI or coronary artery bypass grafting revascularization as an early treatment for high-risk patients and that such an approach also be considered for patients not at high risk.

EARLY PHARMACOTHERAPY FOR ST-SEGMENT-ELEVATION ACS

(Fig. 5–3)

- According to the American College of Cardiology/American Heart Association (ACC/AHA) practice guidelines, early pharmacologic therapy

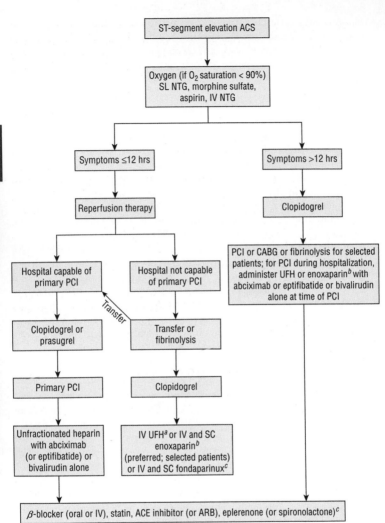

FIGURE 5–3. Initial pharmacotherapy for ST-segment-elevation myocardial infarction. (ACE, angiotensin-converting enzyme; ACS, acute coronary syndromes; ARB, angiotensin receptor blocker; CABG, coronary artery bypass graft surgery; NTG, nitroglycerin; PCI, percutaneous coronary intervention; UFH, unfractionated heparin.) [a]For at least 48 hours. [b]For the duration of hospitalization. [c]For select patients. *(Reprinted (or modified) with permission from the American College of Clinical Pharmacy. Spinler SA. Evolution of antithrombotic therapy used in acute coronary syndromes. In: Richardson MM, Chessman KH, Chant C, et al, eds. Pharmacotherapy Self-assessment Program, Book 1 Cardiology, 7th ed. Lenexa, KS: American College of Clinical Pharmacy; 2010:101.)*

should include (1) intranasal oxygen (if oxygen saturation is <90%), (2) sublingual (SL) nitroglycerin (NTG), (3) aspirin, (4) an anticoagulant, and (5) fibrinolysis in eligible candidates. Morphine is administered to patients with refractory angina as an analgesic and venodilator that lowers preload. These agents should be administered early, while the patient is still in the emergency department. Clopidogrel or prasugrel should be administered to patients undergoing PCI, whereas only clopidogrel is recommended for patients receiving fibrinolytics and those not undergoing reperfusion therapy. An angiotensin-converting enzyme (ACE) inhibitor should be started within 24 hours of presentation, particularly in patients with left ventricular ejection fraction (LVEF) ≤40%, signs of HF, or an anterior wall MI, if there are no contraindications. IV NTG, β-blockers, and an aldosterone antagonist should be administered to select patients. A statin should be initiated prior to hospital discharge if the low-density lipoprotein (LDL) cholesterol is >100 mg/dL.

Fibrinolytic Therapy

- A fibrinolytic agent is indicated in patients with STE MI presenting within 12 hours of the onset of chest discomfort who have at least 1 mm of STE in two or more contiguous ECG leads or a new left bundle-branch block. It should also be considered in patients with those findings and persistent symptoms of ischemia who present within 12 to 24 hours of symptom onset. Fibrinolysis is preferred over primary PCI in patients presenting within 3 hours of symptom onset when there would be a delay in performing primary PCI.
- It is not necessary to obtain the results of biochemical markers before initiating fibrinolytic therapy.
- Absolute contraindications to fibrinolytic therapy include (1) history of hemorrhagic stroke (at any time), (2) ischemic stroke within 3 months, (3) active internal bleeding, (4) known intracranial neoplasm, (5) known structural cerebrovascular lesion, (6) suspected aortic dissection, and (7) significant closed head or facial trauma within 3 months. Primary PCI is preferred in these situations.
- Patients with relative contraindications to fibrinolytics may receive therapy if the perceived risk of death from MI is higher than the risk of major hemorrhage. These situations include (1) severe, uncontrolled hypertension (blood pressure [BP] >180/110 mm Hg); (2) history of prior ischemic stroke more than 3 months prior, dementia, or known intracranial pathology not considered an absolute contraindication; (3) current anticoagulant use; (4) known bleeding diathesis; (5) traumatic or prolonged cardiopulmonary resuscitation or major surgery within 3 weeks; (6) noncompressible vascular puncture; (7) recent (within 2–4 weeks) internal bleeding; (8) pregnancy; (9) active peptic ulcer; (10) history of severe, chronic, poorly controlled hypertension; and (11) for streptokinase, prior administration (>5 days) or prior allergic reactions.
- Practice guidelines indicate that a more fibrin-specific agent (alteplase, reteplase, or tenecteplase) is preferred over the non–fibrin-specific agent streptokinase. Fibrin-specific agents open a greater percentage of infarct arteries, which results in smaller infarcts and lower mortality.

- Eligible patients should be treated as soon as possible, but preferably within 30 minutes from the time they present to the emergency department, with one of the following regimens:
  - ✓ **Alteplase:** 15 mg IV bolus followed by 0.75 mg/kg infusion (maximum 50 mg) over 30 minutes, followed by 0.5 mg/kg infusion (maximum 35 mg) over 60 minutes (maximum dose 100 mg).
  - ✓ **Reteplase:** 10 units IV over 2 minutes, followed 30 minutes later with another 10 units IV over 2 minutes.
  - ✓ **Tenecteplase:** A single IV bolus dose given over 5 seconds based on patient weight: 30 mg if <60 kg; 35 mg if 60 to 69.9 kg; 40 mg if 70 to 79.9 kg; 45 mg if 80 to 89.9 kg; and 50 mg if ≥90 kg.
  - ✓ **Streptokinase:** 1.5 million units in 50 mL of normal saline or 5% dextrose in water IV over 60 minutes.
- ICH and major bleeding are the most serious side effects. The risk of ICH is higher with fibrin-specific agents than with streptokinase. However, the risk of systemic bleeding other than ICH is higher with streptokinase than with fibrin-specific agents.

Aspirin

- **Aspirin** should be administered to all patients without contraindications within the first 24 hours of hospital admission. It provides an additional mortality benefit in patients with STE ACS when given with fibrinolytic therapy.
- In patients experiencing an ACS, non–enteric-coated aspirin, 160 to 325 mg, should be chewed and swallowed as soon as possible after the onset of symptoms or immediately after presentation to the emergency department regardless of the reperfusion strategy being considered.
- A daily maintenance dose of 75 to 162 mg is recommended thereafter and should be continued indefinitely.
- For patients undergoing PCI and receiving stents, the recommended dose is 162 to 325 mg once daily for 1 month after placement of a bare metal stent, for 3 months with a sirolimus-eluting stent, and for 6 months with a paclitaxel-eluting stent, followed by 75 to 162 mg once daily thereafter.
- Low-dose aspirin is associated with a reduced risk of major bleeding, particularly GI bleeding. Other GI disturbances (e.g., dyspepsia and nausea) are infrequent with low-dose aspirin. Other nonsteroidal antiinflammatory drugs (NSAIDs) and cyclooxygenase-2 (COX-2) selective inhibitors should be discontinued at the time of STE MI due to increased risk of mortality, reinfarction, HF, and myocardial rupture.

Thienopyridines

- **Clopidogrel** is recommended for patients with an aspirin allergy. A 300 to 600 mg loading dose is given on the first hospital day, followed by a maintenance dose of 75 mg daily. It should be continued indefinitely.
- For patients treated with fibrinolytics and in those receiving no revascularization therapy, clopidogrel either 75 mg or 300 mg on day 1 followed by 75 mg once daily should be given for at least 14 days and up to 1 year in addition to aspirin.
- For patients undergoing primary PCI, clopidogrel is administered as a 300 to 600 mg loading dose followed by a 75 mg/day maintenance dose,

in combination with aspirin 325 mg once daily, to prevent subacute stent thrombosis and long-term cardiovascular events.

- **Prasugrel** is administered as a loading dose of 60 mg followed by a maintenance dose of 10 mg daily. The recommended duration of therapy for patients undergoing PCI is at least 12 months after bare-metal or drug-eluting stent placement and up to 15 months after bare-metal stent placement in patients at low risk of bleeding.
- The most frequent side effects of clopidogrel and prasugrel are nausea, vomiting, and diarrhea (2–5% of patients). Thrombotic thrombocytopenia purpura has been reported rarely with clopidogrel. The most serious side effect of these drugs is hemorrhage.
- **Ticlopidine** is associated with neutropenia that requires frequent monitoring of the CBC during the first 3 months of use. For this reason, either clopidogrel or prasugrel is the preferred thienopyridine for ACS and PCI patients.

Glycoprotein IIb/IIIa Receptor Inhibitors

- If unfractionated heparin (UFH) is selected for primary PCI in STE MI, a GP IIb/IIIa inhibitor (usually abciximab or eptifibatide) should be added to UFH (in addition to a thienopyridine and aspirin) to reduce the likelihood of reinfarction for patients who have not received fibrinolytics. GP IIb/IIIa inhibitors should not be administered to STE MI patients who will not be undergoing PCI.
- **Abciximab** is typically initiated as a 0.25 mg/kg IV bolus given 10 to 60 minutes before the start of PCI, followed by 0.125 mcg/kg/min (maximum 10 mcg/min) for 12 hours.
- **Eptifibatide** is administered as a 180 mcg/kg IV bolus, which is repeated in 10 minutes, followed by an infusion of 2 mcg/kg/min for 18 to 24 hours after PCI.
- GP IIb/IIIa inhibitors may increase the risk of bleeding, especially if given in the setting of recent (<4 h) administration of fibrinolytic therapy. An immune-mediated thrombocytopenia may occur rarely.

Anticoagulants

- Either **UFH** or **bivalirudin** is preferred for patients undergoing primary PCI, whereas **enoxaparin** is preferred when fibrinolysis reperfusion therapy is chosen for STE MI.
- Anticoagulant therapy should be initiated in the emergency department and continued for at least 48 hours in select patients who will receive chronic warfarin after acute MI. If a patient undergoes PCI, UFH or bivalirudin is discontinued immediately after the procedure.
- The initial UFH dose for primary PCI is 50 to 70 units/kg IV bolus if a GP IIb/IIIa inhibitor is planned and 70 to 100 units/kg IV bolus if no GP IIb/IIIa inhibitor is planned; supplemental IV bolus doses are given to maintain the target activated clotting time (ACT).
- The initial UFH dose for STE MI with fibrinolytics is 60 units/kg IV bolus (maximum 4,000 units), followed by a constant IV infusion of 12 units/kg/h (maximum 1,000 units/h). The dose of the UFH infusion is adjusted frequently to maintain a target activated partial thromboplastin time (aPTT) of 1.5 to 2 times control (50–70 s). The first aPTT should

be measured at 3 hours in patients with STE ACS who are treated with fibrinolytics and at 4 to 6 hours in patients not receiving thrombolytics or undergoing primary PCI.

- The enoxaparin dose for STE MI is 1 mg/kg subcutaneous (SC) every 12 hours (creatinine clearance [Cl_{cr}] ≥30 mL/min) or 24 hours if impaired renal function (Cl_{cr} 15–29 mL/min). For patients with STE MI receiving fibrinolytics, enoxaparin 30 mg IV bolus is followed immediately by 1 mg/kg SC every 12 hours if younger than age 75 years. In patients 75 years and older, the enoxaparin dose is 0.75 mg/kg SC every 12 hours. Enoxaparin should be continued throughout hospitalization or up to 8 days.

- The bivalirudin dose for PCI in STE MI is 0.75 mg/kg IV bolus, followed by 1.75 mg/kg/h infusion. It should be discontinued at the end of PCI or continued at 0.25 mg/kg/h if prolonged anticoagulation is necessary.

Nitrates

- Immediately upon presentation, one SL **NTG** tablet (0.4 mg) should be administered every 5 minutes for up to three doses to relieve chest pain and myocardial ischemia.

- Intravenous NTG is indicated for patients with an ACS who do not have a contraindication and who have persistent ischemic symptoms, HF, or uncontrolled high BP. The usual dose is 5 to 10 mcg/min by continuous infusion, titrated up to 100 mcg/min until relief of symptoms or limiting side effects (e.g., headache or hypotension). Treatment should be continued for ~24 hours after ischemia is relieved.

- NTG causes venodilation, which lowers preload and myocardial oxygen demand. In addition, arterial vasodilation may lower BP, thereby reducing myocardial oxygen demand. Arterial dilation also relieves coronary artery vasospasm and improves myocardial blood flow and oxygenation.

- Oral nitrates play a limited role in ACS because clinical trials have failed to show a mortality benefit for IV followed by oral nitrate therapy in acute MI. Therefore, other life-saving therapy, such as ACE inhibitors and β-blockers, should not be withheld.

- The most significant adverse effects of nitrates are tachycardia, flushing, headache, and hypotension. Nitrates are contraindicated in patients who have taken the oral phosphodiesterase-5 inhibitors sildenafil or vardenafil within the prior 24 hours or tadalafil within the prior 48 hours.

β-Adrenergic Blockers

- If there are no contraindications, a β-blocker should be administered early in the care of patients with STE ACS (within the first 24 h) and continued indefinitely.

- The benefits result from blockade of β_1 receptors in the myocardium, which reduces heart rate, myocardial contractility, and BP, thereby decreasing myocardial oxygen demand. The reduced heart rate increases diastolic time, thus improving ventricular filling and coronary artery perfusion.

- Because of these effects, β-blockers reduce the risk for recurrent ischemia, infarct size, risk of reinfarction, and occurrence of ventricular arrhythmias.

- The usual doses of β-blockers are as follows, with a target resting heart rate of 50 to 60 beats/min:
  - ✓ **Metoprolol:** 5 mg by slow (over 1–2 min) IV bolus, repeated every 5 minutes for a total initial dose of 15 mg. If a conservative regimen is desired, initial doses can be reduced to 1 to 2 mg. This is followed in 1 to 2 hours by 25 to 50 mg orally every 6 hours. If appropriate, initial IV therapy may be omitted.
  - ✓ **Propranolol:** 0.5 to 1 mg slow IV push, followed in 1 to 2 hours by 40 to 80 mg orally every 6 to 8 hours. If appropriate, the initial IV therapy may be omitted.
  - ✓ **Atenolol:** 5 mg IV dose, followed 5 minutes later by a second 5 mg IV dose, then 50 to 100 mg orally once daily beginning 1 to 2 hours after the IV dose. The initial IV therapy may be omitted.
- The most serious side effects early in ACS are hypotension, acute HF, bradycardia, and heart block. Initial acute administration of β-blockers is not appropriate for patients presenting with acute HF but may be attempted in most patients before hospital discharge after treatment of acute HF.

Calcium Channel Blockers

- In the setting of STE MI, calcium channel blockers are reserved for patients who have contraindications to β-blockers. Current data suggest little clinical benefit beyond symptom relief.
- Patients who had been prescribed calcium channel blockers for hypertension who are not receiving β-blockers and who do not have a contraindication should have the calcium channel blocker discontinued and a β-blocker initiated.
- Dihydropyridine channel blockers (e.g., **amlodipine, felodipine,** and **nifedipine**) primarily produce antiischemic effects through peripheral vasodilation with no effects on atrioventricular (AV) node conduction or heart rate. Short-acting dihydropyridines should be avoided because they appear to worsen outcomes. **Diltiazem** and **verapamil** have additional antiischemic effects by reducing contractility and AV conduction and slowing heart rate; their role is limited to relief of ischemia-related symptoms or control of heart rate in patients with supraventricular arrhythmias in whom β-blockers are contraindicated or ineffective.
- Patients with variant (Prinzmetal) angina or cocaine-induced ACS may benefit from calcium channel blockers as initial therapy because they can reverse coronary vasospasm. β-Blockers generally should be avoided in these situations because they may worsen vasospasm through an unopposed β_1-blocking effect on smooth muscle.

EARLY PHARMACOTHERAPY FOR NON–ST-SEGMENT-ELEVATION ACS

(Fig. 5–4)

- Early pharmacotherapy for NSTE ACS is similar to that for STE ACS. According to ACC/AHA practice guidelines, early pharmacotherapy should include (1) **intranasal oxygen** (if oxygen saturation is <90%),

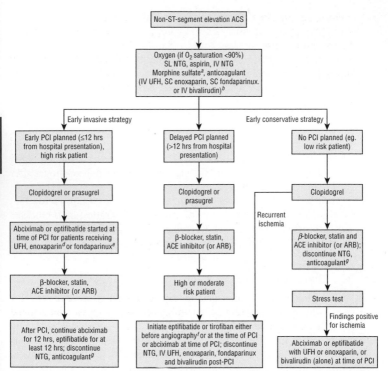

FIGURE 5–4. Initial pharmacotherapy for non–ST-segment-elevation acute coronary syndrome (ACS). (ACE, angiotensin-converting enzyme; ARB, angiotensin receptor blocker; CABG, coronary artery bypass graft surgery; NTG, nitroglycerin; PCI, percutaneous coronary intervention; UFH, unfractionated heparin.) [a]For selected patients. [b]Enoxaparin, UFH, fondaparinux plus UFH, or bivalirudin for early invasive strategy; enoxaparin or fondaparinux if no angiography/PCI planned; fondaparinux or bivalirudin preferred if high risk of bleeding; UFH preferred for patients undergoing CABG. [c]For patients unlikely to undergo CABG. [d]May require an IV supplemental dose of enoxaparin. [e]May require an IV supplemental dose of UFH. [f]For signs and symptoms of recurrent ischemia. [g]SC enoxaparin or UFH can be continued at a lower dose for venous thromboembolism prophylaxis. *(Reprinted (or modified) with permission from the American College of Clinical Pharmacy. Spinler SA. Evolution of antithrombotic therapy used in acute coronary syndromes. In: Richardson MM, Chessman KH, Chant C, et al, eds. Pharmacotherapy Self-assessment Program, Book 1 Cardiology, 7th ed. Lenexa, KS: American College of Clinical Pharmacy; 2010:102.)*

(2) **aspirin,** (3) SL **NTG**, and (4) an **anticoagulant** (**UFH, enoxaparin, fondaparinux,** or **bivalirudin**). These measures should be initiated early, while the patient is still in the emergency department.
- High-risk patients should proceed to early coronary angiography and may also receive a **GP IIb/IIIa inhibitor**.
- **Clopidogrel** or **prasugrel** should be administered to all patients.

- IV **β-blockers** and **IV NTG** should be given to select patients.
- **Morphine** is also administered to patients with refractory angina, as described previously.
- **Fibrinolytic therapy** is never administered to NSTE ACS, even with patients who have positive biochemical markers that indicate infarction. The risk of death from MI is lower in these patients, and the hemorrhagic risks of fibrinolytic therapy outweigh the benefits.

Aspirin

- **Aspirin** reduces the risk of death or developing MI by ~50% compared with no antiplatelet therapy in patients with NSTE ACS. Dosing of aspirin is the same as for STE ACS, and aspirin is continued indefinitely.

Thienopyridines

- Either clopidogrel or prasugrel is indicated for patients managed invasively with early coronary angiography and revascularization, whereas clopidogrel is indicated in patients managed conservatively.
- **Clopidogrel** is initiated as either a 300 or 600 mg loading dose, followed by 75 mg daily.
- **Prasugrel** is initiated as a 60 mg loading dose followed by 10 mg daily.
- Clopidogrel or prasugrel should be administered for at least 12 months for NSTE ACS patients undergoing PCI with placement of either a bare-metal or drug-eluting stent and up to 15 months for patients with a drug-eluting stent when the risk of thrombotic occlusion may be greater. For medical therapy of NSTE ACS, clopidogrel should be administered for up to 12 months for patients not at high risk of bleeding.
- For patients undergoing coronary artery bypass grafting, clopidogrel (but not aspirin) should be withheld at least 5 days and preferably 7 days before the procedure.

Glycoprotein IIb/IIIa Receptor Inhibitors

- Administration of **abciximab** or **eptifibatide** (alternatively **tirofiban**) with aspirin and UFH or enoxaparin is recommended for high-risk NSTE ACS patients undergoing PCI.
- Administration of tirofiban or eptifibatide is also indicated for patients with continued or recurrent ischemia despite treatment with aspirin, clopidogrel, and an anticoagulant.

Anticoagulants

- For patients with NSTE ACS undergoing planned early angiography and revascularization and PCI, **UFH, low-molecular-weight heparin (LMWH, e.g., enoxaparin), low-dose fondaparinux,** or **bivalirudin** should be administered. Therapy should be continued for up to 48 hours for UFH, until the patient is discharged for either enoxaparin or fondaparinux, and until the end of the PCI or angiography procedure (or up to 72 hours after PCI) for bivalirudin.
- For patients initiating warfarin therapy, UFH or LMWH should be continued until the international normalized ratio with warfarin is in the therapeutic range.

- For NSTE ACS, the dose of UFH is 60 units/kg IV bolus (maximum 4,000 units), followed by a continuous IV infusion of 12 units/kg/h (maximum 1,000 units/h). The dose is titrated to maintain the aPTT between 1.5 and 2 times control.

Nitrates

- In the absence of contraindications, SL followed by IV **NTG** should be administered to all patients with NSTE ACS with persistent ischemia, HF symptoms, or hypertension. IV NTG is continued for ~24 hours after ischemia relief.

β-Blockers

- In the absence of contraindications, oral β-blockers should be administered to all patients with NSTE ACS. IV β-blockers should be considered for hemodynamically stable patients who present with persistent ischemia, hypertension, or tachycardia. The drugs are continued indefinitely.

Calcium Channel Blockers

- As described previously for STE ACS, calcium channel blockers should not be administered to most patients with ACS.

SECONDARY PREVENTION AFTER MYOCARDIAL INFARCTION

DESIRED OUTCOME

- The long-term goals after MI are to (1) control modifiable coronary heart disease (CHD) risk factors; (2) prevent development of systolic HF; (3) prevent recurrent MI and stroke; and (4) prevent death, including sudden cardiac death.

PHARMACOTHERAPY

General Approach

- Pharmacotherapy that has been proven to decrease mortality, HF, reinfarction, or stroke should be started before hospital discharge for secondary prevention.
- The ACC/AHA guidelines suggest that after MI from either STE or NSTE ACS, patients should receive indefinite treatment with **aspirin**, a β-**blocker**, and an **ACE inhibitor** (or alternatively an angiotensin receptor blocker [ARB]).
- All patients should receive **SL NTG** or **lingual spray** and instructions for use in case of recurrent ischemic chest discomfort.
- **Clopidogrel** or **prasugrel** should be considered for most patients, but the duration of therapy is individualized according to the type of ACS and whether the patient is treated medically and whether a drug-eluting versus a bare-metal stent is placed.
- All patients should receive annual an **influenza vaccination.**
- Selected patients (e.g., those with atrial fibrillation) should also be treated with long-term **warfarin** anticoagulation in addition to aspirin and a thienopyridine.

- **Eplerenone** should be added to therapy with a β-blocker and an ACE inhibitor for patients with LVEF <40%.
- For all ACS patients, treatment and control of modifiable risk factors such as hypertension, dyslipidemia, and diabetes mellitus are essential.

ASPIRIN

- **Aspirin** decreases the risk of death, recurrent MI, and stroke after MI. All patients should receive aspirin indefinitely (or clopidogrel if there are aspirin contraindications).

THIENOPYRIDINES

- For patients with ACS, **clopidogrel** and **prasugrel** decrease the risk of death, MI, or stroke in patients post-PCI.
- For patients with STE MI treated medically without revascularization, clopidogrel can be given for 14 days and up to 1 year. If a stent has been implanted, clopidogrel or prasugrel should be continued for up to 12 months for patients at low risk for bleeding, with an option of up to 15 months for patients with a drug-eluting stent.

ANTICOAGULATION

- **Warfarin** should be considered in select patients after an ACS, including those with an LV thrombus, extensive ventricular wall motion abnormalities on cardiac echocardiogram, and a history of thromboembolic disease or chronic atrial fibrillation.

β-BLOCKERS, NITRATES, AND CALCIUM CHANNEL BLOCKERS

- After an ACS, patients should receive a β-blocker indefinitely, regardless of whether they have residual symptoms of angina. Therapy should continue indefinitely in the absence of contraindications or intolerance.
- A calcium channel blocker can be used to prevent anginal symptoms in patients who cannot tolerate or have a contraindication to a β-blocker but should not be used routinely in the absence of such findings.
- All patients should be prescribed a short-acting SL NTG or lingual NTG spray to relieve anginal symptoms when necessary. Chronic long-acting nitrates have not been shown to reduce CHD events after MI. Therefore, chronic long-acting oral nitrates are not used in ACS patients who have undergone revascularization unless the patient has chronic stable angina or significant coronary stenosis that was not revascularized.

ACE INHIBITORS AND ANGIOTENSIN RECEPTOR BLOCKERS

- ACE inhibitors should be initiated in all patients after MI to reduce mortality, decrease reinfarction, and prevent the development of HF. Data suggest that most patients with CAD (not just those with ACS or heart failure) benefit from an ACE inhibitor.
- The dose should be low initially and titrated to the dose used in clinical trials if tolerated. Example doses include the following:
  - ✓ **Captopril:** 6.25 to 12.5 mg initially; target dose 50 mg two or three times daily
  - ✓ **Enalapril:** 2.5 to 5 mg initially; target dose 10 mg twice daily

✓ **Lisinopril:** 2.5 to 5 mg initially; target dose 10 to 20 mg once daily
✓ **Ramipril:** 1.25 to 2.5 mg initially; target dose 5 mg twice daily or 10 mg once daily
✓ **Trandolapril:** 1 mg initially; target dose 4 mg once daily

- An angiotensin receptor blocker may be prescribed for patients with ACE inhibitor cough and a low LVEF and HF after MI. Example doses include the following:
  ✓ **Candesartan:** 4 to 8 mg initially; target dose 32 mg once daily
  ✓ **Valsartan:** 40 mg initially; target dose 160 mg twice daily

ALDOSTERONE ANTAGONISTS

- Either **eplerenone** or **spironolactone** should be considered within the first 2 weeks after MI to reduce mortality in all patients already receiving an ACE inhibitor who experienced HF symptoms during hospitalization for MI and have LVEF ≤40%. The drugs are continued indefinitely. Example oral doses include the following:
  ✓ **Eplerenone:** 25 mg initially; target dose 50 mg once daily
  ✓ **Spironolactone:** 12.5 mg initially; target dose 25 to 50 mg once daily

LIPID-LOWERING AGENTS

- All patients with CAD should receive dietary counseling and pharmacotherapy in order to reach an LDL cholesterol concentration <100 mg/dL. The National Cholesterol Education Program recommendations give an optional LDL goal of <70 mg/dL in select patients.
- **Statins** are the preferred agents for lowering LDL cholesterol and should be prescribed at or near discharge in most patients.
- A **fibrate derivative** or **niacin** should be considered in select patients with a low high-density lipoprotein (HDL) cholesterol (<40 mg/dL) and/or a high triglyceride level (>200 mg/dL).

FISH OILS (MARINE-DERIVED OMEGA-3 FATTY ACIDS)

- Eicosapentaenoic acid (EPA) and docosahexaenoic acid (DHA) are omega-3 polyunsaturated fatty acids that are most abundant in fatty fish such as sardines, salmon, and mackerel. A diet high in EPA plus DHA or supplementation with these fish oils reduces the risk of cardiovascular mortality, reinfarction, and stroke in patients who have experienced an MI.
- The AHA recommends that CHD patients consume ~1 g EPA plus DHA per day, preferably from oily fish. Because of variable fish oil content, one would need to consume from 4 to more than 14 6-oz servings of fish per week to provide 7 g of the fish oils. Because the average diet provides only 10% to 20% of that amount, supplements may be considered for some patients. Approximately three 1-g fish oil capsules per day should be consumed to provide 1 g of EPA/DHA, depending on the brand. Alternatively, the prescription drug LOVAZA (omega-3-acid ethyl esters) can be used at a dose of 1 g/day. Higher doses of EPA/DHA (2–4 g/day) may be considered for managing hypertriglyceridemia.
- Adverse effects of fish oils include fishy aftertaste, nausea, and diarrhea.

EVALUATION OF THERAPEUTIC OUTCOMES

- Monitoring parameters for efficacy of therapy for both STE and NSTE ACS include (1) relief of ischemic discomfort, (2) return of ECG changes to baseline, and (3) absence or resolution of HF signs.
- Monitoring parameters for adverse effects are dependent upon the individual drugs used. In general, the most common adverse reactions from ACS therapies are hypotension and bleeding.

See Chapter 24, Acute Coronary Syndromes, authored by Sarah A. Spinler and Simon De Denus, for a more detailed discussion of this topic.

Arrhythmias

DEFINITION

- Arrhythmia is defined as loss of cardiac rhythm, especially irregularity of heartbeat. This chapter covers the group of conditions caused by an abnormality in the rate, regularity, or sequence of cardiac activation.

PATHOPHYSIOLOGY

SUPRAVENTRICULAR ARRHYTHMIAS

- Common supraventricular tachycardias requiring drug treatment are atrial fibrillation (AF) or atrial flutter, paroxysmal supraventricular tachycardia (PSVT), and automatic atrial tachycardias. Other common supraventricular arrhythmias that usually do not require drug therapy are not discussed in this chapter (e.g., premature atrial complexes, wandering atrial pacemaker, sinus arrhythmia, and sinus tachycardia).

Atrial Fibrillation and Atrial Flutter

- AF is characterized as an extremely rapid (400–600 atrial beats/min) and disorganized atrial activation. There is a loss of atrial contraction (atrial kick), and supraventricular impulses penetrate the atrioventricular (AV) conduction system to variable degrees, resulting in irregular ventricular activation and irregularly irregular pulse (120–180 beats/min).
- Atrial flutter is characterized by rapid (270–330 atrial beats/min) but regular atrial activation. The ventricular response usually has a regular pattern and a pulse of 300 beats/min. This arrhythmia occurs less frequently than AF but has similar precipitating factors, consequences, and drug therapy.
- The predominant mechanism of AF and atrial flutter is reentry, which is usually associated with organic heart disease that causes atrial distention (e.g., ischemia or infarction, hypertensive heart disease, and valvular disorders). Additional associated disorders include acute pulmonary embolus and chronic lung disease, resulting in pulmonary hypertension and cor pulmonale, and states of high adrenergic tone such as thyrotoxicosis, alcohol withdrawal, sepsis, and excessive physical exertion.

Paroxysmal Supraventricular Tachycardia Caused by Reentry

- PSVT arising by reentrant mechanisms includes arrhythmias caused by AV nodal reentry, AV reentry incorporating an anomalous AV pathway, sinoatrial (SA) nodal reentry, and intraatrial reentry.

Automatic Atrial Tachycardias

- Automatic atrial tachycardias such as multifocal atrial tachycardia appear to arise from supraventricular foci with enhanced automatic properties.

Severe pulmonary disease is the underlying precipitating disorder in 60% to 80% of patients.

VENTRICULAR ARRHYTHMIAS

Premature Ventricular Complexes

- Premature ventricular complexes (PVCs) are common ventricular rhythm disturbances that occur in patients with or without heart disease and may be elicited experimentally by abnormal automaticity, triggered activity, or reentrant mechanisms.

Ventricular Tachycardia

- Ventricular tachycardia (VT) is defined by three or more repetitive PVCs occurring at a rate >100 beats/min. It is a wide QRS tachycardia that may occur acutely as a result of severe electrolyte abnormalities (hypokalemia or hypomagnesemia), hypoxia, drug toxicity (e.g., digoxin), or (most commonly) during an acute myocardial infarction (MI) or ischemia complicated by heart failure (HF). The chronic recurrent form is almost always associated with underlying organic heart disease (e.g., idiopathic dilated cardiomyopathy or remote MI with left ventricular [LV] aneurysm).
- Sustained VT is that which requires therapeutic intervention to restore a stable rhythm or persists a relatively long time (usually >30 sec). Nonsustained VT self-terminates after a brief duration (usually <30 sec). *Incessant VT* refers to VT occurring more frequently than sinus rhythm, so that VT becomes the dominant rhythm. Monomorphic VT has a consistent QRS configuration, whereas polymorphic VT has varying QRS complexes. Torsades de pointes (TdP) is a polymorphic VT in which the QRS complexes appear to undulate around a central axis.

Ventricular Proarrhythmia

- *Proarrhythmia* refers to development of a significant new arrhythmia, such as VT, ventricular fibrillation (VF), or TdP, or worsening of an existing arrhythmia. Proarrhythmia results from the same mechanisms that cause other arrhythmias or from an alteration in the underlying substrate due to the antiarrhythmic agent. TdP is a rapid form of polymorphic VT associated with evidence of delayed ventricular repolarization due to blockade of potassium conductance. TdP may be hereditary or acquired. Acquired forms are associated with many clinical conditions and drugs, especially class Ia and class III I_{Kr} blockers.

Ventricular Fibrillation

- VF is electrical anarchy of the ventricle resulting in no cardiac output and cardiovascular collapse. Sudden cardiac death occurs most commonly in patients with coronary artery disease and those with LV dysfunction. VF associated with acute MI may be classified as either (1) primary (an uncomplicated MI not associated with HF) or (2) secondary or complicated (an MI complicated by HF).

BRADYARRHYTHMIAS

- Sinus bradyarrhythmias (heart rate <60 beats/min) are common, especially in young, athletically active individuals, and are usually asymptomatic and do not require intervention. However, some patients have sinus node dysfunction (sick sinus syndrome) because of underlying organic heart disease and the normal aging process, which attenuates SA nodal function. Sinus node dysfunction is usually representative of diffuse conduction disease, which may be accompanied by AV block and by paroxysmal tachycardias such as AF. Alternating bradyarrhythmias and tachyarrhythmias are referred to as the tachy–brady syndrome.

- AV block or conduction delay may occur in any area of the AV conduction system. AV block may be found in patients without underlying heart disease (e.g., trained athletes) or during sleep when vagal tone is high. It may be transient when the underlying etiology is reversible (e.g., myocarditis, myocardial ischemia, after cardiovascular surgery, or during drug therapy). β-Blockers, digoxin, or nondihydropyridine calcium antagonists may cause AV block, primarily in the AV nodal area. Class I antiarrhythmics may exacerbate conduction delays below the level of the AV node. AV block may be irreversible if the cause is acute MI, rare degenerative diseases, primary myocardial disease, or congenital heart disease.

CLINICAL PRESENTATION

- Supraventricular tachycardias may cause clinical manifestations ranging from no symptoms to minor palpitations or irregular pulse to severe and even life-threatening symptoms. Patients may experience dizziness or acute syncopal episodes, symptoms of HF, anginal chest pain, or, more often, a choking or pressure sensation during the tachycardia episode.

- AF or atrial flutter may be manifested by the entire range of symptoms associated with other supraventricular tachycardias, but syncope is not a common presenting symptom. An additional complication of AF is arterial embolization resulting from atrial stasis and poorly adherent mural thrombi, which accounts for the most devastating complication: embolic stroke. Patients with AF and concurrent rheumatic heart disease are at particularly high risk for stroke.

- PVCs often cause no symptoms or only mild palpitations. The presentation of VT may vary from totally asymptomatic to pulseless hemodynamic collapse. Consequences of proarrhythmia range from no symptoms to worsening of symptoms to sudden death. VF results in hemodynamic collapse, syncope, and cardiac arrest.

- Patients with bradyarrhythmias experience symptoms associated with hypotension, such as dizziness, syncope, fatigue, and confusion. If LV dysfunction exists, patients may experience worsening HF symptoms.

DIAGNOSIS

- The surface electrocardiogram (ECG) is the cornerstone of diagnosis for cardiac rhythm disturbances.

- Less sophisticated methods are often the initial tools for detecting qualitative and quantitative alterations of heartbeat. For example, direct auscultation can reveal the irregularly irregular pulse that is characteristic of AF.
- Proarrhythmia can be difficult to diagnose because of the variable nature of underlying arrhythmias.
- TdP is characterized by long QT intervals or prominent U waves on the surface ECG.
- Specific maneuvers may be required to delineate the etiology of syncope associated with bradyarrhythmias. Diagnosis of carotid sinus hypersensitivity can be confirmed by performing carotid sinus massage with ECG and blood pressure monitoring. Vasovagal syncope can be diagnosed using the upright body-tilt test.
- On the basis of ECG findings, AV block is usually categorized into three different types: first-, second-, and third-degree AV block.

DESIRED OUTCOME

- The desired outcome depends on the underlying arrhythmia. For example, the ultimate treatment goals of treating AF or atrial flutter are restoring sinus rhythm, preventing thromboembolic complications, and preventing further recurrences.

TREATMENT

GENERAL APPROACH

- The use of antiarrhythmic drugs in the United States is declining because of major trials that showed increased mortality with their use in several clinical situations, the realization of proarrhythmia as a significant side effect, and the advancing technology of nondrug therapies, such as ablation and the implantable cardioverter-defibrillator (ICD).

CLASSIFICATION OF ANTIARRHYTHMIC DRUGS

- Drugs may have antiarrhythmic activity by directly altering conduction in several ways. Drugs may depress the automatic properties of abnormal pacemaker cells by decreasing the slope of phase 4 depolarization and/or by elevating threshold potential. Drugs may alter the conduction characteristics of the pathways of a reentrant loop.
- The most frequently used classification system is that proposed by Vaughan Williams (Table 6–1). Class Ia drugs slow conduction velocity, prolong refractoriness, and decrease the automatic properties of sodium-dependent (normal and diseased) conduction tissue. Class Ia drugs are broad-spectrum antiarrhythmics, being effective for both supraventricular and ventricular arrhythmias.
- Although categorized separately, class Ib drugs probably act similarly to class Ia drugs, except that class Ib agents are considerably more effective in ventricular than supraventricular arrhythmias.

TABLE 6–1	Classification of Antiarrhythmic Drugs				
Class	Drug	Conduction Velocity[a]	Refractory Period	Automaticity	Ion Block
Ia	Quinidine Procainamide Disopyramide	↓	↑	↓	Sodium (intermediate) Potassium
Ib	Lidocaine Mexiletine	0/↓	↓	↓	Sodium (fast on/off)
Ic	Flecainide Propafenone[b]	↓↓	0	↓	Sodium (slow on/off)
II[c]	β-Blockers	↓	↑	↓	Calcium (indirect)
III	Amiodarone[d] Dofetilide Dronedarone[d] Sotalol[b] Ibutilide	0	↑↑	0	Potassium
IV[c]	Verapamil Diltiazem	↓	↑	↓	Calcium

0, no change; ↑, increased; ↓, decreased.
[a]Variables for normal tissue models in ventricular tissue.
[b]Also has β-blocking actions.
[c]Variables for sinoatrial and atrioventricular nodal tissue only.
[d]Also has sodium, calcium, and β-blocking actions.

- Class Ic drugs profoundly slow conduction velocity while leaving refractoriness relatively unaltered. Although effective for both ventricular and supraventricular arrhythmias, their use for ventricular arrhythmias has been limited by the risk of proarrhythmia.
- Collectively, class I drugs can be referred to as sodium channel blockers. Antiarrhythmic sodium channel receptor principles account for drug combinations that are additive (e.g., **quinidine** and **mexiletine**) and antagonistic (e.g., **flecainide** and **lidocaine**), as well as potential antidotes to excess sodium channel blockade (sodium bicarbonate).
- Class II drugs include **β-adrenergic antagonists**; clinically relevant mechanisms result from their antiadrenergic actions. β-Blockers are most useful in tachycardias in which nodal tissues are abnormally automatic or are a portion of a reentrant loop. These agents are also helpful in slowing ventricular response in atrial tachycardias (e.g., AF) by their effects on the AV node.
- Class III drugs specifically prolong refractoriness in atrial and ventricular tissue and include very different drugs that share the common effect of delaying repolarization by blocking potassium channels.
- **Amiodarone** and **sotalol** are effective in most supraventricular and ventricular tachycardias. Amiodarone displays electrophysiologic characteristics consistent with each type of antiarrhythmic drug. It is a sodium channel blocker with relatively fast on-off kinetics, has nonselective

TABLE 6–2	Typical Maintenance Doses of Oral Antiarrhythmic Drugs	
Drug	**Dose**	**Dose Adjusted**
Disopyramide	100–150 mg every 6 hours 200–300 mg every 12 hours (SR form)	HEP, REN
Quinidine	200–300 mg sulfate salt every 6 hours 324–648 mg gluconate salt every 8–12 hours	HEP
Mexiletine	200–300 mg every 8 hours	HEP
Flecainide	50–150 mg every 8 hours	HEP, REN
Propafenone	150–300 mg every 8 hours 225–425 mg every 12 hours (SR form)	HEP
Amiodarone	400 mg two or three times daily until 10 g total, then 200–400 mg daily[a]	
Dofetilide	500 mcg every 12 hours	REN[b]
Dronedarone	400 mg every 12 hours (with meals)[c]	
Sotalol	80–160 mg every 12 hours	REN[d]

HEP, hepatic disease; REN, renal dysfunction; SR, sustained-release.

[a]Usual maintenance dose for atrial fibrillation is 200 mg/day (may further decrease dose to 100 mg/day with long-term use if patient is clinically stable in order to decrease risk of toxicity); usual maintenance dose for ventricular arrhythmias is 300 to 400 mg/day.

[b]Dose should be based on creatinine clearance; should not be used when creatinine clearance <20 mL/min.

[c]Should not be used in severe hepatic impairment.

[d]Should not be used for atrial fibrillation when creatinine clearance <40 mL/min.

β blocking actions, blocks potassium channels, and has slight calcium-blocking activity. The impressive effectiveness and low proarrhythmic potential of amiodarone have challenged the notion that selective ion channel blockade is preferable. Sotalol is a potent inhibitor of outward potassium movement during repolarization and also possesses nonselective β-blocking actions. **Dronedarone**, **ibutilide**, and **dofetilide** are only approved for treatment of supraventricular arrhythmias.

- Class IV drugs inhibit calcium entry into the cell, which slows conduction, prolongs refractoriness, and decreases SA and AV nodal automaticity. **Calcium channel antagonists** are effective for automatic or reentrant tachycardias that arise from or use the SA or AV nodes.
- Recommended doses of the oral antiarrhythmic dosage forms are given in **Table 6–2**; usual IV antiarrhythmic doses are shown in **Table 6–3**; common side effects are listed in **Table 6–4**.

ATRIAL FIBRILLATION OR ATRIAL FLUTTER

- The traditional approach to treatment of AF involves several sequential goals. First, evaluate the need for acute treatment (usually with drugs that slow ventricular rate). Next, consider methods to restore sinus rhythm, considering the risks involved (e.g., thromboembolism). Lastly, consider ways to prevent the long-term complications of AF, such as recurrent arrhythmia and thromboembolism (**Fig. 6–1**).

TABLE 6–3	Intravenous Antiarrhythmic Dosing	
Drug	**Clinical Situation**	**Dose**
Amiodarone	Pulseless VT/VF	300 mg IV/IO push (can give additional 150 mg IV/IO push if persistent VT/VF), followed by infusion of 1 mg/min for 6 hours, then 0.5 mg/min
	Stable VT (with a pulse)	150 mg IV over 10 min, followed by infusion of 1 mg/min for 6 hours, then 0.5 mg/min
	AF (termination)	5 mg/kg IV over 30 min, followed by infusion of 1 mg/min for 6 hours, then 0.5 mg/min
Diltiazem	PSVT; AF (rate control)	0.25 mg/kg IV over 2 min (may repeat with 0.35 mg/kg IV over 2 min), followed by infusion of 5 to 15 mg/hour
Ibutilide	AF (termination)	1 mg IV over 10 min (may repeat if needed)
Lidocaine	Pulseless VT/VF	1 to 1.5 mg/kg IV/IO push (can give additional 0.5–0.75 mg/kg IV/IO push every 5–10 min if persistent VT/VF [maximum cumulative dose = 3 mg/kg]), followed by infusion of 1 to 4 mg/min (1–2 mg/min if liver disease or HF)
	Stable VT (with a pulse)	1 to 1.5 mg/kg IV push (can give additional 0.5–0.75 mg/kg IV push every 5–10 min if persistent VT [maximum cumulative dose = 3 mg/kg]), followed by infusion of 1 to 4 mg/min (1–2 mg/min if liver disease or HF)
Procainamide	AF (termination); stable VT (with a pulse)	15 to 18 mg/kg IV over 60 min, followed by infusion of 1 to 4 mg/min
Sotalol[a]	AF/AFl (SR maintenance) Ventricular arrhythmias	75 to 150 mg IV once or twice daily (infused over 5 hours)[b]
Verapamil	PSVT; AF (rate control)	2.5 to 5 mg IV over 2 min (may repeat up to maximum cumulative dose of 20 mg); can follow with infusion of 2.5 to 10 mg/hour

AF, atrial fibrillation; AFl, atrial flutter; HF, heart failure; IO, intraosseous; PSVT, paroxysmal supraventricular tachycardia; VF, ventricular fibrillation; VT, ventricular tachycardia.
[a]Should be used only when patients are unable to take sotalol daily.
[b]IV sotalol should be administered at the same frequency as oral sotalol (based on creatinine clearance). Oral sotalol may be converted to IV sotalol as follows: 80 mg oral = 75 mg IV; 120 mg oral = 112.5 mg IV; 160 mg oral = 150 mg IV.

- In patients with new-onset AF or atrial flutter with signs and/or symptoms of hemodynamic instability (e.g., severe hypotension, angina, and/or pulmonary edema), direct-current cardioversion (DCC) is indicated to restore sinus rhythm immediately (without regard to the risk of thromboembolism).
- If patients are hemodynamically stable, the focus should be directed toward controlling the ventricular rate. Drugs that slow conduction and increase refractoriness in the AV node should be used as initial therapy. In patients with normal LV function (left ventricular ejection fraction [LVEF] >40%), IV β-blockers (**propranolol, metoprolol,** and **esmolol**),

TABLE 6-4	Side Effects of Antiarrhythmic Drugs
Disopyramide	Anticholinergic symptoms (dry mouth, urinary retention, constipation, and blurred vision), nausea, anorexia, TdP, HF, conduction disturbances, ventricular arrhythmias
Procainamide[a]	Hypotension, TdP, worsening HF, conduction disturbances, ventricular arrhythmias
Quinidine	Cinchonism, diarrhea, abdominal cramps, nausea, vomiting, hypotension, TdP, worsening HF, conduction disturbances, ventricular arrhythmias, fever, hepatitis, thrombocytopenia, hemolytic anemia
Lidocaine	Dizziness, sedation, slurred speech, blurred vision, paresthesia, muscle twitching, confusion, nausea, vomiting, seizures, psychosis, sinus arrest, conduction disturbances
Mexiletine	Dizziness, sedation, anxiety, confusion, paresthesia, tremor, ataxia, blurred vision, nausea, vomiting, anorexia, conduction disturbances, ventricular arrhythmias
Flecainide	Blurred vision, dizziness, dyspnea, headache, tremor, nausea, worsening HF, conduction disturbances, ventricular arrhythmias
Propafenone	Dizziness, fatigue, bronchospasm, headache, taste disturbances, nausea, vomiting, bradycardia or AV block, worsening HF, ventricular arrhythmias
Amiodarone	Tremor, ataxia, paresthesia, insomnia, corneal microdeposits, optic neuropathy/neuritis, nausea, vomiting, anorexia, constipation, TdP (<1%), bradycardia or AV block (IV and oral use), pulmonary fibrosis, liver function test abnormalities, hepatitis, hypothyroidism, hyperthyroidism, photosensitivity, blue-gray skin discoloration, hypotension (IV use), phlebitis (IV use)
Dofetilide	Headache, dizziness, TdP
Dronedarone	Nausea, vomiting, diarrhea, serum creatinine elevations, bradycardia, TdP (<1%)
Ibutilide	Headache, TdP, hypotension
Sotalol	Dizziness, weakness, fatigue, nausea, vomiting, diarrhea, bradycardia, TdP, bronchospasm, worsening HF

AV, atrioventricular; HF, heart failure; TdP, torsades de pointes.
[a]Side effects are listed for the IV formulation only; oral formulations are no longer available.

diltiazem, or **verapamil** is recommended as first-line therapy. If a high adrenergic state is the precipitating factor, IV β-blockers can be highly effective and should be considered first. In patients with LVEF ≤40%, IV diltiazem and verapamil should be avoided, and IV β-blockers should be used with caution. In patients having an exacerbation of HF symptoms, IV **digoxin** or **amiodarone** should be used as first-line therapy for ventricular rate control. IV amiodarone can also be used in patients who are refractory or have contraindications to β-blockers, nondihydropyridine calcium channel blockers, and digoxin.

- After treatment with AV nodal blocking agents and a subsequent decrease in ventricular response, the patient should be evaluated for the possibility of restoring sinus rhythm if AF persists.

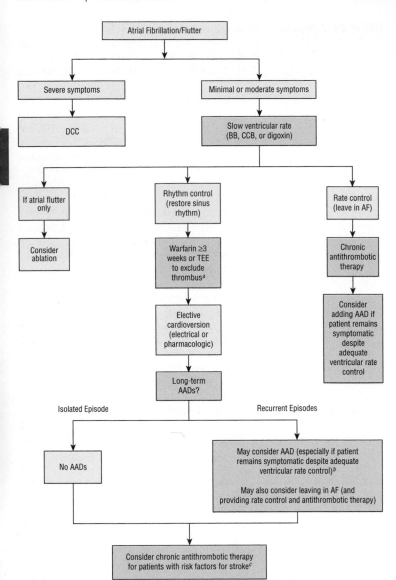

FIGURE 6–1. Algorithm for the treatment of atrial fibrillation (AF) and atrial flutter. (BB, β-blocker; CCB, calcium channel blocker [i.e., verapamil or diltiazem]; DCC, direct-current cardioversion.) [a]If AF <48 hours, anticoagulation prior to cardioversion is unnecessary; may consider transesophageal echocardiogram (TEE) if patient has risk factors for stroke. [b]Ablation may be considered for patients who fail or do not tolerate one or more antiarrhythmic drugs (AADs). [c]Chronic antithrombotic therapy should be considered in all patients with AF and risk factors for stroke regardless of whether or not they remain in sinus rhythm.

- If sinus rhythm is to be restored, anticoagulation should be initiated prior to cardioversion because return of atrial contraction increases risk of thromboembolism. Patients with AF for longer than 48 hours or an unknown duration should receive warfarin (target International Normalized Ratio [INR] 2.5; range 2–3) for at least 3 weeks prior to cardioversion and continuing for at least 4 weeks after effective cardioversion and return of normal sinus rhythm. Patients with AF less than 48 hours in duration do not require warfarin, but it is recommended that these patients receive either IV unfractionated heparin or a low-molecular-weight heparin (subcutaneously at treatment doses) at presentation prior to cardioversion.

- After prior anticoagulation (or after transesophageal echocardiography demonstrated the absence of a thrombus, thereby obviating the need for warfarin), methods for restoring sinus rhythm in patients with AF or atrial flutter are pharmacologic cardioversion and DCC. DCC is quick and more often successful, but it requires prior sedation or anesthesia and has a small risk of serious complications, such as sinus arrest or ventricular arrhythmias. Advantages of initial drug therapy are that an effective agent may be determined in case long-term therapy is required. Disadvantages are significant side effects, such as drug-induced TdP, drug–drug interactions, and lower cardioversion rate for drugs compared with DCC. There is relatively strong evidence for efficacy of class III pure Ik blockers (**ibutilide** and **dofetilide**), class Ic drugs (e.g., **flecainide** and **propafenone**), and amiodarone (oral or IV). With the "pill in the pocket" approach, outpatient, patient-controlled self-administration of a single, oral loading dose of either flecainide or propafenone can be relatively safe and effective for termination of recent-onset AF in select patients without sinus or AV node dysfunction, bundle-branch block, QT interval prolongation, Brugada's syndrome, or structural heart disease. It should only be considered for patients who have been successfully cardioverted with these drugs on an inpatient basis.

- The American College of Chest Physicians Consensus Conference on antithrombotic therapy recommends chronic **warfarin** treatment (target INR 2.5; range 2–3) for all patients with AF who are at high risk for stroke (CHADS2 score ≥2). Those at intermediate risk (CHADS2 [acronym derived from stroke risk factors: congestive heart failure, hypertension, age >75 y, diabetes, and prior stroke or transient ischemic attack] score of 1) should receive either warfarin (target INR 2.5; range 2–3) or **aspirin** 75 to 325 mg/day. Those at low risk for stroke (CHADS2 score of 0) should receive aspirin 75 to 325 mg/day. Chronic antithrombotic therapy should be considered for all patients with AF and risk factors for stroke regardless of whether or not they remain in sinus rhythm.

- AF often recurs after initial cardioversion because most patients have irreversible underlying heart or lung disease. A meta-analysis confirmed that **quinidine** maintained sinus rhythm better than placebo; however, 50% of patients had recurrent AF within 1 year, and more importantly, quinidine increased mortality, presumably due in part to proarrhythmia. Class Ic or III antiarrhythmic agents are reasonable alternatives to consider for maintaining patients in sinus rhythm. Because the class Ic

71

drugs flecainide and propafenone increase the risk of proarrhythmia, they should be avoided in patients with structural heart disease. Amiodarone is the most effective and most frequently used class III agent for preventing AF recurrences despite its potential for significant organ toxicity.

PAROXYSMAL SUPRAVENTRICULAR TACHYCARDIA

- The choice between pharmacologic and nonpharmacologic methods for treating PSVT depends on symptom severity (**Fig. 6–2**). Treatment measures are directed first at terminating the acute episode and then at preventing recurrences. For patients with severe symptoms (e.g., syncope, near syncope, anginal chest pain, oe severe HF), synchronized DCC is the treatment of choice. If symptoms are mild to moderate, nondrug measures that increase vagal tone to the AV node (e.g., unilateral carotid sinus massage and Valsalva maneuver) can be used initially. If these methods fail, drug therapy is the next option.
- The choice among drugs is based on the QRS complex (see **Fig. 6–2**). Drugs can be divided into three broad categories: (1) those that directly or indirectly increase vagal tone to the AV node (e.g., **digoxin**); (2) those that depress conduction through slow, calcium-dependent tissue (e.g., **adenosine, β-blockers,** and **nondihydropyridine calcium channel blockers**); and (3) those that depress conduction through fast, sodium-dependent tissue (e.g., **quinidine, procainamide, disopyramide,** and **flecainide**).
- **Adenosine** has been recommended as the drug of first choice for patients with PSVT because its short duration of action will not cause prolonged hemodynamic compromise in patients with wide QRS complexes who actually have VT rather than PSVT.
- After acute PSVT is terminated, long-term preventive treatment is indicated if frequent episodes necessitate therapeutic intervention or if episodes are infrequent but severely symptomatic. Serial testing of antiarrhythmic agents can be evaluated in the ambulatory setting via ambulatory ECG recordings (Holter monitors) or telephonic transmissions of cardiac rhythm (event monitors) or by invasive electrophysiologic techniques in the laboratory.
- Transcutaneous catheter ablation using radiofrequency current on the PSVT substrate should be considered in any patient who would have previously been considered for chronic antiarrhythmic drug treatment. It is highly effective and curative, rarely results in complications, obviates the need for chronic antiarrhythmic drug therapy, and is cost-effective.

AUTOMATIC ATRIAL TACHYCARDIAS

- Underlying precipitating factors should be corrected by ensuring proper oxygenation and ventilation and by correcting acid–base or electrolyte disturbances.
- If tachycardia persists, the need for additional treatment is determined by symptoms. Patients with asymptomatic atrial tachycardia and relatively slow ventricular response usually require no drug therapy.
- In symptomatic patients, medical therapy can be tailored either to control ventricular response or to restore sinus rhythm. Nondihydropyridine

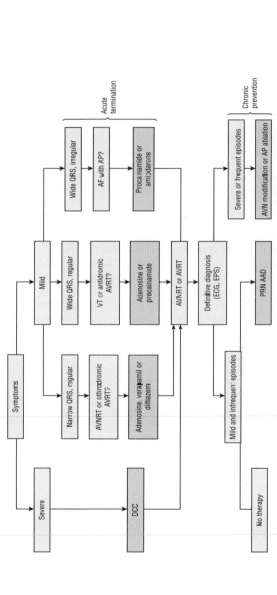

FIGURE 6–2. Algorithm for the treatment of acute *(top portion)* paroxysmal supraventricular tachycardia and chronic prevention of recurrences *(bottom portion)*. *Note:* For empiric bridge therapy prior to radiofrequency ablation procedures, calcium channel blockers (or other atrioventricular [AV] nodal blockers) should not be used if the patient has AV reentry with an accessory pathway. (AAD, antiarrhythmic drugs; AF, atrial fibrillation; AP, accessory pathway; AVN atrioventricular nodal; AVNRT, atrioventricular nodal reentrant tachycardia; AVRT, atrioventricular reentrant tachycardia; DCC, direct-current cardioversion; ECG, electrocardiographic monitoring; EPS, electrophysiologic studies; PRN, as needed; VT, ventricular tachycardia.)

calcium antagonists (e.g., **verapamil**) are considered first-line drug therapy for decreasing ventricular response. Class I agents (e.g., **procainamide** and **quinidine**) are only occasionally effective in restoring sinus rhythm. DCC is ineffective, and β-blockers are usually contraindicated because of coexisting bronchospastic pulmonary disease or decompensated HF.

PREMATURE VENTRICULAR COMPLEXES

- In apparently healthy individuals, drug therapy is unnecessary because PVCs without associated heart disease carry little or no risk. In patients with risk factors for arrhythmic death (recent MI, LV dysfunction, or complex PVCs), chronic drug therapy should be restricted to *β-blockers* because only they have been conclusively proven to prevent mortality in these patients.

VENTRICULAR TACHYCARDIA

Acute Ventricular Tachycardia

- If severe symptoms are present, synchronized DCC should be instituted immediately to restore sinus rhythm. Precipitating factors should be corrected if possible. If VT is an isolated electrical event associated with a transient initiating factor (e.g., acute myocardial ischemia or digitalis toxicity), there is no need for long-term antiarrhythmic therapy after precipitating factors are corrected.
- Patients with mild or no symptoms can be treated initially with antiarrhythmic drugs. IV **procainamide, amiodarone,** or **sotalol** may be considered in this situation; **lidocaine** is an alternative agent. Synchronized DCC should be delivered if the patient's status deteriorates, VT degenerates to VF, or drug therapy fails.

Sustained Ventricular Tachycardia

- Patients with chronic recurrent sustained VT are at extremely high risk for death; trial-and-error attempts to find effective therapy are unwarranted. Neither electrophysiologic studies nor serial Holter monitoring with drug testing is ideal. These findings and the side effect profiles of antiarrhythmic agents have led to nondrug approaches.
- The automatic ICD is a highly effective method for preventing sudden death due to recurrent VT or VF.

Ventricular Proarrhythmia

- The typical form of proarrhythmia caused by the class Ic antiarrhythmic drugs is a rapid, sustained, monomorphic VT with a characteristic sinusoidal QRS pattern that is often resistant to resuscitation with cardioversion or overdrive pacing. Some clinicians have had success with IV **lidocaine** (competes for the sodium channel receptor) or **sodium bicarbonate** (reverses the excessive sodium channel blockade).

Torsades de Pointes

- For an acute episode of TdP, most patients require and respond to DCC. However, TdP tends to be paroxysmal and often recurs rapidly after DCC.

- IV **magnesium sulfate** is considered the drug of choice for preventing recurrences of TdP. If ineffective, strategies to increase heart rate and shorten ventricular repolarization should be instituted (i.e., temporary transvenous pacing at 105–120 beats/min or pharmacologic pacing with **isoproterenol** or **epinephrine** infusion). Agents that prolong the QT interval should be discontinued and exacerbating factors (e.g., hypokalemia and hypomagnesemia) corrected. Drugs that further prolong repolarization (e.g., IV procainamide) are contraindicated. Lidocaine is usually ineffective.

Ventricular Fibrillation

- Patients with pulseless VT or VF (with or without associated myocardial ischemia) should be managed according to the American Heart Association's guidelines for cardiopulmonary resuscitation and emergency cardiovascular care (see Chap. 7).

BRADYARRHYTHMIAS

- Treatment of sinus node dysfunction involves elimination of symptomatic bradycardia and possibly managing alternating tachycardias such as AF. Asymptomatic sinus bradyarrhythmias usually do not require therapeutic intervention.
- In general, the long-term therapy of choice for patients with significant symptoms is a permanent ventricular pacemaker.
- Drugs commonly employed to treat supraventricular tachycardias should be used with caution, if at all, in the absence of a functioning pacemaker.
- Symptomatic carotid sinus hypersensitivity also should be treated with permanent pacemaker therapy. Patients who remain symptomatic may benefit from adding an α-adrenergic stimulant such as **midodrine**.
- Vasovagal syncope has traditionally been treated successfully with oral β-blockers (e.g., **metoprolol**) to inhibit the sympathetic surge that causes forceful ventricular contraction and precedes the onset of hypotension and bradycardia. Other drugs that have been used successfully (with or without β-blockers) include fludrocortisone, anticholinergics (**scopolamine patches** and **disopyramide**), α-adrenergic agonists (**midodrine**), adenosine analogues (**theophylline** and **dipyridamole**), and selective serotonin reuptake inhibitors (**sertraline** and **paroxetine**).

Atrioventricular Block

- If patients with Mobitz II or third-degree AV block develop signs or symptoms of poor perfusion (e.g., altered mental status, chest pain, hypotension, and/or shock) **atropine** (0.5 mg IV given every 3–5 min, up to 3 mg total dose) should be administered. Transcutaneous pacing can be initiated in patients unresponsive to atropine. Infusions of **epinephrine** (2–10 mcg/min) or **dopamine** (2–10 mcg/kg/min) can also be used in the event of atropine failure. These agents usually do not help if the site of the AV block is below the AV node (Mobitz II or trifascicular AV block).
- Chronic symptomatic AV block warrants insertion of a permanent pacemaker. Patients without symptoms can sometimes be followed closely without the need for a pacemaker.

EVALUATION OF THERAPEUTIC OUTCOMES

- The most important monitoring parameters include (1) mortality (total and due to arrhythmic death), (2) arrhythmia recurrence (duration, frequency, and symptoms), (3) hemodynamic consequences (rate, blood pressure, and symptoms), and (4) treatment complications (side effects or need for alternative or additional drugs, devices, or surgery).

See Chapter 25, The Arrhythmias, authored by Cynthia A. Sanoski and Jerry L. Bauman, for a more detailed discussion of this topic.

DEFINITION

- Cardiac arrest is the cessation of cardiac mechanical activity as confirmed by the absence of signs of circulation (e.g., detectable pulse, unresponsiveness, and apnea).

PATHOPHYSIOLOGY

- Coronary artery disease is the most common clinical finding in adults with cardiac arrest and is the cause of ~80% of sudden cardiac deaths. In pediatric patients, cardiac arrest is often the terminal event of respiratory failure or progressive shock.
- Two different pathophysiologic conditions are associated with cardiac arrest:
  ✓ Primary cardiac arrest, in which arterial blood is typically fully oxygenated at the time of arrest.
  ✓ Secondary cardiac arrest, resulting from respiratory failure in which lack of ventilation leads to severe hypoxemia, hypotension, and cardiac arrest.
- Cardiac arrest in adults usually results from arrhythmias. Historically, ventricular fibrillation (VF) and pulseless ventricular tachycardia (PVT) were the most common initial rhythms. The incidence of VF in out-of-hospital arrests is declining, which is of concern because survival rates are substantially higher after VF/PVT compared with cardiac arrest that results from asystole or pulseless electrical activity (PEA). Survival rates for out-of-hospital cardiac arrest due to VF/PVT are 25% to 40%, with higher rates in communities with organized rapid response systems.
- Because in-hospital cardiac arrest is typically preceded by hypoxia or hypotension, asystole or PEA occurs more commonly than VF or PVT. Hospital survival for in-hospital cardiac arrest related to VF/PVT is ~36% and for asystole/PEA ~11%.
- Survival after pediatric out-of-hospital arrest is ~7%, with most survivors having poor neurologic status. Only 14% of pediatric patients with in-hospital arrest present with VF or PFT as the initial rhythm, of which 29% survive to hospital discharge. Most pediatric arrests are respiratory related rather than cardiac related as in adults.

CLINICAL PRESENTATION

- The onset of cardiac arrest may be characterized by symptoms of anxiety, mental status changes, or unconsciousness; cold, clammy extremities; dyspnea, shortness of breath, or no respiration; chest pain; diaphoresis; and nausea or vomiting.

- Physical signs may include hypotension, tachycardia, bradycardia, irregular or no pulse, cyanosis, hypothermia, and distant or absent heart and lung sounds.

DIAGNOSIS

- Rapid diagnosis of cardiac arrest is vital to the success of cardiopulmonary resuscitation (CPR). Patients must receive early intervention to prevent cardiac rhythms from degenerating into less treatable arrhythmias.
- Cardiac arrest is diagnosed initially by observation of clinical manifestations consistent with cardiac arrest. The diagnosis is confirmed by evaluating vital signs, especially heart rate and respirations.
- Electrocardiography (ECG) is useful for determining the cardiac rhythm, which in turn determines drug therapy.
  ✓ VF is electrical anarchy of the ventricle resulting in no cardiac output and cardiovascular collapse.
  ✓ PEA is the absence of a detectable pulse and the presence of some type of electrical activity other than VF or PVT.
  ✓ Asystole is the presence of a flat line on the ECG monitor.

DESIRED OUTCOME

- The goal of treating cardiac arrest is the return of spontaneous circulation (ROSC) with effective ventilation and perfusion by CPR as quickly as possible to minimize hypoxic damage to vital organs.
- After successful resuscitation, the primary goals include optimizing tissue oxygenation, identifying precipitating cause(s) of arrest, and preventing subsequent episodes.

TREATMENT

GENERAL APPROACH

- The most recent American Heart Association (AHA) guidelines for CPR and emergency cardiovascular care (ECC) were published online in *Circulation* in October 2010. The guidelines differ from the previous 2005 guidelines in several important respects.
- The likelihood of a successful outcome is enhanced if each of five critical elements in the "chain of survival" is implemented promptly: (1) immediate recognition of cardiac arrest and activation of the emergency response system, (2) early CPR with an emphasis on chest compressions, (3) rapid defibrillation, (4) effective advanced cardiac life support (ACLS), and (5) integrated post–cardiac arrest care.
- According to the 2010 AHA guidelines, basic life support given by healthcare providers trained in CPR includes the following actions performed in this order:
  ✓ First, determine patient responsiveness. If the victim is unresponsive with no breathing or no normal breathing (i.e., only gasping), activate

the emergency medical response team and obtain an automated external defibrillator (AED) if one is available.

✓ Check for a pulse, but if one is not definitely felt within 10 seconds, begin CPR and use the AED when available.

✓ Begin CPR with 30 chest compressions at a rate of at least 100/min and a compression depth of at least 2 in (5 cm) in adults and at least one third of the anteroposterior chest diameter in infants and children (~1.5 in [4 cm] in infants and 2 in [5 cm] in children).

✓ Open the airway and deliver two rescue breaths, then repeat chest compressions. Follow each cycle of 30 chest compressions by two rescue breaths.

✓ Continue cycles of 30 compressions/2 breaths until an AED arrives and is ready for use or emergency medical service (EMS) providers take over care of the victim.

✓ If an AED is available, check the rhythm to determine if defibrillation is advised. If so, then deliver one shock with the immediate resumption of chest compressions/rescue breaths. After five cycles, reevaluate the rhythm to determine the need for further defibrillation. Repeat this sequence of actions until help arrives or the rhythm is no longer "shockable."

✓ If the rhythm is not shockable, then continue chest compressions/rescue breath cycles until help arrives or the victim recovers spontaneous circulation. If the rhythm is not shockable, it is likely to be either asystole or PEA.

- Once ACLS providers arrive, further definitive therapy is given following the ACLS algorithm shown in **Fig. 7–1.**
- Central venous catheter access results in faster and higher peak drug concentrations than peripheral venous administration, but central line access is not needed in most resuscitation attempts. However, if a central line is already present, it should be the access site of choice. If IV access (either central or peripheral) has not been established, a large peripheral venous catheter should be inserted. If this is not successful, an intraosseous (IO) device should be inserted.
- If neither IV nor IO access can be established, atropine, lidocaine, epinephrine, naloxone, and vasopressin may be administered endotracheally. The endotracheal dose should generally be 2 to 2.5 times larger than the IV/IO dose.

TREATMENT OF VENTRICULAR FIBRILLATION AND VENTRICULAR TACHYCARDIA

Nonpharmacologic Therapy

- Persons in VF or PVT should receive electrical defibrillation with one shock using 360 J (monophasic defibrillator) or 120 to 200 J (biphasic defibrillator). After defibrillation is attempted, CPR should be immediately restarted and continued for about five cycles (~2 min) before analyzing the rhythm or checking a pulse. If there is still evidence of VF/PVT after 2 minutes, then pharmacologic therapy with repeat attempts at single-discharge defibrillation should be attempted.

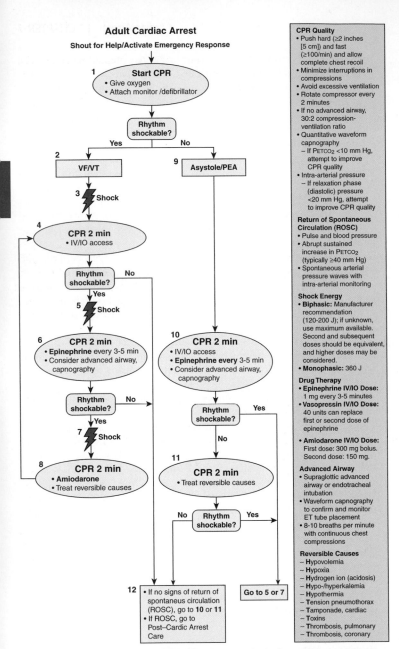

FIGURE 7–1. Advanced cardiac life support (ACLS) cardiac arrest algorithm. (CPR, cardiopulmonary resuscitation; PEA, pulseless electrical activity; VF, ventricular fibrillation; VT, ventricular tachycardia.) *(Reprinted with permission: 2010 American Heart Association Guidelines for Cardiopulmonary Resuscitation and Emergency Cardiovascular Care, Part 8: Adult Advanced Cardiovascular Life Support. Circulation 2010;122(Suppl 3):S729–S767. © 2010 American Heart Association, Inc.)*

- Endotracheal intubation and IV access should be obtained when feasible, but not at the expense of stopping chest compressions. Once an airway is achieved, patients should be ventilated with 100% oxygen.

Pharmacologic Therapy

SYMPATHOMIMETICS

- The goal of sympathomimetic therapy is to augment both coronary and cerebral perfusion pressures during the low-flow state associated with CPR. These agents increase systemic arteriolar vasoconstriction, thereby improving coronary and cerebral perfusion pressure. They also maintain vascular tone, decrease arteriolar collapse, and shunt blood to the heart and brain.
- **Epinephrine** is a drug of first choice for treating VF, PVT, asystole, and PEA. It is an agonist of both α and β receptors, but its effectiveness is primarily due to α effects.
- The recommended adult dose of epinephrine is 1 mg administered by IV or IO injection every 3 to 5 minutes. Although some studies have shown that higher doses (e.g., 5–15 mg) may increase the initial resuscitation rate, overall survival is not significantly improved.

VASOPRESSIN

- **Vasopressin** is a potent nonadrenergic vasoconstrictor that increases blood pressure (BP) and systemic vascular resistance. Its vasoconstrictive properties are due primarily to effects on V_1 receptors. It may have several advantages over epinephrine. First, the metabolic acidosis that frequently accompanies cardiac arrest can blunt the vasoconstrictive effect of epinephrine; this does not occur with vasopressin. Second, stimulation of β receptors by epinephrine can increase myocardial oxygen demand and complicate the postresuscitative phase of CPR. Vasopressin can also have a beneficial effect on blood flow in the kidney, causing vasodilation and increased water reabsorption. Despite these theoretical advantages, clinical trials have not consistently demonstrated results that are superior to epinephrine. The 2010 AHA guidelines indicate that vasopressin 40 units IV/IO can replace the first or second dose of epinephrine.

ANTIARRHYTHMICS

- The purpose of antiarrhythmic drug therapy after unsuccessful defibrillation and vasopressor administration is to prevent the development or recurrence of VF and PVT by raising the fibrillation threshold. However, the role of antiarrhythmics is limited because clinical evidence demonstrating improved survival to hospital discharge is lacking.
- **Amiodarone** is the first-line antiarrhythmic and may be considered for VF/VT unresponsive to CPR, defibrillation, and vasopressors. The dose is 300 mg IV/IO followed by a second dose of 150 mg.
- **Lidocaine** may be used if amiodarone is unavailable, but clinical trials have not shown it to improve rates of ROSC and hospital admission compared with amiodarone. The initial dose is 1 to 1.5 mg/kg IV. Additional doses of 0.5 to 0.75 mg/kg can be administered at 5- to 10-minute intervals to a maximum dose of 3 mg/kg if VF/PVT persists.

THROMBOLYTICS

- The role of thrombolytics during CPR has been investigated because most cardiac arrests are related to either myocardial infarction (MI) or pulmonary embolism (PE). Although several studies demonstrated successful thrombolytic use, few have shown improvements to hospital discharge, and an increase in intracranial hemorrhage was noted. Therefore, fibrinolytic therapy should not be used routinely in cardiac arrest, but it can be considered when PE is the presumed or known cause of the arrest.

MAGNESIUM

- Although severe hypomagnesemia has been associated with VF/PVT, clinical trials have not demonstrated any benefit with routine administration of magnesium during a cardiac arrest. Two trials showed improvement in ROSC in patients with arrest associated with torsades de pointes. Therefore, magnesium administration should be limited to these patients. The dose is 1 to 2 g diluted in 10 mL of 5% dextrose in water administered IV/IO push over 5 to 20 minutes.

Postresuscitative Care

- ROSC from a cardiac arrest may be followed by a post–cardiac arrest syndrome characterized by post–cardiac arrest brain injury, myocardial dysfunction, systemic ischemia/reperfusion response, and persistent precipitating pathology.
- Hypothermia can protect from cerebral injury by suppressing chemical reactions that occur after restoration of blood flow. The 2010 AHA guidelines recommend that comatose (i.e., lack of meaningful response to verbal commands) adult patients with ROSC after out-of-hospital VF cardiac arrest should be cooled to 32–34°C (89.6–93.2°F) for 12 to 24 hours. Cooling may also be considered for comatose adults patients with ROSC after out-of-hospital arrests with an initial rhythm of asystole or PEA or after in-hospital cardiac arrest of any initial rhythm; there is insufficient evidence to recommend therapeutic hypothermia in children. Potential complications of hypothermia include coagulopathy, dysrhythmias, hyperglycemia, increased incidence of pneumonia and sepsis, and profound effects on drug distribution and elimination.

TREATMENT OF PULSELESS ELECTRICAL ACTIVITY AND ASYSTOLE

Nonpharmacologic Therapy

- Successful treatment of PEA and asystole depends almost entirely on the diagnosis of the underlying cause. Potentially reversible causes include (1) hypovolemia, (2) hypoxia, (3) acidosis, (4) hyper- or hypokalemia, (5) hypothermia, (6) hypoglycemia, (7) drug overdose, (8) cardiac tamponade, (9) tension pneumothorax, (10) coronary thrombosis, (11) pulmonary thrombosis, and (12) trauma.
- Treatment of PEA is the same as treatment of asystole. Both conditions require CPR, airway control, and IV access. Defibrillation should be avoided in asystole because the resulting parasympathetic discharge can

reduce the chance of ROSC and worsen the chance of survival. If available, transcutaneous pacing can be attempted.

Pharmacologic Therapy

- The recommended adult dose of epinephrine is 1 mg administered by IV or IO injection every 3 to 5 minutes. Studies comparing **epinephrine** and **vasopressin** in patients with PEA and asystole have not consistently demonstrated an advantage with one agent over the other. Vasopressin 40 units IV/IO can replace the first or second dose of epinephrine.
- **Atropine** is an antimuscarinic agent that blocks the depressant effect of acetylcholine on the sinus and atrioventricular nodes, thereby decreasing parasympathetic tone. During asystole, parasympathetic tone may increase because of vagal stimulation from intubation, hypoxia and acidosis, or alterations in the balance of parasympathetic and sympathetic control. However, available evidence suggests that atropine use during PEA or asystole is not likely to be beneficial. Therefore, the 2010 AHA guidelines have removed atropine from the ACLS cardiac arrest algorithm.

ACID–BASE MANAGEMENT

- Acidosis occurs during cardiac arrest because of decreased blood flow or inadequate ventilation. Chest compressions generate only ~20% to 30% of normal cardiac output, leading to inadequate organ perfusion, tissue hypoxia, and metabolic acidosis. Furthermore, the lack of ventilation causes retention of CO_2, leading to respiratory acidosis. The combined acidosis reduces myocardial contractility and may cause arrhythmias because of a lower fibrillation threshold.
- Sodium bicarbonate administration for cardiac arrest is controversial because there are few clinical data supporting its use, and it may have some detrimental effects. Therefore, routine use of sodium bicarbonate is not recommended for patients in cardiac arrest. It can be used in special circumstances (e.g., preexisting metabolic acidosis, hyperkalemia, and tricyclic antidepressant overdose). The dosage should be guided by laboratory analysis if possible.

EVALUATION OF THERAPEUTIC OUTCOMES

- To measure the success of CPR, therapeutic outcome monitoring should occur both during the resuscitation attempt and in the postresuscitation phase. The optimal outcome following CPR is an awake, responsive, spontaneously breathing patient. Ideally, patients must remain neurologically intact with minimal morbidity after the resuscitation.
- Heart rate, cardiac rhythm, and BP should be assessed and documented throughout the resuscitation attempt and after each intervention. Determination of the presence or absence of a pulse is paramount to deciding which interventions are appropriate.
- Coronary perfusion pressure should be assessed in patients for whom intraarterial monitoring is in place.

- End-tidal CO_2 monitoring is a safe and effective method to assess cardiac output during CPR and has been associated with ROSC.
- Clinicians should consider the precipitating cause of the cardiac arrest, such as MI, electrolyte imbalance, or primary arrhythmia. Prearrest status should be carefully reviewed, particularly if the patient was receiving drug therapy.
- Altered cardiac, hepatic, and renal function resulting from ischemic damage during the arrest warrant special attention.
- Neurologic function should be assessed by the Cerebral Performance Category and the Glasgow Coma Scale.

See Chapter 18, Cardiac Arrest, authored by Jeffrey F. Barletta and Jeffrey L. Wilt, for a more detailed discussion of this topic.

CHAPTER 8

Dyslipidemia

DEFINITION

- Dyslipidemia is defined as elevated total cholesterol, low-density lipoprotein (LDL) cholesterol, or triglycerides; a low high-density lipoprotein (HDL) cholesterol; or a combination of these abnormalities. Hyperlipoproteinemia describes an increased concentration of the lipoprotein macromolecules that transport lipids in the plasma. Abnormalities of plasma lipids can result in a predisposition to coronary, cerebrovascular, and peripheral vascular arterial disease.

PATHOPHYSIOLOGY

- Cholesterol, triglycerides, and phospholipids are transported in the bloodstream as complexes of lipids and proteins known as lipoproteins. Elevated total and LDL cholesterol and reduced HDL cholesterol are associated with the development of coronary heart disease (CHD).
- The response-to-injury hypothesis states that risk factors such as oxidized LDL, mechanical injury to the endothelium, excessive homocysteine, immunologic attack, and infection-induced changes in endothelial and intimal function lead to endothelial dysfunction and a series of cellular interactions that culminate in atherosclerosis. The eventual clinical outcomes may include angina, myocardial infarction (MI), arrhythmias, stroke, peripheral arterial disease, abdominal aortic aneurysm, and sudden death.
- Atherosclerotic lesions are thought to arise from transport and retention of plasma LDL through the endothelial cell layer into the extracellular matrix of the subendothelial space. Once in the artery wall, LDL is chemically modified through oxidation and nonenzymatic glycation. Mildly oxidized LDL recruits monocytes into the artery wall. These monocytes then become transformed into macrophages that accelerate LDL oxidation.
- Oxidized LDL provokes an inflammatory response mediated by a number of chemoattractants and cytokines (e.g., monocyte colony-stimulating factor, intercellular adhesion molecule, platelet-derived growth factor, transforming growth factors, interleukin-1, and interleukin-6).
- Repeated injury and repair within an atherosclerotic plaque eventually lead to a fibrous cap protecting the underlying core of lipids, collagen, calcium, and inflammatory cells, such as T lymphocytes. Maintenance of the fibrous plaque is critical to prevent plaque rupture and subsequent coronary thrombosis.
- Primary or genetic lipoprotein disorders are classified into six categories for the phenotypic description of dyslipidemia. The types and corresponding lipoprotein elevations include the following: I (chylomicrons), IIa (LDL), IIb (LDL + very-low-density lipoprotein[VLDL]), III (intermediate-density lipoprotein), IV (VLDL), and V (VLDL +

chylomicrons). Secondary forms of dyslipidemia also exist, and several drug classes may affect lipid levels (e.g., progestins, thiazide diuretics, glucocorticoids, β-blockers, isotretinoin, protease inhibitors, cyclosporine, mirtazapine, and sirolimus).

- The primary defect in familial hypercholesterolemia is the inability to bind LDL to the LDL receptor (LDL-R) or, rarely, a defect of internalizing the LDL-R complex into the cell after normal binding. This leads to a lack of LDL degradation by cells and unregulated biosynthesis of cholesterol, with total cholesterol and LDL cholesterol (LDL-C) being inversely proportional to the deficit in LDL-Rs.

CLINICAL PRESENTATION

- Familial hypercholesterolemia is characterized by a selective elevation in plasma LDL and deposition of LDL-derived cholesterol in tendons (xanthomas) and arteries (atheromas).
- Familial lipoprotein lipase deficiency is characterized by a massive accumulation of chylomicrons and a corresponding increase in plasma triglycerides or a type I lipoprotein pattern. Presenting manifestations include repeated attacks of pancreatitis and abdominal pain, eruptive cutaneous xanthomatosis, and hepatosplenomegaly beginning in childhood. Symptom severity is proportional to dietary fat intake and consequently to the elevation of chylomicrons. Accelerated atherosclerosis is not associated with this disease.
- Familial type III hyperlipoproteinemia results in the following clinical features after age 20: xanthoma striata palmaris (yellow discolorations of the palmar and digital creases); tuberous or tuberoeruptive xanthomas (bulbous cutaneous xanthomas); and severe atherosclerosis involving the coronary arteries, internal carotids, and abdominal aorta.
- Type IV hyperlipoproteinemia is common and occurs in adults, primarily in patients who are obese, diabetic, and hyperuricemic and do not have xanthomas. It may be secondary to alcohol ingestion and can be aggravated by stress, progestins, oral contraceptives, thiazides, or β-blockers.
- Type V hyperlipoproteinemia is characterized by abdominal pain, pancreatitis, eruptive xanthomas, and peripheral polyneuropathy. These patients are commonly obese, hyperuricemic, and diabetic; alcohol intake, exogenous estrogens, and renal insufficiency tend to be exacerbating factors. The risk of atherosclerosis is increased with this disorder.

DIAGNOSIS

- A fasting lipoprotein profile including total cholesterol, LDL, HDL, and triglycerides should be measured in all adults 20 years of age or older at least once every 5 years.
- Measurement of plasma cholesterol (which is ~3% lower than serum determinations), triglyceride, and HDL levels after a 12-hour or longer

fast is important, because triglycerides may be elevated in nonfasting individuals; total cholesterol is only modestly affected by fasting.

- Two determinations, 1 to 8 weeks apart, with the patient on a stable diet and weight, and in the absence of acute illness, are recommended to minimize variability and to obtain a reliable baseline. If the total cholesterol is >200 mg/dL, a second determination is recommended, and if the values are >30 mg/dL apart, the average of three values should be used.

- After a lipid abnormality is confirmed, major components of the evaluation are the history (including age, gender, and, if female, menstrual and estrogen replacement status), physical examination, and laboratory investigations.

- A complete history and physical examination should assess the (1) presence or absence of cardiovascular risk factors or definite cardiovascular disease in the individual; (2) family history of premature cardiovascular disease or lipid disorders; (3) presence or absence of secondary causes of dyslipidemia, including concurrent medications; and (4) presence or absence of xanthomas, abdominal pain, or history of pancreatitis, renal or liver disease, peripheral vascular disease, abdominal aortic aneurysm, or cerebral vascular disease (carotid bruits, stroke, or transient ischemic attack).

- Diabetes mellitus is regarded as a CHD risk equivalent. That is, the presence of diabetes in patients without known CHD is associated with the same level of risk as patients without diabetes but having confirmed CHD.

- If the physical examination and history are insufficient to diagnose a familial disorder, then agarose-gel lipoprotein electrophoresis is useful to determine which class of lipoproteins is affected. If the triglyceride levels are <400 mg/dL, and neither type III dyslipidemia nor chylomicrons are detected by electrophoresis, then one can calculate VLDL and LDL concentrations: VLDL = triglycerides ÷ 5; LDL = total cholesterol − (VLDL + HDL). Initial testing uses total cholesterol for case finding, but subsequent management decisions should be based on LDL.

- Because total cholesterol is composed of cholesterol derived from LDL, VLDL, and HDL, determination of HDL is useful when total plasma cholesterol is elevated. HDL may be elevated by moderate alcohol ingestion (fewer than two drinks per day), physical exercise, smoking cessation, weight loss, oral contraceptives, phenytoin, and terbutaline. HDL may be lowered by smoking, obesity, a sedentary lifestyle, and drugs such as β-blockers.

- Diagnosis of lipoprotein lipase deficiency is based on low or absent enzyme activity with normal human plasma or apolipoprotein C-II, a cofactor of the enzyme.

DESIRED OUTCOME

- The goals of treatment are to lower total and LDL cholesterol in order to reduce the risk of first or recurrent events such as MI, angina, heart failure, ischemic stroke, or other forms of peripheral arterial disease, such as carotid stenosis and abdominal aortic aneurysm.

TREATMENT

GENERAL APPROACH

- The National Cholesterol Education Program Adult Treatment Panel III (NCEP ATP III) recommends that a fasting lipoprotein profile and risk factor assessment be used in the initial classification of adults.
- If the total cholesterol is <200 mg/dL, then the patient has a desirable blood cholesterol level (Table 8–1). If the HDL is also >40 mg/dL, no further follow-up is recommended for patients without known CHD and who have fewer than two risk factors (Table 8–2).
- In patients with borderline-high blood cholesterol (200–239 mg/dL), assessment of risk factors is needed to more clearly define disease risk.
- Decisions regarding classification and management are based on the LDL cholesterol levels listed in Table 8–3.
- There are four categories of risk that modify the goals and modalities of LDL-lowering therapy. The highest risk category is having known CHD or CHD risk equivalents; the risk for major coronary events is equal to or greater than that for established CHD (i.e., >20% per 10 years, or 2% per year). The next category is moderately high risk, consisting of patients with two or more risk factors in which 10-year risk for CHD is 10% to 20%. Moderate risk is defined as two or more risk factors and a 10-year risk of 10% or less. The lowest risk category is persons with zero to one risk factor, which is usually associated with a 10-year CHD risk of <10%.

TABLE 8–1	Classification of Total, LDL, and HDL Cholesterol and Triglycerides
Total cholesterol	
<200 mg/dL	Desirable
200–239 mg/dL	Borderline high
≥240 mg/dL	High
LDL cholesterol	
<100 mg/dL	Optimal
100–129 mg/dL	Near or above optimal
130–159 mg/dL	Borderline high
160–189 mg/dL	High
≥190 mg/dL	Very high
HDL cholesterol	
<40 mg/dL	Low
≥60 mg/dL	High
Triglycerides	
<150 mg/dL	Normal
150–199 mg/dL	Borderline high
200–499 mg/dL	High
≥500 mg/dL	Very high

HDL, high-density lipoprotein; LDL, low-density lipoprotein.

TABLE 8–2 Major Risk Factors (Exclusive of LDL Cholesterol) That Modify LDL Goals[a]

Age

    Men: ≥45 years

    Women: ≥55 years or premature menopause without estrogen replacement therapy

Family history of premature CHD (definite myocardial infarction or sudden death before 55 years of age in father or other male first-degree relative or before 65 years of age in mother or other female first-degree relative)

Cigarette smoking

Hypertension (≥140/90 mm Hg or on antihypertensive medication)

Low HDL cholesterol (<40 mg/dL)[b]

CHD, coronary heart disease; HDL, high-density lipoprotein; LDL, low-density lipoprotein.

[a]Diabetes is regarded as a CHD risk equivalent.

[b]HDL cholesterol (≥60 mg/dL) counts as a "negative" risk factor; its presence removes one risk factor from the total count.

- ATP III recognizes the metabolic syndrome as a secondary target of risk reduction after LDL-C has been addressed. This syndrome is characterized by abdominal obesity, atherogenic dyslipidemia (elevated triglycerides, small LDL particles, and low HDL cholesterol), increased blood pressure (BP), insulin resistance (with or without glucose intolerance), and

TABLE 8–3 LDL Cholesterol Goals and Cutpoints for Therapeutic Lifestyle Changes (TLCs) and Drug Therapy in Different Risk Categories

Risk Category	LDL Goal (mg/dL)	LDL Level at Which to Initiate TLC (mg/dL)	LDL Level at Which to Consider Drug Therapy (mg/dL)
High risk: CHD or CHD risk equivalents (10-year risk >20%)	<100 (optional goal: <70)	≥100	≥100 (<100: consider drug options)[a]
Moderately high risk: 2+ risk factors (10-year risk 10–20%)	<130	≥130	≥130 (100–129: consider drug options)
Moderate risk: 2+ risk factors (10-year risk <10%)	<130	≥130	≥160
Lower risk: 0 or 1 risk factor[b]	<160	≥160	≥190 (160–189: LDL-lowering drug optional)

CHD, coronary heart disease; LDL, low-density lipoprotein.

[a]Some authorities recommend use of LDL-lowering drugs in this category if LDL cholesterol <100 mg/dL cannot be achieved by TLC. Others prefer to use drugs that primarily modify triglycerides and HDL (e.g., nicotinic acid or fibrates). Clinical judgment also may call for deferring drug therapy in this subcategory.

[b]Almost all people with zero or one risk factor have a 10-year risk <10%; thus, 10-year risk assessment in people with zero or 1 risk factor is not necessary.

prothrombotic and proinflammatory states. If the metabolic syndrome is present, the patient is considered to have a CHD risk equivalent.

- Other targets include non-HDL goals for patients with triglycerides >200 mg/dL. Non-HDL cholesterol is calculated by subtracting HDL from total cholesterol, and the targets are 30 mg/dL greater than LDL for each risk stratum.

NONPHARMACOLOGIC THERAPY

- Therapeutic lifestyle changes (TLCs) are begun on the first visit and include dietary therapy, weight reduction, and increased physical activity. Inducing a weight loss of 10% should be discussed with patients who are overweight. In general, physical activity of moderate intensity 30 minutes a day for most days of the week should be encouraged. All patients should be counseled to stop smoking and to meet the seventh report of the Joint National Committee on Prevention, Detection, Evaluation, and Treatment of High Blood Pressure (JNC7) guidelines for control of hypertension.
- The objectives of dietary therapy are to progressively decrease the intake of total fat, saturated fat, and cholesterol and to achieve a desirable body weight (Table 8–4).
- Increased intake of soluble fiber in the form of oat bran, pectins, certain gums, and psyllium products can reduce total and LDL cholesterol by 5% to 20%, but these dietary alterations or supplements should not be substituted for more active forms of treatment. They have little or no effect on HDL-C or triglyceride concentrations. These products may also be useful in managing constipation associated with the bile acid resins (BARs).
- Fish oil supplementation has a fairly large effect in reducing triglycerides and VLDL cholesterol, but it either has no effect on total and LDL

TABLE 8–4	Macronutrient Recommendations for the Therapeutic Lifestyle Change (TLC) Diet
Component[a]	**Recommended Intake**
Total fat	25–35% of total calories
Saturated fat	<7% of total calories
Polyunsaturated fat	Up to 10% of total calories
Monounsaturated fat	Up to 20% of total calories
Carbohydrates[b]	50–60% of total calories
Cholesterol	<200 mg/day
Dietary fiber	20–30 g/day
Plant sterols	2 g/day
Protein	~15% of total calories
Total calories	To achieve and maintain desirable body weight

[a]Calories from alcohol not included.
[b]Carbohydrates should derive from foods rich in complex carbohydrates, such as whole grains, fruits, and vegetables.

TABLE 8–5	Effects of Drug Therapy on Lipids and Lipoproteins		
Drug	**Mechanism of Action**	**Effects on Lipids**	**Effects on Lipoproteins**
Cholestyramine, colestipol, and colesevelam	↑ LDL catabolism ↓ Cholesterol absorption	↓ Cholesterol	↓ LDL ↑ VLDL
Niacin	↓ LDL and VLDL synthesis	↓ Triglyceride ↓ Cholesterol	↓ VLDL ↓ LDL ↑ HDL
Gemfibrozil, fenofibrate, and clofibrate	↑ VLDL clearance ↓ VLDL synthesis	↓ Triglyceride ↓ Cholesterol	↓ VLDL ↓ LDL ↑ HDL
Lovastatin, pravastatin, simvastatin, fluvastatin, atorvastatin, and rosuvastatin	↑ LDL catabolism ↓ LDL synthesis	↓ Cholesterol	↓ LDL
Ezetimibe	Blocks cholesterol absorption across the intestinal border	↓ Cholesterol	↓ LDL

↑, increased; ↓, decreased.

cholesterol or may cause elevations in these fractions. Other actions of fish oil may account for any cardioprotective effects.

- Ingestion of 2 to 3 g daily of plant sterols will reduce LDL by 6% to 15%. They are usually available in commercial margarines.
- If all recommended dietary changes from the NCEP were instituted, the estimated average reduction in LDL would range from 20% to 30%.

PHARMACOLOGIC THERAPY

- The effect of drug therapy on lipids and lipoproteins is shown in **Table 8–5**.
- Recommended drugs of choice for each lipoprotein phenotype are given in **Table 8–6**.
- Available products and their doses are provided in **Table 8–7**.

Bile Acid Resins

- BARs (**cholestyramine, colestipol,** and **colesevelam**) bind bile acids in the intestinal lumen, with a concurrent interruption of enterohepatic circulation of bile acids, which decreases the bile acid pool size and stimulates hepatic synthesis of bile acids from cholesterol. Depletion of the hepatic pool of cholesterol results in an increase in cholesterol biosynthesis and an increase in the number of LDL-Rs on the hepatocyte membrane, which stimulates an enhanced rate of catabolism from plasma and lowers LDL levels. The increase in hepatic cholesterol biosynthesis may be paralleled by increased hepatic VLDL production; consequently, BARs may aggravate hypertriglyceridemia in patients with combined dyslipidemia.
- BARs are useful in treating primary hypercholesterolemia (familial hypercholesterolemia, familial combined dyslipidemia, and type IIa hyperlipoproteinemia).

TABLE 8-6	Lipoprotein Phenotype and Recommended Drug Treatment	
Lipoprotein Type	**Drug of Choice**	**Combination Therapy**
I	Not indicated	–
IIa	Statins	Niacin or BARs
	Cholestyramine or colestipol	Statins or niacin
	Niacin	Statins or BARs
	Ezetimibe	
IIb	Statins	BARs, fibrates, or niacin
	Fibrates	Statins, niacin, or BARs[a]
	Niacin	Statins or fibrates
	Ezetimibe	
III	Fibrates	Statins or niacin
	Niacin	Statins or fibrates
	Ezetimibe	
IV	Fibrates	Niacin
	Niacin	Fibrates
V	Fibrates	Niacin
	Niacin	Fish oils

BARs, bile acid resins; fibrates include gemfibrozil or fenofibrate.
[a]BARs are not used as first-line therapy if triglycerides are elevated at baseline because hypertriglyceridemia may worsen with BARs alone.

- Common GI complaints include constipation, bloating, epigastric fullness, nausea, and flatulence. They can be managed by increasing fluid intake, modifying the diet to increase bulk, and using stool softeners.
- The gritty texture and bulk may be minimized by mixing the powder with orange drink or juice. Colestipol may have better palatability than cholestyramine because it is odorless and tasteless. Tablet forms should help improve adherence with this form of therapy.
- Other potential adverse effects include impaired absorption of fat-soluble vitamins A, D, E, and K; hypernatremia and hyperchloremia; GI obstruction; and reduced bioavailability of acidic drugs such as warfarin, nicotinic acid, thyroxine, acetaminophen, hydrocortisone, hydrochlorothiazide, loperamide, and possibly iron. Drug interactions may be avoided by alternating administration times with an interval of 6 hours or more between the BARs and other drugs.

Niacin

- **Niacin** (nicotinic acid) reduces the hepatic synthesis of VLDL, which in turn leads to a reduction in the synthesis of LDL. Niacin also increases HDL by reducing its catabolism.
- The principal use of niacin is for mixed dyslipidemia or as a second-line agent in combination therapy for hypercholesterolemia. It is a first-line agent or alternative for the treatment of hypertriglyceridemia and diabetic dyslipidemia.

TABLE 8–7	Comparison of Drugs Used in the Treatment of Dyslipidemia[a]		
Drug	**Dosage Forms**	**Usual Daily Dose**	**Maximum Daily Dose**
Cholestyramine (Questran)	Bulk powder/4 g packets	8 g three times daily	32 g
Cholestyramine (Cholybar)	4 g resin per bar	8 g three times daily	32 g
Colestipol hydrochloride (Colestid)	Bulk powder/5 g packets	10 g twice daily	30 g
Colesevelam (Welchol)	625 mg tablets	1,875 mg twice daily	4,375 mg
Niacin	50, 100, 250, and 500 mg tablets; 125, 250, and 500 mg capsules	0.5–1 g three times daily	6 g
Extended-release niacin (Niaspan)	500, 750, and 1,000 mg tablets	1,000–2,000 mg once daily	2,000 mg
Extended-release niacin + lovastatin (Advicor)	Niacin/lovastatin 500 mg/20 mg tablets Niacin/lovastatin 750 mg/ 20 mg tablets Niacin/lovastatin 1,000 mg/ 20 mg tablets	500 mg/20 mg – –	1,000 mg/ 20 mg – –
Fenofibrate (Tricor)	67, 134, and 200 mg capsules (micronized); 54 and 160 mg tablets; 40 and 120 mg tablets; 50 and 160 mg tablets	54 mg or 67 mg	201 mg
Gemfibrozil (Lopid)	300 mg capsules	600 mg twice daily	1.5 g
Lovastatin (Mevacor)	20 and 40 mg tablets	20–40 mg	80 mg
Pravastatin (Pravachol)	10, 20, 40, and 80 mg tablets	10–20 mg	40 mg
Simvastatin (Zocor)	5, 10, 20, 40, and 80 mg tablets	10–20 mg	80 mg
Atorvastatin (Lipitor)	10, 20, 40, and 80 mg tablets	10 mg	80 mg
Rosuvastatin (Crestor)	5, 10, 20, and 40 mg tablets	5 mg	40 mg
Pitavastatin (Livalo)	1, 2, and 4 mg tablets	2 mg	4 mg
Ezetimibe (Zetia)	10 mg tablet	10 mg	10 mg
Simvastatin/ezetimibe (Vytorin)	Simvastatin/ezetimibe 10 mg/10 mg, 20 mg/10 mg, 40 mg/10 mg, and 80 mg/10 mg	Simvastatin/ ezetimibe 20 mg/10 mg	Simvastatin/ ezetimibe 80 mg/ 10 mg

[a]This table does not include all drugs used for treating dyslipidemia.

- Niacin has many common adverse drug reactions; most of the symptoms and biochemical abnormalities seen do not require discontinuation of therapy.
- Cutaneous flushing and itching appear to be prostaglandin mediated and can be reduced by taking aspirin 325 mg shortly before niacin ingestion. Taking the niacin dose with meals and slowly titrating the dose upward may minimize these effects. Concomitant alcohol and hot drinks may magnify the flushing and pruritus from niacin, and they should be avoided at the time of ingestion. GI intolerance is also a common problem.
- Potentially important laboratory abnormalities occurring with niacin therapy include elevated liver function tests, hyperuricemia, and hyperglycemia. Niacin-associated hepatitis is more common with sustained-release preparations, and their use should be restricted to patients intolerant of regular-release products. Niacin is contraindicated in patients with active liver disease, and it may exacerbate preexisting gout and diabetes.
- **Niaspan** is a prescription-only, extended-release niacin formulation with pharmacokinetics intermediate between prompt- and sustained-release products. Controlled trials have shown it to have fewer dermatologic reactions and a low risk of hepatotoxicity. Combination with statins can produce large reductions in LDL and increases in HDL.
- Nicotinamide should not be used in the treatment of dyslipidemia because it does not effectively lower cholesterol or triglyceride levels.

HMG-CoA Reductase Inhibitors

- Statins (**atorvastatin, fluvastatin, lovastatin, pitavastatin, pravastatin, rosuvastatin,** and **simvastatin**) inhibit 3-hydroxy-3-methylglutaryl coenzyme A (HMG-CoA) reductase, interrupting the conversion of HMG-CoA to mevalonate, the rate-limiting step in de novo cholesterol biosynthesis. Reduced synthesis of LDL and enhanced catabolism of LDL mediated through LDL-Rs appear to be the principal mechanisms for lipid-lowering effects.
- When used as monotherapy, statins are the most potent total and LDL cholesterol–lowering agents and among the best tolerated. Total and LDL cholesterol are reduced in a dose-related fashion by 30% or more when added to dietary therapy.
- Combination therapy with a statin and a BAR is rational because the numbers of LDL-Rs are increased, leading to greater degradation of LDL cholesterol; intracellular synthesis of cholesterol is inhibited; and enterohepatic recycling of bile acids is interrupted.
- Combination therapy with a statin and ezetimibe is also rational because ezetimibe inhibits cholesterol absorption across the gut border and adds 12% to 20% further reduction when combined with a statin or other drug.
- Constipation occurs in <10% of patients taking statins. Other adverse effects include elevated serum aminotransferase levels (primarily alanine aminotransferase), elevated creatine kinase levels, myopathy, and, rarely, rhabdomyolysis.

Fibric Acids

- Fibrate monotherapy (**gemfibrozil**, **fenofibrate**, or **clofibrate**) is effective in reducing VLDL, but a reciprocal rise in LDL may occur, and total cholesterol values may remain relatively unchanged. Plasma HDL concentrations may rise 10% to 15% or more with fibrates.
- Gemfibrozil reduces the synthesis of VLDL and, to a lesser extent, apolipoprotein B with a concurrent increase in the rate of removal of triglyceride-rich lipoproteins from plasma. Clofibrate is less effective than gemfibrozil or niacin in reducing VLDL production.
- GI complaints occur in 3% to 5% of patients, rash in 2%, dizziness in 2.4%, and transient elevations in transaminase levels and alkaline phosphatase in 4.5% and 1.3%, respectively. Gemfibrozil and probably fenofibrate may rarely enhance gallstone formation.
- A myositis syndrome of myalgia, weakness, stiffness, malaise, and elevations in creatine kinase and aspartate aminotransferase may occur and seems to be more common in patients with renal insufficiency.
- Fibrates may potentiate the effects of oral anticoagulants, and the international normalized ratio (INR) should be monitored very closely with this combination.

Ezetimibe

- **Ezetimibe** interferes with the absorption of cholesterol from the brush border of the intestine, a novel mechanism that makes it a good choice for adjunctive therapy. It is approved as monotherapy and for use with a statin. The dose is 10 mg once daily, given with or without food. When used alone, it results in ~18% reduction in LDL cholesterol. When added to a statin, ezetimibe lowers LDL by an additional 12% to 20%. A combination product (Vytorin) containing ezetimibe 10 mg and simvastatin 10, 20, 40, or 80 mg is available. Ezetimibe is well tolerated; ~4% of patients experience GI upset. Because cardiovascular outcomes with ezetimibe have not been evaluated, it should be reserved for patients unable to tolerate statin therapy or those who do not achieve satisfactory lipid lowering with a statin alone.

Fish Oil Supplementation

- Diets high in omega-3 polyunsaturated fatty acids (from fish oil), most commonly eicosapentaenoic acid (EPA), reduce cholesterol, triglycerides, LDL, and VLDL and may elevate HDL cholesterol.
- Fish oil supplementation may be most useful in patients with hypertriglyceridemia, but its role in treatment is not well defined.
- **LOVAZA (omega-3-acid ethyl esters)** is a prescription form of concentrated fish oil EPA 465 mg and docosahexaenoic acid 375 mg. The daily dose is 4 g, which can be taken as four 1-g capsules once daily or two 1-g capsules twice daily. This product lowers triglycerides by 14% to 30% and raises HDL by ~10%.
- Complications of fish oil supplementation such as thrombocytopenia and bleeding disorders have been noted, especially with high doses (EPA 15–30 g/day).

TREATMENT RECOMMENDATIONS

- Treatment of type I hyperlipoproteinemia is directed toward reduction of chylomicrons derived from dietary fat with the subsequent reduction in plasma triglycerides. Total daily fat intake should be no more than 10 to 25 g, or ~15% of total calories. Secondary causes of hypertriglyceridemia should be excluded, and, if present, the underlying disorder should be treated appropriately.
- Primary hypercholesterolemia (familial hypercholesterolemia, familial combined dyslipidemia, and type IIa hyperlipoproteinemia) is treated with **BARs, statins, niacin,** or **ezetimibe**.
- Combined hyperlipoproteinemia (type IIb) may be treated with **statins, niacin,** or **gemfibrozil** to lower LDL-C without elevating VLDL and triglycerides. Niacin is the most effective agent and may be combined with a BAR. A BAR alone in this disorder may elevate VLDL and triglycerides, and their use as single agents for treating combined hyperlipoproteinemia should be avoided.
- Type III hyperlipoproteinemia may be treated with **fibrates** or **niacin**. Although fibrates have been suggested as the drugs of choice, niacin is a reasonable alternative because of the lack of data supporting a cardiovascular mortality benefit from fibrates and because of their potentially serious adverse effects. Fish oil supplementation may be an alternative therapy.
- Type V hyperlipoproteinemia requires stringent restriction of dietary fat intake. Drug therapy with **fibrates** or **niacin** is indicated if the response to diet alone is inadequate. **Medium-chain triglycerides**, which are absorbed without chylomicron formation, may be used as a dietary supplement for caloric intake if needed for both types I and V.

Combination Drug Therapy

- Combination therapy may be considered after adequate trials of monotherapy and for patients documented to be adherent to the prescribed regimen. Two or three lipoprotein profiles at 6-week intervals should confirm the lack of response prior to initiation of combination therapy.
- Contraindications to and drug interactions with combined therapy should be screened carefully, and the extra cost of drug product and monitoring should be considered.
- In general, a **statin** plus a **BAR** or **niacin** plus a **BAR** provides the greatest reduction in total and LDL cholesterol.
- Regimens intended to increase HDL levels should include either **gemfibrozil** or **niacin**, bearing in mind that **statins** combined with either of these drugs may result in a greater incidence of hepatotoxicity or myositis.
- Familial combined dyslipidemia may respond better to a fibrate and a statin than to a fibrate and a BAR.

TREATMENT OF HYPERTRIGLYCERIDEMIA

- Lipoprotein pattern types I, III, IV, and V are associated with hypertriglyceridemia, and these primary lipoprotein disorders should be excluded prior to implementing therapy.

- A family history positive for CHD is important in identifying patients at risk for premature atherosclerosis. If a patient with CHD has elevated triglycerides, the associated abnormality is probably a contributing factor to CHD and should be treated.
- High serum triglycerides (see **Table 8–1**) should be treated by achieving desirable body weight, consumption of a low saturated fat and cholesterol diet, regular exercise, smoking cessation, and restriction of alcohol (in select patients).
- ATP III identifies the sum of LDL and VLDL (termed *non-HDL* [total cholesterol − HDL]) as a secondary therapeutic target in persons with high triglycerides (≥200 mg/dL). The goal for non-HDL with high serum triglycerides is set at 30 mg/dL higher than that for LDL on the premise that a VLDL level ≤30 mg/dL is normal.
- Drug therapy with **niacin** should be considered in patients with borderline-high triglycerides but with accompanying risk factors of established CHD, family history of premature CHD, concomitant LDL elevation or low HDL, and genetic forms of hypertriglyceridemia associated with CHD. Niacin may be used cautiously in persons with diabetes because a clinical trial found only a slight increase in glucose and no change in hemoglobin A1C. Alternative therapies include **gemfibrozil** or **fenofibrate, statins,** and **fish oil.** The goal of therapy is to lower triglycerides and VLDL particles that may be atherogenic, increase HDL, and reduce LDL.
- Very high triglycerides are associated with pancreatitis and other adverse consequences. Management includes dietary fat restriction (10–20% of calories as fat), weight loss, alcohol restriction, and treatment of coexisting disorders (e.g., diabetes). Drug therapy includes **gemfibrozil** or **fenofibrate, niacin,** and higher-potency statins (**atorvastatin, pitavastatin, rosuvastatin,** and **simvastatin**). Successful treatment is defined as reduction in triglycerides to <500 mg/dL.

TREATMENT OF LOW HDL CHOLESTEROL

- Low HDL cholesterol is a strong independent risk predictor of CHD. ATP III redefined low HDL cholesterol as <40 mg/dL but specified no goal for HDL raising. In low HDL, the primary target remains LDL, but treatment emphasis shifts to weight reduction, increased physical activity, and smoking cessation, and to **fibrates** and **niacin** if drug therapy is required.

TREATMENT OF DIABETIC DYSLIPIDEMIA

- Diabetic dyslipidemia is characterized by hypertriglyceridemia, low HDL, and minimally elevated LDL. Small, dense LDL (pattern B) in diabetes is more atherogenic than larger, more buoyant forms of LDL (pattern A).
- ATP III considers diabetes to be a CHD risk equivalent, and the primary target is to lower the LDL to <100 mg/dL. When LDL is >130 mg/dL, most patients require simultaneous TLCs and drug therapy. When LDL is between 100 and 129 mg/dL, intensifying glycemic control, adding drugs for atherogenic dyslipidemia (**fibrates** and **niacin**), and intensifying LDL-lowering therapy are options. **Statins** are considered by many to be the drugs of choice because the primary target is LDL.

EVALUATION OF THERAPEUTIC OUTCOMES

- Short-term evaluation of therapy for dyslipidemia is based on response to diet and drug treatment as measured by total cholesterol, LDL-C, HDL-C, and triglycerides.
- Many patients treated for primary dyslipidemia have no symptoms or clinical manifestations of a genetic lipid disorder (e.g., xanthomas), and monitoring may be solely laboratory based.
- In patients treated for secondary intervention, symptoms of atherosclerotic cardiovascular disease, such as angina and intermittent claudication, may improve over months to years. Xanthomas or other external manifestations of dyslipidemia should regress with therapy.
- Lipid measurements should be obtained in the fasting state to minimize interference from chylomicrons. Monitoring is needed every few months during dosage titration. Once the patient is stable, monitoring at intervals of 6 months to 1 year is sufficient.
- Patients on BAR therapy should have a fasting panel checked every 4 to 8 weeks until a stable dose is reached; triglycerides should be checked at a stable dose to ensure they have not increased.
- Niacin requires baseline tests of liver function (alanine aminotransferase), uric acid, and glucose. Repeat tests are appropriate at doses of 1,000 to 1,500 mg/day. Symptoms of myopathy or diabetes should be investigated and may require creatine kinase or glucose determinations. Patients with diabetes may require more frequent monitoring.
- Patients receiving statins should have a fasting panel 4 to 8 weeks after the initial dose or dose changes. Liver function tests should be obtained at baseline and periodically thereafter based on package insert information. Some experts believe that monitoring for hepatotoxicity and myopathy should be triggered by symptoms.
- Patients with multiple risk factors and established CHD should also be monitored and evaluated for progress in managing their other risk factors such as BP control, smoking cessation, exercise and weight control, and glycemic control (if diabetic).
- Evaluation of dietary therapy with diet diaries and recall survey instruments allows information about diet to be collected in a systematic fashion and may improve patient adherence to dietary recommendations.

See Chapter 28, Dyslipidemia, authored by Robert L. Talbert, for a more detailed discussion of this topic.

CHAPTER 9

Heart Failure

DEFINITION

- Heart failure (HF) is a clinical syndrome caused by the inability of the heart to pump sufficient blood to meet the metabolic needs of the body. HF can result from any disorder that reduces ventricular filling (diastolic dysfunction) and/or myocardial contractility (systolic dysfunction). This chapter focuses primarily on systolic HF.

PATHOPHYSIOLOGY

- Causes of systolic dysfunction (decreased contractility) are reduction in muscle mass (e.g., myocardial infarction [MI]), dilated cardiomyopathies, and ventricular hypertrophy. Ventricular hypertrophy can be caused by pressure overload (e.g., systemic or pulmonary hypertension and aortic or pulmonic valve stenosis) or volume overload (e.g., valvular regurgitation, shunts, and high-output states).
- Causes of diastolic dysfunction (restriction in ventricular filling) are increased ventricular stiffness, ventricular hypertrophy, infiltrative myocardial diseases, myocardial ischemia and MI, mitral or tricuspid valve stenosis, and pericardial disease (e.g., pericarditis and pericardial tamponade).
- The leading causes of HF are coronary artery disease and hypertension.
- As cardiac function decreases after myocardial injury, the heart relies on the following compensatory mechanisms: (1) tachycardia and increased contractility through sympathetic nervous system activation; (2) the Frank–Starling mechanism, whereby increased preload increases stroke volume; (3) vasoconstriction; and (4) ventricular hypertrophy and remodeling. Although these compensatory mechanisms initially maintain cardiac function, they are responsible for the symptoms of HF and contribute to disease progression.
- The neurohormonal model of HF recognizes that an initiating event (e.g., acute MI) leads to decreased cardiac output but that the HF state then becomes a systemic disease whose progression is mediated largely by neurohormones and autocrine/paracrine factors. These substances include angiotensin II, norepinephrine, aldosterone, natriuretic peptides, arginine vasopressin, endothelin peptides, proinflammatory cytokines (e.g., tumor necrosis factor α and various interleukins), and endothelin-1.
- Common precipitating factors that may cause a previously compensated patient to decompensate include myocardial ischemia and MI, atrial fibrillation, pulmonary infections, nonadherence with diet or drug therapy, and inappropriate medication use. Drugs may precipitate or exacerbate HF because of their negative inotropic, cardiotoxic, or sodium- and water-retaining properties.

CLINICAL PRESENTATION

- The patient presentation may range from asymptomatic to cardiogenic shock.
- The primary symptoms are dyspnea (particularly on exertion) and fatigue, which lead to exercise intolerance. Other pulmonary symptoms include orthopnea, paroxysmal nocturnal dyspnea, tachypnea, and cough.
- Fluid overload can result in pulmonary congestion and peripheral edema.
- Nonspecific symptoms may include fatigue, nocturia, hemoptysis, abdominal pain, anorexia, nausea, bloating, ascites, poor appetite, mental status changes, and weight gain.
- Physical examination findings may include pulmonary crackles, an S_3 gallop, cool extremities, Cheyne–Stokes respiration, tachycardia, narrow pulse pressure, cardiomegaly, symptoms of pulmonary edema (extreme breathlessness and anxiety, sometimes with coughing and pink, frothy sputum), peripheral edema, jugular venous distention, hepatojugular reflux, and hepatomegaly.

DIAGNOSIS

- A diagnosis of HF should be considered in patients exhibiting characteristic signs and symptoms. A complete history and physical examination with appropriate laboratory testing are essential in the initial evaluation of patients suspected of having HF.
- Laboratory tests for identifying disorders that may cause or worsen HF include complete blood cell count; serum electrolytes (including calcium and magnesium); renal, hepatic, and thyroid function tests; urinalysis; lipid profile; and hemoglobin A1C. B-type natriuretic peptide (BNP) will generally be >100 pg/mL.
- Ventricular hypertrophy can be demonstrated on chest radiograph or electrocardiogram (ECG). Chest radiograph may also show pleural effusions or pulmonary edema.
- The echocardiogram is the single most useful evaluation procedure because it can identify abnormalities of the pericardium, myocardium, or heart values and quantify the left ventricular ejection fraction (LVEF) to determine if systolic or diastolic dysfunction is present.
- The New York Heart Association Functional Classification System is intended primarily to classify *symptomatic* HF patients according to the physician's subjective evaluation. Functional class (FC)-I patients have no limitation of physical activity, FC-II patients have slight limitation, FC-III patients have marked limitation, and FC-IV patients are unable to carry on physical activity without discomfort.
- The American College of Cardiology/American Heart Association (ACC/AHA) staging system provides a more comprehensive framework for evaluating, preventing, and treating HF (see further discussion below).

DESIRED OUTCOME

- The therapeutic goals for chronic HF are to improve quality of life, relieve or reduce symptoms, prevent or minimize hospitalizations, slow disease progression, and prolong survival.

TREATMENT OF SYSTOLOC HEART FAILURE

GENERAL APPROACH

- The first step in managing chronic HF is to determine the etiology or precipitating factors. Treatment of underlying disorders (e.g., hyperthyroidism) may obviate the need for treating HF.
- Nonpharmacologic interventions include cardiac rehabilitation and restriction of fluid intake (maximum 2 L/day from all sources) and dietary sodium (<2–3 g of sodium/day).
- **ACC/AHA stage A:** These are patients at high risk for developing heart failure. The emphasis is on identifying and modifying risk factors to prevent development of structural heart disease and subsequent HF. Strategies include smoking cessation and control of hypertension, diabetes mellitus, and dyslipidemia according to current treatment guidelines. **Angiotensin-converting enzyme (ACE) inhibitors (or angiotensin receptor blockers [ARBs])** can be useful for antihypertensive therapy in patients with multiple vascular risk factors.
- **ACC/AHA stage B:** In these patients with structural heart disease but no HF signs or symptoms, treatment is targeted at minimizing additional injury and preventing or slowing the remodeling process. In addition to treatment measures outlined for stage A, patients with a previous MI should receive both **ACE inhibitors** (or **ARBs** in patients intolerant of ACE inhibitors) and **β-blockers** regardless of the ejection fraction. Patients with reduced ejection fractions should also receive both agents, regardless of whether they have had an MI.
- **ACC/AHA stage C:** These patients have structural heart disease and previous or current HF symptoms. Most should receive the treatments for stages A and B, as well as initiation and titration of a **diuretic** (if clinical evidence of fluid retention), **ACE inhibitor**, and **β-blocker** (if not already receiving a β-blocker for previous MI, left ventricular [LV] dysfunction, or other indication). If diuresis is initiated, and symptoms improve once the patient is euvolemic, long-term monitoring can begin. If symptoms do not improve, an **aldosterone receptor antagonist, ARB** (in ACE inhibitor intolerant patients), **digoxin**, and/or **hydralazine/isosorbide dinitrate** (ISDN) may be useful with carefully screened patients. Other general measures include moderate sodium restriction, daily weight measurement, immunization against influenza and pneumococcus, modest physical activity, and avoidance of medications that can exacerbate HF.
- **ACC/AHA stage D:** These are patients with refractory HF (i.e., symptoms at rest despite maximal medical therapy). They should be considered for specialized therapies, including mechanical circulatory support,

continuous IV positive inotropic therapy, cardiac transplantation, or hospice care (when no additional treatments are appropriate).

PHARMACOLOGIC THERAPY

Drug Therapies for Routine Use in Stage C Heart Failure
(Fig. 9–1)

DIURETICS

- Compensatory mechanisms in HF stimulate excessive sodium and water retention, often leading to systemic and pulmonary congestion. Consequently, diuretic therapy (in addition to sodium restriction) is recommended for all patients with clinical evidence of fluid retention. However, because they do not alter disease progression or prolong survival, they are not considered mandatory therapy for patients without fluid retention.

- Thiazide diuretics (e.g., **hydrochlorothiazide**) are relatively weak and are used alone infrequently in HF. However, thiazides or the thiazide-like diuretic **metolazone** can be used in combination with a loop diuretic to promote very effective diuresis. Thiazides may be preferred over loop

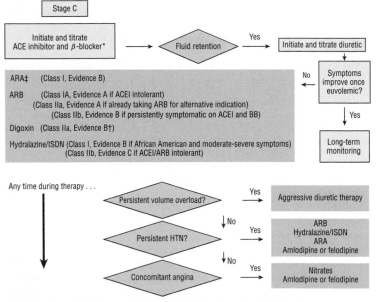

* If not already receiving this therapy for previous MI, LV dysfunction, or other indication.
‡ If moderately severe to severe symptoms.
† Indication is to reduce hospitalization.

FIGURE 9–1. Treatment algorithm for patients with ACC/AHA stage C heart failure. (ACE, angiotensin-converting enzyme; ARA, aldosterone receptor antagonist; ARB, angiotensin receptor blocker; BB, β-blocker; HTN, hypertension; ISDN, isosorbide dinitrate; LV, left ventricular; MI, myocardial infarction.)

TABLE 9-1	Loop Diuretic Use in Heart Failure		
	Furosemide	**Bumetanide**	**Torsemide**
Usual daily dose (oral)	20–160 mg/day	0.5–4 mg/day	10–80 mg/day
Ceiling dose^a			
Normal renal function	80–160 mg	1–2 mg	20–40 mg
CL_{cr} 20–50 mL/min	160 mg	2 mg	40 mg
CL_{cr} <20 mL/min	400 mg	8–10 mg	100 mg
Bioavailability	10–100% Average: 50%	80–90%	80–100%
Affected by food	Yes	Yes	No
Half-life	0.3–3.4 hours	0.3–1.5 hours	3–4 hours

CL_{cr}, creatinine clearance.
^{a}Ceiling dose: single dose above which additional response is unlikely to be observed.

diuretics in patients with only mild fluid retention and elevated blood pressure (BP) because of their more persistent antihypertensive effects.

- Loop diuretics (**furosemide, bumetanide,** and **torsemide**) are usually necessary to restore and maintain euvolemia in HF. In addition to acting in the thick ascending limb of the loop of Henle, they induce a prostaglandin-mediated increase in renal blood flow that contributes to their natriuretic effect. Unlike thiazides, loop diuretics maintain their effectiveness in the presence of impaired renal function, although higher doses may be necessary.

- Doses of loop diuretics above the recommended ceiling doses produce no additional diuresis in HF. Thus, once those doses are reached, more frequent dosing should be used for additional effect, rather than giving progressively higher doses. Ranges of doses and ceiling doses for loop diuretics in patients with varying degrees of renal function are listed in **Table 9–1.**

ANGIOTENSIN-CONVERTING ENZYME INHIBITORS

- ACE inhibitors (**Table 9–2**) decrease angiotensin II and aldosterone, attenuating many of their deleterious effects, including reducing ventricular remodeling, myocardial fibrosis, myocyte apoptosis, cardiac hypertrophy, norepinephrine release, vasoconstriction, and sodium and water retention.

- Clinical trials have produced unequivocal evidence that ACE inhibitors improve symptoms, slow disease progression, and decrease mortality in patients with HF and reduced LVEF (stage C). These patients should receive ACE inhibitors unless contraindications are present. ACE inhibitors should also be used to prevent the development of HF in at-risk patients (i.e., stages A and B).

β-BLOCKERS

- There is overwhelming clinical trial evidence that certain β-blockers slow disease progression, decrease hospitalizations, and reduce mortality in patients with HF.

TABLE 9–2	ACE Inhibitors Routinely Used for Treatment of Heart Failure				
Generic Name	Brand Name	Initial Dose	Target Dosing–Survival Benefit[a]	Prodrug	Elimination[b]
Captopril	Capoten	6.25 mg three times daily	50 mg three times daily	No	Renal
Enalapril	Vasotec	2.5–5 mg twice daily	10 mg twice daily	Yes	Renal
Lisinopril	Zestril, Prinivil	2.5–5 mg daily	20–40 mg daily[c]	No	Renal
Quinapril	Accupril	5 mg twice daily	20–40 mg twice daily[d]	Yes	Renal
Ramipril	Altace	1.25–2.5 mg twice daily	5 mg twice daily	Yes	Renal
Fosinopril	Monopril	5–10 mg daily	40 mg daily[d]	Yes	Renal/hepatic
Trandolapril	Mavik	0.5–1 mg daily	4 mg daily	Yes	Renal/hepatic
Perindopril	Aceon	2 mg daily	8–16 mg daily	Yes	Renal/hepatic

[a]Target doses associated with survival benefits in clinical trials.
[b]Primary route of elimination.
[c]Note that in the ATLAS trial (Circulation 1999;100:2312–2318), no significant difference in mortality was found between low-dose (~5 mg/day) and high-dose (~35 mg/day) lisinopril therapy.
[d]Effects on mortality have not been evaluated.

- Beneficial effects of β-blockers may result from antiarrhythmic effects, slowing or reversing ventricular remodeling, decreasing myocyte death from catecholamine-induced necrosis or apoptosis, preventing fetal gene expression, improving LV systolic function, decreasing heart rate and ventricular wall stress and thereby reducing myocardial oxygen demand, and inhibiting plasma renin release.
- The ACC/AHA guidelines recommend use of β-blockers in all stable patients with HF and a reduced LVEF in the absence of contraindications or a clear history of β-blocker intolerance. Patients should receive a β-blocker even if symptoms are mild or well controlled with ACE inhibitor and diuretic therapy. It is not essential that ACE inhibitor doses be optimized before a β-blocker is started because the addition of a β-blocker is likely to be of greater benefit than an increase in ACE inhibitor dose.
- β-Blockers are also recommended for asymptomatic patients with a reduced LVEF (stage B) to decrease the risk of progression to HF.
- β-Blockers should be initiated in stable patients who have no or minimal evidence of fluid overload. Because of their negative inotropic effects, β-blockers should be started in very low doses with slow upward dose titration to avoid symptomatic worsening or acute decompensation. Patients should be titrated to target doses when possible to provide maximal survival benefits.
- Carvedilol, metoprolol CR/XL, and bisoprolol are the only β-blockers shown to reduce mortality in large HF trials. It cannot be assumed

that immediate-release metoprolol will provide benefits equivalent to metoprolol CR/XL. Because bisoprolol is not available in the necessary starting dose of 1.25 mg, the choice is typically limited to either carvedilol or metoprolol CR/XL. On the basis of regimens proven in large clinical trials to reduce mortality, initial and target oral doses are as follows:

✓ **Carvedilol**, 3.125 mg twice daily initially; target dose 25 mg twice daily (the target dose for patients weighing >85 kg [187 lb] is 50 mg twice daily).

✓ **Carvedilol CR**, 10 mg once daily initially; target dose 80 mg once daily. This product should be considered in patients with difficulty maintaining adherence to the immediate-release carvedilol formulation.

✓ **Metoprolol succinate CR/XL**, 12.5 to 25 mg once daily initially; target dose 200 mg once daily.

✓ **Bisoprolol**, 1.25 mg once daily initially; target dose 10 mg once daily.

- Doses should be doubled no more often than every 2 weeks, as tolerated, until the target dose or the maximally tolerated dose is reached. Patients should understand that dose up-titration is a long, gradual process and that achieving the target dose is important to maximize benefits. Further, the response to therapy may be delayed, and HF symptoms may actually worsen during the initiation period.

Drug Therapies to Consider for Select Patients

ANGIOTENSIN II RECEPTOR BLOCKERS

- The angiotensin II receptor antagonists block the angiotensin II receptor subtype AT_1, preventing the deleterious effects of angiotensin II, regardless of its origin. They do not appear to affect bradykinin and are not associated with the side effect of cough that sometimes results from ACE inhibitor–induced accumulation of bradykinin. Also, direct blockade of AT_1 receptors allows unopposed stimulation of AT_2 receptors, causing vasodilation and inhibition of ventricular remodeling.
- Although some data suggest that ARBs produce equivalent mortality benefits when compared with ACE inhibitors, the ACC/AHA guidelines recommend use of ARBs only in patients with stage A, B, or C HF who are intolerant of ACE inhibitors. Although there are currently seven ARBs on the market in the United States, only candesartan and valsartan are FDA-approved for the treatment of HF and are the preferred agents, whether used alone or in combination with ACE inhibitors.
- Therapy should be initiated at low doses and then titrated to target doses:

✓ **Candesartan**, 4 to 8 mg once daily initially; target dose 32 mg once daily.

✓ **Valsartan**, 20 to 40 mg twice daily initially; target dose 160 mg twice daily.

- BP, renal function, and serum potassium should be evaluated within 1 to 2 weeks after therapy initiation and dose increases, with these endpoints used to guide subsequent dose changes. It is not necessary to reach target ARB doses before adding a β-blocker.
- Cough and angioedema are the most common causes of ACE inhibitor intolerance. Caution should be exercised when ARBs are used in patients

with angioedema from ACE inhibitors because cross-reactivity has been reported. ARBs are not alternatives in patients with hypotension, hyperkalemia, or renal insufficiency due to ACE inhibitors because they are just as likely to cause these adverse effects.

- Combination therapy with an ARB and ACE inhibitor offers a theoretical advantage over either agent alone through more complete blockade of the deleterious effects of angiotensin II. However, clinical trial results indicate that the addition of an ARB to optimal HF therapy (e.g., ACE inhibitors, β-blockers, and diuretics) offers marginal benefits at best with increased risk of adverse effects. The addition of an ARB may be considered with patients who remain symptomatic despite receiving optimal conventional therapy.

ALDOSTERONE ANTAGONISTS

- **Spironolactone** and **eplerenone** block the mineralocorticoid receptor, the target site for aldosterone. In the kidney, aldosterone antagonists inhibit sodium reabsorption and potassium excretion. However, diuretic effects are minimal, suggesting that their therapeutic benefits result from other actions. Effects in the heart attenuate cardiac fibrosis and ventricular remodeling. Recent evidence also suggests an important role in attenuating the systemic proinflammatory state and oxidative stress caused by aldosterone. Spironolactone also interacts with androgen and progesterone receptors, which may lead to gynecomastia and other sexual side effects; these effects are less frequent with eplerenone because of its low affinity for androgen and progesterone receptors.

- Based on clinical trial results demonstrating reduced mortality, low-dose aldosterone antagonists may be appropriate for (1) patients with moderately severe to severe HF who are receiving standard therapy and (2) those with LV dysfunction early after MI.

- Data from clinical practice suggest that the risks of serious hyperkalemia and worsening renal function are much higher than observed in clinical trials. This may be due in part to failure of clinicians to consider renal impairment, reduce or stop potassium supplementation, or monitor renal function and potassium closely once the aldosterone antagonist is initiated. Thus, aldosterone antagonists must be used cautiously and with careful monitoring of renal function and potassium concentration. They should be avoided in patients with renal impairment, recent worsening of renal function, high-normal potassium levels, or a history of severe hyperkalemia.

- Initial doses should be low (spironolactone 12.5 mg/day; eplerenone 25 mg/day), especially in the elderly and those with diabetes or creatinine clearance <50 mL/min. A spironolactone dose of 25 mg/day was used in one major clinical trial. The eplerenone dose should be titrated to the target dose of 50 mg once daily, preferably within 4 weeks as tolerated by the patient.

DIGOXIN

- Although digoxin has positive inotropic effects, its benefits in HF are related to its neurohormonal effects. Digoxin attenuates the excessive sympathetic nervous system activation present in HF patients, perhaps by reducing central sympathetic outflow and improving impaired baroreceptor function. It also increases parasympathetic activity in HF patients and decreases heart rate, thus enhancing diastolic filling. Digoxin does not improve survival in patients with HF but does provide symptomatic benefits.

- In patients with HF and supraventricular tachyarrhythmias such as atrial fibrillation, digoxin should be considered early in therapy to help control ventricular response rate.

- For patients in normal sinus rhythm, effects on symptom reduction and quality-of-life improvement are evident in patients with mild to severe HF. Therefore, it should be used together with standard HF therapies (ACE inhibitors, β-blockers, and diuretics) in patients with symptomatic HF to reduce hospitalizations.

- Doses should be adjusted to achieve plasma digoxin concentration of 0.5 to 1 ng/mL. Higher plasma levels are not associated with additional benefits but may increase the risk of toxicity. Most patients with normal renal function can achieve this level with a dose of 0.125 mg/day. Patients with decreased renal function, the elderly, or those receiving interacting drugs (e.g., amiodarone) should receive 0.125 mg every other day. In the absence of supraventricular tachyarrhythmias, a loading dose is not indicated because digoxin is a mild inotropic agent that produces gradual effects over several hours, even after loading. Blood samples for measuring plasma digoxin concentrations should be collected at least 6 hours, and preferably 12 hours or more, after the last dose.

NITRATES AND HYDRALAZINE

- Nitrates (e.g., **ISDN**) and **hydralazine** were combined originally in the treatment of HF because of their complementary hemodynamic actions. Nitrates are primarily venodilators, producing reductions in preload. Hydralazine is a direct vasodilator that acts predominantly on arterial smooth muscle to reduce systemic vascular resistance (SVR) and increase stroke volume and cardiac output. Evidence also suggests that the combination may provide additional benefits by interfering with the biochemical processes associated with HF progression.

- The combination of nitrates and hydralazine improves the composite endpoint of mortality, hospitalizations for HF, and quality of life in African Americans who receive standard therapy. A fixed-dose combination product is available that contains ISDN 20 mg and hydralazine 37.5 mg (BiDil). Current guidelines recommend the addition of hydralazine and nitrates to self-described African Americans with moderate to severe symptoms despite therapy with ACE inhibitors, diuretics, and β-blockers. The combination may also be reasonable for patients of other ethnicities with persistent symptoms despite optimized therapy with an ACE inhibitor (or ARB) and β-blocker. The combination is also appropriate as first-line therapy in patients unable to tolerate ACE inhibitors or ARBs because of renal insufficiency, hyperkalemia, or possibly hypotension.

- Obstacles to successful therapy with this drug combination include the need for frequent dosing (i.e., three times daily with the fixed-dose combination product), a high frequency of adverse effects (e.g., headache, dizziness, GI distress), and increased cost for the fixed-dose combination product.

TREATMENT OF ACUTE DECOMPENSATED HEART FAILURE

GENERAL APPROACH

- The term *decompensated HF* refers to patients with new or worsening signs or symptoms that are usually caused by volume overload and/or hypoperfusion and lead to the need for additional medical care, such as emergency department visits and hospitalizations.
- The goals of therapy are to relieve congestive symptoms, optimize volume status, treat symptoms of low cardiac output, and minimize the risks of drug therapy so the patient can be discharged in a compensated state on oral drug therapy.
- Hospitalization is *recommended* or *should be considered* depending on each patient's symptoms and physical findings. Admission to an intensive care unit (ICU) may be required if the patient experiences hemodynamic instability requiring frequent monitoring, invasive hemodynamic monitoring, or rapid titration of IV medications with close monitoring.
- Reversible or treatable causes of decompensation should be addressed and corrected. Medications that may aggravate HF should be evaluated carefully and discontinued when possible.
- The first step in managing decompensated HF is to ascertain that optimal treatment with oral medications has been achieved. If there is evidence of fluid retention, aggressive diuresis, often with IV diuretics, should be accomplished. Optimal treatment with an ACE inhibitor should be a priority. Although β-blockers should not be started during this period of instability, they should be continued, if possible, in patients who are already receiving them on a chronic basis. Most patients should be receiving digoxin at a low dose prescribed to achieve a trough serum concentration of 0.5 to 1 ng/mL.
- Appropriate management of decompensated HF is aided by determination of whether the patient has signs and symptoms of fluid overload ("wet" HF) or low cardiac output ("dry" HF) (**Fig. 9–2**).
- Invasive hemodynamic monitoring should be considered in patients who are refractory to initial therapy, whose volume status is unclear, or who have clinically significant hypotension such as systolic BP <80 mm Hg or worsening renal function despite therapy. Such monitoring helps guide treatment and classify patients into four specific hemodynamic subsets based on cardiac index and pulmonary artery occlusion pressure (PAOP). Refer to textbook Chap. 22 (Acute Decompensated Heart Failure) for more information.

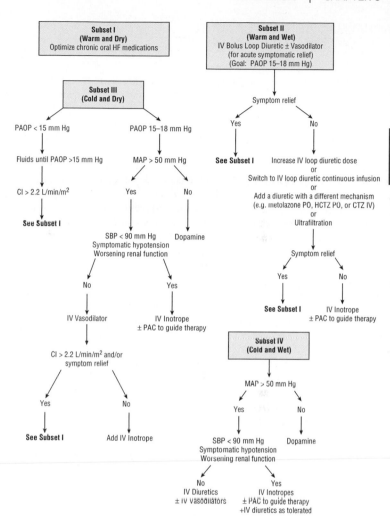

FIGURE 9–2. General treatment algorithm for acute decompensated heart failure (ADHF) based on clinical presentation. IV vasodilators that may be used include nitroglycerin, nesiritide, and nitroprusside. Metolazone or spironolactone may be added if the patient fails to respond to loop diuretics and a second diuretic is required. IV inotropes that may be used include dobutamine and milrinone. (CI, cardiac index; CTZ, chlorothiazide; D/C, discontinue; HCTZ, hydrochlorothiazide; HF, heart failure; MAP, mean arterial pressure; PAC, pulmonary artery catheter; PAOP, pulmonary artery occlusion pressure; SBP, systolic blood pressure.)

PHARMACOTHERAPY OF ACUTE DECOMPENSATED HEART FAILURE

Diuretics

- IV loop diuretics, including **furosemide, bumetanide,** and **torsemide**, are used for acute decompensated HF, with furosemide being the most widely studied and used agent.
- Bolus diuretic administration decreases preload by functional venodilation within 5 to 15 minutes and later (>20 min) via sodium and water excretion, thereby improving pulmonary congestion. However, acute reductions in venous return may severely compromise effective preload in patients with significant diastolic dysfunction or intravascular depletion.
- Because diuretics can cause excessive preload reduction, they must be used judiciously to obtain the desired improvement in congestive symptoms while avoiding a reduction in cardiac output, symptomatic hypotension, or worsening renal function.
- Diuretic resistance may be overcome by administering larger IV bolus doses or continuous IV infusions of loop diuretics. Diuresis may also be improved by adding a second diuretic with a different mechanism of action (e.g., combining a loop diuretic with a distal tubule blocker, e.g., **metolazone** or **hydrochlorothiazide**). The loop diuretic–thiazide combination should generally be reserved for inpatients who can be monitored closely for the development of severe sodium, potassium, and volume depletion. Very low doses of the thiazide-type diuretic should be used in the outpatient setting to avoid serious adverse events.

Positive Inotropic Agents

DOBUTAMINE

- **Dobutamine** is a β_1- and β_2-receptor agonist with some α_1-agonist effects. The net vascular effect is usually vasodilation. It has a potent inotropic effect without producing a significant change in heart rate. Initial doses of 2.5 to 5 mcg/kg/min can be increased progressively to 20 mcg/kg/min on the basis of clinical and hemodynamic responses.
- Dobutamine increases cardiac index because of inotropic stimulation, arterial vasodilation, and a variable increase in heart rate. It causes relatively little change in mean arterial pressure compared with the more consistent increases observed with dopamine.
- Although concern over attenuation of dobutamine's hemodynamic effects with prolonged administration has been raised, some effect is likely retained. Consequently, the dobutamine dose should be tapered rather than abruptly discontinued.

MILRINONE

- **Milrinone** is a bipyridine derivative that inhibits phosphodiesterase III and produces positive inotropic and arterial and venous vasodilating effects; hence, milrinone has been referred to as an inodilator. It has supplanted use of amrinone, which has a higher rate of thrombocytopenia.

- During IV administration, milrinone increases stroke volume (and cardiac output) with little change in heart rate. It also decreases pulmonary capillary wedge pressure (PCWP) by venodilation and thus is particularly useful in patients with a low cardiac index and an elevated LV filling pressure. However, this decrease in preload can be hazardous for patients without excessive filling pressure, leading to further decline in cardiac index.
- Milrinone should be used cautiously as a single agent in severely hypotensive HF patients because it will not increase, and may even decrease, arterial BP.
- The usual loading dose of milrinone is 50 mcg/kg over 10 minutes. If rapid hemodynamic changes are unnecessary, the loading dose should be eliminated because of the risk of hypotension. Most patients are simply started on the maintenance continuous infusion of 0.1 to 0.3 mcg/kg/min (up to 0.75 mcg/kg/min).
- The most notable adverse events are arrhythmia, hypotension, and, rarely, thrombocytopenia. Patients should have platelet counts determined before and during therapy.
- Routine use of milrinone (and perhaps other inotropes) should be discouraged because recent studies suggest a higher in-hospital mortality rate than with some other drugs. However, inotropes may be needed with certain patients, such as those with low cardiac output states with organ hypoperfusion and cardiogenic shock. It may be considered for patients receiving chronic β-blocker therapy because its positive inotropic effect does not involve stimulation of β-receptors.

DOPAMINE

- **Dopamine** should generally be avoided in decompensated HF, but its pharmacologic actions may be preferable to dobutamine or milrinone in patients with marked systemic hypotension or cardiogenic shock in the face of elevated ventricular filling pressures, where dopamine in doses >5 mcg/kg/min may be necessary to raise central aortic pressure.
- Dopamine produces dose-dependent hemodynamic effects because of its relative affinity for α_1, β_1, β_2, and D_1 (vascular dopaminergic) receptors. Positive inotropic effects mediated primarily by β_1-receptors become more prominent with doses of 2 to 5 mcg/kg/min. At doses between 5 and 10 mcg/kg/min, chronotropic and α_1-mediated vasoconstricting effects become more prominent. Dopamine, particularly at higher doses, alters several parameters that increase myocardial oxygen demand and potentially decrease myocardial blood flow, worsening ischemia in some patients with coronary disease.

Vasodilators

- Arterial vasodilators act as impedance-reducing agents, reducing afterload and causing a reflex increase in cardiac output. Venodilators act as preload reducers by increasing venous capacitance, reducing symptoms of pulmonary congestion in patients with high cardiac filling pressures. Mixed vasodilators act on both arterial resistance and venous capacitance vessels, reducing congestive symptoms while increasing cardiac output.

NITROPRUSSIDE

- **Sodium nitroprusside** is a mixed arteriovenous vasodilator that acts directly on vascular smooth muscle to increase cardiac index and decrease venous pressure. Despite its lack of direct inotropic activity, nitroprusside exerts hemodynamic effects that are qualitatively similar to those of dobutamine and milrinone. However, nitroprusside generally decreases PCWP, SVR, and BP more than those agents do.
- Hypotension is an important dose-limiting adverse effect of nitroprusside and other vasodilators. Therefore, nitroprusside is primarily used with patients who have a significantly elevated SVR and often requires invasive hemodynamic monitoring.
- Nitroprusside is effective in the short-term management of severe HF in a variety of settings (e.g., acute MI, valvular regurgitation, after coronary bypass surgery, and decompensated chronic HF). Generally, it will not worsen, and may improve, the balance between myocardial oxygen demand and supply. However, an excessive decrease in systemic arterial pressure can decrease coronary perfusion and worsen ischemia.
- Nitroprusside has a rapid onset and a duration of action <10 minutes, which necessitates use of continuous IV infusions. It should be initiated at a low dose (0.1–0.2 mcg/kg/min) to avoid excessive hypotension, then increased by small increments (0.1–0.2 mcg/kg/min) every 5 to 10 minutes as needed and tolerated. Usual effective doses range from 0.5 to 3 mcg/kg/min. Because of a rebound phenomenon after abrupt withdrawal of nitroprusside in patients with HF, doses should be tapered slowly when stopping therapy. Nitroprusside-induced cyanide and thiocyanate toxicity are unlikely when doses <3 mcg/kg/min are administered for less than 3 days, except in patients with serum creatinine levels >3 mg/dL.

NITROGLYCERIN

- The major hemodynamic effects of IV **nitroglycerin** are decreased preload and PCWP because of functional venodilation and mild arterial vasodilation. It is used primarily as a preload reducer for patients with pulmonary congestion. In higher doses, nitroglycerin displays potent coronary vasodilating properties and beneficial effects on myocardial oxygen demand and supply, making it the vasodilator of choice for patients with severe HF and ischemic heart disease.
- Nitroglycerin should be initiated at 5 to 10 mcg/min (0.1 mcg/kg/min) and increased every 5 to 10 minutes as necessary and tolerated. Maintenance doses usually range from 35 to 200 mcg/min (0.5–3 mcg/kg/min). Hypotension and an excessive decrease in PCWP are important dose-limiting side effects. Some tolerance may develop over 12 to 72 hours of continuous administration.

NESIRITIDE

- **Nesiritide** is manufactured using recombinant techniques and is identical to the endogenous BNP secreted by the ventricular myocardium in response to volume overload. Consequently, nesiritide mimics the vasodilatory and natriuretic actions of the endogenous peptide, resulting in venous and arterial vasodilation; increases in cardiac output; natriuresis and diuresis; and decreased cardiac filling pressures, sympathetic nervous system activity, and renin–angiotensin–aldosterone system activity.

- The precise role of nesiritide in the pharmacotherapy of decompensated HF remains controversial. Compared with nitroglycerin or nitroprusside, it produces little improvement in clinical outcomes and is substantially more expensive. Two meta-analyses suggested an increased risk of renal dysfunction and mortality with nesiritide; these effects were not confirmed in the prospective, randomized ASCEND-HF (Acute Study of Clinical Effectiveness of Nesiritide in Decompensated Heart Failure) trial. However, nesiritide was not associated with statistically significant reductions in dyspnea or 30-day death or rehospitalizations for HF compared with placebo in the ASCEND-HF trial.

Vasopressin Receptor Antagonists

- The vasopressin receptor antagonists currently available affect one or two arginine vasopressin (AVP; antidiuretic hormone) receptors, V_{1A} or V_2. Stimulation of V_{1A} receptors (located in vascular smooth muscle cells and myocardium) results in vasoconstriction, myocyte hypertrophy, coronary vasoconstriction, and positive inotropic effects. V_2 receptors are located in renal tubules, where they regulate water reabsorption.
  - ✓ **Tolvaptan** selectively binds to and inhibits the V_2 receptor. It is an oral agent indicated for hypervolemic and euvolemic hyponatremia in patients with syndrome of inappropriate antidiuretic hormone (SIADH), cirrhosis, and HF. Tolvaptan is typically initiated at 15 mg orally daily and then titrated to 30 or 60 mg daily as needed to resolve hyponatremia. It is a substrate of cytochrome P450-3A4 and is contraindicated with potent inhibitors of this enzyme.
  - ✓ **Conivaptan** nonselectively inhibits both the V_{1A} and V_2 receptors. It is an IV agent indicated for hypervolemic and euvolemic hyponatremia due to a variety of causes; however, it is not indicated for hyponatremia associated with HF.
- Patients receiving either agent must be monitored closely to avoid an excessively rapid rise in serum sodium that could result in hypotension or hypovolemia. The drug should be discontinued if that occurs. Therapy may be restarted at a lower dose if hyponatremia recurs or persists and/or these side effects resolve.
- Tolvaptan was well tolerated in clinical trials, with the most common side effects being dry mouth, thirst, urinary frequency, constipation, and hyperglycemia.
- In clinical trials, tolvaptan improved hyponatremia, diuresis, and signs/symptoms of congestion. However, one study failed to demonstrate improvement in global clinical status at discharge or a reduction in 2-year all-cause mortality, cardiovascular mortality, and HF rehospitalization. Thus, the role of vasopressin receptor antagonists in the long-term management of HF is unclear.

MECHANICAL CIRCULATORY SUPPORT

Intraaortic Balloon Pump

- The intraaortic balloon pump (IABP) is typically employed in patients with advanced HF who do not respond adequately to drug therapy, such as those with intractable myocardial ischemia or patients in cardiogenic shock.
- IABP support increases cardiac index, coronary artery perfusion, and myocardial oxygen supply accompanied by decreased myocardial oxygen demand.
- IV vasodilators and inotropic agents are generally used in conjunction with the IABP to maximize hemodynamic and clinical benefits.

Ventricular Assist Devices

- Ventricular assist devices are surgically implanted and assist, or in some cases replace, the pumping functions of the right and/or left ventricles.
- Ventricular assist devices can be used in the short-term (days to several weeks) for temporary stabilization of patients awaiting an intervention to correct the underlying cardiac dysfunction. They can also be used long term (several months to years) as a bridge to heart transplantation. Permanent device implantation has recently become an option for patients who are not heart transplant candidates.

SURGICAL THERAPY

- Orthotopic cardiac transplantation is the best therapeutic option for patients with chronic irreversible New York Heart Association class IV HF, with a 10-year survival of ~50% in well-screened patients.
- The shortage of donor hearts has prompted development of new surgical techniques, including ventricular aneurysm resection, mitral valve repair, and myocardial cell transplantation, which have resulted in variable degrees of symptomatic improvement.

EVALUATION OF THERAPEUTIC OUTCOMES

SYSTOLIC HEART FAILURE

- Patients should be asked about the presence and severity of symptoms and how the symptoms affect their daily activities.
- The efficacy of diuretic treatment is evaluated by the disappearance of the signs and symptoms of excess fluid retention. Physical examination should focus on body weight, extent of jugular venous distention, presence of hepatojugular reflux, and presence and severity of pulmonary congestion (rales, dyspnea on exertion, orthopnea, and paroxysmal nocturnal dyspnea) and peripheral edema.
- Other outcomes are improvement in exercise tolerance and fatigue, decreased nocturia, and a decrease in heart rate.
- BP should be monitored to ensure that symptomatic hypotension does not develop as a result of drug therapy.

- Body weight is a sensitive marker of fluid loss or retention, and patients should weigh themselves daily and report changes to their healthcare provider so that adjustments can be made in diuretic doses.
- Symptoms may worsen initially on β-blocker therapy, and it may take weeks to months before patients notice symptomatic improvement.
- Routine monitoring of serum electrolytes and renal function is mandatory in patients with HF.

ACUTE DECOMPENSATED HEART FAILURE

- Initial stabilization requires achievement of adequate arterial oxygen saturation and content. Cardiac index and BP must be sufficient to ensure adequate organ perfusion, as assessed by alert mental status, creatinine clearance sufficient to prevent metabolic azotemic complications, hepatic function adequate to maintain synthetic and excretory functions, a stable heart rate and rhythm, absence of ongoing myocardial ischemia or MI, skeletal muscle and skin blood flow sufficient to prevent ischemic injury, and normal arterial pH (7.34–7.47) with a normal serum lactate concentration. These goals are most often achieved with a cardiac index >2.2 L/min/m^2, a mean arterial BP >60 mm Hg, and PCWP ≥15 mm Hg.
- Daily monitoring should include weight, strict fluid intake and output measurements, and HF signs/symptoms to assess the efficacy of drug therapy. Monitoring for electrolyte depletion, symptomatic hypotension, and renal dysfunction should be assessed frequently. Vital signs should be assessed frequently throughout the day.
- Discharge from the ICU requires maintenance of the preceding parameters in the absence of ongoing IV infusion therapy, mechanical circulatory support, or positive-pressure ventilation.

See Chapter 20, Systolic Heart Failure, authored by Robert B. Parker and Larisa H. Cavallari, and Chap. 22, Acute Decompensated Heart Failure, authored by Jo E. Rodgers and Craig R. Lee, for a more detailed discussion of this topic.

Hypertension

CHAPTER 10

DEFINITION

- Hypertension is defined as persistently elevated arterial blood pressure (BP). The seventh report of the Joint National Committee on Prevention, Detection, Evaluation, and Treatment of High Blood Pressure (JNC7) classifies adult BP as shown in **Table 10–1**.
- Patients with diastolic blood pressure (DBP) values <90 mm Hg and systolic blood pressure (SBP) values ≥140 mm Hg have isolated systolic hypertension.
- A hypertensive crisis (BP >180/120 mm Hg) may be categorized as either a hypertensive emergency (extreme BP elevation with acute or progressing target-organ damage) or a hypertensive urgency (high BP elevation without acute or progressing target-organ injury).

PATHOPHYSIOLOGY

- Hypertension is a heterogeneous disorder that may result either from a specific cause (secondary hypertension) or from an underlying pathophysiologic mechanism of unknown etiology (primary or essential hypertension). Secondary hypertension accounts for <10% of cases, and most of these are caused by chronic kidney disease or renovascular disease. Other conditions causing secondary hypertension are Cushing's syndrome, coarctation of the aorta, obstructive sleep apnea, hyperparathyroidism, pheochromocytoma, primary aldosteronism, and hyperthyroidism. Drugs that may increase BP include corticosteroids, estrogens, nonsteroidal antiinflammatory drugs (NSAIDs), amphetamines, sibutramine, cyclosporine, tacrolimus, erythropoietin, and venlafaxine.
- Multiple factors may contribute to the development of primary hypertension, including:
  - ✓ Humoral abnormalities involving the renin–angiotensin–aldosterone system, natriuretic hormone, or insulin resistance and hyperinsulinemia;
  - ✓ A pathologic disturbance in the CNS, autonomic nerve fibers, adrenergic receptors, or baroreceptors;
  - ✓ Abnormalities in either the renal or tissue autoregulatory processes for sodium excretion, plasma volume, and arteriolar constriction;
  - ✓ A deficiency in the local synthesis of vasodilating substances in the vascular endothelium (prostacyclin, bradykinin, and nitric oxide) or excess vasoconstricting substances (angiotensin II andendothelin I);
  - ✓ High sodium intake or lack of dietary calcium.
- The main causes of death in hypertensive subjects are cerebrovascular accidents, cardiovascular (CV) events, and renal failure. The probability of premature death correlates with the severity of BP elevation.

TABLE 10-1	Classification of Blood Pressure in Adults		
Classification	**Systolic (mm Hg)**		**Diastolic (mm Hg)**
Normal	<120	and	<80
Prehypertension	120–139	or	80–89
Stage 1 hypertension	140–159	or	90–99
Stage 2 hypertension	≥160	or	≥100

CLINICAL PRESENTATION

- Patients with uncomplicated primary hypertension are usually asymptomatic initially.
- Patients with secondary hypertension may have symptoms suggestive of the underlying disorder. Patients with pheochromocytoma may have a history of paroxysmal headaches, sweating, tachycardia, palpitations, and orthostatic hypotension. In primary aldosteronism, hypokalemic symptoms of muscle cramps and weakness may be present. Patients with hypertension secondary to Cushing's syndrome may complain of weight gain, polyuria, edema, menstrual irregularities, recurrent acne, or muscular weakness in addition to classic features (moon face, buffalo hump, and hirsutism).

DIAGNOSIS

- Frequently, the only sign of primary hypertension on physical examination is elevated BP. The diagnosis of hypertension should be based on the average of two or more readings taken at each of two or more clinical encounters.
- As hypertension progresses, signs of end-organ damage begin to appear, chiefly related to pathologic changes in the eye, brain, heart, kidneys, and peripheral blood vessels.
- The funduscopic examination may reveal arteriolar narrowing, focal arteriolar constrictions, arteriovenous nicking, retinal hemorrhages and exudates, and disk edema. The presence of papilledema usually indicates a hypertensive emergency requiring rapid treatment.
- Cardiopulmonary examination may reveal an abnormal heart rate or rhythm, left ventricular (LV) hypertrophy, coronary heart disease, and heart failure (HF).
- Peripheral vascular examination can detect evidence of atherosclerosis, which may present as aortic or abdominal bruits, distended veins, diminished or absent peripheral pulses, or lower extremity edema.
- Patients with renal artery stenosis may have an abdominal systolic-diastolic bruit.
- Baseline hypokalemia may suggest mineralocorticoid-induced hypertension. The presence of protein, blood cells, and casts in the urine may indicate renovascular disease.
- Laboratory tests that should be obtained include blood urea nitrogen (BUN)/serum creatinine, fasting lipid panel, fasting blood glucose, serum

electrolytes (sodium and potassium), spot urine albumin-to-creatinine ratio, and estimated glomerular filtration rate (GFR, using the Modification of Diet in Renal Disease [MDRD] equation). A 12-lead electrocardiogram (ECG) should also be obtained.

- Laboratory tests used to diagnose secondary hypertension include plasma norepinephrine and urinary metanephrine levels for pheochromocytoma, plasma and urinary aldosterone concentrations for primary aldosteronism, plasma renin activity, captopril stimulation test, renal vein renin, and renal artery angiography for renovascular disease.

DESIRED OUTCOME

- The overall goal of treating hypertension is to reduce morbidity and mortality by the least intrusive means possible.
- Goal BP values are <140/90 for most patients, but <130/80 for patients with diabetes mellitus, significant chronic kidney disease, known coronary artery disease (myocardial infarction [MI] or angina), noncoronary atherosclerotic vascular disease (ischemic stroke, transient ischemic attack [TIA], peripheral arterial disease [PAD], abdominal aortic aneurysm), or ≥10% Framingham 10-year risk of fatal coronary heart disease or nonfatal MI. Patients with LV dysfunction have a BP goal of <120/80 mm Hg.

TREATMENT

NONPHARMACOLOGIC THERAPY

- All patients with prehypertension and hypertension should be prescribed lifestyle modifications, including (1) weight loss if overweight, (2) adoption of the Dietary Approaches to Stop Hypertension (DASH) eating plan, (3) dietary sodium restriction ideally to 1.5 g/day (3.8 g/day sodium chloride), (4) regular aerobic physical activity, (5) moderate alcohol consumption (two or fewer drinks per day), and (6) smoking cessation.
- Lifestyle modification alone is appropriate therapy for most patients with prehypertension. Lifestyle modification alone is insufficient for patients with hypertension and additional CV risk factors or hypertension-associated target-organ damage.

PHARMACOLOGIC THERAPY

- Initial drug selection depends on the degree of BP elevation and the presence of compelling indications for selected drugs.
- Primary antihypertensive agents that are acceptable as first-line options include **thiazide-type diuretics, angiotensin-converting enzyme (ACE) inhibitors, angiotensin II receptor blockers (ARBs),** and **calcium channel blockers (CCBs)** (**Table 10–2**).
- *β*-**Blockers** are preferred to either treat a specific compelling indication or as combination therapy with a primary antihypertensive agent for patients without a compelling indication.

TABLE 10–2 Primary Antihypertensive Agents

Class/Subclass/Drug (brand name)	Usual Dose Range (mg/day)	Daily Frequency
Diuretics		
Thiazides		
Chlorthalidone (Hygroton)	6.25–25	1
Hydrochlorothiazide (Microzide)	12.5–25	1
Indapamide (Lozol)	1.25–2.5	1
Metolazone (Zaroxolyn)	2.5–10	1
Loops		
Bumetanide (Bumex)	0.5–4	2
Furosemide (Lasix)	20–80	2
Torsemide (Demadex)	5–10	1
Potassium sparing		
Amiloride (Midamor)	5–10	1 or 2
Amiloride/hydrochlorothiazide (Moduretic)	5–10/50–100	1
Triamterene (Dyrenium)	50–100	1 or 2
Triamterene/hydrochlorothiazide (Dyazide)	37.5–75/25–50	1
Aldosterone antagonists		
Eplerenone (Inspra)	50–100	1 or 2
Spironolactone (Aldactone)	25–50	1 or 2
Spironolactone/hydrochlorothiazide (Aldactazide)	25–50/25–50	1
Angiotensin-converting enzyme inhibitors		
Benazepril (Lotensin)	10–40	1 or 2
Captopril (Capoten)	12.5–150	2 or 3
Enalapril (Vasotec)	5–40	1 or 2
Fosinopril (Monopril)	10–40	1
Lisinopril (Prinivil, Zestril)	10–40	1
Moexipril (Univasc)	7.5–30	1 or 2
Perindopril (Aceon)	4–16	1
Quinapril (Accupril)	10–80	1 or 2
Ramipril (Altace)	2.5–10	1 or 2
Trandolapril (Mavik)	1–4	1
Angiotensin II receptor blockers		
Candesartan (Atacand)	8–32	1 or 2
Eprosartan (Teveten)	600–800	1 or 2
Irbesartan (Avapro)	150–300	1
Losartan (Cozaar)	50–100	1 or 2
Olmesartan (Benicar)	20–40	1
Telmisartan (Micardis)	20–80	1
Valsartan (Diovan)	80–320	1
Calcium channel blockers		
Dihydropyridines		
Amlodipine (Norvasc)	2.5–10	1
Felodipine (Plendil)	5–20	1
Isradipine (DynaCirc)	5–10	2
Isradipine SR (DynaCirc SR)	5–20	1
Nicardipine sustained-release (Cardene SR)	60–120	2

(continued)

TABLE 10–2 Primary Antihypertensive Agents *(Continued)*

Class/Subclass/Drug (brand name)	Usual Dose Range (mg/day)	Daily Frequency
Calcium channel blockers *(cont'd)*		
Nifedipine long-acting (Adalat CC, Procardia XL)	30–90	1
Nisoldipine (Sular)	10–40	1
Nondihydropyridines		
Diltiazem sustained-release (Cardizem SR)	180–360	2
Diltiazem sustained-release (Cardizem CD, Cartia XT, Dilacor XR, Diltia XT, Tiazac, Taztia XT)	120–480	1
Diltiazem extended-release (Cardizem LA)	120–540	1 (morning or evening)
Verapamil sustained-release (Calan SR, Isoptin SR, Verelan)	180–480	1 or 2
Verapamil controlled-onset extended-release (Covera HS)	180–420	1 (in the evening)
Verapamil oral drug absorption system (Verelan PM)	100–400	1 (in the evening)
β-Blockers		
Cardioselective		
Atenolol (Tenormin)	25–100	1
Betaxolol (Kerlone)	5–20	1
Bisoprolol (Zebeta)	2.5–10	1
Metoprolol tartrate (Lopressor)	100–400	2
Metoprolol succinate extended-release (Toprol XL)	50–200	1
Nonselective		
Nadolol (Corgard)	40–120	1
Propranolol (Inderal)	160–480	2
Propranolol long-acting (Inderal LA, InnoPran XL)	80–320	1
Timolol (Blocadren)	10–40	1
Intrinsic sympathomimetic activity		
Acebutolol (Sectral)	200–800	2
Carteolol (Cartrol)	2.5–10	1
Penbutolol (Levatol)	10–40	1
Pindolol (Visken)	10–60	2
Mixed α- and β-blockers		
Carvedilol (Coreg)	12.5–50	2
Carvedilol phosphate (Coreg CR)	20–80	1
Labetalol (Normodyne, Trandate)	200–800	2
Cardioselective and vasodilatory		
Nebivolol (Bystolic)	5–20	1

- Most patients with stage 1 hypertension should be treated initially with a first-line antihypertensive drug or the combination of two agents (**Fig. 10–1**). Combination therapy is recommended for patients with stage 2 hypertension, preferably with two first-line agents.
- There are six compelling indications where specific antihypertensive drug classes have shown evidence of unique benefits (**Fig. 10–2**).

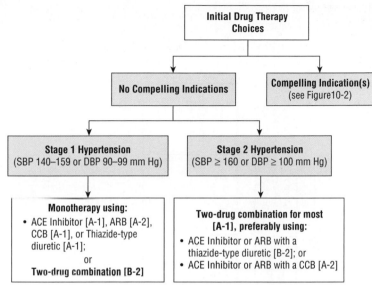

FIGURE 10–1. Algorithm for treatment of hypertension. Drug therapy recommendations are graded with strength of recommendation and quality of evidence in brackets. Strength of recommendations: A, B, C are good, moderate, and poor evidence to support recommendation, respectively. Quality of evidence: (1) evidence from more than one properly randomized, controlled trial; (2) evidence from at least one well-designed clinical trial with randomization, from cohort or case-controlled studies, or dramatic results from uncontrolled experiments or subgroup analyses; (3) evidence from opinions of respected authorities, based on clinical experience, descriptive studies, or reports of expert communities. (ACE, angiotensin-converting enzyme; ARB, angiotensin receptor blocker; CCB, calcium channel blocker; DBP, diastolic blood pressure; SBP, systolic blood pressure.)

- Other antihypertensive drug classes (α_1-blockers, direct renin inhibitors, central α_2-agonists, peripheral adrenergic antagonists, and direct arterial vasodilators) are alternatives that may be used in select patients after first-line agents (Table 10–3).

Diuretics

- **Thiazide-type diuretics** reduce the risk of CV morbidity and mortality and are a preferred drug class according to the 2003 JNC7 guidelines. However, the 2007 American Heart Association (AHA) guidelines do not identify thiazide diuretics as preferred over an ACE inhibitor, ARB, or CCB for first-line therapy in patients without compelling indications. Most evidence continues to support the JNC7 recommendations of using a thiazide-type diuretic as a first-line antihypertensive unless there are contraindications or a compelling indication for another agent.
- **Loop diuretics** are more potent for inducing diuresis but are not ideal antihypertensive agents unless relief of edema is also needed. Loops are

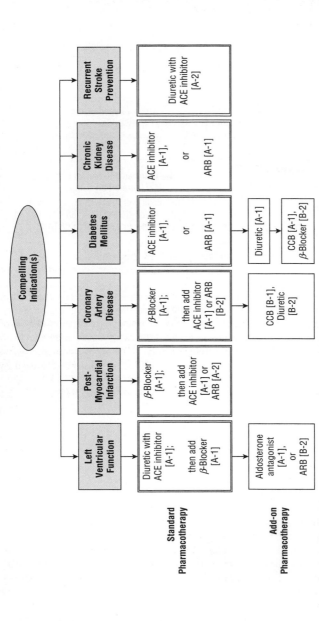

FIGURE 10–2. Compelling indications for individual drug classes. Compelling indications for specific drugs are evidence-based recommendations from outcome studies or existing clinical guidelines. (ACE, angiotensin-converting enzyme; ARB, angiotensin receptor blocker; CCB, calcium channel blocker.)

TABLE 10-3	Alternative Antihypertensive Agents	
Class Drug (Brand Name)	**Usual Dose Range (mg/day)**	**Daily Frequency**
α_1-Blockers		
Doxazosin (Cardura)	1–8	1
Prazosin (Minipress)	2–20	2 or 3
Terazosin (Hytrin)	1–20	1 or 2
Direct renin inhibitor		
Aliskiren (Tekturna)	150–300	1
Central α_2-agonists		
Clonidine (Catapres)	0.1–0.8	2
Clonidine patch (Catapres-TTS)	0.1–0.3	1 weekly
Methyldopa (Aldomet)	250–1,000	2
Peripheral adrenergic antagonist		
Reserpine (generic only)	0.05–0.25	1
Direct arterial vasodilators		
Minoxidil (Loniten)	10–40	1 or 2
Hydralazine (Apresoline)	20–100	2 to 4

often preferred over thiazide-type diuretics in patients with chronic kidney disease when estimated GFR is <30 mL/min/1.73m².

- **Potassium-sparing diuretics** are weak antihypertensives when used alone but provide an additive hypotensive effect when combined with thiazide or loop diuretics. Moreover, they counteract the potassium- and magnesium-losing properties and perhaps glucose intolerance caused by other diuretics.
- **Aldosterone antagonists (spironolactone** and **eplerenone)** are also potassium-sparing diuretics but are more potent antihypertensives with a slow onset of action (up to 6 weeks with spironolactone).
- Acutely, diuretics lower BP by causing diuresis. The reduction in plasma volume and stroke volume associated with diuresis decreases cardiac output and BP. The initial drop in cardiac output causes a compensatory increase in peripheral vascular resistance. With chronic diuretic therapy, the extracellular fluid volume and plasma volume return almost to pretreatment levels, and peripheral vascular resistance falls below its pretreatment baseline. The reduction in peripheral vascular resistance is responsible for the long-term hypotensive effects. Thiazides lower BP by mobilizing sodium and water from arteriolar walls, which may contribute to decreased peripheral vascular resistance.
- When diuretics are combined with other antihypertensive agents, an additive hypotensive effect is usually observed because of independent mechanisms of action. Furthermore, many nondiuretic antihypertensive agents induce sodium and water retention, which is counteracted by concurrent diuretic use.
- Side effects of thiazides include hypokalemia, hypomagnesemia, hypercalcemia, hyperuricemia, hyperglycemia, dyslipidemia, and sexual dysfunction.

Loop diuretics have less effect on serum lipids and glucose, but hypokalemia is more pronounced, and hypocalcemia may occur.

- Hypokalemia and hypomagnesemia may cause muscle fatigue or cramps. Serious cardiac arrhythmias may occur, especially in patients receiving digitalis therapy, patients with LV hypertrophy, and those with ischemic heart disease. Low-dose therapy (e.g., 25 mg **hydrochlorothiazide** or 12.5 mg **chlorthalidone** daily) causes small electrolyte disturbances.

- Potassium-sparing diuretics may cause hyperkalemia, especially in patients with chronic kidney disease or diabetes and in patients receiving concurrent treatment with an ACE inhibitor, ARB, direct renin inhibitor, or potassium supplement. **Eplerenone** has an increased risk for hyperkalemia and is contraindicated in patients with impaired renal function or type 2 diabetes with proteinuria. **Spironolactone** may cause gynecomastia in up to 10% of patients, but this effect occurs rarely with eplerenone.

Angiotensin-converting Enzyme Inhibitors

- ACE inhibitors are a first-line antihypertensive option, and many clinicians feel that if they are not the first agent used in most patients, they should be the second agent tried.

- ACE facilitates production of angiotensin II, which has a major role in regulating arterial BP. ACE is distributed in many tissues and is present in several different cell types, but its principal location is in endothelial cells. Therefore, the major site for angiotensin II production is in the blood vessels, not the kidney. ACE inhibitors block the conversion of angiotensin I to angiotensin II, a potent vasoconstrictor and stimulator of aldosterone secretion. ACE inhibitors also block the degradation of bradykinin and stimulate the synthesis of other vasodilating substances, including prostaglandin E_2 and prostacyclin. The fact that ACE inhibitors lower BP in patients with normal plasma renin activity suggests that bradykinin and perhaps tissue production of ACE are important in hypertension.

- Starting doses of ACE inhibitors should be low with slow dose titration. Acute hypotension may occur at the onset of ACE inhibitor therapy, especially in patients who are sodium- or volume-depleted, in HF exacerbation, very elderly, or on concurrent vasodilators or diuretics. Patients with these risk factors should start with half the normal dose followed by slow dose titration.

- Most ACE inhibitors can be dosed once daily for hypertension. In some patients, especially when higher doses are used, twice-daily dosing is needed to maintain 24-hour effects with enalapril, benazepril, moexipril, quinapril, and ramipril.

- ACE inhibitors decrease aldosterone and can increase serum potassium concentrations. Hyperkalemia occurs primarily in patients with chronic kidney disease or those also taking potassium supplements, potassium-sparing diuretics, ARBs, or a direct renin inhibitor.

- Acute renal failure is a rare but serious side effect of ACE inhibitors; preexisting kidney disease increases the risk. Bilateral renal artery stenosis or unilateral stenosis of a solitary functioning kidney renders patients dependent on the vasoconstrictive effect of angiotensin II on efferent arterioles, making these patients particularly susceptible to acute renal failure.

- The GFR decreases in patients receiving ACE inhibitors because of inhibition of angiotensin II vasoconstriction on efferent arterioles. Serum creatinine concentrations often increase, but modest elevations (e.g., absolute increases <1 mg/dL) do not warrant changes. Therapy should be stopped or the dose reduced if larger increases occur.
- Angioedema is a serious potential complication that occurs in <1% of patients. It may be manifested as lip and tongue swelling and possibly difficulty breathing. Drug withdrawal is necessary for all patients with angioedema, and some patients may also require drug treatment and/or emergent intubation. Cross-reactivity between ACE inhibitors and ARBs does not appear to be a serious concern, and an ARB can be used if needed in patients with a history of ACE inhibitor–induced angioedema, with careful monitoring.
- A persistent dry cough occurs in up to 20% of patients and is thought to be due to inhibition of bradykinin breakdown.
- ACE inhibitors are absolutely contraindicated in pregnancy because of possible major congenital malformations associated with exposure in the first trimester and serious neonatal problems, including renal failure and death in the infant, from exposure during the second and third trimesters.

Angiotensin II Receptor Blockers

- Angiotensin II is generated by the renin–angiotensin pathway (which involves ACE) and an alternative pathway that uses other enzymes such as chymases. ACE inhibitors block only the renin–angiotensin pathway, whereas ARBs antagonize angiotensin II generated by either pathway. The ARBs directly block the angiotensin type 1 receptor that mediates the known effects of angiotensin II (vasoconstriction, aldosterone release, sympathetic activation, antidiuretic hormone release, and constriction of the efferent arterioles of the glomerulus).
- Unlike ACE inhibitors, ARBs do not block the breakdown of bradykinin. Although this accounts for the lack of cough as a side effect, there may be negative consequences because some of the antihypertensive effect of ACE inhibitors may be due to increased levels of bradykinin. Bradykinin may also be important for regression of myocyte hypertrophy and fibrosis, as well as increased levels of tissue plasminogen activator.
- All ARBs have similar antihypertensive efficacy and fairly flat dose-response curves. The addition of low doses of a thiazide diuretic or a CCB significantly increases antihypertensive efficacy.
- ARBs have the lowest incidence of side effects compared with other antihypertensive agents. Because they do not affect bradykinin, they do not cause a dry cough like ACE inhibitors. Like ACE inhibitors, they may cause renal insufficiency, hyperkalemia, and orthostatic hypotension. Patients with a history of ACE inhibitor angioedema can be treated cautiously with an ARB, if needed. ARBs should not be used in pregnancy.

Calcium Channel Blockers

- CCBs cause relaxation of cardiac and smooth muscle by blocking voltage-sensitive calcium channels, thereby reducing the entry of extracellular calcium into cells. Vascular smooth muscle relaxation leads to vasodilation and a corresponding reduction in BP. Dihydropyridine calcium channel antagonists may cause reflex sympathetic activation, and all agents (except amlodipine and felodipine) may demonstrate negative inotropic effects.

- **Verapamil** decreases heart rate, slows atrioventricular (AV) nodal conduction, and produces a negative inotropic effect that may precipitate HF in patients with borderline cardiac reserve. **Diltiazem** decreases AV conduction and heart rate to a lesser extent than verapamil.
- Diltiazem and verapamil can cause cardiac conduction abnormalities such as bradycardia, AV block, and HF. Both can cause anorexia, nausea, peripheral edema, and hypotension. Verapamil causes constipation in ~7% of patients.
- Dihydropyridines cause a baroreceptor-mediated reflex increase in heart rate because of their potent peripheral vasodilating effects. Dihydropyridines do not decrease AV node conduction and are not effective for treating supraventricular tachyarrhythmias.
- Short-acting nifedipine may rarely cause an increase in the frequency, intensity, and duration of angina in association with acute hypotension. This effect may be obviated by using sustained-release formulations of nifedipine or other dihydropyridines. Other side effects of dihydropyridines are dizziness, flushing, headache, gingival hyperplasia, and peripheral edema. Side effects due to vasodilation such as dizziness, flushing, headache, and peripheral edema occur more frequently with dihydropyridines than with verapamil or diltiazem.

β-Blockers

- The exact hypotensive mechanism of β-blockers is not known but may involve decreased cardiac output through negative chronotropic and inotropic effects on the heart and inhibition of renin release from the kidney.
- Even though there are important pharmacodynamic and pharmacokinetic differences among the various β-blockers, there is no difference in clinical antihypertensive efficacy.
- **Atenolol, betaxolol, bisoprolol,** and **metoprolol** are cardioselective at low doses and bind more avidly to β_1-receptors than to β_2-receptors. As a result, they are less likely to provoke bronchospasm and vasoconstriction and may be safer than nonselective β-blockers in patients with asthma, chronic obstructive pulmonary disease (COPD), diabetes, and PAD. Cardioselectivity is a dose-dependent phenomenon, and the effect is lost at higher doses.
- **Acebutolol, carteolol, penbutolol,** and **pindolol** possess intrinsic sympathomimetic activity (ISA) or partial β-receptor agonist activity. When sympathetic tone is low, as in resting states, β-receptors are partially stimulated, so resting heart rate, cardiac output, and peripheral blood flow are not reduced when receptors are blocked. Theoretically, these drugs may have advantages in patients with HF or sinus bradycardia. Unfortunately, they do not reduce CV events as well as other β-blockers and may increase risk after MI or in those with high coronary disease risk. Thus, agents with ISA are rarely needed.
- There are pharmacokinetic differences among β-blockers in first-pass metabolism, serum half-lives, degree of lipophilicity, and route of

elimination. **Propranolol** and **metoprolol** undergo extensive first-pass metabolism. **Atenolol** and **nadolol** have relatively long half-lives and are excreted renally; the dosage may need to be reduced in patients with moderate to severe renal insufficiency. Even though the half-lives of the other β-blockers are much shorter, once-daily administration still may be effective. β-Blockers vary in their lipophilic properties and thus CNS penetration.

- Side effects from β-blockade in the myocardium include bradycardia, AV conduction abnormalities, and acute HF. Blocking β_2-receptors in arteriolar smooth muscle may cause cold extremities and aggravate PAD or Raynaud phenomenon because of decreased peripheral blood flow.

- Abrupt cessation of β-blocker therapy may produce unstable angina, MI, or even death in patients with coronary disease. In patients without heart disease, abrupt discontinuation of β-blockers may be associated with tachycardia, sweating, and generalized malaise in addition to increased BP. For these reasons, it is always prudent to taper the dose gradually over 1 to 2 weeks before discontinuation.

- Increases in serum lipids and glucose appear to be transient and of little clinical importance.

α_1-Receptor Blockers

- **Prazosin, terazosin,** and **doxazosin** are selective α_1-receptor blockers that inhibit catecholamine uptake in smooth muscle cells of the peripheral vasculature, resulting in vasodilation.

- A potentially severe side effect is a first-dose phenomenon characterized by orthostatic hypotension accompanied by transient dizziness or faintness, palpitations, and even syncope within 1 to 3 hours of the first dose or after later dosage increases. These episodes can be obviated by having the patient take the first dose, and subsequent first increased doses, at bedtime. Occasionally, orthostatic dizziness persists with chronic administration.

- Sodium and water retention can occur with chronic administration. These agents are most effective when given with a diuretic to maintain antihypertensive efficacy and minimize potential edema.

- Because data suggest that doxazosin (and probably other α_1-receptor blockers) are not as protective against CV events as other therapies, they should be reserved as alternative agents for unique situations, such as men with benign prostatic hyperplasia. If used to lower BP in this situation, they should only be used in combination with first-line antihypertensives.

Direct Renin Inhibitor

- **Aliskiren** blocks the renin–angiotensin–aldosterone system at its point of activation, which results in reduced plasma renin activity and BP. It provides BP reductions comparable to an ACE inhibitor, ARB, or CCB. It also has additive antihypertensive effects when used in combination with thiazides, ACE inhibitors, ARBs, or CCBs. It is approved for monotherapy or in combination with other agents.

- Many of the cautions and adverse effects seen with ACE inhibitors and ARBs apply to aliskiren. It is contraindicated in pregnancy.

- At this time, aliskiren should be used only as an alternative therapy because of the lack of long-term studies evaluating CV event reduction and its significant cost compared with generic agents with outcomes data.

Central α_2-Agonists

- **Clonidine, guanabenz, guanfacine,** and **methyldopa** lower BP primarily by stimulating α_2-adrenergic receptors in the brain, which reduces sympathetic outflow from the vasomotor center and increases vagal tone. Stimulation of presynaptic α_2-receptors peripherally may contribute to the reduction in sympathetic tone. Consequently, there may be decreases in heart rate, cardiac output, total peripheral resistance, plasma renin activity, and baroreceptor reflexes.
- Chronic use results in sodium and fluid retention. Other side effects may include depression, orthostatic hypotension, dizziness, and anticholinergic effects.
- Abrupt cessation may lead to rebound hypertension, which is thought to result from a compensatory increase in norepinephrine release that follows discontinuation of presynaptic α-receptor stimulation.
- Methyldopa rarely may cause hepatitis or hemolytic anemia. A transient elevation in hepatic transaminases occasionally occurs and is clinically unimportant. However, the drug should be quickly discontinued if persistent increases in serum hepatic transaminases or alkaline phosphatase are detected, as this may herald the onset of a fulminant, life-threatening hepatitis. A Coombs-positive hemolytic anemia occurs in <1% of patients receiving methyldopa, although 20% exhibit a positive direct Coombs test without anemia. For these reasons, methyldopa has limited usefulness in the management of hypertension except in pregnancy.

Reserpine

- **Reserpine** depletes norepinephrine from sympathetic nerve endings and blocks the transport of norepinephrine into its storage granules. When the nerve is stimulated, less than the usual amount of norepinephrine is released into the synapse. This reduces sympathetic tone, decreasing peripheral vascular resistance and BP.
- Reserpine has a long half-life that allows for once-daily dosing, but it may take 2 to 6 weeks before the maximal antihypertensive effect is seen.
- Reserpine can cause significant sodium and fluid retention, and it should be given with a diuretic (preferably a thiazide).
- Reserpine's strong inhibition of sympathetic activity results in parasympathetic activity, which is responsible for side effects of nasal stuffiness, increased gastric acid secretion, diarrhea, and bradycardia.
- A dose-related depression has been reported; this can be minimized by not exceeding 0.25 mg daily.

Direct Arterial Vasodilators

- **Hydralazine** and **minoxidil** cause direct arteriolar smooth muscle relaxation. Compensatory activation of baroreceptor reflexes results in increased sympathetic outflow from the vasomotor center, producing an increase in heart rate, cardiac output, and renin release. Consequently, the hypotensive effectiveness of direct vasodilators diminishes over time unless the patient is also taking a sympathetic inhibitor and a diuretic.

- All patients taking these drugs for long-term hypertension therapy should first receive both a diuretic and a β-blocker. The diuretic minimizes the side effect of sodium and water retention. Direct vasodilators can precipitate angina in patients with underlying coronary artery disease unless the baroreceptor reflex mechanism is completely blocked with a β-blocker. Nondihydropyridine CCBs can be used as an alternative to β-blockers in patients with contraindications to β-blockers.
- Hydralazine may cause a dose-related, reversible lupus-like syndrome, which is more common in slow acetylators. Lupus-like reactions can usually be avoided by using total daily doses <200 mg. Because of side effects, hydralazine has limited usefulness for chronic hypertension management. However, it may be useful in patients with severe chronic kidney disease and in kidney failure with hemodialysis.
- Minoxidil is a more potent vasodilator than hydralazine, and the compensatory increases in heart rate, cardiac output, renin release, and sodium retention are more dramatic. Severe sodium and water retention may precipitate congestive HF. Minoxidil also causes reversible hypertrichosis on the face, arms, back, and chest. Minoxidil is reserved for very difficult to control hypertension and in patients requiring hydralazine who experience drug-induced lupus.

COMPELLING INDICATIONS

- The six compelling indications identified by JNC7 represent specific comorbid conditions for which clinical trial data support using specific antihypertensive drug classes to treat both hypertension and the compelling indication (see **Fig. 10–2**).

Left Ventricular Dysfunction (Systolic Heart Failure)

- Standard therapy for LV dysfunction consists of an ACE inhibitor with diuretic therapy, followed by the addition of an appropriate β-blocker. ACE inhibitors have numerous outcome data showing reduced CV morbidity and mortality. Diuretics provide symptomatic relief of edema by inducing diuresis. Loop diuretics are often needed, especially in patients with more advanced disease.
- Because of the high renin status of patients with HF, ACE inhibitors should be initiated at low doses to avoid orthostatic hypotension.
- β-Blocker therapy is appropriate to further modify disease in LV dysfunction and is a component of standard therapy for these patients. Because of the risk of exacerbating HF, they must be started in very low doses and titrated slowly to high doses based on tolerability. Bisoprolol, carvedilol, and sustained-release metoprolol succinate are the only β-blockers proven to be beneficial in LV dysfunction.
- ARBs are acceptable as alternative therapy for patients who cannot tolerate ACE inhibitors and possibly as add-on therapy for those already receiving a standard three-drug regimen.

- An aldosterone antagonist may be considered in addition to a diuretic, ACE inhibitor or ARB, and β-blocker. Regimens employing both an aldosterone antagonist and ARB are not recommended because of the potential risk of severe hyperkalemia.

Postmyocardial Infarction

- β-Blockers (without ISA) and ACE inhibitor therapy are recommended. β-Blockers decrease cardiac adrenergic stimulation and reduce the risk of a subsequent MI or sudden cardiac death. ACE inhibitors improve cardiac function and reduce CV events after MI. ARBs are alternatives to ACE inhibitors in postmyocardial patients with LV dysfunction.
- The aldosterone antagonist eplerenone reduces CV morbidity and mortality in patients soon after an acute MI (within 3–14 days) in patients with symptoms of acute LV dysfunction. Its use should be limited to select patients, and then with diligent monitoring of serum potassium.

Coronary Artery Disease

- β-Blockers (without ISA) are first-line therapy in chronic stable angina and have the ability to reduce BP, improve myocardial consumption, and decrease demand. Long-acting CCBs are either alternatives (the nondihydropyridines verapamil and diltiazem) or add-on therapy (dihydropyridines) to β-blockers in chronic stable angina. Once ischemic symptoms are controlled with β-blocker and/or CCB therapy, other antihypertensive drugs (e.g., ACE inhibitor or ARB) can be added to provide additional CV risk reduction. Thiazide diuretics may be added thereafter to provide additional BP lowering and further reduce CV risk.
- For acute coronary syndromes, first-line therapy should consist of a β-blocker and ACE inhibitor; the combination lowers BP, controls acute ischemia, and reduces CV risk.

Diabetes Mellitus

- The BP goal in diabetes is <130/80 mm Hg.
- All patients with diabetes and hypertension should be treated with either an ACE inhibitor or an ARB. Both classes provide nephroprotection and reduced CV risk.
- A thiazide-type diuretic is recommended as the second agent to lower BP and provide additional CV risk reduction.
- CCBs are useful add-on agents for BP control in hypertensive patients with diabetes. Limited data suggest that nondihydropyridines may have more renal protective effects than dihydropyridines.
- β-Blockers reduce CV risk in patients with diabetes and should be used when needed as add-on therapy with other standard agents or to treat another compelling indication (e.g., post-MI). However, they may mask most of the symptoms of hypoglycemia (tremor, tachycardia, and palpitations but not sweating) in tightly controlled patients, delay recovery from hypoglycemia, and produce elevations in BP due to vasoconstriction caused by unopposed α-receptor stimulation during the hypoglycemic recovery phase. Despite these potential problems, β-blockers can be used safely in patients with diabetes.

Chronic Kidney Disease

- Either an ACE inhibitor or an ARB is recommended as first-line therapy to control BP and preserve kidney function in chronic kidney disease.
- Because these patients usually require multiple-drug therapy, diuretics and a third antihypertensive drug class (e.g., β-blocker or CCB) are often needed.

Recurrent Stroke Prevention

- One clinical trial showed that the combination of an ACE inhibitor and thiazide diuretic reduces the incidence of recurrent stroke in patients with a history of ischemic stroke or TIAs.

SPECIAL POPULATIONS

- Selection of drug therapy should follow the JNC7 and AHA 2007 recommendations, but the treatment approach in some patient populations may be slightly different. In these situations, alternative agents may have unique properties that benefit a coexisting condition, but the data may not be based on evidence from outcome studies in hypertension.

Older People

- Elderly patients may present with either isolated systolic hypertension or an elevation in both SBP and DBP. Epidemiologic data indicate that CV morbidity and mortality are more closely related to SBP than to DBP in patients 50 years of age and older.
- Diuretics, ACE inhibitors, and ARBs provide significant benefits and can be used safely in the elderly, but smaller-than-usual initial doses must be used for initial therapy.

Children and Adolescents

- Secondary hypertension is more common in children and adolescents than in adults. Kidney disease (e.g., pyelonephritis and glomerulonephritis) is the most common cause of secondary hypertension in children. Coarctation of the aorta can also produce secondary hypertension. Medical or surgical management of the underlying disorder usually normalizes BP.
- Nonpharmacologic treatment (particularly weight loss in obese children) is the cornerstone of therapy of primary hypertension.
- ACE inhibitors, ARBs, β-blockers, CCBs, and thiazide-type diuretics are all acceptable drug therapy choices.
- ACE inhibitors, ARBs, and direct renin inhibitors are contraindicated in sexually active girls because of potential teratogenic effects.

Pregnancy

- Preeclampsia, defined as BP $\geq$140/90 mm Hg that appears after 20 weeks' gestation accompanied by new-onset proteinuria ($\geq$300 mg/24 hours), can lead to life-threatening complications for both the mother and fetus. **Eclampsia,** the onset of convulsions in preeclampsia, is a medical emergency.
- Definitive treatment of preeclampsia is delivery, and this is indicated if pending or frank eclampsia is present. Otherwise, management consists of restricting activity, bedrest, and close monitoring. Salt restriction or other

measures that contract blood volume should be avoided. Antihypertensives are used prior to induction of labor if the DBP is >105 mm Hg, with a target DBP of 95 to 105 mm Hg. IV hydralazine is most commonly used; IV labetalol is also effective.

- Chronic hypertension is defined as elevated BP that was noted before pregnancy began. Methyldopa is considered the drug of choice because of experience with its use. β-Blockers, labetalol, and CCBs are also reasonable alternatives. ACE inhibitors and ARBs are known teratogens and are absolutely contraindicated. The direct renin inhibitor aliskiren also should not be used in pregnancy.

African Americans

- Hypertension is more common and more severe in African Americans than in those of other races. Differences in electrolyte homeostasis, GFR, sodium excretion and transport mechanisms, plasma renin activity, and BP response to plasma volume expansion have been noted.
- Lifestyle modifications are recommended to augment drug therapy. Thiazide diuretics are first-line drug therapy for most patients, but recent guidelines aggressively promote combination therapy. Two drugs are recommended in patients with SBP values ≥15 mm Hg from goal.
- Thiazides and CCBs are particularly effective in African Americans. Antihypertensive response is significantly increased when either class is combined with a β-blocker, ACE inhibitor, or ARB.

Pulmonary Disease and Peripheral Arterial Disease

- Although β-blockers (especially nonselective agents) have generally been avoided in hypertensive patients with asthma and COPD because of fear of inducing bronchospasm, data suggest that cardioselective β-blockers can be used safely. Consequently, cardioselective agents should be used to treat a compelling indication (i.e., post-MI, coronary disease, or HF) in patients with reactive airway disease.
- PAD is considered a coronary artery disease risk equivalent. ACE inhibitors may be ideal in patients with symptomatic lower-extremity PAD; CCBs may also be beneficial. β-Blockers can theoretically be problematic because of possible decreased peripheral blood flow secondary to unopposed stimulation of α-receptors that results in vasoconstriction. If problematic, this can be mitigated by using a β-blocker that also has α-blocking properties (e.g., carvedilol). However, β-blockers are not contraindicated in PAD and have not been shown to adversely affect walking capacity.

HYPERTENSIVE URGENCIES AND EMERGENCIES

- **Hypertensive urgencies** are ideally managed by adjusting maintenance therapy by adding a new antihypertensive and/or increasing the dose of a present medication.
  - ✓ Acute administration of a short-acting oral drug (captopril, clonidine, or labetalol) followed by careful observation for several hours to ensure a gradual BP reduction is an option.
  - ✓ Oral captopril doses of 25 to 50 mg may be given at 1- to 2-hour intervals. The onset of action is 15 to 30 minutes.

✓ For treatment of hypertensive rebound after withdrawal of **clonidine,** 0.2 mg is given initially, followed by 0.2 mg hourly until the DBP falls below 110 mm Hg or a total of 0.7 mg has been administered; a single dose may be sufficient.

✓ Labetalol can be given in a dose of 200 to 400 mg, followed by additional doses every 2 to 3 hours.

- **Hypertensive emergencies** require immediate BP reduction to limit new or progressing target-organ damage. The goal is not to lower BP to normal; instead, the initial target is a reduction in mean arterial pressure of up to 25% within minutes to hours. If BP is then stable, it can be reduced toward 160/100–110 mm Hg within the next 2 to 6 hours. Precipitous drops in BP may cause end-organ ischemia or infarction. If BP reduction is well tolerated, additional gradual decrease toward the goal BP can be attempted after 24 to 48 hours.

✓ Nitroprusside is the agent of choice for minute-to-minute control in most cases. It is usually given as a continuous IV infusion at a rate of 0.25 to 10 mcg/kg/min. Its onset of hypotensive action is immediate and disappears within 1 to 2 minutes of discontinuation. When the infusion must be continued longer than 72 hours, serum thiocyanate levels should be measured, and the infusion should be discontinued if the level exceeds 12 mg/dL. The risk of thiocyanate toxicity is increased in patients with impaired kidney function. Other adverse effects are nausea, vomiting, muscle twitching, and sweating.

✓ Dosing guidelines and adverse effects of parenteral agents for treating hypertensive emergency are listed in **Table 10–4.**

EVALUATION OF THERAPEUTIC OUTCOMES

- Clinic-based BP monitoring is the standard for managing hypertension. BP response should be evaluated 2 to 4 weeks after initiating or making changes in therapy. Once goals BP values are obtained, BP monitoring can be done every 3 to 6 months, assuming no signs or symptoms of acute target-organ disease. More frequent evaluations are required in patients with a history of poor control, nonadherence, progressive target-organ damage, or symptoms of adverse drug effects.

- Self-measurements of BP or automatic ambulatory BP monitoring can be useful to establish effective 24-hour control. These techniques are currently recommended only for select situations such as suspected white coat hypertension.

- Patients should be monitored for signs and symptoms of progressive target-organ disease. A careful history should be taken for chest pain (or pressure), palpitations, dizziness, dyspnea, orthopnea, headache, sudden change in vision, one-sided weakness, slurred speech, and loss of balance to assess for the presence of complications.

- Other clinical parameters that should be monitored periodically include funduscopic changes on eye examination, LV hypertrophy on ECG, proteinuria, and changes in kidney function.

TABLE 10–4	Parenteral Antihypertensive Agents for Hypertensive Emergency			
Drug	**Dose**	**Onset (min)**	**Duration (min)**	**Adverse Effects**
Clevidipine	1–2 mg/hour (32 mg/hour max)	2–4	5–15	Headache, nausea, tachycardia, hypertriglyceridemia
Enalaprilat	1.25–5 mg IV four times daily	15–30	360–720	Precipitous fall in BP in high-renin states; variable response
Esmolol hydrochloride	250–500 mcg/kg/min IV bolus, then 50–100 mcg/kg/min IV infusion; may repeat bolus after 5 min or increase infusion to 300 mcg/min	1–2	10–20	Hypotension, nausea, asthma, first-degree heart block, heart failure
Fenoldopam mesylate	0.1–0.3 mcg/kg/min IV infusion	<5	30	Tachycardia, headache, nausea, flushing
Hydralazine hydrochloride	12–20 mg IV 10–50 mg IM	10–20 20–30	60–240 240–360	Tachycardia, flushing, headache, vomiting, aggravation of angina
Labetalol hydrochloride	20–80 mg IV bolus every 10 min; 0.5–2 mg/min IV infusion	5–10	180–360	Vomiting, scalp tingling, bronchoconstriction, dizziness, nausea, heart block, orthostatic hypotension
Nicardipine hydrochloride	5–15 mg/hour IV	5–10	15–30; may exceed 240	Tachycardia, headache, flushing, local phlebitis
Nitroglycerin	5–100 mcg/min IV infusion	2–5	5–10	Headache, vomiting, methemoglobinemia, tolerance with prolonged use
Sodium nitroprusside	0.25–10 mcg/kg/min IV infusion (requires special delivery system)	Immediate	1–2	Nausea, vomiting, muscle twitching, sweating, thiocyanate and cyanide intoxication

IM, intramuscular.

- Monitoring for adverse drug effects should typically occur 2 to 4 weeks after starting a new agent or dose increases, then every 6 to 12 months in stable patients. Additional monitoring may be needed for other concomitant diseases. Patients taking aldosterone antagonists should have

potassium concentration and kidney function assessed within 3 days and again at 1 week after initiation to detect potential hyperkalemia.
- Patient adherence with the therapeutic regimen should be assessed regularly. Patients should be questioned periodically about changes in their general health perception, energy level, physical functioning, and overall satisfaction with treatment.

See Chapter 19, Hypertension, authored by Joseph J. Saseen and Eric J. MacLaughlin, for a more detailed discussion of this topic.

Ischemic Heart Disease

DEFINITION

- Ischemic heart disease (IHD) is defined as a lack of oxygen and decreased or no blood flow to the myocardium resulting from coronary artery narrowing or obstruction. IHD may present as an acute coronary syndrome (ACS, which includes unstable angina and non–ST-segment elevation or ST-segment elevation myocardial infarction [MI]), chronic stable exertional angina, ischemia without symptoms, or ischemia due to coronary artery vasospasm (variant or Prinzmetal angina).

PATHOPHYSIOLOGY

- The major determinants of myocardial oxygen demand (MVo_2) are heart rate (HR), contractility, and intramyocardial wall tension during systole. Wall tension is thought to be the most important factor. Because the consequences of IHD usually result from increased demand in the face of a fixed oxygen supply, alterations in MVo_2 are important in producing ischemia and for interventions intended to alleviate it.
- A clinically useful indirect estimate of MVo_2 is the double product (DP), which is HR multiplied by systolic blood pressure (SBP) ($DP = HR \times SBP$). The DP does not consider changes in contractility (an independent variable), and because only changes in pressure are considered, volume loading of the left ventricle and increased MVo_2 related to ventricular dilation are underestimated.
- The caliber of the resistance vessels delivering blood to the myocardium and MVo_2 are the prime determinants in the occurrence of ischemia.
- The normal coronary system consists of large epicardial or surface vessels (R_1) that offer little resistance to myocardial flow and intramyocardial arteries and arterioles (R_2), which branch into a dense capillary network to supply basal blood flow (**Fig. 11–1**). Under normal circumstances, the resistance in R_2 is much greater than that in R_1. Myocardial blood flow is inversely related to arteriolar resistance and directly related to the coronary driving pressure.
- Atherosclerotic lesions occluding R_1 increase arteriolar resistance, and R_2 can vasodilate to maintain coronary blood flow. With greater degrees of obstruction, this response is inadequate, and the coronary flow reserve afforded by R_2 vasodilation is insufficient to meet oxygen demand. Relatively severe stenosis (>70%) may provoke ischemia and symptoms at rest, whereas less severe stenosis may allow a reserve of coronary blood flow for exertion.
- The diameter and length of obstructing lesions and the influence of pressure drop across an area of stenosis also affect coronary blood flow and function of the collateral circulation. Dynamic coronary obstruction can occur in normal vessels and vessels with stenosis in which vasomotion or a spasm may be superimposed on a fixed stenosis. Persisting ischemia may promote growth of developed collateral blood flow.

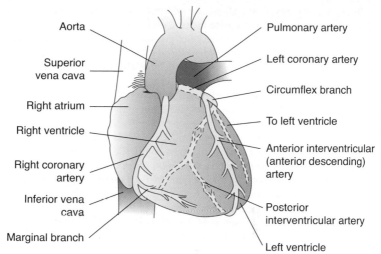

FIGURE 11—1. Coronary artery anatomy. *(From Tintinalli JE, Kelen GD, Stapczynski JR, eds. Tintinalli's Emergency Medicine: A Comprehensive Study Guide. 6th ed. New York: McGraw-Hill, 2004:344.)*

- Critical stenosis occurs when the obstructing lesion encroaches on the luminal diameter and exceeds 70%. Lesions creating obstruction of 50% to 70% may reduce blood flow, but these obstructions are not consistent, and vasospasm and thrombosis superimposed on a "noncritical" lesion may lead to clinical events such as MI. If the lesion enlarges from 80% to 90%, resistance in that vessel is tripled. Coronary reserve is diminished at ~85% obstruction due to vasoconstriction.

- Abnormalities of ventricular contraction can occur, and regional loss of contractility may impose a burden on the remaining myocardial tissue, resulting in heart failure (HF), increased MVo$_2$, and rapid depletion of blood flow reserve. Zones of tissue with marginal blood flow may develop that are at risk for more severe damage if the ischemic episode persists or becomes more severe. Nonischemic areas of myocardium may compensate for the severely ischemic and border zones of ischemia by developing more tension than usual in an attempt to maintain cardiac output. The left or right ventricular dysfunction that ensues may be associated with clinical findings of an S$_3$ gallop, dyspnea, orthopnea, tachycardia, fluctuating blood pressure, transient murmurs, and mitral or tricuspid regurgitation. Impaired diastolic and systolic function leads to elevation of the filling pressure of the left ventricle.

CLINICAL PRESENTATION

- Many episodes of ischemia do not cause symptoms of angina (silent ischemia). Patients often have a reproducible pattern of pain or other symptoms that appear after a specific amount of exertion. Increased symptom frequency, severity, or duration, and symptoms at rest suggest an unstable pattern that requires immediate medical evaluation.

- Symptoms may include a sensation of pressure or burning over the sternum or near it, which often radiates to the left jaw, shoulder, and arm. Chest tightness and shortness of breath may also occur. The sensation usually lasts from 30 seconds to 30 minutes.
- Precipitating factors include exercise, cold environment, walking after a meal, emotional upset, fright, anger, and coitus. Relief occurs with rest and within 45 seconds to 5 minutes of taking nitroglycerin.
- Patients with variant or Prinzmetal angina secondary to coronary spasm are more likely to experience pain at rest and in the early morning hours. Pain is not usually brought on by exertion or emotional stress, nor is it relieved by rest; the electrocardiogram (ECG) pattern is that of current injury with ST-segment elevation rather than depression.
- Unstable angina is stratified into categories of low, intermediate, or high risk for short-term death or nonfatal MI. Features of high-risk unstable angina include (but are not limited to) (1) accelerating tempo of ischemic symptoms in the preceding 48 hours; (2) pain at rest lasting more than 20 minutes; (3) age older than 75 years; (4) ST-segment changes; and (5) clinical findings of pulmonary edema, mitral regurgitation, S_3, rales, hypotension, bradycardia, or tachycardia.
- Episodes of ischemia may also be painless, or "silent," in at least 60% of patients, perhaps due to a higher threshold and tolerance for pain than in patients who have pain more frequently.

DIAGNOSIS

- Important aspects of the clinical history include the nature or quality of the chest pain, precipitating factors, duration, pain radiation, and the response to nitroglycerin or rest. There appears to be little relationship between the historical features of angina and the severity or extent of coronary artery vessel involvement. Ischemic chest pain may resemble pain arising from a variety of noncardiac sources, and the differential diagnosis of anginal pain from other etiologies may be difficult based on history alone.
- The patient should be asked about existing personal risk factors for coronary heart disease (CHD), including smoking, hypertension, and diabetes mellitus.
- A detailed family history should be obtained that includes information about premature CHD, hypertension, familial lipid disorders, and diabetes mellitus.
- There are few signs on physical examination to indicate the presence of coronary artery disease (CAD). Findings on the cardiac examination may include abnormal precordial systolic bulge, decreased intensity of S_1, paradoxical splitting of S_2, S_3, S_4, apical systolic murmur, and diastolic murmur. Elevated HR or blood pressure can yield an increased DP and may be associated with angina. Noncardiac physical findings suggesting significant cardiovascular disease include abdominal aortic aneurysms and peripheral vascular disease.

- Laboratory tests recommended include hemoglobin (to ensure adequate oxygen-carrying capacity), fasting glucose (to exclude diabetes), and fasting lipoprotein panel. Important risk factors in some patients may include C-reactive protein; homocysteine level; evidence of *Chlamydia* infection; and elevations in lipoprotein (a), fibrinogen, and plasminogen activator inhibitor. Cardiac enzymes should all be normal in stable angina. Troponin T or I, myoglobin, and creatinine kinase myocardial band (CK-MB) may be elevated in unstable angina.

- The resting ECG is normal in about one half of patients with angina who are not experiencing an acute attack. Typical ST-T-wave changes include depression, T-wave inversion, and ST-segment elevation. Variant angina is associated with ST-segment elevation, whereas silent ischemia may produce elevation or depression. Significant ischemia is associated with ST-segment depression >2 mm, exertional hypotension, and reduced exercise tolerance.

- Exercise tolerance (stress) testing (ETT) is recommended for patients with an intermediate probability of CAD. Results correlate well with the likelihood of progressing to angina, occurrence of acute MI, and cardiovascular death. Ischemic ST-segment depression during ETT is an independent risk factor for cardiovascular events and mortality. Thallium myocardial perfusion scintigraphy may be used in conjunction with ETT to detect reversible and irreversible defects in blood flow to the myocardium.

- Radionuclide angiocardiography is used to measure ejection fraction (EF), regional ventricular performance, cardiac output, ventricular volumes, valvular regurgitation, asynchrony or wall motion abnormalities, and intracardiac shunts.

- Ultrarapid computed tomography may minimize artifact from heart motion during contraction and relaxation and provides a semiquantitative assessment of calcium content in coronary arteries.

- Echocardiography is useful if the history or physical findings suggest valvular pericardial disease or ventricular dysfunction. In patients unable to exercise, pharmacologic stress echocardiography (e.g., dobutamine, dipyridamole, or adenosine) may identify abnormalities that would occur during stress.

- Cardiac catheterization and coronary angiography are used in patients with suspected CAD to document the presence and severity of disease, as well as for prognostic purposes. Interventional catheterization is used for thrombolytic therapy in patients with acute MI and for managing patients with significant CAD to relieve obstruction through percutaneous transluminal coronary angioplasty, atherectomy, laser treatment, or stent placement.

- A chest radiograph should be done if the patient has HF symptoms.

DESIRED OUTCOME

- The short-term goals of therapy for IHD are to reduce or prevent anginal symptoms that limit exercise capability and impair quality of life. Long-term goals are to prevent CHD events such as MI, arrhythmias, and HF and to extend the patient's life.

TREATMENT

RISK-FACTOR MODIFICATION

- Primary prevention through the modification of risk factors should significantly reduce the prevalence of IHD. Secondary intervention is effective in reducing subsequent morbidity and mortality.
- Risk factors for IHD are additive and can be classified as alterable or unalterable. Unalterable risk factors include gender, age, family history or genetic composition, environmental influences, and, to some extent, diabetes mellitus. Alterable risk factors include smoking, hypertension, hyperlipidemia, obesity, sedentary lifestyle, hyperuricemia, psychosocial factors such as stress and type A behavior patterns, and the use of drugs that may be detrimental (e.g., progestins, corticosteroids, and calcineurin inhibitors). Although thiazide diuretics and β-blockers (nonselective without intrinsic sympathomimetic activity) may elevate both cholesterol and triglycerides by 10% to 20%, and these effects may be detrimental, no objective evidence exists from prospective well-controlled studies to support avoiding these drugs.

PHARMACOLOGIC THERAPY

β-Adrenergic Blockers

- Decreased HR, contractility, and blood pressure reduce MVo_2 and oxygen demand in patients with effort-induced angina. β-Blockers do not improve oxygen supply, and, in certain instances, unopposed α-adrenergic stimulation may lead to coronary vasoconstriction.
- β-Blockers improve symptoms in ~80% of patients with chronic exertional stable angina, and objective measures of efficacy demonstrate improved exercise duration and delay in the time at which ST-segment changes and initial or limiting symptoms occur. β-Blockade may allow angina patients previously limited by symptoms to perform more exercise and ultimately improve overall cardiovascular performance through a training effect.
- Ideal candidates for β-blockers include patients in whom physical activity is a prominent cause of attacks; those with coexisting hypertension, supraventricular arrhythmias, or post-MI angina; and those with anxiety associated with anginal episodes. β-Blockers may be used safely in angina and HF.
- β-Blockade is effective in chronic exertional angina as monotherapy and in combination with nitrates and/or calcium channel blockers (CCBs). β-Blockers are the first-line drugs in chronic angina requiring daily maintenance therapy because they are more effective in reducing episodes of silent ischemia and early morning peak of ischemic activity and improving mortality after Q-wave MI than nitrates or CCBs.
- If β-blockers are ineffective or not tolerated, then monotherapy with a CCB or combination therapy may be instituted. Reflex tachycardia from nitrates can be blunted with β-blocker therapy, making this a useful combination. Patients with severe angina, rest angina, or variant angina may be better treated with CCBs or long-acting nitrates.

- Initial doses of β-blockers should be at the lower end of the usual dosing range and titrated to response. Treatment objectives include lowering the resting HR to 50 to 60 beats/min and limiting maximal exercise HR to ~100 beats/min or less. HR with modest exercise should be no more than ~20 beats/min above resting HR (or a 10% increment over resting HR).
- There is little evidence to suggest the superiority of any particular β-blocker. Those with longer half-lives may be administered less frequently, but even **propranolol** may be given twice daily in most patients. Membrane-stabilizing activity is irrelevant in the treatment of angina. Intrinsic sympathomimetic activity appears to be detrimental in patients with rest or severe angina because the reduction in HR would be minimized, therefore limiting a reduction in MVO_2. Cardioselective β-blockers may be used in some patients to minimize adverse effects such as bronchospasm, intermittent claudication, and sexual dysfunction. Combined nonselective β- and α-blockade with **labetalol** may be useful in some patients with marginal left ventricular (LV) reserve.
- Adverse effects of β-blockade include hypotension, decompensated HF, bradycardia, heart block, bronchospasm, altered glucose metabolism, fatigue, malaise, and depression. Abrupt withdrawal in patients with angina has been associated with increased severity and number of pain episodes and MI. Tapering of therapy over ~2 days should minimize the risk of withdrawal reactions if therapy is to be discontinued.

Nitrates

- The action of nitrates appears to be mediated indirectly through reduction of MVO_2 secondary to venodilation and arterial-arteriolar dilation, leading to a reduction in wall stress from reduced ventricular volume and pressure. Direct actions on the coronary circulation include dilation of large and small intramural coronary arteries, collateral dilation, coronary artery stenosis dilation, abolition of normal tone in narrowed vessels, and relief of spasm.
- Pharmacokinetic characteristics common to nitrates include a large first-pass effect of hepatic metabolism, short to very short half-lives (except for **isosorbide mononitrate** [ISMN]), large volumes of distribution, high clearance rates, and large interindividual variations in plasma or blood concentrations. The half-life of **nitroglycerin** is 1 to 5 minutes regardless of the route, hence the potential advantage of sustained-release and transdermal products. **Isosorbide dinitrate** (ISDN) is metabolized to ISMN. ISMN has a half-life of ~5 hours and may be given once or twice daily, depending on the product chosen.
- Nitrate therapy may be used to terminate an acute anginal attack, to prevent effort- or stress-induced attacks, or for long-term prophylaxis, usually in combination with β-blockers or CCBs. Sublingual, buccal, or spray nitroglycerin products are preferred for alleviation of anginal attacks because of rapid absorption (**Table 11–1**). Symptoms may be prevented by prophylactic oral or transdermal products (usually in combination with β-blockers or CCBs), but development of tolerance may be problematic.
- **Sublingual nitroglycerin,** 0.3 to 0.4 mg, relieves pain in ~75% of patients within 3 minutes, with another 15% becoming pain-free in 5 to 15 minutes.

TABLE 11–1 Nitrate Products

Product	Onset (min)	Duration	Initial Dose
Nitroglycerin			
IV	1–2	3–5 min	5 mcg/min
Sublingual/lingual	1–3	30–60 min	0.3 mg
Oral	40	3–6 hours	2.5–9 mg three times daily
Ointment	20–60	2–8 hours	0.05–1 inch
Patch	40–60	>8 hours	1 patch
Erythritol tetranitrate	5–30	4–6 hours	5–10 mg three times daily
Pentaerythritol tetranitrate	30	4–8 hours	10–20 mg three times daily
Isosorbide dinitrate			
Sublingual/chewable	2–5	1–2 hours	2.5–5 mg three times daily
Oral	20–40	4–6 hours	5–20 mg three times daily
Isosorbide mononitrate	30–60	6–8 hours	20 mg daily, twice daily[a]

[a]Product dependent.

Pain persisting beyond 20 to 30 minutes after use of two or three nitroglycerin tablets suggests ACS, and the patient should be instructed to seek emergency aid.

- Chewable, oral, and transdermal products are acceptable for long-term prophylaxis of angina. Dosing of long-acting preparations should be adjusted to provide a hemodynamic response. This may require doses of oral ISDN ranging from 10 to 60 mg as often as every 3 to 4 hours due to tolerance or first-pass metabolism. Intermittent (10–12 hours on, 12–14 hours off) transdermal nitroglycerin therapy may produce modest but significant improvement in exercise time in chronic stable angina.

- Adverse effects include postural hypotension with associated CNS symptoms, reflex tachycardia, headaches and flushing, and occasional nausea. Excessive hypotension may result in MI or stroke. Noncardiovascular adverse effects include rash (especially with transdermal nitroglycerin), methemoglobinemia with high doses given for extended periods, and measurable ethanol and propylene glycol concentrations with IV nitroglycerin.

- Because both the onset and offset of tolerance to nitrates occur quickly, one strategy to circumvent it is to provide a daily nitrate-free interval of 8 to 12 hours. For example, ISDN should not be used more often than three times daily to avoid tolerance.

- Nitrates may be combined with other drugs with complementary mechanisms of action for chronic prophylactic therapy. Combination therapy is generally used in patients with more frequent symptoms or symptoms that do not respond to β-blockers alone (nitrates plus β-blockers or CCBs), in patients intolerant of β-blockers or CCBs, and in patients having an element of vasospasm leading to decreased supply (nitrates plus CCBs).

Calcium Channel Blockers

- Direct actions include vasodilation of systemic arterioles and coronary arteries, leading to a reduction of arterial pressure and coronary vascular resistance, as well as depression of myocardial contractility and the conduction velocity of the sinoatrial and atrioventricular (AV) nodes. Reflex β-adrenergic stimulation overcomes much of the negative inotropic effect, and depression of contractility becomes clinically apparent only in the presence of LV dysfunction and when other negative inotropic drugs are used concurrently.

- **Verapamil** and **diltiazem** cause less peripheral vasodilation than dihydropyridines such as **nifedipine** but greater decreases in AV node conduction. They must be used with caution in patients with preexisting conduction abnormalities and those taking other drugs with negative chronotropic properties.

- MVo_2 is reduced with all CCBs primarily because of reduced wall tension secondary to reduced arterial pressure. Overall, the benefit provided by CCBs is related to reduced MVo_2 rather than improved oxygen supply.

- In contrast to the β-blockers, CCBs have the potential to improve coronary blood flow through areas of fixed coronary obstruction by inhibiting coronary artery vasomotion and vasospasm.

- Good candidates for CCBs include patients with contraindications or intolerance to β-blockers, coexisting conduction system disease (except for verapamil and diltiazem), Prinzmetal angina, peripheral vascular disease, severe ventricular dysfunction, and concurrent hypertension. **Amlodipine** is probably the CCB of choice in severe ventricular dysfunction, and the others should be used with caution if the EF is <40%.

Ranolazine

- This drug reduces calcium overload in ischemic myocytes through inhibition of the late sodium current. Ranolazine does not affect HR, inotropic state, or hemodynamic state, or increase coronary blood flow.

- Ranolazine is indicated for the treatment of chronic angina. In controlled trials, the drug modestly improved exercise time by 15 to ~45 seconds compared with placebo. In a large ACS trial, ranolazine reduced recurrent ischemia but did not improve the primary efficacy composite end point of cardiovascular death, MI, or recurrent ischemia.

- Because it prolongs the QT interval, ranolazine should be reserved for patients who have not achieved an adequate response to other antianginal drugs. It should be used in combination with amlodipine, β-blockers, or nitrates.

- The most common adverse effects are dizziness, headache, constipation, and nausea. Ranolazine should be started at 500 mg twice daily and increased to 1,000 mg twice daily if needed based on symptoms. Baseline and follow-up ECGs should be obtained to evaluate effects on the QT interval.

TREATMENT OF STABLE EXERTIONAL ANGINA PECTORIS

- **Table 11–2** lists the evidence-based drug therapy recommendations of the American College of Cardiology and American Heart Association. A treatment algorithm is shown in **Fig. 11–2**.

TABLE 11–2	Evidence-based Recommendations for Treatment of Stable Exertional Angina Pectoris

Recommendations	Recommendation Grades[a]
All patients should be given the following unless contraindications exist:	
• Aspirin	Class I, level A
• β-Blockers with prior MI	Class I, level A
• ACE inhibitor to patients with CAD and diabetes or LV systolic dysfunction	Class I, level A
• LDL-lowering therapy with CAD and LDL >130 mg/dL	Class I, level A
• Sublingual nitroglycerin for immediate relief of angina	Class I, level B
• CCBs or long acting nitrates for reduction of symptoms when β-blockers are contraindicated	Class I, level B
• CCBs or long-acting nitrates in combination with β-blockers when initial treatment with β-blockers is unsuccessful	Class I, level C
• CCBs or long-acting nitrates as a substitute for β-blockers if initial treatment with β-blockers leads to unacceptable side effects	Class I, level A
Clopidogrel may be substituted for aspirin when aspirin is absolutely contraindicated	Class IIa, level B
Long-acting nondihydropyridine calcium antagonists instead of β-blockers as initial therapy	Class IIa, level B
ACE inhibitors are recommended in patients with CAD or other vascular disease	Class IIa, level B
Low-intensity anticoagulation with warfarin, in addition to aspirin, is recommended, but bleeding would be increased	Class IIb, level B
Therapies to be avoided include	
• Dipyridamole	Class III, level B
• Chelation therapy	Class III, level B

ACE, angiotensin-converting enzyme; CAD, coronary artery disease; CCBs, calcium channel blockers; LDL, low-density lipoprotein; LV, left ventricular; MI, myocardial infarction.

[a]American College of Cardiology and American Heart Association Evidence Grading System

Recommendation Class:

I = Conditions for which there is evidence or general agreement that a given procedure or treatment is useful and effective.

II = Conditions for which there is conflicting evidence or a divergence of opinion about the usefulness/efficacy of a given procedure or treatment.

IIa = Weight of evidence/opinion is in favor of usefulness or efficacy.

IIb = Usefulness/efficacy is less well established by evidence/opinion.

III = Conditions for which there is evidence or general agreement that a given procedure or treatment is not useful/effective and in some cases may be harmful.

Level of Evidence:

A = Data derived from multiple randomized clinical trials with large numbers of patients.

B = Data derived from a limited number of randomized trials with small numbers of patients, careful analyses of nonrandomized studies, or observational registries.

C = Expert consensus was the primary basis for the recommendation.

- After assessing and manipulating alterable risk factors, a regular exercise program should be undertaken with caution in a graduated fashion and with adequate supervision to improve cardiovascular and muscular fitness.

- Nitrate therapy should be the first step in managing acute attacks of chronic stable angina if the episodes are infrequent (e.g., a few times per month). If angina occurs no more often than once every few days, then sublingual nitroglycerin tablets or spray or buccal products may be sufficient.

- For prophylaxis when undertaking activities that predictably precipitate attacks, nitroglycerin 0.3 to 0.4 mg sublingually may be used ~5 minutes prior to the time of the activity. Nitroglycerin spray may be useful when inadequate saliva is produced to rapidly dissolve sublingual **nitroglycerin** or if a patient has difficulty opening the tablet container. The response usually lasts ~30 minutes.

- When angina occurs more frequently than once a day, a chronic prophylactic regimen using *β*-**blockers** as first-line therapy should be considered. *β*-Blockers may be preferable because of less frequent dosing and other desirable properties (e.g., potential cardioprotective effects, antiarrhythmic effects, lack of tolerance, and antihypertensive efficacy). The appropriate dose should be determined by the goals outlined for HR and DP. An agent should be selected that is well tolerated by individual patients at a reasonable cost. Patients most likely to respond well to *β*-blockade are those with a high resting HR and those with a relatively fixed anginal threshold (i.e., their symptoms appear at the same level of exercise or workload on a consistent basis).

- **Calcium channel blockers** have the potential advantage of improving coronary blood flow through coronary artery vasodilation, as well as decreasing MVo_2, and may be used instead of *β*-blockers for chronic prophylactic therapy. They are as effective as *β*-blockers and are most useful in patients who have a variable threshold for exertional angina. Calcium antagonists may provide better skeletal muscle oxygenation, resulting in decreased fatigue and better exercise tolerance. They can be used safely in many patients with contraindications to *β*-blocker therapy. The available drugs have similar efficacy in the management of chronic stable angina. Patients with conduction abnormalities and moderate to severe LV dysfunction (EF <35%) should not be treated with **verapamil** or **diltiazem,** whereas **amlodipine** may be used safely in many of these patients. **Diltiazem** has significant effects on the AV node and can produce heart block in patients with preexisting conduction disease or when other drugs with effects on conduction (e.g., digoxin and *β*-blockers) are used concurrently. **Nifedipine** may cause excessive HR elevation, especially if the patient is not receiving a *β*-blocker, and this may offset its beneficial effect on MVo_2. The combination of CCBs and *β*-blockers is rational because the hemodynamic effect of calcium antagonists is complementary to *β*-blockade. However, combination therapy may not always be more effective than single-agent therapy.

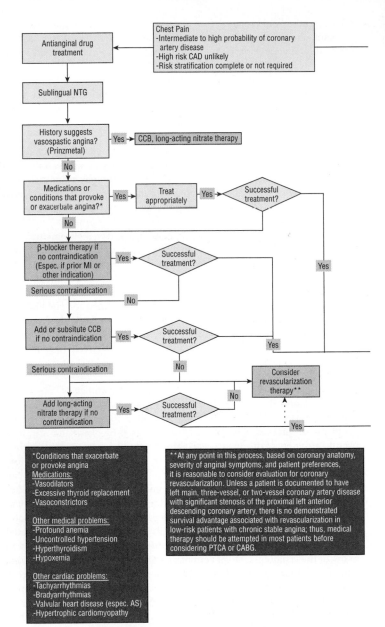

FIGURE 11-2. Treatment of stable angina pectoris. (AS, aortic stenosis; CABG, coronary artery bypass grafting; CAD, coronary artery disease; CCB, calcium channel blocker; JNC VII, Seventh Report of the Joint National Committee on Prevention, Detection, Evaluation, and Treatment of High Blood Pressure; MI, myocardial infarction, NCEP, National Cholesterol Education Program; NTG, nitroglycerin; PTCA, percutaneous transluminal coronary angioplasty; QD, every day.)

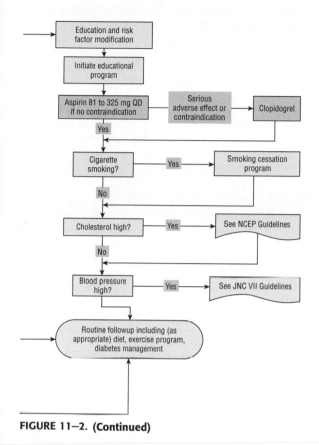

FIGURE 11–2. (Continued)

- Chronic prophylactic therapy with long-acting forms of **nitroglycerin** (oral or transdermal), **ISDN, ISMN,** and **pentaerythritol trinitrate** may also be effective when angina occurs more than once a day, but development of tolerance is a limitation. Monotherapy with nitrates should not be first-line therapy unless β-blockers and CCBs are contraindicated or not tolerated. A nitrate-free interval of 8 hours per day or longer should be provided to maintain efficacy. The choice among nitrate products should be based on experience, cost, and patient acceptance.

TREATMENT OF CORONARY ARTERY SPASM AND VARIANT ANGINA PECTORIS

- All patients should be treated for acute attacks and maintained on prophylactic treatment for 6 to 12 months after the initial episode. Aggravating factors such as alcohol or cocaine use and cigarette smoking should be stopped.

- **Nitrates** are the mainstay of therapy, and most patients respond rapidly to sublingual **nitroglycerin** or **ISDN**. IV and intracoronary nitroglycerin may be useful for patients not responding to sublingual preparations.

- Because CCBs may be more effective, have few serious adverse effects, and can be given less frequently than nitrates, some authorities consider them the agents of choice for variant angina. **Nifedipine, verapamil,** and **diltiazem** are all equally effective as single agents for initial management. Patients unresponsive to CCBs alone may have nitrates added. Combination therapy with nifedipine plus diltiazem or nifedipine plus verapamil is reported to be useful in patients unresponsive to single-drug regimens.

- β-Blockers have little or no role in the management of variant angina as they may induce coronary vasoconstriction and prolong ischemia.

EVALUATION OF THERAPEUTIC OUTCOMES

- Subjective measures of drug response include the number of painful episodes, amount of rapid-acting nitroglycerin consumed, and symptomatic improvement in exercise capacity (i.e., longer duration of exercise or fewer symptoms at the same exercise level). Once patients have been optimized on medical therapy, symptoms should improve over 2 to 4 weeks and remain stable until the disease progresses.

- The Seattle Angina Questionnaire, Specific Activity Scale, and Canadian Cardiovascular Society classification system are instruments that can be used to improve the reproducibility of symptom assessment.

- If the patient is doing well, no other assessment may be necessary. Objective improvement may be assessed by increased exercise duration on ETT and the absence of ischemic changes on ECG or deleterious hemodynamic changes. Use of echocardiography and cardiac imaging is limited to patients who are not doing well to determine if revascularization or other measures should be undertaken.

- Monitoring for major adverse effects should be undertaken; they include headache and dizziness with nitrates; fatigue and lassitude with β-blockers; and peripheral edema, constipation, and dizziness with CCBs.

- A comprehensive plan includes ancillary monitoring of lipid profiles, fasting plasma glucose, thyroid function tests, hemoglobin/hematocrit, and electrolytes.

See Chapter 23, Ischemic Heart Disease, authored by Robert L. Talbert, for a more detailed discussion of this topic.

CHAPTER 12

Shock

DEFINITION

- *Shock* is an acute, generalized state of inadequate perfusion of critical organs that can lead to death if therapy is not optimal. Shock is defined as systolic blood pressure (SBP) <90 mm Hg or reduction of at least 40 mm Hg from baseline with perfusion abnormalities despite adequate fluid resuscitation. Shock may be caused by intravascular volume deficit (hypovolemic shock), myocardial pump failure (cardiogenic shock), or peripheral vasodilation (septic, anaphylactic, or neurogenic shock).

PATHOPHYSIOLOGY

- Shock results in failure of the circulatory system to deliver sufficient oxygen (O_2) to body tissues despite normal or reduced O_2 consumption. General pathophysiologic mechanisms of different forms of shock are similar except for initiating events.
- Hypovolemic shock is characterized by acute intravascular volume deficiency due to external losses or internal redistribution of extracellular water. This type of shock can be precipitated by hemorrhage, burns, trauma, surgery, intestinal obstruction, and dehydration from considerable insensible fluid loss, overaggressive loop-diuretic administration, and severe vomiting or diarrhea. Relative hypovolemia leading to hypovolemic shock occurs during significant vasodilation, which accompanies anaphylaxis, sepsis, and neurogenic shock.
- Regardless of the etiology, fall in blood pressure (BP) is compensated by an increase in sympathetic outflow, activation of the renin–angiotensin system, and other humoral factors that stimulate peripheral vasoconstriction. Compensatory vasoconstriction redistributes blood away from the skin, skeletal muscles, kidneys, and GI tract toward vital organs (e.g., heart and brain) in an attempt to maintain oxygenation, nutrition, and organ function.
- Severe metabolic lactic acidosis often develops secondary to tissue ischemia and causes localized vasodilation, which further exacerbates the impaired cardiovascular state.

CLINICAL PRESENTATION

- Shock presents with a diversity of signs and symptoms. Patients with hypovolemic shock may present with thirst, anxiousness, weakness, lightheadedness, and dizziness. Patients may also report scanty urine output and darkyellow-colored urine.
- Signs of more severe volume loss include tachycardia (>120 beats/min), tachypnea (>30 breaths/min), hypotension (SBP <90 mm Hg), mental status changes or unconsciousness, agitation, and normal or low body

temperature (in the absence of infection) with cold extremities and decreased capillary refill.

- Serum sodium and chloride concentrations are usually high with acute volume depletion. The blood urea nitrogen (BUN): creatinine ratio may be elevated initially, but the creatinine increases with renal dysfunction. Metabolic acidosis results in elevated base deficit and lactate concentrations with decreased bicarbonate and pH.
- The complete blood cell count (CBC) should be normal in the absence of infection. In hemorrhagic shock, the red cell count, hemoglobin, and hematocrit will decrease.
- Urine output is decreased to <0.5 to 1 mL/hour. With more severe volume depletion, dysfunction of other organs may be reflected in laboratory testing (e.g., elevated serum transaminases levels with hepatic dysfunction).

DIAGNOSIS AND MONITORING

- Information from noninvasive and invasive monitoring (**Table 12–1**) and evaluation of past medical history, clinical presentation, and laboratory findings are key components in establishing the diagnosis, as well as in assessing general mechanisms responsible for shock. Regardless of the etiology, consistent findings include hypotension (SBP <90 mm Hg), depressed cardiac index (CI <2.2 L/min/m^2), tachycardia (heart rate >100 beats/min), and low urine output (<20 mL/hour).
- A pulmonary artery (Swan–Ganz) catheter can be used to determine central venous pressure (CVP); pulmonary artery pressure (PAP); cardiac output (CO); and pulmonary artery occlusion pressure (PAOP), an approximate measure of the left ventricular end-diastolic volume and a major determinant of left ventricular preload.
- CO (2.5–3 L/min) and mixed venous O_2 saturation (70–75%) may be very low in a patient with extensive myocardial damage.
- Respiratory alkalosis is associated with low partial pressure of O_2 (25–35 mm Hg) and alkaline pH but normal bicarbonate. The first two values are measured by arterial blood gas, which also yields partial pressure of carbon dioxide (PCO_2) and arterial O_2 saturation. Circulating arterial O_2 saturation can also be measured by an oximeter, which is a noninvasive method that is fairly accurate and useful at the patient's bedside.
- Renal function can be grossly assessed by hourly measurements of urine output, but estimation of creatinine clearance based on isolated serum creatinine values in critically ill patients may yield erroneous results. Decreased renal perfusion and aldosterone release result in sodium retention and thus low urinary sodium (<30 mEq/L).
- In normal individuals, O_2 consumption (VO_2) is dependent on O_2 delivery (DO_2) up to a certain critical level (VO_2 flow dependency). At this point, tissue O_2 requirements have apparently been satisfied, and further increases in DO_2 will not alter VO_2 (flow independency). However, studies in critically ill patients show a continuous, pathologic dependence relationship of VO_2 with DO_2. These indexed parameters are calculated as

$$DO_2 = CI \times (CaO_2) \quad \text{and} \quad VO_2 = CI \times (CaO_2 - CvO_2),$$

TABLE 12-1	Hemodynamic and Oxygen (O_2)-Transport Monitoring Parameters
Parameter	**Normal Value^a**
Blood pressure (systolic/diastolic)	100–130/70–85 mm Hg
Mean arterial pressure (MAP)	80–100 mm Hg
Pulmonary artery pressure (PAP)	25/10 mm Hg
Mean pulmonary artery pressure (MPAP)	12–15 mm Hg
Central venous pressure (CVP)	8–12 mm Hg
Pulmonary artery occlusion pressure (PAOP)	12–15 mm Hg
Heart rate (HR)	60–80 beats/min
Cardiac output (CO)	4–7 L/min
Cardiac index (CI)	2.8–3.6 L/min/m^2
Stroke volume index (SVI)	30–50 mL/m^2
Systemic vascular resistance index(SVRI)	1,300–2,100 dyne • sec/m^2 • cm^5
Pulmonary vascular resistance index (PVRI)	45–225 dyne • sec/m^2 • cm^5
Arterial O_2 saturation (Sao$_2$)	97% (range 95–100%)
Mixed venous O_2 saturation (Svo$_2$)	70–75%
Arterial O_2 content (Cao$_2$)	20.1 vol% (range 19–21%)
Venous O_2 content (Cvo$_2$)	15.5 vol% (range 11.5–16.5%)
O_2 content difference (C[a–v]o$_2$)	5 vol% (range 4–6%)
O_2 consumption index (Vo$_2$)	131 mL/min/m^2 (range 100–180)
O_2 delivery index (Do$_2$)	578 mL/min/m^2 (range 370–730)
O_2 extraction ratio (O$_2$FR)	25% (range 22–30%)
Intramucosal pH (pHi)	7.40 (range 7.35–7.45)
Index (I)	Parameter indexed to body surface area

^{a}Normal values may not be the same as values needed to optimize management of a critically ill patient.

where CI = cardiac index, Cao$_2$ = arterial O_2 content, and Cvo$_2$ = mixed venous O_2 content. Currently available data do not support the concept that patient outcome or survival is altered by treatment measures directed to achieve supranormal levels of Do$_2$ and Vo$_2$.

- The Vo$_2$:Do$_2$ ratio (O_2 extraction ratio) can be used to assess adequacy of perfusion and metabolic response. Patients who are able to increase Vo$_2$ when Do$_2$ is increased are more likely to survive. However, low Vo$_2$ and O_2 extraction ratio values are indicative of poor O_2 utilization and lead to greater mortality.
- Blood lactate concentrations may be used as another measure of tissue oxygenation and may show better correlation with outcome than O_2 transport parameters in some patients.
- Gastric tonometry measures gut luminal Pco$_2$ at equilibrium by placing a saline-filled gas-permeable balloon in the gastric lumen. Increases in mucosal Pco$_2$ and calculated decreases in gastric intramucosal pH (pHi) are associated with mucosal hypoperfusion and perhaps increased mortality. However, the presence of respiratory acid–base disorders, systemic

bicarbonate administration, arterial blood gas measurement errors, enteral feeding products, and blood or stool in the gut may confound pHi determinations. Many clinicians believe that the change in gastric mucosal P_{CO_2} may be more accurate than pHi.

DESIRED OUTCOME

- The initial goal is to support O_2 delivery through the circulatory system by ensuring effective intravascular plasma volume, optimal O_2-carrying capacity, and adequate BP while definitive diagnostic and therapeutic strategies are being determined. The ultimate goals are to prevent further progression of the disease with subsequent organ damage and, if possible, to reverse organ dysfunction that has already occurred.

TREATMENT

GENERAL PRINCIPLES

- Fig. 12–1 and Fig. 12–2 contain algorithms for acute and ongoing management of adults with hypovolemia.
- Supplemental O_2 should be initiated at the earliest signs of shock, beginning with 4 to 6 L/min via nasal cannula or 6 to 10 L/min by face mask.
- Adequate fluid resuscitation to maintain circulating blood volume is essential in managing all forms of shock. Different therapeutic options are discussed in the next section.
- If fluid challenge does not achieve desired end points, pharmacologic support is necessary with inotropic and vasoactive drugs.

FLUID RESUSCITATION FOR HYPOVOLEMIC SHOCK

- Initial fluid resuscitation consists of isotonic crystalloid (**0.9% sodium chloride** or **lactated Ringer solution**), colloid (**5% Plasmanate** or **albumin** and **6% hetastarch**), or **whole blood**. Choice of solution is based on O_2-carrying capacity (e.g., hemoglobin and hematocrit), cause of hypovolemic shock, accompanying disease states, degree of fluid loss, and required speed of fluid delivery.
- Most clinicians agree that crystalloids should be the initial therapy of circulatory insufficiency. Crystalloids are preferred over colloids as initial therapy for burn patients because they are less likely to cause interstitial fluid accumulation. If volume resuscitation is suboptimal following several liters of crystalloid, colloids should be considered. Some patients may require blood products to ensure maintenance of O_2-carrying capacity, as well as clotting factors and platelets for blood hemostasis.

Crystalloids

- Crystalloids consist of electrolytes (e.g., Na^+, Cl^-, and K^+) in water solutions, with or without dextrose. **Lactated Ringer solution** may be preferred because it is unlikely to cause the hyperchloremic metabolic acidosis seen with infusion of large amounts of normal saline.

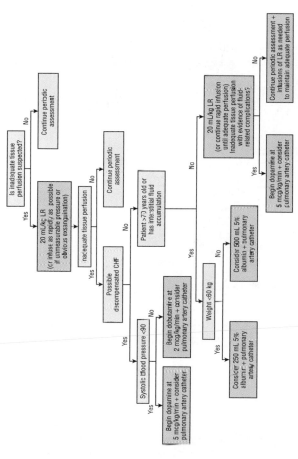

FIGURE 12–1. Hypovolemia protocol for adults. This protocol is not intended to replace or delay therapies such as surgical intervention or blood products for restoring O_2-carrying capacity or hemostasis. If available, some measurements may be used in addition to those listed in the algorithm, such as mean arterial pressure or pulmonary artery catheter recordings. The latter can be used to assist in medication choices (e.g., agents with primary pressor effects may be desirable in patients with normal cardiac outputs, whereas dopamine or dobutamine may be indicated in patients with suboptimal cardiac outputs). Lower maximal doses of the medications in this algorithm should be considered when pulmonary artery catheterization is not available. Colloids that may be substituted for albumin are hydroxyethyl starch 6% and dextran 40. (CHF, congestive heart failure; LR, lactated Ringer's solution.)

153

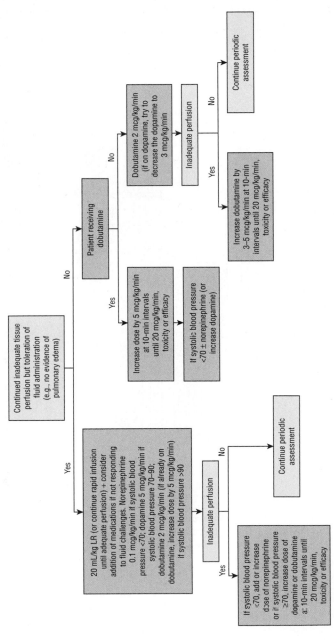

FIGURE 12–2. Ongoing management of inadequate tissue perfusion. (LR, lactated Ringer solution.)

- Crystalloids are administered at a rate of 500 to 2,000 mL/hour, depending on the severity of the deficit, degree of ongoing fluid loss, and tolerance to infusion volume. Usually 2 to 4 L of crystalloid normalizes intravascular volume.
- Advantages of crystalloids include rapidity and ease of administration, compatibility with most drugs, absence of serum sickness, and low cost.
- The primary disadvantage is the large volume necessary to replace or augment intravascular volume. Approximately 4 L of normal saline must be infused to replace 1 L of blood loss. In addition, dilution of colloid oncotic pressure leading to pulmonary edema is more likely to follow crystalloid than colloid resuscitation.

Colloids

- Colloids are larger molecular weight solutions (>30,000 daltons) that have been recommended for use in conjunction with or as replacements for crystalloid solutions. **Albumin** is a monodisperse colloid because all of its molecules are of the same molecular weight, whereas **hydroxyethyl starch** and **dextran** solutions are polydisperse compounds with molecules of varying molecular weights.
- The theoretical advantage of colloids is their prolonged intravascular retention time compared with crystalloid solutions. Isotonic crystalloid solutions have substantial interstitial distribution within minutes of IV administration, but colloids remain in the intravascular space for hours or days, depending on factors such as capillary permeability. However, even with intact capillary permeability, the colloid molecules eventually leak through capillary membranes.
- **Albumin** 5% and 25% concentrations are available. It takes approximately three to four times as much lactated Ringer or normal saline solution to yield the same volume expansion as 5% albumin solution. However, albumin is much more costly than crystalloid solutions. The 5% albumin solution is relatively iso-oncotic, whereas 25% albumin is hyperoncotic and tends to pull fluid into the compartment containing the albumin molecules. In general, 5% albumin is used for hypovolemic states. The 25% solution should not be used for acute circulatory insufficiency unless diluted with other fluids or unless it is being used in patients with excess total body water but intravascular depletion, as a means of pulling fluid into the intravascular space.
- **Hydroxyethyl starch** has comparable plasma expansion to 5% albumin solution but is usually less expensive, which accounts for much of its use. Hetastarch should be avoided in situations in which short-term impairments in hemostasis could have dire consequences (e.g., cardiopulmonary bypass surgery and intracranial hemorrhage), because it may aggravate bleeding. Hetastarch may cause elevations in serum amylase concentrations but does not cause pancreatitis.
- **Dextran 40, dextran 70,** and **dextran 75** are available for use as plasma expanders (the number indicates the average molecular weight × 1,000). These solutions are not used as often as albumin or hetastarch for plasma expansion, possibly due to concerns related to aggravation of bleeding (i.e., anticoagulant actions related to inhibiting stasis of microcirculation)

and anaphylaxis, which is more likely to occur with the higher molecular weight solutions.

- Colloids (especially albumin) are expensive solutions, and a large study involving almost 7,000 critically ill patients found no significant difference in 28–day mortality between patients resuscitated with either normal saline or 4% albumin. For these reasons, crystalloids should be considered first-line therapy in patients with hypovolemic shock.
- Adverse effects of colloids are generally extensions of their pharmacologic activity (e.g., fluid overload and dilutional coagulopathy). **Albumin** and **dextran** may be associated with anaphylactoid reactions or anaphylaxis. Bleeding may occur in certain patients receiving **hetastarch** and **dextran**.

Blood Products

- **Whole blood** could be used for large–volume blood loss, but most institutions use component therapy, with crystalloids or colloids used for plasma expansion.
- **Packed red blood cells** contain hemoglobin that increases the O_2-carrying capacity of blood, thereby increasing O_2 delivery to tissues. This is a function not performed by crystalloids or colloids. Packed red cells are usually indicated in patients with continued deterioration after volume replacement or obvious exsanguination. The product needs to be warmed before administration, especially when used in children.
- **Fresh frozen plasma** replaces clotting factors. Although it is often overused, the product is indicated if there is ongoing hemorrhage in patients with a prothrombin time (PT) or activated partial thromboplastin time (aPTT) >1.5 times normal, severe hepatic disease, or other bleeding disorders.
- **Platelets** are used for bleeding due to severe thrombocytopenia (platelet counts <10,000/mm³) or in patients with rapidly dropping platelet counts, as seen in massive bleeding.
- **Cryoprecipitate** and **factor VIII** are generally not indicated in acute hemorrhage but may be used once specific deficiencies have been identified.
- Risks associated with infusion of blood products include transfusion-related reactions, virus transmission (rare), hypocalcemia resulting from added citrate, elevations in serum potassium and phosphorus concentrations from use of stored blood that has hemolyzed, increased blood viscosity from supranormal hematocrit elevations, and hypothermia from failure to appropriately warm solutions before administration.

PHARMACOLOGIC THERAPY FOR SHOCK

- Inotropic agents and vasopressors are generally not indicated in the initial treatment of hypovolemic shock (assuming that fluid therapy is adequate), as the body's normal response is to increase CO and constrict blood vessels to maintain BP. However, once the cause of circulatory insufficiency has been stopped or treated and fluids have been optimized, medications may be needed in patients who continue to have signs and symptoms of inadequate tissue perfusion. Pressor agents such as **norepinephrine** and **high-dose dopamine** should be avoided if possible because they may increase BP at the expense of peripheral tissue ischemia. In patients with

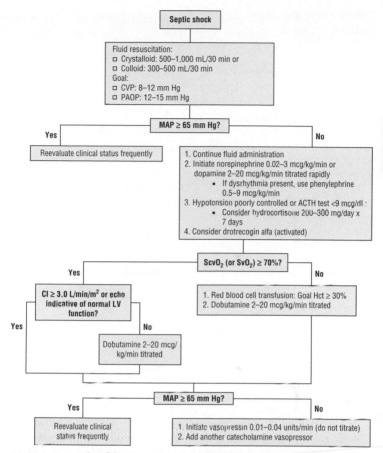

FIGURE 12–3. Algorithmic approach to resuscitative management of septic shock. Algorithmic approach is intended to be used in conjunction with clinical judgment, hemodynamic monitoring parameters, and therapy end points. (ACTH, adrenocorticotropic hormone; CI, cardiac index; CVP, central venous pressure; Hct, hematocrit; MAP, mean arterial pressure; PAOP, pulmonary artery occlusion pressure; ScvO₂, central venous O₂ saturation; SvO₂, mixed venous O₂ saturation.)

unstable BP despite massive fluid replacement and increasing interstitial fluid accumulation, inotropic agents such as **dobutamine** are preferred if BP is adequate (SBP ≥90 mm Hg) because they should not aggravate the existing vasoconstriction. When pressure cannot be maintained with inotropes, or when inotropes with vasodilatory properties cannot be used due to concerns about inadequate BP, pressors may be required as a last resort.

- The choice of vasopressor or inotropic agent in septic shock should be made according to the needs of the patient. An algorithm for the use of fluid resuscitation and these pharmacologic agents in septic shock is shown in **Fig. 12–3.** The traditional approach is to start with **dopamine,**

TABLE 12–2 Receptor Pharmacology of Selected Inotropic and Vasopressor Agents Used in Septic Shock[a]

Agent	α_1	α_2	β_1	β_2	D
Dobutamine (0.5–4 mg/mL D_5W or NS)					
2–10 mcg/kg/min	+	0	++++	++	0
>10–20 mcg/kg/min	++	0	++++	+++	0
Dopamine (0.8–3.2 mg/mL D_5W or NS)					
1–3 mcg/kg/min	0	0	+	0	++++
3–10 mcg/kg/min	0/+	0	++++	++	++++
>10–20 mcg/kg/min	+++	0	++++	+	0
Epinephrine (0.008–0.016 mg/mL D_5W or NS)					
0.01–0.05 mcg/kg/min	++	++	++++	+++	0
>0.05–3 mcg/kg/min	++++	++++	+++	+	0
Norepinephrine (0.016–0.064 mg/mL D_5W)					
0.02–3 mcg/kg/min	+++	+++	+++	+/++	0
Phenylephrine (0.1–0.4 mg/mL D_5W or NS)					
0.5–9 mcg/kg/min	+++	+	+	0	0

[a]Activity ranges from no activity (0) to maximal (++++) activity.

D, dopamine; D_5W, dextrose 5% in water; NS, normal saline.

then **norepinephrine; dobutamine** is added for low CO states, and occasionally **epinephrine** and **phenylephrine** are used when necessary. However, recent observations of improved outcomes with norepinephrine and decreased regional perfusion with dopamine are calling into question the use of dopamine as a first-line agent.

- The receptor selectivities of vasopressors and inotropes are listed in **Table 12–2**. In general, these drugs act rapidly with short durations of action and are given as continuous infusions. Potent vasoconstrictors such as norepinephrine and phenylephrine should be given through central veins due to the possibility of extravasation and tissue damage with peripheral administration. Careful monitoring and calculation of infusion rates are advised because dosing adjustments are made frequently, and varying admixture concentrations are used in volume-restricted patients.

- **Dopamine** is often the initial vasopressor used in septic shock because it increases BP by increasing myocardial contractility and vasoconstriction. Although dopamine has been reported to have dose-related receptor activity at dopamine, β_1, and α_1 receptors, this dose–response relationship has not been confirmed in critically ill patients. In patients with septic shock, there is overlap of hemodynamic effects with doses as low as 3 mcg/kg/min. Doses of 5 to 10 mcg/kg/min are initiated to improve mean arterial pressure (MAP). In septic shock, these doses increase CI by improving ventricular contractility, heart rate, MAP, and systemic vascular resistance (SVR). The clinical utility of dopamine in septic shock is limited because large doses are frequently necessary to maintain CO and MAP. At doses

>20 mcg/kg/min, there is limited further improvement in cardiac performance and regional hemodynamics. The use of dopamine is also hampered frequently by tachycardia and tachydysrhythmias. Other adverse effects limiting its use in septic shock include increases in PAOP, pulmonary shunting, and decreases in Pao_2. Dopamine should be used with caution in patients with elevated preload, as it may worsen pulmonary edema. Low doses of dopamine (1–3 mcg/kg/min) once were advocated for use in patients with septic shock receiving vasopressors with or without oliguria. The goal of therapy is to minimize or reverse renal vasoconstriction caused by other pressors, to prevent oliguric renal failure, or to convert it to nonoliguric renal failure. Based on recent clinical trial results, low-dose dopamine for treatment or prevention of acute renal failure cannot be justified and should be eliminated from routine clinical use.

- **Norepinephrine** is a combined α- and β-agonist, but it primarily produces vasoconstriction, thereby increasing SVR. It generally produces either no change or a slight decrease in CO. Norepinephrine is initiated after vasopressor doses of dopamine (4–20 mcg/kg/min), alone or in combination with dobutamine (5 mcg/kg/min), fail to achieve the desired goals. Doses of dopamine and dobutamine are kept constant or stopped; in some instances, dopamine is kept at low doses for purported renal protection. Norepinephrine, 0.01 to 2 mcg/kg/min, reliably and predictably improves hemodynamic parameters to normal or supranormal values in most patients with septic shock. Recent data suggest that norepinephrine should potentially be repositioned as the vasopressor of choice in septic shock.

- **Dobutamine** is primarily a selective β_1-agonist with mild β_2 and vascular α_1 activity, resulting in strong positive inotropic activity without concomitant vasoconstriction. Dobutamine produces a larger increase in CO and is less arrhythmogenic than dopamine. Clinically, β_2-induced vasodilation and the increased myocardial contractility with subsequent reflex reduction in sympathetic tone lead to a decrease in SVR. Even though dobutamine is optimally used for low CO states with high filling pressures or in cardiogenic shock, vasopressors may be needed to counteract arterial vasodilation. The addition of dobutamine (held constant at 5 mcg/kg/min) to epinephrine regimens can improve gastric mucosal perfusion as measured by improvements in pHi, arterial lactate concentrations, and Pco_2 gap. Dobutamine should be started with doses ranging from 2.5 to 5 mcg/kg/min. Doses >5 mcg/kg/min provide limited beneficial effects on O_2 transport values and hemodynamics and may increase adverse cardiac effects. Infusion rates should be guided by clinical end points and mixed venous O_2 saturation/central venous O_2 saturation. Decreases in partial pressure of O_2, as well as myocardial adverse effects such as tachycardia, ischemic changes on ECG, tachydysrhythmias, and hypotension, are seen.

- **Phenylephrine** is a pure α_1-agonist and is thought to increase BP through vasoconstriction. It may also increase contractility and CO. Phenylephrine may be beneficial in septic shock because of its selective α-agonism, vascular effects, rapid onset, and short duration. Phenylephrine may be a useful alternative in patients who cannot tolerate the tachycardia or tachydysrhythmias with use of dopamine or norepinephrine, in patients with known underlying myocardial dysfunction, and in patients refractory to dopamine or norepinephrine (because of β-receptor desensitization). It is generally initiated at dosages of 0.5 mcg/kg/min and may be titrated every 5 to 15 minutes to desired effects. Adverse effects such as tachydysrhythmias are infrequent when it is used as a single agent or with higher doses.

- **Epinephrine** has combined α- and β-agonist effects and has traditionally been reserved as the vasopressor of last resort because of reports of peripheral vasoconstriction, particularly in the splanchnic and renal beds. At the high infusion rates used in septic shock, α-adrenergic effects are predominantly seen, and SVR and MAP are increased. It is an acceptable single agent in septic shock due to its combined vasoconstrictor and inotropic effects. Epinephrine may be particularly useful when used earlier in the course of septic shock in young patients and those without known cardiac abnormalities. Infusion rates of 0.04 to 1 mcg/kg/min alone increase hemodynamic and O_2 transport variables to supranormal levels without adverse effects in patients without coronary heart disease. Large doses (0.5–1 mcg/kg/min) may be required when epinephrine is added to other agents. Smaller doses (0.1–0.5 mcg/kg/min) are effective if dobutamine and dopamine infusions are kept constant. Although Do_2 increases mainly as a function of consistent increases in CI (and a more variable increase in SVR), Vo_2 may not increase, and the O_2 extraction ratio may fall. Lactate concentrations may rise during the first few hours of epinephrine therapy but normalize over the ensuing 24 hours in survivors. Caution must be used before considering epinephrine for managing hypoperfusion in hypodynamic patients with coronary artery disease to avoid ischemia, chest pain, and myocardial infarction.
- **Vasopressin** causes vasoconstrictive effects that, unlike adrenergic receptor agonists, are preserved during hypoxia and severe acidosis. It also causes vasodilation in the pulmonary, coronary, and selected renal vascular beds that may reduce PAP and preserve cardiac and renal function. However, based on available evidence, vasopressin is not recommended as a replacement for norepinephrine or dopamine in patients with septic shock but may be considered in patients who are refractory to catecholamine vasopressors despite adequate fluid resuscitation. If used, the dose should not exceed .04 unit/min.
- **Corticosteroids** were shown in a meta-analysis to improve hemodynamics and survival and reduce the duration of vasopressor support in septic shock. Corticosteroids can be initiated in septic shock when adrenal insufficiency is present or when weaning of vasopressor therapy proves futile. A daily dose equivalent to 200 to 300 mg hydrocortisone should be continued for 7 days. Adverse events are few because of the short duration of therapy.

EVALUATION OF THERAPEUTIC OUTCOMES

- The initial monitoring of a patient with suspected volume depletion should include vital signs, urine output, mental status, and physical examination.
- Placement of a CVP line provides a useful (although indirect and insensitive) estimate of the relationship between increased right atrial pressure and CO.

- The indications for pulmonary artery catheterization are controversial. Because there is a lack of a well-defined outcome of data associated with this procedure, its use is presently best reserved for complicated cases of shock not responding to conventional fluid and medication therapies. Complications related to catheter insertion, maintenance, and removal include damage to vessels and organs during insertion, arrhythmias, infections, and thromboembolic damage.
- Laboratory tests indicated for the ongoing monitoring of shock include electrolytes and renal function tests (BUN and serum creatinine); CBC to assess possible infection, O_2-carrying capacity of the blood, and ongoing bleeding; PT and aPTT to assess clotting ability; and lactate concentration and base deficit to detect inadequate tissue perfusion.
- Cardiovascular and respiratory parameters should be monitored continuously (see Table 12–1). Trends, rather than specific CVP or PAOP numbers, should be monitored because of interpatient variability in response.
- Successful fluid resuscitation should increase SBP (>90 mm Hg), CI (>2.2 L/min/m²), and urine output (0.5–1 mL/kg/hour) while decreasing SVR to the normal range. MAP >60 mm Hg should be achieved to ensure adequate cerebral and coronary perfusion pressure.
- Intravascular volume overload is characterized by high filling pressures (CVP >12–15 mm Hg, PAOP >20–24 mm Hg) and decreased CO (<3.5 L/min). If volume overload occurs, furosemide, 20 to 40 mg, should be administered by slow IV push to produce rapid diuresis of intravascular volume and "unload" the heart through venous dilation.
- Coagulation problems are primarily associated with low levels of clotting factors in stored blood, as well as dilution of endogenous clotting factors and platelets following administration of the blood. As a result, a coagulation panel (PT, international normalized ratio, and aPTT) should be checked in patients undergoing replacement of 50% to 100% of blood volume in 12 to 24 hours.

See Chapter 30, Use of Vasopressors and Inotropes in the Pharmacotherapy of Shock, authored by Robert MacLaren, Maria I. Rudis, and Joseph F. Dasta, and Chapter 31, Hypovolemic Shock, authored by Brian L. Erstad, for a more detailed discussion of this topic.

Stroke

DEFINITION

- *Stroke* is a term used to describe an abrupt onset of focal neurologic deficit that lasts at least 24 hours and is presumed to be of vascular origin. Stroke can be either ischemic or hemorrhagic in origin. Transient ischemic attacks (TIAs) are focal ischemic neurologic deficits lasting less than 24 hours and usually less than 30 minutes.

PATHOPHYSIOLOGY

RISK FACTORS FOR STROKE

- Nonmodifiable risk factors for stroke include increased age, male gender, race (African Americans, Asian–Pacific Islanders, and Hispanics), family history of stroke, and low birth weight.
- The major modifiable risk factors include hypertension and cardiac disease (especially atrial fibrillation).
- Other major risk factors are diabetes mellitus, dyslipidemia, and cigarette smoking.

ISCHEMIC STROKE

- Ischemic strokes account for 88% of all strokes and are due either to local thrombus formation or to emboli that occlude a cerebral artery. Cerebral atherosclerosis is a causative factor in most cases of ischemic stroke, although 30% are of unknown etiology. Emboli can arise either from intra- or extracranial arteries. Twenty percent of embolic strokes arise from the heart.
- In carotid atherosclerosis, plaques may rupture, resulting in collagen exposure, platelet aggregation, and thrombus formation. The clot may cause local occlusion or may dislodge and travel distally, eventually occluding a cerebral vessel.
- In cardiogenic embolism, stasis of blood flow in the atria or ventricles leads to formation of local clots that can dislodge and travel through the aorta to the cerebral circulation.
- The final result of both thrombus formation and embolism is arterial occlusion, decreasing cerebral blood flow and causing ischemia and ultimately infarction distal to the occlusion.

HEMORRHAGIC STROKE

- Hemorrhagic strokes account for 12% of strokes and include subarachnoid hemorrhage, intracerebral hemorrhage, and subdural hematomas. Subarachnoid hemorrhage may result from trauma or rupture of an intracranial aneurysm or arteriovenous malformation (AVM). Intracerebral hemorrhage occurs when a ruptured blood vessel within the brain parenchyma causes formation of a hematoma. Subdural hematomas are most often caused by trauma.

- The presence of blood in the brain parenchyma causes damage to surrounding tissue through a mass effect and the neurotoxicity of blood components and their degradation products. Much of the early mortality of hemorrhagic stroke is due to an abrupt increase in intracranial pressure that can lead to herniation and death.

CLINICAL PRESENTATION

- The patient may not be able to give a reliable history because of cognitive or language deficits. This information may need to be obtained from family members or other witnesses.
- The patient may experience weakness on one side of the body, inability to speak, loss of vision, vertigo, or falling. Ischemic stroke is not usually painful, but headache may occur and may be severe in hemorrhagic stroke.
- Patients usually have multiple signs of neurologic dysfunction on physical examination. The specific deficits observed depend on the area of the brain involved. Hemi- or monoparesis and hemisensory deficits are common. Patients with posterior circulation involvement may present with vertigo and diplopia. Anterior circulation strokes commonly result in aphasia. Patients may also experience dysarthria, visual field defects, and altered levels of consciousness.

DIAGNOSIS

- Laboratory tests for hypercoagulable states should be done only when the cause of the stroke cannot be determined based on the presence of well-known risk factors. Protein C, protein S, and antithrombin III are best measured in steady state rather than in the acute stage. Antiphospholipid antibodies are of higher yield but should be reserved for patients younger than age 50 and those who have had multiple venous or arterial thrombotic events or livedo reticularis.
- Computed tomography (CT) head scan will reveal an area of hyperintensity (white) in an area of hemorrhage and will be normal or hypointense (dark) in an area of infarction. The area of infarction may not be visible on CT scan for 24 hours (and rarely longer).
- Magnetic resonance imaging (MRI) of the head will reveal areas of ischemia with higher resolution and earlier than the CT scan. Diffusion-weighted imaging will reveal an evolving infarct within minutes.
- Carotid Doppler (CD) studies will determine whether there is a high degree of stenosis in the carotid arteries.
- The electrocardiogram (ECG) will determine whether atrial fibrillation is present as a possible etiologic factor.
- A transthoracic echocardiogram (TTE) can detect valve or wall motion abnormalities that are sources of emboli to the brain.
- A transesophageal echocardiogram (TEE) is a more sensitive test for left atrial thrombus. It is also effective in examining the aortic arch for atheroma, another potential source of emboli.

- Transcranial Doppler (TCD) can determine the presence of intracranial sclerosis (e.g., middle cerebral artery stenosis).

DESIRED OUTCOME

- The goals of treatment for acute stroke are to (1) reduce the ongoing neurologic injury and decrease mortality and long-term disability, (2) prevent complications secondary to immobility and neurologic dysfunction, and (3) prevent stroke recurrence.

TREATMENT

GENERAL APPROACH

- The initial approach is to ensure adequate respiratory and cardiac support and to determine quickly whether the lesion is ischemic or hemorrhagic based on a CT scan.
- Ischemic stroke patients presenting within hours of symptom onset should be evaluated for reperfusion therapy.
- Elevated blood pressure (BP) should remain untreated in the acute period (first 7 days) after ischemic stroke because of the risk of decreasing cerebral blood flow and worsening symptoms. The pressure should be lowered if it exceeds 220/120 mm Hg or there is evidence of aortic dissection, acute myocardial infarction (MI), pulmonary edema, or hypertensive encephalopathy. If BP is treated in the acute phase, short-acting parenteral agents (e.g., labetalol, nicardipine, and nitroprusside) are preferred.
- Patients with hemorrhagic stroke should be assessed to determine whether they are candidates for surgical intervention.
- After the hyperacute phase has passed, attention is focused on preventing progressive deficits, minimizing complications, and instituting appropriate secondary prevention strategies.

NONPHARMACOLOGIC THERAPY

- In acute ischemic stroke, surgical interventions are limited. However, surgical decompression can be lifesaving in cases of significant swelling associated with cerebral infarction. An interdisciplinary approach to stroke care that includes early rehabilitation is very effective in reducing long-term disability. In secondary prevention, carotid endarterectomy is effective in reducing stroke incidence and recurrence in appropriate patients. Carotid stenting may be effective in reducing recurrent stroke risk in patients at high risk of complications from endarterectomy.
- In subarachnoid hemorrhage due to a ruptured intracranial aneurysm or AVM, surgical intervention to clip or ablate the vascular abnormality substantially reduces mortality from rebleeding. The benefits of surgery are less well documented in cases of primary intracerebral hemorrhage. Some patients with intracerebral hematomas may undergo surgical evacuation; insertion of an external ventricular drain with monitoring of intracranial pressure is commonly performed in these patients.

PHARMACOLOGIC THERAPY OF ISCHEMIC STROKE

- The Stroke Council of the American Stroke Association guidelines for the management of acute ischemic stroke give grade I recommendations to only two pharmacologic therapies: (1) IV tissue plasminogen activator (alteplase) within 4.5 hours of onset and (2) aspirin within 48 hours of onset. Evidence-based recommendations for pharmacotherapy of ischemic stroke are given in **Table 13–1**.

- **Alteplase** initiated within 4.5 hours of symptom onset has been shown to reduce the ultimate disability due to ischemic stroke. Adherence to a strict protocol is essential to achieving positive outcomes: (1) activate the stroke team; (2) treat as early as possible within 4.5 hours of onset; (3) obtain CT scan to rule out hemorrhage; (4) meet all inclusion and no exclusion criteria (**Table 13–2**); (5) administer alteplase 0.9 mg/kg (maximum 90 mg) infused IV over 1 hour, with 10% given as initial bolus over 1 minute; (6) avoid anticoagulant and antiplatelet therapy for 24 hours; and (7) monitor the patient closely for elevated BP, response, and hemorrhage.

TABLE 13–1	Recommendations for Pharmacotherapy of Ischemic Stroke	
	Recommendation	**Evidence[a]**
Acute treatment	Alteplase 0.9 mg/kg IV (max 90 mg) over 1 hour in select patients within 3 hours of onset	IA
	Alteplase 0.9 mg/kg IV (max 90 mg) over 1 hour between 3 and 4.5 hours of onset	IB
	Aspirin 160–325 mg daily started within 48 hours of onset	IA
Secondary prevention		
Noncardioembolic	Antiplatelet therapy	IA
	Aspirin 50–325 mg daily	IIa A (all three as initial options
	Clopidogrel 75 mg daily	IIb B (over aspirin)
	Aspirin 25 mg + extended release dipyridamole 200 mg twice daily	IIa A (over aspirin)
Cardioembolic (esp. atrial fibrillation)	Warfarin (INR = 2.5)	IA
All patients	Antihypertensive treatment	IA
Previously hypertensive	ACE inhibitor + diuretic	IA
Previously normotensive	ACE inhibitor + diuretic	IIa B
Dyslipidemic	Statin	IA
Normal lipids	Statin	IB

ACE, angiotensin-converting enzyme; INR, international normalized ratio.
[a]Classes of evidence: I, evidence or general agreement that treatment is useful and effective; II, conflicting evidence about usefulness; IIa, weight of evidence in favor of the treatment; IIb, usefulness less well established. Levels of evidence: A, multiple randomized clinical trials; B, a single randomized trial or nonrandomized studies; C, expert consensus or case studies.

TABLE 13–2	Inclusion and Exclusion Criteria for Alteplase Use in Acute Ischemic Stroke

Inclusion Criteria (all YES boxes must be checked before treatment)

YES

- ❑ Age 18 years or older
- ❑ Clinical diagnosis of ischemic stroke causing a measurable neurologic deficit
- ❑ Time of symptom onset well established to be less than 4.5 hours before treatment would begin

Exclusion Criteria (all NO boxes must be checked before treatment)

NO

- ❑ Evidence of intracranial hemorrhage on noncontrast head CT
- ❑ Only minor or rapidly improving stroke symptoms
- ❑ High clinical suspicion of subarachnoid hemorrhage even with normal CT
- ❑ Active internal bleeding (e.g., GI/GU bleeding within 21 days)
- ❑ Known bleeding diathesis, including but not limited to platelet count <100,000/mm^3
- ❑ Patient has received heparin within 48 hours and had an elevated aPTT
- ❑ Recent use of anticoagulant (e.g., warfarin) and elevated PT (>15 s)/INR
- ❑ Intracranial surgery, serious head trauma, or previous stroke within 3 months
- ❑ Major surgery or serious trauma within 14 days
- ❑ Recent arterial puncture at noncompressible site
- ❑ Lumbar puncture within 7 days
- ❑ History of intracranial hemorrhage, arteriovenous malformation, or aneurysm
- ❑ Witnessed seizure at stroke onset
- ❑ Recent acute myocardial infarction
- ❑ SBP >185 mm Hg or DBP >110 mm Hg at time of treatment

Additional exclusion criteria if within 3–4.5 hours of onset:

- ❑ Age greater than 80 years
- ❑ Current treatment with oral anticoagulants
- ❑ NIH Stroke scale >25 (severe stroke)
- ❑ History of both stroke and diabetes

aPTT, activated partial thromboplastin time; CT, computed tomography; DBP, diastolic blood pressure; GI, gastrointestinal; GU, genitourinary; INR, international normalized ratio; NIH, National Institutes of Health; PT, prothrombin time; SBP, systolic blood pressure.

- **Aspirin** 50 to 325 mg/day started between 24 and 48 hours after completion of alteplase has also been shown to reduce long-term death and disability.
- For secondary stroke prevention, all patients who have had an acute ischemic stroke or TIA should receive long-term antithrombotic therapy. In patients with noncardioembolic stroke, this involves antiplatelet therapy. **Aspirin, clopidogrel,** and **extended-release dipyridamole plus aspirin** are all considered first-line antiplatelet agents (see **Table 13–1**). The combination of aspirin and clopidogrel can only be recommended in patients with ischemic stroke and a recent history of MI or coronary stent placement and then only with ultra-low-dose aspirin to minimize bleeding risk.

TABLE 13-3	Monitoring Hospitalized Acute Stroke Patients		
	Treatment	**Parameter(s)**	**Frequency**
Ischemic stroke	Alteplase	BP, neurologic function, bleeding	Every 15 minutes × 1 hour; every 0.5 hour × 6 hours; every 1 hour × 17 hours; every shift after
	Aspirin	Bleeding	Daily
	Clopidogrel	Bleeding	Daily
	ERDP/ASA	Headache, bleeding	Daily
	Warfarin	Bleeding, INR, Hb/Hct	INR daily × 3 days; weekly until stable; monthly
Hemorrhagic stroke		BP, neurologic function, ICP	Every 2 hours in ICU
	Nimodipine (for SAH)	BP, neurologic function, fluid status	Every 2 hours in ICU
All patients		Temperature, CBC	Temperature every 8 hours; CBC daily
		Pain (calf or chest)	Every 8 hours
		Electrolytes and ECG	Up to daily
	Heparins for DVT prophylaxis	Bleeding, platelets	Bleeding daily, platelets if suspected thrombocytopenia

BP, blood pressure; CBC, complete blood cell count; DVT, deep vein thrombosis; ECG, electrocardiogram; ERDP/ASA, extended-release dipyridamole plus aspirin; Hb, hemoglobin; Hct, hematocrit; ICP, intracranial pressure; ICU, intensive care unit; INR, international normalized ratio; SAH, subarachnoid hemorrhage.

- **Warfarin** is the antithrombotic agent of first choice for secondary prevention in patients with atrial fibrillation and a presumed cardiac source of embolism.
- Elevated BP is common after ischemic stroke, and its treatment is associated with a decreased risk of stroke recurrence. An **angiotensin-converting enzyme (ACE) inhibitor and a diuretic** are recommended for reduction of blood pressure in patients with stroke or TIA after the acute period (first 7 days). **Angiotensin II receptor blockers** have also been shown to reduce the risk of stroke and should be considered in patients unable to tolerate ACE inhibitors after acute ischemic stroke.
- The National Cholesterol Education Program considers ischemic stroke or TIA to be a coronary risk equivalent and recommends the use of **statins** in ischemic stroke patients to achieve a low-density lipoprotein cholesterol concentration <100 mg/dL. It is now recommended that ischemic stroke patients, regardless of baseline cholesterol, be treated with high-dose statin therapy for secondary stroke prevention.
- **Low-molecular-weight heparin** or **low-dose subcutaneous unfractionated heparin** (5,000 units three times daily) is recommended for prevention of deep vein thrombosis in hospitalized patients with decreased mobility due to stroke and should be used in all but the most minor strokes.

- The use of **full-dose unfractionated heparin** in the acute stroke period has not been proven to positively affect stroke outcome, and it significantly increases the risk of intracerebral hemorrhage. Trials of low-molecular-weight heparins and heparinoids have been largely negative and do not support their routine use in stroke patients.

PHARMACOLOGIC THERAPY OF HEMORRHAGIC STROKE

- There are currently no standard pharmacologic strategies for treating intracerebral hemorrhage. Medical guidelines for managing BP, increased intracranial pressure, and other medical complications in acutely ill patients in neurointensive care units should be followed.
- Subarachnoid hemorrhage due to aneurysm rupture is associated with a high incidence of delayed cerebral ischemia in the 2 weeks after the bleeding episode. Vasospasm of the cerebral vasculature is thought to be responsible for the delayed ischemia and occurs between 4 and 21 days after the bleed. The calcium channel blocker **nimodipine** 60 mg every 4 hours for 21 days, along with maintenance of intravascular volume with pressor therapy, is recommended to reduce the incidence and severity of neurologic deficits resulting from delayed ischemia.

EVALUATION OF THERAPEUTIC OUTCOMES

- Patients with acute stroke should be monitored intensely for the development of neurologic worsening (recurrence or extension), complications (thromboembolism, infection), and adverse effects from treatments.
- The most common reasons for clinical deterioration in stroke patients are (1) extension of the original lesion in the brain, (2) development of cerebral edema and raised intracranial pressure, (3) hypertensive emergency, (4) infection (e.g., urinary and respiratory tract), (5) venous thromboembolism, (6) electrolyte abnormalities and rhythm disturbances, and (7) recurrent stroke. The approach to monitoring stroke patients is summarized in **Table 13–3**.

See Chapter 27, Stroke, authored by Susan C. Fagan and David C. Hess, for a more detailed discussion of this topic.

14 Venous Thromboembolism

DEFINITION

- Venous thromboembolism (VTE) results from clot formation in the venous circulation and is manifested as deep vein thrombosis (DVT) and pulmonary embolism (PE). A DVT is a thrombus composed of cellular material (red and white blood cells and platelets) bound together with fibrin strands. A PE is a thrombus that arises from the systemic circulation and lodges in the pulmonary artery or one of its branches, causing complete or partial obstruction of pulmonary blood flow.

PATHOPHYSIOLOGY

- Hemostasis occurs in three overlapping steps: initiation, amplification, and propagation (**Fig. 14–1**).
- The normal hemostatic process is initiated by vascular injury, which allows platelets and factor VIII complexed to von Willebrand factor to come into contact with collagen and tissue factor–bearing cells in the extravascular space. These cells produce small amounts of thrombin via what has traditionally been termed the "extrinsic" coagulation pathway (i.e., the factor VIIa/tissue factor complex and the factor Xa/Va complex).
- Thrombin amplifies the hemostatic process by inducing platelets that were partially activated during adherence to collagen to higher levels of procoagulant activity.
- Thrombin also activates cofactors V, VIII, and XI on platelet surfaces in preparation for large-scale thrombin production. This propagation phase has traditionally been called the "intrinsic" pathway (i.e., factor XIa, the factor IXa/VIIIa complex, and the factor Xa/Va complex) occurring on the surface of activated platelets.
- The final step in hemostasis is the thrombin-mediated conversion of fibrinogen to fibrin monomers, which precipitate and polymerize to form fibrin strands. Factor XIIIa covalently bonds these strands to one another. Local fibrin deposition forms a meshwork that encases aggregated platelets to form a stabilized clot that seals the site of vascular injury and prevents blood loss.
- The coagulation process is controlled by several antithrombotic substances secreted by intact endothelium adjacent to damaged tissue. Thrombomodulin modulates thrombin activity by converting protein C to its activated form (aPC), which joins with protein S to inactivate factors Va and VIIIa. This prevents coagulation reactions from spreading to healthy, uninjured vessel walls. In addition, circulating antithrombin inhibits thrombin and factor Xa. Heparan sulfate is secreted by endothelial cells and accelerates antithrombin activity. Heparin cofactor II also inhibits thrombin.

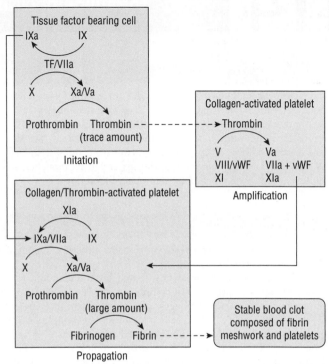

FIGURE 14–1. Coagulation cascade. (TF, tissue factor; vWF, von Willebrand factor.)

- The fibrinolytic system dissolves formed blood clots; plasminogen is converted to plasmin by tissue plasminogen activator and urokinase plasminogen activator. Plasmin degrades the fibrin mesh into soluble end products known as fibrin split products or fibrin degradation products.
- Alterations in any one of three primary components can lead to pathologic clot formation—blood vessels, circulating elements in the blood, and the speed of blood flow (Virchow triad).
- Vascular injury occurs in patients who sustain trauma (especially fractures of the pelvis, hip, or leg), undergo major orthopedic surgery (e.g., knee and hip replacement), or have indwelling venous catheters.
- Hypercoagulable states include malignancy; activated protein C resistance; deficiency of protein C, protein S, or antithrombin; excessively high concentrations of factor VIII, IX, and/or XI or fibrinogen; antiphospholipid antibodies; estrogen use; and other situations.
- Venous stasis favors thrombogenesis in part through reduced clearance of activated clotting factors from sites of thrombus formation. Stasis can result from damage to venous valves, vessel obstruction, prolonged immobility, or increased blood viscosity. Conditions associated with venous stasis include major medical illness (e.g., heart failure and myocardial

infarction), major surgery, paralysis (resulting from, e.g., stroke or spinal cord injury), polycythemia vera, obesity, or varicose veins.

- Although a thrombus can form in any part of the venous circulation, the majority of thrombi begin in the lower extremities. Once formed, a venous thrombus may (1) remain asymptomatic, (2) lyse spontaneously, (3) obstruct the venous circulation, (4) propagate into more proximal veins, (5) embolize, or (6) act in any combination of these ways. Even asymptomatic patients may experience long-term consequences, such as postthrombotic syndrome and recurrent VTE.

CLINICAL PRESENTATION

- Many patients with VTE never develop symptoms from the acute event.
- Symptoms of DVT include unilateral leg swelling, pain, tenderness, erythema, and warmth. Physical signs may include a palpable cord and a positive Homans sign.
- Postthrombotic syndrome (a long-term complication of DVT caused by damage to venous valves) may produce chronic lower extremity swelling, pain, tenderness, skin discoloration, and ulceration.
- Symptoms of PE include dyspnea, tachypnea, pleuritic chest pain, tachycardia, palpitations, cough, diaphoresis, and hemoptysis. Cardiovascular collapse, characterized by cyanosis, shock, and oliguria, is an ominous sign.

DIAGNOSIS

- Assessment of the patient's status should focus on the search for risk factors (e.g., increased age, major surgery, previous VTE, trauma, malignancy, hypercoagulable states, and drug therapy). Signs and symptoms of DVT are nonspecific, and objective tests are required to confirm or exclude the diagnosis.
- Radiographic contrast studies are the most accurate and reliable method for diagnosis of VTE. Contrast venography allows visualization of the entire venous system in the lower extremity and abdomen. Pulmonary angiography allows visualization of the pulmonary arteries. The diagnosis of VTE can be made if there is a persistent intraluminal filling defect on multiple radiographic films.
- Because contrast studies are expensive, invasive, and technically difficult to perform and evaluate, noninvasive tests (e.g., ultrasonography, computed tomography scans, and the ventilation-perfusion scan) are used frequently for the initial evaluation of patients with suspected VTE.
- D-dimer is a degradation product of fibrin blood clots, and blood levels are substantially elevated in patients with acute thrombosis. Although the D-dimer test is a very sensitive marker of clot formation, elevated levels can result from a variety of other conditions (e.g., recent surgery or trauma, pregnancy, and cancer). Therefore, a negative test can help exclude the diagnosis of VTE, but a positive test is not conclusive evidence of the diagnosis.

DESIRED OUTCOME

- The objectives of treating VTE are to prevent the development of PE and postthrombotic syndrome, to reduce morbidity and mortality from the acute event, and to minimize adverse effects and cost of treatment.

TREATMENT

(**Fig. 14–2** and **Table 14–1**)

UNFRACTIONATED HEPARIN

- **Unfractionated heparin (UFH)** is a heterogeneous mixture of sulfated mucopolysaccharides of variable lengths and pharmacologic properties. The molecular weight of these molecules ranges from 3,000 to 30,000 daltons (mean 15,000 daltons).
- The anticoagulant effect of UFH is mediated through a specific pentasaccharide sequence on the heparin molecule that binds to antithrombin, provoking a conformational change. The UFH–antithrombin complex is 100 to 1,000 times more potent as an anticoagulant than antithrombin alone. Antithrombin inhibits the activity of factors IXa, Xa, XIIa, and thrombin (IIa). It also inhibits thrombin-induced activation of factors V and VIII.
- UFH prevents the growth and propagation of a formed thrombus and allows the patient's own thrombolytic system to degrade the clot.
- UFH must be given parenterally, preferably by the IV or subcutaneous (SC) route. Intramuscular administration is discouraged because absorption is erratic, and it may cause large hematomas.
- When immediate and full anticoagulation is required, a weight-based IV bolus dose followed by a continuous IV infusion is preferred (**Table 14–2**). SC UFH (initial dose 333 units/kg followed by 250 units/kg every 12 hours) also provides adequate anticoagulation for treatment of acute VTE.
- The activated partial thromboplastin time (aPTT) with a therapeutic range of 1.5 to 2.5 times the mean normal control value has traditionally been used to determine the degree of therapeutic anticoagulation. Because of interlaboratory variability in aPTT, an institution-specific aPTT therapeutic range that correlates with a plasma heparin concentration of 0.3 to 0.7 unit/mL should be established. The aPTT should be measured prior to initiation of therapy and 6 hours after the start of therapy or a dose change. The dose of heparin should be adjusted promptly based on the patient's response and the institution-specific therapeutic range (see **Table 14–2**).
- Bleeding is the primary adverse effect associated with all anticoagulant drugs. The most common bleeding sites are the GI tract, urinary tract, and soft tissues. Critical areas include intracranial, pericardial, and intraocular sites, as well as the adrenal glands. Symptoms of bleeding may include severe headache, joint pain, chest pain, abdominal pain, swelling, tarry stools, hematuria, or the passing of bright red blood

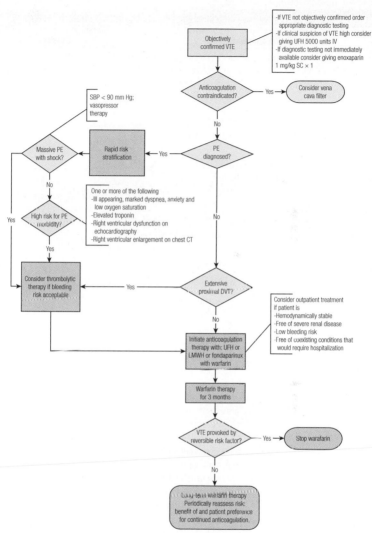

FIGURE 14–2. Treatment of venous thromboembolism (VTE). (DVT, deep vein thrombosis; LMWH, low-molecular-weight heparin; PE, pulmonary embolism; SBP, systolic blood pressure; UFH, unfractionated heparin.)

through the rectum. Minor bleeding occurs frequently (e.g., epistaxis, gingival bleeding, prolonged bleeding from cuts, and bruising from minor trauma).

- If major bleeding occurs, UFH should be discontinued immediately, and IV **protamine sulfate** should be given by slow IV infusion over 10 minutes (1 mg/100 units of UFH infused during the previous 4 hours; maximum 50 mg).

TABLE 14–1	Consensus Guidelines for Venous Thromboembolism Treatment	
	Recommendation	**Grade**[a]
Acute anticoagulation	Acute treatment of DVT or PE should be with SC LMWH, fondaparinux, or fixed-dose UFH; IV UFH; or adjusted-dose SC UFH	1A
	The dose of monitored UFH (SC or IV) should be sufficient to prolong the aPTT to a range that corresponds to a plasma heparin level of 0.3 to 0.7 international units/mL anti-Xa activity	1C
	LMWH (as an outpatient if possible) is recommended rather than IV UFH for patients with acute DVT	1C (outpatient); 1A (inpatient)
	UFH is suggested over LMWH for patients with severe renal failure	2C
Duration of acute treatment	Treatment with UFH, LMWH, or fondaparinux should be overlapped with warfarin for at least 5 days and until the INR is ≥2.0 for 24 hours	1C
	Warfarin should be initiated together with UFH, LMWH, or fondaparinux on the first treatment day	1A
	Patients with cancer should be treated with an LMWH for the first 3 to 6 months	1A
Long-term anticoagulation	Warfarin (target INR 2.5, range 2–3) should be continued for at least 3 months *in all patients*	1A
	All patients with unprovoked VTE should be evaluated for the risk–benefit ratio of long-term anticoagulation	1C
	Patients with a first unprovoked proximal DVT or PE who are at low risk for bleeding and for whom good anticoagulant monitoring is achievable should receive long-term anticoagulation	1A
	Patients with recurrent unprovoked VTE should receive long-term anticoagulation	1A
	Patients receiving long-term anticoagulation should receive periodic reassessment of the risk–benefit ratio of continuing anticoagulation	1C
	In patients with cancer, following 3 to 6 months of LMWH, subsequent anticoagulation with either warfarin or LMWH should continue indefinitely or until the cancer is resolved	1C

aPTT, activated partial thromboplastin time; DVT, deep vein thrombosis; INR, international normalized ratio; IV, intravenous; LMWH, low-molecular-weight heparin; PE, pulmonary embolism; SC, subcutaneous; UFH, unfractionated heparin; VTE, venous thromboembolism.

[a]Refers to grade of recommendation (1A, strong recommendation applying to most patients in most circumstances; 1C, strong recommendation applying to most patients in most circumstances; 2C, weak recommendation in which alternative approaches are likely to be better for some patients under some circumstances).

TABLE 14–2	Weight-based[a] Dosing for Unfractionated Heparin Administered by Continuous IV Infusion	
Indication	**Initial Loading Dose**	**Initial Infusion Rate**
Deep vein thrombosis/pulmonary embolism	80–100 units/kg Maximum = 10,000 units	17–20 units/kg/hour Maximum = 2,300 units/hour
Activated Partial Thromboplastin Time (seconds)	**Maintenance Infusion Rate** **Dose Adjustment**	
<37 (or >12 s below institution-specific therapeutic range)	80 units/kg bolus, then increase infusion by 4 units/kg/hour	
37–47 (or 1–12 s below institution-specific therapeutic range)	40 units/kg bolus, then increase infusion by 2 units/kg/hour	
48–71 (or within institution-specific therapeutic range)	No change	
72–93 (or 1–22 s above institution-specific therapeutic range)	Decrease infusion by 2 units/kg/hour	
>93 (or >22 s above institution-specific therapeutic range)	Hold infusion for 1 hour, then decrease by 3 units/kg/hour	

[a]Use actual body weight for all calculations. Adjusted body weight may be used for obese patients (>130% of ideal body weight).

- Thrombocytopenia (platelet count <150,000/mm³) is common, and two distinct types can occur:
  ✓ Heparin-associated thrombocytopenia (HAT) is a benign, transient, and mild phenomenon that usually occurs within the first few days of treatment. Platelet counts rarely drop below 100,000/mm³ and recover with continued therapy.
  ✓ Heparin-induced thrombocytopenia (HIT) is a serious immune-mediated problem that requires immediate intervention. For patients receiving therapeutic UFH doses, a baseline platelet count should be obtained before therapy is initiated and then every other day for 14 days or until therapy is stopped, whichever occurs first. HIT should be suspected if a patient develops a thromboembolic event during or soon after receiving UFH. The platelet count invariably drops by more than 50% from baseline and is typically <150,000/mm³. Platelet counts typically begin to fall after 5 to 10 days of UFH therapy but may drop sooner if the patient has received UFH in the past 3 months. Laboratory testing to detect heparin antibodies must be performed to confirm the diagnosis of HIT. All sources of heparin (including heparin flushes) should be discontinued immediately, and an alternative anticoagulant should be initiated. Anticoagulants that rapidly inhibit thrombin activity and are devoid of significant cross-reactivity with heparin–PF-4 antibodies are the drugs of choice. The direct thrombin inhibitors **lepirudin** and **argatroban** are FDA approved for this use; **bivalirudin** is also commercially available (see section on direct thrombin inhibitors).

- Bruising, local irritation, mild pain, erythema, histamine-like reactions, and hematoma can occur at the site of injection. Long-term UFH has been reported to cause alopecia, priapism, hyperkalemia, and osteoporosis.

LOW-MOLECULAR-WEIGHT HEPARINS

- Low-molecular-weight heparins (LMWHs) are fragments of UFH that are heterogeneous mixtures of sulfated glycosaminoglycans with approximately one third the molecular weight of UFH.
- Advantages of LMWHs over UFH include (1) predictable anticoagulation dose response, (2) improved SC bioavailability, (3) dose-independent clearance, (4) longer biologic half-life, (5) lower incidence of thrombocytopenia, and (6) less need for routine laboratory monitoring.
- Like UFH, the LMWHs enhance and accelerate the activity of antithrombin and prevent the growth and propagation of formed thrombi. The peak anticoagulant effect is seen in 3 to 5 hours after SC dosing.
- The usefulness of LMWHs has been evaluated extensively for many indications, including acute coronary syndromes, DVT, PE, and prevention of VTE in several high-risk populations.
- LMWHs are given in fixed or weight-based doses based on the product and indication. The recommended doses (based on actual body weight) for treatment of DVT with or without PE are
  - ✓ **Enoxaparin** (Lovenox): 1 mg/kg SC every 12 hours or 1.5 mg/kg every 24 hours
  - ✓ **Dalteparin** (Fragmin): 100 units/kg every 12 hours or 200 units/kg every 24 hours (not approved by the U.S. FDA for this indication)
  - ✓ **Tinzaparin** (Innohep): 175 units/kg SC every 24 hours
- Because the LMWHs achieve predictable anticoagulant response when given subcutaneously, routine laboratory monitoring is unnecessary to guide dosing. The PT and aPTT are minimally affected by LMWH. Prior to the initiation of therapy, a baseline complete blood cell count (CBC) with platelet count and serum creatinine should be obtained. The CBC should be checked every 5 to 10 days during the first 2 weeks of LMWH therapy and every 2 to 4 weeks thereafter to monitor for occult bleeding. Measuring antifactor Xa activity may be helpful in select patients.
- As with UFH, bleeding is the most common adverse effect of the LMWHs, but major bleeding may be less common than with UFH. Minor bleeding occurs frequently, particularly at the site of injection. If major bleeding occurs, **protamine sulfate** should be administered IV, although it cannot neutralize the anticoagulant effect completely. The recommended dose of protamine sulfate is 1 mg per 1 mg of enoxaparin or 1 mg per 100 antifactor Xa units of dalteparin or tinzaparin administered in the previous 8 hours. Smaller protamine doses can be used if the LMWH dose was given in the previous 8 to 12 hours. Protamine sulfate is not recommended if the LMWH was given more than 12 hours earlier.
- Thrombocytopenia can occur with LMWHs, but the incidence of HIT is substantially lower than with UFH. Platelet counts should be monitored periodically in patients receiving LMWH.

FONDAPARINUX

- **Fondaparinux sodium** (Arixtra) indirectly inhibits factor Xa through its interaction with antithrombin. Similar to UFH and the LMWHs, it binds to antithrombin, greatly accelerating its activity. However, it has no direct effect on thrombin activity at therapeutic plasma concentrations.
- It is approved for prevention of VTE in patients undergoing orthopedic (e.g., hip fracture and hip and knee replacement) or abdominal surgery and for treatment of VTE and PE (in conjunction with warfarin). For VTE prevention, the dose is 2.5 mg SC once daily starting 6 to 8 hours after surgery. For treatment of DVT and PE, the usual dose is 7.5 mg SC once daily.
- Patients receiving fondaparinux do not require routine coagulation testing. A CBC should be measured at baseline and periodically thereafter to detect occult bleeding. Signs and symptoms of bleeding should be monitored daily. There is no specific antidote to reverse the antithrombotic activity of fondaparinux.

DIRECT THROMBIN INHIBITORS

- These agents interact directly with thrombin and do not require antithrombin to have antithrombotic activity. They are capable of inhibiting both circulating and clot-bound thrombin, which is a potential advantage over UFH and the LMWHs. They also do not induce immune-mediated thrombocytopenia and are widely used for the treatment of HIT.
- **Lepirudin** (Refludan) is indicated for anticoagulation in patients with HIT and associated thrombosis to prevent further thromboembolic complications. The recommended dose is 0.4 mg/kg as an IV bolus over 15 to 20 seconds, followed by a 0.15-mg/kg/hour continuous IV infusion for 2 to 10 days or longer if needed. After obtaining a baseline aPTT, an aPTT should be obtained at least 4 hours after starting the infusion and then at least daily thereafter. The dose should be titrated to achieve an aPTT 1.5 to 2.5 times control. Dose adjustment is required in patients with impaired renal function. Many patients develop antibodies to lepirudin, which may increase its anticoagulant effect; close monitoring of aPTT is necessary during prolonged therapy. Because fatal anaphylaxis has been reported in patients who developed antibodies, patients should not be treated with lepirudin more than once.
- **Bivalirudin** (Angiomax) is FDA-approved for (1) use as an anticoagulant in patients with unstable angina undergoing percutaneous transluminal coronary angioplasty; (2) with provisional use of glycoprotein IIb/IIIa inhibitor for use as an anticoagulant in patients undergoing percutaneous coronary intervention (PCI); and (3) for patients with, or at risk of, HIT undergoing PCI. For PCI, the recommended dose is an IV bolus of 0.75 mg/kg, followed by a continuous infusion of 1.75 mg/kg/hour for the duration of the PCI procedure. Bivalirudin is intended for use with aspirin 300 to 325 mg/day. The activated clotting time can be used to monitor the anticoagulant effect of bivalirudin; the aPTT has also been used.

- **Argatroban** has two indications: (1) prevention or treatment of thrombosis in patients with HIT; and (2) as an anticoagulant in patients with HIT, or at risk of HIT, who are undergoing PCI. The recommended dose for the treatment of HIT is 2 mcg/kg/min by continuous IV infusion. The first aPTT should be obtained 2 hours after initiation. The dose can be adjusted as clinically indicated to maintain the target aPTT.
- **Desirudin** (Iprivask) is FDA-approved for prevention of DVT in patients undergoing elective hip replacement surgery; it is not commercially available in the United States as of early 2011. The recommended dose is 15 mg SC every 12 hours beginning 5 to 15 minutes prior to surgery and for up to 12 days thereafter. Daily aPTT monitoring is recommended.
- Contraindications to direct thrombin inhibitors are similar to those of other antithrombotic drugs, and hemorrhage is the most common and serious adverse effect. For all agents in this class, a CBC should be obtained at baseline and periodically thereafter to detect potential bleeding. There are no known agents that reverse the activity of direct thrombin inhibitors.

WARFARIN

- **Warfarin** inhibits the enzymes responsible for the cyclic interconversion of vitamin K in the liver. Reduced vitamin K is a cofactor required for the carboxylation of the vitamin K–dependent coagulation proteins prothrombin (II); factors VII, IX, and X; and the endogenous anticoagulant proteins C and S. By reducing the supply of vitamin K available to serve as a cofactor in the production of these proteins, warfarin indirectly slows their rate of synthesis. By suppressing the production of clotting factors, warfarin prevents the initial formation and propagation of thrombi. Warfarin has no direct effect on previously circulating clotting factors or previously formed thrombi. The time required to achieve its anticoagulant effect depends on the elimination half-lives of the coagulation proteins. Because prothrombin has a 2- to 3-day half-life, warfarin's full antithrombotic effect is not achieved for 8 to 15 days after initiation of therapy.
- Warfarin should begin concurrently with UFH or LMWH therapy. For patients with acute VTE, UFH, LMWH, or fondaparinux should be overlapped for at least 5 days, regardless of whether the target international normalized ratio (INR) has been achieved earlier. The UFH or LMWH can then be discontinued once the INR is within the desired range for 2 consecutive days.
- Guidelines for initiating warfarin therapy are given in **Fig. 14–3**. The usual initial dose is 5 to 10 mg. Lower starting doses may be acceptable based on patient factors such as advanced age, malnutrition, liver disease, or heart failure. Starting doses >10 mg should be avoided.
- Warfarin therapy is monitored by the INR; for most indications, the target INR is 2.5, with an acceptable range of 2 to 3. After an acute thromboembolic event, the INR should be measured minimally every 3 days during the first week of therapy. In general, dose changes should not be made more frequently than every 3 days. Doses should be adjusted by calculating the weekly dose and reducing or increasing it by 5% to 25%. The effect

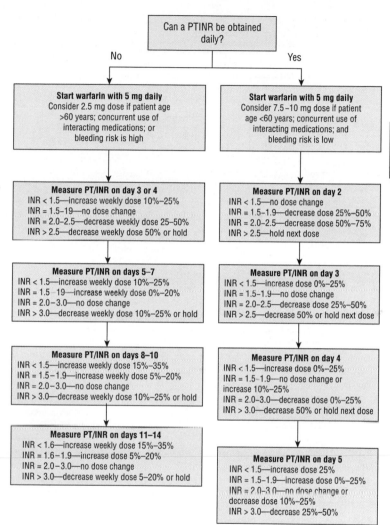

FIGURE 14–3. Initiation of warfarin therapy. (INR, international normalized ratio; PT, prothrombin time.)

of a small dose change may not become evident for 5 to 7 days. Once the patient's dose response is established, an INR should be determined every 7 to 14 days until it stabilizes, then every 4 to 8 weeks thereafter.

- Hemorrhagic complications ranging from mild to severe and life-threatening can occur at any body site. The GI tract and nose are the most frequent sites of bleeding. Intracranial hemorrhage is the most serious complication and often results in permanent disability and death. **Fig. 14–4** outlines guidelines for managing an elevated INR. Patients with a mildly elevated INR (3.5–5) and no signs or symptoms of bleeding can usually be managed

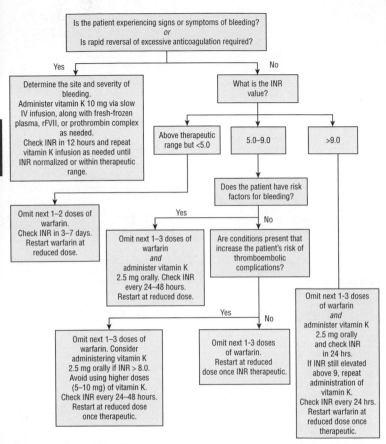

FIGURE 14-4. Management of an elevated international normalized ratio (INR) in patients taking warfarin. Dose reductions should be made by determining the weekly warfarin dose and reducing the weekly dose by 10% to 25% based on the degree of INR elevation. Conditions that increase the risk of thromboembolic complications include history of hypercoagulability disorders (e.g., protein C or S deficiency, presence of antiphospholipid antibodies, antithrombin deficiency, or activated protein C resistance), arterial or venous thrombosis within the previous month, thromboembolism associated with malignancy, and mechanical mitral valve in conjunction with atrial fibrillation, previous stroke, poor ventricular function, or coexisting mechanical aortic valve. (rFVII, recombinant factor VII.)

by either reducing the dose or holding one or two warfarin doses. If rapid reduction of an elevated INR is required, oral or IV administration of vitamin K_1 **(phytonadione)** can be given. Oral administration is preferable in the absence of major bleeding. The IV route produces the most rapid reversal of anticoagulation but has been associated with anaphylactoid reactions. If the INR is 5 to 9, warfarin doses may be withheld or may be

combined with a low dose of oral phytonadione (≤2.5 mg). If the INR is >9, an oral phytonadione dose of 2.5 to 5 mg is recommended. In the event of serious or life-threatening bleeding, IV vitamin K should be administered together with fresh-frozen plasma, clotting factor concentrates, or recombinant factor VII.
- Nonhemorrhagic adverse effects include the rare "purple toe" syndrome and skin necrosis.
- Because of the large number of food–drug and drug–drug interactions with warfarin, close monitoring and additional INR determinations may be indicated whenever other medications are initiated, or discontinued, or an alteration in consumption of vitamin K—containing foods is noted.

THROMBOLYSIS AND THROMBECTOMY

- Thrombolytic agents are proteolytic enzymes that enhance the conversion of plasminogen to plasmin, which subsequently degrades the fibrin matrix.
- Most patients with VTE do not require thrombolytic therapy. Thrombolysis for DVT should be reserved for patients who present with extensive proximal DVT (e.g., iliofemoral) within 14 days of symptom onset, have good functional status, and are at low risk of bleeding.
- Thrombolytic therapy should be administered to patients with massive PE with evidence of hemodynamic compromise (hypotension or shock) unless contraindicated by bleeding risk. Thrombolytic therapy should be considered for select high-risk patients without hypotension provided the risk of bleeding is acceptable.
- Three thrombolytic agents and regimens are available for treatment of DVT and/or PE:
  - ✓ **Alteplase** (Activase): For PE, 100 mg by IV infusion over 2 hours
  - ✓ **Streptokinase** (Streptase): 250,000 units IV over 30 minutes, followed by a continuous IV infusion of 100,000 units/hour for 24 hours (PE) or 24 to 72 hours (DVT)
  - ✓ **Urokinase** (Abbokinase): For PE, 4,400 international units/kg IV over 10 minutes, followed by 4,400 international units/kg/hour for 12 to 24 hours
- During thrombolytic therapy, IV UFH may be either continued or suspended; the most common practice in the United States is to suspend UFH. The aPTT should be measured after the completion of thrombolytic therapy. If the aPTT at that time is <80 seconds, UFH infusion should be started and adjusted to maintain the aPTT in the therapeutic range. If the posttreatment aPTT is >80 seconds, it should be remeasured every 2 to 4 hours and a UFH infusion started when the aPTT is <80 seconds.
- Removal of clot by either catheter-directed interventions or surgery is usually reserved for patients who are not candidates for or have not responded to thrombolysis.

PREVENTION OF VENOUS THROMBOEMBOLISM

- Nonpharmacologic methods improve venous blood flow by mechanical means and include early ambulation, venous foot pumps during

TABLE 14–3 DVT Risk Classification and Suggested Prevention Strategies

Level of Risk	Prevention Strategies
Low	
Patients undergoing minor surgery and fully ambulatory	Early and aggressive ambulation
Patients who are medically ill and fully ambulatory	
Moderate	
Most patients undergoing general, gynecological, or urological surgeries	UFH 5,000 units SC twice daily
	LMWH (at recommended dose)
Most patients who are hospitalized for an acute medical illness (e.g., MI, ischemic stroke, CHF exacerbation, or acute respiratory illness)	Fondaparinux
Patients who are at moderate DVT risk and high risk for bleeding	Mechanical thromboprophylaxis[a]
High	LMWH (at recommended dose)
Patients undergoing major lower extremity orthopedic surgery (e.g., hip or knee arthroplasty or hip fracture repair)	Fondaparinux
	Warfarin (INR goal = 2–3)
	Oral factor Xa inhibitors[b]
Spinal cord injury	Oral direct thrombin inhibitors[b]
Major trauma	Mechanical thromboprophylaxis[a]
Patients who are at high risk for DVT and/or bleeding	

DVT, deep vein thrombosis; CHF, congestive heart failure; INR, international normalized ratio; LMWH, low-molecular-weight heparin; MI, myocardial infarction; SC, subcutaneously; UFH, unfractionated heparin.

[a]Mechanical thromboprophylaxis includes intermittent pneumatic compression, graduated compression stockings, and venous foot pumps.

[b]Oral factor Xa inhibitors and oral direct thrombin inhibitors are investigational agents. These agents have not yet been formally endorsed as appropriate VTE prevention strategies in clinical practice guidelines.

prolonged surgery, graduated compression stockings, intermittent pneumatic compression devices, and inferior vena cava filters.

- Pharmacologic techniques counteract the propensity for thrombosis formation by dampening the coagulation cascade. Appropriately selected therapy can dramatically reduce the incidence of VTE after hip or knee replacement, general surgery, myocardial infarction, and ischemic stroke (Table 14–3).

- The **LMWHs** and **fondaparinux** provide superior protection against VTE compared with **low-dose UFH.** Even so, UFH is a highly effective, cost-conscious choice for many patients, provided that it is given in the appropriate dose. Low-dose UFH (5,000 units SC every 8 or 12 h) reduces the risk of DVT by 55% to 70% in patients undergoing many general surgical procedures and after MI or stroke. Its effectiveness is considerably lower for prevention of DVT after hip and knee replacement surgery. The LMWHs and fondaparinux provide a high degree of protection against DVT in most high-risk populations; the appropriate dose for each product is indication specific. There is no evidence that one LMWH is superior to another for the prevention of VTE. **Warfarin** is commonly used for VTE prevention after orthopedic surgeries of the lower extremities, but evidence is equivocal regarding its relative effectiveness compared with

LMWH for preventing clinically important VTE events in the highest risk populations.

- Prophylaxis should be continued throughout the period of risk. For general surgical procedures and medical conditions, prophylaxis can be discontinued once the patient is able to ambulate regularly and other risk factors are no longer present. Most clinical trials support the use of antithrombotic therapy for 21 to 35 days after total hip replacement and hip fracture repair surgeries.

EVALUATION OF THERAPEUTIC OUTCOMES

- Patients should be monitored for resolution of symptoms, the development of recurrent thrombosis, and symptoms of the postthrombotic syndrome, as well as for adverse effects from the treatments described in this chapter.
- Hemoglobin, hematocrit, and blood pressure should be monitored carefully to detect bleeding from anticoagulant therapy.
- Coagulation tests (aPTT, PT, and INR) should be performed prior to initiating therapy to establish the patient's baseline values and guide later anticoagulation.
- Outpatients taking warfarin should be questioned about medication adherence and symptoms related to bleeding and thromboembolic complications. Any changes in concurrent medications should be carefully explored.

See Chapter 26, Venous Thromboembolism, authored by Daniel M. Witt, Edith A. Nutescu, and Stuart T. Haines, for a more detailed discussion of this topic.

15 Acne Vulgaris

DEFINITION

- Acne vulgaris is a common, usually self-limiting, multifactorial disease involving inflammation of the sebaceous follicles of the face and upper trunk.

PATHOPHYSIOLOGY

- Acne usually begins in the prepubertal period, when the adrenal glands mature, and progresses as androgen production and sebaceous gland activity increase with gonad development.
- The four primary factors involved in the formation of acne lesions are increased sebum production due to hormonal influences, hyperproliferation of ductal epidermis, bacterial colonization of the ducts, and inflammation.
- Circulating androgens cause sebaceous glands to increase their size and activity. There is increased keratinization of epidermal cells and development of an obstructed sebaceous follicle, called a microcomedone. Cells adhere to each other, forming a dense keratinous plug. Sebum, produced in increasing amounts by the active gland, becomes trapped behind the keratin plug and solidifies, contributing to open or closed comedone formation.
- Pooling of sebum in the follicle provides ideal conditions for proliferation of the anaerobic bacterium *Propionibacterium acnes,* which generates a T-cell response resulting in inflammation. *P. acnes* produces a lipase that hydrolyzes sebum triglycerides into free fatty acids that may increase keratinization and lead to microcomedone formation.
- The closed comedone (whitehead) is the first visible lesion of acne. It is almost completely obstructed to drainage and has a tendency to rupture.
- An open comedone (blackhead) is formed as the plug extends to the upper canal and dilates its opening. Its dark color is due to either oxidized lipid and melanin or the impacted mass of horny cells. Acne characterized by open and closed comedones is termed noninflammatory acne.
- Pus formation occurs due to recruitment of neutrophils into the follicle during the inflammatory process and release of *P. acnes*–generated chemokines. *P. acnes* also produces enzymes that increase the permeability of the follicular wall, causing it to rupture, thereby releasing keratin, lipids, and irritating free fatty acids into the dermis. Inflammatory lesions that may form and lead to scarring include pustules, nodules, and cysts.

CLINICAL PRESENTATION

- Acne lesions typically occur on the face, back, upper chest, and shoulders. Severity varies from a mild comedonal form to severe inflammatory acne. The disease is categorized as mild, moderate, or severe, depending on the type and severity of lesions.
- Lesions may take months to heal completely, and fibrosis associated with healing may lead to permanent scarring.

DIAGNOSIS

- The diagnosis of acne vulgaris is established by patient assessment, which includes observation of the lesions and excluding other potential causes (e.g., drug-induced acne). Several different systems are in use to grade acne severity.

DESIRED OUTCOME

- The goals of treatment are to reduce the number and severity of lesions, slow disease progression, limit disease duration, prevent formation of new lesions, and prevent scarring and hyperpigmentation.

TREATMENT

GENERAL APPROACH
(Fig. 15–1)

- Nondrug and pharmacologic measures should address all four mechanisms involved in acne pathogenesis. Therapies should be selected and altered as appropriate for the severity of the clinical presentation.
- Treatment is directed at controlling the disorder, not curing it. Regimens should be tapered over time, adjusting to response.
- The smallest number of agents should be used at the lowest possible doses to ensure efficacy, safety, avoidance of resistance, and patient adherence. Once control is achieved, simplify the regimen, but continue with some suppressive therapy.
- For mild to moderate acne with predominantly noninflammatory lesions (comedones) and no scars, agents of first choice are those that correct the defect in keratinization by producing effective exfoliation (e.g., benzoyl peroxide, topical retinoids, and salicylic acid).
- For moderate to severe acne with predominantly inflammatory lesions and some scars, it is important to reduce the population of *P. acnes* in the follicle and the generation of its extracellular products and inflammatory effects. Drugs of choice include benzoyl peroxide, topical antibiotics (alone or in combination with benzoyl peroxide), and oral antibiotics (e.g., minocycline). Retinoids (tretinoin, adapalene, and tazarotene) and azelaic acid are also recommended.

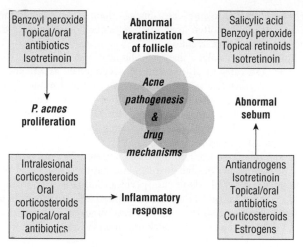

© Debra Sibbald

FIGURE 15–1. Acne pathogenesis and drug mechanisms.

- For severe acne with inflammatory lesions, extensive nodules, cysts, and scars, or acne resistant to other approaches, drugs that decrease sebaceous activity should be added to the regimen (e.g., antiandrogens, isotretinoin, or topical and oral antibiotics).

NONPHARMACOLOGIC THERAPY

- Patients should be encouraged to avoid aggravating factors, maintain a balanced diet, and control stress.
- Patients should wash no more than twice daily with a mild, nonfragranced opaque or glycerin soap or a soapless cleanser. Scrubbing should be minimized to prevent follicular rupture.
- Comedone extraction results in immediate cosmetic improvement but has not been widely tested in clinical trials.

TOPICAL PHARMACOTHERAPY

Exfoliants (Peeling Agents)

- Exfoliants induce continuous mild drying and peeling by primary irritation, damaging the superficial skin layers and inciting inflammation. This stimulates mitosis, thickening the epidermis and increasing horny cells, scaling, and erythema. Decreased sweating results in a dry, less oily surface and may superficially resolve pustular lesions.
- **Salicylic acid** is keratolytic, has mild antibacterial activity against *P. acnes*, and offers slight antiinflammatory activity at concentrations up to 5%. Salicylic acid is recognized by the FDA as safe and effective, but it may be less potent than benzoyl peroxide or topical retinoids. Salicylic acid products are often used as first-line therapy for mild acne because of their availability in concentrations up to 2% without a prescription. Concentrations of 5% to 10% can also be used by prescription, beginning

with a low concentration and increasing as tolerance develops to the irritation. Salicylic acid is often used when patients cannot tolerate topical retinoids because of skin irritation.

- **Resorcinol** is less keratolytic than salicylic acid and when used alone is classified as FDA category II (not generally recognized as safe and effective). The FDA considers resorcinol 2% and resorcinol monoacetate 3% to be safe and effective when used in combination with sulfur 3% to 8%. Resorcinol is an irritant and sensitizer and should not be applied to large areas or on broken skin. It produces a reversible dark brown scale on some dark-skinned individuals.
- **Sulfur** is keratolytic and has antibacterial activity. Its popularity is due to its ability to quickly resolve pustules and papules, mask lesions, and produce irritation that leads to skin peeling. Sulfur is used in the precipitated or colloidal form in concentrations of 2% to 10%. Although it is often combined with salicylic acid or resorcinol to increase its effect, its use is limited by an offensive odor and the availability of more effective agents.

Topical Retinoids

- Retinoids reduce obstruction within the follicle and are useful for both comedonal and inflammatory acne. They reverse abnormal keratinocyte desquamation and are highly active skin peelers. They inhibit microcomedone formation, decreasing the number of mature comedones and, subsequently, inflammatory lesions. Retinoids also increase skin permeability and facilitate absorption of other topical agents (e.g., antimicrobials and benzoyl peroxide) and increase penetration of oral antibiotics into the follicular canal. Combination products with oral or topical antimicrobials have increased efficacy and faster onset and may result in decreased total antibiotic use, less risk of resistance, and shorter duration of treatment.
- Topical retinoids provide safe, effective, and economical means of treating all but the most severe cases of acne vulgaris. They should be the first step in moderate acne, alone or in combination with antibiotics and benzoyl peroxide, reverting to retinoids alone for maintenance once adequate results are achieved. Retinoids tend to produce extended remissions, provided that irritation does not impede patient adherence. Side effects include erythema, xerosis, burning, and peeling.
- Retinoids should be applied at night, a half hour after cleansing, starting with every other night for 1 to 2 weeks to adjust to irritation. Doses can be increased only after beginning with 4 to 6 weeks of the lowest concentration and least irritating vehicle.
- **Tretinoin** (retinoic acid and vitamin A acid) is available as 0.05% solution (most irritating), 0.01% and 0.025% gels, and 0.025%, 0.05%, and 0.1% creams (least irritating). Tretinoin should not be used in pregnant women because of risk to the fetus.
- **Adapalene** (Differin) is a fast-acting agent that is better at reducing inflammatory lesions and total lesion count with less local irritation than tretinoin or tazarotene. Adapalene is available as 0.1% gel, cream, alcoholic solution, and pledgets. A 0.3% gel formulation is also available.

- **Tazarotene** (Tazorac) is as effective as adapalene in reducing noninflammatory and inflammatory lesion counts when applied half as frequently. Compared with tretinoin, it is as effective for comedonal and more effective for inflammatory lesions when applied once daily. The product is available as a 0.05% and 0.1% gel or cream.

Antibacterial Agents

- **Benzoyl peroxide** is a bactericidal agent that also suppresses sebum production and reduces free fatty acids, which are comedogenic and inflammatory triggers. It is useful for both noninflammatory and inflammatory acne. It has a rapid onset and may decrease the number of inflamed lesions within 5 days. Benzoyl peroxide preparations are the single most useful group of topical nonprescription drugs and are the first choice for most patients with mild to moderate acne vulgaris.
- Soaps, lotions, creams, washes, and gels are available in concentrations of 1% to 10%. Preparations are available without prescription in concentrations up to 5%. Gel formulations are usually most potent, whereas lotions, creams, and soaps have weaker potency. Alcohol-based gel preparations generally cause more dryness and irritation. The 4% hydrophase gel product may be a useful option for patients with easily irritated skin who require additional potency.
- Therapy should be initiated with the weakest concentration (2.5%) in a water-based formulation or the 4% hydrophase gel. One method to initiate therapy is to cleanse the skin and apply the preparation for only 15 minutes the first evening, then double the application time each evening thereafter until the product is left on for 4 hours and subsequently all night. Once tolerance is achieved, the strength may be increased to 5% or the base changed to the acetone or alcohol gels, or to paste. It is important to wash the product off in the morning. A sunscreen should be applied during the day.
- Side effects of benzoyl peroxide include dryness, irritation, and, rarely, allergic contact dermatitis. It may bleach hair and clothing.
- **Topical erythromycin** and **clindamycin** have become less effective due to resistance by *P. acnes*. Addition of benzoyl peroxide or topical retinoids to the macrolide is more effective than antibiotic monotherapy and mitigates against survival of resistant *P. acnes* populations. Clindamycin is preferred because of potent action and lack of systemic absorption. It is available as a single-ingredient topical preparation or in combination with benzoyl peroxide. Erythromycin is available alone and in combination with retinoic acid or benzoyl peroxide.
- **Azelaic acid** (Azelex) has antibacterial, antiinflammatory, and comedolytic activity. It is used for mild to moderate inflammatory acne but has limited efficacy compared with other antiacne therapies. However, it is well tolerated, with adverse effects of pruritus, burning, stinging, and tingling occurring in 1% to 5% of patients. Erythema, dryness, peeling, and irritation occur in <1% of patients. Azelaic acid is available in 20% cream and 15% gel formulations, which are usually applied twice daily (morning and evening) on clean, dry skin. Most patients experience improvement within 4 weeks, but treatment may be continued over several months if necessary.

SYSTEMIC PHARMACOTHERAPY

Oral Antibacterials

- Systemic antibiotics are a standard of care for management of moderate and severe acne and treatment-resistant forms of inflammatory acne. Because of increasing bacterial resistance, patients with less severe forms of acne should not be treated with oral antibiotics, and where possible the duration of therapy should be limited.
- **Erythromycin** is effective, but because of bacterial resistance, its use should be limited to patients who cannot use a tetracycline derivative (e.g., pregnant women and children under 8 years old). **Ciprofloxacin, trimethoprim—sulfamethoxazole,** and **trimethoprim** alone are also effective in cases where other antibiotics cannot be used or are ineffective.
- **Tetracyclines** have antibacterial and antiinflammatory effects. **Tetracycline** itself is no longer the drug of choice in this family due to diet-related effects on absorption and lower antibacterial and antiinflammatory efficacy. **Minocycline** and **doxycycline** are tenfold more effective than tetracycline, and there is evidence that minocycline is superior to doxycycline in reducing *P. acnes.*

Antisebum Agents

- **Isotretinoin** decreases sebum production, inhibits *P. acnes* growth, and reduces inflammation. It is approved for the treatment of severe recalcitrant nodular acne. It is also useful for managing less severe acne that is treatment resistant or that is producing either physical or psychological scarring. Isotretinoin is the only drug treatment for acne that produces prolonged remission.
- The approved dose is 0.5 to 2 mg/kg/day, usually given over a 20-week course. Drug absorption is greater when taken with food. Initial flaring can be minimized by starting with 0.5 mg/kg/day or less. Alternatively, lower doses can be used for longer periods, with a total cumulative dose of 120 to 150 mg/kg.
- Adverse effects are frequent and often dose related. About 90% of patients experience mucocutaneous effects; drying of the mouth, nose, and eyes is most common. Cheilitis and skin desquamation occur in >80% of patients. Systemic effects include transient increases in serum cholesterol and triglycerides, increased creatine kinase, hyperglycemia, photosensitivity, pseudotumor cerebri, abnormal liver injury tests, bone abnormalities, arthralgias, muscle stiffness, headache, and a high incidence of teratogenicity. Patients should be counseled about and screened for depression during therapy, although a causal relationship to isotretinoin therapy is controversial.
- Because of teratogenicity, two different forms of contraception must be started in female patients of childbearing potential beginning 1 month before therapy, continuing throughout treatment, and for up to 4 months after discontinuation of therapy. All patients receiving isotretinoin must participate in the iPLEDGE program, which requires pregnancy tests and assurances by prescribers and pharmacists that they will follow required procedures.

- **Oral contraceptives** containing estrogen can be useful for acne in some women. Agents with FDA approval for this indication include **norgestimate with ethinyl estradiol** and **norethindrone acetate with ethinyl estradiol;** other estrogen-containing products may also be effective.
- **Spironolactone** in higher doses is an antiandrogenic compound. Doses of 50 to 200 mg have been shown to be effective in acne.
- **Cyproterone acetate** is an antiandrogen that may be effective for acne in females when combined with ethinyl estradiol (in the form of an oral contraceptive). No cyproterone/estrogen–containing oral contraceptives are available in the United States.
- **Oral corticosteroids** in high doses used for short courses may be of temporary benefit in patients with severe inflammatory acne.

EVALUATION OF THERAPEUTIC OUTCOMES

- Patients with acne should be provided with a monitoring framework that includes specific parameters and frequency of monitoring. They should record the objective response to treatment in a diary. Patients should be contacted within 2 to 3 weeks after the start of therapy to assess progress.
- Lesion counts should decrease by 10% to 15% within 4 to 8 weeks or by more than 50% within 2 to 4 months. Inflammatory lesions should resolve within a few weeks, and comedones should resolve by 3 to 4 months. If anxiety or depression is present at the outset, control or improvement should be achieved within 2 to 4 months.
- Long-term parameters should include no progression of severity, lengthening of acne-free periods throughout therapy, and no further scarring or pigmentation throughout therapy.
- Patients should be monitored regularly for adverse treatment effects, with appropriate dose reduction, alternative treatments, or drug discontinuation considered if these effects become intolerable.

See Chapter 106, Acne Vulgaris, authored by Debra J. Sibbald, for a more detailed discussion of this topic.

Dermatologic Drug Reactions and Common Skin Conditions

DEFINITIONS

- Drug-induced skin reactions can be irritant or allergic in nature. Allergic drug reactions can be classified into exanthematous, urticarial, blistering, and pustular eruptions. The skin disorders discussed in this chapter include contact dermatitis, diaper dermatitis, and atopic dermatitis.

PATHOPHYSIOLOGY (FIG. 16–1)

- **Exanthematous** drug reactions include maculopapular rashes and drug hypersensitivity syndrome. **Urticarial** reactions include urticaria, angioedema, and serum sickness-like reactions. **Blistering** reactions include fixed drug eruptions, Stevens–Johnson syndrome, and toxic epidermal necrolysis. **Pustular** eruptions include acneiform drug reactions and acute generalized exanthematous pustulosis (AGEP) (Fig. 16–1).
- Drug-induced **hyperpigmentation** may be related to increased melanin (e.g., hydantoins), direct deposition (e.g., silver, mercury, tetracyclines, and antimalarials), or other mechanisms (e.g., fluorouracil).
- Drug-induced photosensitivity reactions may be **phototoxic** (a nonimmunologic reaction) or **photoallergic** (an immunologic reaction). Medications associated with phototoxicity include amiodarone, tetracyclines, sulfonamides, psoralens, and coal tar. Common causes of photoallergic reactions include sulfonamides, sulfonylureas, thiazides, nonsteroidal antiinflammatory drugs (NSAIDs), chloroquine, and carbamazepine.
- **Contact dermatitis** is an inflammation of the skin caused by irritants or allergic sensitizers. In **allergic contact dermatitis (ACD)**, an antigenic substance triggers an immunologic response, sometimes several days later. **Irritant contact dermatitis (ICD)** is caused by an organic substance that usually results in a reaction within a few hours of exposure.
- **Diaper dermatitis** (diaper rash) is an acute, inflammatory dermatitis of the buttocks, genitalia, and perineal region. The reaction is a type of contact dermatitis, as it results from direct fecal and moisture contact with the skin in an occlusive environment.
- **Atopic dermatitis** is an inflammatory condition with genetic, environmental, and immunologic mechanisms. Neuropeptides, irritation, or pruritus-induced scratching may cause release of proinflammatory cytokines from keratinocytes. Alternatively, allergens in the epidermal barrier or in food may cause T-cell mediated but immunoglobulin E (IgE)–independent reactions.

CLINICAL PRESENTATION

- **Maculopapular skin reaction** is an afebrile exanthematous eruption that presents with erythematous macules and papules that may be pruritic. It is the most common allergic skin reaction. The lesions usually begin within

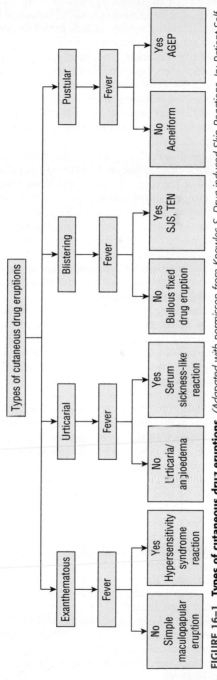

FIGURE 16–1. Types of cutaneous drug eruptions. *(Adapted with permisson from Knowles S. Drug-induced Skin Reactions. In: Patient Self-Care (PSC). Ontario, Canada: Canadian Pharmacists Association, 2002:584–591.)*

7 to 10 days after starting the offending medication and generally resolve within 7 to 14 days after drug discontinuation. Lesions may spread and become confluent. Common culprits include penicillins, cephalosporins, sulfonamides, and some anticonvulsants.

- **Drug hypersensitivity syndrome** is an exanthematous eruption accompanied by fever, lymphadenopathy, and multiorgan involvement (kidneys, liver, lung, bone marrow, heart, and brain). Signs and symptoms begin 1 to 4 weeks after starting the offending drug, and the reaction may be fatal if not promptly treated. Drugs implicated include allopurinol, sulfonamides, some anticonvulsants (barbiturates, phenytoin, carbamazepine, and lamotrigine), and dapsone.

- **Urticaria** and **angioedema** are simple eruptions that are caused by drugs in 5% to 10% of cases. Other causes are foods (most common) and physical factors such as cold or pressure, infections, and latex exposure. The condition may also be idiopathic. Urticaria may be the first sign of an emerging anaphylactic reaction characterized by hives, extremely pruritic red raised wheals, angioedema, and mucous membrane swelling that typically occurs within minutes to hours. Offending drugs include penicillins and related antibiotics, aspirin, sulfonamides, radiograph contrast media, and opioids.

- **Serum sickness-like reactions** are complex urticarial eruptions presenting with fever, rash (usually urticarial), and arthralgias usually within 1 to 3 weeks after starting the offending drug.

- **Fixed drug eruptions** present as pruritic, red, raised lesions that may blister. Symptoms can include burning or stinging. Lesions may evolve into plaques. These so-called fixed eruptions recur in the same area each time the offending drug is given. Lesions appear and disappear within minutes to days, leaving hyperpigmented skin for months. Usual offenders include tetracyclines, barbiturates, sulfonamides, codeine, phenolphthalein, and NSAIDs.

- **Stevens–Johnson syndrome (SJS)** and **toxic epidermal necrolysis (TEN)** are blistering eruptions that are rare but severe and life-threatening conditions. The onset occurs within 7 to 14 days after drug exposure. Patients present with generalized tender/painful bullous formation with fever, headache, and respiratory symptoms leading to rapid clinical deterioration. Lesions show rapid confluence and spread, resulting in extensive epidermal detachment and sloughing. This may result in marked loss of fluids, hypotension, electrolyte imbalances, and secondary infections. Usual offending drugs include sulfonamides, penicillins, some anticonvulsants (hydantoins, carbamazepine, barbiturates, and lamotrigine), NSAIDs, and allopurinol.

- **Acneiform drug reactions** are pustular eruptions caused by medications that induce acne. The onset is within 1 to 3 weeks. Common culprits include corticosteroids, androgenic hormones, some anticonvulsants, isoniazid, and lithium.

- **Acute generalized exanthematous pustulosis (AGEP)** is characterized by an acute onset (within days after starting the offending drug), fever, diffuse erythema, and many pustules. Generalized desquamation occurs 2 weeks later. Usual offending drugs include β-lactam antibiotics, macrolides, and calcium channel blockers.

- **Sun-induced skin reactions** appear similar to a sunburn and present with erythema, papules, edema, and sometimes vesicles. They appear in areas exposed to sunlight (e.g., ears, nose, cheeks, forearms, and hands).
- **Diaper dermatitis** results in an erythematous rash, and severe cases may have vesicles and oozing erosions. The rash may be infected by *Candida* species and present with confluent red plaques, papules, and pustules.
- **Atopic dermatitis** presents differently, depending on age. In infancy, an erythematous, patchy, pruritic, papular skin rash may first appear on the cheeks and chin and progress to red, scaling, oozing lesions. The rash affects the malar region of the cheeks, forehead, scalp, chin, and behind the ears while sparing the nose and paranasal creases. Over several weeks, lesions may spread to extensor surfaces of the lower legs (due to the infant's crawling), and eventually the entire body may be involved with the exception of the diaper area and nose. In childhood, the skin in atopic dermatitis often appears dry, flaky, rough, and cracked; scratching may result in bleeding and lichenification. In adulthood, lesions are more diffuse with underlying erythema. The face is commonly involved and may be dry and scaly. Lichenification may be seen.

DIAGNOSIS

- A comprehensive patient history is important with all skin conditions to obtain the following information:
  - ✓ Signs and symptoms (onset, progression, timeframe, lesion location and description, presenting symptoms, and previous occurrence
  - ✓ Urgency (severity, area, and extent of skin involvement; signs of a systemic/generalized reaction or disease condition)
  - ✓ Medication history
  - ✓ Differential diagnosis
- Lesion assessment includes identifying macules, papules, nodules, blisters, plaques, and lichenification. Some skin conditions cause more than one type of lesion.
- Lesions should be inspected for color, texture, size, and temperature. Areas that are oozing, erythematous, and warm to the touch may be infected.
- Signs and symptoms of atopic dermatitis include pruritus; early age of onset; eczematous skin lesions that vary with age; chronic and relapsing courses; dry and flaky skin; IgE reactivity; and family or personal history of asthma, hay fever, or other atopic diseases. Allergy skin testing may be helpful in identifying factors that trigger flares.

DESIRED OUTCOME

- Treatment goals for patients with skin disorders are to relieve bothersome symptoms, remove precipitating factors, prevent recurrences, avoid adverse treatment effects, and improve quality of life.

TREATMENT

DRUG-INDUCED SKIN REACTIONS

- If a drug-induced skin reaction is suspected, the most important treatment in nearly all cases is discontinuing the suspected drug as quickly as possible and avoiding use of potential cross-sensitizers.
- The next step is to control symptoms (e.g., pruritus). Signs or symptoms of a systemic or generalized reaction may require additional supportive therapy. For high fevers, acetaminophen is a more appropriate antipyretic than aspirin or another NSAID, which may exacerbate some skin lesions.
- Most maculopapular reactions disappear within a few days after discontinuing the agent, so symptomatic control of the affected area is the primary intervention. **Topical corticosteroids** and **oral antihistamines** can relieve pruritus. In severe cases, a short course of **systemic corticosteroids** may be warranted.
- Treatment of fixed drug reactions involves removal of the offending agent. Other therapeutic measures include **topical corticosteroids, oral antihistamines** to relieve itching, and perhaps cool water compresses on the affected area.
- Photosensitivity reactions typically resolve with drug discontinuation. Some patients benefit from **topical corticosteroids** and **oral antihistamines**, but these are relatively ineffective. **Systemic corticosteroids** (e.g., **oral prednisone** 1 mg/kg/day tapered over 3 weeks) is more effective for these patients.
- For life-threatening SJS/TEN, supportive measures such as maintenance of adequate blood pressure, fluid and electrolyte balance, broad-spectrum antibiotics and vancomycin for secondary infections, and IV immunoglobulin (IVIG) may be appropriate. Corticosteroid use is controversial; if used, relatively high doses should be offered initially, followed by rapid tapering as soon as disease progression stops.
- Patients should be informed about the suspected drug and potential drugs to avoid in the future, and which drugs may be used instead. Patients with photosensitivity reactions should be given information about preventive measures, such as use of sunscreens and sun avoidance.

CONTACT DERMATITIS

- The first intervention involves identification, withdrawal, and avoidance of the offending agent.
- The second treatment goal is to provide symptomatic relief while decreasing skin lesions. **Cold compresses** help soothe and cleanse the skin; they are applied to wet or oozing lesions, removed, remoistened, and reapplied every few minutes for a 20- to 30-minute period. If affected areas are already dry or hardened, wet dressings applied as soaks (without removal for up to 20–30 min) will soften and hydrate the skin; soaks should not be used on acute exudating lesions. **Calamine lotion** or **Burow solution (aluminum acetate)** may also be soothing.

- **Topical corticosteroids** help resolve the inflammatory process and are the mainstay of treatment. ACD responds better to topical corticosteroids than does ICD. Generally, higher potency corticosteroids are used initially, switching to medium or lower potency corticosteroids as the condition improves (see Chap. 17, Table 17–1, for topical corticosteroid potencies).
- **Oatmeal baths** or oral **first-generation antihistamines** may provide relief for excessive itching.
- **Moisturizers** may be used to prevent dryness and skin fissuring.

DIAPER DERMATITIS

- Management involves frequent diaper changes, air drying (removing the diaper for as long as practical), gentle cleansing (preferably with nonsoap cleansers and lukewarm water), and the use of barrier products. **Zinc oxide** has astringent and absorbent properties and provides an effective barrier.
- Candidal (yeast) diaper rash should be treated with a topical antifungal agent and then covered by a barrier product. **Imidazoles** are the treatment of choice. The antifungal agents should be stopped once the rash subsides and the barrier product continued.
- In severe inflammatory diaper rashes, a very low potency topical corticosteroid **(hydrocortisone 0.5–1%)** may be used for short periods (1–2 wk).

ATOPIC DERMATITIS

- Nonpharmacologic measures for infants and children include the following:
  ✓ Give lukewarm baths
  ✓ Apply lubricants/moisturizers immediately after bathing
  ✓ Use scent-free moisturizers liberally each day
  ✓ Keep fingernails filed short
  ✓ Select clothing made of soft cotton fabrics
  ✓ Consider sedating oral antihistamines to reduce scratching at night
  ✓ Keep the child cool; avoid situations that cause overheating
  ✓ Learn to recognize skin infections and seek treatment promptly
  ✓ Identify and remove irritants and allergens
- Topical corticosteroids are the drug treatment of choice. Low-potency agents (e.g., **hydrocortisone 1%**) are suitable for the face, and medium-potency products (e.g., **betamethasone valerate 0.1%**) may be used for the body. For longer-duration maintenance therapy, low-potency corticosteroids are recommended. Midstrength and high-potency corticosteroids should be used for short-term management of exacerbations. Ultra-high and high-potency agents (e.g., **betamethasone dipropionate 0.05%** and **clobetasone propionate 0.05%**) are typically reserved for short-term treatment of lichenified lesions in adults. After lesions have improved significantly, a lower-potency corticosteroid should be used for maintenance when necessary. Potent fluorinated corticosteroids should be avoided on the face, genitalia, and intertriginous areas and in infants.
- The topical immunomodulators **tacrolimus** (Protopic) and **pimecrolimus** (Elidel) inhibit calcineurin, which normally initiates T-cell activation. Both agents are approved for atopic dermatitis in adults and children older

than age 2. They can be used on all parts of the body for prolonged periods without producing corticosteroid-induced adverse effects. Tacrolimus ointment 0.03% (for moderate to severe atopic dermatitis in patients ages 2 and older) and 0.1% (for ages 16 and older) is applied twice daily. Pimecrolimus cream 1% is applied twice daily for mild to moderate atopic dermatitis in patients older than age 2. The most common adverse effect is transient burning at the site of application. Both drugs are recommended as second-line treatments due to concerns about a possible risk of cancer. For this reason, sun protection factor (SPF) 30 or higher is recommended on all exposed skin areas.

- Phototherapy may be recommended when the disease is not controlled by calcineurin inhibitors. It may also be steroid sparing, allowing for use of lower-potency corticosteroids, or even eliminating the need for corticosteroids in some cases.
- Coal tar preparations reduce itching and skin inflammation and are available as **crude coal tar** (1–3%) or **liquor carbonis detergens** (5–20%). They have been used in combination with topical corticosteroids, as adjuncts to permit effective use of lower corticosteroid strengths, and in conjunction with ultraviolet light therapies. Patients can apply the product at bedtime and wash it off in the morning. Factors limiting coal tar use include its strong odor and staining of clothing. Coal tar preparations should not be used on acute oozing lesions, which would result in stinging and irritation.
- Systemic therapies that have been used (but not FDA approved) for atopic dermatitis include corticosteroids, cyclosporine, interferon-γ, azathioprine, methotrexate, mycophenolate mofetil, IVIG, and biologic response modifiers.

EVALUATION OF THERAPEUTIC OUTCOMES

- Information regarding causative factors, avoidance of substances that trigger skin reactions, and the potential benefits and limitations of nondrug and drug therapy should be conveyed to patients.
- Patients with chronic skin conditions should be evaluated periodically to assess disease control, the efficacy of current therapy, and the presence of possible adverse effects.

See Chapter 105, Dermatologic Drug Reactions and Common Skin Conditions, by Rebecca M. Law and David T.S. Law; and Chapter 108, Atopic Dermatitis, by Rebecca M. Law and Po Gin Kwa, for a more detailed discussion of these topics.

DEFINITION

- Psoriasis is a common chronic inflammatory disease characterized by recurrent exacerbations and remissions of thickened, erythematous, and scaling plaques.

PATHOPHYSIOLOGY

- Psoriasis is a T-lymphocyte–mediated inflammatory disease. Cutaneous inflammatory T-cell–mediated immune activation requires two T-cell signals mediated via cell–cell interactions by surface proteins and antigen-presenting cells, such as dendritic cells or macrophages. The first signal is the interaction of the T-cell receptor with antigen presented by antigen-presenting cells. The second signal (called costimulation) is mediated through various surface interactions.
- Activated T cells migrate from lymph nodes and the bloodstream into skin and secrete cytokines (e.g., interferon-γ and interleukin 2 [IL-2]) that induce the pathologic changes of psoriasis. Local keratinocytes and neutrophils produce other cytokines, such as tumor necrosis factor-α (TNF-α) and IL-8. T-cell production and activation results in keratinocyte proliferation.
- There is a significant genetic component in psoriasis. Studies of histocompatibility antigens show associations with human leukocyte antigens (HLA)-Cw6, TNF-α, and IL-3.
- Skin injury, infection, drugs, smoking, alcohol consumption, obesity, and psychogenic stress have been implicated in the development of psoriasis. Psoriatic lesions may develop at the site of skin injury, such as rubbing, venipuncture, and insect bites (Koebner response). Lithium, β-blockers, antimalarials, nonsteroidal antiinflammatory drugs, and withdrawal of corticosteroids have been reported to exacerbate psoriasis.

CLINICAL PRESENTATION

- Plaque psoriasis (psoriasis vulgaris) is seen in ~90% of psoriasis patients. Lesions in plaque psoriasis are erythematous, red-violet in color, at least 0.5 cm in diameter, well demarcated, and typically covered with silver flaking scales. They may appear as single lesions at predisposed areas (e.g., knees and elbows) or generalized over a wide body surface area (BSA).
- More than 50% of patients have pruritus, which may be severe and require treatment to minimize excoriations from frequent scratching. Lesions may also be physically debilitating or socially isolating.
- Potential comorbidities include depression, hypertension, obesity, diabetes mellitus, Crohn's disease, anxiety, and alcoholism.
- Psoriatic arthritis involves both psoriatic lesions and inflammatory arthritis-like symptoms. Distal interphalangeal joints and adjacent nails

are most commonly involved, but knees, elbows, wrists, and ankles may also be affected.

DIAGNOSIS

- The diagnosis is based on physical examination findings of the characteristic lesions of psoriasis. Skin biopsies are not diagnostic of psoriasis.
- Classification of psoriasis as mild, moderate, or severe is generally based on BSA and Psoriasis Area and Severity Index (PASI) measurements.

DESIRED OUTCOME

- The goals of therapy are to minimize or eliminate skin lesions, alleviate pruritus, reduce frequency of flare-ups, ensure treatment of comorbid conditions, avoid adverse treatment effects, and provide appropriate counseling (e.g., stress reduction).

TREATMENT

See Figs. 17–1 and 17–2 for psoriasis treatment algorithms based on disease severity.

NONPHARMACOLOGIC THERAPY

- Stress reduction using methods such as guided imagery and stress management can improve the extent and severity of psoriasis.
- Nonmedicated moisturizers help maintain skin moisture, reduce skin shedding, control scaling, and reduce pruritus.
- Oatmeal baths further reduce pruritus, and regular use may reduce the need for systemic antipruritic drugs. Harsh soaps and detergents should be

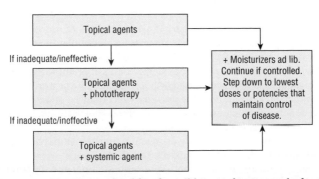

FIGURE 17–1. Treatment algorithm for mild to moderate psoriasis.

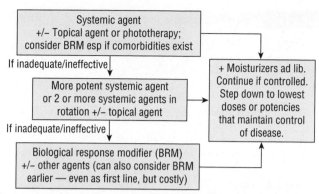

FIGURE 17-2. Treatment algorithm for moderate to severe psoriasis.

avoided. Cleansing should involve tepid water, preferably with lipid- and fragrance-free cleansers.

- Sunscreens (preferably sun protection factor [SPF] 30 or higher) should be used when outdoors.

PHARMACOLOGIC THERAPY

Topical Therapies

- **Corticosteroids** (Table 17-1) have antiinflammatory, antiproliferative, immunosuppressive, and vasoconstrictive effects.
- Lower-potency products should be used for infants and for lesions on the face, intertriginous areas, and areas with thin skin. Mid- to high-potency agents are generally recommended as initial therapy for other areas of the body in adults. The highest potency corticosteroids are generally reserved for patients with very thick plaques or recalcitrant disease, such as plaques on the palms and soles. Potency class I corticosteroids should be used for only 2 to 4 weeks.
- Ointments are the most occlusive and most potent formulations because of enhanced penetration into the dermis. Patients may prefer the less greasy creams or lotions for daytime use.
- Adverse effects include skin atrophy, acne, contact dermatitis, hypertrichosis, folliculitis, hypopigmentation, perioral dermatitis, striae, telangiectasias, and traumatic purpura. Systemic adverse effects may occur with superpotent agents or with extended or widespread use of midpotency agents. Such effects include hypothalamic-pituitary-adrenal axis suppression and less commonly Cushing's syndrome, osteonecrosis of the femoral head, cataracts, and glaucoma. All topical corticosteroids are pregnancy category C.
- **Calcipotriene** (Dovonex) is a synthetic vitamin D_3 analogue that binds to vitamin D receptors, which inhibits keratinocyte proliferation and enhances keratinocyte differentiation. Vitamin D_3 analogues also inhibit T-lymphocyte activity.

TABLE 17–1	Topical Corticosteroid Potency Chart
Potency Rating	**Corticosteroid–Topical Preparations**
Class 1: Superpotent	Betamethasone dipropionate 0.05% ointment (Diprolene and Diprosone ointment)
	Clobetasone propionate 0.05% lotion/spray/shampoo (Clobex lotion/spray/shampoo, OLUX foam)
	Clobetasone propionate 0.05% cream and ointment (Cormax, Temovate)
	Diflorasone diacetate 0.05% ointment (Florone, Psorcon)
	Halobetasol propionate 0.05% cream and ointment (Ultravate)
	Flurandrenolide tape 4 mcg/cm² (Cordran)
Class 2: Potent	Amcinonide 0.1% ointment (Cyclocort ointment)
	Betamethasone dipropionate 0.05% cream/gel (Diprolene cream, gel, and Diprosone cream)
	Desoximetasone 0.25% cream (Topicort)
	Fluocinonide 0.05% cream, gel, ointment (Lidex)
	Halcinonide 0.1% cream (Halog)
Class 3: Upper mid–strength	Amcinonide 0.1% cream (Cyclocort cream)
	Betamethasone valerate 0.1% ointment (Betnovate/Valisone ointment)
	Diflorasone diacetate 0.05% cream (Psorcon cream)
	Fluticasone propionate 0.005% ointment (Cutivate ointment)
	Mometasone furoate 0.1% ointment (Elocon ointment)
	Triamcinolone acetonide 0.5% cream and ointment (Aristocort)
Class 4: Mid–strength	Betamethasone valerate 0.12% foam (Luxiq)
	Clocortolone pivolate 0.1% cream (Cloderm)
	Desoximetasone 0.05% cream and gel (Topicort LP)
	Fluocinolone acetonide 0.025% ointment (Synalar ointment)
	Fluocinolone acetonide 0.2% cream (Synalar–HP)
	Hydrocortisone valerate 0.2% ointment (Westcort ointment)
	Mometasone furoate 0.1% cream (Elocon cream)
	Triamcinolone acetonide 0.1% ointment (Kenalog)
Class 5: Lower mid–strength	Betamethasone dipropionate 0.05% lotion (Diprosone lotion)
	Betamethasone valerate 0.1% cream and lotion (Betnovate/Valisone cream & lotion)
	Desonide 0.05% lotion (DesOwen)
	Fluocinolone acetonide 0.01% shampoo (Capex shampoo)
	Fluocinolone acetonide 0.01%, 0.025%, 0.03% cream (Synalar cream)
	Flurandrenolide 0.05% cream and lotion (Cordran)
	Fluticasone propionate 0.05% cream and lotion (Cutivate cream and lotion)
	Hydrocortisone butyrate 0.1% cream (Locoid)
	Hydrocortisone valerate 0.2% cream (Westcort cream)
	Prednicarbate 0.1% cream (Dermatop)
	Triamcinolone acetonide 0.1% cream and lotion (Kenalog cream and lotion)

(continued)

TABLE 17–1	Topical Corticosteroid Potency Chart *(Continued)*
Potency Rating	**Corticosteroid–Topical Preparations**
Class 6: Mild	Alclometasone dipropionate 0.05% cream and ointment (Aclovate)
	Betamethasone valerate 0.05% cream and ointment
	Desonide 0.05% cream, ointment, gel (DesOwen, Desonate, Tridesilon)
	Desonide 0.05% foam (Verdeso)
	Fluocinonide acetonide 0.01% cream and solution (Synalar)
	Fluocinonide acetonide 0.01% FS oil (Derma–Smoothe)
Class 7: Least Potent	Hydrocortisone 0.5%, 1%, 2%, 2.5% cream, lotion, spray, and ointment (various brands)

Adapted from The National Psoriasis Foundation–Mild Psoriasis: Steroid potency chart, http://www.psoriasis. org/netcommunity/sublearn03_mild_potency. Rosso JD, Friedlander SF. Corticosteroids: Options in the era of steroid-sparing therapy. J Am Acad Dermatol 2005;53:S50–S58; and Leung DYM, Nicklas RA, Li JT, et al. Disease management of atopic dermatitis: An updated practice parameter. Ann Allergy Asthma Immunol 2004;93:S1–S17.

- For mild psoriasis, calcipotriene is more effective than anthralin and comparable to or slightly more effective than class 3 (upper midstrength) topical corticosteroid ointments. Calcipotriene 0.005% cream, ointment, or solution is applied one or two times daily (no more than 100 g/wk).
- Adverse effects of calcipotriene include mild irritant contact dermatitis, burning, pruritus, edema, peeling, dryness, and erythema. Calcipotriene is pregnancy category C.
- **Tazarotene** (Tazorac) is a topical retinoid that normalizes keratinocyte differentiation, diminishes keratinocyte hyperproliferation, and clears the inflammatory infiltrate in psoriatic plaques. It is available as a 0.05% or 0.1% gel and cream and is applied once daily (usually in the evening).
- Adverse effects of tazarotene include a high incidence of dose-dependent irritation at application sites, resulting in burning, stinging, and erythema. Irritation may be reduced by using the cream formulation, lower concentration, alternate-day applications, or short-contact (30–60 min) treatment. Tazarotene is pregnancy category X and should not be used in women of childbearing age unless effective contraception is being used.
- **Anthralin** has a direct antiproliferative effect on epidermal keratinocytes, normalizing keratinocyte differentiation. Short-contact anthralin therapy (SCAT) is usually the preferred regimen, with ointment applied only to the thick plaque lesions for 2 hours or less and then wiped off. Zinc oxide ointment or nonmedicated stiff paste should be applied to the surrounding normal skin to protect it from irritation. Anthralin should be used with caution, if at all, on the face and intertriginous areas due to the potential for severe skin irritation.
- Anthralin concentrations for SCAT range from 1% to 4% or as tolerated. Concentrations for continuous therapy vary from 0.05% to 0.4%.
- In addition to significant and often severe skin irritation, anthralin may cause folliculitis and allergic contact dermatitis, but these are uncommon. Anthralin is pregnancy category C.

- **Coal tar** is keratolytic and may have antiproliferative and antiinflammatory effects. Coal tar formulations include crude coal tar and tar distillates (liquor carbonis detergens) in ointments, creams, and shampoos. Coal tar is infrequently used due to limited efficacy and poor patient adherence and acceptance. It has a slower onset of action than calcipotriene, has an unpleasant odor, and stains clothing.
- Adverse effects of coal tar include folliculitis, acne, local irritation, and phototoxicity. It is carcinogenic in animals, but there are no convincing data for human carcinogenicity with topical use. The risk of teratogenicity when used in pregnancy is likely to be small, if it exists.
- **Salicylic acid** has keratolytic properties and has been used in shampoos or bath oils for scalp psoriasis. It enhances penetration of topical corticosteroids, thereby increasing corticosteroid efficacy. Systemic absorption and toxicity can occur, especially when applied to >20% BSA or in patients with renal impairment.
- Salicylic acid should not be used in children. It may be used for limited and localized plaque psoriasis in pregnancy.

Phototherapy and Photochemotherapy

- Phototherapy consists of nonionizing electromagnetic radiation, either ultraviolet A (UVA) or UVB, as light therapy for psoriatic lesions. UVB is given alone as either broadband or narrowband (NB-UVB). Broadband UVB is also given as photochemotherapy with topical agents such as crude coal tar (Goeckerman regimen) or anthralin (Ingram regimen) for enhanced efficacy. UVA is generally given with a photosensitizer such as an oral psoralen to enhance efficacy; this regimen is called PUVA (psoralen + UVA treatment).
- Adverse effects of phototherapy include erythema, pruritus, xerosis, hyperpigmentation, and blistering. Patients must be provided with eye protection during and for 24 hours after PUVA treatments. PUVA therapy may also cause nausea or vomiting, which may be minimized by taking the oral psoralens with food or milk. Long-term PUVA use can lead to photoaging and cataracts. PUVA is also associated with a dose-related risk of carcinogenesis.

Systemic Therapies

- **Acitretin** (Soriatane) is a retinoic acid derivative and the active metabolite of etretinate. Retinoids may be less effective than methotrexate or cyclosporine when used as monotherapy. Acitretin is more commonly used in combination with topical calcipotriene or phototherapy. The initial recommended dose is 25 or 50 mg; therapy is continued until lesions have resolved. It is better tolerated when taken with meals. Common adverse effects include hypertriglyceridemia and mucocutaneous effects such as dryness of the eyes, nasal and oral mucosa, chapped lips, cheilitis, epistaxis, xerosis, brittle nails, and burning skin. Less commonly, "retinoid dermatitis" may occur. Skeletal abnormalities occur rarely. All retinoids are teratogenic and are pregnancy category X. Acitretin should not be used in women of childbearing age unless they use effective contraception for the duration of therapy and for 3 years after drug discontinuation.

- **Cyclosporine** is a systemic calcineurin inhibitor that is effective for inducing remission and for maintenance therapy of moderate to severe plaque psoriasis. It is also effective in treating pustular, erythrodermic, and nail psoriasis. Clinical trials have shown cyclosporine to be significantly more effective than etretinate and similar or slightly better in efficacy than methotrexate. The usual dose is between 2.5 and 5 mg/kg/day given in two divided doses. After inducing remission, maintenance therapy using low doses (1.25–3 mg/kg/day) may prevent relapse. When discontinuing cyclosporine, a gradual taper of 1 mg/kg/day each week may prolong the time before relapse when compared with abrupt discontinuation. Because more than half of patients stopping cyclosporine relapse within 4 months, patients should be given appropriate alternative treatments shortly before or after discontinuing cyclosporine therapy. Adverse effects include nephrotoxicity, hypertension, hypomagnesemia, hyperkalemia, hypertriglyceridemia, hypertrichosis, and gingival hyperplasia. The risk of skin cancer increases with the duration of treatment and with prior PUVA treatments.

- **Methotrexate** has antiinflammatory effects due to its effects on T-cell gene expression and also has cytostatic effects. It is more effective than acitretin and has similar or slightly less efficacy than cyclosporine. Methotrexate can be administered orally, subcutaneously, or intramuscularly. The starting dose is 7.5 to 15 mg once weekly, increased incrementally by 2.5 mg every 2 to 4 weeks until response; maximal doses are ~25 mg wkly. Adverse effects include nausea, vomiting, stomatitis, macrocytic anemia, and hepatic and pulmonary toxicity. Nausea and macrocytic anemia may be reduced by giving oral folic acid 1 to 5 mg daily. Methotrexate should be avoided in patients with active infections and in those with liver disease. It is an abortifacient and teratogenic and is contraindicated in pregnancy (pregnancy category X).

Systemic Therapy with Biologic Response Modifiers

- Biologic response modifiers (BRMs) are often considered for patients with moderate to severe psoriasis when other systemic agents are inadequate or contraindicated. Cost considerations tend to limit their use as first-line therapy.

- **Adalimumab** (Humira) is a monoclonal TNF-α antibody that provides rapid control of psoriasis. It is indicated for psoriatic arthritis and treatment of adults with moderate to severe chronic plaque psoriasis who are candidates for systemic therapy or phototherapy. The recommended dose for psoriatic arthritis is 40 mg subcutaneously every other week. The recommended dose for adults with plaque psoriasis is an initial dose of 80 mg, followed by 40 mg every other week starting 1 week after the initial dose. The most common adverse reactions are infections (e.g., upper respiratory and sinusitis), injection site reactions, headache, and rash.

- **Etanercept** (Enbrel) is a fusion protein that binds TNF-α, competitively interfering with its interaction with cell-bound receptors. Unlike the chimeric infliximab, etanercept is fully humanized, thereby minimizing the risk of immunogenicity. Etanercept is FDA approved for reducing signs and symptoms and inhibiting the progression of joint damage in patients with psoriatic arthritis. It can be used in combination with methotrexate in patients who do not respond adequately to methotrexate alone. It is also indicated for adult patients with chronic moderate to severe plaque psoriasis. The recommended dose for psoriatic arthritis is 50 mg subcutaneously once per week. For plaque psoriasis, the dose is 50 mg subcutaneously twice weekly (administered 3 or 4 days apart) for 3 months, followed by a maintenance dose of 50 mg once weekly. Adverse effects include local reactions at the injection site (20% of patients), respiratory tract and GI infections, abdominal pain, nausea and vomiting, headaches, and rash. Serious infections (including tuberculosis) and malignancies are rare.

- **Infliximab** (Remicade) is a chimeric monoclonal antibody directed against TNF-α. It is indicated for psoriatic arthritis and chronic severe plaque psoriasis. The recommended dose is 5 mg/kg as an IV infusion at weeks 0, 2, and 6, then every 8 weeks thereafter. For psoriatic arthritis, it may be used with or without methotrexate. Adverse effects include headaches, fever, chills, fatigue, diarrhea, pharyngitis, and upper respiratory and urinary tract infections. Hypersensitivity reactions (urticaria, dyspnea, and hypotension) and lymphoproliferative disorders have been reported.

- **Alefacept** (Amevive) is a dimeric fusion protein that binds to CD2 (cluster of differentiation 2) on T cells to inhibit cutaneous T-cell activation and proliferation. It also produces a dose-dependent decrease in circulating total lymphocytes. Alefacept is approved for treatment of moderate to severe plaque psoriasis and is also effective for treatment of psoriatic arthritis. Significant response is usually achieved after about 3 months of therapy. The recommended dose is 15 mg intramuscularly once weekly for 12 weeks. Adverse effects are mild and include pharyngitis, flu-like symptoms, chills, dizziness, nausea, headache, injection site pain and inflammation, and nonspecific infection.

- **Ustekinumab** (Stelara) is an IL-12/23 monoclonal antibody approved for the treatment of psoriasis in adults 18 years or older with moderate to severe plaque psoriasis. In two large randomized, placebo-controlled trials, ~70% of patients achieved 75% skin clearance after two doses and maintained the response for 1 year with continued treatment. The recommended dose for patients weighing ≤100 kg is 45 mg initially and 4 weeks later, followed by 45 mg every12 weeks. For patients weighing >100 kg, the dose is 90 mg initially and 4 weeks later, followed by 90 mg every 12 weeks. Common adverse effects include upper respiratory infections, headache, and tiredness. Serious adverse effects include those seen with other BRMs, including tubercular, fungal, and viral infections and cancers. One case of reversible posterior leukoencephalopathy syndrome (RPLS) has been reported.

Combination Therapies

- Combination therapy may be used to either enhance efficacy or minimize toxicity. Combinations can include two topical agents, a topical agent plus phototherapy, a systemic agent plus topical therapy, a systemic agent plus phototherapy, two systemic agents used in rotation, or a systemic agent and a BRM (see **Figs. 17–1** and **17–2**).

- The combination of a topical corticosteroid and a topical vitamin D_3 analogue is effective and safe with less skin irritation than monotherapy with either agent. The combination product containing calcipotriene and betamethasone dipropionate ointment (Taclonex) is effective for relatively severe psoriasis and may also be steroid sparing.

- The combination of retinoids with phototherapy (e.g., tazarotene plus broadband UVB, acitretin plus broadband UVB or NB-UVB) also increases efficacy. Because retinoids may be photosensitizing and increase the risk of burning after UV exposure, doses of phototherapy should be reduced to minimize adverse effects. The combination of acitretin and PUVA (RE-PUVA) may be more effective than monotherapy with either treatment.
- Phototherapy has also been used with other topical agents, such as UVB with coal tar (Goeckerman regimen) to increase treatment response, as coal tar is also photosensitizing.
- BRMs used in combination with other therapies are being explored (e.g., alefacept plus NB-UVB, infliximab plus methotrexate).

Alternative Drug Treatments

- **Mycophenolate mofetil** (CellCept) inhibits DNA and RNA synthesis and may have a specific lymphocyte antiproliferative effect. Although not FDA approved for this indication, oral mycophenolate mofetil may be effective in some cases of moderate to severe plaque psoriasis. The usual dose is 500 mg orally four times daily, up to a maximum of 4 g daily. Common adverse effects include GI toxicity (diarrhea, nausea, and vomiting), hematologic effects (anemia, neutropenia, and thrombocytopenia), and viral and bacterial infections. Lymphoproliferative disease or lymphoma has been reported.
- **Hydroxyurea** inhibits cell synthesis in the S phase of the DNA cycle. It is sometimes used for patients with recalcitrant severe psoriasis, but BRMs may be a better option in these patients. The typical dose is 1 g daily, with a gradual increase to 2 g daily as needed and as tolerated. Adverse effects include bone marrow suppression, lesional erythema, localized tenderness, and reversible hyperpigmentation.

EVALUATION OF THERAPEUTIC OUTCOMES

- Patients should understand the general concepts of therapy and the importance of adherence.
- A positive response involves normalization of involved areas of skin, as measured by reduced erythema and scaling, as well as reduction of plaque elevation.
- PASI is a uniform method to determine the extent of BSA affected, along with the degree of erythema, induration, and scaling. Severity scores are rated as <12 (mild), 12 to 18 (moderate), and >18 (severe).
- The Physician Global Assessment can also be used to summarize erythema, induration, scaling, and extent of plaques relative to baseline assessment.
- The National Psoriasis Foundation Psoriasis Score incorporates quality of life and the patient's perception of well-being, as well as induration, extent of involvement, the physician's static global assessment, and pruritus.

- Achievement of efficacy by any therapeutic regimen requires days to weeks. Initial dramatic response may be achieved with some agents, such as corticosteroids. However, sustained benefit with pharmacologically specific antipsoriatic therapy may require 2 to 8 weeks or longer for clinically meaningful response.

See Chapter 107, Psoriasis, authored by Rebecca M. Law and Wayne P. Gulliver, for a more detailed discussion of this topic.

18 Adrenal Gland Disorders

DEFINITIONS

- Hyperfunction of the adrenal glands occurs in Cushing's syndrome, a disorder caused by excessive secretion of cortisol by the adrenal gland (hypercortisolism). Other causes of adrenal gland hyperfunction include primary and secondary aldosteronism (not discussed in this chapter; refer to textbook Chap. 85 for more information on these disorders).
- Adrenal gland hypofunction is associated with primary (Addison's disease) or secondary adrenal insufficiency. Adrenal insufficiency occurs when the adrenal glands do not produce enough cortisol and, in some cases, aldosterone.

CUSHING'S SYNDROME

PATHOPHYSIOLOGY

- Cushing's syndrome results from the effects of supraphysiologic levels of glucocorticoids originating from either exogenous administration or endogenous overproduction by the adrenal gland (adrenocorticotropic hormone [ACTH]-dependent) or by abnormal adrenocortical tissues (ACTH-independent).
- ACTH-dependent Cushing's syndrome (80% of all cases of Cushing's syndrome) is usually caused by overproduction of ACTH by the pituitary gland, causing adrenal hyperplasia. Pituitary adenomas account for ~85% of these cases (Cushing's disease). Ectopic ACTH-secreting tumors and nonneoplastic corticotropin hypersecretion are responsible for the remaining 20% of ACTH-dependent cases.
- Ectopic ACTH syndrome refers to excessive ACTH production resulting from an endocrine or nonendocrine tumor, usually of the pancreas, thyroid, or lung (e.g., small-cell lung cancer).
- ACTH-independent Cushing's syndrome is usually caused by adrenal adenomas and carcinomas.

CLINICAL PRESENTATION

- The most common findings in Cushing's syndrome are central obesity and facial rounding (90% of patients). Peripheral obesity and fat accumulation occur in 50% of patients. Fat accumulation in the dorsocervical area (buffalo hump) is a nonspecific finding, but increased supraclavicular fat pads are more specific for Cushing's syndrome. Patients are often described as having moon facies and a buffalo hump.

- Many patients complain of myopathies (65%) or muscular weakness (85%).
- Striae are usually present along the lower abdomen and take on a red to purple color.
- Hypertension is seen in 75% to 85% of patients, with diastolic blood pressure >119 mm Hg noted in >20% of patients.
- Glucose intolerance is seen in 60% of patients.
- Psychiatric changes can occur in up to 55% of patients.
- Approximately 50% to 60% of patients develop Cushing's-induced osteoporosis; ~40% present with back pain, and 20% will progress to compression fractures of the spine.
- Gonadal dysfunction is common, with amenorrhea seen in up to 75% of women.
- Excess androgen secretion is responsible for 80% of women presenting with hirsutism.

DIAGNOSIS

- The presence of hypercortisolism can be established with a 24-hour urinary free cortisol (UFC), midnight plasma cortisol, late-night (11 PM) salivary cortisol, and/or low-dose dexamethasone suppression test (DST).
- Other diagnostic tests are the plasma ACTH test; adrenal vein catheterization; metyrapone stimulation test; adrenal, chest, or abdominal computed tomography (CT); corticotropin-releasing hormone (CRH) stimulation test; inferior petrosal sinus sampling; and pituitary magnetic resonance imaging (MRI).
- Adrenal nodules and masses are identified using high-resolution CT scanning and perhaps MRI.

DESIRED OUTCOME

- The goals of treatment for Cushing's syndrome are to limit morbidity and mortality and return the patient to a normal functional state by removing the source of hypercortisolism without causing any pituitary or adrenal deficiencies.

TREATMENT

- Treatment plans in Cushing's syndrome based on etiology are included in Table 18–1.

Nonpharmacologic Therapy

- The treatment of choice for both ACTH-dependent and ACTH-independent Cushing's syndrome is surgical resection of offending tumors. Transsphenoidal resection of the pituitary microadenoma is the treatment of choice for Cushing's disease.
- Pituitary irradiation provides clinical improvement in ~50% of patients within 3 to 5 years, but improvement may not be seen for 6 to 12 months, and pituitary-dependent hormone deficiencies can occur.

TABLE 18–1 Possible Treatment Plans in Cushing's Syndrome Based on Etiology

Etiology	Nondrug	Generic (Brand) Drug Name	Initial	Usual	Max
Ectopic ACTH syndrome	Surgery, chemotherapy, irradiation	Metyrapone (Metopirone) 250 mg capsules	0.5–1 g/day, divided every 4 to 6 hours	1–2 g/day, divided every 4 to 6 hours	6 g/day
		Aminoglutethimide (Cytadren) 250 mg tablets	0.5–1 g/day, divided two to four times daily for 2 weeks	1 g/day, divided every 6 hours	2 g/day
Pituitary-dependent	Surgery, irradiation	Cyproheptadine (Periactin) 2 mg/5 mL syrup or 4 mg tablets	4 mg twice daily	24–32 mg/day, divided four times daily	32 mg/day
		Mitotane (Lysodren) 500 mg tablets	0.5–1 g/day, increased by 0.5–1 g/ day every 1 to 4 weeks	1–4 g daily, with food to decrease GI effects	12 g/day
		Metyrapone	See above	See above	See above
Adrenal adenoma	Surgery, postoperative replacement	Ketoconazole (Nizoral) 200 mg tablets	200 mg once or twice a day	200–1,200 mg/day, divided twice daily	1,600 mg/day divided four times daily
Adrenal carcinoma	Surgery	Mitotane	See above	See above	See above

ACTH, adrenocorticotropic hormone.

- Laparoscopic adrenalectomy may be preferred in patients with unilateral adrenal adenomas or for whom transsphenoidal surgery and pituitary radiotherapy have failed or cannot be used.

Pharmacotherapy

- Pharmacologic options are generally used as secondary treatments in preoperative patients or as adjunctive therapy in postoperative patients awaiting a response. Rarely, single-drug therapy is used as a palliative treatment when surgery is not indicated.

STEROIDOGENIC INHIBITORS

- **Metyrapone** inhibits 11 β-hydroxylase, thereby inhibiting cortisol synthesis. Initially, patients can demonstrate an increase in plasma ACTH concentrations because of a sudden drop in cortisol. This can increase androgenic and mineralocorticoid hormones, resulting in hypertension, acne, and hirsutism. Nausea, vomiting, vertigo, headache, dizziness, abdominal discomfort, and allergic rash have been reported after oral administration. Metyrapone is currently available through the manufacturer only for compassionate use.
- **Ketoconazole** inhibits cytochrome P-450 enzymes, including 11 β-hydroxylase and 17 α-hydroxylase. It is effective in lowering serum cortisol levels after several weeks of therapy. It also has antiandrogenic activity, which may be beneficial in women but can cause gynecomastia and decreased libido in men. The most common adverse effects are reversible elevation of hepatic transaminases, GI discomfort, and dermatologic reactions. Ketoconazole may be used concomitantly with metyrapone to achieve synergistic reduction in cortisol levels; in addition, ketoconazole's antiandrogenic actions may offset the androgenic potential of metyrapone.
- **Etomidate** is an imidazole derivative similar to ketoconazole that inhibits 11 β-hydroxylase. Because it is only available in a parenteral formulation, its use is limited to patients with acute hypercortisolemia requiring emergency treatment.
- **Aminoglutethimide** inhibits cortisol synthesis by blocking the conversion of cholesterol to pregnenolone early in the cortisol pathway. The side effects of severe sedation, nausea, ataxia, and skin rashes limit aminoglutethimide use in many patients. Other steroidogenesis inhibitors offer greater efficacy with fewer side effects; if aminoglutethimide is used, it should be coadministered with another steroidogenesis inhibitor (usually metyrapone) due to high relapse rates with aminoglutethimide monotherapy.

ADRENOLYTIC AGENTS

- **Mitotane** is a cytotoxic drug that inhibits the 11-hydroxylation of 11-desoxycortisol and 11-desoxycorticosterone in the adrenal cortex, reducing synthesis of cortisol and corticosterone. Similar to ketoconazole, mitotane takes weeks to months to exert beneficial effects. Sustained cortisol suppression occurs in most patients and may persist after drug discontinuation in up to one third of patients. Mitotane degenerates cells within the zona fasciculata and reticularis; the zona glomerulosa is minimally affected during acute therapy but can become damaged after long-term treatment. Mitotane can cause significant neurologic and GI side effects, and patients should be monitored carefully or hospitalized when initiating therapy. Nausea and diarrhea are common at doses >2 g/day and can be avoided by gradually increasing the dose and/or administering it with food. Lethargy, somnolence, and other CNS effects are also common. Reversible hypercholesterolemia and prolonged bleeding times can occur.

NEUROMODULATORS OF ACTH RELEASE

- Pituitary secretion of ACTH is normally mediated by neurotransmitters such as serotonin, γ-aminobutyric acid (GABA), acetylcholine, and catecholamines. Although ACTH-secreting pituitary tumors (Cushing's disease) self-regulate ACTH production to some degree, these neurotransmitters can still promote pituitary ACTH production. Consequently, agents that target these transmitters have been proposed for treatment of Cushing's disease. Such agents include cyproheptadine, bromocriptine, cabergoline, valproic acid, octreotide, rosiglitazone, and tretinoin. None of these drugs have demonstrated consistent clinical efficacy for treating Cushing's syndrome.
- **Cyproheptadine** can decrease ACTH secretion in some patients with Cushing's disease. However, side effects such as sedation and weight gain significantly limit its use.

GLUCOCORTICOID-RECEPTOR BLOCKING AGENTS

- **Mifepristone** (RU-486) is a progesterone- and glucocorticoid-receptor antagonist that inhibits dexamethasone suppression and increases endogenous cortisol and ACTH values in normal subjects. Limited experience in Cushing's syndrome suggests that mifepristone is highly effective in reversing the manifestations of hypercortisolism. Its use for treatment of Cushing's syndrome remains investigational.

EVALUATION OF THERAPEUTIC OUTCOMES

- Close monitoring of 24-hour UFC and serum cortisol levels are essential to identify adrenal insufficiency in patients with Cushing's syndrome. Steroid secretion should be monitored with all drug therapy and corticosteroid replacement given if needed.

ADRENAL INSUFFICIENCY

PATHOPHYSIOLOGY

- Primary adrenal insufficiency (Addison's disease) most often involves the destruction of all regions of the adrenal cortex. There are deficiencies of cortisol, aldosterone, and the various androgens, and levels of CRH and ACTH increase in a compensatory manner.
- Autoimmune dysfunction is responsible for 80% to 90% of cases in developed countries, whereas tuberculosis is the predominant cause in developing countries.

- Medications that inhibit cortisol synthesis (e.g., ketoconazole) or accelerate cortisol metabolism (e.g., phenytoin, rifampin, and phenobarbital) can also cause primary adrenal insufficiency.
- Secondary adrenal insufficiency most commonly results from exogenous corticosteroid use, leading to suppression of the hypothalamic-pituitary-adrenal axis and decreased release of ACTH, resulting in impaired androgen and cortisol production. Mirtazapine and progestins (e.g., medroxyprogesterone acetate and megestrol acetate) have also been reported to induce secondary adrenal insufficiency. Secondary disease typically presents with normal mineralocorticoid concentrations.

CLINICAL PRESENTATION

- Weight loss, dehydration, hyponatremia, hyperkalemia, and elevated blood urea nitrogen are common in Addison's disease.
- Hyperpigmentation is common in Addison's disease and may involve exposed and nonexposed parts of the body. Hyperpigmentation is usually not seen in secondary adrenal insufficiency because of low amounts of melanocyte-stimulating hormone.

DIAGNOSIS

- The short cosyntropin stimulation test can be used to assess patients with suspected hypocortisolism. An increase to a cortisol level ≥18 mcg/dL (500 nmol/L) rules out adrenal insufficiency.
- Patients with Addison's disease have an abnormal response to the short cosyntropin stimulation test. Plasma ACTH levels are usually 400 to 2,000 pg/mL in primary insufficiency versus normal to low (5–50 pg/mL) in secondary insufficiency. A normal cosyntropin-stimulation test does not rule out secondary adrenal insufficiency.
- Other tests include the insulin hypoglycemia test, the metyrapone test, and the CRH stimulation test.

DESIRED OUTCOME

- The goals of treatment for adrenal insufficiency are to limit morbidity and mortality, return the patient to a normal functional state, and prevent episodes of acute adrenal insufficiency.

TREATMENT

Nonpharmacologic Therapy

- Patients must be informed of treatment complications, expected outcome, proper medication administration and adherence, and possible side effects.

Pharmacotherapy of Adrenal Insufficiency

CORTICOSTEROIDS

- **Hydrocortisone, cortisone**, and **prednisone** are the glucocorticoids of choice, administered twice daily at the lowest effective dose while mimicking the normal diurnal adrenal rhythm of cortisol production.

TABLE 18–2	Relative Potencies of Glucocorticoids			
Glucocorticoid	Antiinflammatory Potency	Equivalent Potency (mg)	Approximate Half-Life (min)	Sodium-retaining Potency
Cortisone	0.8	25	30	2
Hydrocortisone	1	20	90	2
Prednisone	3.5	5	60	1
Prednisolone	4	5	200	1
Triamcinolone	5	4	300	0
Methylprednisolone	5	4	180	0
Betamethasone	25	0.6	100–300	0
Dexamethasone	30	0.75	100–300	0

- Recommended starting total daily doses are hydrocortisone 15 to 25 mg daily, which is approximately equivalent to cortisone acetate 25 to 37.5 mg, or prednisone 2.5 mg (**Table 18–2**). Two thirds of the dose is given in the morning, and one third is given 6 to 8 hours later.
- The patient's symptoms can be monitored every 6 to 8 weeks to assess proper glucocorticoid replacement.
- **Fludrocortisone acetate** 0.05 to 0.2 mg orally once daily can be used to replace mineralocorticoid loss. If parenteral therapy is needed, 2 to 5 mg of deoxycorticosterone trimethylacetate in oil can be administered intramuscularly every 3 to 4 weeks. The major reason for adding the mineralocorticoid is to minimize development of hyperkalemia.
- Because most adrenal crises occur because of glucocorticoid dose reductions or lack of stress-related dose adjustments, patients receiving corticosteroid replacement therapy should add 5 to 10 mg hydrocortisone (or equivalent) to their normal daily regimen shortly before strenuous activities, such as exercise. During times of severe physical stress (e.g., febrile illnesses and after accidents), patients should be instructed to double their daily dose until recovery.
- Treatment of secondary adrenal insufficiency is identical to primary disease treatment, with the exception that mineralocorticoid replacement is usually not necessary.

Pharmacotherapy of Acute Adrenal Insufficiency

- Acute adrenal insufficiency (also known as adrenal crisis or addisonian crisis) represents a true endocrine emergency.
- Stressful situations, surgery, infection, and trauma are potential events that increase adrenal requirements, especially in patients with some underlying adrenal or pituitary insufficiency.
- The most common cause of adrenal crisis is abrupt withdrawal of exogenous glucocorticoids in patients receiving chronic treatment that resulted in hypothalamic-pituitary-adrenal-axis suppression.
- **Hydrocortisone** given parenterally is the corticosteroid of choice because of its combined glucocorticoid and mineralocorticoid activity.

The starting dose is 100 mg IV by rapid infusion, followed by a continuous infusion (usually 10 mg/hour) or intermittent bolus of 100 to 200 mg every 24 hours. IV administration is continued for 24 to 48 hours. If the patient is stable at that time, oral hydrocortisone can be started at a dose of 50 mg every 6 to 8 hours, followed by tapering to the individual's chronic replacement needs.

- **Fluid replacement** often is required and can be accomplished with IV dextrose 5% in normal saline solution at a rate to support blood pressure.
- If hyperkalemia is present after the hydrocortisone maintenance phase, additional mineralocorticoid supplementation can be achieved with **fludrocortisone acetate** 0.1 mg daily.
- Patients with adrenal insufficiency should carry a card or wear a bracelet or necklace that contains information about their condition. They should also have easy access to injectable hydrocortisone or glucocorticoid suppositories in case of an emergency or during times of physical stress, such as febrile illness or injury.

EVALUATION OF THERAPEUTIC OUTCOMES

- The end point of therapy for adrenal insufficiency is difficult to assess in most patients, but a reduction in excess pigmentation is a good clinical marker. Development of features of Cushing's syndrome indicates excessive replacement.

See Chapter 85, Adrenal Gland Disorders, authored by Steven M. Smith and John G. Gums, for a more detailed discussion of this topic.

Diabetes Mellitus

DEFINITION

- Diabetes mellitus (DM) is a group of metabolic disorders characterized by hyperglycemia and abnormalities in carbohydrate, fat, and protein metabolism. It results from defects in insulin secretion, insulin sensitivity, or both. Chronic microvascular, macrovascular, and neuropathic complications may ensue.

PATHOPHYSIOLOGY

- Type 1 DM accounts for 5% to 10% of all diabetes cases. It generally develops in childhood or early adulthood and results from immune-mediated destruction of pancreatic β-cells, resulting in an absolute deficiency of insulin. There is a long preclinical period (9–13 years) marked by the presence of immune markers when β-cell destruction is thought to occur. Hyperglycemia occurs when 80% to 90% of β-cells are destroyed. There is a transient remission ("honeymoon" phase) followed by established disease with associated risks for complications and death. The factors that initiate the autoimmune process are unknown, but the process is mediated by macrophages and T lymphocytes with circulating autoantibodies to various β-cell antigens (e.g., islet cell antibody, insulin antibodies).
- Type 2 DM accounts for up to 90% of DM cases and is usually characterized by the presence of both insulin resistance and relative insulin deficiency. Insulin resistance is manifested by increased lipolysis and free fatty acid production, increased hepatic glucose production, and decreased skeletal muscle uptake of glucose. β-Cell dysfunction is progressive and contributes to worsening blood glucose control over time. Type 2 DM occurs when a diabetogenic lifestyle (excessive calories, inadequate exercise, and obesity) is superimposed upon a susceptible genotype.
- Uncommon causes of diabetes (1–2% of cases) include endocrine disorders (e.g., acromegaly and Cushing's syndrome), gestational diabetes mellitus (GDM), diseases of the exocrine pancreas (e.g., pancreatitis), and medications (e.g., glucocorticoids, pentamidine, niacin, and α-interferon).
- *Impaired fasting glucose* and *impaired glucose tolerance* are terms used to describe patients whose plasma glucose levels are higher than normal but not diagnostic of DM (see Diagnosis). These disorders are risk factors for developing DM and cardiovascular disease and are associated with the insulin-resistance syndrome.
- Microvascular complications include retinopathy, neuropathy, and nephropathy. Macrovascular complications include coronary heart disease, stroke, and peripheral vascular disease.

217

CLINICAL PRESENTATION

TYPE 1 DIABETES MELLITUS

- Individuals with type 1 DM are often thin and are prone to develop diabetic ketoacidosis if insulin is withheld or under conditions of severe stress with an excess of insulin counterregulatory hormones.
- Between 20% and 40% of patients present with diabetic ketoacidosis after several days of polyuria, polydipsia, polyphagia, and weight loss.

TYPE 2 DIABETES MELLITUS

- Patients with type 2 DM are often asymptomatic and may be diagnosed secondary to unrelated blood testing. However, the presence of complications may indicate that they have had DM for several years.
- Lethargy, polyuria, nocturia, and polydipsia can be present on diagnosis; significant weight loss is less common.

DIAGNOSIS

- Criteria for the diagnosis of DM include any one of the following:
  1. Hemoglobin A1C ≥6.5%
  2. Fasting (defined as no caloric intake for at least 8 hours) plasma glucose ≥126 mg/dL (7.0 mmol/L)
  3. Two-hour plasma glucose ≥200 mg/dL (111.1 mmol/L) during an oral glucose tolerance test (OGTT) using a glucose load containing the equivalent of 75 g anhydrous glucose dissolved in water
  4. A random plasma glucose concentration ≥200 mg/dL (111.1 mmol/L) in a patient with classic symptoms of hyperglycemia or hyperglycemic crisis

In the absence of unequivocal hyperglycemia, criteria 1 through 3 should be confirmed by repeat testing.

- The normal fasting plasma glucose (FPG) is <100 mg/dL (5.6 mmol/L).
- Impaired fasting glucose is defined as FPG of 100 to 125 mg/dL (5.6–6.9 mmol/L).
- Impaired glucose tolerance is diagnosed when the 2-hour postload sample of the OGTT is between 140 and 199 mg per dL (7.8–11.0 mmol/L).
- Pregnant women should undergo risk assessment for GDM at their first prenatal visit and proceed with glucose testing if at high risk (e.g., positive family history, personal history of GDM, marked obesity, or member of a high-risk ethnic group).

DESIRED OUTCOME

- The goals of therapy in DM are to ameliorate symptoms of hyperglycemia, reduce the risk of microvascular and macrovascular complications, reduce mortality, and improve quality of life. Desirable plasma glucose and glycosylated hemoglobin (A1C) levels are listed in **Table 19–1**.

TABLE 19–1	Glycemic Goals of Therapy	
Biochemical Index	ADA	ACE and AACE
Hemoglobin A1C	<7%[a]	≤6.5%
Preprandial plasma glucose	70–130 mg/dL	<110 mg/dL
	(3.9–7.2 mmol/L)	(6.1 mmol/L)
Postprandial plasma glucose	<180 mg/dL[b]	<140 mg/dL
	(<10 mmol/L)	(<7.8 mmol/L)

AACE, American Association of Clinical Endocrinologists; ACE, American College of Endocrinology; ADA, American Diabetes Association.

[a]Referenced to a nondiabetic range of 4% to 6% using a Diabetes Control and Complications Trial–based assay. More stringent glycemic goals (i.e., a normal A1C, <6%) may be appropriate if accomplished without significant hypoglycemia or adverse effects. Less stringent goals may also be appropriate in some situations.

[b]Postprandial glucose measurements should be made 1 to 2 hours after the beginning of the meal, generally the time of peak levels in patients with diabetes.

TREATMENT

GENERAL APPROACH

- Near-normal glycemia reduces the risk of microvascular disease complications, but aggressive management of traditional cardiovascular risk factors (i.e., smoking cessation, treatment of dyslipidemia, intensive blood pressure (BP) control, and antiplatelet therapy) is needed to reduce macrovascular disease risk.

- Appropriate care requires goal setting for glycemia, BP, and lipid levels; regular monitoring for complications; dietary and exercise modifications; appropriate self-monitoring of blood glucose (SMBG); and appropriate assessment of laboratory parameters.

NONPHARMACOLOGIC THERAPY

- Medical nutrition therapy is recommended for all patients. For individuals with type 1 DM, the focus is on regulating insulin administration with a balanced diet to achieve and maintain a healthy body weight. A meal plan that is moderate in carbohydrates and low in saturated fat, with a focus on balanced meals, is recommended. Patients with type 2 DM often require caloric restriction to promote weight loss. Bedtime and between-meal snacks are not usually needed if pharmacologic management is appropriate.

- Aerobic exercise improves insulin sensitivity and glycemic control in most patients and may reduce cardiovascular risk factors, contribute to weight loss or maintenance, and improve well-being. Exercise should be started slowly in previously sedentary patients. Older patients and those with atherosclerotic disease should have a cardiovascular evaluation prior to beginning an exercise program.

PHARMACOLOGIC THERAPY: DRUG CLASS INFORMATION

Insulin

(Table 19–2 and 19–3)

- **Regular insulin** has a relatively slow onset of action when given subcutaneously, requiring injection 30 minutes prior to meals to achieve

---

TABLE 19–2	Available Insulins and Other Injectable Preparations	
Generic Name	**Analog**[a]	**Administration Options**
Rapid-acting insulins		
Humalog (insulin lispro)	Yes	Insulin pen 3 mL, vial, and 3 mL pen cartridge
NovoLog (insulin aspart)	Yes	Insulin pen 3 mL, vial, or 3 mL pen cartridge
Apidra (insulin glulisine)	Yes	3 mL pen cartridge or OptiClik pen system
Short-acting insulins		
Humulin R (regular)	No	U-100, 10 mL vial; U-500, 20 mL vial
Novolin R (regular)	No	Insulin pen, vial, or 3 mL pen cartridge, and InnoLet
Intermediate-acting insulins (NPH)		
Humulin N	No	Vial, 3 mL prefilled pen
Novolin N	No	Vial, prefilled pen, and InnoLet
Long-acting insulins		
Lantus (insulin glargine)	Yes	Vial, 3 mL OptiClik pen system
Levemir (insulin detemir)	Yes	Vial, 3 mL pen cartridge and InnoLet
Premixed insulins		
Premixed insulin analog		
Humalog Mix 75/25 (75%	Yes	Vial, prefilled pen
neutral protamine lispro,		Vial, prefilled pen, 3 mL pen cartridge
25% lispro)	Yes	3 mL pen
Novolog Mix 70/30		
(70% aspart protamine		
suspension, 30% aspart)	Yes	
Humalog Mix 50/50 (50%		
neutral protamine lispro,		
50% lispro)		
NPH-regular combinations		
Humulin 70/30	No	Vial, 3 mL prefilled pen
Novolin 70/30	No	Vial, pen cartridge, InnoLet
Other injectable preparations		
Exenatide (Byetta)	No	5 mcg/dose and 10 mcg/dose, 60 doses prefilled pen
Liraglutide (Victoza)	Yes	3 mL pen, can deliver 0.6 mg, 1.2 mg, or 1.8 mg dose
Pramlintide (Symlin)	Yes	5 mL vial, 1.5 mL and 2.7 mL SymlinPen

NPH, neutral protamine Hagedorn.

[a]All insulins available in the United States are made by human recombinant DNA technology. An insulin analog is a modified human insulin molecule that imparts particular pharmacokinetic advantages.

TABLE 19–3	Pharmacokinetics of Various Insulins Administered Subcutaneously				
Type of Insulin	Onset	Peak (hours)	Duration (hours)	Maximum Duration (hours)	Appearance
Rapid-acting					
Aspart	15–30 min	1–2	3–5	5–6	Clear
Lispro	15–30 min	1–2	3–4	4–6	Clear
Glulisine	15–30 min	1–2	3–4	5–6	Clear
Short-acting					
Regular	30–60 min	2–3	3–6	6–8	Clear
Intermediate-acting					
NPH	2–4 hours	4–6	8–12	14–18	Cloudy
Long-acting					
Detemir	2 hours	6–9	14–24	24	Clear
Glargine	4–5 hours	–	22–24	24	Clear

NPH, neutral protamine Hagedorn.

optimal postprandial glucose control and to prevent delayed postmeal hypoglycemia.

- **Lispro, aspart**, and **glulisine insulins** are analogs that are more rapidly absorbed, peak faster, and have shorter durations of action than regular insulin. This permits more convenient dosing within 10 minutes of meals (rather than 30 min prior), produces better efficacy in lowering postprandial blood glucose than regular insulin in type 1 DM, and minimizes delayed postmeal hypoglycemia.

- **Neutral protamine Hagedorn (NPH)** is intermediate-acting. Variability in absorption, inconsistent preparation by the patient, and inherent pharmacokinetic differences may contribute to a labile glucose response, nocturnal hypoglycemia, and fasting hyperglycemia.

- **Glargine** and **detemir** are long-acting "peakless" human insulin analogs that result in less nocturnal hypoglycemia than NPH insulin when given at bedtime.

- In type 1 DM, the average daily insulin requirement is 0.5 to 0.6 units/kg. Requirements may fall to 0.1 to 0.4 units/kg in the honeymoon phase. Higher doses (0.5–1 unit/kg) are warranted during acute illness or ketosis. In type 2 DM, a dosage range of 0.7 to 2.5 units/kg is often required for patients with significant insulin resistance.

- Hypoglycemia and weight gain are the most common adverse effects of insulin. Treatment of hypoglycemia is as follows:
  - ✓ **Glucose** (10–15 g) given orally is the recommended treatment in conscious patients.
  - ✓ **Dextrose** IV may be required in individuals who have lost consciousness.
  - ✓ **Glucagon**, 1 g intramuscularly, is the treatment of choice in unconscious patients when IV access cannot be established.

Glucagon-like Peptide 1 (GLP-1) Agonists

- **Exenatide** (Byetta) is a synthetic analog of exendin-4, a 39-amino acid peptide isolated from the saliva of the Gila monster that enhances glucose-dependent insulin secretion and reduces hepatic glucose production. It also decreases appetite and slows gastric emptying, which may reduce caloric intake and cause weight loss. It significantly decreases postprandial glucose excursions but has only a modest effect on FPG values. The average A1C reduction is ~0.9%. The most common adverse effects are nausea, vomiting, and diarrhea. The initial dose is 5 mcg subcutaneously twice daily, titrated to 10 mcg twice daily in 1 month if needed and as tolerated. It should be injected 0 to 60 minutes before the morning and evening meals.

- **Liraglutide** (Victoza) is produced through recombinant DNA technology and has 97% amino acid sequence homology to endogenous GLP-1. Its pharmacologic and adverse effects are similar to exenatide. Its longer half-life permits once-daily dosing. The average A1C reduction is ~1.1%. Dosing of liraglutide should be 0.6 mg subcutaneously once daily for at least 1 week, then increased to 1.2 mg daily for at least 1 week. Patients may be maintained on the 1.2 mg dose or increased to the maximum dose of 1.8 mg daily after at least 1 week of therapy. Dosing can be given independent of meals.

Amylinomimetic

- **Pramlintide** (Symlin) is a synthetic analog of amylin, a neurohormone cosecreted from β-cells with insulin. Pramlintide suppresses inappropriately high postprandial glucagon secretion, increases satiety (which can cause weight loss), and slows gastric emptying. The average A1C reduction is ~0.6%, but optimization of concurrent insulin therapy may result in further A1C decreases. Pramlintide decreases prandial glucose excursions but has little effect on FPG concentrations. The most common adverse effects are nausea, vomiting, and anorexia. It does not cause hypoglycemia when used alone, but it is indicated only in patients receiving insulin, so hypoglycemia can occur. If a prandial insulin dose is used, it should be reduced by 30% to 50% when pramlintide is started to minimize severe hypoglycemic reactions. In type 2 DM, the starting dose is 60 mcg subcutaneously prior to major meals; the dose is titrated up to 120 mcg per dose as tolerated and as warranted based on postprandial plasma glucose levels. In type 1 DM, dosing starts at 15 mcg prior to each meal, titrated up in 15 mcg increments to a maximum of 60 mcg prior to each meal if tolerated and warranted.

Sulfonylureas

(Table 19–4)

- Sulfonylureas exert a hypoglycemic action by stimulating pancreatic secretion of insulin. All sulfonylureas are equally effective in lowering blood glucose when administered in equipotent doses. On average, the A1C will fall by 1.5% to 2% with FPG reductions of 60 to 70 mg/dL (3.3–3.9 mmol/L).

TABLE 19-4 Oral Agents for the Treatment of Type 2 Diabetes Mellitus

Generic Name (generic version available? Y = yes, N = no)	Brand	Dosage Strengths (mg)	Recommended Starting Dosage (mg/day) Nonelderly	Recommended Starting Dosage (mg/day) Elderly	Equivalent Therapeutic Dose (mg)	Maximum Dose (mg/day)	Duration of Action	Metabolism or Therapeutic Notes
Sulfonylureas								
Acetohexamide (Y)	Dymelor	250, 500	250	125–250	500	1,500	Up to 16 hours	Metabolized in liver; metabolite potency equal to parent compound; renally eliminated
Chlorpropamide (Y)	Diabinese	100, 250	250	100	250	500	Up to 72 hours	Metabolized in liver; also excreted unchanged renally
Tolazamide (Y)	Tolinase	100, 250, 500	100–250	100	250	1,000	Up to 24 hours	Metabolized in liver; metabolite less active than parent compound; renally eliminated
Tolbutamide (Y)	Orinase	250, 500	1,000–2,000	500–1,000	1,000	3,000	Up to 12 hours	Metabolized in liver to inactive metabolites that are renally excreted
Glipizide (Y)	Glucotrol	5, 10	5	2.5–5	5	40	Up to 20 hours	Metabolized in liver to inactive metabolites
Glipizide (Y)	Glucotrol XL	2.5, 5, 10, 20	5	2.5–5	5	20	24 hours	Slow-release form; do not cut tablet
Glyburide (Y)	DiaBeta, Micronase	1.25, 2.5, 5	5	1.25–2.5	5	20	Up to 24 hours	Metabolized in liver; elimination one half renal, one half feces
Glyburide, micronized (Y)	Glynase	1.5, 3, 6	3	1.5–3	3	12	Up to 24 hours	Equal control, but better absorption from micronized preparation
Glimepiride (Y)	Amaryl	1, 2, 4	1–2	0.5–1	2	8	24 hours	Metabolized in liver to inactive metabolites

(continued)

223

TABLE 19–4 Oral Agents for the Treatment of Type 2 Diabetes Mellitus (Continued)								
Short-acting insulin secretagogues								
Nateglinide (N)	Starlix	60, 120	120 with meals		NA	120 mg three times daily	Up to 4 hours	Metabolized by cytochrome (CYP) -2C9 and -3A4 to weakly active metabolites; renally eliminated
Repaglinide (N)	Prandin	0.5, 1, 2	0.5–1 with meals		NA	16	Up to 4 hours	Metabolized by CYP-3A4 to inactive metabolites; excreted in bile
Biguanides								
Metformin (Y)	Glucophage	500, 850, 1,000	500 mg twice daily		Assess renal function	2,550	Up to 24 hours	No metabolism; renally secreted and excreted
Metformin extended-release (Y)	Glucophage XR	500, 750, 1,000	500–1,000 mg with evening meal		Assess renal function	2,550	Up to 24 hours	Take with evening meal or may split dose; may consider trial if intolerant to immediate-release
Thiazolidinediones								
Pioglitazone (N)	Actos	15, 30, 45	15	15	NA	45	24 hours	Metabolized by CYP-2C8 and -3A4; two metabolites have longer half-lives than parent compound
Rosiglitazone (N)	Avandia	2, 4, 8	2–4	2	NA	8 mg/day or 4 mg twice daily	24 hours	Metabolized by CYP- 2C8 and -2C9 to inactive metabolites that are renally excreted
α-Glucosidase inhibitors								
Acarbose (N)	Precose	25, 50, 100	25 mg 1–3 times daily	25 mg 1–3 times daily	NA	25–100 mg three times a day	1–3 hours	Eliminated in bile

Miglitol (N)	Glyset	25, 50, 100	25 mg 1-3 times daily	NA	25 mg 1-3 times daily	25-100 mg 3 times daily	1-3 hours	Eliminated renally

Dipeptidyl peptidase-4 (DPP-4) inhibitors

Sitagliptin (N)	Januvia	25, 50, 100	100 mg daily	NA	25-100 mg daily based on renal function	100 mg daily	24 hours	50 mg daily if creatinine clearance >30 to <50 mL/min; 25 mg daily if creatinine clearance <30 mL/min
Saxagliptin (N)	Onglyza	2.5, 5	5 mg daily	NA	2.5-5 mg daily based on renal function	5 mg daily	24 hours	2.5 mg daily if creatinine clearance <50 mL/min or if on strong inhibitors of CYP-3A4/5

Example combination products

Glyburide/metformin (Y)	Glucovance	1.25/250, 2.5/500, 5/500	2.5-5/500 mg twice daily	NA	1.25/250 mg twice daily; assess renal function	20 mg of glyburide, 2,000 mg of metformin	Combination medication	Used as initial therapy: 1.25/250 mg twice daily
Glipizide/metformin (N)	Metaglip	2.5/250, 2.5/500, 5/500	2.5-5/500 mg twice daily	NA	2.5/250 mg; assess renal function	20 mg of glipizide, 2,000 mg of metformin	Combination medication	Used as initial therapy: 2.5/250 mg twice daily
Rosiglitazone/metformin (N)	Avandamet	1/500, 2/500, 4/500, 2/1,000, 4/1,000	1-2/500 mg twice daily	NA	1/500 mg twice daily; assess renal function	8 mg of rosiglitazone, 2,000 mg of metformin	Combination medication	Can use as initial therapy

NA, not available.

- The most common side effect is hypoglycemia, which is more problematic with long half-life drugs. Individuals at high risk include the elderly, those with renal insufficiency or advanced liver disease, and those who skip meals, exercise vigorously, or lose a substantial amount of weight. Weight gain is common; less common adverse effects include skin rash, hemolytic anemia, GI upset, and cholestasis. Hyponatremia is most common with chlorpropamide but has also been reported with tolbutamide.
- The recommended starting doses (see **Table 19-4**) should be reduced in elderly patients who may have compromised renal or hepatic function. Dosage can be titrated every 1 to 2 weeks (longer interval with chlorpropamide) to achieve glycemic goals.

Short-acting Insulin Secretagogues (Meglitinides)

- Similar to sulfonylureas, meglitinides lower glucose by stimulating pancreatic insulin secretion, but insulin release is glucose dependent and diminishes at low blood glucose concentrations. Hypoglycemic risk appears to be less with meglitinides than with sulfonylureas. The average reduction in A1C is ~0.8% to 1%. These agents can be used to provide increased insulin secretion during meals (when it is needed) in patients who are close to glycemic goals. They should be administered before each meal (up to 30 min prior). If a meal is skipped, the medication should also be skipped.
- **Repaglinide** (Prandin) is initiated at 0.5 to 2 mg with a maximum dose of 4 mg per meal (up to four meals daily or 16 mg/day).
- **Nateglinide** (Starlix) dosing is 120 mg three times daily before each meal. The dose may be lowered to 60 mg per meal in patients who are near goal A1C when therapy is initiated.

Biguanides

- **Metformin** is the only biguanide available in the United States. It enhances insulin sensitivity of both hepatic and peripheral (muscle) tissues. This allows for increased uptake of glucose into these insulin-sensitive tissues. Metformin consistently reduces A1C levels by 1.5% to 2%, FPG levels by 60 to 80 mg/dL, and retains the ability to reduce FPG levels when they are very high (>300 mg/dL). It reduces plasma triglycerides and low-density lipoprotein (LDL) cholesterol by 8% to 15% and modestly increases high-density lipoprotein (HDL) cholesterol (2%). It does not induce hypoglycemia when used alone.
- Metformin is logical in overweight/obese type 2 DM patients (if tolerated and not contraindicated) because it is the only oral antihyperglycemic medication proven to reduce the risk of total mortality and is available generically.
- The most common adverse effects are abdominal discomfort, stomach upset, diarrhea, and anorexia. These effects can be minimized by titrating the dose slowly and taking it with food. Extended-release metformin (Glucophage XR) may reduce some of the GI side effects. Lactic acidosis occurs rarely and can be minimized by avoiding its use in patients with renal insufficiency (serum creatinine ≥1.4 mg/dL in

women and ≥1.5 mg/dL in men), congestive heart failure, or conditions predisposing to hypoxemia or inherent lactic acidosis. Metformin should be withheld staring the day of IV radiographic dye procedures and resumed in 2 or 3 days, after normal renal function has been documented.

- **Metformin immediate-release** is usually initiated at 500 mg twice daily with the largest meals and increased by 500 mg weekly until glycemic goals or 2,500 mg/day is achieved. Metformin 850 mg can be dosed once daily and then increased every 1 to 2 weeks to a maximum of 850 mg three times daily (2,550 mg/day).

- **Metformin extended-release** (Glucophage XR) can be initiated with 500 mg with the evening meal and increased by 500 mg weekly to a maximum single evening dose of 2,000 mg/day. Administration two or three times daily may help minimize GI side effects and improve glycemic control. The 750 mg tablets can be titrated weekly to the maximum dose of 2,250 mg/day.

Thiazolidinediones (Glitazones)

- These agents activate PPAR-γ, a nuclear transcription factor important in fat cell differentiation and fatty acid metabolism. PPAR-γ agonists enhance insulin sensitivity in muscle, liver, and fat tissues indirectly. Insulin must be present in significant quantities for these actions to occur.

- When given for ~6 months, pioglitazone and rosiglitazone reduce A1C values by ~1.5% and FPG levels by ~60 to 70 mg/dL at maximal doses. Maximal glycemic-lowering effects may not be seen until 3 to 4 months of therapy.

- Pioglitazone decreases plasma triglycerides by 10% to 20%, whereas rosiglitazone tends to have no effect. Pioglitazone does not cause significant increases in LDL cholesterol, whereas LDL cholesterol may increase by 5% to 15% with rosiglitazone.

- Fluid retention may occur, perhaps as a result of peripheral vasodilation and/or improved insulin sensitization with a resultant increase in renal sodium and water retention. A dilutional anemia may result, which does not require treatment. Edema is reported in 4% to 5% of patients when glitazones are used alone or with other oral agents. When used in combination with insulin, the incidence of edema is ~15%. Glitazones are contraindicated in patients with New York Heart Association class III or IV heart failure and should be used with great caution in patients with class I or II heart failure or other underlying cardiac disease.

- Weight gain is dose related, and an increase of 1.5 to 4 kg is not uncommon. Rarely, rapid gain of a large amount of weight may necessitate discontinuation of therapy. Weight gain positively predicts a larger A1C reduction but must be balanced with the potential adverse effects of long-term weight gain.

- Several case reports of hepatotoxicity with pioglitazone or rosiglitazone have been reported, but improvement in alanine aminotransferase (ALT) was consistently observed upon drug discontinuation. Baseline ALT should be obtained prior to therapy and then periodically thereafter at the practitioner's discretion. Neither drug should be started if the baseline

ALT exceeds 2.5 times the upper limit of normal. The drugs should be discontinued if the ALT is more than three times the upper limit of normal.

- Glitazones have been associated with an increased fracture rate in the upper and lower limbs; women appear to have a higher risk than men. Most fractures occur in the wrists, forearms, ankles, or feet rather than in the common osteoporosis fracture sites (e.g., spine and hip). Although the underlying pathophysiology is not conclusively known, a patient's risk factors for fractures should be considered if glitazone therapy is contemplated.
- **Pioglitazone** (Actos) is started at 15 mg once daily. The maximum dose is 45 mg/day.
- **Rosiglitazone** (Avandia) is initiated with 2 to 4 mg once daily. The maximum dose is 8 mg/day. A dose of 4 mg twice daily can reduce A1C by 0.2% to 0.3% more than a dose of 8 mg taken once daily.

α-Glucosidase Inhibitors

- These agents prevent the breakdown of sucrose and complex carbohydrates in the small intestine, thereby prolonging the absorption of carbohydrates. The net effect is a reduction in the postprandial glucose concentrations (40–50 mg/dL) while fasting glucose levels are relatively unchanged (~10% reduction). Efficacy on glycemic control is modest, with average reductions in A1C of 0.3% to 1%. Good candidates for these drugs are patients who are near target A1C levels with near-normal FPG levels but high postprandial levels.
- The most common side effects are flatulence, bloating, abdominal discomfort, and diarrhea, which can be minimized by slow dosage titration. If hypoglycemia occurs when used in combination with a hypoglycemic agent (sulfonylurea or insulin), oral or parenteral glucose (dextrose) products or glucagon must be given because the drug will inhibit the breakdown and absorption of more complex sugar molecules (e.g., sucrose).
- **Acarbose** (Precose) and **miglitol** (Glyset) are dosed similarly. Therapy is initiated with a very low dose (25 mg with one meal a day) and increased very gradually (over several months) to a maximum of 50 mg three times daily for patients weighing ≥60 kg, or 100 mg three times daily for patients >60 kg. The drugs should be taken with the first bite of the meal so that the drug is present to inhibit enzyme activity.

Dipeptidyl Peptidase-4 (DPP-4) Inhibitors

- DPP-4 inhibitors prolong the half-life of endogenously produced GLP-1. These agents partially reduce the inappropriately elevated glucagon postprandially and stimulate glucose-dependent insulin secretion. The average reduction in A1C is ~0.7% to 1% at maximum dose.
- The drugs are well tolerated, weight neutral, and do not cause GI side effects. Mild hypoglycemia may occur, but DPP-4 inhibitors do not increase the risk of hypoglycemia when used as monotherapy or in combination with medications that have a low incidence of hypoglycemia. Urticaria and/or facial edema may occur in 1% of patients, and discontinuation is warranted. Rare cases of Stevens–Johnson syndrome

have been reported. Saxagliptin causes a dose-related reduction in absolute lymphocyte count; discontinuation should be considered if prolonged infection occurs.

- **Sitagliptin** (Januvia) is usually dosed at 100 mg orally once daily. In patients with renal impairment, the daily dose should be reduced to 50 mg (creatinine clearance 30–50 mL/min) or 25 mg (creatinine clearance <30 mL/min).
- **Saxagliptin** (Onglyza) is usually dosed 5 mg orally daily. The recommended dose should be reduced to 2.5 mg daily if the creatinine clearance is <50 mL/min or strong CYP-3A4/5 inhibitors are used concurrently.

Bile Acid Sequestrants

- **Colesevelam** (Welchol) binds bile acid in the intestinal lumen, decreasing the bile acid pool for reabsorption. Its precise mechanism of action in lowering plasma glucose levels is unknown.
- A1C reductions from baseline were ~0.4% when colesevelam 3.8 g/day was added to stable metformin, sulfonylureas, or insulin. The FPG was modestly reduced by ~5 to 10 mg/dL. It may also reduce LDL cholesterol by 12% to 16%. Triglycerides may increase when combined with sulfonylureas or insulin, but not with metformin. Colesevelam is weight neutral.
- The most common side effects are constipation and dyspepsia; it should be taken with a large amount of water. Colesevelam has multiple absorption-related drug–drug interactions.
- The dose of colesevelam for type 2 DM is six 625 mg tablets daily (total 3.75 g/day), which may be split into three tablets twice daily if desired. Each dose should be administered with meals because colesevelam binds to bile released during the meal.

PHARMACOTHERAPY OF TYPE 1 DIABETES MELLITUS

- All patients with type 1 DM require insulin, but the type and manner of delivery differ considerably among individual patients and clinicians.
- Therapeutic strategies should attempt to match carbohydrate intake with glucose-lowering processes (usually insulin) and exercise. Dietary intervention should allow the patient to live as normal a life as possible.
- **Fig. 19–1** depicts the relationship between glucose concentrations and insulin secretion over the course of a day and how various insulin and amylinomimetic regimens may be given.
- The timing of insulin onset, peak, and duration of effect must match meal patterns and exercise schedules to achieve near-normal blood glucose values throughout the day.
- A regimen of two daily injections that may roughly approximate physiologic insulin secretion is split-mixed injections of a morning dose of intermediate-duration insulin (e.g., NPH) and regular insulin before breakfast and again before the evening meal (see **Fig. 19–1**, no. 1). This assumes that the morning intermediate-acting insulin provides basal insulin for the day and covers the midday meal, the morning regular insulin covers breakfast, the evening intermediate-acting insulin gives basal insulin for the rest of the day, and the evening regular insulin

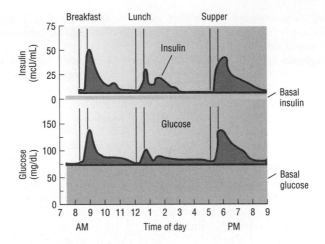

Intensive insulin therapy regimens

	7AM (meal)	11 AM (meal)	5 PM (meal)	Bedtime
1. 2 doses,[a] R or rapid acting + N	R, L, A, GLU + N		R, L, A, GLU + N	
2. 3 doses, R or rapid acting + N	R, L, A, GLU + N	R, L, A, GLU	R, L, A, GLU + N	
3. 4 doses, R or rapid acting + N	R, L, A, GLU	R, L, A, GLU	R, L, A, GLU	N
4. 4 doses R or rapid acting + N	R, L, A, GLU + N	R, L, A, GLU	R, L, A, GLU	N
5. 4 doses,[b] R or rapid acting + long acting	R, L, A, GLU	R, L, A, GLU	R, L, A, GLU	G or D[b] (G may be given anytime every 24 hours)
6. CS-II pump	Bolus	Bolus	Bolus	←——— Adjusted basal ———→
7. 3 doses pramlintide added to regimens above	P	P	P	

[a]Many clinicians may not consider this intensive insulin therapy

[b]May be given BID in type 1 DM = 5 doses

FIGURE 19–1. Relationship between insulin and glucose over the course of a day and how various insulin and amylinomimetic regimens could be given. (A, aspart; CS-II, continuous subcutaneous insulin infusion; D, detemir; G, glargine; GLU, glulisine; L, lispro; N, neutral protamine Hagedorn; P, pramlintide; R, regular.)

covers the evening meal. Patients may be started on 0.6 units/kg/day, with two thirds given in the morning and one third in the evening. Intermediate-acting insulin (e.g., NPH) should comprise two thirds of the morning dose and one half of the evening dose. However, most patients are not sufficiently predictable in their schedule and food intake to allow tight glucose control with this approach. If the fasting glucose in the morning is too high, the evening NPH dose may be moved to bedtime (now three total injections per day). This may provide sufficient intensification of therapy for some patients.

- The basal-bolus injection concept attempts to replicate normal insulin physiology by giving intermediate- or long-acting insulin as the basal component and short-acting insulin as the bolus portion (see Fig. 19–1, nos. 2, 3, 4, and 5). Intensive therapy using this approach is recommended for all adult patients at the time of diagnosis to reinforce the importance of glycemic control from the outset of treatment. Occasional patients with an extended honeymoon period may need less intensive therapy initially but should be converted to basal-bolus therapy at the onset of glycemic lability.

- The basal insulin component may be provided by once- or twice-daily **NPH** or **detemir**, or once-daily **insulin glargine**. Most type 1 DM patients require two injections of all insulins except insulin glargine. Insulin glargine or insulin detemir is a feasible basal insulin supplement for most patients.

- The bolus insulin component is given before meals with **regular insulin, insulin lispro, insulin aspart,** or **insulin glulisine**. The rapid onset and short duration of rapid-acting insulin analogs more closely replicate normal physiology than regular insulin, allowing the patient to vary the amount of insulin injected based on the preprandial SMBG level, upcoming activity level, and anticipated carbohydrate intake. Most patients have a prescribed dose of insulin preprandially that they vary based on an insulin algorithm. Carbohydrate counting is an effective tool for determining the amount of insulin to be injected preprandially.

- As an example, patients may begin on ~0.6 units/kg/day of insulin, with basal insulin 50% of the total dose and prandial insulin 20% of the total dose before breakfast, 15% before lunch, and 15% before dinner. Most patients require total daily doses between 0.5 and 1 unit/kg/day.

- Continuous subcutaneous insulin infusion pump therapy (generally using **insulin lispro** or **aspart** to diminish aggregation) is the most sophisticated form of basal-bolus insulin delivery (see Fig. 19–1, no. 6). The basal insulin dose may be varied, consistent with changes in insulin requirements throughout the day. In select patients, this feature of continuous subcutaneous insulin infusion allows greater glycemic control. However, it requires greater attention to detail and frequency of SMBG more than four injections daily.

- Pramlintide may be appropriate in type 1 DM patients who continue to have erratic postprandial control despite implementation of these strategies (see Fig. 19–1, no. 7). At initiation of therapy, each dose of prandial insulin must be reduced by 30% to 50% to avoid severe hypoglycemic reactions.

Pramlintide should be judiciously titrated based on GI adverse effects and postprandial glycemic goals.

- All patients receiving insulin should have extensive education in the recognition and treatment of hypoglycemia.

PHARMACOTHERAPY OF TYPE 2 DIABETES MELLITUS

(Fig. 19–2)

- Symptomatic patients may initially require insulin or combination oral therapy to reduce glucose toxicity (which may reduce β-cell insulin secretion and worsen insulin resistance).
- Patients with A1C ≤7% are usually treated with therapeutic lifestyle measures and an agent that will not cause hypoglycemia. Those with A1C >7% but <8.5% could be initially treated with a single oral agent or low-dose combination. Patients with higher initial A1C values may benefit from initial therapy with two oral agents or insulin. Patients with higher initial A1C values may benefit from initial therapy with two oral agents or even insulin.
- Obese patients (>120% ideal body weight) without contraindications should be started on metformin initially, titrated to ~2,000 mg/day. A glitazone may be used in patients intolerant of or having a contraindication to metformin.
- Near-normal-weight patients may be better treated with insulin secretagogues, although metformin will work in this population.
- When the disease progresses on metformin therapy, an insulin secretagogue such as a sulfonylurea is often added; however, better choices to sustain A1C reductions would be a glitazone or GLP-1 agonist.
- When initial therapy is no longer keeping the patient at the goal, adding one agent may be appropriate if the A1C is close to the goal. If the A1C is >1 to 1.5% above the goal, multiple oral agents or insulin therapy may be appropriate.
- Triple therapy often consists of metformin, a sulfonylurea, and a glitazone or DPP-4 inhibitor. A good alternative is metformin, a glitazone, and a GLP-1 agonist.
- Insulin therapy should be considered if the A1C is >8.5 to 9% on multiple therapies. Sulfonylureas are often stopped when insulin is added and insulin sensitizers are continued.
- Virtually all patients ultimately become insulinopenic and require insulin therapy. Patients are often transitioned to insulin by using a bedtime injection of an intermediate- or long-acting insulin with oral agents used primarily for glycemic control during the day. This results in less hyperinsulinemia during the day and less weight gain than starting prandial insulin or split-mix twice-daily insulin. Insulin sensitizers are commonly used with insulin because most patients are insulin resistant.
- When the combination of bedtime insulin plus daytime oral medications fails, a conventional multiple daily dose insulin regimen with an insulin sensitizer can be tried. If this is unsuccessful, a bolus injection can be given with the second largest meal of the day, for a total of three injections. After

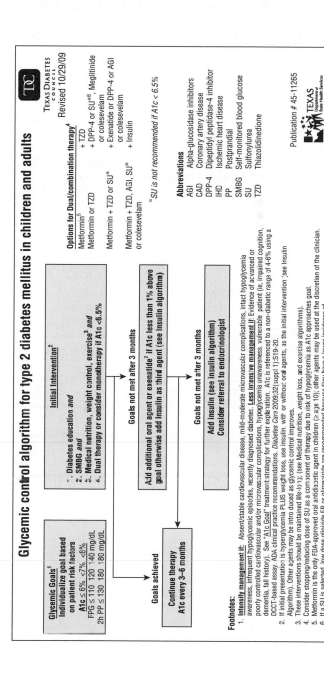

FIGURE 19–2. Glycemic control algorithm for type 2 diabetes mellitus in children and adults. See www.texasdiabetescouncil.org for current algorithms. *(Reprinted with permission from the Texas Diabetes Council.)*

this, the standard basal-bolus model is followed. Other treatment options are also available.

- Because of the variability of insulin resistance, insulin doses may range from 0.7 to 2.5 units/kg/day or more.

TREATMENT OF COMPLICATIONS

Retinopathy

- Patients with established retinopathy should be examined by an ophthalmologist at least every 6 to 12 months.
- Early background retinopathy may reverse with improved glycemic control. More advanced disease will not regress with improved control and may actually worsen with short-term improvements in glycemia.
- Laser photocoagulation has markedly improved sight preservation in diabetic patients.

Neuropathy

- Peripheral neuropathy is the most common complication in patients with type 2 DM. Paresthesias, numbness, or pain may be predominant symptoms. The feet are involved far more often than the hands. Improved glycemic control may alleviate some of the symptoms. Pharmacologic therapy is symptomatic and empiric, including low-dose **tricyclic antidepressants,** anticonvulsants (e.g., **gabapentin, pregabalin, carbamazepine,** and **topiramate**), **duloxetine, venlafaxine, topical capsaicin,** and various analgesics, including **tramadol** and **nonsteroidal antiinflammatory drugs**.
- Gastroparesis can be severe and debilitating. Improved glycemic control, discontinuation of medications that slow gastric motility, and use of **metoclopramide** (preferably for only a few days at a time) or **erythromycin** may be helpful.
- Patients with orthostatic hypotension may require mineralocorticoids or adrenergic agonists.
- Diabetic diarrhea is commonly nocturnal and frequently responds to a 10- to 14-day course of an antibiotic such as **doxycycline** or **metronidazole**. **Octreotide** may be useful in unresponsive cases.
- Erectile dysfunction is common, and initial treatment should include one of the oral medications available (e.g., **sildenafil, vardenafil,** or **tadalafil**).

Nephropathy

- Glucose and BP control are most important for prevention of nephropathy, and BP control is most important for retarding the progression of established nephropathy.
- Angiotensin-converting enzyme (ACE) inhibitors and angiotensin receptor blockers have shown efficacy in preventing the clinical progression of renal disease in patients with type 2 DM. Diuretics are frequently necessary due to volume-expanded states and are recommended second-line therapy.

Peripheral Vascular Disease and Foot Ulcers

- Claudication and nonhealing foot ulcers are common in type 2 DM. Smoking cessation, correction of dyslipidemia, and antiplatelet therapy are important treatment strategies.
- **Cilostazol** (Pletal) may be useful in select patients. Revascularization is successful with some patients.
- Local debridement and appropriate footwear and foot care are important in the early treatment of foot lesions. Topical treatments may be beneficial in more advanced lesions.

Coronary Heart Disease

- Multiple-risk-factor intervention (treatment of dyslipidemia and hypertension, smoking cessation, and antiplatelet therapy) reduces macrovascular events.
- The National Cholesterol Education Program Adult Treatment Panel III guidelines (see Chap. 8) classify the presence of DM as a coronary heart disease risk equivalent, and the goal LDL cholesterol is <100 mg/dL. An optional LDL goal in high-risk patients is <70 mg/dL. After the LDL goal is reached (usually with a **statin**), treatment of high triglycerides (≥200 mg/dL) is considered. The non-HDL goal for patients with DM is <130 mg/dL. **Niacin** or a **fibrate** can be added to reach that goal if triglycerides are 201 to 499 mg/dL.
- The American Diabetes Association recommends a goal BP <130/80 mm Hg in patients with DM. **ACE inhibitors** and **angiotensin receptor blockers** are generally recommended for initial therapy. Many patients require multiple agents, so **diuretics, calcium channel blockers**, and **β-blockers** are useful as second and third agents.

EVALUATION OF THERAPEUTIC OUTCOMES

- The A1C is the current standard for following long-term glycemic control for the previous 3 months. It should be measured at least twice a year in patients meeting treatment goals on a stable therapeutic regimen.
- Regardless of the insulin regimen chosen, gross adjustments in the total daily insulin dose can be made based on A1C measurements and symptoms such as polyuria, polydipsia, and weight gain or loss. Finer insulin adjustments can be determined on the basis of the results of frequent SMBG.
- Patients receiving insulin should be questioned about the recognition of hypoglycemia at least annually. Documentation of frequency of hypoglycemia and the treatment required should be recorded.
- Patients receiving bedtime insulin should be monitored for hypoglycemia by asking about nocturnal sweating, palpitations, and nightmares, as well as the results of SMBG.
- Patients with type 2 DM should have a routine urinalysis at diagnosis as the initial screening test for albuminuria. If positive, a 24-hour urine test for quantitative assessment will assist in developing a treatment plan. If the urinalysis is negative for protein, a test to evaluate the presence of microalbuminuria is recommended.

- Fasting lipid profiles should be obtained at each follow-up visit if not at goal, annually if stable and at goal, or every 2 years if the profile suggests low risk.
- Regular frequency of foot exams (each visit), urine albumin assessment (annually), and dilated ophthalmologic exams (yearly or more frequently with abnormalities) should also be documented.
- Assessment for influenza and pneumococcal vaccine administration and assessment and management of other cardiovascular risk factors (e.g., smoking and antiplatelet therapy) are components of sound preventive medicine strategies.

See Chapter 83, Diabetes Mellitus, authored by Curtis L. Triplitt and Charles A. Reasner, for a more detailed discussion of this topic.

Thyroid Disorders

DEFINITION

- Thyroid disorders encompass a variety of disease states affecting thyroid hormone production or secretion that result in alterations in metabolic stability. Hyperthyroidism and hypothyroidism are the clinical and biochemical syndromes resulting from increased and decreased thyroid hormone production, respectively.

THYROID HORMONE PHYSIOLOGY

- The thyroid hormones thyroxine (T_4) and triiodothyronine (T_3) are formed on thyroglobulin, a large glycoprotein synthesized within the thyroid cell. Inorganic iodide enters the thyroid follicular cell and is oxidized by thyroid peroxidase and covalently bound (organified) to tyrosine residues of thyroglobulin.
- The iodinated tyrosine residues monoiodotyrosine (MIT) and diiodotyrosine (DIT) combine (couple) to form iodothyronines in reactions catalyzed by thyroid peroxidase. Thus, two molecules of DIT combine to form T_4, and MIT and DIT join to form T_3.
- Thyroid hormone is liberated into the bloodstream by the process of proteolysis within thyroid cells. T_4 and T_3 are transported in the bloodstream by three proteins: thyroid-binding globulin (TBG), transthyretin, and albumin. Only the unbound (free) thyroid hormone is able to diffuse into the cell, elicit a biologic effect, and regulate thyroid-stimulating hormone (TSH) secretion from the pituitary.
- T_4 is secreted solely from the thyroid gland, but <20% of T_3 is produced there; the majority of T_3 is formed from the breakdown of T_4 catalyzed by the enzyme 5'-monodeiodinase found in peripheral tissues. T_3 is about five times more active than T_4.
- T_4 may also be acted on by the enzyme 5'-monodeiodinase to form reverse T_3, which has no significant biologic activity.
- Thyroid hormone production is regulated by TSH secreted by the anterior pituitary, which in turn is under negative feedback control by the circulating level of free thyroid hormone and the positive influence of hypothalamic thyrotropin-releasing hormone (TRH). Thyroid hormone production is also regulated by extrathyroidal deiodination of T_4 to T_3, which can be affected by nutrition, nonthyroidal hormones, drugs, and illness.

THYROTOXICOSIS (HYPERTHYROIDISM)

PATHOPHYSIOLOGY

- Thyrotoxicosis results when tissues are exposed to excessive levels of T_4, T_3, or both.

- TSH-secreting pituitary tumors release biologically active hormone that is unresponsive to normal feedback control. The tumors may cosecrete prolactin or growth hormone; therefore, patients may present with amenorrhea, galactorrhea, or signs of acromegaly.
- In Graves' disease, hyperthyroidism results from the action of thyroid-stimulating antibodies (TSAb) directed against the thyrotropin receptor on the surface of the thyroid cell. These immunoglobulins bind to the receptor and activate the enzyme adenylate cyclase in the same manner as TSH.
- An autonomous thyroid nodule (toxic adenoma) is a discrete thyroid mass whose function is independent of pituitary control. Hyperthyroidism usually occurs with larger nodules (i.e., those >3 cm in diameter).
- In multinodular goiters (Plummer's disease), follicles with autonomous function coexist with normal or even nonfunctioning follicles. Thyrotoxicosis occurs when the autonomous follicles generate more thyroid hormone than is required.
- Painful subacute (granulomatous or de Quervain) thyroiditis often develops after a viral syndrome, but rarely has a specific virus been identified in thyroid parenchyma.
- Painless (silent, lymphocytic, or postpartum) thyroiditis is a common cause of thyrotoxicosis; its etiology is not fully understood and may be heterogeneous; autoimmunity may underlie most cases.
- Thyrotoxicosis factitia is hyperthyroidism produced by the ingestion of exogenous thyroid hormone. This may occur when thyroid hormone is used for inappropriate indications, when excessive doses are used for accepted medical indications, or when it is used surreptitiously by patients.
- Amiodarone may induce thyrotoxicosis (2–3% of patients) or hypothyroidism. It interferes with type I 5′-deiodinase, leading to reduced conversion of T_4 to T_3, and iodide release from the drug may contribute to iodine excess. Amiodarone also causes a destructive thyroiditis with loss of thyroglobulin and thyroid hormones.

CLINICAL PRESENTATION

- Symptoms of thyrotoxicosis include nervousness, anxiety, palpitations, emotional lability, easy fatigability, heat intolerance, weight loss concurrent with increased appetite, increased frequency of bowel movements, proximal muscle weakness (noted on climbing stairs or arising from a sitting position), and scanty or irregular menses in women.
- Physical signs of thyrotoxicosis may include warm, smooth, moist skin and unusually fine hair; separation of the ends of the fingernails from the nail beds (onycholysis); retraction of the eyelids and lagging of the upper lid behind the globe upon downward gaze (lid lag); tachycardia at rest, a widened pulse pressure, and a systolic ejection murmur; occasional gynecomastia in men; a fine tremor of the protruded tongue and outstretched hands; and hyperactive deep tendon reflexes.
- Graves' disease is manifested by hyperthyroidism, diffuse thyroid enlargement, and the extrathyroidal findings of exophthalmos, pretibial

myxedema, and thyroid acropachy. The thyroid gland is usually diffusely enlarged, with a smooth surface and consistency varying from soft to firm. In severe disease, a thrill may be felt and a systolic bruit may be heard over the gland.

- In subacute thyroiditis, patients complain of severe pain in the thyroid region, which often extends to the ear on the affected side. Systemic symptoms may include fever, malaise, myalgia, and the signs and symptoms of thyrotoxicosis. The thyroid gland is firm and exquisitely tender on physical examination.
- Painless thyroiditis has a triphasic course that mimics that of painful subacute thyroiditis. Most patients present with mild thyrotoxic symptoms; lid retraction and lid lag are present, but exophthalmos is absent. The thyroid gland may be diffusely enlarged, but thyroid tenderness is absent.
- Thyroid storm is a life-threatening medical emergency characterized by decompensated thyrotoxicosis, high fever (often >39.4°C [103°F]), tachycardia, tachypnea, dehydration, delirium, coma, nausea, vomiting, and diarrhea. Precipitating factors include infection, trauma, surgery, radioactive iodine (RAI) treatment, and withdrawal from antithyroid drugs.

DIAGNOSIS

- An elevated 24-hour radioactive iodine uptake (RAIU) indicates true hyperthyroidism: the patient's thyroid gland is overproducing T_4, T_3, or both (normal RAIU 10–30%). Conversely, a low RAIU indicates that the excess thyroid hormone is not a consequence of thyroid gland hyperfunction but is likely caused by thyroiditis or hormone ingestion.
- TSH-induced hyperthyroidism is diagnosed by evidence of peripheral hypermetabolism, diffuse thyroid gland enlargement, elevated free thyroid hormone levels, and elevated serum immunoreactive TSH concentrations. Because the pituitary gland is extremely sensitive to even minimal elevations of free T_4, a "normal" or elevated TSH level in any thyrotoxic patient indicates inappropriate production of TSH.
- TSH-secreting pituitary adenomas are diagnosed by demonstrating lack of TSH response to TRH stimulation, inappropriate TSH levels, elevated TSH α-subunit levels, and radiologic imaging.
- In thyrotoxic Graves' disease, there is an increase in the overall hormone production rate with a disproportionate increase in T_3 relative to T_4 (**Table 20–1**). Saturation of TBG is increased due to the elevated levels of serum T_4 and T_3, which is reflected in an elevated T_3 resin uptake. As a result, the concentrations of free T_4, free T_3, and the free T_4 and T_3 indices are increased to an even greater extent than are the measured serum total T_4 and T_3 concentrations. The TSH level is undetectable due to negative feedback by elevated levels of thyroid hormone at the pituitary. In patients with manifest disease, measurement of the serum free T_4 concentration (or total T_4 and T_3 resin uptake), total T_3, and TSH will confirm the diagnosis of thyrotoxicosis. If the patient is not pregnant, an increased 24-hour RAIU documents that the thyroid gland is inappropriately using the iodine to produce more thyroid hormone when the patient is thyrotoxic.

TABLE 20–1	Thyroid Function Test Results in Different Thyroid Conditions					
	Total T$_4$	Free T$_4$	Total T$_3$	T$_3$ Resin Uptake	Free Thyroxine Index	TSH
Normal	4.5–10.9 mcg/dL	0.8–2.7 ng/dL	60–181 ng/dL	22–34%	1.0–4.3 units	0.5–4.7 milli-international units/L
Hyperthyroid	↑↑	↑↑	↑↑↑	↑	↑↑↑	↓↓
Hypothyroid	↓↓	↓↓	↓	↓↓	↓↓↓	↑↑
Increased TBG	↑	Normal	↑	↓	Normal	Normal

TBG, thyroid-binding globulin; TSH, thyroid-stimulating hormone; T$_3$, triiodothyronine; T$_4$, thyroxine.

- Toxic adenomas may result in hyperthyroidism with larger nodules. Because there may be isolated elevation of serum T$_3$ with autonomously functioning nodules, a T$_3$ level must be measured to rule out T$_3$ toxicosis if the T$_4$ level is normal. If autonomous function is suspected, but the TSH is normal, the diagnosis can be confirmed by failure of the autonomous nodule to decrease its iodine uptake during exogenous T$_3$ administration sufficient to suppress TSH.
- In multinodular goiters, a thyroid scan shows patchy areas of autonomously functioning thyroid tissue.
- A low RAIU indicates the excess thyroid hormone is not a consequence of thyroid gland hyperfunction. This may be seen in painful subacute thyroiditis, painless thyroiditis, struma ovarii, follicular cancer, and factitious ingestion of exogenous thyroid hormone.
- In subacute thyroiditis, thyroid function tests typically run a triphasic course in this self-limited disease. Initially, serum T$_4$ levels are elevated due to release of preformed thyroid hormone from disrupted follicles. The 24-hour RAIU during this time is <2% because of thyroid inflammation and TSH suppression by the elevated T$_4$ level. As the disease progresses, intrathyroidal hormone stores are depleted, and the patient may become mildly hypothyroid with an appropriately elevated TSH level. During the recovery phase, thyroid hormone stores are replenished, and serum TSH elevation gradually returns to normal.
- During the thyrotoxic phase of painless thyroiditis, the 24-hour RAIU is suppressed to <2%. Antithyroglobulin and antithyroid peroxidase antibody levels are elevated in >50% of patients.
- Thyrotoxicosis factitia should be suspected in a thyrotoxic patient without evidence of increased hormone production, thyroidal inflammation, or ectopic thyroid tissue. The RAIU is low because thyroid gland function is suppressed by the exogenous thyroid hormone. Measurement of plasma thyroglobulin reveals the presence of very low levels.

DESIRED OUTCOME

- The therapeutic objectives for hyperthyroidism are to eliminate the excess thyroid hormone; minimize symptoms and long-term consequences; and provide individualized therapy based on the type and severity of disease, patient age and gender, existence of nonthyroidal conditions, and response to previous therapy.

TREATMENT

Nonpharmacologic Therapy

- Surgical removal of the thyroid gland should be considered in patients with a large gland (>80 g), severe ophthalmopathy, or a lack of remission on antithyroid drug treatment.
- If thyroidectomy is planned, **propylthiouracil** (PTU) or **methimazole** is usually given until the patient is biochemically euthyroid (usually 6–8 weeks), followed by the addition of **iodides** (500 mg/day) for 10 to 14 days before surgery to decrease the vascularity of the gland. **Levothyroxine** may be added to maintain the euthyroid state while the thionamides are continued.
- **Propranolol** has been used for several weeks preoperatively and 7 to 10 days after surgery to maintain a pulse rate <90 beats/min. Combined pretreatment with propranolol and 10 to 14 days of **potassium iodide** also has been advocated.
- Complications of surgery include persistent or recurrent hyperthyroidism (0.6–18%), hypothyroidism (up to ~49%), hypoparathyroidism (up to 4%), and vocal cord abnormalities (up to 5%). The frequent occurrence of hypothyroidism requires periodic follow-up for identification and treatment.

Pharmacologic Therapy

THIOUREAS (THIONAMIDES)

- **PTU** and **methimazole** block thyroid hormone synthesis by inhibiting the peroxidase enzyme system of the thyroid gland, thus preventing oxidation of trapped iodide and subsequent incorporation into iodotyrosines and ultimately iodothyronine ("organification"); and by inhibiting coupling of MIT and DIT to form T_4 and T_3. PTU (but not methimazole) also inhibits the peripheral conversion of T_4 to T_3.
- Usual initial doses include PTU 300 to 600 mg daily (usually in three or four divided doses) or methimazole 30 to 60 mg daily given in three divided doses. Evidence exists that both drugs can be given as a single daily dose.
- Improvement in symptoms and laboratory abnormalities should occur within 4 to 8 weeks, at which time a tapering regimen to maintenance doses can be started. Dosage changes should be made on a monthly basis because the endogenously produced T_4 will reach a new steady-state concentration in this interval. Typical daily maintenance doses are PTU 50 to 300 mg and methimazole 5 to 30 mg.
- Antithyroid drug therapy should continue for 12 to 24 months to induce long-term remission.
- Patients should be monitored every 6 to 12 months after remission. If a relapse occurs, alternate therapy with RAI is preferred to a second course of antithyroid drugs, as subsequent courses of therapy are less likely to induce remission.

- Minor adverse reactions include pruritic maculopapular rashes, arthralgias, fever, and a benign transient leukopenia (white blood cell count <4,000/mm³). The alternate thiourea may be tried in these situations, but cross-sensitivity occurs in ~50% of patients.
- Major adverse effects include agranulocytosis (with fever, malaise, gingivitis, oropharyngeal infection, and a granulocyte count <250/mm³), aplastic anemia, a lupus-like syndrome, polymyositis, GI intolerance, hepatotoxicity, and hypoprothrombinemia. If it occurs, agranulocytosis usually develops in the first 3 months of therapy; routine monitoring is not recommended because of its sudden onset. Patients who have experienced a major adverse reaction to one thiourea should not be converted to the alternate drug because of cross-sensitivity.

IODIDES

- **Iodide** acutely blocks thyroid hormone release, inhibits thyroid hormone biosynthesis by interfering with intrathyroidal iodide use, and decreases the size and vascularity of the gland.
- Symptom improvement occurs within 2 to 7 days of initiating therapy, and serum T_4 and T_3 concentrations may be reduced for a few weeks.
- Iodides are often used as adjunctive therapy to prepare a patient with Graves' disease for surgery, to acutely inhibit thyroid hormone release and quickly attain the euthyroid state in severely thyrotoxic patients with cardiac decompensation, or to inhibit thyroid hormone release after RAI therapy.
- **Potassium iodide** is available as a saturated solution (**SSKI,** 38 mg iodide per drop) or as **Lugol solution,** containing 6.3 mg of iodide per drop.
- The typical starting dose of SSKI is 3 to 10 drops daily (120–400 mg) in water or juice. When used to prepare a patient for surgery, it should be administered 7 to 14 days preoperatively.
- As an adjunct to RAI, SSKI should not be used before but rather 3 to 7 days after RAI treatment so that the RAI can concentrate in the thyroid.
- Adverse effects include hypersensitivity reactions (skin rashes, drug fever, rhinitis, and conjunctivitis), salivary gland swelling, "iodism" (metallic taste, burning mouth and throat, sore teeth and gums, symptoms of a head cold, and sometimes stomach upset and diarrhea), and gynecomastia.

ADRENERGIC BLOCKERS

- β-Blockers have been used widely to ameliorate thyrotoxic symptoms such as palpitations, anxiety, tremor, and heat intolerance. They have no effect on peripheral thyrotoxicosis and protein metabolism and do not reduce TSAb or prevent thyroid storm. **Propranolol** and **nadolol** partially block the conversion of T_4 to T_3, but this contribution to the overall therapeutic effect is small.
- β-Blockers are usually used as adjunctive therapy with antithyroid drugs, RAI, or iodides when treating Graves' disease or toxic nodules; in preparation for surgery; or in thyroid storm. The only conditions

for which β-blockers are primary therapy for thyrotoxicosis are those associated with thyroiditis.

- **Propranolol** doses required to relieve adrenergic symptoms vary, but an initial dose of 20 to 40 mg four times daily is effective for most patients (heart rate <90 beats/min). Younger or more severely toxic patients may require as much as 240 to 480 mg/day.
- β-Blockers are contraindicated in patients with decompensated heart failure unless it is caused solely by tachycardia (high output). Other contraindications are sinus bradycardia, concomitant therapy with mono-amine oxidase inhibitors or tricyclic antidepressants, and patients with spontaneous hypoglycemia. Side effects include nausea, vomiting, anxiety, insomnia, lightheadedness, bradycardia, and hematologic disturbances.
- Centrally acting sympatholytics (e.g., **clonidine**) and calcium channel antagonists (e.g., **diltiazem**) may be useful for symptom control when contraindications to β-blockade exist.

RADIOACTIVE IODINE

- **Sodium iodide–131** is an oral liquid that concentrates in the thyroid and initially disrupts hormone synthesis by incorporating into thyroid hormones and thyroglobulin. Over a period of weeks, follicles that have taken up RAI and surrounding follicles develop evidence of cellular necrosis and fibrosis of the interstitial tissue.
- RAI is the agent of choice for Graves' disease, toxic autonomous nodules, and toxic multinodular goiters. Pregnancy is an absolute contraindication to the use of RAI.
- β-Blockers are the primary adjunctive therapy to RAI, as they may be given anytime without compromising RAI therapy.
- Patients with cardiac disease and elderly patients are often treated with thionamides prior to RAI ablation because thyroid hormone levels will transiently increase after RAI treatment due to release of preformed thyroid hormone.
- Antithyroid drugs are not routinely used after RAI because their use is associated with a higher incidence of posttreatment recurrence or persistent hyperthyroidism.
- If iodides are administered, they should be given 3 to 7 days after RAI to prevent interference with the uptake of RAI in the thyroid gland.
- The goal of therapy is to destroy overactive thyroid cells, and a single dose of 4,000 to 8,000 rad results in a euthyroid state in 60% of patients at 6 months or sooner. A second dose of RAI should be given 6 months after the first RAI treatment if the patient remains hyperthyroid.
- Hypothyroidism commonly occurs months to years after RAI. The acute, short-term side effects include mild thyroidal tenderness and dysphagia. Long-term follow-up has not revealed an increased risk for development of thyroid carcinoma, leukemia, or congenital defects.

Treatment of Thyroid Storm

- The following therapeutic measures should be instituted promptly: (1) suppression of thyroid hormone formation and secretion, (2) antiadrenergic

TABLE 20-2	Drug Dosages Used in the Management of Thyroid Storm
Drug	**Regimen**
Propylthiouracil	900–1,200 mg/day orally in four or six divided doses
Methimazole	90–120 mg/day orally in four or six divided doses
Sodium iodide	Up to 2 g/day IV in single or divided doses
Lugol solution	5–10 drops three times daily in water or juice
Saturated solution of potassium iodide	1–2 drops three times daily in water or juice
Propranolol	40–80 mg every 6 hours
Dexamethasone	5–20 mg/day orally or IV in divided doses
Prednisone	25–100 mg/day orally in divided doses
Methylprednisolone	20–80 mg/day IV in divided doses
Hydrocortisone	100–400 mg/day IV in divided doses

therapy, (3) administration of corticosteroids, and (4) treatment of associated complications or coexisting factors that may have precipitated the storm (**Table 20–2**).

- **PTU** in large doses is the preferred thionamide because it interferes with the production of thyroid hormones and blocks the peripheral conversion of T_4 to T_3.
- **Iodides,** which rapidly block the release of preformed thyroid hormone, should be administered after PTU is initiated to inhibit iodide utilization by the overactive gland.
- Antiadrenergic therapy with the short-acting agent **esmolol** is preferred because it can be used in patients with pulmonary disease or at risk for cardiac failure and because its effects can be rapidly reversed.
- **Corticosteroids** are generally recommended, but there is no convincing evidence of adrenocortical insufficiency in thyroid storm; their benefits may be attributed to their antipyretic action and stabilization of blood pressure (BP).
- General supportive measures, including **acetaminophen** as an antipyretic (aspirin or other nonsteroidal antiinflammatory drugs may displace bound thyroid hormone), **fluid and electrolyte replacement, sedatives, digoxin, antiarrhythmics, insulin,** and **antibiotics** should be given as indicated. Plasmapheresis and peritoneal dialysis have been used to remove excess hormone in patients not responding to more conservative measures.

EVALUATION OF THERAPEUTIC OUTCOMES

- After therapy (thionamides, RAI, or surgery) for hyperthyroidism has been initiated, patients should be evaluated on a monthly basis until they reach a euthyroid condition.
- Clinical signs of continuing thyrotoxicosis or the development of hypothyroidism should be noted.
- After T_4 replacement is initiated, the goal is to maintain both the free T_4 level and the TSH concentration in the normal range. Once a stable dose of T_4 is identified, the patient may be followed every 6 to 12 months.

HYPOTHYROIDISM

PATHOPHYSIOLOGY

- The vast majority of patients have primary hypothyroidism due to thyroid gland failure from chronic autoimmune thyroiditis (Hashimoto's disease). Evidence suggests that defects in suppressor T lymphocyte function lead to the survival of a randomly mutating clone of helper T lymphocytes that are directed against normally occurring antigens on the thyroid membrane. Once these T lymphocytes interact with the thyroid membrane antigen, B lymphocytes are stimulated to produce thyroid antibodies.
- Iatrogenic hypothyroidism follows exposure to excessive amounts of radiation (radioiodine or external radiation) or after total thyroidectomy.
- Other causes of primary hypothyroidism include iodine deficiency, enzymatic defects within the thyroid gland, thyroid hypoplasia, and maternal ingestion of goitrogens during fetal development.
- Secondary hypothyroidism due to pituitary failure is uncommon. Pituitary insufficiency may be caused by destruction of thyrotrophs by pituitary tumors, surgical therapy, external pituitary radiation, post-partum pituitary necrosis (Sheehan's syndrome), trauma, and infiltrative processes of the pituitary (e.g., metastatic tumors and tuberculosis).

CLINICAL PRESENTATION

- Common symptoms of hypothyroidism include dry skin, cold intolerance, weight gain, constipation, weakness, lethargy, fatigue, muscle cramps, myalgia, stiffness, and loss of ambition or energy. In children, thyroid hormone deficiency may manifest as growth or intellectual retardation.
- Physical signs include coarse skin and hair, cold or dry skin, periorbital puffiness, bradycardia, and slowed or hoarse speech. Objective weakness (with proximal muscles being affected more than distal muscles) and slow relaxation of deep tendon reflexes are common. Reversible neurologic syndromes such as carpal tunnel syndrome, polyneuropathy, and cerebellar dysfunction may also occur.
- Most patients with secondary hypothyroidism due to inadequate TSH production have clinical signs of generalized pituitary insufficiency, such as abnormal menses and decreased libido, or evidence of a pituitary adenoma, such as visual field defects, galactorrhea, or acromegaloid features.
- Myxedema coma is a rare consequence of decompensated hypothyroidism manifested by hypothermia, advanced stages of hypothyroid symptoms, and altered sensorium ranging from delirium to coma. Mortality rates of 60 to 70% necessitate immediate and aggressive therapy.

DIAGNOSIS

- A rise in the TSH level is the first evidence of primary hypothyroidism. Many patients have a free T_4 level within the normal range (compensated hypothyroidism) and few, if any, symptoms of hypothyroidism. As the disease progresses, the free T_4 concentration drops below the normal level. The T_3 concentration is often maintained in the normal range despite a low T_4. Antithyroid peroxidase antibodies and antithyroglobulin antibodies are likely to be elevated. The RAIU is not a useful test in the evaluation of hypothyroidism because it can be low, normal, or even elevated.

- Pituitary failure (secondary hypothyroidism) should be suspected in patients with decreased T_4 levels and inappropriately normal or low TSH levels.

DESIRED OUTCOME

- The treatment goals for hypothyroidism are to restore thyroid hormone concentrations in tissue, provide symptomatic relief, prevent neurologic deficits in newborns and children, and reverse the biochemical abnormalities of hypothyroidism.

TREATMENT OF HYPOTHYROIDISM

(Table 20–3)

- **Levothyroxine** (L-thyroxine, T_4) is the drug of choice for thyroid hormone replacement and suppressive therapy because it is chemically stable, relatively inexpensive, free of antigenicity, and has uniform potency. Other commercially available thyroid preparations can be used but are not preferred therapy. Once a particular product is selected, therapeutic interchange is discouraged.
- Because T_3 (and not T_4) is the biologically active form, levothyroxine administration results in a pool of thyroid hormone that is readily and consistently converted to T_3.
- Young patients with long-standing disease and patients older than 45 years without known cardiac disease should be started on 50 mcg daily of levothyroxine and increased to 100 mcg daily after 1 month.
- The recommended initial daily dose for older patients or those with known cardiac disease is 25 mcg/day titrated upward in increments of 25 mcg at monthly intervals to prevent stress on the cardiovascular system.
- The average maintenance dose for most adults is ~125 mcg/day, but there is a wide range of replacement doses, necessitating individualized therapy and appropriate TSH monitoring to determine an appropriate dose.
- Although the treatment of subclinical hypothyroidism is controversial, patients presenting with marked elevations in TSH (>10 mIU/L) and high titers of thyroid peroxidase antibody or prior treatment with sodium iodide–131 may be most likely to benefit from treatment.
- Levothyroxine is the drug of choice for pregnant women, and the objective of the treatment is to decrease TSH to 1 mIU/L and to maintain free T_4 concentrations in the normal range.
- Cholestyramine, calcium carbonate, sucralfate, aluminum hydroxide, ferrous sulfate, soybean formula, and dietary fiber supplements may impair the absorption of levothyroxine from the GI tract. Drugs that increase nondeiodinative T_4 clearance include rifampin, carbamazepine, and possibly phenytoin. Amiodarone may block the conversion of T_4 to T_3.

TABLE 20–3	Thyroid Preparations Used in the Treatment of Hypothyroidism	
Drug/Dosage Form	**Content**	**Relative Dose**
Thyroid USP Armour Thyroid (T_4:T_3 ratio) 9.5 mcg:2.25 mcg, 19 mcg:4.5 mcg, 38 mcg:9 mcg, 57 mcg:13.5 mcg, 76 mcg:18 mcg, 114 mcg:27 mcg, 152 mcg:36 mcg, 190 mcg:45 mcg tablets	Desiccated beef or pork thyroid gland	1 grain (equivalent to 60 mcg of T_4)
Thyroglobulin Proloid 32, 65, 100, 130, 200 mg tablets	Partially purified pork thyroglobulin	1 grain
Levothyroxine Synthroid, Levothroid, Levoxyl, Unithroid, and other generics 25, 50, 75, 88, 100, 112, 125, 137, 150, 175, 200, 300 mcg tablets; 200 and 500 mcg/vial injection	Synthetic T_4	50–60 mcg
Liothyronine Cytomel 5, 25, and 50 mcg tablets	Synthetic T_3	15–37.5 mcg
Liotrix Thyrolar ¼-, ½-, 1-, 2-, and 3-strength tablets	Synthetic T_4:T_3 in 4:1 ratio	50–60 mcg T_4 and 12.5–15 mcg T_3

T_3, triiodothyronine; T_4, thyroxine.

- **Thyroid USP** (or desiccated thyroid) is derived from hog, beef, or sheep thyroid gland. It may be antigenic in allergic or sensitive patients. Inexpensive generic brands may not be bioequivalent.
- **Thyroglobulin** is a purified hogland extract that is standardized biologically to give a T_4:T_3 ratio of 2.5:1. It has no clinical advantages and is not widely used.
- **Liothyronine** (synthetic T_3) has uniform potency but has a higher incidence of cardiac adverse effects, higher cost, and difficulty in monitoring with conventional laboratory tests.
- **Liotrix** (synthetic T_4:T_3 in a 4:1 ratio) is chemically stable, pure, and has a predictable potency but is expensive. It lacks therapeutic rationale because ~35% of T_4 is converted to T_3 peripherally.
- Excessive doses of thyroid hormone may lead to heart failure, angina pectoris, and myocardial infarction (MI). Allergic or idiosyncratic reactions

can occur with the natural animal-derived products, such as desiccated thyroid and thyroglobulin, but they are extremely rare with the synthetic products used today. Hyperthyroidism leads to reduced bone density and increased risk of fracture.

TREATMENT OF MYXEDEMA COMA

- Immediate and aggressive therapy with IV bolus **levothyroxine**, 300 to 500 mcg, has traditionally been used. Initial treatment with IV **liothyronine** or a combination of both hormones has also been advocated because of impaired conversion of T_4 to T_3.
- Glucocorticoid therapy with IV **hydrocortisone** 100 mg every 8 hours should be given until coexisting adrenal suppression is ruled out.
- Consciousness, lowered TSH concentrations, and normal vital signs are expected within 24 hours.
- Maintenance levothyroxine doses are typically 75 to 100 mcg IV until the patient stabilizes and oral therapy is begun.
- Supportive therapy must be instituted to maintain adequate ventilation, euglycemia, BP, and body temperature. Underlying disorders such as sepsis and MI must be diagnosed and treated.

EVALUATION OF THERAPEUTIC OUTCOMES

- Serum TSH concentration is the most sensitive and specific monitoring parameter for adjustment of levothyroxine dose. Concentrations begin to fall within hours and are usually normalized within 2 to 6 weeks.
- TSH and T_4 concentrations should both be checked every 6 weeks until a euthyroid state is achieved. An elevated TSH level indicates insufficient replacement. Serum T_4 concentrations can be useful in detecting noncompliance, malabsorption, or changes in levothyroxine product bioequivalence. TSH may also be used to help identify noncompliance.
- In patients with hypothyroidism caused by hypothalamic or pituitary failure, alleviation of the clinical syndrome and restoration of serum T_4 to the normal range are the only criteria available for estimating the appropriate replacement dose of levothyroxine.

See Chapter 84, Thyroid Disorders, authored by Jacqueline Jonklaas and Robert L. Talbert, for a more detailed discussion of this topic.

CHAPTER

21 Cirrhosis and Portal Hypertension

CIRRHOSIS

- Cirrhosis is a diffuse injury to the liver characterized by fibrosis and a conversion of the normal hepatic architecture into structurally abnormal nodules. The end result is destruction of hepatocytes and their replacement by fibrous tissue.

- The resulting resistance to blood flow results in portal hypertension and the development of varices and ascites. Hepatocyte loss and intrahepatic shunting of blood result in diminished metabolic and synthetic function, which leads to hepatic encephalopathy (HE) and coagulopathy.

- Cirrhosis has many causes (Table 21-1). In the United States, excessive alcohol intake and chronic viral hepatitis (types B and C) are the most common causes.

- Cirrhosis results in elevation of portal blood pressure because of fibrotic changes within the hepatic sinusoids, changes in the levels of vasodilatory and vasoconstrictor mediators, and an increase in blood flow to the splanchnic vasculature. The pathophysiologic abnormalities that cause it result in the commonly encountered problems of ascites, portal hypertension and esophageal varices, HE, and coagulation disorders.

- **Portal hypertension** is characterized by hypervolemia, increased cardiac index, hypotension, and decreased systemic vascular resistance.

- Ascites is the pathologic accumulation of lymph fluid within the peritoneal cavity. It is one of the earliest and most common presentations of cirrhosis.

- The development of ascites is related to systemic arterial vasodilation that leads to the activation of the baroreceptors in the kidney and an activation of the renin–angiotensin–aldosterone system, activation of the sympathetic nervous system, and release of antidiuretic hormone in response to the arterial hypotension. These changes cause sodium and water retention.

PORTAL HYPERTENSION AND VARICES

- The most important sequelae of portal hypertension are the development of varices and alternative routes of blood flow resulting in acute variceal bleeding. Patients with cirrhosis are at risk for varices when portal pressures exceed the vena cava pressure by ≥12 mm Hg.

- Hemorrhage from varices occurs in 25% to 40% of patients with cirrhosis and is the cause of death for one third.

TABLE 21–1	Etiology of Cirrhosis

Chronic alcohol consumption

Chronic viral hepatitis (types B, C, and D)

Metabolic liver disease
    Hemochromatosis
    Wilson's disease
    α_1-Antitrypsin deficiency
    Nonalcoholic steatohepatitis ("fatty liver")
    Cystic fibrosis

Immunologic disease
    Autoimmune hepatitis
    Primary biliary cirrhosis
    Primary sclerosing cholangitis (90% associated
        with ulcerative colitis)

Vascular disease
    Budd–Chiari syndrome
    Cardiac failure

Drugs
    Isoniazid, methyldopa, amiodarone, methotrexate, tamoxifen, retinol (vitamin A),
        propylthiouracil, and didanosine

HEPATIC ENCEPHALOPATHY

- HE is a CNS disturbance with a wide range of neuropsychiatric symptoms associated with hepatic insufficiency and liver failure.
- The symptoms of HE are thought to result from an accumulation of gut-derived nitrogenous substances in the systemic circulation as a consequence of shunting through portosystemic collaterals bypassing the liver. These substances then enter the CNS and result in alterations of neurotransmission that affect consciousness and behavior.
- Altered ammonia, glutamate, benzodiazepine receptor agonists, and manganese are associated with HE. However, an established correlation between blood ammonia levels and mental status does not exist.
- Type A HE is induced by acute liver failure, type B results from portal-systemic bypass without intrinsic liver disease, and type C occurs with cirrhosis. HE may be classified as episodic, persistent, or minimal.

COAGULATION DEFECTS

- Complex coagulation derangements can occur in cirrhosis. These derangements include the reduction in the synthesis of coagulation factors, excessive fibrinolysis, disseminated intravascular coagulation, thrombocytopenia, and platelet dysfunction.
- Vitamin K–dependent clotting factor levels are decreased, with factor VII affected first because it has a short half-life. The net effect of these events is the development of bleeding diathesis.

TABLE 21–2	Clinical Presentation of Cirrhosis

Signs and symptoms
  Asymptomatic
  Hepatomegaly and splenomegaly
  Pruritus, jaundice, palmar erythema, spider angiomata, and hyperpigmentation
  Gynecomastia and reduced libido
  Ascites, edema, pleural effusion, and respiratory difficulties
  Malaise, anorexia, and weight loss
  Encephalopathy

Laboratory tests
  Hypoalbuminemia
  Elevated prothrombin time
  Thrombocytopenia
  Elevated alkaline phosphatase
  Elevated aspartate transaminase, alanine transaminase, and γ-glutamyl transpeptidase

CLINICAL PRESENTATION

- The range of presentation of patients with cirrhosis may be from asymptomatic, with abnormal laboratory or radiographic tests, to decompensated with ascites, spontaneous bacterial peritonitis, HE, or variceal bleeding.
- Some presenting characteristics with cirrhosis are anorexia, weight loss, weakness, fatigue, jaundice, pruritis, GI bleeding, coagulopathy, increased abdominal girth with shifting flank dullness, mental status changes, and vascular spiders. **Table 21–2** describes the presenting signs and symptoms of cirrhosis.
- A thorough history including risk factors that predispose patients to cirrhosis should be taken. Quantity and duration of alcohol intake should be determined. Risk factors for hepatitis B and C transmission should be determined.

LABORATORY ABNORMALITIES

- There are no laboratory or radiographic tests of hepatic function that can accurately diagnose cirrhosis. Routine liver assessment tests include alkaline phosphatase, bilirubin, aspartate transaminase (AST), alanine aminotransferase (ALT), and γ-glutamyl transpeptidase (GGT). Additional markers of hepatic synthetic activity include albumin and prothrombin time. The substances are typically elevated in chronic inflammatory liver diseases such as hepatitis C but may be normal in others with resolved infectious processes.
- The aminotransferases, AST and ALT, are enzymes that have increased concentrations in plasma following hepatocellular injury. The highest concentrations are seen in acute viral infections and ischemic or toxic liver injury.
- Alkaline phosphatase levels and GGT are elevated in plasma with obstructive disorders that disrupt the flow of bile from hepatocytes to the bile ducts or from the biliary tree to the intestines in conditions such as

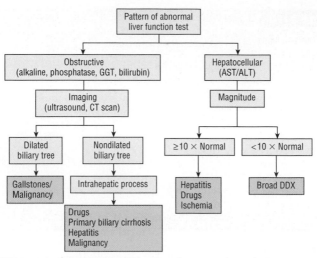

FIGURE 21–1. Interpretation of liver function tests. (ALT, alanine transaminase; AST, aspartate transaminase; CT, computed tomography; DDX, differential diagnosis; GGT, γ-glutamyl transpeptidase.)

primary biliary cirrhosis, sclerosing cholangitis, drug-induced cholestasis, bile duct obstruction, autoimmune cholestatic liver disease, and metastatic cancer of the liver.

- Elevations in serum conjugated bilirubin indicate that the liver has lost at least half its excretory capacity. When alkaline phosphatase is elevated, and aminotransferase levels are normal, elevated conjugated bilirubin is a sign of cholestatic disease or possible cholestatic drug reactions.
- **Fig. 21–1** describes a general algorithm for the interpretation of liver function tests.
- Albumin and coagulation factors are markers of hepatic synthetic activity and are used to estimate hepatocyte functioning in cirrhosis.
- Thrombocytopenia is a relatively common feature in chronic liver disease and is found in 15% to 70% of cirrhotic patients.
- The Child–Pugh classification system uses a combination of physical and laboratory findings to assess and define the severity of cirrhosis and is a predictor of patient survival, surgical outcome, and risk of variceal bleeding (**Table 21–3**).
- The Model for End-Stage Liver Disease (MELD) is a newer scoring system:

$$\text{MELD score} = 0.957 \times \log (\text{serum creatinine mg/dL}) + 0.378 \\ \times \log (\text{bilirubin mg/dL}) + 1.120 \times \log (\text{INR}) + 0.643,$$

where International Normalized Ratio (INR) is TK.

- In MELD, laboratory values <1 are rounded up to 1. The formula's score is multiplied by 10 and rounded to the nearest whole number.

TABLE 21–3	Criteria and Scoring for the Child–Pugh Grading of Chronic Liver Disease		
Score	**1**	**2**	**3**
Total bilirubin (mg/dL)	1–2	2–3	>3
Albumin (g/dL)	>3.5	2.8–3.5	<2.8
Ascites	None	Mild	Moderate
Encephalopathy (grade)	None	1 and 2	3 and 4
Prothrombin time (sec prolonged)	1–4	4–6	>6

Grade A, 1–6 points; grade B, 7–9 points; grade C, 10–15 points.

TREATMENT

DESIRED OUTCOME

- Treatment goals are clinical improvement or resolution of acute complications, such as variceal bleeding, and resolution of hemodynamic instability for an episode of acute variceal hemorrhage.
- Other goals are prevention of complications, adequate lowering of portal pressure with medical therapy using β-adrenergic blocker therapy, and support of abstinence from alcohol.

GENERAL APPROACHES

Approaches to treatment include the following:

1. Identify and eliminate the causes of cirrhosis (e.g., alcohol abuse).
2. Assess the risk for variceal bleeding and begin pharmacologic prophylaxis where indicated, reserving endoscopic therapy for high-risk patients or acute bleeding episodes.

- The patient should be evaluated for clinical signs of ascites and managed with pharmacologic treatment (e.g., diuretics) and paracentesis. Careful monitoring for spontaneous bacterial peritonitis (SBP) should be employed in patients with ascites who undergo acute deterioration.
- HE is a common complication of cirrhosis and requires clinical vigilance and treatment with dietary restriction, elimination of CNS depressants, and therapy to lower ammonia levels.
- Frequent monitoring for signs of hepatorenal syndrome, pulmonary insufficiency, and endocrine dysfunction is necessary.

MANAGEMENT OF PORTAL HYPERTENSION AND VARICEAL BLEEDING

- The management of varices involves three strategies: (1) primary prophylaxis to prevent rebleeding, (2) treatment of variceal hemorrhage, and (3) secondary prophylaxis to prevent rebleeding in patients who have already bled.

Primary Prophylaxis

- All patients with cirrhosis and portal hypertension should be considered for endoscopic screening.
- The mainstay of primary prophylaxis is the use of a nonselective β-adrenergic blocking agent such as **propranolol** or **nadolol**. These agents reduce portal pressure by reducing portal venous inflow via two mechanisms: decrease in cardiac output and decrease in splanchnic blood flow. They prevent bleeding, and there is a trend toward reduced mortality.
- Therapy should be initiated with **propranolol**, 20 mg twice daily, or **nadolol**, 40 mg once daily, and titrated to maximal tolerated dose. In most studies, the dose was titrated to a reduction in resting heart rate by 25. β-Adrenergic blocker therapy should be continued for life, unless it is not tolerated, because bleeding can occur when therapy is abruptly discontinued.
- Endoscopic variceal ligation (EVL) should be considered as alternative prophylactic therapy in patients with contraindications or intolerance to β-adrenergic blockers. EVL is equivalent to nadolol or propranolol for prevention of first variceal bleeding.
- There is insufficient evidence to recommend nitrates in addition to β-adrenergic blockers to further lower portal pressure.

Acute Variceal Hemorrhage

- **Fig. 21–2** presents an algorithm for the management of variceal hemorrhage. Evidence-based recommendations for selected treatments are presented in **Table 21–4**.
- Initial treatment goals include (1) adequate blood volume resuscitation, (2) protection of the airway from aspiration of blood, (3) correction of significant coagulopathy and thrombocytopenia, (4) prophylaxis against spontaneous bacterial peritonitis and other infections, (5) control of bleeding, (4) prevention of rebleeding, and (5) preservation of liver function.
- Prompt stabilization of blood volume to maintain hemoglobin of 8 g/dL with volume expansion to maintain systolic blood pressure of 90 to 100 mm Hg and heart rate <100 beats/min is recommended. Airway management is critical. Fluid resuscitation involves colloids initially and subsequent blood products.
- Combination pharmacologic therapy plus EVL or sclerotherapy (when EVL is not technically feasible) is the most rational approach to treatment of acute variceal bleeding.
- Vasoactive drug therapy (usually octreotide) to stop or slow bleeding is routinely employed early in patient management to allow stabilization of the patient. Treatment with octreotide should be initiated early to control bleeding and facilitate endoscopy. Octreotide is administered as an IV bolus of 50 mcg followed by a continuous infusion of 50 mcg/hour. It should be continued for 5 days after acute variceal bleeding. Patients should be monitored for hypo- or hyperglycemia.
- **Vasopressin**, alone or in combination with nitroglycerin, can no longer be recommended as first-line therapy for the management of variceal hemorrhage. Vasopressin causes nonselective vasoconstriction and can result in myocardial ischemia or infarction, arrhythmias, mesenteric ischemia, ischemia of the limbs, or cerebrovascular accidents.

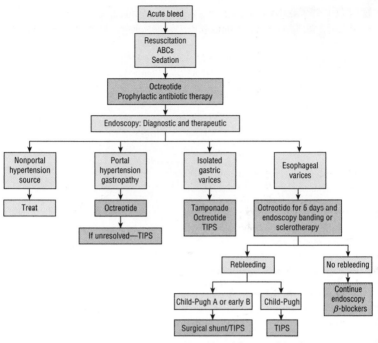

FIGURE 21–2. Management of acute variceal hemorrhage. (ABCs, airway, breathing, and circulation; TIPS, transjugular intrahepatic portosystemic shunt.)

- Antibiotic therapy should be used early to prevent sepsis in patients with signs of infection or ascites. A short course (up to 7 days) of oral **norfloxacin** 400 mg twice daily or IV **ciprofloxacin** is recommended.
- EVL is the recommended form of endoscopic therapy for acute variceal bleeding, although endoscopic injection sclerotherapy (injection of 1–4 mL of a sclerosing agent into the lumen of the varices) may be used.
- If standard therapy fails to control bleeding, a salvage procedure such as balloon tamponade (with a Sengstaken–Blakemore tube) or transjugular intrahepatic portosystemic shunt (TIPS) is necessary.

Prevention of Rebleeding

- A nonselective β-adrenergic blocker along with EVL is the best treatment option for prevention of rebleeding.
- **Propranolol** may be given at 20 mg twice daily (or **nadolol**, 20 mg once daily) and titrated weekly to achieve a goal of heart rate 55 to 60 beats/min or the maximal tolerated dose. Patients should be monitored for evidence of heart failure, bronchospasm, or glucose intolerance. A decrease in hepatic venous pressure gradient to <12 mm Hg and a reduction of >20% from baseline are considered therapeutic targets.
- The combination therapy of a nonselective β-blocker with **isosorbide mononitrate** can be used in patients unable to undergo EVL.

TABLE 21–4	Evidence-Based Table of Selected Treatment Recommendations: Variceal Bleeding in Portal Hypertension

Recommendation	Grade
Prevention of variceal bleeding	
Nonselective β-blocker therapy should be initiated in:	
Patients with small varices and criteria for increased risk of hemorrhage	IIaC
Patients with medium/large varices without high risk of hemorrhage	IA
Endoscopic variceal ligation (EVL) should be offered to patients who have contraindications or intolerance to nonselective β-blockers	IA
EVL may be recommended for prevention in patients with medium/large varices at high risk of hemorrhage instead of nonselective β-blocker therapy	IA
Treatment of variceal bleeding	
Short-term antibiotic prophylaxis should be instituted upon admission	IA
Vasoactive drugs should be started as soon as possible, prior to endoscopy, and maintained for 3–5 days	IA
Endoscopy should be performed within 12 hours to diagnose variceal bleeding and to treat bleeding with either sclerotherapy or EVL	IA
Secondary prophylaxis of variceal bleeding	
Nonselective β-blocker therapy plus EVL is the best therapeutic option for prevention of recurrent variceal bleeding	IA

Recommendation grading:

Class I—Conditions for which there is evidence and/or general agreement

Class II—Conditions for which there is conflicting evidence and/or a divergence of opinion

Class IIa—Weight of evidence/opinion is in favor of efficacy

Class IIb—Efficacy less well established

Class III—Conditions for which there is evidence and/or general agreement that treatment is not effective and/or potentially harmful

Level A—Data from multiple randomized trials or meta-analyses

Level B—Data derived from single randomized trial or nonrandomized studies

Level C—Only consensus opinion, case studies, or standard of care

Data from Garcia-Tsao G, Sanyal AJ, Grace ND, et al. Prevention and management of gastroesophageal varices and variceal hemorrhage in cirrhosis. Hepatology 2007;46(3):922–938.

ASCITES

- The therapeutic goals for patients with ascites are to control the ascites, prevent or relieve ascites-related symptoms (dyspnea and abdominal pain and distention), and prevent SBP and hepatorenal syndrome.
- For patients with ascites, a serum–ascites albumin gradient should be determined. If the serum–ascites albumin gradient is >1.1, portal hypertension is most likely present.
- The treatment of ascites secondary to portal hypertension includes abstinence from alcohol, sodium restriction (to 2 g/day), and diuretics.
- Diuretic therapy should be initiated with single morning doses of **spironolactone**, 100 mg, and **furosemide**, 40 mg, titrated every 3 to 5 days, with a goal of 0.5 kg maximum daily weight loss. The dose of each can be increased together, maintaining the 100:40 mg ratio, to a maximum daily dose of 400 mg spironolactone and 160 mg furosemide.
- If tense ascites is present, paracentesis should be performed prior to institution of diuretic therapy and salt restriction.

TABLE 21–5	Treatment Goals: Episodic and Persistent Hepatic Encephalopathy
Episodic HE	**Persistent HE**
Control precipitating factor	Reverse encephalopathy
Reverse encephalopathy	Avoid recurrence
Hospital/inpatient therapy	Home/outpatient therapy
Maintain fluid and hemodynamic support	Manage persistent neuropsychiatric abnormalities
	Manage chronic liver disease
Expect normal mentation after recovery	High prevalence of abnormal mentation after recovery

- Patients who experience encephalopathy, severe hyponatremia despite fluid restriction, or renal insufficiency should have diuretic therapy discontinued.
- Liver transplantation should be considered in patients with refractory ascites.

SPONTANEOUS BACTERIAL PERITONITIS

- Antibiotic therapy for prevention of SBP should be considered in all patients who are at high risk for this complication (those who experience a prior episode of SBP or variceal hemorrhage and those with low-protein ascites).
- Patients with documented or suspected SBP should receive broad-spectrum antibiotic therapy to cover *Escherichia coli, Klebsiella pneumoniae,* and *Streptococcus pneumoniae.*
- **Cefotaxime**, 2 g every 8 hours, or a similar third-generation cephalosporin for 5 days is considered the drug of choice. **Oral ofloxacin**, 400 mg every 12 hours for 8 days, is equivalent to IV cefotaxime.
- Patients who survive an episode of SBP should receive long-term antibiotic prophylaxis with daily norfloxacin 400 mg or double-strength trimethoprim-sulfamethoxazole.

Hepatic Encephalopathy
- **Table 21–5** describes the treatment goals for HE.
- The first approach to treatment of HE is to identify any precipitating causes. Precipitating factors and therapy alternatives are presented in **Table 21–6**.
- Treatment approaches include (1) reduction of blood ammonia concentrations by dietary restrictions, with drug therapy aimed at inhibiting ammonia production or enhancing its removal (lactulose and antibiotics); and (2) inhibition of γ-aminobutyric acid–benzodiazepine receptors by flumazenil.
- To reduce blood ammonia concentrations in patients with episodic HE, protein intake is limited or withheld (while maintaining caloric intake) until the clinical situation improves. Protein intake can be titrated back up based on tolerance to a total of 1 to 1.5 g/kg/day.
- To reduce blood ammonia concentrations in episodic HE, lactulose is initiated at 45 mL orally every hour (or 300 mL lactulose syrup with 700 mL water given as a retention enema held for 60 minutes) until

TABLE 21–6	Portosystemic Encephalopathy: Precipitating Factors and Therapy
Factor	**Therapy Alternatives**
GI bleeding	
Variceal	Band ligation/sclerotherapy
	Octreotide
Nonvariceal	Endoscopic therapy
	Proton pump inhibitors
Infection/sepsis	Antibiotics
	Paracentesis
Electrolyte abnormalities	Discontinue diuretics
	Fluid and electrolyte replacement
Sedative ingestion	Discontinue sedatives/tranquilizers
	Consider reversal (flumazenil/naloxone)
Dietary excesses	Limit daily protein
	Lactulose
Constipation	Cathartics
	Bowel cleansing/enema
Renal insufficiency	Discontinue diuretics
	Discontinue nonsteroidal antiinflammatory drugs, nephrotoxic antibiotics
	Fluid resuscitation

TABLE 21–7	Cirrhosis: Management Approach and Outcome Assessments		
Complication	**Treatment Approach**	**Monitoring Parameter**	**Outcome Assessment**
Ascites	Diet, diuretics, paracentesis, TIPS	Daily assessment of weight	Prevent or eliminate ascites and secondary complications
Spontaneous bacterial peritonitis	Antibiotic therapy, prophylaxis if undergoing paracentesis	Evidence of clinical deterioration (e.g., abdominal pain, fever, anorexia, malaise, fatigue)	Prevent/treat infection to decrease mortality
Variceal bleeding	Pharmacologic prophylaxis	Child–Pugh score, endoscopy, CBC	Appropriate reduction in heart rate and portal pressure
	Endoscopy, vasoactive drug therapy (octreotide), sclerotherapy, volume resuscitation, pharmacologic prophylaxis	CBC, evidence of overt bleeding	Acute: control acute bleed. Chronic: variceal obliteration, reduce portal pressures

(continued)

		TABLE 21-7	Cirrhosis: Management Approach and Outcome Assessments *(Continued)*

Complication	Treatment Approach	Monitoring Parameter	Outcome Assessment
Coagulation disorders	Blood products (PPF, platelets), vitamin K	CBC, prothrombin time, platelet count	Normalize PT, maintain/improve hemostasis
Hepatic encephalopathy	Ammonia reduction (lactulose, cathartics), elimination of drugs causing CNS depression, limit excess protein in diet	Grade of encephalopathy, EEG, psychological testing, mental status changes, concurrent drug therapy	Maintain functional capacity, prevent hospitalization for encephalopathy, decrease ammonia levels, provide adequate nutrition
Hepatorenal syndrome	Eliminate concurrent nephrotoxins (NSAIDs), decrease or discontinue diuretics, volume resuscitation, liver transplantation	Serum and urine electrolytes, concurrent drug therapy	Prevent progressive renal injury by preventing dehydration and avoiding other nephrotoxins Liver transplantation for refractory hepatorenal syndrome
Hepatopulmonary syndrome	Paracentesis, O_2 therapy	Dyspnea, presence of ascites	Acute: relief of dyspnea and hypoxia. Chronic: manage ascites as above

CBC, complete blood cell count; CNS, central nervous system; EEG, electroencephalogram; NSAIDs, nonsteroidal antiinflammatory drugs; O_2, oxygen; PPF, plasma protein fraction; PT, prothrombin time; TIPS, transjugular intrahepatic portosystemic shunt.

catharsis begins. The dose is then decreased to 15 to 30 mL orally every 8 to 12 hours and titrated to produce two or three soft stools per day.
- Antibiotic therapy with **metronidazole** or **neomycin** is reserved for patients who have not responded to diet and lactulose. **Rifaximin** 400 mg three times daily can be used for patients with inadequate response to lactulose.
- Zinc acetate supplementation (220 mg twice daily) is recommended for long-term management in patients with cirrhosis who are zinc deficient.

EVALUATION OF THERAPEUTIC OUTCOMES

- **Table 21-7** summarizes the management approach for patients with cirrhosis, including monitoring parameters and therapeutic outcomes.

See Chapter 44, Portal Hypertension and Cirrhosis, authored by Julie M. Sease, for a more detailed discussion of this topic.

Constipation

22 CHAPTER

DEFINITION

- Constipation does not have a single, generally agreed upon definition. Normal people pass at least three stools per week. Some of the definitions of constipation are fewer than three stools per week for women and five for men despite a high-residue diet or a period of more than 3 days without a bowel movement, straining at stool >25% of the time and/or two or fewer stools per week, and straining at defecation and less than one stool daily with minimal effort. The American Gastroenterological Association defines functional constipation as a bowel disorder characterized by difficult, infrequent, or seemingly incomplete defecation that does not meet criteria for irritable bowel syndrome (IBS).

PATHOPHYSIOLOGY

- Constipation may be primary (occurs without an underlying identifiable cause) or secondary (the result of constipating drugs, lifestyle factors, or medical disorders).
- Constipation is not a disease but a symptom of an underlying disease or problem.
- Disorders of the GI tract, metabolic disorders, and endocrine disorders may cause constipation.
- Constipation commonly results from a diet low in fiber or from use of constipating drugs such as opiates. Constipation may sometimes be psychogenic in origin.
- Diseases or conditions that may cause constipation include the following:
  - ✓ GI disorders: IBS, diverticulitis, upper and lower GI tract diseases, hemorrhoids, anal fissures, ulcerative proctitis, tumors, hernia, volvulus of the bowel, syphilis, tuberculosis, lymphogranuloma venereum, and Hirschsprung's disease
  - ✓ Metabolic and endocrine disorders: diabetes mellitus with neuropathy, hypothyroidism, panhypopituitarism, pheochromocytoma, hypercalcemia, and enteric glucagon excess
  - ✓ Pregnancy
  - ✓ Cardiac disorders (e.g., heart failure)
  - ✓ Neurogenic constipation: head trauma, CNS tumors, spinal cord injury, cerebrospinal accidents, and Parkinson's disease
  - ✓ Psychiatric disorders
  - ✓ Inappropriate bowel habits
- Causes of drug-induced constipation are listed in Table 22-1. All opiate derivatives are associated with constipation, but the degree of intestinal inhibitory effects seems to differ among agents. Orally administered opiates appear to have greater inhibitory effect than parenterally administered agents; oral codeine is well known as a potent antimotility agent.

TABLE 22–1 Drugs Causing Constipation

Analgesics
  Inhibitors of prostaglandin synthesis
  Opiates
Anticholinergics
  Antihistamines
  Antiparkinsonian agents (e.g., benztropine or trihexyphenidyl)
  Phenothiazines
  Tricyclic antidepressants
Antacids containing calcium carbonate or aluminum hydroxide
Barium sulfate
Calcium channel blockers
Clonidine
Diuretics (nonpotassium-sparing)
Ganglionic blockers
Iron preparations
Muscle blockers (D-tubocurarine, succinylcholine)
Nonsteroidal antiinflammatory agents
Polystyrene sodium sulfonate

CLINICAL PRESENTATION

- The laxative abuser may present with contradictory findings, sometimes diarrhea or weight loss. Laxative abusers may also have vomiting, abdominal pain, lassitude, thirst, edema, and bone pain (due to osteomalacia). With prolonged abuse, patients may have fluid and electrolyte imbalances (most commonly hypokalemia), protein-losing gastroenteropathy with hypoalbuminemia, and syndromes resembling colitis. Laxative abusers frequently deny laxative use (**Table 22–2**).

DESIRED OUTCOME

- A major goal for treatment of constipation is prevention of constipation by alteration of lifestyle (particularly diet) to prevent further episodes of constipation. For acute constipation, the goal is to relieve symptoms and restore normal bowel function.

TREATMENT

GENERAL APPROACH TO TREATMENT

- The patient should be asked about the frequency of bowel movements and the chronicity of constipation. The patient should also be carefully questioned about usual diet and laxative regimens. Does the patient have

TABLE 22–2	Clinical Presentation of Constipation

History and physical examination

Clarify what the patient means by constipation and identify specific signs and symptoms.

Ask about the presence of alarm signs and symptoms (see below).

Evaluate general health, psychological status, medications, diet, comorbidities, onset of symptoms, and previous treatments.

Rectal examination should be performed for the presence of anatomical abnormalities, stricture, rectal mass, or fecal impaction.

Signs and symptoms

Infrequent bowel movements; stools that are hard, small, or dry; difficulty or pain on defecation; feeling of abdominal discomfort; incomplete evaluation

Alarm signs and symptoms: hematochezia, melena, family history of colon cancer or inflammatory bowel disease, anemia, weight loss, anorexia, nausea and vomiting, severe persistent constipation refractory to treatment, or new onset or worsening of constipation in elderly patients without evidence of a primary cause

Laboratory tests

There is no routine laboratory testing recommended.

A series of examinations, including proctoscopy, sigmoidoscopy, colonoscopy, and barium enema, may be necessary to determine the presence of colorectal pathology.

Thyroid function studies, electrolytes, and blood glucose may be performed to determine the presence of metabolic or endocrine disorders.

a diet consistently deficient in high-fiber items and containing mainly highly refined foods? What laxatives or cathartics has the patient used to attempt relief of constipation? The patient should be questioned about other concurrent medications, with interest toward agents that might cause constipation.

- General measures believed to be beneficial in managing constipation include dietary modification to increase the amount of fiber consumed daily, exercise, adjustment of bowel habits so that a regular and adequate time is made to respond to the urge to defecate, and increased fluid intake.

- If an underlying disease is recognized as the cause of constipation, attempts should be made to correct it. GI malignancies may be removed through a surgical resection. Endocrine and metabolic derangements are corrected by the appropriate methods.

- Potential drug causes of constipation should be identified. For some medications (e.g., antacids), nonconstipating alternatives exist. If no reasonable alternatives exist to the medication thought to be responsible for constipation, consideration should be given to lowering the dose. If a patient must remain on constipating medications, then more attention must be paid to general measures for prevention of constipation, as discussed in Dietary Modification and Bulk-Forming Agents below.

DIETARY MODIFICATION AND BULK-FORMING AGENTS

- The most important aspect of the therapy for constipation for the majority of patients is dietary modification to increase the amount of fiber consumed. Patients should be advised to gradually increase daily fiber intake to 20 to 25 g, either through dietary changes or through fiber supplements. Fruits, vegetables, and cereals have the highest fiber content.

- A trial of dietary modification with high-fiber content should be continued for at least 1 month before the effects on bowel function are determined. Most patients begin to notice effects on bowel function 3 to 5 days after beginning a high-fiber diet.
- The patient should be cautioned that abdominal distention and flatus may be particularly troublesome in the first few weeks, particularly with high bran consumption.

PHARMACOLOGIC THERAPY

- The various types of laxatives are discussed in this section. The agents are divided into three general classifications: (1) those causing softening of feces in 1 to 3 days (bulk-forming laxatives, **docusates,** and **lactulose**), (2) those that result in soft or semifluid stool in 6 to 12 hours (bisacodyl and senna), and (3) those causing water evacuation in 1 to 6 hours (**saline cathartics, castor oil,** and **polyethylene glycol (PEG)–electrolyte lavage solution**).
- Dosage recommendations for laxatives and cathartics are provided in Table 22–3.

Recommendations

- The basis for treatment and prevention of constipation should consist of bulk-forming agents in addition to dietary modifications that increase dietary fiber.
- For most nonhospitalized persons with acute constipation, the infrequent use (less often than every few weeks) of most laxative products is acceptable; however, before more potent laxative or cathartics are used, relatively simple measures may be tried. For example, acute constipation may be relieved by the use of a **tap water enema** or a **glycerin** suppository; if neither is effective, the use of oral sorbitol, low doses of bisacodyl or senna, low-dose polyethylene PEG solutions, or saline laxatives (e.g., **milk of magnesia**) may provide relief.
- If laxative treatment is required for longer than 1 week, the person should be advised to consult a physician to determine if there is an underlying cause of constipation that requires treatment with agents other than laxatives.
- For some bedridden or geriatric patients, or others with chronic constipation, bulk-forming laxatives remain the first line of treatment, but the use of more potent laxatives may be required relatively frequently. Agents that may be used in these situations include **sorbitol, lactulose,** low-dose PEG solutions, and **milk of magnesia.**
- In the hospitalized patient without GI disease, constipation may be related to the use of general anesthesia and/or opiate substances. Most orally or rectally administered laxatives may be used. For prompt initiation of a bowel movement, a **tap water enema** or **glycerin** suppository is recommended, or **milk of magnesia.**

TABLE 22–3 Dosage Recommendations for Laxatives and Cathartics

Agent	Recommended Dose
Agents that cause softening of feces in 1–3 days	
Bulk-forming agents/osmotic laxatives	
Methylcellulose	4–6 g/day
Polycarbophil	4–6 g/day
Psyllium	Varies with product
Emollients	
Docusate sodium	50–360 mg/day
Docusate calcium	50–360 mg/day
Docusate potassium	100–300 mg/day
Lactulose	15–30 mL orally
Sorbitol	30–50 g/day orally
Mineral oil	15–30 mL orally
Agents that result in soft or semifluid stool in 6–12 hours	
Bisacodyl (oral)	5–15 mg orally
Senna	Dose varies with formulation
Magnesium sulfate (low dose)	<10 g orally
Agents that cause watery evacuation in 1–6 hours	
Magnesium citrate	18 g in 300 mL water
Magnesium hydroxide	2.4–4.8 g orally
Magnesium sulfate (high-dose)	10–30 g orally
Sodium phosphates	Varies with salt used
Bisacodyl	10 mg rectally
Polyethylene glycol–electrolyte preparations	4 L

- The approach to the treatment of constipation in infants and children should consider neurologic, metabolic, or anatomical abnormalities when constipation is a persistent problem. When not related to an underlying disease, the approach to constipation is similar to that in an adult. A high-fiber diet should be emphasized.

Emollient Laxatives (Docusates)

- These surfactant agents, **docusate** in its various salts, work by facilitating the mixing of aqueous and fatty materials within the intestinal tract. They may increase water and electrolyte secretion in the small and large bowel and result in a softening of stools within 1 to 3 days.
- Emollient laxatives are not effective in treating constipation but are used mainly to prevent constipation. They may be helpful in situations where straining at stool should be avoided, such as after recovery from myocardial infarction, with acute perianal disease, or after rectal surgery.
- It is unlikely that these agents are effective in preventing constipation if major causative factors (e.g., heavy opiate use, uncorrected pathology, and inadequate dietary fiber) are not concurrently addressed.

Mineral Oil

- **Mineral oil** is the only lubricant laxative in routine use and acts by coating stool and allowing easier passage. It inhibits colonic absorption of water, thereby increasing stool weight and decreasing stool transit time. Generally, the effect on bowel function is noted after 2 or 3 days of use.

- Mineral oil is helpful in situations similar to those suggested for docusates: to maintain a soft stool and avoid straining for relatively short periods of time (a few days to 2 weeks) but should be avoided in bedridden patients because of the risk of aspiration and lipoid pneumonia.
- Mineral oil may be absorbed systemically and cause a foreign-body reaction in lymphoid tissue.

Lactulose and Sorbitol

- **Lactulose** is a disaccharide that causes an osmotic effect retained in the colon. It is generally not recommended as a first-line agent for the treatment of constipation because it is costly and may cause flatulence, nausea, and abdominal discomfort or bloating. It may be justified as an alternative for acute constipation and has been found to be particularly useful in elderly patients.
- **Sorbitol,** a monosaccharide, has been recommended as a primary agent in the treatment of functional constipation in cognitively intact patients. It is as effective as lactulose, may cause less nausea, and is much less expensive.

Saline Cathartics

- Saline cathartics are composed of relatively poorly absorbed ions such as magnesium, sulfate, phosphate, and citrate, which produce their effects primarily by osmotic action to retain fluid in the GI tract. These agents may be given orally or rectally.
- A bowel movement may result within a few hours of oral doses and in 1 hour or sooner after rectal administration.
- These agents should be used primarily for acute evacuation of the bowel, which may be necessary before diagnostic examinations, after poisonings, and in conjunction with some anthelmintics to eliminate parasites.
- Agents such as **milk of magnesia** (an 8% suspension of magnesium hydroxide) may be used occasionally (every few weeks) to treat constipation in otherwise healthy adults.
- Saline cathartics should not be used on a routine basis to treat constipation. With fecal impactions, the enema formulations of these agents may be helpful.

Glycerin

- This agent is usually administered as a 3 g suppository and exerts its effect by osmotic action in the rectum. As with most agents given as suppositories, the onset of action is usually <30 minutes. Glycerin is considered a safe laxative, although it may occasionally cause rectal irritation. Its use is acceptable on an intermittent basis for constipation, particularly in children.

Polyethylene Glycol–Electrolyte Lavage Solution

- Whole-bowel irrigation with **PEG–electrolyte lavage solution** has become popular for colon cleansing before diagnostic procedures or colorectal operations.

- Four liters of this solution is administered over 3 hours to obtain complete evacuation of the GI tract. The solution is not recommended for the routine treatment of constipation, and its use should be avoided in patients with intestinal obstruction.
- Low doses of PEG solution (10–30 g or 17–34 g per 120–240 mL) once or twice daily may be used for treatment of constipation.

Lubiprostone

- Lubiprostone is a chloride channel activator that acts locally on the gut to accelerate genitourinary transit time and delay gastric emptying. It is approved for chronic idiopathic constipation and constipation-predominant IBS in adults. The dose is 24 mg capsule twice daily with food. Lubiprostone may cause headache, diarrhea, and nausea.

Opioid-Receptor Antagonists

- Alvimopan is an oral GI-specific mu-receptor antagonist for short-term use in hospitalized patients to accelerate recovery of bowel function after large or small bowel resection. It is given 12 mg (capsule) 30 minutes to 5 hours before surgery and then 12 mg twice daily for up to 7 days or until hospital discharge (maximum 15 doses).
- Methylnaltrexone is another mu-receptor antagonist approved for opioid-induced constipation in patients with advanced disease receiving palliative care or when response to laxative therapy has been insufficient.

Other Agents

- Tap water enemas may be used to treat simple constipation. The administration of 200 mL of water by enema to an adult often results in a bowel movement within 1.5 hours. Soapsuds are no longer recommended in enemas because their use may result in proctitis or colitis.

See Chapter 43, Diarrhea, Constipation, and Irritable Bowel Syndrome, authored by Patricia H. Powell and Virginia H. Fleming, for a more detailed discussion of this topic.

DEFINITION

- Diarrhea is an increased frequency and decreased consistency of fecal discharge as compared with an individual's normal bowel pattern. Frequency and consistency are variable within and between individuals. For example, some individuals defecate as many as three times a day, whereas others defecate only two or three times per week. Most cases of acute diarrhea are caused by infections with viruses, bacteria, or protozoa and are generally self-limited.

PATHOPHYSIOLOGY

- Diarrhea is an imbalance in absorption and secretion of water and electrolytes. It may be associated with a specific disease of the GI tract or with a disease outside the GI tract.
- Four general pathophysiologic mechanisms disrupt water and electrolyte balance, leading to diarrhea. These four mechanisms are the basis of diagnosis and therapy. They are (1) a change in active ion transport by either decreased sodium absorption or increased chloride secretion, (2) a change in intestinal motility, (3) an increase in luminal osmolarity, and (4) an increase in tissue hydrostatic pressure. These mechanisms have been related to four broad clinical diarrheal groups: secretory, osmotic, exudative, and altered intestinal transit.
- Secretory diarrhea occurs when a stimulating substance (e.g., vasoactive intestinal peptide [VIP], laxatives, or bacterial toxin) increases secretion or decreases absorption of large amounts of water and electrolytes.
- Poorly absorbed substances retain intestinal fluids, resulting in osmotic diarrhea.
- Inflammatory diseases of the GI tract can cause exudative diarrhea by discharge of mucus, proteins, or blood into the gut.
- In **altered intestinal transit,** intestinal motility is altered by reduced contact time in the small intestine, premature emptying of the colon, or bacterial overgrowth.

CLINICAL PRESENTATION

- The clinical presentation of diarrhea is shown in **Table 23–1**.
- Many agents, including antibiotics and other drugs, cause diarrhea (**Table 23–2**). Laxative abuse for weight loss may also result in diarrhea.

DESIRED OUTCOME

- The therapeutic goals of diarrhea treatment are to manage the diet; prevent excessive water, electrolyte, and acid–base disturbances; provide

TABLE 23–1	Clinical Presentation of Diarrhea

General

Usually, acute diarrheal episodes subside within 72 hours of onset, whereas chronic diarrhea involves frequent attacks over extended time periods.

Signs and symptoms

Abrupt onset of nausea, vomiting, abdominal pain, headache, fever, chills, and malaise

Bowel movements are frequent and never bloody, and diarrhea lasts 12 to 60 hours.

Intermittent periumbilical or lower right quadrant pain with cramps and audible bowel sounds is characteristic of small intestinal disease.

When pain is present in large intestinal diarrhea, it is a gripping, aching sensation with tenesmus (straining, ineffective, and painful stooling). Pain localizes to the hypogastric region, right or left lower quadrant, or sacral region.

In chronic diarrhea, a history of previous bouts, weight loss, anorexia, and chronic weakness are important findings.

Physical examination

Typically demonstrates hyperperistalsis with borborygmi and generalized or local tenderness

Laboratory tests

Stool analysis studies include examination for microorganisms, blood, mucus, fat, osmolality, pH, electrolyte and mineral concentration, and cultures.

Stool test kits are useful for detecting GI viruses, particularly rotavirus.

Antibody serologic testing shows rising titers over a 3- to 6-day period, but this test is not practical and is nonspecific.

Occasionally, total daily stool volume is also determined.

Direct endoscopic visualization and biopsy of the colon may be undertaken to assess for the presence of conditions such as colitis or cancer.

Radiographic studies are helpful in neoplastic and inflammatory conditions.

symptomatic relief; treat curable causes of diarrhea; and manage secondary disorders causing diarrhea. Clinicians must clearly understand that diarrhea, like a cough, may be a body defense mechanism for ridding itself of harmful substances or pathogens. The correct therapeutic response is not necessarily to stop diarrhea at all costs. If diarrhea is secondary to another illness, controlling the primary condition is necessary.

TREATMENT

GENERAL PRINCIPLES

- Management of the diet is a first priority for treatment of diarrhea (**Figs. 23–1** and **23–2**). Most clinicians recommend stopping solid foods for 24 hours and avoiding dairy products.
- When nausea or vomiting is mild, a digestible low-residue diet is administered for 24 hours.
- If vomiting is present and is uncontrollable with antiemetics, nothing is taken by mouth. As bowel movements decrease, a bland diet is begun. Feeding should continue in children with acute bacterial diarrhea.

TABLE 23–2	Drugs Causing Diarrhea

Laxatives
Antacids containing magnesium
Antineoplastics
Auranofin (gold salt)
Antibiotics
   Clindamycin
   Tetracyclines
   Sulfonamides
   Any broad-spectrum antibiotic
Antihypertensives
   Reserpine
   Guanethidine
   Methyldopa
   Guanabenz
   Guanadrel
   Angiotensin-converting enzyme inhibitors
Cholinergics
   Bethanechol
   Neostigmine
Cardiac agents
   Quinidine
   Digitalis
   Digoxin
Nonsteroidal antiinflammatory drugs
Misoprostol
Colchicine
Proton pump inhibitors
H_2-receptor blockers

- Rehydration and maintenance of water and electrolytes are the primary treatment measures until the diarrheal episode ends. If vomiting and dehydration are not severe, enteral feeding is the less costly and preferred method. In the United States, many commercial oral rehydration preparations are available (**Table 23–3**).

PHARMACOLOGIC THERAPY

- Various drugs have been used to treat diarrhea (**Table 23–4**). These drugs are grouped into several categories: antimotility, adsorbents, antisecretory compounds, antibiotics, enzymes, and intestinal microflora. Usually, these drugs are not curative but palliative.
- Opiates and opioid derivatives delay the transit of intraluminal content or increase gut capacity, prolonging contact and absorption. The limitations of the opiates are addiction potential (a real concern with long-term use) and worsening of diarrhea in selected infectious diarrheas.

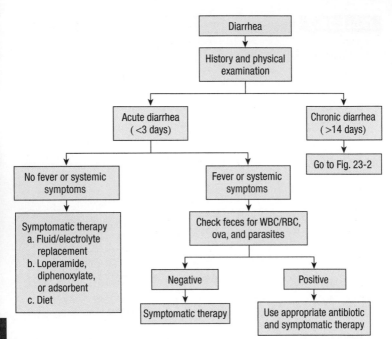

FIGURE 23–1. Recommendations for treating acute diarrhea. Follow these steps: (1) Perform a complete history and physical examination. (2) Is the diarrhea acute or chronic? If chronic diarrhea, go to Fig. 23–2. (3) If acute diarrhea, check for fever and/or systemic signs and symptoms (i.e., toxic patient). If systemic illness (fever, anorexia, or volume depletion), check for an infectious source. If positive for infectious diarrhea, use the appropriate antibiotic/anthelmintic drug and symptomatic therapy. If negative for infectious cause, use only symptomatic treatment. (4) If no systemic findings, then use symptomatic therapy based on severity of volume depletion, oral or parenteral fluid/electrolytes, antidiarrheal agents (see Table 23–4), and diet. (RBC, red blood cells; WBC, white blood cells.)

- **Loperamide** is often recommended for managing acute and chronic diarrhea. Diarrhea lasting 48 hours beyond initiating loperamide warrants medical attention.
- Adsorbents (such as **kaolin-pectin**) are used for symptomatic relief (see **Table 23–4**). Adsorbents are nonspecific in their action; they adsorb nutrients, toxins, drugs, and digestive juices. Coadministration with other drugs reduces their bioavailability.
- **Bismuth subsalicylate** is often used for treatment or prevention of diarrhea (traveler's diarrhea) and has antisecretory, antiinflammatory, and antibacterial effects. Bismuth subsalicylate contains multiple components that might be toxic if given in excess to prevent or treat diarrhea.
- *Lactobacillus* preparation is intended to replace colonic microflora. This supposedly restores intestinal functions and suppresses the growth of

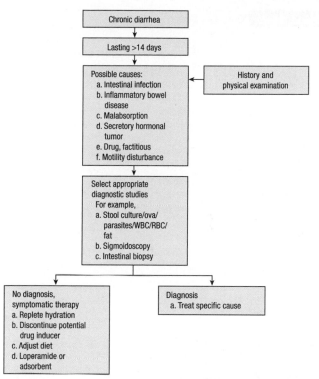

FIGURE 23–2. Recommendations for treating chronic diarrhea. Follow these steps: (1) Perform a careful history and physical examination. (2) The possible causes of chronic diarrhea are many. These can be classified into intestinal infections (bacterial or protozoal), inflammatory disease (Crohn's disease or ulcerative colitis), malabsorption (lactose intolerance), secretory hormonal tumor (intestinal carcinoid tumor or vasoactive intestinal peptide–secreting tumors), drug (antacid), factitious (laxative abuse), or motility disturbance (diabetes mellitus, irritable bowel syndrome, or hyperthyroidism) (3) If the diagnosis is uncertain, appropriate diagnostic studies should be ordered. (4) Once diagnosed, treatment is planned for the underlying cause with symptomatic antidiarrheal therapy. (5) If no specific cause can be identified, symptomatic therapy is prescribed. (RBC, red blood cells; WBC, white blood cells.)

pathogenic microorganisms. However, a dairy product diet containing 200 to 400 g of lactose or dextrin is equally effective in recolonization of normal flora.

- Anticholinergic drugs, such as **atropine**, block vagal tone and prolong gut transit time. Their value in controlling diarrhea is questionable and limited by side effects.

- **Octreotide**, a synthetic octapeptide analogue of endogenous somatostatin, is prescribed for the symptomatic treatment of carcinoid tumors and VIP-secreting tumors. It is used in select patients with carcinoid syndrome.

TABLE 23–3 Oral Rehydration Solutions

	WHO-ORS	Pedialyte[a] (Ross)	Rehydralyte[a] (Ross)	Infalyte (Mead Johnson)	Resol[a] (Wyeth)
Osmolality (mOsm/L)	311	249	304	200	269
Carbohydrates[a] (g/L)	13.5	25	25	30[b]	20
Calories (cal/L)	65	100	100	126	80
Electrolytes (mEq/L)					
Sodium	75	45	75	50	50
Potassium	20	20	20	25	20
Chloride	65	35	65	45	50
Citrate	–	30	30	34	34
Bicarbonate	30	–	–	–	–
Calcium	–	–	–	–	4
Magnesium	–	–	–	–	4
Sulfate	–	–	–	–	–
Phosphate	–	–	–	–	5

WHO-ORS, World Health Organization Oral Rehydration Solution.
[a]Carbohydrate is glucose.
[b]Rice syrup solids are a carbohydrate source.

TABLE 23–4 Selected Antidiarrheal Preparations

	Dose Form	Adult Dose
Antimotility		
Diphenoxylate	2.5 mg/tablet 2.5 mg/5 mL	5 mg four times daily; do not exceed 20 mg/day
Loperamide	2 mg/capsule 2 mg/capsule	Initially 4 mg, then 2 mg after each loose stool; do not exceed 16 mg/day
Paregoric	2 mg/5 mL (morphine)	5–10 mL one to four times daily
Opium tincture	10 mg/mL (morphine)	0.6 mL four times daily
Difenoxin	1 mg/tablet	2 tablets, then 1 tablet after each loose stool; up to 8 tablets/day
Adsorbents		
Kaolin-pectin mixture	5.7 g kaolin + 130.2 mg pectin/30 mL	30–120 mL after each loose stool
Polycarbophil	500 mg/tablet	Chew 2 tablets four times daily or after each loose stool; do not exceed 12 tablets/day
Attapulgite	750 mg/15 mL 300 mg/7.5 mL 750 mg/tablet 600 mg/tablet 300 mg/tablet	1200–1500 mg after each loose bowel movement or every 2 hours; up to 9000 mg/day

(continued)

TABLE 23–4	Selected Antidiarrheal Preparations *(Continued)*	
Antisecretory		
Bismuth subsalicylate	1050 mg/30 mL 262 mg/15 mL 524 mg/15 mL 262 mg/tablet	Two tablets or 30 mL every 30 min to 1 hour as needed up to 8 doses/day
Enzymes (lactase)	1,250 neutral lactase units/4 drops 3,300 FCC lactase units per tablet	3–4 drops taken with milk or dairy product
Bacterial replacement (*Lactobacillus acidophilus, Lactobacillus bulgaricus*)		2 tablets or 1 granule packet three to four times daily; give with milk, juice, or water
Octreotide	0.05 mg/mL 0.1 mg/mL 0.5 mg/mL	Initial: 50 mcg subcutaneously One to two times per day and titrate dose based on indication up to 600 mcg/day in two to four divided doses

Octreotide blocks the release of serotonin and other active peptides and is effective in controlling diarrhea and flushing. The dosage range for managing diarrhea associated with carcinoid tumors is 100 to 600 mcg daily in two to four divided doses, subcutaneously, for 2 weeks. Octreotide is associated with adverse effects such as cholelithiasis, nausea, diarrhea, and abdominal pain.

EVALUATION OF THERAPEUTIC OUTCOMES

- Therapeutic outcomes are directed to key symptoms, signs, and laboratory studies. The constitutional symptoms usually improve within 24 to 72 hours.
- One should check the frequency and character of bowel movements each day along with the vital signs and improving appetite.
- The clinician also needs to monitor body weight, serum osmolality, serum electrolytes, complete blood cell count, urinalysis, and cultures (if appropriate). With an urgent or emergency situation, any change in the volume status of the patient is the most important outcome.
- Toxic patients (those with fever, dehydration, and hematochezia and those who are hypotensive) require hospitalization; they need IV electrolyte solutions and empiric antibiotics while awaiting cultures. With quick management, they usually recover within a few days.

See Chapter 43, Diarrhea, Constipation, and Irritable Bowel Syndrome, authored by Patricia H. Powell and Virginia H. Fleming, for a more detailed discussion of this topic.

CHAPTER 24

Gastroesophageal Reflux Disease

DEFINITION

- *Gastroesophageal reflux disease (GERD)* occurs when refluxed stomach contents lead to troublesome symptoms and/or complications. Episodic heartburn that is not frequent or painful enough to be bothersome is not included in the definition of GERD.
- Symptom-based GERD may exist without or without esophageal injury, and tissue injury–based GERD may exist with or without symptoms (see Clinical Presentation). Esophagitis occurs when the esophagus is repeatedly exposed to refluxed gastric contents for prolonged periods. This can progress to erosion of the squamous epithelium of the esophagus (erosive esophagitis).

PATHOPHYSIOLOGY

- The key factor in the development of GERD is abnormal reflux of gastric contents from the stomach into the esophagus.
- In some cases, gastroesophageal reflux is associated with defective lower esophageal sphincter (LES) pressure or function. Patients may have decreased LES pressure related to spontaneous transient LES relaxations, transient increases in intraabdominal pressure, or an atonic LES. A variety of foods and medications may decrease LES pressure (Table 24–1).
- Problems with other normal mucosal defense mechanisms may also contribute to the development of GERD, including abnormal esophageal anatomy, improper esophageal clearance of gastric fluids, reduced mucosal resistance to acid, delayed or ineffective gastric emptying, inadequate production of epidermal growth factor, and reduced salivary buffering of acid.
- Substances that may promote esophageal damage upon reflux into the esophagus include gastric acid, pepsin, bile acids, and pancreatic enzymes. The composition and volume of the refluxate and the duration of exposure are the most important factors in determining the consequences of gastroesophageal reflux.
- Complications from long-term acid exposure may include esophagitis, esophageal strictures, Barrett esophagus, and esophageal adenocarcinoma.

CLINICAL PRESENTATION

- Symptom-based GERD (with or without esophageal tissue injury) typically presents with heartburn, usually described as a substernal sensation of warmth or burning rising up from the abdomen that may radiate to the neck. It may be waxing and waning in character and aggravated by activities that worsen gastroesophageal reflux (e.g., recumbent position, bending over, or eating a high-fat meal). Other symptoms are water brash (hypersalivation), belching, and regurgitation. Alarm symptoms that may

| TABLE 24–1 | Foods and Medications That May Worsen GERD Symptoms |

Decreased lower esophageal sphincter pressure

Foods	Medications
Fatty meal	Anticholinergics
Carminatives (peppermint and spearmint)	Barbiturates
Chocolate	Caffeine
Coffee, cola, and tea	Dihydropyridine calcium channel blockers
Garlic	Dopamine
Onions	Estrogen
Chili peppers	Ethanol
	Nicotine
	Nitrates
	Progesterone
	Tetracycline
	Theophylline

Direct irritants to the esophageal mucosa

Foods	Medications
Spicy foods	Alendronate
Orange juice	Aspirin
Tomato juice	Nonsteroidal antiinflammatory drugs
Coffee	Iron
	Quinidine
	Potassium chloride

indicate complications include dysphagia, odynophagia, and unexplained weight loss.

- Tissue injury–based GERD (with or without esophageal symptoms) may present with esophagitis, esophageal strictures, Barrett esophagus, or esophageal carcinoma. Alarm symptoms may also be present.
- Extracsophageal symptoms may include chronic cough, laryngitis, asthma, and dental enamel erosion.

DIAGNOSIS

- The most useful diagnostic tool is the clinical history, including both presenting symptoms and associated risk factors. Patients with mild, typical reflux symptoms do not usually require invasive evaluation; a clinical diagnosis of GERD can be assumed in patients who respond to appropriate therapy.
- Diagnostic tests should be performed in patients who do not respond to therapy or who present with alarm symptoms.
- Endoscopy is the preferred technique for assessing the mucosa for esophagitis, identifying Barrett esophagus, and diagnosing complications. Unfortunately, the presence or absence of mucosal damage does not prove that symptoms are reflux related.

- A camera-containing capsule swallowed by the patient can visualize the esophageal mucosa (PillCamESO, Given Imaging Ltd., Yoqneam, Israel). The procedure is less invasive than endoscopy and takes less than 15 minutes to perform in the clinician's office. Images of the esophagus are downloaded through sensors placed on the patient's chest that are connected to a data collector. The camera-containing capsule is passed in the stool.
- Ambulatory pH monitoring helps to correlate symptoms with abnormal esophageal acid exposure and is useful in patients not responding to acid-suppression therapy. A small pH probe is passed transnasally and placed ~5 cm above the LES. Patients keep a diary of symptoms that are later correlated with pH measurements when symptoms were reported. Combined impedance-pH monitoring measures both acid and nonacid reflux.
- Esophageal manometry is used to evaluate esophageal peristalsis and motility prior to antireflux surgery.
- An empiric trial of a proton pump inhibitor as a diagnostic test for GERD is less expensive and more convenient than ambulatory pH monitoring, but there is no standard dosing regimen or trial duration.
- Barium radiography is not routinely used to diagnose GERD because it lacks sensitivity and specificity and cannot identify Barrett esophagus.

DESIRED OUTCOME

- The goals of treatment are to reduce or eliminate symptoms, decrease the frequency and duration of gastroesophageal reflux, promote healing of the injured mucosa, and prevent the development of complications.

TREATMENT

GENERAL APPROACH

- Therapy is directed to decreasing the acidity of the refluxate, decreasing the gastric volume available to be refluxed, improving gastric emptying, increasing LES pressure, enhancing esophageal acid clearance, and protecting the esophageal mucosa (**Fig. 24–1**).
- Treatment is categorized using the following modalities:
  ✓ Lifestyle changes and patient-directed therapy with **antacids** and/or nonprescription acidsuppression therapy (**histamine$_2$-receptor antagonists [H$_2$RAs]** and/or **proton pump inhibitors [PPIs]**)
  ✓ Pharmacologic intervention with prescription-strength acidsuppression therapy
  ✓ Antireflux surgery
- The initial intervention depends in part on the patient's condition (symptom frequency, degree of esophagitis, and presence of complications). In the past, a step-up approach was used, starting with noninvasive lifestyle modifications and patient-directed therapy and progressing to pharmacologic management or antireflux surgery (**Table 24–2**). A step-down approach is also effective, starting with a PPI given once or twice daily

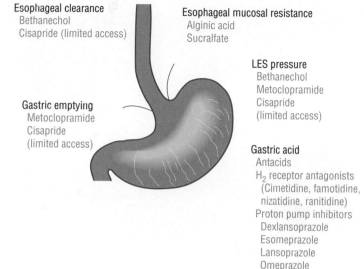

FIGURE 24–1. Therapeutic interventions in the management of gastroesophageal reflux disease. Pharmacologic interventions are targeted at improving defense mechanisms or decreasing aggressive factors. (LES, lower esophageal sphincter.)

instead of an H_2RA, then stepping down to the lowest dose of acid suppression needed to control symptoms (using either an H_2RA or PPI).

- Education on lifestyle modifications should be tailored to the individual needs of the patient (Table 24–3).

ANTACIDS AND ANTACID–ALGINIC ACID PRODUCTS

- Antacids provide immediate symptomatic relief for mild GERD and are often used concurrently with acid suppression therapies. Patients who require frequent use for chronic symptoms should receive prescription-strength acid suppression therapy instead.
- An antacid with alginic acid (Gaviscon) is not a potent acid-neutralizing agent and does not enhance LES pressure, but it does form a viscous solution that floats on the surface of the gastric contents. This serves as a protective barrier for the esophagus against reflux of gastric contents and reduces the frequency of reflux episodes. The combination product may be superior to antacids alone in relieving GERD symptoms, but efficacy data indicating endoscopic healing are lacking.
- Antacids have a short duration, which necessitates frequent administration throughout the day to provide continuous acid neutralization. Taking antacids after meals can increase duration of action from ~1 to 3 hours; however, nighttime acid suppression cannot be maintained with bedtime doses.

TABLE 24–2 Therapeutic Approach to GERD in Adults

Patient Presentation	Recommended Treatment Regimen	Comments
Intermittent, mild heartburn	**Lifestyle modifications** **plus** **patient-directed therapy** Antacids • Maalox or Mylanta 30 mL as needed or after meals and at bedtime • Gaviscon two tablets after meals and at bedtime • Calcium carbonate 500 mg, two to four tablets as needed **and/or** Nonprescription H$_2$RA (taken up to twice daily) • Cimetidine 200 mg • Famotidine 10 mg • Nizatidine 75 mg • Ranitidine 75 mg **or** Nonprescription PPI (taken once daily) • Omeprazole 20 mg • Lansoprazole 15 mg	Lifestyle modifications should be individualized for each patient. Weight loss in obese patients and elevation of the head of the bed have been proven most beneficial. If symptoms are unrelieved with lifestyle modifications and nonprescription medications after 2 weeks, patient should seek medical attention.
Symptomatic relief of GERD	**Lifestyle modifications** **plus** **prescription-strength acid-suppression therapy** H$_2$RA (for 6–12 wk) • Cimetidine 400 mg twice daily • Famotidine 20 mg twice daily • Nizatidine 150 mg twice daily • Ranitidine 150 mg twice daily	For typical symptoms, treat empirically with prescription-strength acid suppression therapy. If symptoms recur, consider MT. *Note:* Most patients will require standard doses for MT. Mild GERD can usually be treated effectively with H$_2$RAs.

	or PPIs (for 4–8 wk); all are given once daily • Dexlansoprazole 30 mg • Esomeprazole 20 mg • Lansoprazole 15 mg • Omeprazole 20 mg • Pantoprazole 40 mg • Rabeprazole 20 mg	Patients with moderate to severe symptoms should receive a PPI as initial therapy.
Healing of erosive esophagitis or treatment of patients presenting with moderate to severe symptoms or complications	Lifestyle modifications plus PPI for 4–16 weeks (up to twice daily) • Dexlansoprazole 60 mg • Esomeprazole 20–40 mg daily • Lansoprazole 30 mg daily • Omeprazole 20 mg daily • Rabeprazole 20 mg daily • Pantoprazole 40 mg daily or High-dose H₂RA (for 8–12 wk) • Cimetidine 400 mg four times daily or 800 mg twice daily • Famotidine 40 mg twice daily • Nizatidine 150 mg four times daily • Ranitidine 150 mg four times daily	For atypical or alarm symptoms, obtain endoscopy (if possible) to evaluate mucosa. Give a trial of a PPI. If symptoms are relieved, consider MT. PPIs are the most effective MT in patients with atypical symptoms, complications, and erosive disease.
Interventional therapies	Antireflux surgery	Patients not responding to pharmacologic therapy, including those with persistent atypical symptoms, should be evaluated via ambulatory reflux monitoring to confirm the diagnosis of GERD (if possible).

H₂RA, histamine₂-receptor antagonist; MT, maintenance therapy; PPI, proton pump inhibitor.

TABLE 24–3	Nonpharmacologic Treatment of GERD with Lifestyle Modifications

Recommended lifestyle modifications for all GERD patients
- Elevate the head of the bed (increases esophageal clearance). Use 6 to 8in blocks under the head of the bed. Sleep on a foam wedge.
- Recommend weight reduction (reduces symptoms) for obese patients.

Recommended lifestyle modifications that should be individualized to specific patients
- Avoid foods that may decrease LES pressure (fats, chocolate, alcohol, peppermint, and spearmint).
- Include protein-rich meals in diet (augments LES pressure).
- Avoid foods that have a direct irritant effect on the esophageal mucosa (spicy foods, orange juice, tomato juice, and coffee).
- Behaviors that may reduce esophageal acid exposure
  - Eat small meals and avoid eating immediately prior to sleeping (within 3 hours if possible; decreases gastric volume).
  - Stop smoking (decreases spontaneous esophageal sphincter relaxation).
  - Avoid alcohol (increases amplitude of the LES, peristaltic waves, and frequency of contraction).
  - Avoid tight-fitting clothes.
  - Take drugs that have a direct irritant effect on the esophageal mucosa with plenty of liquid if they cannot be avoided (bisphosphonates, tetracyclines, quinidine, potassium chloride, iron salts, aspirin, and NSAIDs).

LES, lower esophageal sphincter; NSAIDs, nonsteroidal antiinflammatory drugs.

H_2-RECEPTOR ANTAGONISTS

- The H_2RAs **cimetidine, ranitidine, famotidine,** and **nizatidine** in divided doses are effective for treating mild to moderate GERD. Low-dose non-prescription H_2RAs or standard doses given twice daily may be beneficial for symptomatic relief of mild GERD. Patients not responding to standard doses may be hypersecretors of gastric acid and require higher doses (see Table 24–2).
- The efficacy of H_2RAs in GERD is highly variable and frequently lower than desired. Although standard doses produce symptomatic improvement in ~60% of patients after 12 weeks of therapy, endoscopic healing rates average only ~50%. Prolonged courses (6–12 wk) are frequently required.
- The H_2RAs are generally well tolerated. The most common adverse effects are headache, somnolence, fatigue, dizziness, and either constipation or diarrhea. Cimetidine may inhibit the metabolism of theophylline, warfarin, phenytoin, nifedipine, and propranolol, among other drugs.
- Because all of the H_2RAs are equally efficacious, selection of the specific agent should be based on differences in pharmacokinetics, safety profile, and cost.

PROTON PUMP INHIBITORS

- PPIs (**dexlansoprazole, esomeprazole, lansoprazole, omeprazole, pantoprazole,** and **rabeprazole**) block gastric acid secretion by inhibiting hydrogen potassium adenosine triphosphatase in gastric parietal cells, which results in profound and long-lasting antisecretory effects.

- PPIs are superior to H_2RAs in patients with moderate to severe GERD, including those with esophageal tissue injury (Barrett esophagus, strictures, or esophagitis), and those with symptom-based GERD. Symptomatic relief is achieved in ~83% of patients with endoscopic evidence of injury, and endoscopic healing rates are ~78% at 8 weeks.

- PPIs are usually well tolerated. Potential adverse effects include headache, dizziness, somnolence, diarrhea, constipation, nausea, and vitamin B_{12} deficiency. PPIs may play a role in the acquisition of *Clostridium difficile* infection during acid suppression. All PPIs can decrease the absorption of drugs such as **ketoconazole** and **itraconazole** that require an acidic environment for absorption. Inhibition of cytochrome 2C19 (CYP2C19) by PPIs (especially omeprazole) may decrease the effectiveness of clopidogrel, causing cardiovascular events; until more data are available, it may be prudent to consider using an alternative agent (e.g., an H_2RA) with these patients.

- The PPIs degrade in acidic environments and are therefore formulated in delayed-release capsules or tablets. **Lansoprazole, esomeprazole,** and **omeprazole** contain enteric-coated (pH-sensitive) granules in a capsule form. For patients unable to swallow the capsules, the contents can be mixed in applesauce or placed in orange juice. In patients with nasogastric tubes, the contents should be mixed in 8.4% sodium bicarbonate solution. **Esomeprazole** granules can be dispersed in water. Lansoprazole is also available in packets for oral suspension and delayed-release orally disintegrating tablets; the packet for oral suspension should not be placed through nasogastric tubes. Patients taking **pantoprazole** or **rabeprazole** should be instructed not to crush, chew, or split the delayed-release tablets. **Dexlansoprazole** is available in a dual delayed-release capsule, with the first release occurring 1 to 2 hours after the dose, and the second release occurring 4 to 5 hours after the dose; the clinical significance of this dual release is unknown.

- **Zegerid®** is a combination product containing omeprazole 20 or 40 mg with sodium bicarbonate in immediate-release oral capsules and powder for oral suspension. It should be taken on an empty stomach at least 1 hour before a meal. Zegerid® offers an alternative to the delayed-release capsules or the IV formulation in adult patients with nasogastric tubes.

- **Lansoprazole, esomeprazole,** and **pantoprazole** are available in IV formulations for patients who cannot take oral medications, but they are not more effective than oral preparations and are significantly more expensive.

- Patients should take oral PPIs in the morning 15 to 30 minutes before breakfast to maximize efficacy, because these agents inhibit only actively secreting proton pumps. Dexlansoprazole can be taken without regard to meals. If dosed twice daily, the second dose should be taken ~10 to 12 hours after the morning dose and prior to a meal or snack.

PROMOTILITY AGENTS

- Promotility agents may be useful adjuncts to acid suppression therapy in patients with a known motility defect (e.g., LES incompetence, decreased esophageal clearance, or delayed gastric emptying). However, these agents are generally not as effective as acid suppression therapy and have undesirable side effects.

- **Cisapride** has comparable efficacy to H$_2$RAs in patients with mild esophagitis. It is no longer available for routine use because of life-threatening arrhythmias when combined with certain medications and other disease states.
- **Metoclopramide,** a dopamine antagonist, increases LES pressure in a dose-related manner and accelerates gastric emptying. Unlike cisapride, it does not improve esophageal clearance. Metoclopramide provides symptomatic improvement for some patients with GERD, but substantial evidence of endoscopic healing is lacking. Tachyphylaxis and side effects limit its usefulness. Common adverse reactions include somnolence, nervousness, fatigue, dizziness, weakness, depression, diarrhea, and rash.
- **Bethanechol** has very limited value and is not routinely recommended for the treatment of GERD because of side effects.

MUCOSAL PROTECTANTS

- **Sucralfate** is a nonabsorbable aluminum salt of sucrose octasulfate that has very limited value and is not recommended routinely for treatment of GERD.

COMBINATION THERAPY

- Combination therapy with an acid-suppressing agent and a promotility agent or mucosal protectant seems logical, but data supporting such therapy are limited. This approach should not be recommended routinely unless a patient has GERD with motor dysfunction.

MAINTENANCE THERAPY

- Although healing and/or symptomatic improvement may be achieved via many different therapeutic modalities, a large percentage of patients relapse after discontinuation of therapy, especially those with more severe disease.
- Long-term maintenance therapy should be considered to prevent complications and worsening of esophageal function in patients who have symptomatic relapse after discontinuation of therapy or dosage reduction, including patients with Barrett esophagus, strictures, or esophagitis.
- Most patients require standard doses to prevent relapses. **H$_2$RAs** may be effective maintenance therapy in patients with mild disease. **PPIs** are the drugs of choice for maintenance treatment of moderate to severe esophagitis or symptoms. Usual once-daily doses are **omeprazole** 20 mg, **lansoprazole** 30 mg, **rabeprazole** 20 mg, or **esomeprazole** 20 mg. Low doses of a PPI or alternate-day regimens may be effective in some patients with milder symptoms.
- "On-demand" maintenance therapy, by which patients take their PPI only when they have symptoms, may be effective for patients with endoscopy-negative GERD.

EVALUATION OF THERAPEUTIC OUTCOMES

- The short-term goals are to relieve symptoms such as heartburn and regurgitation so they do not impair the patient's quality of life.
- The frequency and severity of GERD symptoms should be monitored, and patients should be counseled on symptoms that suggest the presence of complications requiring immediate medical attention, such as dysphagia or odynophagia. Patients with persistent symptoms should be evaluated for the presence of strictures or other complications.
- Patients should be monitored for the presence of atypical symptoms such as laryngitis, asthma, or chest pain. These symptoms require further diagnostic evaluation.

See Chapter 39, Gastroesophageal Reflux Disease, authored by Dianne B. Williams and Robert R. Schade, for a more detailed discussion of this topic.

DEFINITION

- *Viral hepatitis* refers to the clinically important hepatotropic viruses responsible for hepatitis A (HAV), hepatitis B (HBV), delta hepatitis, hepatitis C (HCV), and hepatitis E.

HEPATITIS A

- HAV infection usually produces a self-limited disease and acute viral infection, with a low fatality rate, and confers lifelong immunity. International travel is a major risk factor for infection.
- HAV infection primarily occurs through transmission by the fecal-oral route, person-to-person, or by ingestion of contaminated food or water. The incidence of HAV correlates directly with low socioeconomic status, poor sanitary conditions, and overcrowding. Rates of HAV infection have increased among international travelers, injection drug users, and men who have sex with men.
- The disease exhibits three phases: incubation (averaging 28 days, range 15–50 days), acute hepatitis (generally lasting 2 months), and convalescence. Most patients have full clinical and biochemical recovery within 12 weeks. Nearly all individuals will have clinical resolution within 6 months of the infection. HAV does not lead to chronic infections.
- The clinical presentation of HAV infection is given in **Table 25–1**. Children under 6 years of age are typically asymptomatic.
- The diagnosis of acute HAV infection is based on clinical criteria of acute onset of fatigue, abdominal pain, loss of appetite, intermittent nausea and vomiting, jaundice or elevated serum aminotransferase levels, and serologic testing for immunoglobulin (Ig) M anti-HAV.

TREATMENT

- The goal of therapy is complete clinical resolution, including avoidance of complications, normalization of liver function, and reduction of infectivity and transmission. No specific treatment options exist for HAV. Management of HAV infection is primarily supportive. Steroid use is not recommended.

PREVENTION

- The spread of HAV can be best controlled by avoiding exposure. The most important measures to avoid exposure include good hand-washing techniques and good personal hygiene practices.
- The current vaccination strategy in the United States includes vaccinating all children at 1 year of age. Groups who should receive HAV vaccine are shown in **Table 25–2**.

| TABLE 25–1 | Clinical Presentation of Acute Hepatitis A |

Signs and symptoms

- The preicteric phase brings nonspecific influenza-like symptoms consisting of anorexia, nausea, fatigue, and malaise.
- Abrupt onset of anorexia, nausea, vomiting, malaise, fever, headache, and right upper quadrant abdominal pain with acute illness
- Icteric hepatitis is generally accompanied by dark urine, acholic (light-colored) stools, and worsening of systemic symptoms.
- Pruritus is often a major complaint of icteric patients.

Physical examination

- Icteric sclera, skin, and secretions
- Mild weight loss of 2 to 5 kg
- Hepatomegaly

Laboratory tests

- Positive serum immunoglobulin M anti–hepatitis A virus
- Mild elevations of serum bilirubin, γ-globulin, and hepatic transaminase (ALT and aspartate transaminase) values to about twice normal in acute anicteric disease
- Elevations of alkaline phosphatase, γ-glutamyl transferase, and total bilirubin in patients with cholestatic illness

- Two inactivated virus vaccines are currently licensed in the United States, Havrix and Vaqta. Approved dosing recommendations are shown in **Table 25–3**. Seroconversion rates ≥94% are achieved with the first dose.
- IG is used when pre- or postexposure prophylaxis against HAV infection is needed in persons for whom vaccination is not an option. It is most effective if given during the incubation phase of infection. A single dose of IG of

| TABLE 25–2 | Recommendations for Hepatitis A Vaccination |

All children at 1 year of age

Children and adolescents ages 2 to 18 years who live in states or communities where routine hepatitis A vaccination has been implemented because of high disease incidence

Persons traveling to or working in countries that have high or intermediate endemicity of infection[a]

Men who have sex with men

Illegal-drug users

Persons who have occupational risk for infection (e.g., persons who work with HAV-infected primates or HAV in a research laboratory setting)

Persons who have clotting factor disorders

Persons who have chronic liver disease (e.g., persons with chronic liver disease caused by hepatitis B or C and persons awaiting liver transplants)

HAV, hepatitis A virus.

[a]Travelers to Canada, Western Europe, Japan, Australia, or New Zealand are at no greater risk for HAV infection than they are while in the United States. All other travelers should be assessed for hepatitis A risk.

Source: Centers for Disease Control and Prevention. www.cdc.gov.

TABLE 25–3 Recommended Dosing of Havrix and Vaqta

Vaccine	Vaccinee's Age (years)	Dose	Volume (mL)	Number Doses	Schedule (months)
Havrix	2–18	720 ELISA units	0.5	2	0, 6–12
	≥19	1,440 ELISA units	1	2	0, 6–12
Vaqta	1–18	25 units	0.5	2	0, 6–18
	≥19	50 units	1	2	0, 6–18

ELISA, enzyme-linked immunosorbent assay.

Source: Centers for Disease Control and Prevention. Prevention of hepatitis A through active or passive immunizations: Recommendations of the Advisory Committee on Immunization Practices (ACIP). MMWR Morb Mortal Wkly Rep 2006;55(RR-7):1–23.

0.02 mL/kg is given intramuscularly for postexposure prophylaxis or short-term (≤5 months) preexposure prophylaxis. For lengthy stays, a single dose of 0.06 mL/kg is used. HAV vaccine may also be given with IG.

- For people recently exposed to HAV and not previously vaccinated, IG is indicated for
  ✓ Those in close contact with an HAV-infected person; all staff and attendees of daycare centers when HAV is documented; if involved in a common source exposure (e.g., a food-borne outbreak); classroom contacts of an index case patient; and schools, hospitals, and work settings where close personal contact occurred with the case patient

- Common vaccine side effects include soreness and warmth at the injection site, headache, malaise, and pain.

HEPATITIS B

- HBV is a leading cause of chronic hepatitis, cirrhosis, and hepatocellular carcinoma.
- Transmission of HBV occurs sexually, parenterally, and perinatally. In the United States, transmission occurs predominantly through sexual contact or injection-drug use. International travel is also an important risk factor.
- Approximately 20% of patients with chronic HBV infection develop complications of decompensated cirrhosis, including hepatic insufficiency and portal hypertension. HBV is a risk factor for development of hepatocellular carcinoma.
- There are three phases of HBV infection. The incubation period for HBV is 4 to 10 weeks during which patients are highly infective. This is followed by a symptomatic phase with intermittent flares of hepatitis and marked increases in aminotransferase serum levels. The final phase is seroconversion to anti–hepatitis B core antigen (anti-HbcAg). Patients who continue to have detectable hepatitis B surface antigen (HbsAg) and HBcAg and a high serum titer of HBV DNA for longer than 6 months have chronic HBV.
- The interpretation of serologic markers for HBV is given in **Table 25–4.**

TABLE 25–4	Interpretation of Serologic Tests in Hepatitis B Virus	
Tests	**Result**	**Interpretation**
HBsAg	(–)	
Anti-HB$_c$	(–)	Susceptible
Anti-HB$_s$	(–)	
HBsAg	(–)	
Anti-HB$_c$	(+)	Immune because of natural infection
Anti-HB$_s$	(+)	
HBsAg	(–)	Immune because of vaccination (valid only if test performed 1–2 months after third vaccine dose)
Anti-HB$_c$	(–)	
Anti-HB$_s$	(+)	
HBsAg	(+)	
Anti-HB$_c$	(+)	Acute infection
IgM anti-HB$_c$	(+)	
HBsAg	(+)	
Anti-HB$_c$	(+)	Chronic infection
IgM anti-HB$_c$	(–)	
Anti-HB$_s$	(–)	
HBsAg	(–)	Four interpretations possible:
Anti-HB$_c$	(+)	1. Recovery from acute infection
Anti-HB$_s$	(–)	2. Distant immunity and test not sensitive enough to detect low level of HB$_s$ in serum
		3. Susceptible with false-positive anti-HB$_c$
		4. May have undetectable level of HBsAg in serum and be chronically infected

HB$_c$, hepatitis B core; HB$_s$, hepatitis B surface; HB$_s$A, hepatitis B surface associated; HBsAg, hepatitis B surface antigen; IgM, immunoglobulin M.

Source: Centers for Disease Control and Prevention. Hepatitis B Serology. http://www.cdc.gov/ncidod/diseases/hepatitis/b/Bserology.htm.

- Clinical manifestations of acute HBV infection are age dependent. Infants infected with HBV are generally asymptomatic, whereas ~85% to 95% of children ages 1 to 5 years are asymptomatic.
- The clinical presentation of chronic HBV is given in Table 25–5.

PREVENTION

- Prophylaxis of HBV can be achieved by vaccination or by passive immunity in postexposure cases with HBV Ig.
- Two products are available for prevention of HBV infection: **HBV vaccine**, which provides active immunity, and **HBV Ig**, which provides temporary passive immunity.

TABLE 25–5	Clinical Presentation of Chronic Hepatitis B[a]

Signs and symptoms

- Easy fatigability, anxiety, anorexia, and malaise
- Ascites, jaundice, variceal bleeding, and hepatic encephalopathy can manifest with liver decompensation.
- Hepatic encephalopathy is associated with hyperexcitability, impaired mentation, confusion, obtundation, and eventually coma.
- Vomiting and seizures

Physical examination

- Icteric sclera, skin, and secretions
- Decreased bowel sounds, increased abdominal girth, and detectable fluid wave
- Asterixis
- Spider angiomata

Laboratory tests

- Presence of hepatitis B surface antigen for at least 6 months.
- Intermittent elevations of hepatic transaminase (ALT and aspartate transaminase) and hepatitis B virus DNA >20,000 IU/mL (10^5 copies/mL)
- Liver biopsies for pathologic classification as chronic persistent hepatitis, chronic active hepatitis, or cirrhosis

[a]Chronic hepatitis B can be present even without all the signs, symptoms, and physical examination findings listed being apparent.

- The goal of immunization against viral hepatitis is prevention of the short-term viremia that can lead to transmission of infection, clinical disease, and chronic HBV infection.
- Persons who should receive HBV vaccine are listed in Table 25–6.
- Side effects of the vaccines are soreness at the injection site, headache, fatigue, irritability, and fever.

TREATMENT

- The key goals of therapy are to increase the likelihood of seroclearance of the virus, prevent disease progression to cirrhosis or hepatocellular carcinoma, and minimize further liver injury. Successful therapy is associated with loss of HBeAg status and seroconversion to anti-HBeAg.
- Some patients with chronic HBV infection should be treated. Recommendations for treatment consider the patient's age, serum HBV DNA and ALT levels, and histologic evidence and clinical progression of the disease. A suggested treatment algorithm for chronic HBV is shown for patients without (Fig. 25–1). and with cirrhosis (Fig. 25–2).
- All patients with chronic HBV infection should be counseled on preventing disease transmission, to avoid alcohol, and to be immunized against HBV.
- Drug therapy is used to suppress viral replication by immune mediating or antiviral effects. **Interferon α2b** (IFN-α2b), **lamivudine, telbivudine, adefovir entecavir, pegylated IFN-α2a** (PEG-IFN), and tenofovir are approved in the United States for first-line treatment of chronic HBV.

TABLE 25-6	Recommendations for Hepatitis B Virus (HBV) Vaccination

Infants

Adolescents, including all previously unvaccinated children <19 years old

All unvaccinated adults at risk for infection

All unvaccinated adults seeking vaccination (specific risk factor not required)

Men and women with a history of other sexually transmitted diseases and persons with a history of multiple sex partners (>1 partner/6 months)

Men who have sex with men

Injection-drug users

Household contacts and sex partners of persons with chronic HBV infection and healthcare and public safety workers with exposure to blood in the workplace

Clients and staff of institutions for the developmentally disabled

International travelers to regions with high or intermediate levels (HBsAg prevalence ≥2%) of endemic HBV infection

Recipients of clotting factor concentrates

Sexually transmitted disease clinic patients

HIV patient/HIV-testing patients

Drug abuse treatment and prevention clinic patients

Correctional facilities inmates

Chronic dialysis/ESRD patients

Persons with chronic liver disease

ESRD, end-stage renal disease; HBsAg, hepatitis B surface antigen; HIV, human immunodeficiency virus.
Source: Centers for Disease Control and Prevention. A comprehensive immunization strategy to eliminate transmission of hepatitis B virus infection in the United States: Recommendations of the Advisory Committee on Immunization Practices (ACIP) Part 1: Immunization of infants, children, and adolescents. MMWR Morb Mortal Wkly Rep 2005;54(RR-16):1–31.

- Several factors correlate with improved response to IFN therapy, including increased ALT and HBV DNA levels, high histologic activity score at biopsy, and being non-Asian. Treatment for a minimum of 12 months is associated with greater sustained virologic response rates than treatment for 4 to 6 months. Conventional IFN therapy has been virtually replaced with PEG-IFN, because of the ease of administration (once-weekly injections), fewer side effects, and improved efficacy.
- Lamivudine (100 mg daily given orally) in combination with PEG-IFN resulted in greater HBV DNA suppression.

HEPATITIS C

- HCV is the most common blood-borne pathogen. Screening for HCV infection is recommended in groups who are at high risk for infection (Table 25–7).

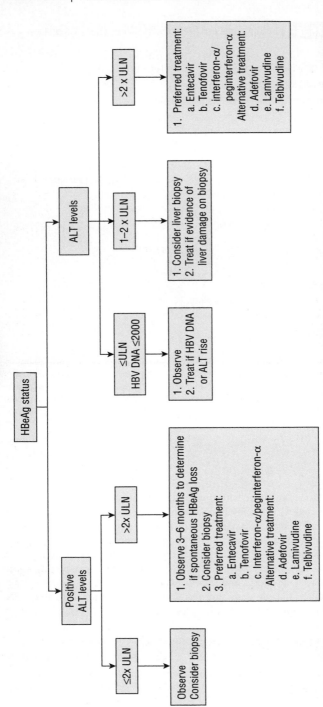

FIGURE 25–1. Suggested treatment algorithm for chronic hepatitis B virus infection based on the recommendations of the American Association for the Study of Liver Diseases. (ALT, alanine transaminases; HBeAg, hepatitis B e antigen; PegIFN, pegylated interferon.) *(Adapted from Lok ASF, McMahon BJ. AASLD practice guidelines: Chronic hepatitis B. Hepatology 2001;34:1225–1241.)*

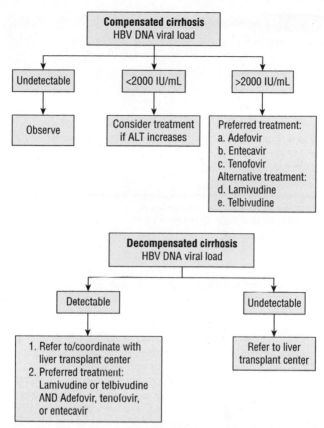

FIGURE 25-2. Suggested treatment algorithm based on the recommendations of the American Association for the Study of Liver Diseases for chronic hepatitis B virus-infected patients with cirrhosis. *(Adapted from Lok ASF, McMahon BJ. AASLD practice guidelines: Chronic hepatitis B. Hepatology 2001;34:1225–1241.)*

- HCV is most often acquired through injection drug use. Other illicit drug use is also a risk factor. Transmission may occur by sexual contact; hemodialysis; or household, occupational, or perinatal exposure.
- In the vast majority of patients (up to 85%), acute HCV infection leads to chronic infection defined by persistently detectable HCV RNA for 6 months or more.
- Patients with acute HCV are often asymptomatic and undiagnosed. One third of adults will experience some mild and nonspecific symptoms, including fatigue, anorexia, weakness, jaundice, abdominal pain, and dark urine.
- The most common symptom of chronic HCV infection is persistent fatigue. An estimated 20% of patients with chronic HCV infection will develop cirrhosis, and half of those patients will progress to decompensated cirrhosis or hepatocellular carcinoma.

TABLE 25–7	Recommendations for Hepatitis C Virus (HCV) Screening

Current or past injection drug use

Coinfection with HIV

Received blood transfusions or organ transplantations before 1992

Received clotting factors before 1987

Ever on chronic hemodialysis

Patients with unexplained elevated ALT levels or evidence of liver disease

Healthcare and public safety workers after a needlestick or mucosal exposure to HCV-positive blood

Children born to HCV-positive mothers

Sexual partners of HCV-positive patients

ALT, alanine transaminase; HIV, human immunodeficiency virus.
Source: Data from Hoofnagle JH. Course and outcome of hepatitis C. Hepatology 2002;36(5 Suppl 1):S21–S29.

- The diagnosis of HCV infection is confirmed with a reactive enzyme immunoassay for anti-HCV. Serum transaminase values are elevated within 4 to 12 weeks after exposure.

TREATMENT

- The goal of treating HCV is to eradicate HCV infection, which prevents the development of chronic HCV infection and sequelae.
- Treatment for HCV infection is necessary because a high percentage of acutely infected patients develop chronic infections. Treatment is indicated in patients previously untreated who have chronic HCV, circulating HCV RNA, increased ALT levels, evidence on biopsy of moderate to severe hepatic grade and stage, and compensated liver disease.
- The current standard of care for chronic HCV patients is combination therapy of a once-weekly injection of PEG-IFN and a daily oral dose of

TABLE 25–8	Recommended Hepatitis C Virus Treatment Dosing		
Genotype	**Peg-IFN Dose**	**Ribavirin Dose**	**Duration[a]**
1, 4	Peginterferon-α2a 180 mcg/wk or	≤75 kg[b] 1,000 mg	48 weeks
		>75 kg 1,200 mg	
	Peginterferon-α2b 1.5 mcg/wk	≤65 kg 800 mg	48 weeks
		>65–85 kg 1000 mg	
		>85–105 kg 1200 mg	
		>105 kg 1,400 mg	
2, 3	Peginterferon-α2a 180 mcg/wk or	800 mg	24 weeks
	Peginterferon-α2b 1.5 mcg/wk	800 mg	24 weeks

[a]Actual treatment duration may be different depending on virological response.
[b]Patient weight.

ribavirin. Therapy is optimized based on genotype, patient weight, and response to therapy. Sustained virologic response rates are 54% to 56%.

- Treatment response is best in patients with HCV genotype 1 and those who take at least 80% of their medications for at least 80% of the treatment time.
- All patients with chronic HCV infection should be vaccinated for HAV and HBV. Patients should be advised to maintain good overall health, stop smoking, and avoid alcohol and illicit drugs.
- Recommended treatment regimens for HCV infection are given in Table 25–8 and Fig. 25–3.

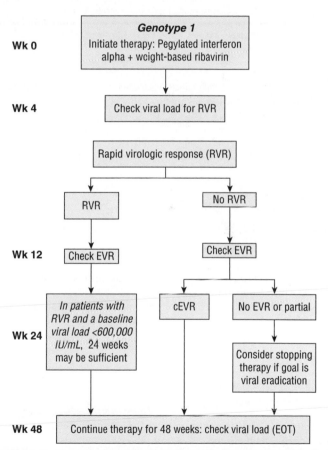

FIGURE 25–3. Suggested response-optimized chronic hepatitis C virus infection treatment regimens based on the recommendations of the American Association for the Study of Liver Diseases. 70EOT, end of treatment. *(Adapted from Ghany, MG, Strader DB, Thomas DL, et al. American Association for the Study of Liver Diseases Practice Guidelines: Diagnosis, management, and treatment of hepatitis C. Hepatology 2009;49:1335–1174.)*

TABLE 25–9	Pegylated Interferon (PEG-IFN) Comparison	
	Pegasys	**PEG-IFN**
Interferon	Alpha-2a	Alpha-2b
Indications	HBV, HCV	HCV
PEG moiety (weight)	Branched (40 kDa)	Linear (12 kDa)
Distribution	8–12 L; highest concentration in liver, spleen, and kidneys	Body weight dependent: 1 L/kg; distributes throughout body
Metabolism	Liver	Liver
Excretion	Renal	Renal
Dosing	Fixed: 180 mcg/wk subcutaneously	Weight dependent: 1.5 mcg/kg/wk subcutaneously

HBV, hepatitis B virus; HCV, hepatitis C virus.

TABLE 25–10	Common Side Effects Associated with Pegylated Interferon Therapy (Experienced by >20% of Patients)	
Fatigue		Arthralgia
Fever		Musculoskeletal pain
Headache		Insomnia
Nausea		Depression
Anorexia		Anxiety/emotional lability
Rigors		Alopecia
Myalgia		Injection site reactions

- Two PEG-IFNs are available, Pegasys and PEG-Intron (Table 25–9). It is unclear which is superior.
- Common side effects of PEG-IFN are given in Table 25–10. Common side effects of ribavirin are fatigue, flu-like symptoms, neutropenia, thrombocytopenia, and anemia.

PREVENTION

- No HCV vaccine is currently available.

See Chapter 47, Viral Hepatitis, authored by Paulina Deming, for a more detailed discussion of this topic.

26 Inflammatory Bowel Disease

DEFINITION

- There are two forms of idiopathic inflammatory bowel disease (IBD): ulcerative colitis (UC), a mucosal inflammatory condition confined to the rectum and colon, and Crohn's disease, a transmural inflammation of GI mucosa that may occur in any part of the GI tract. The etiologies of both conditions are unknown, but they may have a common pathogenetic mechanism.

PATHOPHYSIOLOGY

- The major theories of the cause of IBD involve a combination of infectious, genetic, and immunologic causes. The inflammatory response with IBD may indicate abnormal regulation of the normal immune response or an autoimmune reaction to self-antigens. Microflora of the GI tract may provide a trigger to activate inflammation. Crohn's disease may involve a T lymphocyte disorder that arises in genetically susceptible individuals as a result of a breakdown in the regulatory constraints on mucosal immune responses to enteric bacteria. Proposed etiologies for IBD are found in Table 26–1.
- Antineutrophil cytoplasmic antibodies are found in a high percentage of patients with UC.
- Smoking appears to be protective for ulcerative colitis but associated with increased frequency of Crohn's disease. The use of nonsteroidal antiinflammatory drugs (NSAIDs) may trigger disease occurrence or lead to disease flares.
- UC and Crohn's disease differ in two general respects: anatomical sites and depth of involvement within the bowel wall. There is, however, overlap between the two conditions, with a small fraction of patients showing features of both diseases (Table 26–2).

ULCERATIVE COLITIS

- UC is confined to the colon and rectum and affects primarily the mucosa and the submucosa. The primary lesion occurs in the crypts of the mucosa (crypts of Lieberkühn) in the form of a crypt abscess.
- Local complications (involving the colon) occur in the majority of patients with UC. Relatively minor complications include hemorrhoids, anal fissures, and perirectal abscesses.
- A major complication is toxic megacolon, a severe condition that occurs in up to 7.9% of UC patients admitted to hospitals. The patient with toxic megacolon usually has a high fever, tachycardia, distended abdomen, elevated white blood cell count, and a dilated colon.
- The risk of colonic carcinoma is much greater in patients with UC as compared with the general population.

TABLE 26–1	Proposed Etiologies for Inflammatory Bowel Disease

Infectious agents
  Viruses (e.g., measles) and protozoa
  L-form bacteria
  Mycobacterium paratuberculosis or *avium*
  Listeria monocytogenes
  Chlamydia

Genetics
  Metabolic defects
  Connective tissue disorders
  Select genes and single nucleotide polymorphisms

Environmental factors
  Diet
  Smoking (Crohn's disease)

Immune defects
  Altered host susceptibility
  Immune-mediated mucosal damage

Psychological factors
  Stress
  Emotional or physical trauma
  Occupation

- Approximately 11% of patients with UC have hepatobiliary complications, including fatty liver, pericholangitis, chronic active hepatitis, cirrhosis, sclerosing cholangitis, cholangiocarcinoma, and gallstones.
- Arthritis commonly occurs in patients with IBD and is typically asymptomatic and migratory. Arthritis typically involves one or a few large joints, such as the knees, hips, ankles, wrists, and elbows.
- Ocular complications (iritis, episcleritis, and conjunctivitis) occur in up to 10% of patients. Five percent to 10% of patients experience dermatologic or mucosal complications (erythema nodosum, pyoderma gangrenosum, or aphthous stomatitis).

CROHN'S DISEASE

- Crohn's disease is a transmural inflammatory process. The terminal ileum is the most common site of the disorder, but it may occur in any part of the GI tract. About two thirds of patients have some colonic involvement, and 15% to 25% of patients have only colonic disease. Patients often have normal bowel separating segments of diseased bowel; that is, the disease is often discontinuous.
- Complications of Crohn's disease may involve the intestinal tract or organs unrelated to it. Small bowel stricture with subsequent obstruction is a complication that may require surgery. Fistula formation is common and occurs much more frequently than with UC.
- Systemic complications of Crohn's disease are common and similar to those found with UC. Arthritis, iritis, skin lesions, and liver disease often accompany Crohn's disease.

TABLE 26–2 Comparison of the Clinical and Pathologic Features of Crohn's Disease and Ulcerative Colitis

Feature	Crohn's Disease	Ulcerative Colitis
Clinical		
Malaise, fever	Common	Uncommon
Rectal bleeding	Common	Common
Abdominal tenderness	Common	May be present
Abdominal mass	Common	Absent
Abdominal pain	Common	Unusual
Abdominal wall and internal fistula	Common	Absent
Distribution	Discontinuous	Continuous
Aphthous or linear ulcers	Common	Rare
Pathologic		
Rectal involvement	Rare	Common
Ileal involvement	Very common	Rare
Strictures	Common	Rare
Fistulas	Common	Rare
Transmural involvement	Common	Rare
Crypt abscesses	Rare	Very common
Granulomas	Common	Rare
Linear clefts	Common	Rare
Cobblestone appearance	Common	Absent

- Nutritional deficiencies are common with Crohn's disease (weight loss, iron deficiency anemia, vitamin B_{12} deficiency, folate deficiency, hypoalbuminemia, hypokalemia, and osteomalacia).

CLINICAL PRESENTATION

ULCERATIVE COLITIS

- There is a wide range of UC presentations. Symptoms may range from mild abdominal cramping with frequent small-volume bowel movements to profuse diarrhea (Table 26–3). Many patients have disease confined to the rectum (proctitis).
- Most patients with UC experience intermittent bouts of illness after varying intervals of no symptoms.
- Mild disease, which afflicts two thirds of patients, has been defined as fewer than four stools daily, with or without blood, with no systemic disturbance and a normal erythrocyte sedimentation rate (ESR).
- Patients with moderate disease have more than four stools per day but with minimal systemic disturbance.

TABLE 26–3	Clinical Presentation of Ulcerative Colitis

Signs and symptoms
- Abdominal cramping
- Frequent bowel movements, often with blood in the stool
- Weight loss
- Fever and tachycardia in severe disease
- Blurred vision, eye pain, and photophobia with ocular involvement
- Arthritis
- Raised, tender red nodules that vary in size from 1 cm to several centimeters

Physical examination
- Hemorrhoids, fissures, or perirectal abscesses may be present.
- Iritis, uveitis, episcleritis, and conjunctivitis with ocular involvement
- Dermatologic findings with erythema nodosum, pyoderma gangrenosum, or aphthous ulceration

Laboratory tests
- Decreased hematocrit/hemoglobin
- Increased erythrocyte sedimentation rate
- Leukocytosis and hypoalbuminemia with severe disease
- (+) perinuclear antineutrophil cytoplasmic antibodies

- With severe disease, the patient has more than six stools per day with blood, with evidence of systemic disturbance as shown by fever, tachycardia, anemia, or ESR >30.

CROHN'S DISEASE

- As with UC, the presentation of Crohn's disease is highly variable (Table 26–4). A single episode may not be followed by further episodes, or the patient may experience continuous, unremitting disease. A patient

TABLE 26–4	Clinical Presentation of Crohn's Disease

Signs and symptoms
- Malaise and fever
- Abdominal pain
- Frequent bowel movements
- Hematochezia
- Fistula
- Weight loss and malnutrition
- Arthritis

Physical examination
- Abdominal mass and tenderness
- Perianal fissure or fistula

Laboratory tests
- Increased white blood cell count and erythrocyte sedimentation rate
- anti-*Saccharomyces cerevisiae* antibodies

may present with diarrhea and abdominal pain or a perirectal or perianal lesion.

- The course of Crohn's disease is characterized by periods of remission and exacerbation. Some patients may be free of symptoms for years, whereas others experience chronic problems despite medical therapy.
- Disease activity may be assessed and correlated by evaluation of serum C-reactive protein concentrations.

DESIRED OUTCOME

- The goals of treatment include resolution of acute inflammatory processes, resolution of attendant complications (e.g., fistulas or abscesses), alleviation of systemic manifestations (e.g., arthritis), maintenance of remission from acute inflammation, or surgical palliation or cure.

TREATMENT

NONPHARMACOLOGIC TREATMENT

Nutritional Support

- Patients with moderate to severe IBD are often malnourished. No specific diets have gained widespread acceptance.
- The nutritional needs of the majority of patients can be adequately addressed with enteral supplementation. Patients who have severe disease may require a course of parenteral nutrition.
- Probiotic formulas have been effective in maintaining remission in UC, but the data are not conclusive.

Surgery

- For UC, colectomy may be performed when the patient has disease uncontrolled by maximum medical therapy or when there are complications of the disease, such as colonic perforation, toxic dilation (megacolon), uncontrolled colonic hemorrhage, or colonic strictures.
- The indications for surgery with Crohn's disease are not as well established as they are for UC, and surgery is usually reserved for the complications of the disease. There is a high recurrence rate of Crohn's disease after surgery.

PHARMACOLOGIC THERAPY

- The major types of drug therapy used in IBD are **aminosalicylates, glucocorticoids,** immunosuppressive agents (**azathioprine, mercaptopurine, cyclosporine,** and **methotrexate**), antimicrobials (**metronidazole** and **ciprofloxacin**), agents to inhibit tumor necrosis factor-α (TNF-α) (anti–TNF-α antibodies), and leukocyte adhesion and migration (natalizumab).
- **Sulfasalazine** combines a sulfonamide (sulfapyridine) antibiotic and mesalamine (5-aminosalicylic acid) in the same molecule. Mesalamine-based products are listed in **Table 26–5.**

TABLE 26–5 Mesalamine Derivatives for Treatment of Inflammatory Bowel Disease

Product	Trade Name(s)	Formulation	Dose/Day	Site of Action
Sulfasalazine	Azulfidine Azulfidine EN-tablets Sulfazine Sulfazine EC	Tablet	4–6 g	Colon
Mesalamine	Rowasa	Enema	1–4 g	Rectum, terminal colon
	Asacol Asacol HD	Mesalamine tablet coated with Eudragit-S (delayed-release acrylic resin)	2.4–4.8 g	Distal ileum and colon
	Pentasa	Mesalamine capsules encapsulated in ethylcellulose microgranules	2–4 g	Small bowel and colon
	Lialda	Mesalamine tablet formulated with Multi Matrix System delayed-release technology, allows for once-daily dosing	2.4–4.8 g	Colon
	Apriso	Mesalamine capsule formulated with enteric-coated granules in a delayed-release polymer matrix; allows once daily dosing	1.5 g	Colon
	Canasa	Mesalamine suppository	500–1,000 mg	Rectum
Olsalazine	Dipentum	Dimer of 5-aminosalicylic acid oral capsule	1.5–3 g	Colon
Balsalazide	Colazal	Capsule	6.75 g	Colon

- Corticosteroids and adrenocorticotropic hormone have been widely used for the treatment of UC and Crohn's disease and are used in moderate to severe disease. Prednisone is most commonly used. Budesonide is an oral controlled-release formulation that minimizes systemic effects.
- Immunosuppressive agents such as **azathioprine** and **mercaptopurine** (a metabolite of azathioprine) are sometimes used for the treatment of IBD. These agents are generally reserved for cases that are refractory to steroids and may be associated with serious adverse effects, such as lymphomas, pancreatitis, and nephrotoxicity. Cyclosporine has been of short-term benefit in acute, severe UC when used in a continuous infusion.

- Methotrexate given 25 mg intramuscularly once weekly is useful for treatment and maintenance of Crohn's disease.
- Antimicrobial agents, particularly **metronidazole**, are frequently used in attempts to control Crohn's disease, particularly when it involves the perineal area or fistulas. **Ciprofloxacin** has also been used for treatment of Crohn's disease.
- Infliximab is an anti-TNF antibody that is useful in moderate to severe active disease and steroid-dependent or fistulizing disease, but the cost far exceeds that of other regimens. Adalimumab is another anti-TNF antibody that is an option for patients with moderate to severe active Crohn's disease previously treated with infliximab who have lost response. **Certolizumab** is a pegylated Fab fragment against TNF that is used for patients with Crohn's disease. **Natalizumab** is a leukocyte adhesion and migration inhibitor that is used for patients with Crohn's disease who are unresponsive to other therapies.

Ulcerative Colitis

MILD TO MODERATE DISEASE

- The first line of drug therapy for the patient with mild to moderate colitis is oral **sulfasalazine** or an oral **mesalamine** derivative, or topical mesalamine or steroids for distal disease (**Fig. 26–1**). When given orally, usually 4 g/day, up to 8 g/day of sulfasalazine is required to attain control of active inflammation. **Sulfasalazine** therapy should be instituted at 500 mg/day and increased every few days up to 4 g/day or the maximum tolerated.
- Oral **mesalamine** derivatives (such as those listed in **Table 26–5**) are reasonable alternatives to sulfasalazine for treatment of UC, but they are not more effective than sulfasalazine.

MODERATE TO SEVERE DISEASE

- Steroids have a place in the treatment of moderate to severe UC that is unresponsive to maximal doses of oral and topical mesalamine. **Prednisone** up to 1 mg/kg/day or 40 to 60 mg daily may be used for patients who do not have an adequate response to sulfasalazine or mesalamine.
- Steroids and sulfasalazine appear to be equally efficacious; however, the response to steroids may be evident sooner. Rectally administered steroids or mesalamine can be used as initial therapy for patients with ulcerative proctitis or distal colitis.
- **Infliximab** is another viable option for patients with moderate to severe active UC who are unresponsive to steroids or other immunosuppressive agents.
- Transdermal **nicotine** improved symptoms of patients with mild to moderate active UC in daily doses of 15 to 25 mg.

SEVERE OR INTRACTABLE DISEASE

- Patients with uncontrolled severe colitis or incapacitating symptoms require hospitalization for effective management. Most medication is given by the parenteral route.

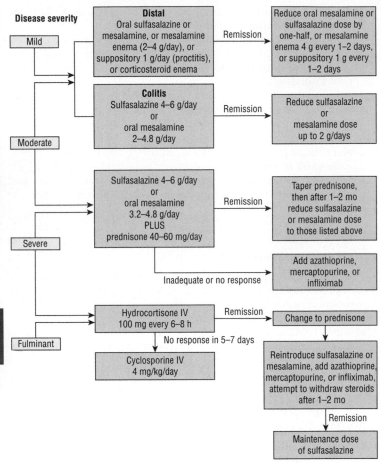

FIGURE 26–1. Treatment approaches for ulcerative colitis.

- With severe colitis, there is a much greater reliance on parenteral steroids and surgical procedures. Sulfasalazine or mesalamine derivatives have not been proven beneficial for the treatment of severe colitis.
- Steroids have been valuable in the treatment of severe disease because the use of these agents may allow some patients to avoid colectomy. A trial of steroids is warranted in most patients before proceeding to colectomy, unless the condition is grave or rapidly deteriorating.
- Continuous IV infusion of **cyclosporine** (4 mg/kg/day) is recommended for patients with acute severe UC refractory to steroids.

MAINTENANCE OF REMISSION

- Once remission from active disease has been achieved, the goal of therapy is to maintain the remission.

Disease severity

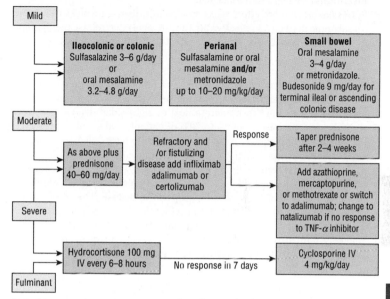

FIGURE 26–2. Treatment approaches for Crohn's disease.

- The major agents used for maintenance of remission are **sulfasalazine** (2 g/day) and the **mesalamine** derivatives, although mesalamine is not as effective as sulfasalazine.
- Steroids do not have a role in the maintenance of remission with UC because they are ineffective. Steroids should be gradually withdrawn after remission is induced (over 3–4 wk). If they are continued, the patient will be exposed to steroid side effects without likelihood of benefits.
- **Azathioprine** is effective in preventing the relapse of UC for periods exceeding 4 years. However, 3 to 6 months may be required for beneficial effect. For steroid-dependent patients who initially respond to infliximab, continued administration of 5 mg/kg every 8 weeks as maintenance therapy is an alternative.

Crohn's Disease

(Fig. 26–2)

ACTIVE CROHN'S DISEASE

- The goal of treatment for active Crohn's disease is to achieve remission; however, in many patients, the reduction of symptoms so that the patient may carry out normal activities or the reduction of the steroid dose required for control is a significant accomplishment.
- In the majority of patients, active Crohn's disease is treated **with sulfasalazine, mesalamine** derivatives, or **steroids,** although

azathioprine, mercaptopurine, methotrexate, biologic agents, and **metronidazole** are frequently used.

- **Sulfasalazine** is more effective when Crohn's disease involves the colon. Mesalamine derivatives (e.g., **Pentasa** and **Asacol**) that release mesalamine in the small bowel may be more effective than sulfasalazine for ileal involvement.

- **Steroids** are frequently used for the treatment of active Crohn's disease, particularly with moderate to severe presentations, or in those patients unresponsive to aminosalicylates. Budesonide is a viable first-line option for patients with mild to moderate ileal or right-sided disease. Systemic steroids induce remission in up to 70% of patients and should be reserved for patients with moderate to severe disease who have failed aminosalicylates or budesonide.

- **Metronidazole** (given orally up to 20 mg/kg/day) may be useful in some patients with Crohn's disease, particularly in patients with colonic or ileocolonic involvement or those with perineal disease. The combination of metronidazole with ciprofloxacin is efficacious in some patients.

- The immunosuppressive agents **azathioprine** and **mercaptopurine** are generally limited to use in patients not achieving adequate response to standard medical therapy or to reduce steroid doses when toxic doses are required. The usual dose of azathioprine is 2 to 3 mg/kg/day and 1 to 1.5 mg/kg/day for mercaptopurine. Up to 3 to 4 months may be required to observe a response. Starting doses are typically 50 mg/day and increased at 2-week intervals while monitoring complete blood count with differential.

- Patients deficient in thiopurine S-methyltransferase (TPMT) are at greater risk of bone marrow suppression from azathioprine and mercaptopurine. Determination of TPMT or TPMT genotype is recommended to guide dosage.

- **Cyclosporine** is not recommended for Crohn's disease except for patients with symptomatic and severe perianal or cutaneous fistulas. The dose of cyclosporine is important in determining efficacy. An oral dose of 5 mg/kg/day was not effective, whereas 7.9 mg/kg/day was effective. However, toxic effects limit application of the higher dosage. Dosage should be guided by cyclosporine whole-blood concentrations.

- **Methotrexate**, given as a weekly injection of 25 mg, has demonstrated efficacy for induction of remission in Crohn's disease, as well as for maintenance therapy. The risks are bone marrow suppression, hepatotoxicity, and pulmonary toxicity.

- **Infliximab** is used for moderate to severe active Crohn's disease in patients failing immunosuppressive therapy, in those who are corticosteroid dependent, and for treatment of fistulizing disease. A single, 5 mg/kg infusion is effective when given every day for 8 weeks. Additional doses at 2 and 6 weeks following the initial dose results in higher response rates. Patients may develop antibodies to infliximab, which can result in serious infusion reactions and loss of drug response.

- **Adalimumab** is effective in 54% of patients with moderate to severe Crohn's disease who have lost response to infliximab. **Natalizumab** is reserved for patients who do not respond to steroids or the TNF inhibitors.

MAINTENANCE OF REMISSION

- Prevention of recurrence of disease is clearly more difficult with Crohn's disease than with ulcerative colitis. **Sulfasalazine** and oral **mesalamine** derivatives are effective in preventing acute recurrences in quiescent Crohn's disease.
- **Systemic steroids** also have no place in the prevention of recurrence of Crohn's disease; these agents do not appear to alter the long-term course of the disease. Budesonide in doses of 6 mg daily is effective in maintaining remission for 3 months but loses efficacy after that time.
- Although the published data are not consistent, there is evidence to suggest that **azathioprine, mercaptopurine, methotrexate, infliximab,** and **adalimumab** are effective in maintaining remission in Crohn's disease.

SELECTED COMPLICATIONS

Toxic Megacolon

- The treatment required for toxic megacolon includes general supportive measures to maintain vital functions, consideration for early surgical intervention, and antimicrobials.
- Aggressive fluid and electrolyte management are required for dehydration.
- When the patient has lost significant amounts of blood (through the rectum), blood replacement is also necessary.
- Steroids in high dosages (hydrocortisone 100 mg every 8 hours) should be administered IV to reduce acute inflammation.
- Antimicrobial regimens that are effective against enteric aerobes and anaerobes should be administered as preemptive therapy in the event that perforation occurs.

Systemic Manifestations

- The common systemic manifestations of IBD include arthritis, anemia, skin manifestations such as erythema nodosum and pyoderma gangrenosum, uveitis, and liver disease.
- Anemia may be a common problem where there is significant blood loss from the GI tract. When the patient can consume oral medication, **ferrous sulfate** should be administered. Vitamin B_{12} or folic acid may also be required.

SPECIAL CONSIDERATIONS

PREGNANCY

- Drug therapy for IBD is not a contraindication for pregnancy, and most pregnancies are well managed in patients with these diseases. The indications for medical and surgical treatment are similar to those in the nonpregnant patient. If a patient has an initial bout of IBD during pregnancy, a standard approach to treatment with sulfasalazine or steroids should be initiated.

- Folic acid supplementation, 1 mg twice daily, should be given.
- **Metronidazole** may be used for short courses to treat trichomoniasis, but **methotrexate** should not be used during pregnancy. **Azathioprine** and **mercaptopurine** may be associated with fetal deformities. **Infliximab, adalimumab,** and **certolizumab** are classified as pregnancy category B and appear to be relatively safe for pregnant patients.

ADVERSE DRUG REACTIONS TO AGENTS USED FOR TREATMENT OF INFLAMMATORY BOWEL DISEASE

- Sulfasalazine is often associated with either dose-related or idiosyncratic adverse drug effects. Dose-related side effects usually include GI disturbances such as nausea, vomiting, diarrhea, or anorexia, but they may also include headache and arthralgia.
- Patients receiving sulfasalazine should receive oral **folic acid** supplementation, as sulfasalazine inhibits folic acid absorption.
- Non-dose-related adverse effects of sulfasalazine include rash, fever, or hepatotoxicity most commonly, as well as relatively uncommon but serious reactions such as bone marrow suppression, thrombocytopenia, pancreatitis, pneumonitis, interstitial nephritis, and hepatitis.
- Oral mesalamine derivatives may impose a lower frequency of adverse effects compared with sulfasalazine. Up to 90% of patients who are intolerant to sulfasalazine will tolerate oral mesalamine derivatives. Olsalazine may cause watery diarrhea in up to 25% of patients.
- The well-appreciated adverse effects of glucocorticoids include hyperglycemia, hypertension, osteoporosis, fluid retention and electrolyte disturbances, myopathies, psychosis, and reduced resistance to infection. In addition, glucocorticoid use may cause adrenocortical suppression. Specific regimens for withdrawal of glucocorticoid therapy have been suggested.
- Immunosuppressants such as azathioprine and mercaptopurine have a significant potential for adverse reactions, including bone marrow suppression, and have been associated with lymphomas (in renal transplant patients) and pancreatitis. Myelosuppression resulting in leukopenia is related to a deficiency in TPMT in some patients.
- Infliximab has been associated with infusion reactions, serum sickness, sepsis, and reactivation of latent tuberculosis. Adalimumab carries risks similar to infliximab. Full prescribing information should be consulted on these products.

EVALUATION OF THERAPEUTIC OUTCOMES

- The success of therapeutic regimens to treat IBDs can be measured by patient-reported complaints, signs and symptoms, direct physician examination (including endoscopy), history and physical examination, selected laboratory tests, and quality of life measures.
- To create more objective measures, disease-rating scales or indices have been created. The Crohn's Disease Activity Index is a commonly used scale, particularly for evaluation of patients during clinical trials. The

scale incorporates eight elements: (1) number of stools in the past 7 days, (2) sum of abdominal pain ratings from the past 7 days, (3) rating of general well-being in the past 7 days, (4) use of antidiarrheals, (5) body weight, (6) hematocrit, (7) finding of abdominal mass, and (8) a sum of symptoms present in the past week. Elements of this index provide a guide for those measures that may be useful in assessing the effectiveness of treatment regimens. The Perianal CD Activity Index is used for perianal Crohn's disease.

- Standardized assessment tools have also been constructed for UC. Elements in these scales include (1) stool frequency; (2) presence of blood in the stool; (3) mucosal appearance (from endoscopy); and (4) physician's global assessment based on physical examination, endoscopy, and laboratory data.

See Chapter 41, Inflammatory Bowel Disease, authored by Brian A. Hemstreet, for a more detailed discussion of this topic.

Nausea and Vomiting

DEFINITION

- Nausea is usually defined as the inclination to vomit or as a feeling in the throat or epigastric region alerting an individual that vomiting is imminent. Vomiting is defined as the ejection or expulsion of gastric contents through the mouth, often requiring a forceful event.

ETIOLOGY AND PATHOPHYSIOLOGY

- Specific etiologies associated with nausea and vomiting are presented in **Table 27–1**.
- **Table 27–2** presents specific cytotoxic agents categorized by their emetogenic potential. Although some agents may have greater emetogenic potential than others, combinations of agents, high doses, clinical settings, psychological conditions, prior treatment experiences, and unusual stimuli to sight, smell, or taste may alter a patient's response to a drug treatment.
- A variety of other common etiologies have been proposed for the development of nausea and vomiting in cancer patients. These are presented in **Table 27–3**.
- The three consecutive phases of emesis are nausea, retching, and vomiting. Nausea, the imminent need to vomit, is associated with gastric stasis. Retching is the labored movement of abdominal and thoracic muscles before vomiting. The final phase of emesis is vomiting, the forceful expulsion of gastric contents due to GI retroperistalsis.
- Vomiting is triggered by afferent impulses to the vomiting center, a nucleus of cells in the medulla. Impulses are received from sensory centers, such as the chemoreceptor trigger zone (CTZ), cerebral cortex, and visceral afferents from the pharynx and GI tract. When excited, afferent impulses are integrated by the vomiting center, resulting in efferent impulses to the salivation center, respiratory center, and the pharyngeal, GI, and abdominal muscles, leading to vomiting.
- Numerous neurotransmitter receptors are located in the vomiting center, CTZ, and GI tract, including cholinergic and histaminic, dopaminergic, opiate, serotonin, neurokinin, and benzodiazepine receptors.

CLINICAL PRESENTATION

- The clinical presentation of nausea and vomiting is given in **Table 27-4**. Nausea and vomiting may be classified as either simple or complex.

DESIRED OUTCOME

- The overall goal of antiemetic therapy is to prevent or eliminate nausea and vomiting; this should be accomplished without adverse effects or with clinically acceptable adverse effects.

TABLE 27–1	Specific Etiologies of Nausea and Vomiting

GI mechanisms	**Metabolic disorders**
Mechanical obstruction	Diabetes mellitus (diabetic ketoacidosis)
Gastric outlet obstruction	Addison's disease
Small bowel obstruction	Renal disease (uremia)
Functional GI disorders	**Psychiatric causes**
Gastroparesis	Psychogenic vomiting
Nonulcer dyspepsia	Anxiety disorders
Chronic intestinal pseudo-obstruction	Anorexia nervosa
Irritable bowel syndrome	**Therapy-induced causes**
Organic GI disorders	Cytotoxic chemotherapy
Peptic ulcer disease	Radiation therapy
Pancreatitis	Theophylline preparations
Pyelonephritis	Anticonvulsant preparations
Cholecystitis	Digitalis preparations
Cholangitis	Opiates
Hepatitis	Antibiotics
Acute gastroenteritis	Volatile general anesthetics
Viral	**Drug withdrawal**
Bacterial	Opiates
Cardiovascular diseases	Benzodiazepines
Acute myocardial infarction	**Miscellaneous causes**
Congestive heart failure	Pregnancy
Radiofrequency ablation	Noxious odors
Neurologic processes	Operative procedures
Increased intracranial pressure	
Migraine headache	
Vestibular disorders	

Source: Adapted from Hasler WL, Chey WD. Gastroenterol 2003;25:1860–1867.

TREATMENT

GENERAL APPROACH TO TREATMENT

- Treatment options for nausea and vomiting include drug and nondrug modalities and depend on associated medical conditions. For patients with simple complaints, perhaps related to food or beverage consumption, avoidance or moderation of dietary intake may be preferable. Patients with symptoms of systemic illness may improve dramatically as their underlying condition improves. Patients in whom these symptoms result from labyrinth changes produced by motion may benefit quickly by assuming a stable physical position.

TABLE 27–2	Emetogenicity of Chemotherapeutic Agents
Emetic Risk (if no Prophylactic Medication is Administered)	**Cytotoxic Agent (in Alphabetical Order)**
High (>90%)	Carmustine
	Cisplatin
	Cyclophosphamide ≥1,500 mg/m^2
	Dacarbazine
	Dactinomycin
	Mechlorethamine
	Streptozotocin
Moderate (30–90%)	Carboplatin
	Cytarabine >1 g/m^2
	Cyclophosphamide <1,500 mg/m^2
	Daunorubicin
	Doxorubicin
	Epirubicin
	Idarubicin
	Ifosfamide
	Irinotecan
	Oxaliplatin
	Procarbazine
Low (10–30%)	Bortezomib
	Cetuximab
	Cytarabine ≤1 g/m^2
	Docetaxel
	Erlotinib
	Etoposide
	Fluorouracil
	Gemcitabine
	Lapatinib
	Methotrexate
	Mitomycin
	Mitoxantrone
	Paclitaxel
	Pemetrexed
	Sorafenib
	Sunitinib
	Temozolamide
	Topotecan
	Trastuzumab
Minimal (<10%)	Bevacizumab
	Bleomycin
	Busulfan
	2-Chlorodeoxyadenosine
	Fludarabine

(continued)

TABLE 27–2	Emetogenicity of Chemotherapeutic Agents *(Continued)*
Emetic Risk (if no Prophylactic Medication is Administered)	**Cytotoxic Agent (in Alphabetical Order)**
	Rituximab
	Vinblastine
	Vincristine
	Vinorelbine

Source: Adapted from Results of the 2004 Perugia International Antiemetic Consensus Conference. Ann Oncol 2006;17:20–28 by permission of Oxford University.

- Nonpharmacologic interventions include behavioral interventions such as relaxation, biofeedback, self-hypnosis, cognitive distraction, guided imagery, and systematic desensitization.
- Psychogenic vomiting may benefit from psychological interventions.

PHARMACOLOGIC MANAGEMENT

- Information concerning commonly available antiemetic preparations is compiled in Table 27–5. Treatment of simple nausea or vomiting usually requires minimal therapy.
- For most conditions, a single-agent antiemetic is preferred; however, for those patients not responding to such therapy and those receiving highly emetogenic chemotherapy, multiple-agent regimens are usually required.

TABLE 27–3	Nonchemotherapy Etiologies of Nausea and Vomiting in Cancer Patients

Fluid and electrolyte abnormalities
  Hypercalcemia
  Volume depletion
  Water intoxication
  Adrenocortical insufficiency
Drug-induced
  Opiates
  Antibiotics
  Antifungals
GI obstruction
Increased intracranial pressure
Peritonitis
Metastases
  Brain
  Meninges
  Hepatic
Uremia
Infections (septicemia, local)
Radiation therapy

TABLE 27–4	Presentation of Nausea and Vomiting

General
    Depending on severity of symptoms, patients may present in mild to severe distress.

Symptoms
    Simple: Self-limiting, resolves spontaneously and requires only symptomatic therapy
    Complex: Not relieved after administration of antiemetics; progressive deterioration of patient secondary to fluid–electrolyte imbalances; usually associated with noxious agents or psychogenic events

Signs
    Simple: Patient complaint of queasiness or discomfort
    Complex: Weight loss, fever, and abdominal pain

Laboratory tests
    Simple: None
    Complex: Serum electrolyte concentrations; upper/lower GI evaluation

Other information
    Fluid input and output
    Medication history
    Recent history of behavioral or visual changes, headache, pain, or stress
    Family history positive for psychogenic vomiting

- The treatment of simple nausea and vomiting usually requires minimal therapy. Both nonprescription and prescription drugs useful in the treatment of simple nausea and vomiting are usually effective in small, infrequently administered doses.
- The management of complex nausea and vomiting, for example, in patients who are receiving cytotoxic chemotherapy, may require combination therapy.

Drug Class Information

ANTACIDS

- Single or combination nonprescription antacid products, especially those containing magnesium hydroxide, aluminum hydroxide, and/or calcium carbonate, may provide sufficient relief from simple nausea or vomiting, primarily through gastric acid neutralization. Common antacid dosage regimens for the relief of nausea and vomiting include one or more 15 to 30 mL doses of single- or multiple-agent products.

HISTAMINE$_2$-RECEPTOR ANTAGONISTS

- Histamine$_2$-receptor antagonists (cimetidine, famotidine, nizatidine, and ranitidine) may be used in low doses to manage simple nausea and vomiting associated with heartburn or gastroesophageal reflux.

ANTIHISTAMINE-ANTICHOLINERGIC DRUGS

- Antiemetic drugs from the antihistaminic-anticholinergic category may be appropriate in the treatment of simple symptomatology.

TABLE 27–5 Common Antiemetic Preparations and Adult Dosage Regimens

Drug	Adult Dosage Regimen	Dosage Form/Route	Availability
Antacids			
Antacids (various)	15–30 mL every 2–4 hours prn	Liquid/oral	OTC
Antihistaminic–anticholinergic agents			
Cyclizine (Marezine)	50 mg before departure; may repeat in 4–6 hours prn	Tab	OTC
Dimenhydrinate (Dramamine)	50–100 mg every 4–6 hours prn	Tab, chew tab, cap	OTC
Diphenhydramine (Benadryl)	25–50 mg every 4–6 hours prn	Tab, cap, liquid	Rx/OTC
	10–50 mg every 2–4 hours prn	IM, IV	
Hydroxyzine (Vistaril, Atarax)	25–100 mg every 4–6 hours prn	IM (unlabeled use)	Rx
Meclizine (Bonine, Antivert)	12.5–25 mg 1 hours before travel; repeat every 12–24 hours prn	Tab, chew tab	Rx/OTC
Scopolamine (Transderm Scop)	1.5 mg every 72 hours	Transdermal patch	Rx
Trimethobenzamide (Tigan)	300 mg 3–4 times daily	Cap	Rx
	200 mg 3–4 times daily	IM	Rx
Benzodiazepines			
Alprazolam (Xanax)	0.5–2 mg three times daily prior to chemotherapy	Tab	Rx (C-IV)
Lorazepam (Ativan)	0.5–2 mg on night before and morning of chemotherapy	Tab	Rx (C-IV)
Butyrophenones			
Haloperidol (Haldol)	1–5 mg every 12 hours prn	Tab, liquid, IM, IV	Rx
Droperidol (Inapsine)[a]	2.5 mg; additional 1.25 mg may be given	IM, IV	Rx

(continued)

TABLE 27–5 Common Antiemetic Preparations and Adult Dosage Regimens *(Continued)*

Drug	Adult Dosage Regimen	Dosage Form/Route	Availability
Cannabinoids			
Dronabinol (Marinol)	5–15 mg/m^2 every 2–4 hours prn	Cap	Rx (C-III)
Nabilone (Cesamet)	1–2 mg twice daily	Cap	Rx (C-II)
Histamine (H$_2$) antagonists			
Cimetidine (Tagamet HB)	200 mg twice daily prn	Tab	OTC
Famotidine (Pepcid AC)	10 mg twice daily prn	Tab	OTC
Nizatidine (Axid AR)	75 mg twice daily prn	Tab	OTC
Ranitidine (Zantac 75)	75 mg twice daily prn	Tab	OTC
5-hydroxytryptamine-3 receptor antagonists (see Tables 27–6 for CINV dosing and 27–7 for PONV dosing)			
Miscellaneous agents			
Metoclopramide (Reglan), for delayed CINV	20–40 mg 3–4 daily	Tab	Rx
Olanzapine (Zyprexa)	2.5–5 mg twice daily	Tab	Rx
Phenothiazines			
Chlorpromazine (Thorazine)	10–25 mg every 4–6 hours prn	Tab, liquid	Rx
	25–50 mg every 4–6 hours prn	IM, IV	
Prochlorperazine (Compazine)	5–10 mg 3–4 daily prn	Tab, liquid	Rx
	5–10 mg every 3–4 hours prn	IM	
	2.5–10 mg every 3–4 hours prn	IV	Rx
	25 mg twice daily prn	Supp	Rx
Promethazine (Phenergan)	12.5–25 mg every 4–6 hours prn	Tab, liquid, IM, IV, supp	Rx

C-II, C-III, C-IV, controlled substance schedule 2, 3, and 4, respectively; cap, capsule; chew tab, chewable tablet; CINV, chemotherapy-induced nausea and vomiting; liquid, oral syrup, concentrate, or suspension; OTC, nonprescription; PONV, postoperative nausea and vomiting; Rx, prescription; supp, rectal suppository; tab, tablet.
*See text for current warnings.

- Adverse reactions that may be apparent with the use of the antihistaminic-anticholinergic agents primarily include drowsiness or confusion, blurred vision, dry mouth, urinary retention, and possibly tachycardia, particularly in elderly patients.

PHENOTHIAZINES

- **Phenothiazines** are most useful in patients with simple nausea and vomiting. Rectal administration is a reasonable alternative in patients in whom oral or parenteral administration is not feasible.
- Problems associated with these drugs are troublesome and potentially dangerous side effects, including extrapyramidal reactions, hypersensitivity reactions with possible liver dysfunction, marrow aplasia, and excessive sedation.

CORTICOSTEROIDS

- **Dexamethasone** has been used successfully in the management of chemotherapy-induced nausea and vomiting (CINV) and postoperative nausea and vomiting (PONV), either as a single agent or in combination with 5-hydroxytriptamine-3 receptor antagonists (5-HT3-RAs). For CINV, dexamethasone is effective in the prevention of both cisplatin-induced acute emesis and when used alone or in combination for the prevention of delayed nausea and vomiting associated with CINV.

METOCLOPRAMIDE

- **Metoclopramide** increases lower esophageal sphincter tone, aids gastric emptying, and accelerates transit through the small bowel, possibly through the release of acetylcholine.
- Metoclopramide is used for its antiemetic properties in patients with diabetic gastroparesis and with dexamethasone for prophylaxis of delayed nausea and vomiting associated with chemotherapy administration.

CANNABINOIDS

- When compared with conventional antiemetics, oral **nabilone** and oral **dronabinol** were slightly more effective than active comparators in patients receiving moderately emetogenic chemotherapy regimens. The efficacy of cannabinoids as compared with 5-HT3-RAs for CINV has not been studied. They should be considered for the treatment of refractory nausea and vomiting in patients receiving chemotherapy.

SUBSTANCE P/NEUROKININ 1 RECEPTOR ANTAGONISTS

- Substance P is a peptide neurotransmitter in the neurokinin family whose preferred receptor is the neurokinin 1 (NK_1) receptor. Substance P is believed to be the primary mediator of the delayed phase of CINV and one of two mediators of the acute phase of CINV.
- **Aprepitant** is the first approved member of this class of drugs and is indicated as part of a multiple drug regimen for prophylaxis of nausea and vomiting associated with high-dose cisplatin-based chemotherapy.

- Numerous potential drug interactions are possible; clinically significant drug interactions with oral contraceptives, warfarin, and oral dexamethasone have been described.

5-HYDROXYTRIPTAMINE-3 RECEPTOR ANTAGONISTS

- 5-HT3-RAs (**dolasetron, granisetron, ondansetron,** and **palonosetron**) act by blocking presynaptic serotonin receptors on sensory vagal fibers in the gut wall. The most common side effects associated with these agents are constipation, headache, and asthenia.

CHEMOTHERAPY-INDUCED NAUSEA AND VOMITING

- Nausea and vomiting that occur within 24 hours of chemotherapy administration are defined as acute; nausea and vomiting that starts more than 24 hours after chemotherapy administration are defined as delayed. The emetogenic potential of the chemotherapeutic agent or regimen (see **Table 27–2**) is the primary factor to consider when selecting an antiemetic for **prophylaxis** of CINV.
- Recommendations for antiemetics in patients receiving chemotherapy are presented in **Table 27–6**.

Prophylaxis of Chemotherapy-Induced Nausea and Vomiting

- Patients receiving chemotherapy that is classified as being of high emetic risk should receive a combination antiemetic regimen containing three drugs on the day of chemotherapy administration (day 1)—a 5-HT3-RA plus dexamethasone plus aprepitant.
- Patients receiving regimens that are classified as being of moderate emetic risk should receive a combination antiemetic regimen containing a 5-HT3-RA plus dexamethasone on day 1.
- Dexamethasone alone is recommended for prophylaxis prior to regimens of low emetic risk; also recommended are any of the following: prochlorperazine, metoclopramide, and/or diphenhydramine, and/or lorazepam alone.
- For prophylaxis of delayed CINV, administration of aprepitant and dexamethasone on days 2 and 3 and dexamethasone with or without lorazepam on day 4 is recommended for high emetic risk. For moderate emetic risk, one recommendation is to give aprepitant or any of the following: dexamethasone, a 5-HT3-RA, and/or lorazepam on days 2 and 3.

POSTOPERATIVE NAUSEA AND VOMITING

- A variety of pharmacologic approaches are available and may be prescribed as single or combination therapy for prophylaxis of PONV. See **Table 27–7** for doses of specific agents. Most patients undergoing an operative procedure do not require preoperative prophylactic antiemetic therapy, and universal PONV prophylaxis is not cost effective. Patients at high risk of PONV should receive prophylactic antiemetics.
- Patients at moderate risk of PONV should receive one or two prophylactic antiemetics, and those at high risk should receive two prophylactic antiemetics from different classes.

TABLE 27–6	Dosage Recommendations for CINV for Adult Patients	
Emetic Risk	Prophylaxis of Acute Phase of CINV (One Dose Administered Prior to Chemotherapy)	Prophylaxis of Delayed Phase of CINV
High (including the AC regimen[a])	5-HT$_3$ receptor antagonists (5-HT$_3$-RA): Dolasetron 100 mg orally or 100 mg IV or 1.8 mg/kg IV Granisetron 2 mg orally or 1 mg IV or 0.01 mg/kg IV or 34.3 mg transdermal patch Ondansetron 16–24 mg orally or 8–12 mg IV (maximum 32 mg) Palonosetron 0.25 mg IV and Dexamethasone 12 mg orally or IV and Aprepitant 125 mg orally or Fosaprepitant 115 mg IV	 Dexamethasone 8–12 mg orally days 2–4 Aprepitant 80 mg orally days 2 and 3 after chemotherapy
Moderate	5-HT$_3$-RA: Dolasetron 100 mg orally or 100 mg IV or 1.8 mg/kg IV Granisetron 2 mg orally or 1 mg IV or 0.01 mg/kg IV or 34.3 mg transdermal patch Ondansetron 16–24 mg orally or 8–12 mg IV (max. 32 mg) Palonosetron 0.25 mg IV Palonosetron 0.5 mg orally and Dexamethasone 8–12 mg orally or IV and in select patients[c] Aprepitant 125 mg orally or Fosaprepitant 115 mg IV	 5-HT$_3$ RA : Dolasetron 100 mg orally daily[b] Granisetron 1–2 mg orally daily[b] Ondansetron 8 mg orally daily or twice daily[b] Dexamethasone 8–12 mg orally daily[b] Aprepitant 80 mg orally days 2 and 3 if used on day 1
Low	Dexamethasone 8–12 mg orally or IV	None
Minimal	None	None

[a]Kris MG, Hesketh PJ, Somerfield MR, et al. American Society of Clinical Oncology guideline for antiemetics in oncology: Update 2006. J Clin Oncol 2006;24:2932–2947.

[b]For 2–3 days following chemotherapy.

[c]Patients receiving other chemotherapies of moderate emetic risk, for example, carboplatin, cisplatin, doxorubicin, epirubicin, ifosfamide, irinotecan, or methotrexate. Doses included in the above table reflect the recommendations from published guidelines (Prevention of chemotherapy and radiotherapy-induced emesis. Results of the 2004 Perugia International Antiemetic Consensus Conference. Ann Oncol 2006;17:20–28; National Comprehensive Cancer Network. Clinical Practice Guidelines in Oncology. Antiemesis. Version 2; 2010. http://www.nccn.org/professionals/physician_gls/PDF/antiemesis.pdf; and Kris MG, Hesketh PJ, Somerfield MR, et al. American Society of Clinical Oncology guideline for antiemetics in oncology: Update 2006. J Clin Oncol 2006;24:2932–2947). These doses may differ from manufacturer labeling; they reflect the consensus of the guideline participants.

CINV, chemotherapy-induced nausea and vomiting.

TABLE 27—7	Recommended Prophylactic Doses of Selected Antiemetics for Postoperative Nausea and Vomiting in Adults and Postoperative Vomiting in Children		
Drug	**Adult Dose**	**Pediatric Dose (IV)**	**Timing of Dose**[a]
Aprepitant[b]	40 mg orally	Not labeled for use in pediatrics	Within 3 hours prior to induction
Dexamethasone	4–5 mg IV	150 mcg/kg up to 5 mg	At induction
Dimenhydrinate	1 mg/kg IV	0.5 mg/kg up to 25 mg	Not specified
Dolasetron	12.5 mg IV	350 mcg/kg up to 12.5 mg	At end of surgery
Droperidol[d]	0.625–1.25 mg IV	10–15 mcg/kg up to 1.25 mg	At end of surgery
Granisetron	0.35–1.5 mg IV	40 mcg/kg up to 0.6 mg	At end of surgery
Haloperidol	0.5–2 mg (IM or IV)	[c]	Not specified
Ondansetron	4 mg IV	50–100 mcg/kg up to 4 mg	At end of surgery
Palonosetron[b]	0.075 mg IV	Not labeled for patients < 18 y	At induction
Prochlorperazine	5–10 mg IM or IV	[c]	At end of surgery
Promethazine[b]	6.25–25 mg IV	[c]	At induction
Scopolamine	Transdermal patch	[c]	Prior evening or 4 hours before surgery
Tropisetron	2 mg IV	0.1 mg/kg up to 2 mg	At end of surgery

[a]Based on recommendations from consensus guidelines; may differ from manufacturer's recommendations.
[b]Labeled for use in PONV but not included in consensus guidelines.
[c]Pediatric dosing not included in consensus guidelines.
[d]See Food and Drug Administration (FDA) "black box" warning.
Gan TJ, Meyer TA, Apfel CC, et al. Society for ambulatory anesthesia guidelines for the management of postoperative nausea and vomiting. Anesth Analg 2007;105:1615–1628.

RADIATION-INDUCED NAUSEA AND VOMITING

• Patients receiving single-exposure, high-dose radiation therapy to the upper abdomen or total- or hemibody irradiation should receive prophylactic antiemetics. Preventive therapy with a 5-HT3-RA and dexamethasone is recommended in patients receiving total-body irradiation.

DISORDERS OF BALANCE

• Beneficial therapy for patients with nausea and vomiting associated with disorders of balance can reliably be found among the antihistaminic-anticholinergic agents. Neither the antihistaminic nor the anticholinergic potency appears to correlate well with the ability of these agents to prevent or treat the nausea and vomiting associated with motion sickness.
• Scopolamine is commonly used to prevent nausea or vomiting caused by motion.

ANTIEMETIC USE DURING PREGNANCY

• Initial management of nausea and vomiting of pregnancy often involves dietary changes and/or lifestyle modifications.

- Pyridoxine (10–25 mg one to four times daily) is recommended as first-line therapy with or without doxylamine (12.5–20 mg one to four times daily). If symptoms persist, addition of a histamine-1 receptor antagonist, such as dimenhydrinate, diphenhydramine, or meclizine, is recommended.

ANTIEMETIC USE IN CHILDREN

- For children receiving chemotherapy of high or moderate risk, a corticosteroid plus 5-HT3-RAs should be administered. The best doses or dosing strategy has not been determined.
- For nausea and vomiting associated with pediatric gastroenteritis, there is greater emphasis on rehydration measures than on pharmacologic intervention.

See Chapter 42, Nausea and Vomiting, authored by Cecily V. DiPiro and Robert J. Ignoffo, for a more detailed discussion of this topic.

Pancreatitis

DEFINITION

- Acute pancreatitis (AP) is an inflammatory disorder of the pancreas characterized by severe pain in the upper abdomen and elevations of pancreatic enzymes in the blood. In most patients, it is a mild, self-limiting disease that resolves spontaneously without complications.
- Chronic pancreatitis (CP) is a progressive disease characterized by long-standing pancreatic inflammation that eventually leads to loss of pancreatic exocrine and endocrine function.

ACUTE PANCREATITIS

PATHOPHYSIOLOGY

- Gallstones and alcohol abuse account for most cases in the United States. A cause cannot be identified in some patients (idiopathic pancreatitis).
- Many medications have been implicated (Table 28–1), but a causal association is difficult to confirm because ethical and practical considerations prevent rechallenge.
- AP is initiated by premature activation of trypsinogen to trypsin within the pancreas, leading to activation of other digestive enzymes and autodigestion of the gland.
- Activated pancreatic enzymes released into the pancreas and surrounding tissues produce damage and necrosis to the pancreatic tissue, the surrounding fat, the vascular endothelium, and adjacent structures. Lipase damages fat cells, producing noxious substances that cause further pancreatic and peripancreatic injury.
- Release of cytokines by acinar cells injures those cells and enhances the inflammatory response. Injured acinar cells liberate chemoattractants that attract neutrophils, macrophages, and other cells to the area of inflammation, causing systemic inflammatory response syndrome (SIRS). Vascular damage and ischemia cause release of kinins, which make capillary walls permeable and promote tissue edema.
- Pancreatic infection may result from increased intestinal permeability and translocation of colonic bacteria.
- Local complications in severe AP may include acute fluid collection, pancreatic necrosis, infection, abscess, pseudocyst formation, and pancreatic ascites.
- Systemic complications may include cardiovascular, renal, pulmonary, metabolic, hemorrhagic, and CNS abnormalities.

CLINICAL PRESENTATION

- The clinical presentation depends on the severity of the inflammatory process and whether damage is confined to the pancreas or involves local and systemic complications.

TABLE 28–1	Medications Associated with Acute Pancreatitis	
Class I: Definite Association	**Class II: Probable Association**	**Class III: Possible Association**
5-Aminosalicylic acid	Acetaminophen	Aldesleukin	Indomethacin
Asparaginase	Carbamazepine	Amiodarone	Infliximab
Azathioprine	Cisplatin	Calcium	Ketoprofen
Corticosteroids	Erythromycin	Celecoxib	Ketorolac
Cytarabine	Hydrochlorothiazide	Clozapine	Lipid emulsion
Didanosine	Interferon α_{2b}	Cholestyramine	Lisinopril
Enalapril	Lamivudine	Cimetidine	Mefenamic acid
Estrogens	Octreotide	Ciprofloxacin	Metformin
Furosemide	Sitagliptin	Clarithromycin	Methyldopa
Mercaptopurine		Clonidine	Metolazone
Opiates		Cyclosporine	Metronidazole
Pentamidine		Danazol	Nitrofurantoin
Pentavalent antimonials		Diazoxide	Omeprazole
Sulfasalazine		Etanercept	Ondansetron
Sulfamethoxazole and trimethoprim		Ethacrynic acid	Oxyphenbutazone
Sulindac		Exenatide	Paclitaxel
Tetracycline		Famciclovir	Pravastatin
Valproic acid/salts		Glyburide	Propofol
		Gold therapy	Propoxyphene
		Granisetron	Rifampin
		Ibuprofen	Sertraline
		Indinavir	Zalcitabine

- The initial presentation ranges from moderate abdominal discomfort to excruciating pain, shock, and respiratory distress. Abdominal pain occurs in 95% of patients and is usually epigastric, often radiating to the upper quadrants or back. The onset is usually sudden, and the intensity is often described as "knife-like" or "boring." The pain usually reaches its maximum intensity within 30 minutes and may persist for hours or days. Nausea and vomiting occur in 85% of patients and usually follow the onset of pain.
- Clinical signs associated with widespread pancreatic inflammation and necrosis include marked epigastric tenderness, abdominal distention, hypotension, tachycardia, and low-grade fever. In severe disease, bowel sounds are diminished or absent. Dyspnea and tachypnea are signs of acute respiratory complications.

DIAGNOSIS

- The diagnosis should be made within 48 hours based on characteristics of abdominal pain and elevation of amylase, lipase, or both to at least three times the upper limit of normal.

- Contrast-enhanced computed tomography (CECT) of the abdomen may be used to confirm the diagnosis; ultrasonography may be an acceptable alternative to CECT.
- AP may be associated with leukocytosis, hyperglycemia, and hypoalbuminemia. Hepatic transaminases, alkaline phosphatase, and bilirubin are usually elevated in gallstone pancreatitis and in patients with intrinsic liver disease.
- The serum amylase concentration usually rises 4 to 8 hours after symptom onset, peaks at 24 hours, and returns to normal over the next 8 to 14 days. Serum amylase concentrations greater than three times the upper limit of normal are highly suggestive of AP.
- Serum lipase is specific to the pancreas, and concentrations are elevated and parallel the serum amylase elevations. The increases persist longer than serum amylase elevations and can be detected after the amylase has returned to normal.
- Marked hypocalcemia indicates severe necrosis and is a poor prognostic sign.
- The hematocrit may be normal, but hemoconcentration results from multiple factors (e.g., vomiting). A hematocrit level >47% predicts severe AP, and a hematocrit level <44% predicts mild disease.
- C-reactive protein levels >150 mg/dL at 48 to 72 hours predict severe AP.
- Thrombocytopenia and increased international normalized ratio (INR) occur in some patients with severe AP and associated liver disease.

DESIRED OUTCOME

- The goals of AP treatment are to relieve abdominal pain and nausea; replace fluids; correct electrolyte, glucose, and lipid abnormalities; minimize systemic complications; and prevent pancreatic necrosis and infection.

NONPHARMACOLOGIC TREATMENT

- **Nutritional support** is important because AP creates a catabolic state that promotes nutritional depletion. Patients with mild AP can begin oral feeding when bowel sounds have returned, and pain has resolved. Nutritional support should begin when it is anticipated that oral nutrition will be withheld for longer than 1 week. Enteral feeding in severe AP is as safe and effective as parenteral nutrition (PN), attenuates the acute inflammatory response, and improves disease severity. Thus, the enteral route is preferred over PN in severe AP, if it can be tolerated. The nasojejunal route may be preferred, but the nasogastric route also appears to be safe and effective.
- **Endoscopic retrograde cholangiopancreatography (ERCP)** is performed to remove any biliary tract stones.
- **Surgery** is indicated in patients with pancreatic pseudocyst or abscess or to drain the pancreatic bed if hemorrhagic or necrotic material is present.

PHARMACOLOGIC TREATMENT

(Fig. 28–1)

- Patients predicted to follow a severe course require treatment of cardiovascular, respiratory, renal, and metabolic complications. Aggressive

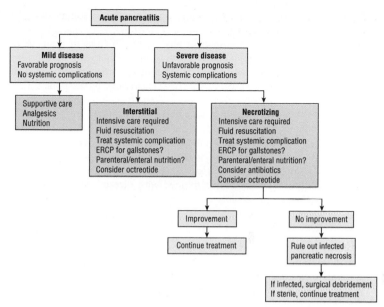

FIGURE 28-1. Algorithm of guidelines for evaluation and treatment of acute pancreatitis. (ERCP, endoscopic retrograde cholangiopancreatography.)

fluid resuscitation is essential to correct intravascular volume depletion. However, specific recommendations cannot be made from the current literature. **IV colloids** may be required to maintain intravascular volume and blood pressure because fluid losses are rich in protein. Patients with AP and SIRS should be treated according to SIRS guidelines. IV **potassium, calcium,** and **magnesium** are used to correct electrolyte deficiency states. **Insulin** is used to treat hyperglycemia. Patients with necrotizing pancreatitis may require antibiotics and surgical intervention. Medications listed in **Table 28-1** should be discontinued if possible.

- Parenteral opioid analgesics are used to control abdominal pain. In the past, parenteral **meperidine** (50–100 mg every 3–4 hours) was used because it did not significantly alter the function of the sphincter of Oddi. Meperidine is not recommended as a first-line agent today because of the risk of adverse effects (e.g., seizures) and dosing limitations. Parenteral **morphine** has a longer duration of action than meperidine and has less risk of seizures, but it is sometimes avoided in AP because it is thought to cause spasm of the sphincter of Oddi, increases in serum amylase, and, rarely, pancreatitis. **Hydromorphone** may also be used because it has a longer half-life than meperidine. Patient-controlled analgesia should be considered in patients who require frequent opioid dosing (e.g., every 2–3 hours).

- There is no evidence that antisecretory drugs such as histamine$_2$-receptor antagonists (H$_2$RAs) or proton pump inhibitors (PPIs) prevent exacerbations of abdominal pain.

- There are insufficient data to support routine use of somatostatin or octreotide for treatment of AP.
- Prophylactic antibiotics do not offer any benefit in cases of mild AP or when there is no necrosis. In patients with severe AP but without infection, use of antibiotics is not supported by randomized, controlled trials. This is true whether or not pancreatic necrosis is present. Because the source of bacterial contamination in AP is most likely the colon, broad-spectrum antibiotics that cover the range of enteric aerobic gram-negative bacilli and anaerobic organisms should be started within the first 48 hours and continued for 2 to 3 weeks when infection is present. **Imipenem–cilastatin** (500 mg IV every 8 hours) has been widely used but has been replaced on many formularies by newer carbapenems. A fluoroquinolone (e.g., **ciprofloxacin** or **levofloxacin**) combined with **metronidazole** should be considered for penicillin-allergic patients.

EVALUATION OF THERAPEUTIC OUTCOMES

- In patients with mild AP, pain control, fluid and electrolyte status, and nutrition should be assessed periodically depending on the degree of abdominal pain and fluid loss.
- Patients with severe AP should be transferred to an intensive care unit for close monitoring of vital signs, fluid and electrolyte status, white blood cell count, blood glucose, lactate dehydrogenase, aspartate aminotransferase, serum albumin, hematocrit, blood urea nitrogen, serum creatinine, and INR. Continuous hemodynamic and arterial blood gas monitoring is essential. Serum lipase, amylase, and bilirubin require less frequent monitoring. The patient should be monitored for signs of infection, relief of abdominal pain, and adequate nutritional status. Severity of disease and patient response should be assessed using an evidence-based method such as APACHE II.

CHRONIC PANCREATITIS

PATHOPHYSIOLOGY

- CP results from long-standing pancreatic inflammation and leads to irreversible destruction of pancreatic tissue with fibrin deposition and loss of exocrine and endocrine function.
- Chronic ethanol consumption accounts for 70% to 80% of all cases in Western society; 10% result from other causes, and 20% are idiopathic.
- The exact mechanism for the pathogenesis of CP is unknown. Regardless of the mechanism, activation of pancreatic stellate cells by toxins, oxidative stress, and/or inflammatory mediators appears to be the cause of fibrin deposition.
- Abdominal pain may be caused in part by increased pancreatic parenchymal pressure from obstruction, inflammation, and necrosis. Compression of pancreatic nerve fibers after a meal, along with continuous firing of peripheral and central neurons, may explain the burning and shooting pain of CP.
- Malabsorption of protein and fat occurs when the capacity for enzyme secretion is reduced by 90%. A minority of patients develop complications,

including pancreatic pseudocyst, abscess, and ascites or common bile duct obstruction, leading to cholangitis or secondary biliary cirrhosis.

CLINICAL PRESENTATION

- The main features of CP are abdominal pain, malabsorption, weight loss, and diabetes. Jaundice occurs in ~10% of patients.
- Patients typically report deep, penetrating epigastric or abdominal pain that may radiate to the back. The pain often occurs with meals and at night and may be associated with nausea and vomiting.
- Steatorrhea (excessive loss of fat in the feces) and azotorrhea (excessive loss of protein in the feces) are seen in most patients. Steatorrhea is often associated with diarrhea and bloating. Weight loss may occur.
- Pancreatic diabetes is usually a late manifestation that is commonly associated with pancreatic calcification.

DIAGNOSIS

- The diagnosis of CP is based primarily on the clinical presentation in combination with either imaging or pancreatic function studies. Noninvasive imaging studies include abdominal ultrasound, computed tomography (CT), and magnetic resonance cholangiopancreatography (MRCP). Invasive imaging tests include endoscopic ultrasonography (EUS) and ERCP. Although histology would be the best diagnostic test, it is difficult and hazardous to perform and is generally not recommended.
- Serum amylase and lipase are usually normal or only slightly elevated but may be increased in acute exacerbations.
- Total bilirubin, alkaline phosphatase, and hepatic transaminases may be elevated with ductal obstruction. Serum albumin and calcium may be low with malnutrition.
- Pancreatic function tests include
  - ✓ Serum trypsinogen (<20 ng/mL is abnormal)
  - ✓ Fecal elastase (<200 mcg/g of stool is abnormal)
  - ✓ Fecal fat estimation (>7 g/day is abnormal; stool must be collected for 72 hours)
  - ✓ Secretin stimulation (evaluates duodenal bicarbonate secretion)
  - ✓ ^{13}C mixed triglyceride breath test

DESIRED OUTCOME

- The goals of treating uncomplicated CP are to relieve abdominal pain, treat the associated complications of malabsorption and glucose intolerance, and improve quality of life.

NONPHARMACOLOGIC TREATMENT

- Lifestyle modifications should include abstinence from alcohol and smoking cessation.
- Patients with steatorrhea should be advised to eat smaller, more frequent meals and reduce dietary fat intake.
- Patients who do not consume adequate calories from their normal diet may be given whole protein or peptide-based oral nutritional supplements.

- Invasive procedures and surgery are used primarily to treat uncontrolled pain and the complications of chronic pancreatitis.

PHARMACOLOGIC TREATMENT

- Pain management should begin with nonopioid analgesics such as **acetaminophen** or a **nonsteroidal antiinflammatory drug** administered on a scheduled basis before meals to help decrease postprandial pain.
- A trial of **pancreatic enzyme supplementation** for pain relief may be given prior to addition of opioids, although data from clinical trials are mixed.
- If these measures fail, low-potency opioids (e.g., **hydrocodone**) should be added to nonopioid analgesics. **Tramadol** has also been used. Severe pain unresponsive to these therapies necessitates use of other opioids (e.g., **codeine, morphine sulfate, oxycodone,** or **hydromorphone**). Unless contraindicated, oral opioids should be used before parenteral, transdermal, or other dosage forms. In patients with pain that is difficult to manage, nonopioid modulators of chronic pain (e.g., **selective serotonin reuptake inhibitors** and **tricyclic antidepressants**) may be considered.

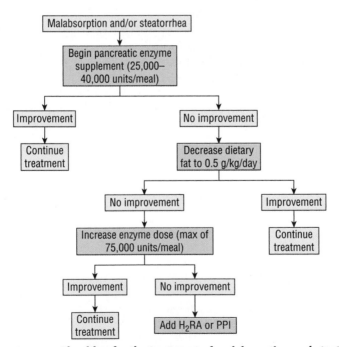

FIGURE 28–2. Algorithm for the treatment of malabsorption and steatorrhea in chronic pancreatitis. (H_2RA, histamine$_2$ receptor antagonist; PPI, proton pump inhibitor.)

TABLE 28–2	Commercially Available Pancreatic Enzyme (Pancrelipase) Preparations		
	Enzyme Content per Unit Dose (USP Units)		
Product	**Lipase**	**Amylase**	**Protease**
Enteric-coated microspheres Ultrase	4,500	20,000	25,000
Enteric-coated microspheres with bicarbonate buffer			
Pancrecarb MS-4	4,000	25,000	25,000
Pancrecarb MS-8	8,000	40,000	45,000
Pancrecarb MS-16	16,000	52,000	52,000
Enteric-coated minimicrospheres			
Creon 6,000 lipase units[a]	6,000	30,000	19,000
Creon 12,000 lipase units[a]	12,000	60,000	38,000
Creon 24,000 lipase units[a]	24,000	120,000	76,000
Enteric-coated minitablets			
Ultrase MT 12	12,000	39,000	39,000
Ultrase MT 18	18,000	58,500	58,500
Ultrase MT 20	20,000	65,000	65,000

USP, United States Pharmacopeia.
[a]FDA-approved product.

- Pancreatic enzyme supplementation and reduction in dietary fat intake are the primary treatments for malabsorption due to CP (Fig. 28–2). This combination enhances nutritional status and reduces steatorrhea. The enzyme dose required to minimize malabsorption is 25,000 to 40,000 units of lipase administered with each meal. The dose may be increased to a maximum of 75,000 units per meal. Products containing enteric-coated microspheres or minimicrospheres may be more effective than other dosage forms (Table 28–2).
- Adverse effects from pancreatic enzyme supplements are generally benign, but high doses can lead to nausea, diarrhea, and intestinal upset. A more serious but uncommon adverse effect is fibrosing colonopathy. Deficiencies in fat-soluble vitamins have been associated with pancreatic enzymes, and appropriate monitoring (especially of vitamin D) is warranted.
- Addition of an H_2RA or PPI may increase the effectiveness of pancreatic enzyme therapy by increasing gastric and duodenal pH.

EVALUATION OF THERAPEUTIC OUTCOMES

- The severity and frequency of abdominal pain should be assessed periodically to determine the efficacy of the analgesic regimen. Patients receiving opioids should be prescribed scheduled bowel regimens and be monitored for constipation.

- Patients receiving pancreatic enzymes for malabsorption should have their weight and stool frequency and consistency monitored periodically.
- Blood glucose must be monitored carefully in diabetic patients.

See Chapter 46, Pancreatitis, authored by Scott Bolesta and Patricia A. Montgomery, for a more detailed discussion of this topic.

CHAPTER 29

Peptic Ulcer Disease

DEFINITION

- Peptic ulcer disease (PUD) refers to a group of ulcerative disorders of the upper GI tract that require acid and pepsin for their formation. PUD differs from gastritis and erosions in that ulcers extend deeper into the muscularis mucosa. The three common forms of peptic ulcers are *Helicobacter pylori* (HP)–positive ulcers, nonsteroidal antiinflammatory drug (NSAID)–induced ulcers, and stress-related mucosal damage (SRMD; also referred to as stress ulcers).

PATHOPHYSIOLOGY

- The pathogenesis of duodenal and gastric ulcers is multifactorial and reflects a combination of pathophysiologic abnormalities and environmental and genetic factors.
- Most peptic ulcers occur in the presence of acid and pepsin when HP, NSAIDs, or other factors disrupt normal mucosal defense and healing mechanisms. Acid is an independent factor that contributes to disruption of mucosal integrity. Increased acid secretion has been observed in patients with duodenal ulcers and may result from HP infection. Patients with gastric ulcers usually have normal or reduced rates of acid secretion.
- Alterations in mucosal defense induced by HP or NSAIDs are the most important cofactors in peptic ulcer formation. Mucosal defense and repair mechanisms include mucus and bicarbonate secretion, intrinsic epithelial cell defense, and mucosal blood flow. Maintenance of mucosal integrity and repair is mediated by endogenous prostaglandin production.
- HP infection causes gastric mucosal inflammation in all infected individuals, but only a minority develop an ulcer or gastric cancer. Mucosal injury is produced by elaborating bacterial enzymes (urease, lipases, and proteases), adherence, and HP virulence factors. HP induces gastric inflammation by altering the host inflammatory response and damaging epithelial cells directly by cell-mediated immune mechanisms or indirectly by activated neutrophils or macrophages attempting to phagocytose bacteria or bacterial products.
- Nonselective NSAIDs (including aspirin) cause gastric mucosal damage by two mechanisms: (1) a direct or topical irritation of the gastric epithelium and (2) systemic inhibition of endogenous mucosal prostaglandin synthesis.
- Use of corticosteroids alone does not increase the risk of ulcer or complications, but ulcer risk is doubled in corticosteroid users taking NSAIDs concurrently.
- Epidemiologic evidence links cigarette smoking to PUD, impaired ulcer healing, and ulcer-related GI complications. The risk is proportional to the amount smoked per day.

- Although clinical observation suggests that ulcer patients are adversely affected by stressful life events, controlled studies have failed to document a cause-and-effect relationship.
- Coffee, tea, cola beverages, beer, milk, and spices may cause dyspepsia but do not increase PUD risk. Ethanol ingestion in high concentrations is associated with acute gastric mucosal damage and upper GI bleeding but is not clearly the cause of ulcers.

CLINICAL PRESENTATION

- Abdominal pain is the most frequent symptom of PUD. The pain is often epigastric and described as burning but can present as vague discomfort, abdominal fullness, or cramping. A typical nocturnal pain may awaken patients from sleep, especially between 12 AM and 3 AM.
- Pain from duodenal ulcers often occurs 1 to 3 hours after meals and is usually relieved by food, whereas food may precipitate or accentuate ulcer pain in gastric ulcers. Antacids provide rapid pain relief in most ulcer patients.
- Heartburn, belching, and bloating often accompany the pain. Nausea, vomiting, and anorexia are more common in gastric than duodenal ulcers.
- The severity of symptoms varies from patient to patient and may be seasonal, occurring more frequently in the spring or fall.
- The presence or absence of epigastric pain does not define an ulcer. Ulcer healing does not necessarily render the patient asymptomatic. Conversely, the absence of pain does not preclude an ulcer diagnosis, especially in the elderly who may present with a "silent" ulcer complication.
- Complications of ulcers caused by HP and NSAIDs include upper GI bleeding, perforation into the peritoneal cavity, penetration into an adjacent structure (e.g., pancreas, biliary tract, or liver), and gastric outlet obstruction. Bleeding may be occult or present as melena or hematemesis. Perforation is associated with sudden, sharp, severe pain, beginning first in the epigastrium but quickly spreading over the entire abdomen. Symptoms of gastric outlet obstruction typically occur over several months and include early satiety, bloating, anorexia, nausea, vomiting, and weight loss.

DIAGNOSIS

- The physical examination may reveal epigastric tenderness between the umbilicus and the xiphoid process that less commonly radiates to the back.
- Routine laboratory tests are not helpful in establishing a diagnosis of PUD. The hematocrit, hemoglobin, and stool guaiac tests are used to detect bleeding.
- The diagnosis of HP infection can be made using endoscopic or nonendoscopic tests. The tests that require upper endoscopy are invasive, more expensive, and usually require a mucosal biopsy for histology, culture,

or detection of urease activity. The nonendoscopic tests include the urea breath test (UBT), serologic antibody detection tests, and stool antigen test. These tests are less invasive, more convenient, and less expensive than endoscopic tests.

- Testing for HP is recommended only if eradication therapy is planned. If endoscopy is not planned, serologic antibody testing is reasonable to determine HP status. The UBT is the preferred nonendoscopic method to verify HP eradication but must be delayed at least 4 weeks after completion of treatment to avoid confusing bacterial suppression with eradication.
- The diagnosis of PUD depends on visualizing the ulcer crater either by upper GI radiography or endoscopy. Endoscopy has largely replaced radiography because it provides a more accurate diagnosis and permits direct visualization of the ulcer.

DESIRED OUTCOME

- The goals of treatment are to relieve ulcer pain, heal the ulcer, prevent ulcer recurrence, and reduce ulcer-related complications. In HP-positive patients with an active ulcer, a previously documented ulcer, or a history of an ulcer-related complication, the goals are to eradicate the organism, heal the ulcer, and cure the disease with a cost-effective drug regimen.

TREATMENT

NONPHARMACOLOGIC TREATMENT

- Patients with PUD should eliminate or reduce psychological stress, cigarette smoking, and the use of NSAIDs (including aspirin). If possible, alternative agents such as **acetaminophen** or a nonacetylated salicylate (e.g., **salsalate**) should be used for pain relief.
- Although there is no need for a special diet, patients should avoid foods and beverages that cause dyspepsia or exacerbate ulcer symptoms (e.g., spicy foods, caffeine, and alcohol).
- Elective surgery is rarely performed because of highly effective medical management. Emergency surgery may be required for bleeding, perforation, or obstruction.

PHARMACOLOGIC TREATMENT

- An algorithm for the evaluation and management of a patient with dyspeptic or ulcer-like symptoms is presented in **Fig. 29–1**.
- Established indications for treatment of HP include gastric or duodenal ulcer, mucosa-associated lymphoid tissue (MALT) lymphoma, postendoscopic resection of gastric cancer, and uninvestigated dyspepsia. Treatment should be effective, well tolerated, convenient, and cost-effective.
- Table 29–1 lists regimens used to eradicate HP infection. First-line eradication therapy is usually initiated with a proton pump inhibitor (PPI)–based, three-drug regimen for 10 to 14 days. If a second treatment course is required, the PPI-based three-drug regimen should contain different

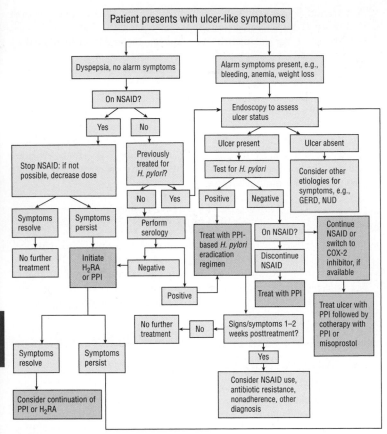

FIGURE 29–1. Algorithm. Guidelines for the evaluation and management of a patient who presents with dyspeptic or ulcer-like symptoms. (COX-2, cyclooxygenase-2; GERD, gastroesophageal reflux disease; *H. pylori, Helicobacter pylori*; H_2RA, histamine$_2$-receptor antagonist; NSAID, nonsteroidal antiinflammatory drug; NUD, nonulcer dyspepsia; PPI, proton pump inhibitor.)

antibiotics, or a four-drug regimen with a bismuth salt, metronidazole, tetracycline, and a PPI should be used.

- Bismuth-based quadruple therapy is recommended as an alternative for patients allergic to penicillin. All medications except the PPI should be taken with meals and at bedtime.
- In sequential therapy, the antibiotics are administered in a sequence rather than all together. The rationale is to treat initially with antibiotics that rarely promote resistance (e.g., amoxicillin) to reduce bacterial load and preexisting resistant organisms and then to follow with different antibiotics (e.g., clarithromycin and metronidazole) to kill the remaining organisms. The potential advantage of superior eradication rates requires

TABLE 29–1	Drug Regimens to Eradicate *Helicobacter pylori*		
Drug #1	**Drug #2**	**Drug #3**	**Drug #4**
Proton pump inhibitor–based triple therapy[a]			
PPI once or twice daily[b]	Clarithromycin 500 mg twice daily	Amoxicillin 1 g twice daily *or* metronidazole 500 mg twice daily	
Bismuth-based quadruple therapy[a]			
PPI or H$_2$RA once or twice daily[b,c]	Bismuth subsalicylate[d] 525 mg 4 times daily	Metronidazole 250–500 mg 4 times daily	Tetracycline 500 mg 4 times daily
Sequential therapy[e]			
PPI once or twice daily on days 1–10[b]	Amoxicillin 1 g twice daily on days 1–5	Metronidazole 250–500 mg twice daily on days 6–10	Clarithromycin 250–500 mg twice daily on days 6–10
Second-line (salvage) therapy for persistent infections			
PPI or H$_2$RA once or twice daily[b,c]	Bismuth subsalicylate[d] 525 mg 4 times daily	Metronidazole 250–500 mg 4 times daily	Tetracycline 500 mg 4 times daily
PPI once or twice daily[b,f]	Amoxicillin 1 g twice daily	Levofloxacin 250 mg twice daily	

H$_2$RA, H$_2$-receptor antagonist; PPI, proton pump inhibitor.

[a]Although treatment is minimally effective if used for 7 days, 10–14 days is recommended. The antisecretory drug may be continued beyond antimicrobial treatment for patients with a history of a complicated ulcer, e.g., bleeding, or in heavy smokers.

[b]Standard PPI peptic ulcer healing dosages given once or twice daily (see Table 29–2).

[c]Standard H$_2$RA peptic ulcer healing dosages may be used in place of a PPI (see Table 29–2).

[d]Bismuth subcitrate potassium (biskalcitrate) 140 mg, as the bismuth salt, is contained in a prepackaged capsule (Pylera), along with metronidazole 125 mg and tetracycline 125 mg; three capsules are taken with each meal and at bedtime; a standard PPI dosage is added to the regimen and taken twice daily. All medications are taken for 10 days.

[e]Requires validation as first-line therapy in the United States.

[f]Requires validation as rescue therapy in the United States.

confirmation in the United States before this regimen can be recommended as first-line therapy.

- If the initial treatment fails to eradicate HP, second-line (salvage) treatment should (1) use antibiotics that were not included in the initial regimen, (2) use antibiotics that are not associated with resistance, (3) use a drug that has a topical effect (e.g., bismuth), and (4) extend the treatment duration to 14 days. A 14-day course of the PPI-based quadruple regimen is the most commonly used second-line therapy after failure of a PPI–amoxicillin–clarithromycin regimen.

- Patients with NSAID-induced ulcers should be tested to determine their HP status. If HP positive, treatment should be initiated with a PPI-based three-drug regimen. If HP negative, the NSAID should

TABLE 29–2	Oral Drug Regimens Used to Heal Peptic Ulcers and Maintain Ulcer Healing		
Generic Name	**Prescription Brand Name**	**Duodenal or Gastric Ulcer Healing (mg/dose)**	**Maintenance of Ulcer Healing (mg/dose)**
Proton pump inhibitors			
Omeprazole	Prilosec, various	20–40 daily	20–40 daily
Omeprazole sodium bicarbonate	Zegerid	20–40 daily	20–40 daily
Lansoprazole	Prevacid, various	15–30 daily	15–30 daily
Rabeprazole	Aciphex	20 daily	20 daily
Pantoprazole	Pantoprazole, various	40 daily	40 daily
Esomeprazole	Nexium	20–40 daily	20–40 daily
Dexlansoprazole	Dexilant	30–60 daily	30 daily
H_2-receptor antagonists			
Cimetidine	Tagamet, various	300 four times daily 400 twice daily 800 at bedtime	400–800 at bedtime
Famotidine	Pepcid, various	20 twice daily 40 at bedtime	20–40 at bedtime
Nizatidine	Axid, various	150 twice daily 300 at bedtime	150–300 at bedtime
Ranitidine	Zantac, various	150 twice daily 300 at bedtime	150–300 at bedtime
Promote mucosal defense			
Sucralfate	Carafate, various	1 g 4 times daily 2 g twice daily	1–2 g twice daily 1 g 4 times daily

be discontinued and the patient treated with either a PPI, H_2RA, or sucralfate (Table 29–2). If the NSAID must be continued despite ulceration, treatment should be initiated with a PPI (if HP negative) or with a PPI-based three-drug regimen (if HP positive). Cotherapy with a PPI or misoprostol or switching to a selective cyclooxygenase-2 (COX-2) inhibitor is recommended for patients at risk of developing an ulcer-related complication.

- Maintenance therapy with a PPI or H_2RA (see Table 29–2) should be limited to high-risk patients with ulcer complications, patients who fail HP eradication, and those with HP-negative ulcers.
- Patients with ulcers refractory to treatment should undergo upper endoscopy to confirm a nonhealing ulcer, exclude malignancy, and assess HP status. HP-positive patients should receive eradication therapy. In HP-negative patients, higher PPI doses (e.g., omeprazole 40 mg/day) heal the majority of ulcers. Continuous PPI treatment is often necessary to maintain healing. Patients with refractory gastric ulcer may require surgery because of the possibility of malignancy.

EVALUATION OF THERAPEUTIC OUTCOMES

- Patients should be monitored for symptomatic relief of ulcer pain, as well as potential adverse effects and drug interactions related to drug therapy.
- Ulcer pain typically resolves in a few days when NSAIDs are discontinued and within 7 days upon initiation of antiulcer therapy. Most patients with uncomplicated PUD will be symptom free after treatment with any of the recommended antiulcer regimens.
- The persistence or recurrence of symptoms within 14 days after the end of treatment suggests failure of ulcer healing or HP eradication, or an alternative diagnosis such as gastroesophageal reflux disease.
- Most patients with uncomplicated HP-positive ulcers do not require confirmation of ulcer healing or HP eradication.
- Patients taking NSAIDs should be closely monitored for signs and symptoms of bleeding, obstruction, penetration, and perforation.
- Follow-up endoscopy is justified in patients with frequent symptomatic recurrence, refractory disease, complications, or suspected hypersecretory states.

See Chapter 40, Peptic Ulcer Disease, authored by Rosemary R. Berardi and Randolph V. Fugit, for a more detailed discussion of this topic.

CHAPTER

30

Contraception

DEFINITION

- Contraception is the prevention of pregnancy following sexual intercourse by inhibiting sperm from reaching a mature ovum (i.e., methods that act as barriers or prevent ovulation) or by preventing a fertilized ovum from implanting in the endometrium (i.e., mechanisms that create an unfavorable uterine environment).
- Method failure (perfect use failure) is a failure inherent to the proper use of the contraceptive alone.
- User failure (typical use failure) takes into account the user's ability to follow directions correctly and consistently.

THE MENSTRUAL CYCLE

- The median length of the menstrual cycle is 28 days (range 21–40 days). The first day of menses is day 1 of the follicular phase. Ovulation usually occurs on day 14 of the menstrual cycle. After ovulation, the luteal phase lasts until the beginning of the next cycle.
- Epinephrine and norepinephrine stimulate the hypothalamus to secrete gonadotropin-releasing hormone, which stimulates the anterior pituitary to secrete bursts of gonadotropins, follicle-stimulating hormone (FSH), and luteinizing hormone (LH).
- In the follicular phase, FSH levels increase and cause recruitment of a small group of follicles for continued growth. Between 5 and 7 days, one of these becomes the dominant follicle, which later ruptures to release the oocyte. The dominant follicle develops, increasing amounts of estradiol and inhibin, which cause a negative feedback on the secretion of gonadotropin-releasing hormone and FSH, causing atresia of the remaining follicles recruited earlier.
- The dominant follicle continues to grow and synthesizes estradiol, progesterone, and androgen. Estradiol stops the menstrual flow from the previous cycle, thickens the endometrial lining, and produces thin, watery cervical mucus. FSH regulates aromatase enzymes that induce conversion of androgens to estrogens in the follicle.
- The pituitary releases a midcycle LH surge that stimulates the final stages of follicular maturation and ovulation. Ovulation occurs 24 to 36 hours after the estradiol peak and 10 to 16 hours after the LH peak.
- The LH surge, occurring 28 to 32 hours before a follicle ruptures, is the most clinically useful predictor of approaching ovulation. Conception is

most successful when intercourse takes place from 2 days before ovulation to the day of ovulation.

- After ovulation, the remaining luteinized follicles become the corpus luteum, which synthesizes androgen, estrogen, and progesterone (Fig. 30–1).
- If pregnancy occurs, human chorionic gonadotropin prevents regression of the corpus luteum and stimulates continued production of estrogen and progesterone. If pregnancy does not occur, the corpus luteum degenerates, and progesterone declines. As progesterone levels decline, menstruation occurs.

TREATMENT

NONPHARMACOLOGIC THERAPY

- A comparison of methods of nonhormonal contraception is shown in Table 30–1.

Periodic Abstinence

- The abstinence (rhythm) method is not well accepted, as it is associated with relatively high pregnancy rates and necessitates avoidance of intercourse for several days in each cycle.

Barrier Techniques

- The effectiveness of the diaphragm depends on its function as a barrier and on the spermicidal cream or jelly placed in the diaphragm before insertion.
- The cervical cap, smaller and less messy than the diaphragm, fits over the cervix like a thimble. Caps can be inserted 6 hours prior to intercourse, and women should not wear the cap for longer than 48 hours to reduce the risk of toxic shock syndrome.
- Most condoms made in the United States are latex rubber, which is impermeable to viruses, but ~5% are made from lamb intestine, which is not impermeable to viruses. Mineral oil–based vaginal drug formulations (e.g., Cleocin vaginal cream, Premarin vaginal cream, Vagistat 1, Femstat, and Monistat vaginal suppositories) can decrease the barrier strength of latex. Condoms with spermicides are no longer recommended, as they provide no additional protection against pregnancy or sexually transmitted diseases (STDs) and may increase vulnerability to human immunodeficiency virus (HIV).
- The female condom (Reality) covers the labia, as well as the cervix; thus, it may be more effective than the male condom in preventing transmission of STDs. However, the pregnancy rate is reported to be 21% in the first year of use.

PHARMACOLOGIC THERAPY

Spermicides

- Spermicides, most of which contain nonoxynol-9, are surfactants that destroy sperm cell walls. They offer no protection against STDs, and when

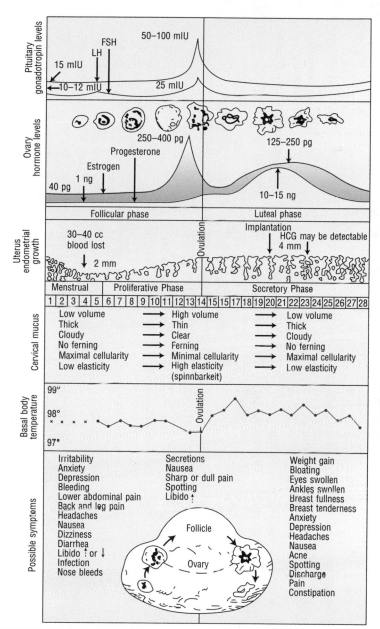

FIGURE 30–1. Menstrual cycle events, idealized 28-day cycle. (FSH, follicle-stimulating hormone; HCG, human chorionic gonadotropin; LH, luteinizing hormone.) (*From Hatcher RA, Nelson AL. Contraceptive Technology. 19th ed. New York: Ardent Media; 2007. This figure may be reproduced at no cost to the reader.*)

TABLE 30–1 Comparison of Methods of Nonhormonal Contraception

Method	Absolute Contraindications	Advantages	Disadvantages	Percentage of Women with Pregnancy[a] Perfect Use	Percentage of Women with Pregnancy[a] Typical Use
Condoms, male	Allergy to latex or rubber	Inexpensive STD protection, including HIV (latex only)	High user failure rate Poor acceptance Possibility of breakage Efficacy decreased by oil-based lubricants Possible allergic reactions to latex in either partner	2	15
Condoms, female	Allergy to polyurethane History of TSS	Can be inserted just before intercourse or ahead of time STD protection, including HIV	High user failure rate Dislike ring hanging outside vagina Cumbersome	5	21
Diaphragm with spermicide	Allergy to latex, rubber, or spermicide Recurrent UTIs History of TSS Abnormal gynecologic anatomy	Low cost Decreased incidence of cervical neoplasia Some protection against STDs	High user failure rate Decreased efficacy with increased frequency of intercourse Increased incidence of vaginal yeast UTIs, TSS Efficacy affected by oil-based lubricants Cervical irritation	6	16

Method	Contraindications	Advantages	Disadvantages		
Cervical cap (FemCap, Lea's Shield)	Allergy to spermicide History of TSS Abnormal gynecologic anatomy Abnormal Papanicolaou smear	Low cost Latex-free Some protection against STDs FemCap reusable for up to 2 years	High user failure rate Decreased efficacy with parity Cannot be used during menses	9	16[b]
Spermicides alone	Allergy to spermicide	Inexpensive	High user failure rate Must be reapplied before each act of intercourse May enhance HIV transmission No protection against STDs	18	29
Sponge (Today)	Allergy to spermicide Recurrent UTIs History of TSS Abnormal gynecologic anatomy	Inexpensive	High user failure rate Decreased efficacy with parity Cannot be used during menses No protection against STDs	9[c]	16[d]

HIV, human immunodeficiency virus; STD, sexually transmitted disease; TSS, toxic shock syndrome; UTI, urinary tract infection.

[a] Failure rates in the United States during first year of use.

[b] Failure rate with FemCap reported to be 29% per package insert.

[c] Failure rate with Today sponge reported to be 20% in parous women.

[d] Failure rate with Today sponge reported to be 32% in parous women.

Data from Hatcher RA, Nelson AL. Contraceptive Technology, 13th ed. New York: Ardent Media, 2007; and Dickey RP. Managing Contraceptive Pill Patients, 13th ed. Dallas, TX: EMIS Inc., 2007.

used more than twice daily, they may increase the transmission of HIV. Women at high risk for HIV or who are HIV infected should not use spermicides.

Spermicide-implanted Barrier Techniques

- The **vaginal contraceptive sponge (Today)** contains 1 g of nonoxynol-9 and provides protection for 24 hours. After intercourse, the sponge must be left in place for at least 6 hours before removal. It should not be left in place for more than 24 to 30 hours to reduce the risk of toxic shock syndrome. It is available without a prescription.

Hormonal Contraception

COMPOSITION AND FORMULATIONS

- Hormonal contraceptives contain either a combination of synthetic estrogen and synthetic progestin or a progestin alone.
- Progestins thicken cervical mucus, delay sperm transport, and induce endometrial atrophy. They also block the LH surge and thus inhibit ovulation. Estrogens suppress FSH release, which may contribute to blocking the LH surge and also stabilizes the endometrial lining and provides cycle control.

COMPONENTS

- Two synthetic estrogens are used in hormonal contraceptives in the United States, **ethinyl estradiol (EE)** and **mestranol**. Mestranol must be converted to EE in the liver to be active. It is ~50% less potent than EE. Most combined oral contraceptives (OCs) contain estrogen at doses of 20 to 50 mcg of EE daily.
- Progestins vary in their progestational activity and differ with respect to inherent estrogenic, antiestrogenic, and androgenic effects. Their estrogenic and antiestrogenic properties occur because progestins are metabolized to estrogenic substances. Androgenic properties occur because of the structural similarity of the progestin to testosterone.
- Progestins include **desogestrel, drospirenone, ethynodiol diacetate, norgestimate, norethindrone, norethindrone acetate, norethynodrel, norgestrel,** and **levonorgestrel,** the active isomer of norgestrel. The patch contains norelgestromin, the active metabolite of norgestimate. The vaginal ring contains **etonogestrel,** the metabolite of desogestrel.
- **Table 30–2** lists available OCs by brand name and hormonal composition.

CONSIDERATIONS WITH ORAL CONTRACEPTIVE USE

- The recommendation of the American College of Obstetricians and Gynecologists is to allow provision of hormonal contraception after a simple medical history and blood pressure measurement.
- Noncontraceptive benefits of OCs include decreased menstrual cramps and ovulatory pain; decreased menstrual blood loss; improved menstrual regularity; increased hemoglobin concentration; improvement in acne; reduced risk of ovarian and endometrial cancer; and reduced risk of ovarian cysts, ectopic pregnancy, pelvic inflammatory disease, endometriosis, uterine fibroids, and benign breast disease.

TABLE 30–2 Composition of Orally Prescribed Oral Contraceptives[a]

Product	Estrogen	Micrograms[b]	Progestin	Milligrams[b]	Spotting and Breakthrough Bleeding
50 mcg estrogen					
Necon 1/50, Norinyl 1+50, Ortho-Novum 1/50	Mestranol	50	Norethindrone	1	10.6
Ovcon 50	Ethinyl estradiol	50	Norethindrone	1	11.9
Ovral, Ogestrel 0.5/50	Ethinyl estradiol	50	Norgestrel	0.5	4.5
Demulen 1/50, Zovia 1/50	Ethinyl estradiol	50	Ethynodiol diacetate	1	13.9
Sub-50 mcg estrogen monophasic					
Aviane, Lessina, Levlite, Lutera, Sronyx	Ethinyl estradiol	20	Levonorgestrel	0.1	26.5
Brevicon, Modicon, Necon 0.5/35, Nortrel 0.5/35	Ethinyl estradiol	35	Norethindrone	0.5	24.6
Demulen 1/35, Zovia 1/35, Kelnor	Ethinyl estradiol	37.4	Ethynodiol diacetate	1	37.4
Apri, Desogen, Ortho-Cept, Reclipsen, Solia	Ethinyl estradiol	30	Desogestrel	0.15	13.1
Levlen, Levora, Nordette, Portia	Ethinyl estradiol	30	Levonorgestrel	0.15	14
Junel 1/20, Junel Fe 1/20, Loestrin 1/20, Microgestin 1/20; Fe 1/20	Ethinyl estradiol	20	Norethindrone 1 mg	1	26.5
Junel 1.5/30, Junel Fe 1.5/30, Loestrin Fe 1.5/30, Microgestin 1.5/30, Microgestin Fe 1.5/30	Ethinyl estradiol	30	Norethindrone acetate	1.5	25.2
Cryselle, Lo-Ovral, Low-Ogestrel	Ethinyl estradiol	30	Norgestrel	0.3	9.6
Necon 1/35, Norinyl 1+35, Norethin 1/35, Nortrel 1/35, Ortho-Novum 1/35	Ethinyl estradiol	35	Norethindrone	1	14.7
Ortho-Cyclen, Mononessa, Previfem, Sprintec	Ethinyl estradiol	35	Norgestimate	0.25	14.3
Ovcon-35, Baziva, Femcon Fe chewable, Zenchent	Ethinyl estradiol	35	Norethindrone	0.4	11
Yasmin	Ethinyl estradiol	30	Drospirenone	3	14.5

(continued)

TABLE 30–2 Composition of Orally Prescribed Oral Contraceptives[a] (Continued)

Product	Estrogen	Micrograms[b]	Progestin	Milligrams[b]	Spotting and Breakthrough Bleeding
Sub-50 mcg estrogen monophasic extended cycle					
Loestrin-24 FE[c]	Ethinyl estradiol	20	Norethindrone	1	50[e]
Lybrel	Ethinyl estradiol	20	Levonorgestrel	0.09	52[e]
Seasonale, Jolessa, Quasense[d]	Ethinyl estradiol	30	Levonorgestrel	0.15	58.5[e]
Yaz[c]	Ethinyl estradiol	20	Drospirenone	3	52.5[e]
Beyaz[f]	Ethinyl estradiol	20	Drospirenone	3	52.5[e]
Sub-50 mcg estrogen multiphasic					
Cyclessa, Cesia, Velivet	Ethinyl estradiol	25 (7) 25 (7) 25 (7)	Desogestrel	0.1 (7) 0.125 (7) 0.15 (7)	11.1
Estrostep Fe, Tilia Fe, Tri-Legest Fe	Ethinyl estradiol	20 (5) 30 (7) 35 (9)	Norethindrone acetate Norethindrone acetate Norethindrone acetate	1 (5) 1 (7) 1 (9)	21.7
Kariva, Mircette	Ethinyl estradiol	20 (21) 10 (5)	Desogestrel Desogestrel	0.15 (21)	19.7
Gencept 10/11, Necon 10/11, Ortho-Novum 10/11	Ethinyl estradiol	35 (10) 35 (11)	Norethindrone Norethindrone	0.5 (10) 1 (11)	17.6
Ortho-Novum 7/7/7, Nortrel 7/7/7, Necon 7/7/7	Ethinyl estradiol	35 (7) 35 (7) 35 (7)	Norethindrone Norethindrone Norethindrone	0.5 (7) 0.75 (7) 1 (7)	14.5

Ortho Tri-Cyclen, Trinessa, Tri-Previfem, Tri-Sprintec	Ethinyl estradiol	35 (7)	Norgestimate	0.18 (7)	17.7
	Ethinyl estradiol	35 (7)	Norgestimate	0.215 (7)	
	Ethinyl estradiol	35 (7)	Norgestimate	0.25 (7)	
Ortho Tri-Cyclen Lo	Ethinyl estradiol	25 (7)	Norgestimate	0.18 (7)	11.5
	Ethinyl estradiol	25 (7)	Norgestimate	0.215 (7)	
	Ethinyl estradiol	25 (7)	Norgestimate	0.25 (7)	
Aranelle, Leena, Tri-Norinyl	Ethinyl estradiol	35 (7)	Norethindrone	0.5 (7)	25.5
	Ethiny estradiol	35 (9)	Norethindrone	1 (9)	
	Ethinyl estradiol	35 (5)	Norethindrone	0.5 (5)	
Enpresse, Tri-Levlen, Triphasil, Trivora	Ethinyl estradiol	30 (6)	Levonorgestrel	0.05 (6)	
	Ethinyl estradiol	40 (5)	Levonorgestrel	0.075 (5)	
	Ethinyl estradiol	30 (10)	Levonorgestrel	0.125 (10)	
Sub-50 mcg estrogen multiphasic extended cycle					
Seasonique	Ethinyl estradiol	30 (84)	Levonorgestrel	0.15 (84)	42.5[e]
	Ethinyl estradiol	10 (7)	Levonorgestrel	0.15 (7)	
Progestin only					
Camila, Errin, Jolivette, Micronor, Nor-QD, Nora-BE	Ethinyl estradiol	–	Norethindrone	0.35	42.3

[a]28-day regimens (21-day active pills, then 7-day pill-free interval) unless otherwise noted.

[b]Number in parentheses refers to the number of days the dose is received in multiphasic oral contraceptives.

[c]28-day regimen (24-day active pills, then 4-day pill-free interval).

[d]91-day regimen (84-day active pills, then 7-day pill-free interval).

[e]Percentage reporting after 6–12 months of use.

[f]Contains folate supplementation (levomefolate calcium 0.451 mg).

Data from Hatcher RA, Nelson AL. Contraceptive Technology, 19th ed. New York: Ardent Media, 2007; Dickey RP. Managing Contraceptive Pill Patients, 13th ed. Dallas, TX: EMIS Inc, 2007; and Anonymous. Hormonal Contraception. Pharmacist's/Prescriber's Letter 2007:23.

TABLE 30–3 Adverse Effects of Combined Hormonal Contraception and Their Management[a]

Adverse Effects	Management
Estrogen excess	
Nausea, breast tenderness, headaches, cyclic weight gain due to fluid retention	Decrease estrogen content in CHC Consider progestin-only methods or IUD
Dysmenorrhea, menorrhagia, uterine fibroid growth	Decrease estrogen content in CHC Consider extended-cycle or continuous regimen OC Consider progestin-only methods or IUD NSAIDs for dysmenorrhea
Estrogen deficiency	
Vasomotor symptoms, nervousness, decreased libido	Increase estrogen content in CHC
Early-cycle (days 1–9) breakthrough bleeding and spotting	Increase estrogen content in CHC
Absence of withdrawal bleeding (amenorrhea)	Exclude pregnancy Increase estrogen content in CHC if menses is desired Continue current CHC if amenorrhea acceptable
Progestin excess	
Increased appetite, weight gain, bloating, constipation	Decrease progestin content in CHC
Acne, oily skin, hirsutism	Decrease progestin content in CHC Choose less androgenic progestin in CHC
Depression, fatigue, irritability	Decrease progestin content in CHC
Progestin deficiency	
Dysmenorrhea, menorrhagia	Increase progestin content in CHC Consider extended-cycle or continuous regimen OC Consider progestin-only methods or IUD NSAIDs for dysmenorrhea
Late-cycle (days 10–21) breakthrough bleeding and spotting	Increase progestin content in CHC

CHC, combined hormonal contraceptive; IUD, intrauterine device; NSAID, nonsteroidal antiinflammatory drug; OC, oral contraceptive.

[a]CHC regimens should be continued for at least 3 months before adjustments are made based on adverse effects.
Data from Hatcher RA, Nelson AL. Contraceptive Technology, 19th ed. New York: Ardent Media, 2007; and Dickey RP. Managing Contraceptive Pill Patients, 13th ed. Dallas, TX: EMIS Inc., 2007.

- The transdermal patch may cause less breast discomfort and dysmenorrhea than OCs.
- Adverse effects associated with combined hormonal contraceptives (CHCs) and their management are shown in Table 30–3.
- The CHC vaginal ring may be uncomfortable and cause vaginal discharge.
- The CHC patch may cause irritation and increase the risk for thromboembolism.
- The main safety concern about CHCs is their lack of protection against STDs.
- The World Health Organization (WHO) developed a graded list of precautions for clinicians to consider when initiating CHCs (Table 30–4).

TABLE 30–4 World Health Organization Precautions in the Provision of Combined Hormonal Contraceptives (CHCs)

Category 4: Refrain from providing CHCs to women with the following diagnoses

- Thrombophlebitis or thromboembolic disorder or a history of these conditions
- Cerebrovascular disease, coronary artery disease, peripheral vascular disease
- Valvular heart disease with thrombogenic complications (e.g., pulmonary hypertension, atrial fibrillation, history of endocarditis)
- Diabetes with vascular involvement (e.g., nephropathy, retinopathy, neuropathy, other vascular disease or diabetes >20 years' duration)
- Migraine headaches with focal aura
- Uncontrolled hypertension (≥160 mm Hg systolic or ≥90 mm Hg diastolic)
- Major surgery with prolonged immobilization
- Thrombogenic mutations (e.g., factor V Leiden, protein C or S deficiency, antithrombin III deficiency, prothrombin deficiency)
- Breast cancer
- Acute or chronic hepatocellular disease with abnormal liver function, cirrhosis, hepatic adenomas, or hepatic carcinomas
- Age >35 years and currently smoking ≥15 cigarettes per day
- Known or suspected pregnancy
- Breastfeeding women <6 weeks postpartum

Category 3: Conditions may be adversely impacted by CHCs, and the risks generally outweigh the benefits; providers should exercise caution if combined CHCs are used in these situations, and patients should be carefully monitored for adverse effects

- Multiple risk factors for arterial cardiovascular disease
- Known hyperlipidemia
- Migraine headache without aura in women ≥35 years old
- History of hypertension (140–159 mm Hg systolic or 90–99 mm Hg diastolic)
- History of cancer, but no evidence of current disease for 5 years
- Cirrhosis, mild and compensated
- Symptomatic gallbladder disease
- Cholestatic jaundice with prior pill use
- Age >35 years and currently smoking <15 cigarettes per day
- Postpartum <21 days, not breastfeeding
- Breast-feeding women 6 weeks to 6 months postpartum
- Commonly used drugs that induce liver enzymes (rifampin, phenytoin, carbamazepine, barbiturates, primidone, topiramate) and reduce efficacy of CHC

(continued)

TABLE 30–4 World Health Organization Precautions in the Provision of Combined Hormonal Contraceptives (CHCs) *(Continued)*

Category 2: Some conditions may trigger potential concerns with CHCs, but benefits usually outweigh risks	Category 1: Do not restrict use of combined oral contraceptives for the following conditions
• Family history of thromboembolism	• Varicose veins
• Superficial thrombophlebitis	• History of gestational diabetes
• Uncomplicated valvular heart disease	• Nonmigrainous headaches
• Diabetes without vascular disease	• Thyroid disease
• Sickle cell disease	• Thalassemia
• Migraine headaches without aura in women <35 years old	• Iron deficiency anemia
• Hypertension during pregnancy, resolved postpartum	• Depression
• Major surgery without prolonged immobilization	• Epilepsy
• Gallbladder disease (symptomatic and treated by cholecystectomy or asymptomatic)	• Infectious diseases (HIV, schistosomiasis, tuberculosis, malaria)
• Cholestatic jaundice of pregnancy	• Minor surgery without immobilization
• Undiagnosed breast mass	• Benign ovarian tumors
• Undiagnosed abnormal genital bleeding	• Endometriosis
• Cervical intraepithelial neoplasia or cervical cancer	• Irregular or heavy vaginal bleeding, severe dysmenorrhea
• Obesity (body mass index ≥30 kg/m²)	• Sexually transmitted diseases
• Age <35 years and currently smoking	• Uterine fibroids
• Breastfeeding women ≥6 months postpartum	• Pelvic inflammatory disease
• Age ≥40 years	• Endometrial cancer
• Drugs that may induce metabolism of CHC and reduce efficacy (griseofulvin, antiretroviral therapy)	• Ovarian cancer
	• History of pelvic surgery
	• Trophoblast disease
	• History of ectopic pregnancy
	• Postabortion
	• Postpartum women ≥21 weeks, not breastfeeding
	• Menarche to 40 years of age
	• Drug interactions with antibiotics other than rifampin and griseofulvin

CHC, combined hormonal contraception; HIV, human immunodeficiency virus.

Data from Hatcher RA, Nelson AL. Contraceptive Technology, 19th ed. New York: Ardent Media, 2007; Dickey RP. Managing Contraceptive Pill Patients, 13th ed. Dallas, TX: EMIS Inc, 2007; World Health Organization. Medical Eligibility Criteria for Contraceptive Use, 3rd ed; 2004. http://www.who.int/reproductivehealth/publications/mec/index.htm; and World Health Organization. Medical Eligibility Criteria for Contraceptive Use, 2008 update; 2008. http://whqlibdoc.who.int/hq/2008/WHO_RHR_08.19_eng.pdf.

Women over 35 Years of Age

- CHCs containing <50 mcg EE are an acceptable form of contraception for healthy nonsmoking women older than 35 years.
- Women older than 35 years with migraine, hypertension, dyslipidemia, or diabetes mellitus should not take CHCs.
- Studies have not demonstrated an increased risk of cardiovascular disease with low-dose CHCs in healthy, nonobese women.

Women Who Smoke

- Women older than 35 years who smoke and take OCs have an increased risk of myocardial infarction; therefore, clinicians should prescribe CHCs with caution, if at all, in these patients. The WHO states that smoking 15 or more cigarettes per day by women over 35 years is a contraindication to the use of CHCs, and that the risks generally outweigh the benefits even in those who smoke fewer than 15 cigarettes per day. Progestin-only contraceptive methods should be considered for women in this group.

Hypertension

- CHCs, even those with <35 mcg estrogen, can cause small increases in blood pressure (6–8 mm Hg) in both normotensive and hypertensive women. In women with hypertension, OCs have been associated with an increased risk of MI and stroke. Use of low-dose CHCs is acceptable in women younger than 35 years with well-controlled and monitored hypertension. Hypertensive women with end-organ disease or who smoke should not use CHCs.

Diabetes

- The new progestins are believed to have little, if any, effect on carbohydrate metabolism. Women younger than 35 years with diabetes but no vascular disease who do not smoke can safely use CHCs, but diabetic women with vascular disease or diabetes of more than 20 years' duration should not use CHCs.

Dyslipidemia

- Generally, synthetic progestins decrease high-density lipoprotein (HDL) and increase low-density lipoprotein (LDL). Estrogens decrease LDL but increase HDL and may moderately increase triglycerides. Most low-dose CHCs (with the possible exception of levonorgestrel pills, which may reduce HDL levels in some patients) have no significant impact on HDL, LDL, triglycerides, or total cholesterol.
- However, the mechanism for the increased incidence of cardiovascular disease in CHC users is believed to be thromboembolic and thrombotic changes, not atherosclerosis.
- Women with controlled dyslipidemias can use low-dose CHCs, with periodic monitoring of fasting lipid profiles. Women with uncontrolled dyslipidemia (LDL >160 mg/dL [4.14 mmol/L], HDL <35 mg/dL [0.91 mmol/L], triglycerides >250 mg/dL [2.83 mmol/L]) and additional risk factors (e.g., coronary artery disease, diabetes, hypertension,

smoking, or a positive family history) should use an alternative method of contraception.

Thromboembolism

- Estrogens have a dose-related effect in the development of venous thromboembolism (VTE) and pulmonary embolism. This is especially true in women with underlying hypercoagulable states or who have acquired conditions (e.g., obesity, pregnancy, immobility, trauma, surgery, and certain malignancies).
- The risk of VTE in women using low-dose OCs (<50 mcg EE with norethindrone or levonorgestrel) was four times the risk in nonusers. However, this risk is less than the risk of thromboembolic events during pregnancy. OCs containing desogestrel have been associated with a 1.7 to 19 times higher risk of VTE than OCs containing levonorgestrel.
- CHCs are contraindicated in women with a history of thromboembolic events and in those at risk due to prolonged immobilization with major surgery unless they are taking anticoagulants.
- Emergency contraception has not been associated with an increased risk of thromboembolic events.

Migraine Headache

- Women with migraines may experience a decreased or increased frequency of migraine headaches when using CHCs.
- CHCs may be considered for healthy, nonsmoking women with migraines without aura; however, women of any age who have migraine with aura should not use CHCs. Women who develop migraines (with or without aura) while receiving CHCs should immediately discontinue their use and consider a progestin-only option.

Breast Cancer

- A U.S. study found no association between overall breast cancer and current or past OC use. Although some studies have found differences in the risk of breast cancer based on the presence of *BRCA1* and *BRCA2* mutations, the most recent cohort study found no association with low-dose OCs and the presence of either mutation.
- The choice to use CHCs should not be affected by the presence of benign breast disease or a family history of breast cancer with either mutation. The WHO precautions state that women with a recent personal history of breast cancer should not use CHCs, but that CHCs can be considered in women without evidence of disease for 5 years.

Systemic Lupus Erythematosus

- OCs do not increase the risk of flare among women with stable systemic lupus erythematosus (SLE) and without antiphospholipid/anticardiolipin antibodies.
- CHCs should be avoided in women with SLE and antiphospholipid antibodies or vascular complications. Progestin-only contraceptives can be used in these women.

Obesity

- OCs have lower efficacy in obese women, and low-dose OCs may be especially problematic. The American College of Obstetrics and Gynecology recommends that the transdermal contraceptive patches not be used as a first choice in women weighing >90 kg (198 lb).
- Obese women are also at risk of VTE.

GENERAL CONSIDERATIONS FOR ORAL CONTRACEPTIVES

- With perfect use, their efficacy is >99%, but with typical use, up to 8% of women may experience unintended pregnancy.
- Monophasic OCs contain the same amounts of estrogen and progestin for 21 days, followed by 7 days of placebo. Biphasic and triphasic pills contain variable amounts of estrogen and progestin for 21 days and are followed by a 7-day placebo phase.
- Extended-cycle pills and continuous combination regimens may offer some side effect benefits. One particular extended-cycle OC increases the number of hormone-containing pills from 21 to 84 days, followed by a 7-day placebo phase, resulting in four menstrual cycles per year. Another product provides hormone-containing pills daily throughout the year. Continuous combination regimens provide OCs for 21 days, then very-low-dose estrogen and progestin for an additional 4 to 7 days.
- Third-generation OCs contain newer progestins (e.g., desogestrel, drospirenone, gestodene, and norgestimate). These potent progestins have no estrogenic effects and are less androgenic than levonorgestrel, and thus are thought to have fewer side effects (e.g., less likelihood or severity of acne). Drospirenone may also cause less weight gain compared with levonorgestrel.
- The progestin-only "minipills" tend to be less effective than combination OCs, and they are associated with irregular and unpredictable menstrual bleeding. They must be taken every day of the menstrual cycle at approximately the same time of day to maintain contraceptive efficacy. They are associated with more ectopic pregnancies than other hormonal contraceptives.
- In the "quick start" method for initiating OCs, the woman takes the first pill on the day of her office visit (after a negative urine pregnancy test). In the first-day start method, women take the first pill on the first day of the next menstrual cycle. The Sunday start method was used for many years, whereby the first pill was taken on the first Sunday after starting the menstrual cycle.
- Specific instructions should be provided about what to do if a pill is missed. The WHO's Selected Practice Recommendations for Contraceptive Use can be used for guidance.

CHOICE OF AN ORAL CONTRACEPTIVE

- In women without coexisting medical conditions, an OC containing ≤35 mcg of EE and <0.5 mg of norethindrone is recommended.
- Adolescents, underweight women (<50 kg [110 lb]), women older than 35 years, and those who are perimenopausal may have fewer side effects

with OCs containing 20 to 25 mcg of EE. However, these low-estrogen OCs are associated with more breakthrough bleeding and an increased risk of contraceptive failure if doses are missed.

- Overweight and obese women may have higher contraceptive failure rates with low-dose OCs and may benefit from pills containing at least 35 mcg of EE.
- Women with migraine headaches, history of thromboembolic disease, heart disease, cerebrovascular disease, and SLE with vascular disease are good candidates for progestin-only methods (e.g., minipills, **depot medroxyprogesterone acetate [DMPA]**, and the levonorgestrel intrauterine system). Also, women with a history of estrogen-dependent cancer, smokers over the age of 35, and those who are postpartum and/or breast-feeding should use progestin only or nonhormonal methods.

MANAGING SIDE EFFECTS

- Many symptoms occurring in the first cycle of OC use (e.g., breakthrough bleeding, nausea, and bloating), improve by the second or third cycle of use. Table 30–3 shows side effects of CHCs and their management.
- Table 30–5 shows symptoms of a serious or potentially serious nature associated with CHC.
- Women should be instructed to immediately discontinue CHCs if they experience warning signs referred to by the mnemonic ACHES (*a*bdominal pain, *c*hest pain, *h*eadaches, *e*ye problems, and *s*evere leg pain).

TABLE 30–5	Serious Symptoms That May Be Associated with Combined Hormonal Contraception	
Serious Symptoms	**Possible Underlying Problem**
Blurred vision, diplopia, flashing lights, blindness, papilledema	Stroke, hypertension, temporary vascular problem of many possible sites, retinal artery thrombosis
Numbness, weakness, tingling in extremities, slurred speech	Hemorrhagic or thrombotic stroke
Migraine headaches	Vascular spasm, stroke
Breast mass, pain, or swelling	Breast cancer
Chest pain (radiating to left arm or neck), shortness of breath, coughing up blood	Pulmonary embolism, myocardial infarction
Abdominal pain, hepatic mass or tenderness, jaundice, pruritus	Gallbladder disease, hepatic adenoma, pancreatitis, thrombosis of abdominal artery or vein
Excessive spotting, breakthrough bleeding	Endometrial, cervical, or vaginal cancer
Severe leg pain (calf, thigh), tenderness, swelling, warmth	Deep-vein thrombosis

Data from Hatcher RA, Nelson AL. Contraceptive Technology, 19th ed. New York: Ardent Media, 2007; and Dickey RP. Managing Contraceptive Pill Patients, 13th ed. Dallas, TX: EMIS Inc., 2007.

DRUG INTERACTIONS

- Women should be told to use an alternative method of contraception if there is a possibility of a drug interaction compromising OC efficacy.
- Rifampin reduces the efficacy of OCs.
- Case reports have shown a reduction in EE levels when CHCs are taken with tetracyclines and penicillin derivatives. The Council on Scientific Affairs of the American Medical Association recommends that women be informed about the small risk of interactions with antibiotics, and, if desired, appropriate additional nonhormonal contraceptive agents should be considered. Women who develop breakthrough bleeding during concomitant use of antibiotics and CHCs should be told to use an alternate method of contraception during the period of concomitant use.
- **Phenobarbital, carbamazepine,** and **phenytoin** potentially reduce the efficacy of OCs, and many anticonvulsants are known teratogens. Intrauterine devices (IUDs), injectable medroxyprogesterone, implants, or nonhormonal options may be considered for women taking these drugs.

DISCONTINUATION OF THE ORAL CONTRACEPTIVE, RETURN OF FERTILITY

- Traditionally, women are advised to allow two or three normal menstrual periods after discontinuing CHCs before becoming pregnant. However, in several large cohort and case-controlled studies, infants conceived in the first month after an OC was discontinued had no greater chance of miscarriage or a birth defect than those born in the general population. The average delay in ovulation after discontinuing OCs is 1 to 2 weeks.

EMERGENCY CONTRACEPTION

- A progestin-only formulation containing levonorgestrel (available in **Plan B, Plan B One-Step,** and **Next Choice**) is approved for emergency contraception in the United States.
- Plan B and Next Choice comprise two tablets, each containing 0.75 mg levonorgestrel. The first tablet is to be taken within 72 hours of unprotected intercourse (the sooner, the more effective); the second dose is taken 12 hours later. Plan B One-Step contains one tablet of 1.5 mg levonorgestrel taken within 72 hours of unprotected intercourse. Plan B is available without a prescription for women at least 17 years old and for those younger than 17 years old by prescription. It is sold only in pharmacies and must be kept behind the counter.
- CHCs and progestin-only products can be used for emergency contraception, and the FDA has approved a long list of products and specific regimens for such use.
- Common side effects, specifically, nausea and vomiting, occur significantly less often with progestin-only emergency contraception.

TRANSDERMAL CONTRACEPTIVES

- A combination contraceptive is available as a transdermal patch (**Ortho Evra**), which may have improved adherence compared with OCs. Efficacy seems to be compromised in women >90 kg (198 lb). The patch should be applied to the abdomen, buttocks, upper torso, or upper arm at the beginning of the menstrual cycle and replaced every week for 3 weeks.

- Women using the patch are exposed to ~60% more estrogen than if they were taking an OC containing 35 mg of EE, but controversy exists correlating the increased exposure to increased risk of thromboembolism or cardiovascular or cerebrovascular events.

CONTRACEPTIVE RINGS

- The first vaginal ring (**NuvaRing**) releases ~15 mcg/day of EE and 120 mcg/day of etonogestrel over a 3-week period. On first use, the ring should be inserted on or prior to the fifth day of the cycle, remain in place for 3 weeks, then be removed. One week should lapse before the new ring is inserted on the same day of the week as it was for the last cycle. A second form of contraception should be used for the first 7 days of ring use or if the ring has been expelled for more than 3 hours.

LONG-ACTING INJECTABLE AND IMPLANTABLE CONTRACEPTIVES

- Women who particularly benefit from progestin-only methods, including minipills, are those who are breast-feeding, those who are intolerant to estrogens, and those with concomitant medical conditions in which estrogen is not recommended. Injectable and implantable contraceptives are also beneficial for women with compliance issues.
- Pregnancy failure rates with long-acting progestin contraception are comparable to that of female sterilization.

Injectable Progestins

- **DMPA** 150 mg administered by deep intramuscular injection in the gluteal or deltoid muscle within 5 days of the onset of menstrual bleeding inhibits ovulation for more than 3 months, and the dose should be repeated every 12 weeks to ensure continuous contraception. A new formulation contains 104 mg of DMPA (Depo-SubQ Provera 104), which is injected subcutaneously into the thigh or abdomen. The manufacturer recommends excluding pregnancy in women more than 1 week late for repeat injection of the intramuscular formulation or 2 weeks late for repeat injection of the subcutaneous formulation.
- DMPA can be given immediately postpartum in women who are not breast-feeding, but in women who are breast-feeding, it should not be given until 6 weeks postpartum.
- Women using DMPA have a lower incidence of *Candida* vulvovaginitis, ectopic pregnancy, pelvic inflammatory disease, and endometrial and ovarian cancer compared with women using no contraception. The median time to conception from the first omitted dose is 10 months.
- The most frequent adverse effect of DMPA is menstrual irregularities, which decrease after the first year. Breast tenderness, weight gain, and depression occur less frequently.
- DMPA has been associated with a reduction in bone mineral density (BMD), but it has not been associated with the development of osteoporosis or fractures. Recent evidence suggests that BMD loss may slow after

1 to 2 years of DMPA use, and effects on BMD may not be completely reversible when DMPA is discontinued.

- DMPA should be continued for more than 2 years only if other contraceptive methods are inadequate.

Subdermal Progestin Implants

- **Implanon** is a single, 4 cm implant, containing 68 mg of etonogestrel that is placed under the skin of the upper arm. It releases 60 mcg daily for the first month, decreasing gradually to 30 mcg/daily at the end of the 3 years of recommended use. With perfect use, efficacy approaches 100%, but it may be less in women weighing >130% of their ideal body weight.
- The major adverse effect is irregular menstrual bleeding. Other side effects are headache, vaginitis, weight gain, acne, and breast and abdominal pain. Implanon does not appear to decrease BMD.
- As fertility returns soon after removal, and because Implanon does not affect bone health, it may be preferred over DMPA.

INTRAUTERINE DEVICES

- IUDs cause low-grade intrauterine inflammation and increased prostaglandin formation. In addition, endometrial suppression is caused by progestin-releasing IUDs. They are spermicidal and also interfere with implantation of the fertilized ovum. Efficacy rates are >99% with both perfect use and typical use.
- The risk of pelvic inflammatory disease among users ranges from 1% to 2.5%; the risk is highest during the first 20 days after the insertion procedure.
- Ideal patients for an IUD are nulligravid women who are monogamous and are not at risk for STDs or pelvic inflammatory disease.
- **ParaGard** (copper) can be left in place for 10 years. A disadvantage of ParaGard is increased menstrual blood flow and dysmenorrhea. The average monthly blood loss increased by 35% in clinical trials.
- **Mirena** releases levonorgestrel over 5 years. It causes a reduction in menstrual blood loss.

EVALUATION OF THERAPEUTIC OUTCOMES

- All CHC users should have at least annual blood pressure monitoring.
- Glucose levels should be monitored closely when CHCs are started or stopped in patients with a history of glucose intolerance or diabetes mellitus.
- Contraceptive users should have at least annual cytologic screening (more often if they are at risk for STDs), and they should also be regularly evaluated for problems that may relate to the CHCs (e.g., breakthrough bleeding, amenorrhea, weight gain, and acne).
- Women using Implanon should be monitored annually for menstrual cycle disturbances, weight gain, local inflammation or infection at the implant site, acne, breast tenderness, headaches, and hair loss.

- Women using DMPA should be evaluated every 3 months for weight gain, menstrual cycle disturbances, and STD risks.
- Patients on DMPA should be weighed, have their blood pressure monitored, and have a physical examination, Papanicolaou smear, and a mammogram yearly as indicated based on the patient's age.

See Chapter 88, Contraception, authored by Sarah P. Shrader, Kelly R. Ragucci, and Vanessa A. Diaz, for a more detailed discussion of this topic.

CHAPTER 31

Menopause & Perimenopausal & Postmenopausal Hormone Therapy

DEFINITION

- Menopause is the permanent cessation of menses following the loss of ovarian follicular activity. Perimenopause is the period immediately prior to menopause and the first year after menopause.

PHYSIOLOGY

- The hypothalamic-pituitary-ovarian axis controls reproductive physiology through the reproductive years. Follicle-stimulating hormone (FSH) and luteinizing hormone, produced by the pituitary in response to gonadotropin-releasing hormone from the hypothalamus, regulate ovarian function. Gonadotropins are also influenced by negative feedback from the sex steroids estradiol (produced by the dominant follicle) and progesterone (produced by the corpus luteum). Other sex steroids are androgens, primarily testosterone and androstenedione, secreted by the ovarian stroma and the adrenal gland.
- Pathophysiologic changes associated with menopause are caused by loss of ovarian follicular activity. The postmenopausal ovary is no longer the primary site of estradiol or progesterone synthesis.
- As women age, circulating FSH progressively rises, and ovarian inhibin declines. When ovarian function has ceased, serum FSH concentrations are greater than 40 international units/L. Menopause is characterized by a 10- to 15-fold increase in circulating FSH concentrations compared with concentrations of FSH in the follicular phase, a four- to fivefold increase in luteinizing hormone, and a >90% decrease in circulating estradiol concentrations.

CLINICAL PRESENTATION

- Vasomotor symptoms (e.g., hot flushes and night sweats) are common short-term symptoms of estrogen withdrawal, which usually disappear within 1 to 2 years but sometimes persist for 20 years.
- Other symptoms of perimenopause and menopause are vaginal dryness, dyspareunia, urogenital atrophy, sleep disturbances, sexual dysfunction, and impaired concentration and memory.
- Other symptoms, including anxiety, mood swings, depression, insomnia, migraine, arthralgia, and urinary frequency, are attributed to menopause, but the relationship between these symptoms and estrogen deficiency is controversial.
- Long-term morbidity associated with menopause includes accelerated bone loss and osteoporosis (see Chap. 3, Osteoporosis).
- Dysfunctional uterine bleeding may occur during perimenopause.

DIAGNOSIS

- Menopause is determined retrospectively after 12 consecutive months of amenorrhea. FSH on day 2 or 3 of the menstrual cycle greater than 10 to 12 international units/L suggests the presence of perimenopause.
- The diagnosis of menopause should include a comprehensive medical history and physical examination, complete blood count, and measurement of serum FSH. When ovarian function has ceased, serum FSH concentrations exceed 40 international units/L. Altered thyroid function and pregnancy must be excluded.

TREATMENT

- Mild vasomotor and/or vaginal symptoms can often be alleviated by lifestyle modification, weight control, smoking cessation, exercise, and a healthy diet.
- Mild vaginal dryness can sometimes be relieved by nonestrogenic vaginal creams, but significant vaginal dryness often requires local or systemic estrogen therapy.
- Little evidence supports the use of nonprescription herbal remedies or soy-based supplements.
- Fig. 31–1 outlines the approach for women with menopausal symptoms requiring pharmacologic treatment.
- Hormone therapy is contraindicated in women with endometrial cancer, breast cancer, undiagnosed vaginal bleeding, coronary heart disease, thromboembolism, stroke or transient ischemic attack, and active liver disease. Relative contraindications are uterine leiomyoma, migraine headaches, and seizure disorder.
- For women with hypertriglyceridemia, liver disease, or gallbladder disease, transdermal estrogen can be used, but oral estrogen should be avoided.
- When hormone therapy is used, it should be used at the lowest effective dose and for the shortest duration needed for symptom control.
- Approved indications for hormone therapy are vasomotor symptoms, urogenital atrophy, and prevention of osteoporosis. For the latter, **raloxifene** and **bisphosphonates** are considered first.
- As new data are continuously published, the most current guidelines should always be consulted.

HORMONE THERAPY

- Hormone therapy is the most effective treatment option for vasomotor and vaginal symptoms. In women with an intact uterus, hormone therapy consists of an estrogen plus a progestogen. In women who have undergone hysterectomy, estrogen therapy is given unopposed by a progestogen.
- The **continuous combined oral estrogen–progestogen** arm of the Women's Health Initiative (WHI) study was terminated early after a mean of 5.2-year follow-up because of the occurrence of a prespecified level of

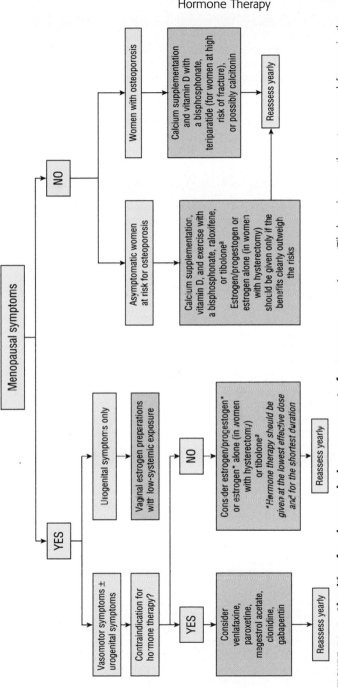

FIGURE 31–1. Algorithm for pharmacologic management of menopause symptoms. [a]Tibolone is currently not approved for use in the United States.

invasive breast cancer. The study also found increased coronary disease events, stroke, and pulmonary embolism. Beneficial effects included decreases in hip fracture and colorectal cancer.

- The oral estrogen-alone arm was stopped early after a mean of 7 year follow-up. Estrogen-only therapy had no effect on coronary heart disease risk and caused no increase in breast cancer risk, but the risk of stroke and hip fracture was increased.

- A subsequent large epidemiologic study found a greater risk for breast cancer with combined estrogen–progestogen use, as well as increased risk for estrogen-only therapy, but selection bias was found in the study population.

Estrogens

- Preparations suitable for replacement therapy are shown in **Table 31–1**. The oral and transdermal routes are used most frequently. There is no evidence that one estrogen compound is more effective than another in relieving menopausal symptoms or preventing osteoporosis.

- **Conjugated equine estrogens** are composed of **estrone sulfate** (50–60%) and other estrogens such as **equilin** and 17 α-**dihydroequilin**.

- **Estradiol** is the predominant and most active form of endogenous estrogens. Given orally, it is metabolized by intestinal mucosa and liver (10% reaches the circulation as free estradiol), and resultant estrone concentrations are three to six times those of estradiol.

- **Ethinyl estradiol** is a semisynthetic estrogen that has similar activity following administration by the oral and parenteral routes.

- **Parenteral estrogens**, including transdermal, intranasal, and vaginal, avoid first-pass metabolism and result in a more physiologic estradiol:estrone ratio (i.e., estradiol concentrations greater than estrone concentrations). These routes also are less likely to affect sex hormone–binding globulin, circulating lipids, coagulation parameters, or C-reactive protein levels.

- Variability in absorption is common with the **percutaneous preparations** (gels, creams, and emulsions).

- **Estradiol pellets** (implants available in the United States) contain pure **crystalline 17 β-estradiol** and are placed subcutaneously into the anterior abdominal wall or buttock. They are difficult to remove.

- **Vaginal creams, tablets,** and **rings** are used for treatment of urogenital atrophy. Systemic estrogen absorption is lower with the vaginal tablets and rings, compared with the vaginal creams.

- New evidence indicates that lower doses of estrogens are effective in controlling postmenopausal symptoms and reducing bone loss (**Table 31–2**). Even ultralow doses of 17 β-estradiol delivered by vaginal ring improved serum lipid profiles and prevented bone loss in elderly women.

- Adverse effects of **estrogen** include nausea, headache, breast tenderness, and heavy bleeding. More serious adverse effects include increased risk for coronary heart disease, stroke, venous thromboembolism, breast cancer, and gallbladder disease. Transdermal estrogen is less likely than oral estrogen to cause nausea, headache, breast tenderness, gallbladder disease, and deep vein thrombosis.

TABLE 31–1 Systemic and Topical Estrogen Products[a,b,c]

Estrogen	Dosage Strength	Comments
Oral estrogens		
Conjugated equine estrogens (Premarin)	0.3, 0.45, 0.625, 0.9, 1.25 mg	Orally administered estrogens stimulate
Synthetic conjugated estrogens (Cenestin, Enjuvia)	0.3, 0.45, 0.625, 0.9, 1.25 mg	synthesis of hepatic proteins and
Esterified estrogens (Menest)	0.3, 0.625, 1.25, 2.5 mg	increase circulating
Estropipate (piperazine estrone sulfate) (Ogen, Ortho-Est, generics)	0.625, 1.25, 2.5, 5[d] mg	concentrations of sex hormone-binding
Micronized 17 β-estradiol (Estrace, generics)	0.5, 1,1.5[d], 2 mg	globulin, which, in turn, may compromise
Estradiol acetate (Femtrace)	0.45, 0.9, 1.8 mg	the bioavailability of androgens and estrogens
Transdermal estrogens[e]		
17β-estradiol transdermal patch (Alora, Climara, Esclim, Menostar, Vivelle, Vivelle Dot, generics)	14, 25, 37.5, 50, 60, 75, 100 mcg per 24 hours	Administered once or twice weekly depending on product
Topical estrogens[e]		
17β-estradiol topical emulsion (Estrasorb)	4.35 mg of estradiol hemihydrate per foil-laminated pouch	Single approved dose is 8.7 mg of estradiol hemihydrate per day (two pouches), which delivers 0.05 mg of estradiol per day. Apply to legs.
17β-estradiol topical gel (EsroGel, Elestrin, Divigel)	0.25 to 1 mg of estradiol per dose	Apply to either arm or thigh (depending on product) once daily
17β-estradiol transdermal spray (Evamist)	1.53 mg of estradiol per spray	1–3 sprays on inner surface of forearm once daily
Vaginal estrogens[e]		
Conjugated equine estrogens vaginal cream (Premarin)	0.625 mg conjugated equine estrogens per g	0.5–2 g per day
17β-estradiol vaginal cream (Estrace)	0.1 mg of estradiol per g	Maintenance dose is 1 g per day
17β-estradiol vaginal ring (Estring)	0.0075 mg per 24 hours	Replaced every 90 days
Estradiol acetate vaginal ring (Femring)	0.05, 0.1 mg per 24 hours	Replaced every 90 days
Estradiol hemihydrate vaginal tablet (Vagifem)	0.01, 0.025 mcg estradiol per tablet	Maintenance dose is 1 tablet twice weekly

[a]Systemic oral and transdermal estrogen and progestogen combination products are available in the United States.
[b]Systemic oral estrogen and androgen combination products are available in the United States.
[c]U.S. brand names.
[d]Not available in the United States.
[e]Women with elevated triglyceride concentrations or significant liver function abnormalities are candidates for non-oral estrogen therapy.

TABLE 31–2	Systemic Estrogen Products for Treatment of Menopausal Symptoms			
Regimen	**Standard Dose**	**Low Dose**	**Route**	**Frequency**
Conjugated equine estrogens	0.625 mg	0.3 or 0.45 mg	Oral	Once daily
Synthetic conjugated estrogens	0.625 mg	0.3 mg	Oral	Once daily
Esterified estrogens	0.625 mg	0.3 mg	Oral	Once daily
Estropipate (piperazine estrone sulfate)	1.25 mg	0.625 mg	Oral	Once daily
Estradiol acetate	0.9 mg	0.45 mg	Oral	Once daily
Micronized 17β-estradiol	1–2 mg	0.25–0.5 mg	Oral	Once daily
Transdermal 17β-estradiol patch	50 mcg	25 mcg	Transdermal	Once or twice weekly
Implanted 17β-estradiol[a]	50–100 mg pellets	25 mg pellets	Pellets implanted subcutaneously	Every 6 months
17β-estradiol topical emulsion	2 pouches	–	Topical	Once daily
17β-estradiol topical gel	0.5–0.75 mg (depends on product)	Depends on product	Topical	Once daily
17β-estradiol transdermal spray	2–3 sprays	1 spray	Topical	Once daily
Estradiol acetate vaginal ring	12.4 mg ring (delivers 0.05 mg per day)	–	Intravaginally	Every 3 months

[a]Not available in the United States.

Progestogens

- In women who have not undergone hysterectomy, a **progestogen** should be added because estrogen monotherapy is associated with endometrial hyperplasia and cancer.
- The most commonly used oral progestogens are **medroxyprogesterone acetate, micronized progesterone,** and **norethisterone acetate**.
- Several progestogen regimens to prevent endometrial hyperplasia are shown in **Table 31–3**.
- Four **combination estrogen and progestogen** regimens are shown in **Table 31–4**.
  - ✓ Continuous-cyclic (sequential): results in scheduled vaginal withdrawal bleeding in ~90% of women, but it may be scant or absent in older women.

TABLE 31–3	Progestogen Doses for Endometrial Protection (Oral Cyclic Administration)
Progestogen	**Dose**
Dydrogesterone[a]	10–20 mg for 12–14 days per calendar month
Medroxyprogesterone acetate	5–10 mg for 12–14 days per calendar month
Micronized progesterone	200 mg for 12–14 days per calendar month
Norethindrone (norethisterone)[b]	0.7–1 mg for 12–14 days per calendar month
Norethindrone acetate	5 mg for 12–14 days per calendar month
Norgestrel[c]	0.15 mg for 12–14 days per calendar month
Levonorgestrel[d]	150 mcg for 12–14 days per calendar month

[a]Not available in the United States.
[b]In the United States, available in a progestogen-only oral dosage form as 0.35 mg tablets approved for prevention of pregnancy.
[c]Not available in a progestogen-only oral dosage form in the United States.
[d]In the United States, available in a progestogen-only oral dosage form as 75 mcg tablets approved for emergency contraception.

✓ Continuous-combined: prevents monthly bleeding. It may initially cause unpredictable spotting or bleeding; thus, it is best reserved for women who are at least 2 years postmenopause.

✓ Continuous long-cycle (cyclic withdrawal): reduces monthly bleeding. Estrogen is given daily, and progestogen is given six times yearly (every other month) for 12 to 14 days, resulting in six periods per year.

TABLE 31–4	Common Combination Postmenopausal Hormone Therapy Regimens
Regimen	**Doses**
Oral continuous-cyclic regimens	
CEE + MPA[a]	0.625 mg + 5 mg; 0.625 mg + 10 mg
Oral continuous-combined regimens	
CEE + MPA	0.625 mg + 2.5 mg; 0.625 mg + 5 mg; 0.45 mg + 2.5 mg; 0.3 mg + 1.5 mg/day
17β-Estradiol + NETA	1 mg + 0.1 mg;1 mg + 0.25 mg; 1 mg + 0.5 mg/day
Ethinyl estradiol + NETA	1 mcg + 0.2 mg; 2.5 mcg + 0.5 mg; 5 mcg + 1 mg; 10 mcg + 1 mg/day
Transdermal continuous-cyclic regimens	
17β-Estradiol + NETA[a]	50 mcg + 0.14 mg; 50 mcg + 0.25 mg
Transdermal continuous-combined regimens	
17β-Estradiol + NETA	50 mcg + 0.14 mg; 50 mcg + 0.25 mg; 25 mcg + 0.125 mg

CEE, conjugated equine estrogens; MPA, medroxyprogesterone acetate; NETA, norethindrone acetate.
Other oral (drospirenone and norgestimate) and transdermal (levonorgestrel) progestogens also are available in combination with an estrogen.
[a]Estrogen alone for days 1–14, followed by estrogen–progestogen on days 15–28.

✓ Intermittent-combined (continuous-pulsed): prevents monthly bleeding. It consists of 3 days of estrogen therapy alone, followed by 3 days of combined estrogen and progestogen, which is then repeated without interruption. It causes fewer side effects than regimens with higher progestogen doses.

- Adverse effects of progestogens are irritability, depression, headache, mood swings, fluid retention, and sleep disturbance.
- Low-dose hormone therapy (**conjugated equine estrogen 0.45 mg and medroxyprogesterone acetate 1.5 mg/day**) has demonstrated equivalent symptom relief and bone density preservation without an increase in endometrial hyperplasia. Whether such lower doses will be safer (cause less venous thromboembolism and breast cancer) remains to be seen.

ALTERNATIVE DRUG TREATMENTS

- Alternatives to estrogen treatment of hot flashes are shown in **Table 31–5**.
- For women with contraindications to hormone therapy, selective serotonin reuptake inhibitors may be used, but the lack of long-term efficacy or drug interactions may be a problem.

TABLE 31–5	Alternatives to Estrogen for Treatment of Hot Flashes		
Drug	**Dose (Oral)**	**Interval**	**Comments**
Tibolone[a]	2.5–5 mg	Once daily	Tibolone is not recommended during the perimenopause because it may cause irregular bleeding
Venlafaxine	37.5–150 mg	Once daily	Side effects include dry mouth, decreased appetite, nausea, and constipation
Paroxetine	12.5–25 mg	Once daily	12.5 mg is an adequate, well-tolerated starting dose for most women; adverse effects include headache, nausea, and insomnia
Fluoxetine	20 mg	Once daily	Modest improvement seen in hot flushes
Megestrol acetate	20–40 mg	Once daily	Progesterone may be linked to breast cancer etiology; also, there is concern regarding the safety of progestational agents in women with preexisting breast cancer
Clonidine	0.1 mg	Once daily	Can be administered orally or transdermally; drowsiness and dry mouth can occur, especially with higher doses
Gabapentin	900 mg	Divided in 3 daily doses	Adverse effects include somnolence and dizziness; these symptoms often can be obviated with a gradual increase in dosing

[a]Not available in the United States.

TABLE 31–6	Androgen Regimens Used for Women		
Regimen	**Dose**	**Frequency**	**Route**
Methyltestosterone in combination with esterified estrogen	1.25–2.5 mg	Daily	Oral
Mixed testosterone esters	50–100 mg	Every 4–6 weeks	Intramuscular
Testosterone pellets	50 mg	Every 6 months	Subcutaneous (implanted)
Transdermal testosterone system[a]	150–300 mcg/day	Every 3–4 days	Transdermal patch
Nandrolone decanoate	50 mg	Every 8–12 weeks	Intramuscular

[a]Undergoing clinical trials in the United States.

Androgens

- The therapeutic use of **testosterone** in women, although controversial, is becoming more widespread, even in the absence of an androgen deficiency. Evidence from several studies shows that testosterone, with or without estrogen, improves the quality of the sexual experience in postmenopausal women.
- Androgen regimens are shown in **Table 31–6**.
- Absolute contraindications to androgen therapy include pregnancy or lactation and known or suspected androgen-dependent neoplasia. Relative contraindications are concurrent use of conjugated equine estrogens (for parenteral testosterone therapy), low sex hormone–binding globulin level, moderate to severe acne, clinical hirsutism, and androgenic alopecia.
- Adverse effects from excessive dosage include virilization, fluid retention, and potentially adverse lipoprotein lipid effects, which are more likely with oral administration. Further study is required to determine the long-term safety of testosterone in women.

SELECTIVE ESTROGEN–RECEPTOR MODULATORS

- These are nonsteroidal compounds that act as estrogen agonists in some tissues such as bone and as estrogen antagonists in other tissues such as breast through high-affinity binding to the estrogen receptor.
- **Tamoxifen** is an antagonist in breast tissue and an agonist on bone and endometrium (see Chap. 62).
- **Raloxifene** is approved for prevention of osteoporosis and reduction of risk of invasive breast cancer in postmenopausal women with osteoporosis. The dose is 60 mg once daily. Raloxifene may worsen vasomotor symptoms, and it increases the risk of venous thromboembolism and fatal stroke (see Chap. 3).

TIBOLONE

- **Tibolone** has combined estrogenic, progestogenic, and androgenic activity. Its effects depend on metabolism and activation in peripheral tissues.

Tibolone has beneficial effects on mood and libido and improves menopausal symptoms and vaginal atrophy. It protects against bone loss and reduces the risk of vertebral fractures. It reduces total cholesterol, triglyceride, lipoprotein (a), and, unfortunately, high-density lipoprotein concentrations. It may increase stroke risk and endometrial cancer risk. It may decrease the risk of breast and colon cancer in women ages 60 to 85 years.

- Major adverse effects include weight gain and bloating. Tibolone may increase the risk of stroke in elderly women.

BENEFITS OF HORMONE THERAPY

- Most women with vasomotor symptoms need hormone treatment for less than 5 years. Without treatment, hot flushes usually disappear within 1 to 2 years. Hormone therapy can usually be tapered and stopped after about 2 or 3 years.
- **Estrogen** is more effective than any other therapy in relieving vasomotor symptoms, and all types and routes of systemic administration are equally effective in a dose-dependent fashion. If treatment can be tapered and stopped within 5 years, no evidence of increased risk of breast cancer is seen.
- Most women with significant vaginal dryness because of vaginal atrophy require local or systemic estrogen therapy. It can be treated with topical estrogen cream, tablets, or the vaginal ring. Vaginal estrogen appears to be better than systemic estrogen for these symptoms and avoids high levels of circulating estrogen.
- Concomitant progestogen therapy generally is unnecessary with **low-dose micronized 17 β-estradiol**, but regular use of **conjugated equine estrogen creams** and other products that may promote endometrial proliferation in women with an intact uterus requires intermittent progestogen challenges (i.e., for 10 days every 12 weeks).
- The benefits of hormone therapies for osteoporosis prevention are discussed in Chap. 3. Hormone therapy should be considered for osteoporosis prevention only in women at significant risk for osteoporosis who cannot take nonestrogen regimens, such as bisphosphonates.
- The WHI study was the first randomized, controlled trial to confirm that hormone therapy reduces the risk of colon cancer.

RISKS OF HORMONE THERAPY

- The American Heart Association recommends against postmenopausal hormone therapy for reducing the risk of coronary heart disease.
- The WHI trial showed an overall increase in the risk of coronary heart disease in healthy postmenopausal women ages 50 to 79 years taking **estrogen–progestogen therapy** compared with those taking placebo. The estrogen-alone arm of the WHI showed no effect (either increase or decrease) in the risk of coronary heart disease. Recent analysis showed that women who started hormone therapy 10 years or more after the time of menopause tended to have increased coronary heart disease risk compared with women who started therapy within 10 years of menopause.

- In the estrogen plus progestogen arm, the increased risk for ischemic stroke and venous thromboembolism continued throughout the 5 years of therapy. In the estrogen-alone arm, there was a similar increase in risk for stroke.

- In the WHI study, **estrogen plus progestogen therapy** had an increased risk for invasive breast cancer, which did not appear until after 3 years of study participation. The estrogen-only arm of the WHI showed no increase in risk for breast cancer during the 7-year follow-up.

- The Million Women Study reported that current use of hormone therapy increased breast cancer risk and breast cancer mortality. Increased incidence was observed for **estrogen only, estrogen plus progestogen,** and **tibolone.**

- In a reanalysis of 51 studies, less than 5 years of therapy with **combined estrogen and progestogen** was associated with a 15% increase in risk for breast cancer, and the risk increased with greater duration of treatment. Five years after discontinuation of hormone replacement therapy, the risk of breast cancer was no longer increased.

- The addition of progestogen to estrogen may increase breast cancer risk beyond that observed with estrogen alone.

- **Estrogen alone** given to women with an intact uterus increases uterine cancer risk; this increased risk begins within 2 years of treatment and persists for many years after estrogen is discontinued. The sequential addition of **progestin** to estrogen for at least 10 days of the cycle or continuous combined estrogen–progestogen does not increase the risk of endometrial cancer. A 4-year trial of **raloxifene** in women with osteoporosis showed no increased risk of endometrial cancer.

- **Combined hormone therapy** and estrogen monotherapy may increase the risk of ovarian cancer.

- Women taking **combined estrogen–progestogen hormone therapy** have a twofold increase in the risk for thromboembolic events, with the highest risk occurring in the first year of use. The increased risk is dose dependent. Oral administration increases the risk compared with transdermal administration.

- Women taking **estrogen** or **combined estrogen–progestogen** hormone therapy are at increased risk for cholecystitis, cholelithiasis, and cholecystectomy. Transdermal estrogen is an alternative to oral therapy for women at high risk for cholelithiasis.

OTHER EFFECTS OF HORMONE THERAPY

- Women with vasomotor symptoms taking hormone therapy have better mental health and fewer depressive symptoms compared with those taking placebo, but hormone therapy may worsen quality of life in women without vasomotor symptoms.

- The WHI study found that postmenopausal women 65 years or older taking **estrogen plus progestogen** therapy had twice the rate of dementia, including Alzheimer disease. Combined therapy also did not prevent mild cognitive impairment.

EVALUATION OF THERAPEUTIC OUTCOMES

- After initiating hormone therapy, follow-up at 6 weeks is advisable to assess for efficacy, side effects, and patterns of withdrawal bleeding.
- With estrogen-based therapy, there should be yearly breast exams, monthly breast self-examinations, and periodic mammograms. Women on hormone therapy should undergo annual monitoring, including pelvic examination, blood pressure checks, and routine endometrial cancer surveillance.
- Bone mineral density should be measured in women older than 65 years and in women younger than 65 years with risk factors for osteoporosis. Repeat testing should be done as clinically indicated.

See Chapter 91, Hormone Therapy in Women, authored by Sophia N. Kalantaridou, Devra K. Dang, Susan R. Davis, and Karim Anton Calis, for a more detailed discussion of this topic.

CHAPTER 32

Pregnancy and Lactation: Therapeutic Considerations

DEFINITION

- Therapeutic considerations associated with pregnancy and lactation encompass many complex issues that affect both the mother and her child, from planning for pregnancy through lactation. Resources on the use of drugs in pregnancy and lactation include the FDA categorization system, the primary literature, tertiary compendia, textbooks, and computerized databases (e.g., *www.motherisk.org* and *www.toxnet.nlm.nih.gov*).

PHYSIOLOGIC AND PHARMACOKINETIC FACTORS

- The duration of pregnancy is ~280 days; this time period extends from the first day of the last menstrual period to birth. Pregnancy is divided into three periods of 3 calendar months; each 3-month period is called a trimester.
- Drug absorption during pregnancy may be altered by delayed gastric emptying and vomiting. An increased gastric pH may affect absorption of weak acids and bases. Higher estrogen and progesterone levels may alter liver enzyme activity and increase elimination of some drugs but cause accumulation of others.
- Maternal plasma volume, cardiac output, and glomerular filtration increase by 30% to 50% or higher during pregnancy, possibly lowering the plasma concentration of renally cleared drugs. Body fat increases; thus, volume of distribution of fat-soluble drugs may increase. Plasma albumin concentrations decrease; thus, volume of distribution of highly protein-bound drugs may increase. However, there may be little change in serum concentration, as these unbound drugs are more rapidly cleared by the liver and kidneys.
- The placenta is the organ of exchange between the mother and fetus for a number of substances, including drugs. Drug molecular weights affect drug transfer across the placenta:
  - ✓ Molecular weights >500 daltons (D) cross readily.
  - ✓ Molecular weights from 600 to 1,000 D cross more slowly.
  - ✓ Molecular weights >1,000 D (e.g., insulin and heparin) do not cross in significant amounts.
- Lipophilic drugs (e.g., opiates and antibiotics) cross more easily than do water-soluble drugs. Certain protein-bound drugs may achieve higher plasma concentrations in the fetus than in the mother.

DRUG SELECTION DURING PREGNANCY

- The incidence of congenital malformation is ~3% to 5%, and it is estimated that 1% of all birth defects are caused by medication exposure.
- Adverse fetal drug effects depend on dosage, route of administration, concomitant exposure to other agents, and stage of pregnancy when the exposure occurred.

- Exposure to the fetus in the first 2 weeks after conception may have an "all or nothing" effect (i.e., could destroy the embryo or have no ill effect). Exposure during the period of organogenesis (18–60 days postconception) may result in structural anomalies (e.g., **methotrexate, cyclophosphamide, diethylstilbestrol, lithium, retinoids, thalidomide,** certain **antiepileptic drugs,** and **coumarin derivatives**).
- Exposure after this point may result in growth retardation, central nervous system (CNS) or other abnormalities, or death. **Nonsteroidal antiinflammatory drugs (NSAIDs)** and **tetracycline derivatives** are more likely to exhibit effects in the second or third trimester.
- Principles for selecting medications for use during pregnancy include
  ✓ Select drugs that have been used safely for long periods of time.
  ✓ Prescribe doses at the lower end of the dosing range.
  ✓ Eliminate nonessential medication and discourage self-medication.
  ✓ Avoid medications known to be harmful.

PRECONCEPTION PLANNING

- Preconception interventions have been shown to improve pregnancy outcomes.
- Neural tube defects occur within the first month of conception. Ingestion of **folic acid** by all women of childbearing potential should be encouraged, as it reduces the risk for neural tube defects in offspring. Women at low risk should take 400 mcg/day throughout the reproductive years. Women at high risk (e.g., those who take certain seizure medications or who have had a previously affected pregnancy) should take 4 mg/day.
- Assessment and reduction in the use of alcohol, tobacco, and other substances prior to pregnancy improve outcomes. For smoking cessation, behavioral interventions are preferred. If **nicotine replacement therapy** is used, intermittent delivery formulations are preferred over the patches. If patches are used, 16-hour patches are preferred over 24-hour patches.

PREGNANCY-INFLUENCED ISSUES

GASTROINTESTINAL TRACT

Constipation

- Constipation commonly occurs during pregnancy. Nondrug modalities such as education, physical exercise, biofeedback, and increased intake of dietary fiber and fluid should be instituted first.
- If additional therapy is warranted, the use of **supplemental fiber** and/or a stool softener is appropriate. **Polyethylene glycol, lactulose, sorbitol, bisacodyl,** or **senna** can be used occasionally.
- **Castor oil** and **mineral oil** should be avoided.

Gastroesophageal Reflux Disease

- Therapy includes lifestyle and dietary modifications, such as small, frequent meals; alcohol, tobacco, and caffeine avoidance; food avoidance 3 hours before bedtime; and elevation of the head of the bed.

- Drug therapy, if necessary, may be initiated with **aluminum, calcium,** or **magnesium antacids; sucralfate;** or **cimetidine** or **ranitidine**. Proton pump inhibitors and **metoclopramide** are also options if the patient does not respond to histamine$_2$-receptor blockers.
- **Sodium bicarbonate** and **magnesium trisilicate** should be avoided.

Hemorrhoids

- Hemorrhoids during pregnancy are common.
- Therapy includes high intake of dietary fiber, adequate oral fluid intake, and use of sitz baths; topical anesthetics, skin protectants, and astringents may also be used. Treatment for refractory hemorrhoids includes rubber band ligation, sclerotherapy, and surgery.

Nausea and Vomiting

- Up to 90% of all pregnant women experience some degree of nausea and vomiting. Hyperemesis gravidarum (i.e., severe nausea and vomiting causing weight loss >5% of prepregnancy weight and ketonuria) occurs in only ~1% to 3% of pregnant women.
- Nonpharmacologic treatments include eating small, frequent meals; avoiding fatty foods; acupressure; and acustimulation. Pharmacotherapy may include the following: antihistamines (e.g., **doxylamine**), **multivitamins, pyridoxine, anticholinergics** (e.g., **dicyclomine**), and **dopamine antagonists** (e.g., **metoclopramide**). **Ondansetron** can be used when other agents have failed, and **ginger** is considered safe and effective. **Dexamethasone** and **prednisolone** have been effective for hyperemesis gravidarum, but the risk of oral clefts is increased.

GESTATIONAL DIABETES MELLITUS

- Groups at high risk for gestational diabetes mellitus (GDM) are African Americans, Native Americans, Asian Americans, Hispanic Americans, and Pacific Islanders.
- First-line therapy for all women with GDM includes dietary modification and caloric restrictions for obese women. Daily self-monitoring of blood glucose is required in these women. If nutritional intervention fails to achieve fasting plasma glucose levels <90 to 99 mg/dL (5–5.5 mmol/L), 1-hour postprandial plasma glucose concentrations ≤140 mg/dL (7.8 mmol/L), or 2-hour postprandial levels <120 to 127 mg/dL (6.7–7 mmol/L), then therapy with **recombinant human insulin** should be instituted; **glyburide** may be considered an alternative. Metformin may also be considered, but it crosses the placenta and is less studied.
- Goals for self-monitored blood glucose levels while on insulin therapy are a preprandial plasma glucose level between 80 and 110 mg/dL (4.4–6.1 mmol/L), and a 2-hour postprandial plasma glucose level <155 mg/dL (8.6 mmol/L).

HYPERTENSION

- Hypertension during pregnancy includes gestational hypertension (pregnancy-induced hypertension without proteinuria), preeclampsia (hypertension with proteinuria), and chronic hypertension (diagnosed prior to pregnancy with or without overlying preeclampsia). Eclampsia, a medical emergency, is preeclampsia with seizures.

- For women at risk for preeclampsia, low-dose **aspirin** (75–81 mg/day) after 12 weeks' gestation reduces the risk for preeclampsia by 17%. Aspirin also reduces the risk of preterm birth by 8% and fetal and neonatal death by 14%. **Calcium**, 1 g/day, is recommended for all pregnant women, as it may help prevent hypertension and reduces the risk of preeclampsia by 31% to 67%.

- Antihypertensive drug therapy for mild to moderate hypertension in pregnancy has not been shown to improve pregnancy outcomes, except in the case of hypertensive crisis. Drug therapy is indicated for women with blood pressure ≥160/110 mm Hg. Commonly used drugs for hypertension in pregnancy include **methyldopa, labetalol,** and calcium channel blockers. Angiotensin-converting enzyme (ACE) inhibitors, angiotensin receptor antagonists, and renin inhibitors should probably be avoided throughout pregnancy. Drugs to avoid are magnesium sulfate (except for eclampsia prevention), high-dose diazoxide, nimodipine, and chlorpromazine.

- The cure for preeclampsia is delivery of the fetus if the pregnancy is at term. Drug therapy for hypertension in preeclampsia includes methyldopa, labetalol, and **calcium channel blockers. Magnesium sulfate** is used to prevent eclampsia and to treat eclamptic seizures. **Diazepam** and **phenytoin** should be avoided.

VENOUS THROMBOEMBOLISM

- Risk factors for venous thromboembolism in pregnancy include increasing age, history of thromboembolism, hypercoagulable conditions, operative vaginal delivery or cesarean section, obesity, and a family history of thrombosis.

- For treatment of acute thromboembolism, adjusted-dose **low-molecular-weight heparin** (preferred) or **unfractionated heparin** should be used for the duration of pregnancy and for 6 weeks after delivery. **Warfarin** should be avoided because it may cause fetal bleeding, malformations of the nose, stippled epiphyses, or CNS anomalies.

ACUTE CARE ISSUES IN PREGNANCY

HEADACHE

- For tension headaches during pregnancy, nonpharmacologic approaches are first-line therapies, including exercise, biofeedback, and massage. If drug therapy is needed, **acetaminophen** or **ibuprofen** is used. Opioids are rarely used.

- Acetaminophen (with or without **codeine** or other narcotic analgesics) may be used for headaches that do not respond to nonpharmacologic treatments. **Caffeine** may be added to simple analgesics to improve response, but overuse can cause withdrawal headaches.

- **Ergotamine** and **dihydroergotamine** are contraindicated.

- Chronic preventive treatment may be used in women with three or four severe episodes per month that are nonresponsive to other treatments. β-Blockers are commonly used, but they may cause intrauterine growth retardation. Calcium channel blockers and antidepressants are alternatives.
- NSAIDs and aspirin are contraindicated in the third trimester. For refractory migraines, narcotics may be used. The use of sumatriptan is controversial. Nausea of migraines may be treated with metoclopramide.

URINARY TRACT INFECTION

- The principal infecting organism is *Escherichia coli*, but *Proteus mirabilis*, *Klebsiella pneumoniae*, and group B *Streptococcus* cause some infections. Untreated bacteriuria may result in pyelonephritis, preterm labor, preeclampsia, transient renal failure, and low birth weight.
- Treatment of asymptomatic bacteriuria is necessary to reduce the risk of pyelonephritis and premature delivery. A course of 7 to 14 days of treatment is common. Repeat urine cultures are recommended monthly for the remainder of gestation when asymptomatic bacteriuria is diagnosed.
- Cephalexin is considered safe and effective for asymptomatic bacteriuria. Nitrofurantoin should not be used after week 37 due to concern for hemolytic anemia in the newborn. Sulfa-containing drugs may increase the risk for kernicterus in the newborn and should be avoided during the last weeks of gestation. Folate antagonists, such as trimethoprim, are relatively contraindicated during the first trimester because of their association with cardiovascular malformations. Fluoroquinolones and tetracyclines are contraindicated.

SEXUALLY TRANSMITTED DISEASES

Chlamydia

- *Chlamydia* infection can be transmitted at birth to the neonate and cause conjunctivitis and a subacute, afebrile pneumonia with onset at 1 to 3 months.
- The current recommendation for the treatment of *Chlamydia* cervicitis is azithromycin, 1 g orally as a single dose, or amoxicillin, 500 mg three times daily for 7 days.
- Other options are erythromycin base and ethylsuccinate.

Syphilis

- Penicillin is the drug of choice, and it is effective for preventing transmission to the fetus and treating the already infected fetus. No alternatives to penicillin are available for the pregnant woman who is allergic to penicillin.

Neisseria Gonorrhoeae

- *Neisseria gonorrhoeae* is a risk factor for preterm delivery. Symptoms in the neonate usually start within 2 to 5 days of birth.
- The treatment of choice is ceftriaxone, 125 mg intramuscularly (IM) as a single dose, or cefixime, 400 mg orally in a single dose. Spectinomycin, 2 g IM as a single dose, is appropriate as a second choice.

Genital Herpes

- The overriding concern with genital herpes is transmission of the virus to the neonate during birth.
- Maternal use of **acyclovir** during the first trimester is not associated with an increased risk of birth defects. **Valacyclovir** is an alternative. For **famciclovir**, safety data are more limited.

Bacterial Vaginosis

- Bacterial vaginosis is a risk factor for premature rupture of membranes, preterm labor, preterm birth, spontaneous abortion, and postpartum endometritis.
- For symptomatic and asymptomatic women at high risk for preterm delivery, the recommended regimen is **metronidazole**, 500 mg twice daily for 7 days; metronidazole, 250 mg three times daily for 7 days; or **clindamycin**, 300 mg twice daily for 7 days.

CHRONIC ILLNESSES IN PREGNANCY

ALLERGIC RHINITIS AND ASTHMA

- Treatment of asthma is divided into six steps based on symptom control.
- As step 1, all pregnant patients with asthma should have access to a short-acting inhaled β_2-agonist (**albuterol** is the preferred agent).
- Treatment of persistent asthma usually begins with step 2, but treatment may be started at step 3 for severely uncontrolled asthma.
- For persistent asthma, step-appropriate doses (low, medium, or high) of inhaled corticosteroids form the foundation of the controller medication regimen. **Budesonide** is preferred during pregnancy, but other inhaled corticosteroids used before pregnancy can be used.
- Long-acting β_2-**agonists** are considered safe.
- **Cromolyn, leukotriene receptor antagonists,** and **theophylline** are considered alternative agents, but they are not preferred.
- For severe, persistent asthma, the inhaled corticosteroid dose should be increased to the high-dose range, and addition of systemic corticosteroids may be needed to gain control of symptoms in the most severe disease.
- **Intranasal corticosteroids** are the most effective treatment for allergic rhinitis during pregnancy. **Beclomethasone** and **budesonide** have been used most. **Nasal cromolyn** and first-generation antihistamines (**chlorpheniramine** and **hydroxyzine**) are also considered first-line therapy. **Loratadine** and **cetirizine** have not been as extensively studied.
- Use of an external nasal dilator, short-term **topical oxymetazoline**, or **inhaled corticosteroids** may be preferred over oral decongestants, especially during early pregnancy.

DERMATOLOGIC CONDITIONS

- Topical agents with minimal pregnancy risk include **bacitracin, benzoyl peroxide, ciclopirox, clindamycin, erythromycin, metronidazole, mupirocin, permethrin,** and **terbinafine**.

- **Topical corticosteroids** are considered to have minimal pregnancy risk, but they should be applied at the lowest possible dose for the shortest time.
- Systemic agents that are considered safe in pregnancy include **acyclovir, amoxicillin, azithromycin, cephalosporins, cyproheptadine, dicloxacillin, diphenhydramine, erythromycin** (except **estolate**), **nystatin,** and **penicillin.**
- **Lidocaine** and **lidocaine with epinephrine** are also considered safe during pregnancy.
- **Acitretin, fluorouracil, isotretinoin, methotrexate,** and **thalidomide** should be avoided during pregnancy because of teratogenic potential.

DIABETES

- **Insulin** is the drug treatment of choice for patients with either type 1 or type 2 diabetes during pregnancy; **glyburide** can be used for type 2 diabetes after the eleventh week of gestation. **Metformin** is also an option.
- Goals for self-monitoring of blood glucose are the same as for GDM.

EPILEPSY

- Major malformations are two to three times more likely to occur in children born to women taking antiepileptic drugs than to those who do not.
- Major malformations with valproic acid therapy are dose related and range from 6.2% to 10.7%. **Valproic acid** should be avoided if possible during pregnancy to minimize the risk of neural tube defects, facial clefts, and cognitive teratogenicity.
- Rates of major malformations associated with monotherapy of other antiepileptic drugs are 2.9% to 3.6%.
- **Carbamazepine** and **lamotrigine** may be the safest.
- **Phenytoin, lamotrigine,** and **carbamazepine** may cause cleft palate, and **phenobarbital** may cause cardiac malformations.
- Drug therapy should be optimized prior to conception, and antiepileptic drug monotherapy is recommended when possible.
- If drug withdrawal is planned, it should be done at least 6 months prior to conception.
- All women with epilepsy should take a **folic acid** supplement, 4 or 5 mg daily, starting before pregnancy and continuing through at least the first trimester. The American Academy of Pediatrics recommends that all neonates receive vitamin K at delivery.

HUMAN IMMUNODEFICIENCY VIRUS INFECTIONS

- Newly diagnosed pregnant women should receive highly active antiretroviral therapy (HAART), selected from those recommended for nonpregnant adults (with consideration given to the teratogenic profiles of each drug).
- **Zidovudine** is the mainstay of antiretroviral therapy and is recommended during pregnancy, labor and delivery, and the postpartum period.
- **Lamivudine** should be used with zidovudine as the nucleoside reverse transcriptase inhibitor.

- For HAART, two nucleoside reverse transcriptase inhibitors plus either a nonnucleoside reverse transcriptase inhibitor or a protease inhibitor are recommended. Current guidelines recommend **nevirapine** or **lopinavir/ritonavir**.
- **Efavirenz** should be avoided during the first trimester and if possible through the entire pregnancy.
- If therapy is discontinued during the first trimester, reintroduction of all medications should occur only when the ability to tolerate drug therapy is certain, and they should all be started at the same time.
- Current zidovudine dosing recommendations during pregnancy are 200 mg three times daily or 300 mg twice daily. IV dosing is recommended during labor.
- The infant should receive zidovudine beginning 6 to 12 hours after birth and continued for the first 6 weeks of life.

HYPERTENSION

- For women with 140 to 179 mm Hg systolic or 90 to 109 mm Hg diastolic, the decision to continue or stop antihypertensive therapy during pregnancy is controversial. Antihypertensive drugs may be continued during pregnancy except for **ACE inhibitors** and **angiotensin II receptor blockers**.
- If discontinued, therapy should be restarted if blood pressure exceeds 150 to 160 mm Hg systolic or 100 to 110 mm Hg diastolic or if target-organ damage is present.
- **Diuretic** use (except **spironolactone**) is acceptable but controversial for chronic hypertension.
- No evidence exists for the superior efficacy of one antihypertensive agent versus another. Women with severe hypertension (systolic blood pressure >170 mm Hg or diastolic blood pressure >110 mm Hg) should receive drug therapy.

DEPRESSION

- If antidepressants are used, the lowest possible dose should be used for the shortest possible time to minimize adverse fetal and maternal pregnancy outcomes.
- In one study, pregnant women who stopped taking antidepressants were five times more likely to have a relapse than women who completed treatment.
- The **selective serotonin reuptake inhibitors (SSRIs)** are widely used by pregnant women. About one or two babies per 1,000 exposed to SSRIs in utero develop persistent pulmonary hypertension. The risk is six times greater in infants born to women who took SSRIs after week 20 of pregnancy. Another risk of using SSRIs late in pregnancy is a withdrawal reaction in the infant (e.g., irritability and difficulty feeding and breathing). An epidemiologic study suggests that first-trimester use of **paroxetine** may be associated with a 1.5- to 2-fold increased risk for cardiac defects in the infant.
- The risk of major malformations with SSRIs is small (~2 in 1,000 births).

LABOR AND DELIVERY

PRETERM LABOR

- Preterm labor is labor that occurs before 37 weeks of gestation.

Tocolytic Therapy

- The goals of tocolytic therapy are (1) to postpone delivery long enough to allow for administration of antenatal corticosteroids to improve pulmonary maturity and for transportation of the mother to a facility equipped to deal with high-risk deliveries, and (2) to prolong pregnancy when there are underlying self-limited conditions that can cause labor.
- Drugs most commonly used for acute tocolysis include **magnesium sulfate, NSAIDs,** and **calcium channel blockers**. All three have similar effectiveness in prolonging pregnancy 2 to 7 days, but this prolongation is not associated with significant reduction in rates of respiratory distress syndrome or neonatal death.
- The FDA recently announced that clinicians should not use **injectable terbutaline** to prevent preterm labor or treat it beyond 48 to 72 hours because of the risk for maternal death and heart problems, including cardiac arrhythmias, myocardial infarction, pulmonary edema, and tachycardia. It should not be used outside of the hospital setting. **Oral terbutaline** should not be used at all for the prevention or treatment of preterm labor, as it has the same risks as the injectable form and has not been shown to be effective.
- **Nifedipine** is associated with fewer side effects than magnesium. Five to 10 mg nifedipine may be administered sublingually every 15 to 20 minutes for three doses. Once stabilized, 10 to 20 mg may be administered by mouth every 4 to 6 hours for preterm contractions.

Antenatal Glucocorticoids

- A Cochrane meta-analysis shows the benefit of antenatal **corticosteroids** for fetal lung maturation to prevent respiratory distress syndrome, intraventricular hemorrhage, and death in infants delivered prematurely.
- Current recommendations are to administer **betamethasone**, 12 mg IM every 24 hours for two doses, or **dexamethasone**, 6 mg IM every 12 hours for four doses, to pregnant women between 26 and 34 weeks' gestation who are at risk for preterm delivery within the next 7 days. Benefits from antenatal glucocorticoid administration are believed to begin within 24 hours.

GROUP B *STREPTOCOCCUS* INFECTION

- The Centers for Disease Control and Prevention recommends prenatal screening (vaginal/rectal cultures) for group B *Streptococcus* colonization of all pregnant women at 35 to 37 weeks' gestation. If cultures are positive, or if the woman had a previous infant with invasive group B *Streptococcus* disease, or if the woman had group B *Streptococcus* bacteriuria, antibiotics are given.

- The currently recommended regimen for group B *Streptococcus* disease is **penicillin G**, 5 million units IV, followed by 2.5 million units IV every 4 hours until delivery. Alternatives include **ampicillin**, 2 g IV, followed by 1 g IV every 4 hours; **cefazolin**, 2 g IV, followed by 1 g every 8 hours; **clindamycin**, 900 mg IV every 8 hours; or **erythromycin**, 500 mg IV every 6 hours. In women who are penicillin-allergic and in whom sensitivity testing shows the organism to be resistant to clindamycin and erythromycin, **vancomycin**, 1 g IV every 12 hours until delivery, can be used.

CERVICAL RIPENING AND LABOR INDUCTION

- Prostaglandin E_2 analogues (e.g., **dinoprostone [Prepidil gel** and **Cervidil vaginal insert]**) are commonly used pharmacologic agents for cervical ripening. Fetal heart rate monitoring is required when Cervidil is used. **Misoprostol**, a prostaglandin E_1 analogue, is an effective and inexpensive drug used for cervical ripening and labor induction, but it is not approved for cervical ripening and has been associated with uterine rupture.
- **Oxytocin** is the most commonly used agent for labor induction after cervical ripening.

LABOR ANALGESIA

- The IV or IM administration of narcotics (**meperidine, morphine,** and **fentanyl**) is commonly used to treat the pain associated with labor. Compared with epidural analgesia, parenteral opioids are associated with lower rates of oxytocin augmentation, shorter stages of labor, and fewer instrumental deliveries.
- Epidural analgesia involves administering an opioid and/or an anesthetic (e.g., fentanyl and/or bupivacaine) through a catheter into the epidural space to provide pain relief. Epidural analgesia is associated with longer stages of labor and more instrumental deliveries than parenteral narcotic analgesia.
- Other options for labor analgesia include spinal analgesia and nerve blocks.

POSTPARTUM ISSUES

DRUG USE DURING LACTATION

- Medications enter breast milk via passive diffusion of nonionized and non-protein-bound medication. Drugs with high molecular weights, lower lipid solubility, and higher protein binding are less likely to cross into breast milk or transfer more slowly or in smaller amounts. The higher the serum concentration of drug in the mother's serum, the higher the concentration will be in the breast milk. Drugs with longer half-lives are more likely to maintain higher levels in breast milk. The timing and frequency of feedings and the amount of milk ingested by the infant are important considerations.
- Strategies for reducing risk to the infant from drugs transferred through breast milk include selecting medications for the mother that would be

considered safe for use in the infant; choosing medications with shorter half-lives; and selecting those that are more protein bound, have lower bioavailability, and have lower lipid solubility.

MASTITIS

- Mastitis is usually caused by *Staphylococcus aureus, E. coli,* and *Streptococcus.*
- Treatment includes 10 to 14 days of antibiotic therapy for the mother (**cloxacillin, dicloxacillin, oxacillin,** or **cephalexin**), bed rest, adequate oral fluid intake, analgesia, and frequent evacuation of breast milk.

POSTPARTUM DEPRESSION

- Nondrug therapies include emotional support from family and friends, education about the condition, and psychotherapy.
- **Sertraline** is considered first-line and **paroxetine** and **nortriptyline** are considered second-line treatments.

RELACTATION

- Recommended pharmacologic therapy for relactation is **metoclopramide**, 10 mg three times daily for 7 to 14 days. It should be used only if nondrug therapy is ineffective.

See Chapter 87, Pregnancy and Lactation: Therapeutic Considerations, authored by Kristina E. Ward and Barbara M. O'Brien, for a more detailed discussion of this topic.

CHAPTER 33 | Anemias

DEFINITION

- Anemias are a group of diseases characterized by a decrease in hemoglobin (Hb) or red blood cells (RBCs), resulting in decreased oxygen-carrying capacity of blood. The World Health Organization defines anemia as Hb <13 g/dL (<130 g/L; <8.07 mmol/L) in men or <12 g/dL (<120 g/L; <7.45 mmol/L) in women.

PATHOPHYSIOLOGY

- Anemias can be classified on the basis of RBC morphology, etiology, or pathophysiology (Table 33–1). The most common anemias are included in this chapter.
- Morphologic classifications are based on cell size. Macrocytic cells are larger than normal and are associated with deficiencies of vitamin B_{12} or folic acid. Microcytic cells are smaller than normal and are associated with iron deficiency, whereas normocytic anemia may be associated with recent blood loss or chronic disease.
- Iron-deficiency anemia can be caused by inadequate dietary intake, inadequate GI absorption, increased iron demand (e.g., pregnancy), blood loss, and chronic diseases.
- Vitamin B_{12}– and folic acid–deficiency anemias can be caused by inadequate dietary intake, decreased absorption, and inadequate utilization. Deficiency of intrinsic factor can cause decreased absorption of vitamin B_{12} (i.e., pernicious anemia). Folic acid–deficiency anemia can be caused by hyperutilization due to pregnancy, hemolytic anemia, myelofibrosis, malignancy, chronic inflammatory disorders, long-term dialysis, or growth spurt. Drugs can cause anemia by reducing absorption of folate (e.g., **phenytoin**) or through folate antagonism (e.g., **methotrexate**).
- Anemia of chronic disease is a hypoproliferative anemia associated with chronic infectious or inflammatory processes, tissue injury, or conditions that release proinflammatory cytokines. The pathogenesis is based on shortened RBC survival and impaired marrow response due to blocked release of iron. For information on anemia of chronic kidney disease, see Chap. 77.
- In anemia of critical illness, the mechanism for RBC replenishment and homeostasis is altered by, for example, blood loss or cytokines, which can blunt the erythropoietic response and inhibit RBC production.

TABLE 33–1 Classification Systems for Anemias

Morphology

Macrocytic anemias
  Megaloblastic anemias
    Vitamin B_{12} deficiency
    Folic acid deficiency

Microcytic hypochromic anemias
  Iron deficiency
  Genetic anomaly
    Sickle cell anemia
    Thalassemia
    Other hemoglobinopathies
      (abnormal hemoglobins)

Normocytic anemias
  Recent blood loss
  Hemolysis
  Bone marrow failure
  Anemia of chronic disease

Renal failure

Endocrine disorders

Myelodysplastic anemias

Etiology

Deficiency
  Iron
  Vitamin B_{12}
  Folic acid
  Pyridoxine
  Central, caused by impaired bone
    marrow function
  Anemia of chronic disease
  Anemia of the elderly
  Malignant bone marrow disorders

Peripheral
  Bleeding (hemorrhage)
  Hemolysis (hemolytic anemias)

Pathophysiology

Excessive blood loss
  Recent hemorrhage
  Trauma
  Peptic ulcer

  Gastritis
  Hemorrhoids

Chronic hemorrhage
  Vaginal bleeding
  Peptic ulcer
  Intestinal parasites
  Aspirin and other nonsteroidal
    antiinflammatory agents

Excessive RBC destruction
  Extracorpuscular (outside the cell) factors
    RBC antibodies
    Drugs
    Physical trauma to RBC (artificial valves)
    Excessive sequestration in the spleen

Intracorpuscular factors
  Heredity
  Disorders of hemoglobin synthesis

Inadequate production of mature RBCs
  Deficiency of nutrients (vitamin B_{12}, folic
    acid, iron, or protein)
  Deficiency of erythroblasts
    Aplastic anemia
    Isolated (often transient) erythroblastopenia
    Folic acid antagonists
    Antibodies
  Conditions with infiltration of bone marrow
    Lymphoma
    Leukemia
    Myelofibrosis
    Carcinoma
  Endocrine abnormalities
    Hypothyroidism
    Adrenal insufficiency
    Pituitary insufficiency
  Chronic renal disease
  Chronic inflammatory disease
    Granulomatous diseases
    Collagen vascular diseases
  Hepatic disease

RBC, red blood cell.

- Age-related reductions in bone marrow reserve can render the elderly patient more susceptible to anemia that is caused by multiple minor and often unrecognized diseases (e.g., nutritional deficiencies) that negatively affect erythropoiesis.

- Anemias in children are often due to a primary hematologic abnormality. The risk of iron-deficiency anemia is increased by rapid growth spurts and dietary deficiency.
- Hemolytic anemia results from decreased RBC survival time due to destruction in the spleen or circulation. The most common etiologies are RBC membrane defects (e.g., hereditary spherocytosis), altered Hb solubility or stability (e.g., sickle cell anemia [see Chap. 34] and thalassemias), and changes in intracellular metabolism (e.g., glucose-6-phosphate dehydrogenase deficiency). Some drugs cause direct oxidative damage to RBCs (see Appendix 3).

CLINICAL PRESENTATION

- Signs and symptoms depend on the rate of development and the age and cardiovascular status of the patient. Acute-onset anemia is characterized by cardiorespiratory symptoms such as tachycardia, lightheadedness, and breathlessness. Chronic anemia is characterized by weakness, fatigue, headache, symptoms of heart failure, vertigo, faintness, cold sensitivity, pallor, and loss of skin tone.
- Iron-deficiency anemia is characterized by glossal pain, smooth tongue, reduced salivary flow, pica (compulsive eating of nonfood items), and pagophagia (compulsive eating of ice). These symptoms are not usually seen until the Hb concentration is <9 g/dL (90 g/L; 5.59 mmol/L).
- Neurologic effects (e.g., numbness and ataxia) of vitamin B_{12} deficiency may occur in the absence of anemia. Psychiatric findings, including irritability, depression, and memory impairment, may also occur with vitamin B_{12} deficiency. Anemia with folate deficiency is not associated with neurologic or psychiatric symptoms.

DIAGNOSIS

- Rapid diagnosis is essential because anemia is often a sign of underlying pathology.
- Initial evaluation of anemia involves a complete blood cell count (Table 33–2), reticulocyte index, and examination of the stool for occult blood. Fig. 33–1 shows a broad, general algorithm for the diagnosis of anemia based on laboratory data.
- The earliest and most sensitive laboratory change for iron-deficiency anemia is decreased serum ferritin (storage iron), which should be interpreted in conjunction with decreased transferrin saturation and increased total iron-binding capacity (TIBC). Hb, hematocrit, and RBC indices usually remain normal until later stages of iron-deficiency anemia.
- In macrocytic anemias, mean corpuscular volume is usually elevated >100 fL. One of the earliest and most specific indications of macrocytic anemia is hypersegmented polymorphonuclear leukocytes on the peripheral blood smear. Vitamin B_{12} and folate concentrations can be measured to differentiate between the two deficiency anemias. A vitamin B_{12} value

TABLE 33–2 Normal Hematologic Values

Test	Reference Range (years)			
	2–6	*6–12*	*12–18*	*18–49*
Hemoglobin (g/dL)	11.5–15.5	11.5–15.5	M 13.0–16.0 F 12.0–16.0	M 13.5–17.5 F 12.0–16.0
Hematocrit (%)	34–40	35–45	M 37–49 F 36–46	M 41–53 F 36–46
MCV (fL)	75–87	77–95	M 78–98 F 78–102	80–100
MCHC (%)	–	31–37	31–37	31–37
MCH (pg)	24–30	25–33	25–35	26–34
RBC (million/mm³)	3.9–5.3	4.0–5.2	M 4.5–5.3	M 4.5–5.9
Reticulocyte count, absolute (%)				0.5–1.5
Serum iron (mcg/dL)		50–120	50–120	M 50–160 F 40–150
TIBC (mcg/dL)	250–400	250–400	250–400	250–400
RDW (%)				11–16
Ferritin (ng/mL)	7–140	7–140	7–140	M 15–200 F 12–150
Folate (ng/mL)				1.8–16.0[a]
Vitamin B$_{12}$ (pg/mL)				100–900[a]
Erythropoietin (milliunits/mL)				0–19

F, female; M, male; MCH, mean corpuscular hemoglobin; MCHC, mean corpuscular hemoglobin concentration; MCV, mean corpuscular volume; RBC, red blood cell (count); RDW, red blood cell distribution; TIBC, total iron-binding capacity.
[a]Varies by assay method.

<150 pg/mL (<111 pmol/L), together with appropriate peripheral smear and clinical symptoms, is diagnostic of vitamin B$_{12}$–deficiency anemia. A decreased RBC folate concentration (<150 ng/mL [<340 nmol/L]) appears to be a better indicator of folate-deficiency anemia than a decreased serum folate concentration (<3 ng/mL [7 nmol/L]).

- The diagnosis of anemia of chronic disease is usually one of exclusion, with consideration of coexisting iron and folate deficiencies. Serum iron is usually decreased but, unlike iron-deficiency anemia, serum ferritin is normal or increased, and TIBC is decreased. The bone marrow reveals an abundance of iron; the peripheral smear reveals normocytic anemia.
- Laboratory findings of anemia of critical illness disease are similar to those of anemia of chronic disease.
- Elderly patients with symptoms of anemia should undergo a complete blood cell count with peripheral smear and reticulocyte count and other laboratory studies as needed to determine the etiology of anemia.
- The diagnosis of anemia in pediatric populations requires the use of age- and gender-adjusted norms for laboratory values.

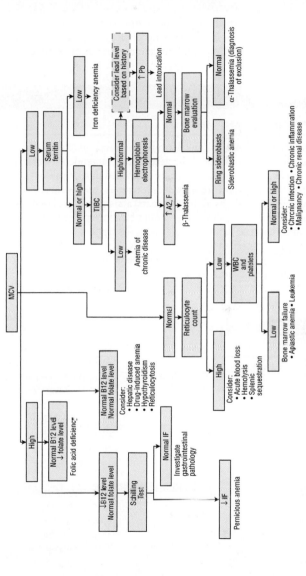

FIGURE 33–1. General algorithm for diagnosis of anemias. (↑, increased; ↓, decreased; A₂, hemoglobin A₂; F, hemoglobin F; IF, intrinsic factor; MCV, mean corpuscular volume; Pb, lead; TIBC, total iron-binding capacity; WBC, white blood cells.)

- Hemolytic anemias tend to be associated with increased levels of reticulocytes, lactic dehydrogenase, and indirect bilirubin.

DESIRED OUTCOME

- The ultimate goals of treatment in the anemic patient are to alleviate signs and symptoms, correct the underlying etiology (e.g., restore substrates needed for RBC production), and prevent recurrence of anemia.

TREATMENT

IRON-DEFICIENCY ANEMIA

- **Oral iron** therapy with soluble ferrous iron salts, which are not enteric coated and not slow- or sustained-release, is recommended at a daily dosage of 200 mg elemental iron in two or three divided doses (Table 33–3).
- Diet plays a significant role because iron is poorly absorbed from vegetables, grain products, dairy products, and eggs; iron is best absorbed from meat, fish, and poultry. Iron should be administered at least 1 hour before meals because food interferes with absorption, but administration with food may be needed to improve tolerability.
- **Parenteral iron** may be required for patients with iron malabsorption, intolerance of oral iron therapy, or noncompliance. Parenteral

TABLE 33–3	Oral Iron Products	
Salt	**Elemental Iron (%)**	**Elemental Iron Provided**
Ferrous sulfate	20	60–65 mg/324–325 mg tablet 18 mg iron/5 mL syrup 44 mg iron/5 mL elixir 15 mg iron/0.6 mL drop
Ferrous sulfate (exsiccated)	30	65 mg/200 mg tablet 60 mg/187 mg tablet 50 mg/160 mg tablet
Ferrous gluconate	12	36 mg/325 mg tablet 27 mg/240 mg tablet
Ferrous fumarate	33	33 mg/100 mg tablet 63–66 mg/200 mg tablet 106 mg/324–325 mg tablet 15 mg/0.6 mL drop 33 mg/5 mL suspension
Polysaccharide iron complex	100	150 mg capsule 50 mg tablet 100 mg/5 mL elixir
Carbonyl iron	100	50 mg caplet

TABLE 33–4	Equations for Calculating Doses of Parenteral Iron

In patients with iron-deficiency anemia:

Adults and children >15 kg (33 lb)

Dose (mL) = 0.0442 (desired Hb − observed Hb) × LBW + (0.26 × LBW)

LBW males = 50 kg + (2.3 × [inches over 5 ft])

LBW females = 45.5 kg + (2.3 × [inches over 5 ft])

Children 5–15 kg (11–33 lb)

Dose (mL) = 0.0442 (desired Hb − observed Hb) × W + (0.26 × W)

In patients with anemia secondary to blood loss (hemorrhagic diathesis or long-term dialysis):

mg of iron = blood loss × hematocrit

where blood loss is in milliliters and hematocrit is expressed as a decimal fraction.

Hb, hemoglobin; LBW, lean body weight; W, weight.

administration, however, does not hasten the onset of hematologic response. The replacement dose depends on the etiology of anemia and Hb concentration (Table 33–4).

- Available parenteral iron preparations have similar efficacy but different pharmacologic, pharmacokinetic, and safety profiles (Table 33–5). Newer products, such as **sodium ferric gluconate**, **ferumoxytol**, and **iron sucrose**, appear to be better tolerated than **iron dextran.**

VITAMIN B_{12}–DEFICIENCY ANEMIA

- Oral vitamin B_{12} supplementation appears to be as effective as parenteral, even in patients with pernicious anemia, because the alternate vitamin B_{12} absorption pathway is independent of intrinsic factor. Oral **cobalamin** is initiated at 1 to 2 mg daily for 1 to 2 weeks, followed by 1 mg daily.
- Parenteral therapy is more rapid acting than oral therapy and should be used if neurologic symptoms are present. A popular regimen is **cyano-cobalamin**, 1,000 mcg daily for 1 week, then weekly for 1 month, and then monthly. When symptoms resolve, daily oral administration can be initiated.
- Adverse events are rare with vitamin B_{12} therapy.

FOLATE-DEFICIENCY ANEMIA

- Oral **folate**, 1 mg daily for 4 months, is usually sufficient for treatment of folic acid deficiency anemia, unless the etiology cannot be corrected. If malabsorption is present, a dose of 1 to 5 mg daily may be necessary.

ANEMIA OF CHRONIC DISEASE

- Treatment of anemia of chronic disease is less specific than that of other anemias and should focus on correcting reversible causes. Iron therapy is not effective when inflammation is present. RBC transfusions are effective but should be limited to episodes of inadequate oxygen transport and Hb of 8 to 10 g/dL (80–100 g/L; 4.97–6.21 mmol/L).

TABLE 33–5 Comparison of Parenteral Iron Preparations

	Ferumoxytol	Sodium Ferric Gluconate	Iron Dextran	Iron Sucrose
Amount of elemental iron	30 mg/mL	62.5 mg iron/5 mL	50 mg iron/mL	20 mg iron/mL
Molecular weight	Feraheme: 75, 000 Da	Ferrlecit: 289,000–444,000 Da	InFeD: 165,000 Da DexFerrum: 267,000 Da	Venofer: 34,000–60,000 Da
Composition	Superparamagnetic iron oxide that is coated with a carbohydrate shell	Ferric oxide hydrate bonded to sucrose chelates with gluconate in a molar rate of 2 iron molecules to 1 gluconate molecule	Complex of ferric hydroxide and dextran	Complex of polynuclear iron hydroxide in sucrose
Preservative	None	Benzyl alcohol 9 mg/5 mL 20% (975 mg in 62.5 mg iron)	None	None
Indication	Treatment of iron deficiency anemia for adult patients with chronic kidney disease (CKD)	Treatment of iron-deficiency anemia for patients undergoing chronic hemodialysis who are receiving supplemental erythropoietin therapy	Treatment of patients with documented iron deficiency in whom oral therapy is unsatisfactory or impossible	Treatment of iron-deficiency anemia for patients undergoing chronic hemodialysis who are receiving supplemental epoetin alfa therapy
Warning	No black-box warning: hypersensitivity reactions	No black-box warning: hypersensitivity reactions	Black-box warning: anaphylactic-type reactions	Black-box warning: anaphylactic-type reactions

IM injection	No	No	Yes	No
Usual dose	Initial 510 mg intravenous injection followed by a second 510 mg intravenous injection 3 to 8 days later (rate 30 mg/s)	125 mg (10 mL) diluted in 100 mL normal saline, infused over 60 minutes; also can be administered as a slow IV injection (rate of 12.5 mg/min).	100 mg undiluted at a rate not to exceed 50 mg (1 mL) per minute	100 mg into the dialysis line at a rate of 1 mL (20 mg of iron) undiluted solution per minute
Treatment	2 doses × 510 mg = 1,020 mg	8 doses × 125 mg = 1,000 mg	10 doses × 100 mg = 1,000 mg	Up to 10 doses × 100 mg = 1,000 mg
Common adverse effects	Diarrhea, constipation, nausea, dizziness, hypotension, peripheral edema,	Cramps, nausea and vomiting, flushing, hypotension, rash, pruritus	Pain and brown staining at injection site, flushing, hypotension, fever, chills, myalgia, anaphylaxis	Leg cramps, hypotension

- **Erythropoiesis-stimulating agents (ESAs)** can be considered, but the response can be impaired in patients with anemia of chronic disease (off-label use). The initial dosage for **epoetin alfa** is 50 to 100 units/kg three times weekly and **darbepoetin alfa** 0.45 mcg/kg once weekly. Iron deficiency can occur in patients treated with ESAs, so many practitioners routinely supplement ESA therapy with oral iron therapy.
- Potential toxicities of exogenous ESA administration include increases in blood pressure, nausea, headache, fever, bone pain, and fatigue. Hb must be monitored during ESA therapy. An increase in Hb >12 g/dL (120 g/L; 7.45 mmol/L) with treatment or a rise of >1 g/dL (>10 g/L; >0.62 mmol/L) every 2 weeks have been associated with increased mortality and cardiovascular events.

OTHER TYPES OF ANEMIAS

- Patients with other types of anemias require appropriate supplementation depending on the etiology of anemia.
- In patients with anemia of critical illness, parenteral iron is often used but is associated with a theoretical risk of infection. Routine use of ESAs or RBC transfusions is not supported by clinical studies.
- Anemia of prematurity is usually treated with RBC transfusions. ESA use is controversial because it has not been shown to clearly reduce transfusion requirements.
- For infants ages 9 to 12 months, the dose of elemental iron, administered as iron sulfate, is 3 mg/kg once or twice daily for 4 weeks. If a response is seen, iron should be continued for 2 months to replace storage iron pools. The dose and schedule of vitamin B_{12} should be titrated according to the clinical and laboratory response. The daily dose of folate is 1 to 3 mg.
- Treatment of hemolytic anemia should focus on correcting the underlying cause. There is no specific therapy for glucose-6-phosphate dehydrogenase deficiency, so treatment consists of avoiding oxidant medications and chemicals. Steroids, other immunosuppressants, and even splenectomy can be indicated to reduce RBC destruction.

EVALUATION OF THERAPEUTIC OUTCOMES

- In iron-deficiency anemia, **iron** therapy should cause reticulocytosis in a few days with an increase in Hb seen at 2 weeks. The patient should be reevaluated if reticulocytosis does not occur or if Hb does not increase by 2 g/dL (20 g/L; <1.24 mmol/L) within 3 weeks. Hb should return to normal after 2 months, but iron therapy is continued until iron stores are replenished, which usually requires at least 3 to 6 months.
- In megaloblastic anemia, signs and symptoms usually improve within a few days after starting **vitamin B_{12}** or **folate** therapy. Neurologic symptoms can take longer to improve or can be irreversible, but they should not progress during therapy. Reticulocytosis should occur within 3 to 5 days. Hb begins to rise a week after starting vitamin B_{12} therapy and should normalize in 1 to 2 months. Hematocrit should rise within 2 weeks after starting folate therapy and should normalize within 2 months.

• In anemia of chronic disease, reticulocytosis should occur a few days after starting ESA therapy. Iron, TIBC, transferrin saturation, and ferritin levels should be monitored at baseline and periodically because iron depletion is a major reason for treatment failure. The optimal form and schedule of iron supplementation are unknown. If a clinical response does not occur by 8 weeks, ESAs should be discontinued.

See Chapter 109, Anemias, authored by Kristen Cook, Beata A. Ineck, and William L. Lyons, for a more detailed discussion of this topic.

Sickle Cell Disease

DEFINITION

- Sickle cell syndromes are hereditary disorders characterized by the presence of sickle hemoglobin (HbS) in red blood cells (RBCs).

PATHOPHYSIOLOGY

- The most common abnormal hemoglobin in the United States is hemoglobin S (HbS). Homozygous HbS (HbSS) is called sickle cell disease (SCD) or sickle cell anemia. Sickle cell trait is the heterozygous inheritance of one normal cell and one sickle cell hemoglobin gene. Hemoglobin C and other rare phenotypes occur when heterozygous inheritance of HbS is compounded with another mutation. SCD most commonly affects people of African heritage.
- Clinical manifestations of SCD are attributable to impaired circulation, RBC destruction, and stasis of blood flow. These problems are attributable to disturbances in RBC polymerization and to membrane damage.
- Polymerization allows deoxygenated hemoglobin to exist as a semisolid gel that protrudes into the cell membrane, distorting RBCs into sickle shapes. Sickle-shaped RBCs increase blood viscosity and encourage sludging in the capillaries and small vessels. Such obstructive events lead to local tissue hypoxia and accentuate the pathologic process.
- Repeated cycles of sickling, upon deoxygenation, and unsickling, upon oxygenation, damage the RBC membrane and cause irreversible sickling. Rigid, sickled RBCs are easily trapped, shortening their circulatory survival and resulting in chronic hemolysis.
- Additional contributing factors are functional asplenia (and increased risk of bacterial infection), deficient opsonization, and coagulation abnormalities.

CLINICAL PRESENTATION

- SCD involves multiple organ systems. Clinical manifestations depend on the genotype (Table 34–1).
- Feature presentations of SCD are hemolytic anemia and vasoocclusion. Symptoms are delayed until 4 to 6 months of age when HbS replaces fetal hemoglobin (HbF). Common findings include pain with fever, pneumonia, splenomegaly, and, in infants, pain and swelling of the hands and feet (e.g., hand-and-foot syndrome or dactylitis).
- Usual clinical signs and symptoms of SCD are chronic anemia; fever; pallor; arthralgia; scleral icterus; abdominal pain; weakness; anorexia; fatigue; enlarged liver, spleen, and heart; and hematuria.

TABLE 34–1	Clinical Features of Sickle Cell Trait and Common Types of Sickle Cell Disease
Type	**Clinical Features**
Sickle cell trait (SCT)	Rare painless hematuria; normal Hb level; heavy exercise under extreme conditions can provoke gross hematuria and complications
Sickle cell anemia (SCA)	Pain crises, microvascular disruption of organs (spleen, liver, bone marrow, kidney, brain, and lung), gallstones, priapism, leg ulcers, anemia (Hb 7–10 g/dL [70–100 g/L; 4.34–6.21 mmol/L])
Sickle cell hemoglobin C	Painless hematuria and rare aseptic necrosis of bone; vasoocclusive crises are less common and occur later in life; other complications are ocular disease and pregnancy-related problems; mild anemia (Hb 10–12 g/dL [100–120 g/L; 6.21–7.45 mmol/L])
Sickle cell β^+-thalassemia	Rare crises; milder severity than sickle cell disease because of production of HbA; Hb 10–14 g/dL (100–140 g/L; 6.21–8.69 mmol/L) with microcytosis
Sickle cell β^0-thalassemia	No HbA production; severity similar to SCA; Hb 7–10 g/dL (70–100 g/L; 4.34–6.21 mmol/L) with microcytosis

Hb, hemoglobin; HbA, hemoglobin A.

- Children experience delayed growth and sexual maturation, as well as characteristic physical findings such as protuberant abdomen and exaggerated lumbar lordosis.
- Acute complications of SCD include fever and infection (e.g., sepsis caused by encapsulated pathogens such as *Streptococcus pneumoniae*), stroke, acute chest syndrome, and priapism. Acute chest syndrome is characterized by pulmonary infiltration, respiratory symptoms, and equivocal response to antibiotic therapy.
- Sickle cell crisis can be precipitated by fever, infection, dehydration, hypoxia, acidosis, sudden temperature change, or a combination of factors. The most common type is vasoocclusive crisis, which is manifested by pain over the involved areas without change in hemoglobin. Aplastic crisis is characterized by decreased reticulocyte count and rapidly developing severe anemia, with or without pain. Splenic sequestration crisis is a massive enlargement of the spleen leading to hypotension, shock, and sudden death in young children. Repeated infarctions lead to autosplenectomy as the disease progresses, therefore, incidence declines as adolescence approaches.
- Chronic complications involve many organs and include pulmonary hypertension, bone and joint destruction, ocular problems, cholelithiasis, cardiovascular abnormalities, and hematuria and other renal complications.
- Patients with sickle cell trait are usually asymptomatic, except for rare painless hematuria.

DIAGNOSIS

- SCD is usually identified by routine neonatal screening programs using isoelectric focusing, high-performance liquid chromatography, or electrophoresis.
- Laboratory findings include low hemoglobin; increased reticulocyte, platelet, and white blood cell counts; and sickle forms on the peripheral smear.

DESIRED OUTCOME

- The goal of treatment is to reduce hospitalizations, complications, and mortality.

TREATMENT

GENERAL PRINCIPLES

- Patients with SCD require lifelong multidisciplinary care. Interventions include general measures, preventive strategies, and treatment of complications and acute crises.
- Patients with SCD should receive routine immunizations plus influenza, meningococcal, and pneumococcal vaccinations.
- Prophylactic **penicillin** is recommended for children with SCD until they are 5 years old. Beginning at age 2 months or earlier, the dosage is penicillin V potassium, 125 mg orally twice daily until 3 years of age and then 250 mg twice daily until age 5 years, or benzathine penicillin, 600,000 units intramuscularly every 4 weeks from age 6 months to 6 years.
- **Folic acid**, 1 mg daily, is recommended in adult patients, pregnant women, and patients of all ages with chronic hemolysis.

FETAL HEMOGLOBIN INDUCERS

- HbF directly effects polymer formation. Increases in HbF correlate with decreased RBC sickling and adhesion. Patients with low HbF levels have more frequent crises and higher mortality.
- **Hydroxyurea**, a chemotherapeutic agent, has many effects on blood cells, including the stimulation of HbF production. It is indicated for patients with frequent painful episodes, severe symptomatic anemia, acute chest syndrome, or other severe vasoocclusive complications. The starting dose is 10 to 15 mg/kg daily as a single daily dose (Fig. 34–1).
- Strategies being investigated to induce HbF include **butyrate** and **5-aza-2-deoxycytidine (decitabine)**.
- Chronic transfusion is indicated to prevent stroke and stroke recurrence in children. Transfusion frequency is usually every 3 to 4 weeks and should be adjusted to maintain HbS <30% of total hemoglobin. The optimal duration is unknown. Risks include alloimmunization, hyperviscosity, viral transmission (requiring hepatitis A and B vaccination), volume and iron overload, and transfusion reactions.

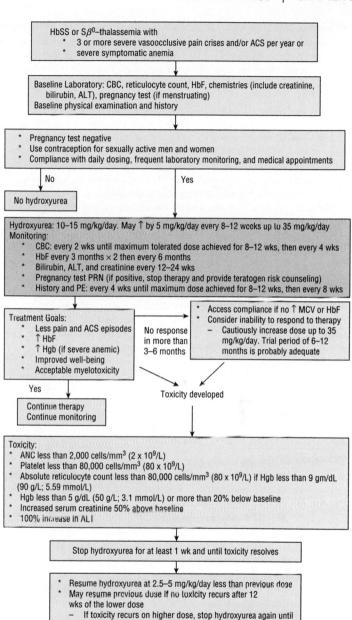

FIGURE 34-1. Hydroxyurea use in sickle cell disease. (ACS, acute chest syndrome; ALT, alanine aminotransferase; ANC, absolute neutrophil count; CBC, complete blood cell count; Hgb, hemoglobin; HbF, fetal hemoglobin; HbSS, homozygous sickle cell hemoglobin; HbSSβ⁰, sickle cell β⁰-thalassemia; MCV, mean corpuscular volume; PE, physical examination; PRN, as needed; RBC, red blood cell.)

- Allogeneic hematopoietic stem cell transplantation is the only therapy that is curative. The best candidates are younger than 16 years of age, have severe complications, and have human leukocyte antigen–matched donors. Risks must be carefully considered and include mortality, graft rejection, and secondary malignancies.

TREATMENT OF COMPLICATIONS

- Patients should be educated to recognize conditions that require urgent evaluation. To avoid exacerbation during acute illness, patients should maintain balanced fluid status and oxygen saturation of at least 92%.
- RBC transfusions are indicated for acute exacerbation of baseline anemia (e.g., aplastic crisis, hepatic or splenic sequestration, or severe hemolysis), severe vasoocclusive episodes, and procedures requiring general anesthesia or ionic contrast. Transfusions can be useful in patients with complicated obstetric problems, refractory leg ulcers, refractory and protracted painful episodes, and severe priapism.
- Fever of 38.5°C (101.3°F) or higher should be evaluated promptly. Empiric antibiotic therapy with coverage against encapsulated organisms is recommended (e.g., **ceftriaxone** for outpatients and **cefotaxime** for inpatients).
- Patients with acute chest syndrome should receive incentive spirometry; appropriate fluid therapy; broad-spectrum antibiotics, including a **macrolide** or **quinolone**; and, for hypoxia or acute distress, oxygen therapy. Steroids and nitric oxide are being evaluated.
- Priapism has been treated with analgesics, antianxiety agents, and vasoconstrictors to force blood out of the corpus cavernosum (e.g., **phenylephrine** and **epinephrine**), and vasodilators to relax smooth muscle (e.g., **terbutaline** and **hydralazine**).

TREATMENT OF SICKLE CELL CRISIS

- Treatment of *aplastic crisis* is primarily supportive. Blood transfusions may be indicated for severe or symptomatic anemia. Antibiotic therapy is not warranted because the most common etiology is viral, not bacterial, infection.
- Treatment options for *splenic sequestration* include observation alone, especially for adults because they tend to have milder episodes; chronic transfusion to delay splenectomy; and splenectomy after a life-threatening crisis, after repetitive episodes, or for chronic hypersplenism.
- Hydration and analgesics are the mainstays of treatment for *vasoocclusive (painful) crisis*. Fluid replacement should be 1.5 times the maintenance requirement, can be administered IV or orally, and should be monitored to avoid volume overload. An infectious etiology should be considered; if appropriate, empiric therapy should be initiated.
- Analgesic therapy should be tailored to the individual because of the variable frequency and severity of pain. Pain scales should be used to quantify the degree of pain.
- Mild to moderate pain should be treated with nonsteroidal antiinflammatory drugs or acetaminophen.

- Severe pain should be treated aggressively with an opioid, such as **morphine, hydromorphone, fentanyl,** or **methadone**. Moderate pain should be treated with a weak opioid, such as **codeine** or **hydrocodone**. **Meperidine** should be avoided because accumulation of the normeperidine metabolite can cause neurotoxicity, especially in patients with impaired renal function.
- Severe pain should be treated with an IV opioid titrated to pain relief and then administered on a scheduled basis with as-needed dosing for breakthrough pain. Patient-controlled analgesia is commonly utilized.
- Suspicion of addiction commonly leads to suboptimal pain control. Factors that minimize dependence include aggressive pain control, frequent monitoring, and tapering medication according to response.
- Omega-3 fatty acids are under investigation for vasoocclusive crisis. Their antiadhesion activity potentially can reduce or ameliorate clinical manifestations of SCD.

EVALUATION OF THERAPEUTIC OUTCOMES

- All patients should be evaluated regularly to establish baseline, monitor changes, and provide age-appropriate education.
- Laboratory evaluations include complete blood cell and reticulocyte counts and HbF level. Renal, hepatobiliary, and pulmonary function should be evaluated. Patients should be screened for retinopathy.
- The efficacy of hydroxyurea can be assessed by monitoring the number, severity, and duration of sickle cell crises.

See Chapter 111, Sickle Cell Disease, authored by C. Y. Jennifer Chan and Reginald Moore, for a more detailed discussion of this topic.

CHAPTER 35

Antimicrobial Regimen Selection

INTRODUCTION

- A systematic approach to the selection and evaluation of an antimicrobial regimen is shown in Table 35–1. An "empiric" antimicrobial regimen is begun before the offending organism is identified and sometimes prior to the documentation of the presence of infection, whereas a "definitive" regimen is instituted when the causative organism is known.

CONFIRMING THE PRESENCE OF INFECTION

FEVER

- Fever is defined as a controlled elevation of body temperature above the normal range of 36.7 to 37°C (98.1–98.6°F) (measured orally). Fever is a manifestation of many disease states other than infection.
- Many drugs have been identified as causes of fever. Drug-induced fever is defined as persistent fever in the absence of infection or other underlying condition. The fever must coincide temporally with the administration of the offending agent and disappear promptly upon its withdrawal, after which the temperature remains normal.

SIGNS AND SYMPTOMS

White Blood Cell Count

- Most infections result in elevated white blood cell (WBC) counts (leukocytosis) because of the mobilization of granulocytes and/or lymphocytes to destroy invading microbes. The generally accepted range of normal values for WBC counts is between 4,000 and 10,000 cells/mm³.
- Bacterial infections are associated with elevated granulocyte counts (neutrophils and basophils), often with increased numbers of immature forms (band neutrophils) seen in peripheral blood smears (left-shift). With infection, peripheral leukocyte counts may be very high, but they are rarely higher than 30,000 to 40,000 cells/mm³. Low neutrophil counts (neutropenia) after the onset of infection indicate an abnormal response and are generally associated with a poor prognosis for bacterial infection.
- Relative lymphocytosis, even with normal or slightly elevated total WBC counts, is generally associated with tuberculosis and viral or fungal infections. Many types of infections, however, may be accompanied by a completely normal WBC count and differential.

| **TABLE 35–1** | Systematic Approach for Selection of Antimicrobials |

Confirm the presence of infection
    Careful history and physical
    Signs and symptoms
    Predisposing factors
Identify the pathogen
    Collection of infected material
    Stains
    Serologies
    Culture and sensitivity
Select the presumptive therapy considering every infected site
    Host factors
    Drug factors
Monitor therapeutic response
    Clinical assessment
    Laboratory tests
    Assess therapeutic failure

Pain and Inflammation

- Pain and inflammation may accompany infection and are sometimes manifested by swelling, erythema, tenderness, and purulent drainage. Unfortunately, these signs may be apparent only if the infection is superficial or in a bone or joint.
- The manifestations of inflammation with deep-seated infections such as meningitis, pneumonia, endocarditis, and urinary tract infection must be ascertained by examining tissues or fluids. For example, the presence of polymorphonuclear leukocytes (neutrophils) in spinal fluid, lung secretions (sputum), and urine is highly suggestive of bacterial infection.

IDENTIFICATION OF THE PATHOGEN

- Infected body materials must be sampled, if at all possible or practical, before the institution of antimicrobial therapy, for two reasons. First, a Gram stain of the material may reveal bacteria, or an acid-fast stain may detect mycobacteria or actinomycetes. Second, a delay in obtaining infected fluids or tissues until after therapy is started may result in false-negative culture results or alterations in the cellular and chemical composition of infected fluids.
- Blood cultures should be performed in the acutely ill, febrile patient. Less accessible fluids or tissues are obtained when needed to assess localized signs or symptoms (e.g., spinal fluid in meningitis and joint fluid in arthritis). Abscesses and cellulitic areas should also be aspirated.
- Caution must be used in the evaluation of positive culture results from normally sterile sites (e.g., blood, cerebrospinal fluid [CSF], and joint fluid). The recovery of bacteria normally found on the skin in large

quantities (e.g., coagulase-negative staphylococci and diphtheroids) from one of these sites may be a result of contamination of the specimen rather than a true infection.

SELECTION OF PRESUMPTIVE THERAPY

- To select rational antimicrobial therapy for a given infection, a variety of factors must be considered, including the severity and acuity of the disease, host factors, factors related to the drugs used, and the necessity for use of multiple agents.
- There are generally accepted drugs of choice for the treatment of most pathogens (Table 35–2). The drugs of choice are compiled from a variety of sources and are intended as guidelines rather than specific rules for antimicrobial use.
- When selecting antimicrobial regimens, local susceptibility data should be considered whenever possible rather than information published by other institutions or national compilations.

HOST FACTORS

- When evaluating a patient for initial or empiric therapy, the following factors should be considered:
  - ✓ Allergy or history of adverse drug reactions
  - ✓ Age of patient
  - ✓ Pregnancy
  - ✓ Metabolic abnormalities
  - ✓ Renal and hepatic function. Patients with diminished renal and/or hepatic function will accumulate certain drugs unless the dosage is adjusted.
  - ✓ Concomitant drug therapy. Any concomitant therapy the patient is receiving may influence the selection of drug therapy, the dose, and monitoring. A list of selected drug interactions involving antimicrobials is provided in Table 35–3.
  - ✓ Concomitant disease states

DRUG FACTORS

- Integration of both pharmacokinetic and pharmacodynamic properties of an agent is important when choosing antimicrobial therapy to ensure efficacy and prevent resistance. Antibiotics may demonstrate concentration-dependent (aminoglycosides and fluoroquinolones) or time-dependent (β-lactams) bactericidal effects.
- The importance of tissue penetration varies with the site of infection. The CNS is one body site where the importance of antimicrobial penetration is relatively well defined, and correlations with clinical outcomes are established. Drugs that do not reach significant concentrations in CSF should either be avoided or instilled directly when treating meningitis.
- Apart from the bloodstream, other body fluids where drug concentration data are clinically relevant are urine, synovial fluid, and peritoneal fluid.

| **TABLE 35–2** | Drugs of Choice, First Choice, and Alternative(s) |

Gram-positive cocci

Enterococcus faecalis (generally not as resistant to antibiotics as *Enterococcus faecium*)
- Serious infection (endocarditis, meningitis, pyelonephritis with bacteremia)
  - Ampicillin (or penicillin G) + (gentamicin or streptomycin)
  - *Vancomycin + (gentamicin or streptomycin), daptomycin, linezolid, telavancin, tigecycline[a]*
- Urinary tract infection (UTI)
  - Ampicillin, amoxicillin
  - *Fosfomycin or nitrofurantoin*

E faecium (generally more resistant to antibiotics than *E faecalis*)
- Recommend consultation with infectious disease specialist
  - Linezolid, quinupristin/dalfopristin, daptomycin, tigecycline[a]

Staphylococcus aureus/Staphylococcus epidermidis
- Methicillin (oxacillin)-sensitive
  - Nafcillin or oxacillin
  - *FGC,[b,c] trimethoprim-sulfamethoxazole, clindamycin, BL/BLI[j]*
- Hospital-acquired methicillin (oxacillin)–resistant
  - Vancomycin ± (gentamicin or rifampin)
  - *Daptomycin, linezolid, telavancin, tigecycline,[a] trimethoprim-sulfamethoxazole,* or quinupristin-dalfopristin
- Community-acquired methicillin (oxacillin)-resistant
  - Clindamycin, trimethoprim-sulfamethoxazole, doxycycline[a]
  - *Daptomycin, linezolid, telavancin, tigecycline,[a] or vancomycin*

Streptococcus (groups A, B, C, G, and *Streptococcus bovis*)
- Penicillin G or V or ampicillin
- *FGC,[b,c] erythromycin, azithromycin, clarithromycin*

Streptococcus pneumoniae
- Penicillin-sensitive (MIC <0.1 mcg/mL)
  - Penicillin G or V or ampicillin
  - *FGC,[b,c] doxycycline,[a] azithromycin, clarithromycin, erythromycin*
- Penicillin intermediate (MIC 0.1–1.0 mcg/mL)
  - High-dose penicillin (12 million units/day for adults) or ceftriaxone[c] or cefotaxime[c]
  - *Levofloxacin,[a] moxifloxacin,[a] gemifloxacin,[a] or vancomycin*
- Penicillin-resistant (MIC ≥1.0 mcg/mL)
  - Recommend consultation with infectious disease specialist.
    - Vancomycin ± rifampin
    - *Per sensitivities: cefotaxime,[c] ceftriaxone,[c] levofloxacin,[a] moxifloxacin,[a] or gemifloxacin[a]*

Streptococcus, viridans group
- Penicillin G ± gentamicin[d]
- *Cefotaxime,[c] ceftriaxone,[c] erythromycin, azithromycin, clarithromycin,* or *vancomycin ± gentamicin*

Gram-negative cocci

Moraxella (Branhamella) catarrhalis
- Amoxicillin-clavulanate, ampicillin-sulbactam
- *Trimethoprim-sulfamethoxazole, erythromycin, azithromycin, clarithromycin, doxycycline,[a] SGC,[c,e] cefotaxime,[c] ceftriaxone,[c] or TGC PO[c,f]*

(continued)

TABLE 35–2 Drugs of Choice, First Choice, and Alternative(s) *(Continued)*

Neisseria gonorrhoeae (also give concomitant treatment for *Chlamydia trachomatis*)
- Disseminated gonococcal infection
  - *Ceftriaxone[c]* or *cefotaxime[c]*
  - *Oral follow-up: cefpodoxime,[c] ciprofloxacin,[a]* or *levofloxacin[a]*
- Uncomplicated infection
  - Ceftriaxone,[c] cefotaxime,[c] or cefpodoxime[c]
  - *Ciprofloxacin[a]* or *levofloxacin[a]*

Neisseria meningitides
- Penicillin G
- *Cefotaxime[c]* or *ceftriaxone[c]*

Gram-positive bacilli

Clostridium perfringens
- Penicillin G ± clindamycin
- *Metronidazole,[a]* clindamycin, doxycycline,[a] cefazolin,[c] carbapenemg,[g,h]

Clostridium difficile
- Oral metronidazole[a]
- *Oral vancomycin*

Gram-negative bacilli

Acinetobacter spp
- Doripenem, imipenem or meropenem ± aminoglycoside[i] (amikacin usually most effective)
- *Ampicillin-sulbactam, colistin,[h]* or *tigecycline[a]*

Bacteroides fragilis (and others)
- Metronidazole[a]
- *BL/BLI,[j]* clindamycin, cefoxitin,[c] cefotetan,[c] or *carbapenemg,[g,h]*

Enterobacter spp
- Carbapenem,[g] or cefepime ± aminoglycoside[i]
- *Ciprofloxacin,[a] levofloxacin,[a] piperacillin-tazobactam, ticarcillin-clavulanate*

Escherichia coli
- Meningitis
  - Cefotaxime,[c] ceftriaxone,[c] meropenem
- Systemic infection
  - Cefotaxime[c] or ceftriaxone[c]
  - *BL/BLI,[j] fluoroquinolone,[a,k] carbapenemg,[g,h]*
- Urinary tract infection
  - Most oral agents: check sensitivities
  - Ampicillin, amoxicillin-clavulanate, doxycyline,[a] or cephalexin[c]
  - *Aminoglycoside,[i] FGC[b,c] nitrofurantoin, fluoroquinolone[a,k]*

Gardnerella vaginalis
- Metronidazole[a]
- *Clindamycin*

Haemophilus influenzae
- Meningitis
  - Cefotaxime[c] or ceftriaxone[c]
  - *Meropenem[h]*
- Other infections
  - BL/BLI,[j] or if β-lactamase-negative, ampicillin or amoxicillin
  - *Trimethoprim-sulfamethoxazole, cefuroxime,[c] azithromycin, clarithromycin,* or *fluoroquinolone[a,k]*

(continued)

TABLE 35–2 Drugs of Choice, First Choice, and Alternative(s) *(Continued)*

Klebsiella pneumoniae
- BL/BLI,[i] cefotaxime,[c] ceftriaxone,[c] cefepime[c]
- *Carbapenem,[g,h] fluoroquinolone[a,k]*

Legionella spp
- Azithromycin, erythromycin ± rifampin, or fluoroquinolone[a,k]
- *Trimethoprim-sulfamethoxazole, clarithromycin, or doxycycline[a]*

Pasteurella multocida
- Penicillin G, ampicillin, amoxicillin
- *Doxycycline,[a] BL/BLI,[i] trimethoprim-sulfamethoxazole or ceftriaxone[c]*

Proteus mirabilis
- Ampicillin
- *Trimethoprim-sulfamethoxazole*

Proteus (indole-positive) (including *Providencia rettgeri*, *Morganella morganii*, and *Proteus vulgaris*)
- Cefotaxime,[c] ceftriaxone,[c] or fluoroquinolone[a,k]
- *BL/BLI,[i] aztreonam,[l] aminoglycosides,[j] carbapenem[g,h]*

Providencia stuartii
- Amikacin, cefotaxime,[c] ceftriaxone,[c] fluoroquinolone[a,k]
- *Trimethoprim-sulfamethoxazole, aztreonam,[l] carbapenem[g,h]*

Pseudomonas aeruginosa
- UTI only
  - Aminoglycoside[j]
  - *Ciprofloxacin,[a] levofloxacin[a]*
- Systemic infection
  - Cefepime,[c] ceftazidime,[c] doripenem,[h] imipenem,[h] meropenem,[h] piperacillin-tazobactam, or ticarcillin-clavulanate + aminoglycoside[j]
  - *Aztreonam,[l] ciprofloxacin,[a] levofloxacin,[a] colistin[h]*

Salmonella typhi
- Ciprofloxacin,[a] levofloxacin,[a] ceftriaxone,[c] cefotaxime[c]
- *Trimethoprim-sulfamethoxazole*

Serratia marcescens
- Ceftriaxone,[c] cefotaxime,[c] cefepime,[c] ciprofloxacin,[a] levofloxacin[a]
- *Aztreonam,[l] carbapenem,[g,h] piperacillin-tazobactam, ticarcillin-clavulanate*

Stenotrophomonas (Xanthomonas) maltophilia (generally very resistant to all antimicrobials)
- Trimethoprim-sulfamethoxazole
- *Check sensitivities to ceftazidime,[c] doxycycline,[a] minocycline,[a] and ticarcillin-clavulanate*

Miscellaneous microorganisms

Chlamydia pneumoniae
- Doxycycline[a]
- *Azithromycin, clarithromycin, erythromycin, or fluoroquinolone[a,k]*

Chlamydia trachomatis
- Azithromycin or doxycycline[a]
- *Levofloxacin,[a] erythomycin*

Mycoplasma pneumoniae
- Azithromycin, clarithromycin, erythromycin, fluoroquinolone[a,k]
- *Doxycycline[a]*

(continued)

TABLE 35–2 Drugs of Choice, First Choice, and Alternative(s) *(Continued)*

Spirochetes

Treponema pallidum
- Neurosyphilis
  - Penicillin G
  - *Ceftriaxone[c]*
- Primary or secondary
  - Benzathine penicillin G
  - *Ceftriaxone[c] or doxycycline[a]*

Borrelia burgdorferi (choice depends on stage of disease)
- Ceftriaxone[c] or cefuroxime axetil,[c] doxycycline,[a] amoxicillin
- *High-dose penicillin, cefotaxime[c]*

MIC, minimal inhibitory concentration; PO, orally.

[a]Not for use in pregnant patients or children.

[b]First-generation cephalosporins—IV: cefazolin; PO: cephalexin, cephradine, or cefadroxil.

[c]Some penicillin-allergic patients may react to cephalosporins.

[d]Gentamicin should be added if tolerance or moderately susceptible (MIC >0.1 g/mL) organisms are encountered; streptomycin is used but can be more toxic.

[e]Second-generation cephalosporins—IV: cefuroxime; PO: cefaclor, cefditoren, cefprozil, cefuroxime axetil, and loracarbef.

[f]Third-generation cephalosporins—PO: cefdinir, cefixime, cefetamet, cefpodoxime proxetil, and ceftibuten.

[g]Carbapenem: doripenem, ertapenem, imipenem/cilastatin, meropenem.

[h]Reserve for serious infection.

[i]Aminoglycosides: gentamicin, tobramycin, and amikacin; use per sensitivities.

[j]β-lactam/β-lactamase inhibitor combination—IV: ampicillin-sulbactam, piperacillin-tazobactam, ticarcillin-clavulanate; PO: amoxicillin- clavulanate.

[k]Fluoroquinolones - IV/PO: ciprofloxacin, levofloxacin, and moxifloxacin.

[l]Generally reserved for patients with hypersensitivity reactions to penicillin.

- Pharmacokinetic parameters such as area under the concentration-time curve (AUC) and maximal plasma concentration can be predictive of treatment outcome when specific ratios of AUC or maximal plasma concentration to the minimum inhibitory concentration (MIC) are achieved. For some agents, the ratio of AUC to MIC, peak-to-MIC ratio, or the time that the drug concentration is above the MIC may predict efficacy.
- The most important pharmacodynamic relationship for antimicrobials that display time-dependent bactericidal effects is the duration that drug concentrations exceed the MIC.

COMBINATION ANTIMICROBIAL THERAPY

- Combinations of antimicrobials are generally used to broaden the spectrum of coverage for empiric therapy, achieve synergistic activity against the infecting organism, and prevent the emergence of resistance.
- Increasing the coverage of antimicrobial therapy is generally necessary in mixed infections where multiple organisms are likely to be present, such as intraabdominal and female pelvic infections in which a variety of aerobic and anaerobic bacteria may produce disease. Another clinical situation in which increased spectrum of activity is desirable is with nosocomial infection.

TABLE 35-3 Major Drug Interactions with Antimicrobials

Antimicrobial	Other Agent(s)	Mechanism of Action/Effect	Clinical Management
Aminoglycosides	Neuromuscular blocking agents	Additive adverse effects	Avoid
	Nephrotoxins (N) or ototoxins (O) (e.g., amphotericin B (N) cisplatin (N/O), cyclosporine (N), furosemide (O), NSAIDs (N), radio contrast (N), vancomycin (N)	Additive adverse effects	Monitor aminoglycoside SDC and renal function
Amphotericin B	Nephrotoxins (e.g., aminoglycosides, cidofovir, cyclosporine, foscarnet, pentamidine)	Additive adverse effects	Monitor renal function
Azoles	See Chap. 38		
Chloramphenicol	Phenytoin, tolbutamide, ethanol	Decreased metabolism of other agents	Monitor phenytoin SDC, blood glucose
Foscarnet	Pentamidine IV	Increased risk of severe nephrotoxicity/hypocalcemia	Monitor renal function/serum calcium
Isoniazid	Carbamazepine, phenytoin	Decreased metabolism of other agents (nausea, vomiting, nystagmus, ataxia)	Monitor drug SDC
Macrolides/azalides	Digoxin	Decreased digoxin bioavailability and metabolism	Monitor digoxin SDC; avoid if possible
	Theophylline	Decreased metabolism of theophylline	Monitor theophylline SDC
Metronidazole	Ethanol (drugs containing ethanol)	Disulfiram-like reaction	Avoid
Penicillins and cephalosporins	Probenecid, aspirin	Blocked excretion of β-lactams	Use if prolonged high concentration of β-lactam desirable

Ciprofloxacin/norfloxacin	Theophylline	Decreased metabolism of theophylline	Monitor theophylline
Quinolones	Classes Ia and III Antiarrhythmics	Increased Q-T interval	Avoid
	Multivalent cations (antacids, iron, sucralfate, zinc, vitamins, dairy, citric acid) didanosine	Decreased absorption of quinolone	Separate by 2 hours
Rifampin	Azoles, cyclosporine, methadone propranolol, PIs, oral contraceptives, tacrolimus warfarin	Increased metabolism of other agent	Avoid if possible
Sulfonamides	Sulfonylureas, phenytoin, warfarin	Decreased metabolism of other agent	Monitor blood glucose, SDC, PT
Tetracyclines	Antacids, iron, calcium, sucralfate	Decreased absorption of tetracycline	Separate by 2 hours
	Digoxin	Decreased digoxin bioavailability and metabolism	Monitor digoxin SDC; avoid if possible

PI, protease inhibitor; PT, prothrombin time; SDC, serum drug concentrations.

Azalides: azithromycin; azoles: fluconazole, itraconazole, ketoconazole, and voriconazole; macrolides: erythromycin, clarithromycin; protease inhibitors: amprenavir, indinavir, lopinavir/ritonavir, nelfinavir, ritonavir, and saquinavir; quinolones: ciprofloxacin, gemifloxacin, levofloxacin, moxifloxacin.

Synergism

- The achievement of synergistic antimicrobial activity is advantageous for infections caused by gram-negative bacilli in immunosuppressed patients.
- Traditionally, combinations of aminoglycosides and β-lactams have been used because these drugs together generally act synergistically against a wide variety of bacteria. However, the data supporting superior efficacy of synergistic over nonsynergistic combinations are weak.
- Synergistic combinations may produce better results in infections caused by *Pseudomonas aeruginosa*, as well as in certain infections caused by *Enterococcus* spp.
- The use of combinations to prevent the emergence of resistance is widely applied but not often realized. The only circumstance where this has been clearly effective is in the treatment of tuberculosis.

Disadvantages of Combination Therapy

- Although there are potentially beneficial effects from combining drugs, there are also potential disadvantages, including increased cost, greater risk of drug toxicity, and superinfection with even more resistant bacteria.
- Some combinations of antimicrobials are potentially antagonistic. For example, agents that are capable of inducing β-lactamase production in bacteria (e.g., cefoxitin) may antagonize the effects of enzyme-labile drugs such as penicillins or imipenem.

MONITORING THERAPEUTIC RESPONSE

- After antimicrobial therapy has been instituted, the patient must be monitored carefully for a therapeutic response. Culture and sensitivity reports from specimens collected must be reviewed.
- Use of agents with the narrowest spectrum of activity against identified pathogens is recommended.
- Patient monitoring should include a variety of parameters, including WBC count, temperature, signs and symptoms of infection, appetite, radiologic studies as appropriate, and determination of antimicrobial concentrations in body fluids.
- As the patient improves, the route of antibiotic administration should be reevaluated. Switching to oral therapy is an accepted practice for many infections. Criteria favoring the switch to oral therapy include

  ✓ Overall clinical improvement
  ✓ Lack of fever for 8 to 24 hours
  ✓ Decreased WBC
  ✓ A functioning GI tract

FAILURE OF ANTIMICROBIAL THERAPY

- A variety of factors may be responsible for the apparent lack of response to therapy. It is possible that the disease is not infectious or nonbacterial in origin, or there is an undetected pathogen. Other factors include those directly related to drug selection, the host, or the pathogen. Laboratory error in identification and/or susceptibility testing errors are rare.

Failures Caused by Drug Selection

- Factors directly related to the drug selection include an inappropriate selection of drug, dosage, or route of administration. Malabsorption of a drug product because of GI disease (e.g., short-bowel syndrome) or a drug interaction (e.g., complexation of fluoroquinolones with multivalent cations resulting in reduced absorption) may lead to potentially subtherapeutic serum concentrations.
- Accelerated drug elimination is also a possible reason for failure and may occur in patients with cystic fibrosis or during pregnancy, when more rapid clearance or larger volumes of distribution may result in low serum concentrations, particularly for aminoglycosides.
- A common cause of failure of therapy is poor penetration into the site of infection. This is especially true for the so-called privileged sites, such as the CNS, the eye, and the prostate gland.

Failures Caused by Host Factors

- Patients who are immunosuppressed (e.g., granulocytopenia from chemotherapy and acquired immunodeficiency syndrome) may respond poorly to therapy because their own defenses are inadequate to eradicate the infection despite seemingly adequate drug regimens.
- Other host factors are related to the necessity for surgical drainage of abscesses or removal of foreign bodies and/or necrotic tissue. If these situations are not corrected, they result in persistent infection and, occasionally, bacteremia, despite adequate antimicrobial therapy.

Failures Caused by Microorganisms

- Factors related to the pathogen include the development of drug resistance during therapy. Primary resistance refers to the intrinsic resistance of the pathogens producing the infection. However, acquisition of resistance during treatment has become a major problem as well.
- The increase in resistance among pathogenic organisms is believed to be due, in large part, to continued overuse of antimicrobials in the community, as well as in hospitals, and the increasing prevalence of immunosuppressed patients receiving long-term suppressive antimicrobials for the prevention of infections.

See Chapter 114, Antimicrobial Regimen Selection, authored by David S. Burgess, for a more detailed discussion of this topic.

Central Nervous System Infections

DEFINITION

- CNS infections include a wide variety of clinical conditions and etiologies: meningitis, meningoencephalitis, encephalitis, brain and meningeal abscesses, and shunt infections. The focus of this chapter is meningitis.

ETIOLOGY AND PATHOPHYSIOLOGY

- Infections are the result of hematogenous spread from a primary infection site, seeding from a parameningeal focus, reactivation from a latent site, trauma, or congenital defects in the CNS.
- Passive and active exposure to cigarette smoke and the presence of a cochlear implant that includes a positioner both increase the risk of bacterial meningitis.
- CNS infections may be caused by a variety of bacteria, fungi, viruses, and parasites. The most common causes of bacterial meningitis are *Streptococcus pneumoniae, Neisseria meningitidis, Listeria monocytogenes,* and *Haemophilus influenzae.*
- The critical first step in the acquisition of acute bacterial meningitis is nasopharyngeal colonization of the host by the bacterial pathogen. The bacteria first attach themselves to nasopharyngeal epithelial cells and are then phagocytized into the host's bloodstream.
- A common characteristic of most CNS bacterial pathogens (e.g., *H. influenzae, Escherichia coli,* and *N. meningitidis*) is the presence of an extensive polysaccharide capsule that is resistant to neutrophil phagocytosis and complement opsonization.
- The neurologic sequelae of meningitis occur due to the activation of host inflammatory pathways. Bacterial cell death causes the release of cell wall components such as lipopolysaccharide, lipid A (endotoxin), lipoteichoic acid, teichoic acid, and peptidoglycan, depending on whether the pathogen is gram-positive or gram-negative. These cell wall components cause capillary endothelial cells and CNS macrophages to release cytokines (interleukin-1, tumor necrosis factor, and other inflammatory mediators). Proteolytic products and toxic oxygen radicals cause an alteration of the blood–brain barrier, whereas platelet-activating factor activates coagulation, and arachidonic acid metabolites stimulate vasodilation. These events lead to cerebral edema, elevated intracranial pressure, cerebrospinal fluid (CSF) pleocytosis, decreased cerebral blood flow, cerebral ischemia, and death.

CLINICAL PRESENTATION

- Meningitis causes CSF fluid changes, and these changes can be used as diagnostic markers of infection (Table 36–1).

TABLE 36-1	Mean Values of the Components of Normal and Abnormal Cerebrospinal Fluid				
Type	Normal	Bacterial	Viral	Fungal	Tuberculosis
WBC (cells/mm^3)	<5	1,000–5,000	100–1,000	40–400	100–500
Differential (%)	>90^a	≥80 PMNs	50^{b,c}	>50^b	>80^{b,c}
Protein (mg/dL)	<50	100–500	30–150	40–150	≤40–150
Glucose (mg/dL)	50–66% simultaneous serum value	<40 (<60% simultaneous serum value)	<30–70	<30–70	<30–70

^{a}Monocytes.
^{b}Lymphocytes.
^{c}In the initial cerebrospinal fluid assessment, the white blood cell (WBC) count may reveal a predominance of polymorphonuclear neutrophils (PMNs).

- Clinical presentation varies with age; generally, the younger the patient, the more atypical and the less pronounced is the clinical picture.
- Up to 50% of patients may receive antibiotics before a diagnosis of meningitis is made, delaying presentation to the hospital. Prior antibiotic therapy may cause the Gram stain and CSF culture to be negative, but the antibiotic therapy rarely affects CSF protein or glucose.
- Classic signs and symptoms include fever, nuchal rigidity, altered mental status, chills, vomiting, photophobia, and severe headache. Kernig and Brudzinski signs may be present but are poorly sensitive and frequently absent in children. Other signs and symptoms include irritability, delirium, drowsiness, lethargy, and coma. Seizures occur more commonly in children (20–30%) than in adults (0–12%).
- Clinical signs and symptoms in young children may include bulging fontanelle, apneas, purpuric rash, and convulsions, in addition to those just mentioned.

SIGNS AND SYMPTOMS AND LABORATORY TESTS

- Purpuric and petechial skin lesions typically indicate meningococcal involvement, although the lesions may be present with *H. influenzae* meningitis. Rashes rarely occur with pneumococcal meningitis.
- *H. influenzae* meningitis and meningococcal meningitis both can cause involvement of the joints during the illness.
- A history of head trauma with or without skull fracture or the presence of a chronically draining ear is associated with pneumococcal involvement.
- Several tubes of CSF are collected via lumbar puncture for chemistry, microbiology, and hematology tests.
- An elevated CSF protein ≥100 mg/dL and a CSF glucose concentration <50% of the simultaneously obtained peripheral value suggest bacterial meningitis (see Table 36–1).
- The values for CSF glucose, protein, and WBC concentrations found with bacterial meningitis overlap significantly with those for viral, tuberculous,

411

and fungal meningitis (see **Table 36–1**) and cannot always distinguish the different etiologies of meningitis.

- Blood and other specimens should be cultured according to clinical judgment because meningitis frequently can arise via hematogenous dissemination or can be associated with infections at other sites.

- Gram stain and culture of the CSF are the most important laboratory tests performed for bacterial meningitis. When performed before antibiotic therapy is initiated, Gram stain is both rapid and sensitive and can confirm the diagnosis of bacterial meningitis in 75% to 90% of cases.

- Polymerase chain reaction (PCR) techniques can be used to diagnose meningitis caused by *N. meningitidis, S. pneumoniae,* and *H. influenzae* type b (Hib). PCR is considered to be highly sensitive and specific.

- Latex fixation, latex coagglutination, and enzyme immunoassay tests provide for the rapid identification of several bacterial causes of meningitis, including *S. pneumoniae, N. meningitidis,* and Hib. The rapid antigen tests should be used in situations in which the Gram stain is negative.

- Diagnosis of tuberculosis meningitis employs acid-fast staining, culture, and PCR of the CSF.

DESIRED OUTCOME

- The goals of treatment are eradication of infection with amelioration of signs and symptoms and prevention of neurologic sequelae, such as seizures, deafness, coma, and death.

TREATMENT

- The administration of fluids, electrolytes, antipyretics, analgesia, and other supportive measures are particularly important for patients presenting with acute bacterial meningitis.

- Antibiotic dosages for treatment of CNS infections must be maximized to optimize penetration to the site of infection.

- Meningitis caused by *S. pneumoniae* is successfully treated with 10 to 14 days of antibiotic therapy. Meningitis caused by *N. meningitidis* usually can be treated with a 7-day course. A longer course, ≥21 days, is recommended for patients infected with *L. monocytogenes.* Therapy should be individualized, and some patients may require longer courses.

PHARMACOLOGIC TREATMENT

- Empiric antimicrobial therapy should be instituted as soon as possible to eradicate the causative organism (**Table 36–2**). Antimicrobial therapy should last at least 48 to 72 hours or until the diagnosis of bacterial meningitis can be ruled out. Continued therapy should be based on the assessment of clinical improvement, cultures, and susceptibility testing results. Once a pathogen is identified, antibiotic therapy should be tailored to the specific pathogen. The first dose of antibiotic should not be withheld even when lumbar puncture is delayed or neuroimaging is being performed.

TABLE 36–2	Bacterial Meningitis: Most Likely Pathogens and Empirical Therapy by Age Group		
Age Commonly Affected	Most Likely Organisms	Empirical Therapy	Risk Factors for All Age Groups
Newborn–1 month	Group B *Streptococcus* Gram-negative enterics[a] *Listeria monocytogenes*	Ampicillin plus cefotaxime or ceftriaxone or aminoglycoside	Respiratory tract infection Otitis media Mastoiditis
1 month–4 years	*S. pneumoniae* *N. meningitidis* *H. influenzae*	Vancomycin[b] and cefotaxime or ceftriaxone	Head trauma Alcoholism High-dose steroids
5–29 years	*N. meningitidis* *S. pneumoniae* *H. influenzae*	Vancomycin[b] and cefotaxime or ceftriaxone	Splenectomy Sickle cell disease Immunoglobulin deficiency
30–60 years	*S. pneumoniae* *N. meningitidis*	Vancomycin[b] and cefotaxime or ceftriaxone	Immunosuppression
>60 years	*S. pneumoniae* Gram-negative enterics *L. monocytogenes*	Vancomycin[b] plus ampicillin plus cefotaxime or ceftriaxone	

[a]*Escherichia coli, Klebsiella* species, and *Enterobacter* species are common.
[b]Vancomycin use should be based on local incidence of penicillin-resistant *S. pneumoniae* and until cefotaxime or ceftriaxone minimum inhibitory concentration results are available.

- With increased meningeal inflammation, there will be greater antibiotic penetration (Table 36–3). Problems of CSF penetration may be overcome by direct instillation of antibiotics by intrathecal, intracisternal, or intra-ventricular routes of administration (Table 36–4).

Dexamethasone as an Adjunctive Treatment for Meningitis

- In addition to antibiotics, **dexamethasone** is a commonly used therapy for the treatment of pediatric meningitis. Several studies have shown that dexamethasone causes a significant improvement in CSF concentrations of proinflammatory cytokines, glucose, protein, and lactate, as well as a significantly lower incidence of neurologic sequelae commonly associated with bacterial meningitis. However, there are conflicting results.
- The American Academy of Pediatrics suggests that the use of dexamethasone be considered for infants and children ages 2 months and older with pneumococcal meningitis and that it be given to those with *H. influenzae* meningitis. The commonly used IV dexamethasone dose is 0.15 mg/kg every 6 hours for 4 days. Alternatively, dexamethasone given 0.15 mg/kg every 6 hours for 2 days or 0.4 mg/kg every 12 hours for 2 days is equally effective and a potentially less toxic regimen.
- Dexamethasone should be administered prior to the first antibiotic dose and not after antibiotics have already been started. Serum hemoglobin and stool guaiac should be monitored for evidence of GI bleeding.

TABLE 36–3	Penetration of Antimicrobial Agents into the Cerebrospinal Fluid (CSF)
Therapeutic levels in CSF with or without inflammation	
Chloramphenicol	Pyrazinamide
Cycloserine	Rifampin
Ethionamide	Sulfonamides
Isoniazid	Trimethoprim
Metronidazole	
Therapeutic levels in CSF with inflammation of meninges	
Acyclovir	Ganciclovir
Ampicillin ± sulbactam	Imipenem
Aztreonam	Levofloxacin
Carbenicillin	Linezolid
Cefotaxime	Meropenem
Ceftazidime	Mezlocillin
Ceftizoxime	Moxifloxacin
Ceftriaxone	Nafcillin
Cefuroxime	Ofloxacin
Ciprofloxacin	Penicillin G
Colistin	Piperacillin
Daptomycin	Pyrimethamine
Ethambutol	Quinupristin/dalfopristin
Fluconazole	Ticarcillin ± clavulanic acid
Flucytosine	Vancomycin
Foscarnet	Vidarabine
Nontherapeutic levels in CSF with or without inflammation	
Aminoglycosides	Cephalosporins (second-generation)[a]
Amphotericin B	Clindamycin[b]
Cefoperazone	Itraconazole[c]
Cephalosporins (first-generation)	Ketoconazole

[a]Cefuroxime is an exception.
[b]Achieves therapeutic brain tissue concentrations.
[c]Achieves therapeutic concentrations for *Cryptococcus neoformans* therapy.

Neisseria meningitidis (Meningococcus)

- *N. meningitidis* meningitis is the leading cause of bacterial meningitis in children and young adults in the United States. Most cases occur in the winter or spring, at a time when viral meningitis is relatively uncommon.

CLINICAL PRESENTATION

- Approximately 10 to 14 days after the onset of the disease and despite successful treatment, the patient develops a characteristic immunologic reaction of fever, arthritis (usually involving large joints), and

	TABLE 36–4	Intraventricular and Intrathecal Antibiotic Dosage Recommendation

Antibiotic	Dose (mg)	Expected CSF Concentration[a] (mg/L)
Ampicillin	10–50	60–300
Methicillin	25–100	160–600
Nafcillin	75	500
Cephalothin	25–100	160–600
Chloramphenicol	25–100	160–600
Gentamicin	1–10	6–60
Quinupristin/dalfopristin	1–2	7–13
Tobramycin	1–10	6–60
Vancomycin	5	30
Amphotericin B	0.05–0.25 mg/day to 0.05–1 mg 1–3 times weekly	–

CSF, cerebrospinal fluid.
[a]Assumes adult CSF volume = 150 mL.

pericarditis. The synovial fluid is characterized by a large number of polymorphonuclear cells, elevated protein concentrations, normal glucose concentrations, and sterile cultures.

- Deafness unilaterally, or more commonly bilaterally, may develop early or late in the disease course.
- Approximately 50% of patients with meningococcal meningitis have purpuric lesions, petechiae, or both. Patients may have an obvious or subclinical picture of disseminated intravascular coagulation, which may progress to infarction of the adrenal glands and renal cortex and cause widespread thrombosis.

TREATMENT AND PREVENTION

- Aggressive, early intervention with high-dose IV crystalline penicillin G, 50,000 units/kg every 4 hours, is usually recommended for treatment of *N. meningitidis* meningitis.
- **Chloramphenicol** may be used in place of penicillin G. Several third-generation cephalosporins (e.g., **cefotaxime, ceftizoxime, ceftriaxone, and cefuroxime**) approved for the treatment of meningitis are acceptable alternatives to penicillin G (Table 36–5). Meropenem and fluoroquinolones are suitable alternatives for treatment of penicillin-nonsusceptible meningococci.
- Close contacts of patients contracting *N. meningitidis* meningitis are at an increased risk of developing meningitis. Prophylaxis of contacts should be started only after consultation with the local health department.
- For prophylaxis of close contacts, adult patients should receive 600 mg of *rifampin* orally every 12 hours for four doses. Children 1 month to 12 years of age should receive 10 mg/kg of rifampin orally every 12 hours

TABLE 36–5 Antimicrobial Agents of First Choice and Alternative Choice for Treatment of Meningitis Caused by Gram-Positive and Gram-Negative Microorganisms

Organism	Antibiotic of First Choice	Alternative Antibiotics	Recommended Duration of Therapy
Gram-positive			
Streptococcus pneumoniae			
Penicillin susceptible	Penicillin G or ampicillin (A-III)	Cefotaxime (A-III), ceftriaxone (A-III), chloramphenicol (A-III)	10–14 days
Penicillin intermediate	Cefotaxime or ceftriaxone (A-III)	Cefepime (B-II), meropenem (B-II), moxifloxacin (B-II), linezolid (C-III)	
Penicillin resistant	Vancomycin^e plus cefotaxime or ceftriaxone (A-III)	Cefepime (B-II), meropenem (B-II), moxifloxacin (B-II), linezolid (C-III)	
Group B *Streptococcus*	Penicillin G or ampicillin ± gentamicin^e (A-III)	Cefotaxime (B-III), ceftriaxone (B-III), chloramphenicol (B-III)	14–21 days
Staphylococcus aureus			14–21 days^e
Methicillin susceptible	Nafcillin or oxacillin (A-III)	Vancomycin^e (A-III), meropenem (B-III)	
Methicillin resistant	Vancomycin^e (A-III)	Trimethoprim-sulfamethoxazole (A-III), linezolid (B-III)	14–21 days^e
Staphylococcus epidermidis	Vancomycin^e (A-III)	Linezolid (B-III)	≥21 days
Listeria monocytogenes	Penicillin G or ampicillin ± gentamicin^e (A-III)	Trimethoprim-sulfamethoxazole (A-III), meropenem (B-III)	
Gram-negative			
Neisseria meningitidis			7 days
Penicillin susceptible	Penicillin G or ampicillin (A-III)	Cefotaxime (A-III), ceftriaxone (A-III), chloramphenicol (A-III)	

Penicillin resistant	Cefotaxime or ceftriaxone (A-III)	Chloramphenicol (A-III), meropenem (A-III), fluoroquinolone (A-III)	
Haemophilus influenzae			
β-Lactamase negative	Ampicillin (A-III)	Cefotaxime (A-III), ceftriaxone (A-III), chloramphenicol (A-III), cefepime (A-III), fluoroquinolone (A-III)	7 days
β-Lactamase positive	Cefotaxime or ceftriaxone (A-I)	Cefepime (A-I), fluoroquinolone (A-III), chloramphenicol (A-III)	
Enterobacteriaceae[d]	Cefotaxime or ceftriaxone (A-II)	Cefepime (A-III), fluoroquinolone (A-III), meropenem (A-III), aztreonam (A-II)	21 days
Pseudomonas aeruginosa	Cefepime or ceftazidime (A-II) ± tobramycin[a,b] (A-III)	Ciprofloxacin (A-III), meropenem (A-III), piperacillin plus tobramycin[a,b] (A-III), colistin sulfomethate[a,c] (B-III), aztreonam (A-III)	21 days

Strength of recommendation: A, good evidence to support a recommendation for use; should always be offered; B, moderate evidence to support a recommendation for use; should generally be offered.

Quality of evidence: I, evidence from ≥1 properly randomized controlled trial; II, evidence from ≤1 well-designed clinical trial, without randomization; from cohort or case-controlled analytic studies (preferably from >1 center) or from multiple time-series; III, evidence from opinions of respected authorities, based on clinical experience, descriptive studies, or reports of expert committees.

[a] Monitor drug levels in serum.

[b] Direct CNS administration may be added; see Table 36-4 for dosage.

[c] Should be reserved for multidrug-resistant pseudomonal or *Acinetobacter* infections for which all other therapeutic options have been exhausted.

[d] Includes *Escherichia coli* and *Klebsiella* species.

[e] Based on clinical experience; no clear recommendations.

for four doses, and children younger than 1 month should receive 5 mg/kg orally every 12 hours for four doses.

Streptococcus pneumoniae (Pneumococcus or Diplococcus)

* *S. pneumoniae* is the leading cause of meningitis in adults. Pneumococcal meningitis occurs in the very young (younger than 2 years of age) and the very old.
* Neurologic complications, such as coma and seizures, are common.

TREATMENT

(See Tables 36–5 and 36–6.)

TABLE 36–6	Dosing of Antimicrobial Agents by Age Group	
Antimicrobial Agent	**Infants and Children**	**Adults**
Antibacterials		
Ampicillin	75 mg/kg every 6 hours	2 g every 4 hours
Aztreonam		2 g every 6–8 hours
Cefepime	50 mg/kg every 8 hours	2 g every 8 hours
Cefotaxime	75 mg/kg every 6–8 hours	2 g every 4–6 hours
Ceftazidime	50 mg/kg every 8 hours	2 g every 8 hours
Ceftriaxone	100 mg/kg once daily	2 g every 12–24 hours
Chloramphenicol	25 mg/kg every 6 hours	1–1.5 g every 6 hours
Ciprofloxacin	10 mg/kg every 8 hours	400 mg every 8–12 hours
Colistin[a,c]	5 mg/kg once daily	5 mg/kg once daily
Gentamicin[a,b]	2.5 mg/kg every 8 hours	2 mg/kg every 8 hours
Levofloxacin	10 mg/kg once daily	750 mg once daily
Linezolid	10 mg/kg every 8 hours	600 mg every 12 hours
Meropenem	40 mg/kg every 8 hours	2 mg every 8 hours
Moxifloxacin		400 mg once daily
Oxacillin/nafcillin	50 mg/kg every 6 hours	2 mg every 4 hours
Penicillin G	0.05 million units/kg every 4–6 hours	4 million units every 4 hours
Piperacillin	50 mg/kg every 4–6 hours	3 g every 4–6 hours
Tobramycin[a,b]	2.5 mg/kg every 8 hours	2 mg/kg every 8 hours
Trimethoprim–sulfamethoxazole[d]	5 mg/kg every 6–12 hours	5 mg/kg every 6–12 hours
Vancomycin[a]	15 mg/kg every 6 hours	15 mg/kg every 8–12 hours
Antimycobacterials		
Isoniazide[e]	10–15 mg/kg once daily	5 mg/kg once daily
Rifampin	10–20 mg/kg once daily	600 mg once daily
Pyrazinamide	15–30 mg/kg once daily	15–30 mg/kg once daily
Ethambutol	15–25 mg/kg once daily	15–25 mg/kg once daily
		(continued)

TABLE 36–6 Dosing of Antimicrobial Agents by Age Group *(Continued)*

Antimicrobial Agent	Infants and Children	Adults
Antifungals		
Amphotericin B		0.7–1 mg/kg once daily
Lipid amphotericin B		4 mg/kg once daily
Flucytosine		25 mg/kg every 6 hours
Fluconazole		400–800 mg once daily
Voriconazole		6 mg/kg every 12 hours × 2 doses, then 4 mg/kg every 12 hours
Antivirals		
Acyclovir	20 mg/kg every 8 hours	10 mg/kg every 8 hours
Foscarnet		60 mg/kg every 8–12 hours

[a]Monitor drug levels in serum.
[b]Direct CNS administration may be added; see Table 36–4 eighth edition, for dosage.
[c]Should be reserved for multidrug-resistant pseudomonal or *Acinetobacter* infections for which all other therapeutic options have been exhausted.
[d]Dosing based on trimethoprim component.
[e]Supplemental pyridoxine hydrochloride (vitamin B$_6$) 50 mg/day is recommended.

- The treatment of choice until susceptibility of the organism is known is the combination of **vancomycin** plus **ceftriaxone.** Penicillin may be used for drug-susceptible isolates with minimum inhibitory concentrations ≤0.06 mcg/mL, but for intermediate isolates ceftriaxone is used, and for highly drug-resistant isolates a combination of ceftriaxone and vancomycin should be used. A high percent of *S. pneumoniae* is either intermediately or highly resistant to penicillin. Meropenem is recommended as an alternative to a third-generation cephalosporin in penicillin nonsusceptible isolates.
- Virtually all serotypes of *S. pneumoniae* exhibiting intermediate or complete resistance to penicillin are found in the current 23 serotype pneumococcal vaccine. A heptavalent conjugate vaccine is available for use in infants between 2 months and 9 years of age. Current recommendations are for all healthy infants younger than 2 years of age to be immunized with the heptavalent vaccine at 2, 4, 6, and 12 to 15 months.
- The Centers for Disease Control and Prevention (CDC) recommends use of pneumococcal vaccine for persons over 65 years of age; persons 2 to 64 years of age who have achronic illness, who live in high-risk environments, and who lack a functioning spleen; and immunocompromised persons over 2 years, including those with human immunodeficiency virus (HIV) infection.

Haemophilus influenzae

- In the past, *H. influenzae* was the most common cause of meningitis in children 6 months to 3 years of age, but this has declined dramatically since the introduction of effective vaccines.

- Approximately 30% to 40% of *H. influenzae* are ampicillin resistant. For this reason, many clinicians use a third-generation cephalosporin (**cefotaxime** or **ceftriaxone**) for initial antimicrobial therapy. Once bacterial susceptibilities are available, ampicillin may be used if the isolate proves ampicillin sensitive. Cefepime and fluoroquinolones are suitable alternatives regardless of β-lactamase activity.
- Secondary cases may occur within 30 days of the index case, so treatment of close contacts (household members, individuals sharing sleeping quarters, crowded confined populations, daycare attendees, and nursing home residents) of patients is usually recommended to eliminate nasopharyngeal and oropharyngeal carriage of *H. influenzae.*
- Prophylaxis of close contacts should be started only after consultation with the local health department and the CDC. In general, children should receive 20 mg/kg (maximum 600 mg) and adults 600 mg daily in one dose for 4 days. Fully vaccinated individuals should not receive prophylaxis.
- Vaccination with Hib conjugate vaccines is usually begun in children at 2 months.
- The vaccine should be considered in patients older than 5 years with sickle cell disease, asplenia, or immunocompromising diseases.

Listeria monocytogenes

- *L. monocytogenes* is a gram-positive, diphtheroid-like organism and is responsible for 8% of all reported cases of meningitis. The disease affects primarily neonates, alcoholics, immunocompromised patients, and the elderly.
- The combination of **penicillin G** or **ampicillin** with an aminoglycoside results in a bactericidal effect. Patients should be treated for 2 to 3 weeks after defervescence to prevent the possibility of relapse. Combination therapy is given for at least 10 days with the remainder completed with penicillin G or ampicillin alone.
- **Trimethoprim–sulfamethoxazole** may be an effective alternative because adequate CSF penetration is achieved with these agents.

Gram-Negative Bacillary Meningitis

- Gram-negative bacteria (excluding *H. influenzae*) are the fourth leading cause of meningitis.
- Optimal antibiotic therapies for gram-negative bacillary meningitis have not been fully defined. Meningitis caused by *Pseudomonas aeruginosa* is initially treated with **ceftazidime** or **cefepime, piperacillin** plus **tazobactam,** or **meropenem** plus an aminoglycoside, usually **tobramycin** (see Table 36–5).
- If the pseudomonad is suspected to be antibiotic resistant or becomes resistant during therapy, an intraventricular aminoglycoside (preservative-free) should be considered along with IV aminoglycoside. Intraventricular aminoglycoside dosages are adjusted to the estimated CSF volume (0.03 mg of tobramycin or **gentamicin** per mL of CSF and 0.1 mg of **amikacin** per mL of CSF every 24 hours). Ventricular levels of aminoglycoside are monitored every 2 or 3 days, just prior to the next intraventricular dose, and "trough levels" should approximate 2 to

10 mg/L. Intraventricular administration of aminoglycosides to infants is not recommended.

- Gram-negative organisms, other than *P. aeruginosa,* that cause meningitis can be treated with a third- or fourth-generation cephalosporin such as **cefotaxime, ceftriaxone, ceftazidime,** or **cefepime**. In adults, daily doses of 8 to 12 g/day of these third-generation cephalosporins or 2 g of ceftriaxone twice daily should produce CSF concentrations of 5 to 20 mg/L.
- Therapy for gram-negative meningitis is continued for a minimum of 21 days. CSF cultures may remain positive for several days or more on a regimen that will eventually be curative.

Bacillus anthracis

- *B. anthracis* may cause meningitis following cutaneous or inhalational infection. It is typically susceptible to penicillin, ampicillin, erythromycin, doxycycline, ciprofloxacin, and chloramphenicol. Ciprofloxacin is recommended for treatment of meningitis.

Mycobacterium tuberculosis

- *Mycobacterium tuberculosis* var. *hominis* is the primary cause of tuberculous meningitis. Tuberculous meningitis may exist in the absence of disease in the lung or extrapulmonary sites. Upon initial examination, CSF usually contains 100 to 1,000 WBC/mm^3, which may be 75% to 80% polymorphonuclear cells. Over time, the pattern of WBCs in the CSF will shift to lymphocytes and monocytes.
- The CDC recommends a regimen of four drugs for empiric treatment of *M. tuberculosis*. This regimen should consist of **isoniazid, rifampin, pyrazinamide,** and **ethambutol,** 15 to 20 mg/kg/day (maximum 1.6 g/day) for the first 2 months, generally followed by isoniazid plus rifampin for the duration of therapy.
- **Isoniazid** is the mainstay in virtually any regimen to treat *M. tuberculosis*. In children, the usual dose of isoniazid is 10 to 15 mg/kg/day (maximum 300 mg/day). Adults usually receive 5 mg/kg/day or a daily dose of 300 mg. Supplemental doses of **pyridoxine hydrochloride (vitamin B$_6$)**, 50 mg/day, are recommended to prevent the peripheral neuropathy associated with isoniazid administration.
- Concurrent administration of rifampin is recommended at doses of 10 to 20 mg/kg/day (maximum 600 mg/day) for children and 600 mg/day for adults. The addition of pyrazinamide (children and adults 15 to 30 mg/kg/day; maximum in both 2 g/day) to the regimen of isoniazid and rifampin is now recommended. The duration of concomitant pyrazinamide therapy should be limited to 2 months to avoid hepatotoxicity.
- Patients with *M. tuberculosis* meningitis should be treated for a duration of 9 months or longer with multiple-drug therapy, and patients with rifampin-resistant strains should receive 18 to 24 months of therapy.
- The use of glucocorticoids for tuberculous meningitis remains controversial. The administration of steroids such as oral **prednisone,** 60 to 80 mg/day (1–2 mg/kg/day in children), or 0.2 mg/kg/day of IV **dexamethasone**, tapered over 4 to 8 weeks, improves neurologic sequelae and survival in

adults and decreases mortality, long-term neurologic complications, and permanent sequelae in children.

Cryptococcus neoformans

- In the United States, cryptococcal meningitis is the most common form of fungal meningitis and is a major cause of morbidity and mortality in immunosuppressed patients.
- Fever and a history of headaches are the most common symptoms of cryptococcal meningitis, although altered mentation and evidence of focal neurologic deficits may be present. Diagnosis is based on the presence of a positive CSF, blood, sputum, or urine culture for *C. neoformans*.
- CSF cultures are positive in >90% of cases.
- **Amphotericin B** is the drug of choice for treatment of acute *C. neoformans* meningitis. Amphotericin B, 0.5 to 1 mg/kg/day, combined with **flucytosine**, 100 mg/kg/day, is more effective than amphotericin alone. In the acquired immune deficiency syndrome (AIDS) population, flucytosine is often poorly tolerated, causing bone marrow suppression and GI distress.
- Due to the high relapse rate following acute therapy for *C. neoformans*, AIDS patients require lifelong maintenance or suppressive therapy. The standard of care for AIDS-associated cryptococcal meningitis is primary therapy, generally using amphotericin B with or without flucytosine, followed by maintenance therapy with fluconazole for the life of the patient.

See Chapter 115, Central Nervous System Infections, authored by Isaac F. Mitropoulos, Elizabeth D. Hermsen, and John C. Rotschafer, for a more detailed discussion of this topic.

CHAPTER 37

Endocarditis

DEFINITION

- **Endocarditis** is an inflammation of the endocardium, the membrane lining the chambers of the heart and covering the cusps of the heart valves. *Infective endocarditis* (IE) refers to infection of the heart valves by microorganisms, primarily bacteria.
- Endocarditis is often referred to as either acute or subacute depending on the clinical presentation. Acute bacterial endocarditis is a fulminating infection associated with high fevers, systemic toxicity, and death within days to weeks if untreated. Subacute infectious endocarditis is a more indolent infection, usually occurring in a setting of prior valvular heart disease.

ETIOLOGY

- Most patients with IE have risk factors, such as preexisting cardiac valve abnormalities. Many types of structural heart disease resulting in turbulence of blood flow will increase the risk for IE. Some of the most important risk factors include
  - ✓ Presence of a prosthetic valve (highest risk)
  - ✓ Previous endocarditis (highest risk)
  - ✓ Congenital heart disease
  - ✓ Chronic intravenous access
  - ✓ Diabetes mellitus
  - ✓ Healthcare-related exposure
  - ✓ Acquired valvular dysfunction (e.g., rheumatic heart disease)
  - ✓ Hypertrophic cardiomyopathy
  - ✓ Mitral valve prolapse with regurgitation
  - ✓ IV drug abuse
- Three groups of organisms cause most cases of IE: streptococci, staphylococci, and enterococci (Table 37–1).

CLINICAL PRESENTATION

- The clinical presentation of patients with IE is highly variable and nonspecific (Table 37–2). Fever is the most common finding. The mitral and aortic valves are most often affected.
- Important clinical signs, especially prevalent in subacute illness, may include the following peripheral manifestations ("stigmata") of endocarditis:
  - ✓ Osler nodes
  - ✓ Janeway lesions
  - ✓ Splinter hemorrhages
  - ✓ Petechiae

TABLE 37–1	Etiologic Organisms in Infective Endocarditis
Agent	**Percentage of Cases (%)**
Streptococci	25–35
Viridans streptococci	10–20
Other streptococci	5–10
Staphylococci	45–70
Coagulase positive	30–60
Coagulase negative	3–25
Enterococci	5–18
Gram-negative aerobic bacilli	1.5–13
Fungi	1–4
Miscellaneous bacteria	<5
Mixed infections	1–2
Culture negative	<5–24

Data from Moreillon P, Que YA. Infective endocarditis. Lancet 2004;363:139–149 and Murdoch DR, Corey GR, Hoen B, et al. Clinical presentation, etiology, and outcome of infective endocarditis in the 21st century: The International Collaboration on Endocarditis–Prospective Cohort Study. Arch Intern Med 2009;169:463–473.

- ✓ Clubbing of the fingers
- ✓ Roth's spots
- ✓ Emboli

- Without appropriate antimicrobial therapy and surgery, IE is usually fatal. With proper management, recovery can be expected in most patients.

TABLE 37–2	Clinical Presentation of Infective Endocarditis

Symptoms

The patient may complain of fever, chills, weakness, dyspnea, night sweats, weight loss, and/or malaise.

Signs

Fever is common, as well as a heart murmur (sometimes new or changing). The patient may or may not have embolic phenomenon, splenomegaly, or skin manifestations (e.g., Osler nodes or Janeway lesions).

Laboratory tests

The patient's white blood cell count may be normal or only slightly elevated. Nonspecific findings include anemia (normocytic or normochromic), thrombocytopenia, an elevated erythrocyte sedimentation rate or C-reactive protein, and altered urinary analysis (proteinuria/microscopic hematuria).

The hallmark laboratory finding is continuous bacteremia; three sets of blood cultures should be collected over 24 hours.

Other diagnostic tests

An electrocardiogram, chest radiograph, and echocardiogram are commonly performed. Echocardiography to determine the presence of valvular vegetations plays a key role in the diagnosis of infective endocarditis; it should be performed in all suspected cases.

- Factors associated with increased mortality include the following:
  - ✓ Congestive heart failure
  - ✓ Culture-negative endocarditis
  - ✓ Endocarditis caused by resistant organisms such as fungi and gram-negative bacteria
  - ✓ Left-sided endocarditis caused by *Staphylococcus aureus*
  - ✓ Prosthetic valve endocarditis (PVE)

LABORATORY AND DIAGNOSTIC FINDINGS

- Ninety percent to 95% of patients with IE have a positive blood culture when three samples are obtained during a 24-hour period. Anemia may be present.
- Transesophageal echocardiography is important in identifying and localizing valvular lesions in patients suspected of having IE. It is more sensitive for detecting vegetations (90–100%), compared with transthoracic echocardiography (58–63%).
- The Modified Duke criteria, encompassing major findings of persistent bacteremia and echocardiographic findings and other minor findings, are used to categorize patients as "definite IE" or "possible IE."

DESIRED OUTCOME

- Relieve the signs and symptoms of disease
- Decrease morbidity and mortality associated with infection
- Eradicate the causative organism with minimal drug exposure
- Provide cost-effective antimicrobial therapy
- Prevent IE in high-risk patients with appropriate prophylactic antimicrobials

TREATMENT

- The most important approach to treatment of IE is isolation of the infecting pathogen and determination of antimicrobial susceptibilities, followed by high-dose, bactericidal antibiotics for an extended period.
- Treatment usually is started in the hospital, but in some patients, it may be completed in the outpatient setting.
- Large doses of parenteral antimicrobials usually are necessary to achieve bactericidal concentrations within vegetations.
- An extended duration of therapy is required, even for susceptible pathogens, because microorganisms are enclosed within valvular vegetations and fibrin deposits.

NONPHARMACOLOGIC THERAPY

- Surgery is an important adjunct to management of endocarditis in certain patients. In most cases, valvectomy and valve replacement are performed to remove infected tissues and restore hemodynamic function. The most important indications for surgical intervention in the past have been heart failure in left-sided IE and persistent infections in right-sided IE.

STREPTOCOCCAL ENDOCARDITIS

- Streptococci are a common cause of IE, with most isolates being viridans streptococci.
- Most viridans streptococci are exquisitely sensitive to penicillin G with minimum inhibitory concentrations (MICs) ≤0.12 mcg/mL. The MIC should be determined for all viridans streptococci and the results used to guide therapy. Approximately 10% to 20% are moderately susceptible (MIC 0.12–0.5 mcg/mL).
- Recommended therapy in the uncomplicated case caused by fully suscep-tible strains is 4 weeks of either high-dose **penicillin G** or **ceftriaxone**, or 2 weeks of combined therapy with high-dose penicillin G plus **gentamicin** (**Table 37–3**).
- The following conditions should all be present to consider a 2-week treatment regimen:
  - ✓ The isolate is penicillin sensitive (MIC ≤0.1 mcg/mL).
  - ✓ There are no cardiovascular risk factors such as heart failure, aortic insufficiency, or conduction abnormalities.
  - ✓ No evidence of thrombotic disease
  - ✓ Native valve infection
  - ✓ No vegetation >5 mm diameter
  - ✓ Clinical response is evident within 7 days.
- Vancomycin is effective and is the drug of choice for the patient with a history of immediate-type hypersensitivity reaction to penicillin. When vancomycin is used, the addition of gentamicin is not recommended.
- For patients with complicated infection (e.g., extracardiac foci) or when the organism is relatively resistant (MIC = 0.12–0.5 mcg/mL), combi-nation therapy with an aminoglycoside and penicillin (higher dose) or ceftriaxone for the first 2 weeks is recommended (**Table 37–4**).
- In patients with endocarditis of prosthetic valves or other prosthetic mate-rial caused by viridans streptococci and *Streptococcus bovis*, treatment courses are extended to 6 weeks (**Table 37–5**).

STAPHYLOCOCCAL ENDOCARDITIS

- *S. aureus* has become more prevalent as a cause of endocarditis because of increased IV drug abuse, frequent use of peripheral and central venous catheters, and valve replacement surgery. Coagulase-negative staphylococci (usually *S. epidermidis*) are prominent causes of PVE.
- The recommended therapy for patients with left-sided IE caused by meth-icillin-sensitive *S. aureus* (MSSA) is 6 weeks of **nafcillin** or **oxacillin**, often combined with a short course of gentamicin (**Table 37–6**).
- If a patient has a mild, delayed allergy to penicillin, **first-generation cephalosporins** are effective alternatives but should be avoided in patients with an immediate-type hypersensitivity reaction.

TABLE 37–3 Therapy of Native Valve Endocarditis Caused by Highly Penicillin-Susceptible Viridans Group Streptococci and *Streptococcus bovis*

Regimen	Dosage[a] and Route	Duration (weeks)	Strength of Recommendation	Comments
Aqueous crystalline penicillin G sodium	12–18 million units/24 hours IV either continuously or in four or six equally divided doses	4	I A	Preferred in most patients older than age 65 years or patients with impairment of eighth cranial nerve (CN 8) function or renal function
or				
Ceftriaxone sodium	2 g/24 hours IV/IM in one dose *Pediatric dose[b]*: penicillin 200,000 units/kg per 24 hours IV in four to six equally divided doses; ceftriaxone 100 mg/kg per 24 hours IV/IM in one dose	4	I A	
Aqueous crystalline penicillin G sodium	12–18 million units/24 hours IV either continuously or in six equally divided doses	2	I B	2-week regimen not intended for patients with known cardiac or extracardiac abscess or for those with creatinine clearance <20 mL/min, impaired CN 8 function, or *Abiotrophia*, *Granulicatella*, or *Gemella* spp. infection; gentamicin dosage should be adjusted to achieve peak serum concentration of 3–4 mcg/mL and trough serum concentration <1 mcg/mL when three divided doses are used (second option to single daily dose)
or				
Ceftriaxone sodium	2 g/24 hours IV/IM in one dose	2	I B	
plus				
Gentamicin sulfate[c]	3 mg/kg per 24 hours IV/IM in one dose	2		

(continued)

TABLE 37-3 Therapy of Native Valve Endocarditis Caused by Highly Penicillin-Susceptible Viridans Group Streptococci and *Streptococcus bovis* (Continued)

Regimen	Dosage[a] and Route	Duration (weeks)	Strength of Recommendation	Comments
	Pediatric dose: penicillin 200,000 units/kg per 24 hours IV in four to six equally divided doses; ceftriaxone 100 mg/kg per 24 hours IV/IM in one dose; gentamicin 3 mg/kg per 24 hours IV/IM in one dose or three equally divided doses[d]			
Vancomycin hydrochloride[e]	30 mg/kg per 24 hours IV in two equally divided doses not to exceed 2 g/24 hours unless concentrations are inappropriately low	4	I B	Vancomycin therapy recommended only for patients unable to tolerate penicillin or ceftriaxone; vancomycin dosage should be adjusted to obtain peak (1 hour after infusion completed) serum concentration of 30–45 mcg/mL and a trough concentration range of 15–20 mcg/ml
	Pediatric dose: 40 mg/kg per 24 hours IV in two to three equally divided doses			

MIC <0.12 mcg/mL.

[a]Dosages recommended are for patients with normal renal function.

[b]Pediatric dose should not exceed that of a normal adult.

[c]Other potentially nephrotoxic drugs (e.g., nonsteroidal antiinflammatory drugs) should be used with caution in patients receiving gentamicin therapy.

[d]Data for once-daily dosing of aminoglycosides for children exist, but no data for treatment of infective endocarditis exist.

[e]Vancomycin dosages should be infused during the course of at least 1 hour to reduce the risk of histamine-release "red man" syndrome.

From Circulation 2005;111:e394–e453, with permission. Copyright 2005, American Medical Association. Modified based on Circulation 2005;112:2374.

TABLE 37–4 Therapy of Native Valve Endocarditis Caused by Strains of Viridans Group Streptococci and *Streptococcus bovis* Relatively Resistant to Penicillin

Regimen	Dosage[a] and Route	Duration (weeks)	Strength of Recommendation	Comments
Aqueous crystalline penicillin G sodium	24 million units/24 hours IV either continuously or in four to six equally divided doses	4	I B	Patients with endocarditis caused by penicillin-resistant (MIC >0.5 mcg/mL) strains should be treated with regimen recommended for enterococcal endocarditis (see Table 37–8)
or				
Ceftriaxone sodium	2 g/24 hours IV/IM in one dose	4	I B	
plus				
Gentamicin sulfate[b]	3 mg/kg per 24 hours IM/IV in one dose *Pediatric dose:[c]* penicillin 300,000 units/24 hours IV in four to six equally divided doses; ceftriaxone 100 mg/kg per 24 hours IV/IM in one dose; gentamicin 3 mg/kg per 24 hours IV/IM in one dose or three equally divided doses	2	I B	Although it is preferred that gentamicin (3 mg/kg) be given as a single daily dose to adult patients, as a second option, gentamicin can be administered daily in three equally divided doses
Vancomycin hydrochloride[c]	30 mg/kg per 24 hours IV in two equally divided doses not to exceed 2 g/24 hours unless serum concentrations are inappropriately low *Pediatric dose:* 40 mg/kg 24 hours in two or three equally divided doses	4	I B	Vancomycin[d] therapy recommended only for patients unable to tolerate penicillin or ceftriaxone therapy

MIC >0.12 mcg/mL to ≤0.5 mcg/mL.

[a]Dosages recommended are for patients with normal renal function.

[b]See Table 37–3 for appropriate dosage of gentamicin.

[c]Pediatric dose should not exceed that of a normal adult.

[d]See Table 37–3 for appropriate dosage of vancomycin.

Reprinted with permission from Baddour LM, Wilson WR, Bayer AS, et al. Infective endocarditis diagnosis, antimicrobial therapy, and management of complications. Circulation 2005;111:e394–e434. Copyright 2005, American Heart Association, Inc.

TABLE 37–5 Therapy for Endocarditis of Prosthetic Valves or Other Prosthetic Material Caused by Viridans Group Streptococci and *Streptococcus bovis*

Regimen	Dosage[a] and Route	Duration (weeks)	Strength of Recommendation	Comments
Penicillin-susceptible strain (MIC ≤ 0.12 mcg/mL)				
Aqueous crystalline penicillin G sodium	24 million units/24 hours IV either continuously or in four to six equally divided doses	6	I B	Penicillin or ceftriaxone together with gentamicin has not demonstrated superior cure rates compared with monotherapy with penicillin or ceftriaxone for patients with highly susceptible strain; gentamicin therapy should not be administered to patients with creatinine clearance <30 mL/min
or				
Ceftriaxone sodium	2 g/24 hours IV/IM in one dose	6	I B	
with or without				
Gentamicin sulfate[b]	3 mg/kg per 24 hours IM/IV in one dose *Pediatric dose:[c]* penicillin 300,000 units/24 hours IV in four to six equally divided doses; ceftriaxone 100 mg/kg per 24 hours IV/IM in one dose; gentamicin 3 mg/kg per 24 hours IV/IM in one dose or three equally divided doses	2		
Vancomycin hydrochloride[d]	30 mg/kg per 24 hours IV in two equally divided doses *Pediatric dose:* 40 mg/kg 24 hours in two or three equally divided doses	6	I B	Vancomycin therapy recommended only for patients unable to tolerate penicillin or ceftriaxone therapy

Penicillin relatively or fully resistant strain (MIC >0.12 mcg/mL)

Aqueous crystalline penicillin sodium	24 million units/24 hours IV either continuously or in four to six equally divided doses	6	I B
or			
Ceftriaxone	2 g/24 hours IV/IM in one dose	6	I B
plus			
Gentamicin sulfate	3 mg/kg per 24 hours IV/IM in one dose *Pediatric dose:* penicillin 300,000 units/kg per 24 hours IV in four to six equally divided doses	6	I B
Vancomycin hydrochloride	30 mg/kg per 24 hours IV in two equally divided doses *Pediatric dose:* 40 mg/kg per 24 hours IV in two or three equally divided doses	6	I B	Vancomycin therapy recommended only for patients unable to tolerate penicillin or ceftriaxone therapy

[a]Dosages recommended are for patients with normal renal function.
[b]See Table 37–3 for appropriate dosage of gentamicin.
[c]Pediatric dose should not exceed that of a normal adult.
[d]See text and Table 37–3 for appropriate dosage of vancomycin

Reprinted with permission from Baddour LM, Wilson WR, Bayer AS, et al. Infective endocarditis diagnosis, antimicrobial therapy, and management of complications. Circulation 2005;111:e394–e434. Copyright 2005, American Heart Association, Inc.

TABLE 37–6 Therapy for Endocarditis Caused by Staphylococci in the Absence of Prosthetic Materials

Regimen	Dosage[a] and Route	Duration	Strength of Recommendation	Comments
Oxacillin-susceptible strains				
Nafcillin or oxacillin[b]	12 g/24 hours IV in four to six equally divided doses	6 weeks	I A	For complicated right-sided IE and for left-sided IE; for uncomplicated right-sided IE, 2 weeks
with				
Optional addition of gentamicin sulfate[c]	3 mg/kg per 24 hours IV/IM in two or three equally divided doses	3–5 days		Clinical benefit of aminoglycosides has not been established
For penicillin-allergic (nonanaphylactoid type) patients:				Consider skin testing for oxacillin-susceptible staphylococci and questionable history of immediate-type hypersensitivity to penicillin
Cefazolin	6 g/24 hours IV in three equally divided doses	6 weeks	I B	Cephalosporins should be avoided in patients with anaphylactoid-type hypersensitivity to β-lactams; vancomycin should be used in these cases[d]

with			
Optional addition of gentamicin sulfate	3 mg/kg per 24 hours IV/IM in two or three equally divided doses *Pediatric dose:* cefazolin 100 mg/kg per 24 hours IV in three equally divided doses; gentamicin 3 mg/kg per 24 hours IV/IM in three equally divided doses	3–5 days	Clinical benefit of aminoglycosides has not been established
Oxacillin-resistant strains			
Vancomycin[e]	30 mg/kg per 24 hours IV in two equally divided doses *Pediatric dose:* 40 mg/kg per 24 hours IV in two or three equally divided doses	6 weeks	I B	Adjust vancomycin dosage to achieve 1-hours serum concentration of 30–45 mcg/mL and trough concentration of 15–20 mcg/Ml

IE, infective endocarditis.

[a]Dosages recommended are for patients with normal renal function.

[b]Penicillin G 24 million units/24 hours IV in four to six equally divided doses may be used in place of nafcillin or oxacillin if the strain is penicillin susceptible (MI ≤0.1 mcg/mL) and does not produce β-lactamase.

[c]Gentamicin should be administered in close temporal proximity to vancomycin, nafcillin, or oxacillin dosing. See Table 37–3 for appropriate dosage of gentamicin.

[d]Pediatric dose should not exceed that of a normal adult.

[e]For specific dosing adjustment and issues concerning vancomycin, see Table 37–3 footnotes.

Reprinted with permission from Badour LM, Wilson WR, Bayer AS, et al. Infective endocarditis diagnosis, antimicrobial therapy, and management of complications. Circulation 2005;111:e394–e434.
Copyright 2005, American Heart Association, Inc.

- In a patient with a positive penicillin skin test or a history of immediate hypersensitivity to penicillin, **vancomycin** is the agent of choice. Vancomycin, however, kills *S. aureus* slowly and is generally regarded as inferior to penicillinase-resistant penicillins for MSSA. Penicillin-allergic patients who fail on vancomycin therapy should be considered for penicillin desensitization.
- **Vancomycin** is the drug of choice for methicillin-resistant staphylococci because most methicillin-resistant *S. aureus* (MRSA) and most coagulase-negative staphylococci are susceptible. Reports of *S. aureus* strains resistant to vancomycin are emerging.

Treatment of *Staphylococcus* Endocarditis in IV Drug Abusers

- IE in IV drug abusers is most frequently (60–70%) caused by *S. aureus*, although other organisms may be more common in certain geographic locations.
- Standard treatment for MSSA consists of 4 weeks of therapy with a **penicillinase-resistant penicillin** (see Table 37–6).
- A 2-week course of **nafcillin** or **oxacillin** plus an aminoglycoside may be effective. Short-course vancomycin, in place of nafcillin or oxacillin, appears to be ineffective.

Treatment of Staphylococcal Prosthetic Valve Endocarditis

- PVE that occurs within 2 months of cardiac surgery is usually caused by staphylococci implanted at the time of surgery. Methicillin-resistant organisms are common. Vancomycin is the cornerstone of therapy.
- Because of the high morbidity and mortality associated with PVE and refractoriness to therapy, combinations of antimicrobials are usually recommended.
- For methicillin-resistant staphylococci (both MRSA and coagulase-negative staphylococci), **vancomycin** is used with rifampin for 6 weeks or more (Table 37–7). An **aminoglycoside** is added for the first 2 weeks if the organism is susceptible.
- For methicillin-susceptible staphylococci, a **penicillinase-stable penicillin** is used in place of vancomycin. If an organism is identified other than staphylococci, the treatment regimen should be guided by susceptibilities and should be at least 6 weeks in duration.

ENTEROCOCCAL ENDOCARDITIS

- Enterococci cause 5% to 18% of endocarditis cases and are noteworthy for the following reasons: (1) no single antibiotic is bactericidal; (2) MICs to penicillin are relatively high (1–25 mcg/mL); (3) they are intrinsically resistant to all cephalosporins and relatively resistant to aminoglycosides (i.e., "low-level" aminoglycoside resistance); (4) combinations of a cell wall–active agent, such as a penicillin or vancomycin, plus an aminoglycoside are necessary for killing; and (5) resistance to all available drugs is increasing.
- Enterococcal endocarditis ordinarily requires 4 to 6 weeks of high-dose **penicillin G** or **ampicillin**, plus **gentamicin** for cure (Table 37–8). A 6-week course is recommended for patients with symptoms lasting longer than 3 months and those with PVE.

TABLE 37–7 Therapy for Prosthetic Valve Endocarditis Caused by Staphylococci

Regimen	Dosage[a] and Route	Duration (weeks)	Strength of Recommendation	Comments
Oxacillin-susceptible strains				
Nafcillin or oxacillin	12 g/24 hours IV in four to six equally divided doses	≥6	I B	Penicillin G 24 million units/24 hours IV in four to six equally divided doses may be used in place of nafcillin or oxacillin if strain is penicillin susceptible (MIC ≤0.1 mcg/mL) and does not produce β-lactamase; vancomycin should be used in patients with immediate-type hypersensitivity reactions to betalactam antibiotics (see Table 37–3 for dosing guidelines); cefazolin may be substituted for nafcillin or oxacillin in patients with non-immediate-type hypersensitivity reactions to penicillins
plus				
Rifampin	900 mg per 24 hours IV/orally in three equally divided doses	≥6		
plus				
Gentamicin[b]	3 mg/kg per 24 hours IV/IM in two or three equally divided doses *Pediatric dose*[c]: nafcillin or oxacillin 200 mg/kg per 24 hours IV in four to six equally divided doses; rifampin 20 mg/kg per 24 hours IV/orally in three equally divided doses; gentamicin 3 mg/kg per 24 hours IV/IM in three equally divided doses	2		

(continued)

TABLE 37–7 Therapy for Prosthetic Valve Endocarditis Caused by Staphylococci *(Continued)*

Regimen	Dosage^a and Route	Duration (weeks)	Strength of Recommendation	Comments
Oxacillin-resistant strains				
Vancomycin	30 mg/kg per 24 hours in two equally divided doses	≥6	I B	Adjust vancomycin to achieve 1 hour serum concentration of 30–45 mcg/mL and trough concentration of 15–20 mcg/Ml
plus				
Rifampin	900 mg/24 hours IV/orally in three equally divided doses	≥6		
plus				
Gentamicin	3 mg/kg per 24 hours IV/IM in two or three equally divided doses Pediatric dose: vancomycin 40 mg/kg per 24 hours IV in two or three equally divided doses; rifampin 20 mg/kg per 24 hours IV/orally in three equally divided doses (up to adult dose); gentamicin 3 mg/kg per 24 hours IV or IM in three equally divided doses	2		

^aDosages recommended are for patients with normal renal function.
^bGentamic n should be administered in close proximity to vancomycin, nafcillin, or oxacillin dosing. See Table 37–3 for appropriate dosage of gentamicin.
^cPediatric dose should not exceed that of a normal adult.

Reprinted with permission from Baddour LM, Wilson WR, Bayer AS, et al. Infective endocarditis diagnosis, antimicrobial therapy, and management of complications. Circulation 2005;111:e394–e434. Copyright 2005, American Heart Association, Inc.

TABLE 37–8 Therapy for Native Valve or Prosthetic Valve Enterococcal Endocarditis Caused by Strains Susceptible to Penicillin, Gentamicin, and Vancomycin

Regimen	Dosage[a] and Route	Duration (weeks)	Strength of Recommendation	Comments
Ampicillin sodium *or*	12 g/24 hours IV in six equally divided doses	4–6	I A	Native valve: 4 wk therapy recommended for patients with symptoms of illness <3 months; 6 wk therapy recommended for patients with symptoms >3 months Prosthetic valve or other prosthetic cardiac material: minimum of 6 wk of therapy recommended
Aqueous crystalline penicillin G sodium	18–30 million units/24 hours IV either continuously or in six equally divided doses	4–6	I A	
plus Gentamicin sulfate[b]	3 mg/kg per 24 hours IV/IM in three equally divided doses	4–6		
Vancomycin hydrochloride[d]	30 mg/kg per 24 hours IV in 2 equally divided doses	6	I B	Vancomycin therapy recommended only for patients unable to tolerate penicillin or ampicillin
plus Gentamicin sulfate	3 mg/kg per 24 hours IV/IM in three equally divided doses *Pediatric dose:[c]* vancomycin 40 mg/kg per 24 hours IV in two or three equally divided doses; gentamicin 3 mg/kg per 24 hours IV/IM in three equally divided doses	6		6 wk of vancomycin therapy recommended because of decreased activity against enterococci

[a]Dosages recommended are for patients with normal renal function.

[b]Dosage of gentamicin should be adjusted to achieve peak serum concentration of 3 to 4 mcg/mL and a trough concentration <1 mcg/mL. See Table 37–3 for appropriate dosage of gentamicin.

[c]Pediatric dose should not exceed that of a normal adult.

[d]See text and Table 37–3 for appropriae dosing of vancomycin.

Reprinted with permission from Baddour LM, Wilson WR, Bayer AS, et al. Infective endocarditis diagnosis, antimicrobial therapy, and management of complications. *Circulation* 2005;111:e394-e434. Copyright 2005, American Heart Association, Inc.

- In addition to isolates with high-level aminoglycoside resistance, β-lactamase-producing enterococci (especially *Enterococcus faecium*) are increasingly reported. If these organisms are discovered, use of vancomycin or ampicillin–sulbactam in combination with gentamicin should be considered.
- Vancomycin-resistant enterococci, particularly *E. faecium,* are becoming more common.

EVALUATION OF THERAPEUTIC OUTCOMES

- The evaluation of patients treated for IE includes assessment of signs and symptoms, blood cultures, microbiologic tests (e.g., MIC, minimum bactericidal concentration [MBC], or serum bactericidal titers), serum drug concentrations, and other tests to evaluate organ function.
- Persistence of fever beyond 1 week may indicate ineffective antimicrobial therapy, emboli, infections of intravascular catheters, or drug reactions. In some patients, low-grade fever may persist even with appropriate antimicrobial therapy.
- With effective therapy, blood cultures should be negative within a few days, although microbiologic response to vancomycin may be unusually slower. After the initiation of therapy, blood cultures should be rechecked until they are negative. During the remainder of the therapy, frequent blood culturing is not necessary.
- If bacteria continue to be isolated from blood beyond the first few days of therapy, it may indicate that the antimicrobials are inactive against the pathogen or that the doses are not producing adequate concentrations at the site of infection.
- For all isolates from blood cultures, MICs (not MBCs) should be determined.
- When aminoglycosides are used for endocarditis caused by gram-positive cocci with a traditional three-times daily regimen, peak serum concentrations are recommended to be on the low side of the traditional ranges (3–4 mcg/mL for gentamicin).
- Serum bactericidal titers may be useful only when the causative organisms are moderately susceptible to antimicrobials, when less well-established regimens are used, or when response to therapy is suboptimal and dosage escalation is considered.
- Serum concentrations of the antimicrobial should generally exceed the MBC of the organism; however, in practice this principle is usually not helpful in monitoring patients with endocarditis.

PREVENTION OF ENDOCARDITIS

- Antimicrobial prophylaxis is used to prevent IE in patients believed to be at high risk.
- The use of antimicrobials for this purpose requires consideration of the types of patients who are at risk; the procedures causing bacteremia; the organisms that are likely to cause endocarditis; and the pharmacokinetics,

TABLE 37–9 Cardiac Conditions Associated with the Highest Risk of Adverse Outcome from Endocarditis for Which Prophylaxis with Dental Procedures Is Recommended

Prosthetic cardiac valves

Previous infective endocarditis

Congenital heart disease (CHD)[a]

  Unrepaired cyanotic CHD, including palliative shunts and conduits

  Completely repaired congenital heart defect with prosthetic material or device, whether placed by surgery or by catheter intervention, during the first 6 months after the procedure[b]

  Repaired CHD with residual defects at the site or adjacent to the site of a prosthetic patch or prosthetic device

Cardiac transplantation recipients who develop cardiac valvulopathy

[a]Except for the conditions listed above, antibiotic prophylaxis is no longer recommended for any other form of CHD.

[b]Prophylaxis is recommended because endothelialization of prosthetic material occurs within 6 months after the procedure.

From Wilson W, Taubert KA, Gewitz M, et al. Prevention of infective endocarditis. Circulation 2007:116: 1736–1754 with permission. Copyright 2007, American Medical Association.

TABLE 37–10 Antibiotic Regimens for a Dental Procedure

| Situation | Agent | Regimen: Single Dose 30 to 60 Minutes before Procedure | |
		Adult	Children
Oral	Amoxicillin	2 g	50 mg/kg
Unable to take oral medication	Ampicillin or	2 g IM or IV	50 mg/kg IM or IV
	Cefazolin or ceftriazone	1 g IM or IV	50 mg/kg IM or IV
Allergic to penicillins or ampicillin oral	Cephalexin[a,b] or	2 g	50 mg/kg
	Clindamycin or	600 mg	20 mg/kg
	Azithromycin or clarithromycin	500 mg	15 mg/kg
Allergic to penicillins or ampicillin and unable to take oral medication	Cefazolin or ceftriaxone[b] or	1 g IM or IV	50 mg/kg IM or IV
	Clindamycin	600 mg IM or IV	20 mg/kg IM or IV

[a]Or other first- or second-generation oral cephalosporin in equivalent adult or pediatric dosage.

[b]Cephalosporins should not be used in an individual with a history of anaphylaxis, angioedema, or urticaria with penicillins or ampicillin.

From Wilson W, Taubert KA, Gewitz M, et al. Prevention of infective endocarditis. Circulation 2007:116: 1736–1754 with permission. Copyright 2007, American Medical Association.

spectrum, cost, and ease of administration of available agents. The objective of prophylaxis is to diminish the likelihood of IE in high-risk individuals who are undergoing procedures that cause transient bacteremia. Cardiac conditions associated with the highest risk of adverse outcome from endocarditis are listed in **Table 37–9**.

- Endocarditis prophylaxis is recommended for all dental procedures that involve manipulation of the gingival tissue of the periapical region of teeth or perforation of the oral mucosa.
- Antibiotic regimens for a dental procedure are given in **Table 37–10**.
- When antibiotic prophylaxis is appropriate, a single 2 g dose of **amoxicillin** for adult patients at risk, given 30 to 60 minutes before undergoing procedures associated with bacteremia.

See Chapter 120, Infective Endocarditis, authored by Angie Veverka and Michael A. Crouch, for a more detailed discussion of this topic.

INTRODUCTION

- Systemic mycoses, such as histoplasmosis, coccidioidomycosis, cryptococcosis, blastomycosis, paracoccidioidomycosis, and sporotrichosis, are caused by primary or "pathogenic" fungi that can cause disease in both healthy and immunocompromised individuals. In contrast, mycoses caused by opportunistic fungi such as *Candida albicans*, *Aspergillus* spp., *Trichosporon*, *Candida glabrata*, *Fusarium*, *Alternaria*, and *Mucor* are generally found only in the immunocompromised host. Advances in medical technology, including organ and bone marrow transplantation, cytotoxic chemotherapy, the widespread use of indwelling IV catheters, and the increased use of potent, broad-spectrum antimicrobial agents, have all contributed to the dramatic increase in the incidence of fungal infections worldwide.

SPECIFIC FUNGAL INFECTIONS

HISTOPLASMOSIS

- Histoplasmosis is caused by inhalation of dust-borne microconidia of the dimorphic fungus *Histoplasma capsulatum*. In the United States, most disease is localized along the Ohio and Mississippi river valleys.

Clinical Presentation and Diagnosis

- In the vast majority of patients, low-inoculum exposure to *H. capsulatum* results in mild or asymptomatic pulmonary histoplasmosis. The course of disease is generally benign, and symptoms usually abate within a few weeks of onset. Patients exposed to a higher inoculum during a primary infection or reinfection may experience an acute, self-limited illness with flu-like pulmonary symptoms, including fever, chills, headache, myalgia, and nonproductive cough.

- Chronic pulmonary histoplasmosis generally presents as an opportunistic infection imposed on a preexisting structural abnormality, such as lesions resulting from emphysema. Patients demonstrate chronic pulmonary symptoms and apical lung lesions that progress with inflammation, calcified granulomas, and fibrosis. Progression of disease over a period of years, seen in 25% to 30% of patients, is associated with cavitation, bronchopleural fistulas, extension to the other lung, pulmonary insufficiency, and often death.

- In patients exposed to a large inoculum and in immunocompromised hosts, progressive illness, disseminated histoplasmosis, occurs. The clinical severity of the diverse forms of disseminated histoplasmosis (**Table 38–1**) generally parallels the degree of macrophage parasitization observed.

- Acute (infantile) disseminated histoplasmosis is seen in infants and young children and (rarely) in adults with Hodgkin's disease or other

TABLE 38–1 Clinical Manifestations and Therapy of Histoplasmosis

Type of Disease and Common Clinical Manifestations	Approximate Frequency (%)[a]	Therapy/Comments
Nonimmunosuppressed host		
Acute pulmonary histoplasmosis		
Asymptomatic or mild-moderate disease	50–99	*Asymptomatic, mild, or symptoms <4 weeks:* No therapy generally required. Itraconazole (200 mg 3 times daily for 3 days and then 200 mg once or twice daily for 6–12 weeks) is recommended for patients who continue to have symptoms for 11 months
		Symptoms >4 weeks: Itraconazole 200 mg once daily × 6–12 weeks[b]
Self-limited disease	1–50	*Self-limited disease:* Amphotericin B[c] 0.3–0.5 mg/kg/day × 2–4 weeks (total dose 500 mg) or ketoconazole 400 mg orally daily × 3–6 months can be beneficial in patients with severe hypoxia following inhalation of large inocula; Antifungal therapy generally not useful for arthritis or pericarditis; NSAIDs or corticosteroids can be useful in some cases
Mediastinal granulomas	1–50	Most lesions resolve spontaneously; surgery or antifungal therapy with amphotericin B 40–50 mg/day × 2–3 weeks or itraconazole 400 mg/day orally × 6–12 months can be beneficial in some severe cases; mild to moderate disease can be treated with itraconazole for 6–12 months
Moderately severe–severe diffuse pulmonary disease		Lipid amphotericin B 3–5 mg/kg/day followed by itraconazole 200 mg twice daily for 3 days then twice daily for a total of 12 weeks of therapy; Alternatively, in patients at low risk for nephrotoxicity, amphotericin B deoxycholate 0.7–1 mg/kg/day can be utilized; Methylprednisolone (0.5–1.0 mg/kg daily IV) during the first 1–2 weeks of antifungal therapy is recommended for patients who develop respiratory complications, including hypoxemia or significant respiratory distress
Inflammatory/fibrotic disease	0.02	*Fibrosing mediastinitis:* The benefit of antifungal therapy (itraconazole 200 mg twice daily × 3 months) is controversial but should be considered, especially in patients with elevated ESR or CF titers ≤1:32; surgery can be of benefit if disease is detected early; late disease cannot respond to therapy
		Sarcoid-like: NSAIDs or corticosteroids[d] can be of benefit for some patients
		Pericarditis: Severe disease: corticosteroids 1 mg/kg/day or pericardial drainage procedure

Chronic cavitary pulmonary histoplasmosis	0.05	Antifungal therapy generally recommended for all patients to halt further lung destruction and reduce mortality *Mild–moderate disease:* Itraconazole (200 mg 3 times daily for 3 days and then 1 or 2 times daily for at least 1 year; Some clinicians recommend therapy for 18–24 months due to the high rate of relapse; Itraconazole plasma concentrations should be obtained after the patient has been receiving this agent for at least 2 weeks *Severe disease:* Amphotericin B 0.7 mg/kg/day for a minimum total dose of 25–35 mg/kg is effective in 59–100% of cases and should be used in patients who require hospitalization or are unable to take itraconazole because of drug interactions, allergies, failure to absorb drug, or failure to improve clinically after a minimum of 12 weeks of itraconazole therapy
Histoplasma endocarditis		Amphotericin B (lipid formulations may be preferred, due to their lower rate of renal toxicity) plus a valve replacement is recommended; If the valve cannot be replaced, lifelong suppression with itraconazole is recommended
Central nervous system histoplasmosis		Amphotericin B should be used as initial therapy (lipid formulations at 5 mg/kg/day, for a total dosage of 175 mg/kg may be preferred, due to their lower rate of renal toxicity) for 4–6 weeks, followed by an oral azole (fluconazole or itraconazole 200 mg 2 or 3 times daily) for at least a year; Some patients may require lifelong therapy; Response to therapy should be monitored by repeat lumbar punctures to assess *Histoplasma* antigen levels. WBC, and CF antibody titers; Blood levels of itraconazole should be obtained to ensure adequate drug exposure
Immunosuppressed host		
Disseminated histoplasmosis	0.02–0.05	*Disseminated histoplasmosis:* Untreated mortality 83–93%; relapse 5–23% in non-AIDS patients; therapy is recommended for all patients
Acute (Infantile)		*Nonimmunosuppressed patients:* Ketoconazole 400 mg/day orally × 6–12 months or amphotericin B 35 mg/kg IV
Subacute		*Immunosuppressed patients (non-AIDS) or endocarditis or CNS disease:* Amphotericin B >35 mg/kg × 3 months followed by fluconazole or itraconazole 200 mg orally twice daily × 12 months

(continued)

TABLE 38–1 Clinical Manifestations and Therapy of Histoplasmosis (*Continued*)

Type of Disease and Common Clinical Manifestations	Approximate Frequency (%)[a]	Therapy/Comments
Immunosuppressed host		
Progressive histoplasmosis (immunocompetent patients and immunosuppressed patients without AIDS)		*Moderately severe to severe:* Liposomal amphotericin B (3.0 mg/kg daily), amphotericin B lipid complex (5.0 mg/kg daily), or deoxycholate amphotericin B (0.7–1.0 mg/kg daily) for 1–2 weeks, followed by itraconazole (200 mg twice daily for at least 12 months) *Mild to moderate:* Itraconazole (200 mg twice daily for at least 12 months)
Progressive disease of AIDS	25–50[e]	Amphotericin B 15–30 mg/kg (1–2 g over 4–10 weeks)[c] or itraconazole 200 mg three times daily for 3 days then twice daily for 12 weeks, followed by lifelong suppressive therapy with itraconazole 200–400 mg orally daily; Although patients receiving secondary prophylaxis (chronic maintenance therapy) might be at low risk for recurrence of systemic mycosis when their CD4+ T-lymphocyte counts increase to >100 cells/microliter in response to HAART, the number of patients who have been evaluated is insufficient to warrant a recommendation to discontinue prophylaxis

AIDS, acquired immunodeficiency syndrome; CF, complement fixation; ESR, erythrocyte sedimentation rate; HAART, highly active antiretroviral therapy; NSAIDs, nonsteroidal antiinflammatory drugs; PO, orally.

[a]As a percentage of all patients presenting with histoplasmosis.

[b]Itraconazole plasma concentrations should be measured during the second week of therapy to ensure that detectable concentrations have been achieved. If the concentration is below 1 mcg/mL, the dose may be insufficient or drug interactions can be impairing absorption or accelerating metabolism, requiring a change in dosage. If plasma concentrations are greater than 10 mcg/mL, the dosage can be reduced.

[c]Desoxycholate amphotericin B.

[d]Effectiveness of corticosteroids is controversial.

[e]As a percentage of AIDS patients presenting with histoplasmosis as the initial manifestation of their disease.

[f]Liposomal amphotericin B (AmBisome) may be more appropriate for disseminated disease.

Data from Deepe GS. Histoplasma capsulatum. In: Mandell GL, Bennett JE, Dolin R, eds. Principles and Practice of Infectious Diseases, 6th ed. Philadelphia, PA: Churchill Livingstone, 2005:3012–3026; Wheat LJ, Freifeld AG, Kleiman MB, et al. Clinical practice guidelines for the management of patients with histoplasmosis: 2007 update by the Infectious Diseases Society of America. Clin Infect Dis 2007;45(7):807–825; and Kauffman CA. Histoplasmosis: a clinical and laboratory update. Clin Microbiol Rev 2007;20(1):15–132.

lymphoproliferative disorders. It is characterized by unrelenting fever; anemia; leukopenia or thrombocytopenia; enlargement of the liver, spleen, and visceral lymph nodes; and GI symptoms, particularly nausea, vomiting, and diarrhea. Untreated disease is uniformly fatal in 1 to 2 months.

- Most adults with disseminated histoplasmosis demonstrate a mild, chronic form of the disease. Untreated patients are often ill for 10 to 20 years, with long asymptomatic periods interrupted by relapses characterized by weight loss, weakness, and fatigue.
- Adult patients with acquired immunodeficiency syndrome (AIDS) demonstrate an acute form of disseminated disease that resembles the syndrome seen in infants and children. Progressive disseminated histoplasmosis can occur as the direct result of initial infection or because of reactivation of dormant foci.
- Identification of mycelial isolates from clinical cultures can be made by conversion of the mycelium to the yeast form (requires 3-6 wk) or by the more rapid (2 hours) and 100% sensitive DNA probe that recognizes ribosomal DNA.
- In most patients, serologic evidence remains the primary method in the diagnosis of histoplasmosis. Results obtained from complement fixation, immunodiffusion, and latex antigen agglutination antibody tests are used alone or in combination.
- In the AIDS patient with progressive disseminated histoplasmosis, the diagnosis is best established by bone marrow biopsy and culture, which yield positive cultures in 90% of patients.

Treatment

- Recommended therapy for the treatment of histoplasmosis is summarized in **Table 38-1**.
- Asymptomatic or mildly ill patients and patients with sarcoid-like disease generally do not benefit from antifungal therapy. Therapy may be helpful in symptomatic patients whose conditions have not improved during the first month of infection.
- Patients with mild, self-limited disease, chronic disseminated disease, or chronic pulmonary histoplasmosis who have no underlying immunosuppression can usually be treated with either oral **itraconazole** or IV **amphotericin B**.
- In AIDS patients, intensive 12-week primary (induction and consolidation therapy) antifungal therapy is followed by lifelong suppressive (maintenance) therapy with **itraconazole**. **Amphotericin B** should be administered in patients who require hospitalization. Itraconazole 200 mg twice daily may be used to complete a 12-week course or for a full 12-week course in patients who do not require hospitalization.
- Response to therapy should be measured by resolution of radiologic, serologic, and microbiologic parameters and improvement in signs and symptoms of infection.
- Once the initial course of therapy for histoplasmosis is completed, lifelong suppressive therapy with oral azoles or **amphotericin B** (1-1.5 mg/kg weekly or biweekly) is recommended, because of the frequent recurrence of infection.

- Relapse rates in AIDS patients not receiving preventive maintenance are 50% to 90%.

BLASTOMYCOSIS

- North American blastomycosis is a systemic fungal infection caused by *Blastomyces dermatitidis*. Pulmonary disease probably occurs by inhalation conidia, which convert to the yeast forms in the lungs. It may be acute or chronic and can mimic infection with tuberculosis (TB), pyogenic bacteria, other fungi, or malignancy.
- Blastomycosis can disseminate to virtually every other body organ, including skin, bones, and joints, or the genitourinary tract, without any evidence of pulmonary disease.

Clinical Presentation and Diagnosis

- Acute pulmonary blastomycosis is generally an asymptomatic or self-limited disease characterized by fever, shaking chills, and a productive, purulent cough, with or without hemoptysis in immunocompetent individuals.
- Sporadic pulmonary blastomycosis may present as a more chronic or subacute disease, with low-grade fever, night sweats, weight loss, and a productive cough resembling that of TB rather than bacterial pneumonia. Chronic pulmonary blastomycosis is characterized by fever, malaise, weight loss, night sweats, chest pain, and productive cough.
- The simplest and most successful method of diagnosing blastomycosis is by direct microscopic visualization of the large, multinucleated yeast with single, broad-based buds in sputum or other respiratory specimens, following digestion of cells and debris with 10% potassium hydroxide.
- Histopathologic examination of tissue biopsies and culture of secretions should be used to identify *B. dermatitidis*.

Treatment

- In patients with mild pulmonary blastomycosis, the clinical presentation of the patient, the immune competence of the patient, and the toxicity of the antifungal agents are the main determinants of whether or not to administer antifungal therapy. All immunocompromised patients and patients with progressive disease or with extrapulmonary disease should be treated (Table 38–2).
- Some authors recommend **ketoconazole** therapy for the treatment of self-limited pulmonary disease, with the hope of preventing late extrapulmonary disease.
- **Itraconazole**, 200 to 400 mg/day, demonstrated 90% efficacy as a first-line agent in the treatment of non-life-threatening, non-CNS blastomycosis and 95% success rate for compliant patients who completed at least 2 months of therapy.
- All patients with disseminated blastomycosis and those with extrapulmonary disease require therapy (**ketoconazole**, 400 mg/day orally for 6 months). CNS disease should be treated with **amphotericin B** for a total cumulative dose >1 g.

- Patients infected with human immunodeficiency virus (HIV) should receive induction therapy with **amphotericin B** and chronic suppressive therapy with an oral azole antifungal. **Itraconazole** is the drug of choice for non-life-threatening histoplasmosis in HIV-infected patients.

COCCIDIOIDOMYCOSIS

- Coccidioidomycosis is caused by infection with *Coccidioides immitis*. The endemic regions encompass the semiarid areas of the southwestern United States from California to Texas, known as the Lower Sonoran Zone. It encompasses a spectrum of illnesses ranging from primary uncomplicated respiratory tract infection that resolves spontaneously to progressive pulmonary or disseminated infection.

TABLE 38–2	Therapy of Blastomycosis	
Type of Disease	**Preferred Treatment**	**Comments**
Pulmonary[a]		
Life-threatening	Amphotericin B[b] IV 0.7–1 mg/kg/day IV (total dose 1.5–2.5 g)	Patients may be initiated on amphotericin B and changed to oral itraconazole 200–400 mg daily once clinically stabilized and a minimum dose of 500 mg of amphotericin B has been administered.
Mild to moderate	Itraconazole 200 mg orally twice daily for ≥6 months[c]	Alternative therapy: Ketoconazole 400–800 mg orally daily for ≥6 months or fluconazole 400–800 mg orally daily for ≥6 months[d] In patients intolerant of azoles or in whom disease progresses during azole therapy: Amphotericin B 0.5–0.7 mg/kg/day IV (total dose 1.5–2.5 g)
Disseminated or extrapulmonary		
CNS	Amphotericin B 0.7–1 mg/kg/day IV (total dose 1.5–2.5 g)	For patients unable to tolerate a full course of amphotericin B, consider lipid formulations of amphotericin B or fluconazole ≥800 mg orally daily.
Non-CNS, non-life-threatening	Amphotericin B 0.7–1 mg/kg/day IV (total dose 1.5–2.5 g)	Patients may be initiated on amphotericin B and changed to oral itraconazole 200–400 mg daily once stabilized.
Mild to moderate	Itraconazole 200–400 mg orally daily for ≥6 months	Ketoconazole 400–800 mg orally daily or fluconazole 400–800 mg orally daily for≥6 months.

(continued)

TABLE 38–2	Therapy of Blastomycosis *(Continued)*	
Type of Disease	**Preferred Treatment**	**Comments**
Disseminated or extrapulmonary		
		Bone disease: Therapy with azoles should be continued for 12 months.
Immunocompromised host (including patients with acquired immunodeficiency syndrome, transplants, or receiving chronic glucocorticoid therapy)		
Acute disease	Amphotericin B 0.7–1 mg/kg/day IV (total dose 1.5–2.5 g)	Patients without CNS infection may be switched to itraconazole once clinically stabilized and a minimum dose of 1 g of amphotericin B has been administered; long-term suppressive therapy with an azole is advised.
Suppressive therapy	Itraconazole 200–400 mg orally daily	For patients with CNS disease or those intolerant of itraconazole, consider fluconazole 800 mg orally daily.

*a*Some patients with acute pulmonary infection may have a spontaneous cure. Patients with progressive pulmonary disease should be treated.

*b*Deoxycholate amphotericin B.

*c*In patients not responding to 400 mg, dosage should be increased by 200 mg increments every 4 weeks to a maximum of 800 mg daily.

*d*Therapy with ketoconazole is associated with relapses, and fluconazole therapy achieves a lower response rate than itraconazole.

Clinical Presentation and Diagnosis

- Most of those infected are asymptomatic or have nonspecific symptoms that are often indistinguishable from those of ordinary upper respiratory infections, including fever, cough, headache, sore throat, myalgias, and fatigue. A fine, diffuse rash may appear during the first few days of illness. Chronic, persistent pneumonia or persistent pulmonary coccidioidomycosis (primary disease lasting >6 wk) is complicated by hemoptysis, pulmonary scarring, and the formation of cavities or bronchopleural fistulas.
- "Valley fever" is a syndrome characterized by erythema nodosum and erythema multiforme of the upper trunk and extremities in association with diffuse joint aches or fever. It occurs in ~25% of infected persons, although, more commonly, a diffuse mild erythroderma or maculopapular rash is observed.
- Disseminated infection occurs in <1% of infected patients. Dissemination may occur to the skin, lymph nodes, bone, meninges, spleen, liver, kidney, and adrenal gland. CNS infection occurs in ~16% of patients with disseminated infection.
- Infection is characterized by the development of immunoglobulin M to *C. immitis*, which peaks within 2 to 3 weeks of infection and then declines

rapidly, and immunoglobulin G, which peaks in 4 to 12 weeks and declines over months to years.

- Recovery of *C. immitis* from infected tissues or secretions for direct examination and culture provides an accurate and rapid method of diagnosis. Most patients develop a positive skin test within 3 weeks of the onset of symptoms.

Treatment

- Therapy of coccidioidomycosis is difficult, and the results are unpredictable. Only 5% of infected persons require therapy. Candidates for therapy include those with severe primary pulmonary infection or concurrent risk factors (e.g., HIV infection, organ transplant, or high doses of glucocorticoids), particularly patients with high complement fixation antibody titers in whom dissemination is likely.
- Specific antifungals (and their usual dosages) for the treatment of coccidioidomycosis include **amphotericin B** IV (0.5–1.5 mg/kg/day), **ketoconazole** (400 mg orally daily), IV or oral **fluconazole** (usually 400–800 mg daily, although dosages as high as 1,200 mg/day have been used without complications), and **itraconazole** (200–300 mg orally twice daily as either capsules or solution). If itraconazole is used, measurement of serum concentrations may be helpful to ascertain whether oral bioavailability is adequate.
- Amphotericin B is generally preferred as initial therapy in patients with rapidly progressive disease, whereas azoles are generally preferred in patients with subacute or chronic presentations. Lipid formulations of amphotericin B have not been extensively studied for coccidioidomycosis but can offer a means of giving more drug with less toxicity. Treatments for primary respiratory disease (mainly symptomatic patients) are 3- to 6-month courses of therapy.
- Patients with disease outside the lungs should be treated with 400 mg/day of an oral azole. For meningeal disease, fluconazole 400 mg/day orally should be used; however, some clinicians initiate therapy with 800 or 1,000 mg/day, and itraconazole doses of 400 to 600 mg/day are comparable.

CRYPTOCOCCOSIS

- Cryptococcosis is a noncontagious, systemic mycotic infection caused by the ubiquitous encapsulated soil yeast *Cryptococcus neoformans*.

Clinical Presentation and Diagnosis

- Primary cryptococcosis in humans almost always occurs in the lungs. Symptomatic infections are usually manifested by cough, rales, and shortness of breath that generally resolve spontaneously.
- Disease may remain localized in the lungs or disseminate to other tissues, particularly the CNS, although the skin can also be affected.
- In the non-AIDS patient, the symptoms of cryptococcal meningitis are nonspecific. Headache, fever, nausea, vomiting, mental status changes, and neck stiffness are generally observed. In AIDS patients, fever and

headache are common, but meningismus and photophobia are much less common than in non-AIDS patients.

- Examination of cerebrospinal fluid (CSF) in patients with cryptococcal meningitis generally reveals an elevated opening pressure, CSF pleocytosis (usually lymphocytes), leukocytosis, a decreased CSF glucose, an elevated CSF protein, and a positive cryptococcal antigen.
- Antigens to *C. neoformans* can be detected by latex agglutination. *C. neoformans* can be detected in ~60% of patients by India ink smear of CSF and cultured in >96% of patients.

Treatment

- Treatment of cryptococcosis is detailed in **Table 38–3**. For asymptomatic, immunocompetent persons with isolated pulmonary disease and no evidence of CNS disease, careful observation may be warranted. With symptomatic infection, **fluconazole** or **amphotericin B** is warranted.
- The combination of **amphotericin B** with **flucytosine** for 6 weeks is often used for treatment of cryptococcal meningitis. An alternative is amphotericin B for 2 weeks, followed by **fluconazole** for an additional 8 to 10 weeks. Suppressive therapy with fluconazole 200 mg/day for 6 to 12 months is optional.
- The use of intrathecal **amphotericin B** is not recommended for the treatment of cryptococcal meningitis except in very ill patients or in those with recurrent or progressive disease despite aggressive IV amphotericin B therapy. The dosage of amphotericin B employed is usually 0.5 mg administered via the lumbar, cisternal, or intraventricular (via an Ommaya reservoir) route two or three times weekly.
- **Amphotericin B** with **flucytosine** is the initial treatment of choice for acute therapy of cryptococcal meningitis in AIDS patients. Many clinicians will initiate therapy with amphotericin B, 0.7 mg/kg/day IV (with flucytosine, 100 mg/kg/day). After 2 weeks, consolidation therapy with either itraconazole 400 mg/day orally or **fluconazole** 400 mg/day orally can be administered for 8 weeks or until CSF cultures are negative. Lifelong therapy with fluconazole is then recommended.
- Relapse of *C. neoformans* meningitis occurs in ~50% of AIDS patients after completion of primary therapy. **Fluconazole** (200 mg daily) is currently recommended for chronic suppressive therapy of cryptococcal meningitis in AIDS patients.

CANDIDA INFECTIONS

- Eight species of *Candida* are regarded as clinically important pathogens in human disease: *C. albicans, C. tropicalis, C. parapsilosis, C. krusei, C. stellatoidea, C. guilliermondii, C. lusitaniae,* and *C. glabrata.*

HEMATOGENOUS CANDIDIASIS

- Hematogenous candidiasis describes the clinical circumstances in which hematogenous seeding to deep organs such as the eye, brain, heart, and kidney occurs.

TABLE 38–3 Therapy of Cryptococcocosis[a,b]

Type of Disease and Common Clinical Manifestations	Therapy/Comments
Nonimmunocompromised host	Comparative trials for amphotericin B[c] versus azoles not available
Isolated pulmonary disease (without evidence of CNS infection)	*Asymptomatic disease:* Drug therapy generally not required; observe carefully or fluconazole 400 mg orally daily for 3 to 6 months
	Mild to moderate symptoms: Fluconazole 200–400 mg orally daily for 3 to 6 months; severe disease or inability to take azoles: amphotericin B 0.4–0.7 mg/kg/day (total dose 1–2 g)
Cryptococcemia with positive serum antigen titer (>1:8), cutaneous infection, a positive urine culture, or prostatic disease	Clinician must decide whether to follow the pulmonary therapeutic regimen or the CNS (disseminated) regimen
Recurrent or progressive disease not responsive to amphotericin B	Amphotericin B[d] IV 0.5–0.75 mg/kg/day ± intrathecal amphotericin B 0.5 mg two or three times weekly
Isolated pulmonary disease (without evidence of CNS infection)	*Mild to moderate symptoms or asymptomatic with a positive pulmonary specimen:* Fluconazole 200–400 mg orally daily lifelong
	or
	Itraconazole 200–400 mg orally daily lifelong
	or
	Fluconazole 400 mg orally daily + flucytosine 100–150 mg/kg/day orally for 10 weeks
	Severe disease: Amphotericin B until symptoms are controlled, followed by fluconazole
CNS disease	Amphotericin B[d] IV 0.7–1 mg/kg/day orally for ≥2 weeks, then fluconazole 400 mg orally daily for ≥8 weeks[e]
Acute (induction/consolidation therapy) (follow all regimens with suppressive therapy)	
	or
	Amphotericin B[d] IV 0.7–1 mg/kg/day + flucytosine 100 mg/kg/day orally for 6 to 10 weeks[e]
	or
	Amphotericin B[d] IV 0.7–1 mg/kg/day for 6 to 10 weeks[e]
	or
	Fluconazole 400–800 mg orally daily for 10 to 12 weeks
	or
	Itraconazole 400–800 mg orally daily for 10 to 12 weeks
	or
	Fluconazole 400–800 mg orally daily + flucytosine 100–150 mg/kg/day orally for 6 weeks[e]

(continued)

451

TABLE 38–3 Therapy of Cryptococcocosis[a,b] *(Continued)*

Type of Disease and Common Clinical Manifestations	Therapy/Comments
Nonimmunocompromised host	
	or
	Lipid formulation of amphotericin B IV 3–6 mg/kg/day for 6 to 10 weeks (Note: Induction therapy with azoles alone is discouraged.)
CNS disease	Amphotericin B[d] IV 0.7–1 mg/kg/day + flucytosine 100 mg/kg/day orally for 2 weeks, followed by fluconazole 400 mg orally daily for a minimum of 10 weeks (in patients intolerant to fluconazole, substitute itraconazole 200–400 mg orally daily)
	or
	Amphotericin B[d] IV 0.7–1 mg/kg/day + 5-flucytosine 100 mg/kg/day orally for 6 to 10 weeks
	or
	Amphotericin B[d] IV 0.7–1 mg/kg/day for 10 weeks
	Refractory disease: Intrathecal or intraventricular amphotericin B
Immunocompromised patients	
Non-CNS pulmonary and extrapulmonary disease	Same as nonimmunocompromised patients with CNS disease
CNS disease	Amphotericin B[d] IV 0.7–1 mg/kg/day for 2 weeks, followed by fluconazole 400–800 mg orally daily 8 to 10 weeks, followed by fluconazole 200 mg orally daily for 6 to 12 months (in patients intolerant to fluconazole, substitute itraconazole 200–400 mg orally daily)
	Refractory disease: Intrathecal or intraventricular amphotericin B
HIV-infected patients	
Suppressive/maintenance therapy	Fluconazole 200–400 mg orally daily lifelong
	or
	Itraconazole 200 mg orally twice daily lifelong
	or
	Amphotericin B IV 1 mg/kg 1 to 3 times weekly lifelong

HIV, human immunodeficiency virus.
[a]When more than one therapy is listed, they are listed in order of preference.
[b]See text for definitions of induction, consolidation, suppressive/maintenance therapy, and prophylactic therapy.
[c]Deoxycholate amphotericin B.
[d]In patients with significant renal disease, lipid formulations of amphotericin B can be substituted for deoxycholate amphotericin B during the induction.
[e]Or until cerebrospinal fluid cultures are negative.

- *Candida* is generally acquired via the GI tract, although organisms may also enter the bloodstream via indwelling IV catheters. Immunosuppressed patients, including those with lymphoreticular or hematologic malignancies, diabetes, immunodeficiency diseases, or those receiving immunosuppressive therapy with high-dose corticosteroids, immunosuppressants, antineoplastic agents, or broad-spectrum antimicrobial agents are at high risk for invasive fungal infections. Major risk factors include the use of central venous catheters, total parenteral nutrition, receipt of multiple antibiotics, extensive surgery and burns, renal failure and hemodialysis, mechanical ventilation, and prior fungal colonization.

- Several distinct presentations of disseminated *C. albicans* have been recognized: (1) the acute onset of fever, tachycardia, tachypnea, and occasionally chills or hypotension (similar to bacterial sepsis); (2) intermittent fevers; (3) progressive deterioration with or without fever; and (4) hepatosplenic candidiasis manifested only as fever while the patient is neutropenic.

- No test has demonstrated reliable accuracy in the clinical setting for diagnosis of disseminated *Candida* infection. Blood cultures are positive in only 25% to 45% of neutropenic patients with disseminated candidiasis. Fluorescence in situ hybridization has excellent sensitivity and specificity in the identification of *C. albicans* from blood.

- Treatment of candidiasis is presented in **Table 38–4**. Amphotericin B may be switched to fluconazole (IV or oral) for completion of therapy. Azoles and deoxycholate amphotericin B are similarly effective; however, fewer adverse effects are observed with azoles. Echinocandins are at least as effective as amphotericin B or fluconazole in nonneutropenic adult patients with candidemia.

- In patients with an intact immune system, removal of all existing central venous catheters should be considered.

- Lipid-associated formulations of amphotericin B, liposomal amphotericin B (AmBisome) and amphotericin B lipid complex (Abelcet), have been approved for use in proven cases of candidiasis; however, patients with invasive candidiasis have also been treated successfully with amphotericin B colloid dispersion (Amphotec or Amphocil). The lipid-associated formulations are less toxic but as effective as deoxycholate amphotericin B.

- Many clinicians advocate early institution of empiric IV **amphotericin B** in patients with neutropenia and persistent fever (>5–7 days). Suggested criteria for the empiric use of amphotericin B include (1) fever of 5 to 7 days' duration that is unresponsive to antibacterial agents, (2) neutropenia of more than 7 days' duration, (3) no other obvious cause for fever, (4) progressive debilitation, (5) chronic adrenal corticosteroid therapy, and (6) indwelling intravascular catheters.

ASPERGILLUS INFECTIONS

- Of more than 300 species of *Aspergillus*, three are most commonly pathogenic: *A. fumigatus*, *A. flavus*, and *A. niger*.

TABLE 38–4 Therapy of Invasive Candidiasis

Type of Disease and Common Clinical Manifestations	Therapy/Comments
Prophylaxis of candidemia	
Nonneutropenic patients*a*	Not recommended except for severely ill/high-risk patients in whom fluconazole IV/PO 400 mg daily should be used (see text)
Neutropenic patients*a*	The optimal duration of therapy is unclear but at a minimum should include the period at risk for neutropenia: Fluconazole IV/PO 400 mg daily *or* itraconazole solution 2.5 mg/kg every 12 hours PO *or* micafungin 50 mg (1 mg/kg in patients under 50 kg) intravenously daily
Solid-organ transplantation, liver transplantation	*Patients with two or more key risk factors*b: Amphotericin B IV 10–20 mg daily *or* liposomal amphotericin B (AmBisome) 1 mg/kg/day *or* fluconazole 400 mg orally daily
Empirical antifungal therapy (unknown *Candida* species)	
Suspected disseminated candidiasis in febrile nonneutropenic patients	None recommended; data are lacking defining subsets of patients who are appropriate for therapy (see text)
Febrile neutropenic patients with prolonged fever despite 4–6 days of empirical antibacterial therapy	*Treatment duration:* Until resolution of neutropenia An echinocandin*d* is a reasonable alternative; Voriconazole can be used in selected situations (see text)
Less critically ill patients with no recent azole exposure	An echinocandin*d* or fluconazole (loading dose of 800 mg [12 mg/kg], then 400 mg [6 mg/kg] daily)
Additional mold coverage is desired	Voriconazole
Empirical therapy of candidemia and acute hematogenously disseminated candidiasis	
Nonimmunocompromised host*c*	*Treatment duration:* 2 weeks after the last positive blood culture and resolution of signs and symptoms of infection *Remove existing central venous catheters when feasible plus* *fluconazole (loading dose of 800 mg [12 mg/kg], then 400 mg [6 mg/kg] daily) or an echinocandin*d
Patients with recent azole exposure, moderately severe or severe illness, or who are at high risk of infection due to *C. glabrata* or *C. krusei*	An echinocandin*d* Transition from an echinocandin to fluconazole is recommended for patients who are clinically stable and have isolates (eg, *C. albicans*) likely to be susceptible to fluconazole
Patients who are less critically ill and who have had no recent azole exposure	Fluconazole

(continued)

TABLE 38–4 Therapy of Invasive Candidiasis *(Continued)*

Type of Disease and Common Clinical Manifestations	Therapy/Comments
Therapy of specific pathogens	
Candida albicans, Candida tropicalis, Candida parapsilosis	Fluconazole IV/PO 6 mg/kg/day *or* an echinocandin[d] *or* amphotericin B IV 0.7 mg/kg/day plus fluconazole IV/PO 800 mg/day; Amphotericin B deoxycholate 0.5–1.0 mg/kg daily or a lipid formulation of amphotericin B (3–5 mg/kg daily) are alternatives in patients who are intolerant to other antifungals; Transition from Amphotericin B deoxycholate or a lipid formulation of amphotericin B to fluconazole is recommended in patients who are clinically stable and whose isolates are likely to be susceptible to fluconazole (eg *C. albicans*); Voriconazole (400 mg [6 mg/kg] twice daily x 2 doses then 200 mg [3mg/kg] twice daily thereafter is efficacious, but offers little advantage over fluconazole; It may be utilized as stepdown oral therapy for selected cases of candidiasis due to *C. krusei* or voriconazole-susceptible *C. glabrata* *Patients intolerant or refractory to other therapy*[e]: Amphotericin B lipid complex IV 5 mg/kg/day Liposomal amphotericin B IV 3–5 mg/kg/day Amphotericin B colloid dispersion IV 2–6 mg/kg/day
Candida krusei	Amphotericin B IV ≤1 mg/kg/day *or* an echinocandin[d]
Candida lusitaniae	Fluconazole IV/PO 6 mg/kg/day
Candida glabrata	An echinocandin[d] (Transition to fluconazole or voriconazole therapy is not recommended without confirmation of isolate susceptibility)
Neutropenic host[f]	*Treatment duration:* Until resolution of neutropenia *Remove existing central venous catheters when feasible, plus:* Amphotericin B IV 0.7–1 mg/kg/day (total dosages 0.5–1 g) *or Patients failing therapy with traditional amphotericin B:* Lipid formulation of amphotericin B IV 3–5 mg/kg/day
Chronic disseminated candidiasis (hepatosplenic candidiasis)	*Treatment duration:* Until calcification or resolution of lesions *Stable patients:* Fluconazole IV/PO 6 mg/kg/day *Acutely ill or refractory patients:* Amphotericin B IV 0.6–0.7 mg/kg/day

(continued)

TABLE 38–4 Therapy of Invasive Candidiasis *(Continued)*

Type of Disease and Common Clinical Manifestations	Therapy/Comments
Therapy of specific pathogens	
Urinary candidiasis	*Asymptomatic disease:* Generally no therapy is required
	Symptomatic or high-risk patients[g]: Removal of urinary tract instruments, stents, and Foley catheters, + 7–14 days therapy with fluconazole 200 mg orally daily *or* amphotericin B IV 0.3–1 mg/kg/day

PO, orally.

[a]Patients at significant risk for invasive candidiasis include those receiving standard chemotherapy for acute myelogenous leukemia, allogeneic bone marrow transplants, or high-risk autologous bone marrow transplants. However, among these populations, chemotherapy or bone marrow transplant protocols do not all produce equivalent risk, and local experience should be used to determine the relevance of prophylaxis.

[b]Risk factors include retransplantation, creatinine of more than 2 mg/dL, choledochojejunostomy, intraoperative use of 40 units or more of blood products, and fungal colonization detected within the first 3 days after transplantation.

[c]Therapy is generally the same for acquired immunodeficiency syndrome (AIDS)/non-AIDS patients except where indicated and should continued for 2 weeks after the last positive blood culture and resolution of signs and symptoms of infection. All patients should receive an ophthalmologic examination. Amphotericin B can be switched to fluconazole (intravenous or oral) for the completion of therapy. Susceptibility testing of the infecting isolate is a useful adjunct to species identification during selection of a therapeutic approach because it can be used to identify isolates that are unlikely to respond to fluconazole or amphotericin B. However, this is not currently available at most institutions.

[d]Echinocandin = caspofungin 70 mg loading dose, then 50 mg IV daily maintenance dose, or micafungin 100 mg daily, or anidulafungin 200 mg loading dose, then 100 mg daily maintenance dose.

[e]Often defined as failure of ≥500 mg amphotericin B, initial renal insufficiency (creatinine ≥2.5 mg/dL or creatinine clearance <25 mL/min), a significant increase in creatinine (to 2.5 mg/dL for adults or 1.5 mg/dL for children), or severe acute administration-related toxicity.

[f]Patients who are neutropenic at the time of developing candidemia should receive a recombinant cytokine (granulocyte colony-stimulating factor or granulocyte-monocyte colony-stimulating factor) that accelerates recovery from neutropenia.

[g]Patients at high risk for dissemination include neutropenic patients, low-birth-weight infants, patients with renal allografts, and patients who will undergo urologic manipulation.

Data from National Committee for Clinical Laboratory Standards (NCCLS). Reference method for broth dilution antifungal susceptibility testing of yeasts: Approved Standard. Wayne, PA: NCCLS, 1997. NCCLS document M27-A; Pappas PG, Kauffman CA, Andes D, et al. Clinical practice guidelines for the management of candidiasis: 2009 update by the Infectious Diseases Society of America. Clin Infect Dis 2009;48(5):503–535; Lam SW, Eschenauer GA, Carver PL. Evolving role of early antifungals in the adult intensive care unit. Crit Care Med 2009;37(5):1580–1593; and Pappas, PG, Rex JH, Lee J, et al. A prospective observational study of candidemia: Epidemiology, therapy, and influences on mortality in hospitalized adult and pediatric patients. Clin Infect Dis 2003;37:634–643.

- Aspergillosis is generally acquired by inhalation of airborne conidia that are small enough (2.5–3 mm) to reach the alveoli or the paranasal sinuses.
- Superficial or locally invasive infections of the ear, skin, or appendages can often be managed with topical antifungal therapy.

Allergic Bronchopulmonary Aspergillosis

- Allergic manifestations of *Aspergillus* range in severity from mild asthma to allergic bronchopulmonary aspergillosis characterized by severe asthma with wheezing, fever, malaise, weight loss, chest pain, and a cough productive of blood-streaked sputum.
- Therapy is aimed at minimizing the quantity of antigenic material released in the tracheobronchial tree.
- Antifungal therapy is generally not indicated in the management of allergic manifestations of aspergillosis, although some patients have demonstrated a decrease in their glucocorticoid dose following therapy with itraconazole. Itraconazole 200 mg twice daily for 16 weeks resulted in reduced corticosteroid dose and improvement in exercise tolerance and pulmonary function.

Aspergilloma

- In the nonimmunocompromised host, *Aspergillus* infections of the sinuses most commonly occur as saprophytic colonization (aspergillomas, or "fungus balls") of previously abnormal sinus tissue. Treatment consists of removal of the aspergilloma. Therapy with glucocorticoids and surgery is generally successful.
- Although IV amphotericin B is generally not useful in eradicating aspergillomas, intracavitary instillation of amphotericin B has been employed successfully in a limited number of patients. Hemoptysis generally ceases when the aspergilloma is eradicated.

Invasive Aspergillosis

- Patients often present with classic signs and symptoms of acute pulmonary embolus: pleuritic chest pain, fever, hemoptysis, a friction rub, and a wedge-shaped infiltrate on chest radiographs.
- Demonstration of *Aspergillus* by repeated culture and microscopic examination of tissue provides the most firm diagnosis.
- In the immunocompromised host, aspergillosis is characterized by vascular invasion leading to thrombosis, infarction, and necrosis of tissue.

TREATMENT

- Antifungal therapy should be instituted in any of the following conditions: (1) persistent fever or progressive sinusitis unresponsive to antimicrobial therapy; (2) an eschar over the nose, sinuses, or palate; (3) the presence of characteristic radiographic findings, including wedge-shaped infarcts, nodular densities, or new cavitary lesions; or (4) any clinical manifestation suggestive of orbital or cavernous sinus disease or an acute vascular event associated with fever. Isolation of *Aspergillus* spp. from nasal or respiratory tract secretions should be considered confirmatory evidence in any of the previously mentioned clinical settings.
- Voriconazole is the drug of choice for primary therapy of most patients with aspergillosis as it provided improved survival and fewer side effects.
- In patients who cannot tolerate voriconazole, amphotericin B can be used. Full doses (1–1.5 mg/kg/day) are generally recommended, with

response measured by defervescence and radiographic clearing. The lipid-based formulations may be preferred as initial therapy in patients with marginal renal function or in patients receiving other nephrotoxic drugs. The optimal duration of treatment is unknown.

- **Caspofungin** is indicated for treatment of invasive aspergillosis in patients who are refractory to or intolerant of other therapies such as amphotericin B.
- The use of prophylactic antifungal therapy to prevent primary infection or reactivation of aspergillosis during subsequent courses of chemotherapy is controversial.

See Chapter 130, Invasive Fungal Infections, authored by Peggy L. Carver, for a more detailed discussion of this topic.

INTRODUCTION

- GI infections are among the more common causes of morbidity and mortality around the world. Most are caused by viruses, and some are caused by bacteria or other organisms. In underdeveloped and developing countries, acute gastroenteritis involving diarrhea is the leading cause of mortality in infants and children younger than 5 years of age. In the United States, there are ~211 million episodes of acute gastroenteritis each year, causing over 900,000 hospitalizations and over 6,000 deaths.
- Public health measures such as clean water supply and sanitation facilities, as well as quality control of commercial products, are important for the control of most enteric infections. Sanitary food handling and preparation practices significantly decrease the incidence of enteric infections.

REHYDRATION THERAPY

- Treatment of dehydration includes rehydration, replacement of ongoing losses, and continuation of normal feeding. Fluid replacement is the cornerstone of therapy for diarrhea regardless of etiology.
- Initial assessment of fluid loss is essential for rehydration. Weight loss is the most reliable means of determining the extent of water loss. Clinical signs such as changes in skin turgor, sunken eyes, dry mucous membranes, decreased tearing, decreased urine output, altered mentation, and changes in vital signs can be helpful in determining approximate deficits (**Table 39–1**).
- The necessary components of oral rehydration solution (ORS) include glucose, sodium, potassium, chloride, and water (**Table 39–2**). ORS should be given in small frequent volumes (5 mL every 2–3 min) in a teaspoon or oral syringe.
- Severely dehydrated patients should be resuscitated initially with lactated Ringer solution or normal IV saline.
- Early refeeding as tolerated is recommended. Age-appropriate diet may be resumed as soon as dehydration is corrected. Early initiation of feeding shortens the course of diarrhea. Initially, easily digested foods, such as bananas, applesauce, and cereal, may be added as tolerated. Foods high in fiber, sodium, and sugar should be avoided.

BACTERIAL INFECTIONS

- The bacterial species most commonly associated with GI infection and infectious diarrhea in the United States are *Shigella* spp., *Salmonella* spp., *Campylobacter* spp., *Yersinia* spp., *Escherichia* spp., *Clostridium* spp., and *Staphylococcus* spp.

| | **TABLE 39–1** | Clinical Assessment of Degree of Dehydration in Children Based on Percentage of Body Weight Loss[a] | |

Variable	Minimal or No Dehydration (<3% Loss of Body Weight)	Mild to Moderate (3–9% Loss of Body Weight)	Severe (≥10% Loss of Body Weight)
Blood pressure	Normal	Normal	Normal to reduced
Quality of pulses	Normal	Normal or slightly decreased	Weak, thready, or not palpable
Heart rate	Normal	Normal to increased	Increased (bradycardia in severe cases)
Breathing	Normal	Normal to fast	Deep
Mental status	Normal	Normal to listless	Apathetic, lethargic, or comatose
Eyes	Normal	Sunken orbits/ decreased tears	Deeply sunken orbits/ absent tears
Mouth and tongue	Moist	Dry	Parched
Thirst	Normal	Eager to drink	Drinks poorly; too lethargic to drink
Skin fold	Normal	Recoil in <2 seconds	Recoil in >2 seconds
Extremities	Warm, normal capillary refill	Cool, prolonged capillary refill	Cold, mottled, cyanotic, prolonged capillary refill
Urine output	Normal to decreased	Decreased	Minimal
Hydration therapy	None	ORS 50–100 mL/ kg over 3–4 hours	Lactated Ringer's solution or normal saline 20 mL/kg in 15–30 minutes intravenously until mental status or perfusion improve; Followed by 5% dextrose ½ normal saline intravenously at twice maintenance rates or ORS 100 mL/kg over 4 hours.
Replacement of ongoing losses	<10kg body weight: 60–120 mL ORS per >10kg body weight: 120–240 mL ORS per diarrheal stool or emesis	Same	If unable to tolerate ORS, administer through nasogastric tube or administer 5% dextrose ½ normal saline with 20 mEq/L potassium chloride intravenously

ORS, oral rehydration solution.

[a]Percentages vary among authors for each dehydration category; hemodynamic and perfusion status is most important; when unsure of category, therapy for more severe category is recommended.

Data from King CK, Glass R, Bresee JS, Duggan C. Managing acute gastroenteritis among children: oral rehydration, maintenance, and nutritional therapy. MMWR Recomm Rep. 2003;52(RR-16):1–16; and World Health Organization. The treatment of diarrhoea: a manual for physicians and other senior health workers http:// whqlibdoc.who. int/publications/2005/9241593180.pdf >. Geneva, Switzerland: World Health Organization; 2005.

	Na (mEq/L)	K (mEq/L)	Base (mEq/L)	Carbohydrate (mmol/L)	Osmolality (mOsm/L)
TABLE 39–2	**Comparison of Common Solutions Used in Oral Rehydration and Maintenance**				
Product					
WHO/UNICEF (2002)	75	20	30	75	245
Naturalyte	45	20	48	140	265
Pedialyte	45	20	30	140	250
Infalyte	50	25	30	70	200
Rehydralyte	75	20	30	140	250
Cola	2	0	13	700	750
Apple juice[a]	5	32	0	690	730
Chicken broth[a]	250	8	0	0	500
Sports beverage[a]	20	3	3	255	330

WHO/UNICEF, World Health Organization/United Nations (International) Children's Fund.
[a]These solutions should be avoided in dehydration.

- Antibiotics are not essential in the treatment of most mild diarrheas, and empirical therapy for acute GI infections may result in unnecessary antibiotic courses. Antibiotic choices for bacterial infections are given in **Table 39–3**.

ENTEROTOXIGENIC (CHOLERA-LIKE) DIARRHEA

Cholera (*Vibrio cholerae*)

- *Vibrio cholerae* 01 is the serogroup that most often causes human epidemics and pandemics. Four mechanisms for transmission have been proposed: animal reservoirs, chronic carriers, asymptomatic or mild disease victims, and water reservoirs.
- Most pathology of cholera is thought to result from an enterotoxin that increases cyclic adenosine monophosphate–mediated secretion of chloride ion into the intestinal lumen, which results in isotonic secretion (primarily in the small intestine) exceeding the absorptive capacity of the intestinal tract (primarily the colon).
- The incubation period of *V. cholerae* is 1 to 3 days.
- Cholera is characterized by a spectrum from the asymptomatic state to the most severe typical cholera syndrome. Patients may lose up to 1 L of isotonic fluid every hour. The onset of diarrhea is abrupt and is followed rapidly or sometimes preceded by vomiting. Fever occurs in <5% of patients. In the most severe state, this disease can progress to death in a matter of 2 to 4 hours if not treated.

TREATMENT

- The goal of treatment is rapid restoration of fluid losses, correction of metabolic acidosis, and replacement of potassium deficiency. The mainstay of treatment for cholera consists of fluid and electrolyte replacement with ORS to restore fluid and electrolyte losses. Rice-based rehydration

TABLE 39–3 Recommendations for Antibiotic Therapy

Pathogen	First-Line Agents	Alternative Agents
Enterotoxigenic (cholera-like) diarrhea		
Vibrio cholerae O1 or O139	Doxycycline 300 mg orally × 1	Tetracycline 500 mg orally four times daily × 3 days; ciprofloxacin 500 mg orally every 12 hours × 3 days or 1 g orally single dose; norfloxacin 400 mg orally every 12 hours × 3 days; levofloxacin 500 mg orally once daily × 3 days; trimethoprim-sulfamethoxazole DS tablet twice daily × 3 days; erythromycin 250–500 mg orally every 6–8 hours; azithromycin 1,000 mg orally × 1
Enterotoxigenic Escherichia coli	Ciprofloxacin 500 mg orally every 12 hours, norfloxacin 400 mg orally every 12 hours, levofloxacin 500 mg orally once daily × 3 days	Rifaximin 200 mg 3 times daily × 3 days; azithromycin 1,000 mg orally × 1 or 500 mg orally daily × 3 days
Invasive (dysentery-like) diarrhea		
Shigella species[a]	Ciprofloxacin 500 mg orally every 12 hours, norfloxacin 400 mg orally every 12 hours, levofloxacin 500 mg orally 1 daily × 5 days	Azithromycin 500 mg orally × 1, then 250 mg orally daily × 4 days
Salmonella Nontyphoidal[a]	Gastroenteritis: Ciprofloxacin 500 mg every 12 hours × 5–7 days Bacteremia: Ceftriaxone 2 g IV daily × 7–14 days Chronic carriers: Ciprofloxacin 750 mg orally every 12 hours × 1 month	Gastroenteritis: Azithromycin 1,000 mg orally × 1 day, followed by 500 mg orally once daily × 6 days; trimethoprim-sulfamethoxazole DS orally every 12 hours × 5–7 days Chronic carriers: amoxicillin 1,000 mg orally every 8 hours × 3 months; trimethoprim-sulfamethoxazole DS orally every 12 hours × 3 months
Campylobacter[a]	Erythromycin 500 mg orally twice daily, azithromycin 1,000 mg orally × 1 day followed by 500 mg daily or clarithromycin 500 mg orally twice daily × 5 days	Ciprofloxacin 500 mg or norfloxacin 400 mg orally twice daily × 5 days

Yersinia species[a]	A combination therapy with doxycycline, aminoglycosides, trimethoprim-sulfamethoxazole, or fluoroquinolones
Clostridium difficile	Mild to moderate disease: Metronidazole 250 mg every 6 hours to 500 mg every 8 hours orally or intravenously daily × 10–14 days Severe disease: Vancomycin 125 mg every 6 hours orally × 10–14 days First relapse: same as above Subsequent relapses: Tapered pulse dose of oral vancomycin (125 mg every 6 hours × 2 weeks, every 12 hours × 1 week, every 24 hours × 1 week, every 48 hours × 8 days (4 doses), every 72 hours × 15 days (5 doses)	Subsequent relapses: Oral vancomycin 125 mg every 6 hours × 10–14 days followed by rifaximin 400 mg every 12 hours orally × 2 weeks; Nitazoxanide 500 mg every 12 hours × 10 days
Traveler's diarrhea		
Prophylaxis[a]	Norfloxacin 400 mg or ciprofloxacin 750 mg orally daily	Rifaximin 200 mg one to three times daily up to 2 weeks
Treatment	Norfloxacin 800 mg orally × 1 or 400 mg orally every 12 hours × 3 days, or Ciprofloxacin 750 mg orally ×1 or 500 mg orally every 12 hours × 3 days, or Levofloxacin 1,000 mg orally × 1 or 500 mg orally daily × 3 days Azithromycin 1,000 mg orally × 1 or 500 mg orally daily × 3 days	Rifaximin 200 mg 3 times daily × 3 days

[a]For high-risk patients only. See the preceding text for the high-risk patients in each infection.

formulations are the preferred ORS for cholera patients. In patients who cannot tolerate ORS, IV therapy with Ringer lactate can be used.

- Antibiotics are not necessary in most cholera cases. In severe cases, antibiotics shorten the duration of diarrhea, decrease the volume of fluid lost, and shorten the duration of the carrier state (see **Table 39–3**). A single dose of oral **doxycycline** is the preferred agent. In children and pregnant women, **erythromycin** and **azithromycin** may be used. In areas of high tetracycline resistance, fluoroquinolones are effective.

ESCHERICHIA COLI

- *Escherichia coli* GI disease may be caused by enterotoxigenic *E. coli* (ETEC), enteroinvasive *E. coli* (EIEC), enteropathogenic *E. coli* (EPEC), enteroadhesive *E. coli* (EAEC), and enterohemorrhagic *E. coli* (EHEC). ETEC is now incriminated as being the most common cause of traveler's diarrhea.
- ETEC is capable of producing either of two plasmid-mediated enterotoxins: heat-labile toxin and heat-stable toxin. The net effect of either toxin on the mucosa is production of a cholera-like secretory diarrhea.
- Nausea and watery stools, with or without abdominal cramping, are characteristic of the disease caused by ETEC. Most ETEC diarrhea is typically abrupt in onset and resolves within 24 to 48 hours without complication.
- The cornerstone of management is to prevent dehydration by correcting fluid and electrolyte imbalances. Most cases respond readily to ORS. Antibiotics are effective in preventing the development of ETEC diarrhea and shortening the duration of disease, but they are not recommended.
- Fluid and electrolyte replacement should be initiated at the onset of diarrhea.
- Antibiotics used for treatment are found in **Table 39–3**.
- **Loperamide** and **bismuth subsalicylate** are effective in decreasing the severity of ETEC diarrhea.

CLOSTRIDIUM DIFFICILE

- *C. difficile* is the most common cause of infectious diarrhea in hospitalized patients in North America and Europe. It is associated most often with broad-spectrum antimicrobials, including clindamycin, ampicillin, cephalosporins, and fluoroquinolones.
- Pseudomembranous colitis may result in a spectrum of disease, from mild diarrhea to life-threatening toxic megacolon and pseudomembranous enterocolitis. In colitis without pseudomembranes, patients present with malaise, abdominal pain, nausea, anorexia, watery diarrhea, low-grade fever, and leukocytosis. Fulminant disease is characterized by severe abdominal pain, perfuse diarrhea, high fever, marked leukocytosis, and classic pseudomembrane formation.
- *C. difficile* infection should be suspected in patients experiencing diarrhea with a recent history of antibiotic use (within the previous 3 mo) or in those whose diarrhea began 72 hours after hospitalization.
- Diagnosis is established by detection of toxin A or B in the stool, stool culture for *C. difficile,* or endoscopy.

- Initial therapy should include discontinuation of the offending agent. The patient should be supported with fluid and electrolyte replacement.
- Both vancomycin and metronidazole are effective, but **metronidazole,** 250 mg orally four times daily, is the drug of choice. Oral **vancomycin,** 125 mg orally four times daily, is reserved for patients not responding to metronidazole.
- Relapse can occur in 20% of patients. Management of a first relapse is identical to the primary episode. The optimal management of multiple relapses is not clear. Fecal transplantation is sometimes used.
- Drugs that inhibit peristalsis, such as **diphenoxylate,** are contraindicated.

INVASIVE (DYSENTERY-LIKE) DIARRHEA

BACILLARY DYSENTERY (SHIGELLOSIS)

- Four species of *Shigella* are most often associated with disease: *S. dysenteriae* type I, *S. flexneri, S. boydii,* and *S. sonnei.*
- Poor sanitation, poor personal hygiene, inadequate water supply, malnutrition, and increased population density are associated with increased risk of *Shigella* gastroenteritis epidemics, even in developed countries. The majority of cases are thought to result from fecal-oral transmission.
- *Shigella* spp. cause dysentery upon penetrating the epithelial cells lining the colon. Microabscesses may eventually coalesce, forming larger abscesses. Some *Shigella* species produce a cytotoxin, or shigatoxin, the pathogenic role of which is unclear, although it is thought to damage endothelial cells of the lamina propria, resulting in microangiopathic changes that can progress to hemolytic uremic syndrome. Watery diarrhea commonly precedes the dysentery and may be a result of these toxins.
- Initial signs and symptoms include abdominal pain, cramping, and fever, followed by frequent watery stools. Within a few days, patients experience a decrease in fever, severe abdominal pain, and tenderness prior to the development of bloody diarrhea and other signs of dysentery. If untreated, bacillary dysentery usually lasts ~1 week (range 1–30 days).
- Shigellosis is usually a self-limiting disease. Most patients recover in 4 to 7 days. Treatment of bacillary dysentery generally includes correction of fluid and electrolyte disturbances and, occasionally, antimicrobials.
- Antimicrobials are indicated in the infirm, those who are immunocompromised, children in daycare centers, the elderly, malnourished children, and healthcare workers. Antimicrobials may shorten the period of fecal shedding and attenuate the clinical illness.
- The preferred agents of choice are fluoroquinolones (**ciprofloxacin, levofloxacin,** or **norfloxacin**). A single dose is reasonable, but 5 days is recommended for *S. dysenteriae* type I.
- Fluid and electrolyte losses can generally be replaced with oral therapy, as dysentery is generally not associated with significant fluid loss. IV replacement is necessary only for children or the elderly.
- Antimotility agents such as diphenoxylate are not recommended because they can worsen dysentery.

SALMONELLOSIS

- Human disease caused by *Salmonella* generally falls into four categories—acute gastroenteritis (enterocolitis), bacteremia, extraintestinal localized infection, and enteric fever (typhoid and paratyphoid fever)—along with a chronic carrier state. Salmonellosis is a disease primarily of infants, children, and adolescents.
- Conditions that predispose to infection include those that decrease gastric acidity, antibiotic use, malnutrition, and immunodeficiency states. Contaminated food or water is implicated in most cases.
- With enterocolitis, patients often complain of nausea and vomiting within 72 hours of ingestion, followed by crampy abdominal pain, fever, and diarrhea, although the actual presentation is variable.
- Stool cultures inevitably yield the causative organism, if obtained early. However, recovery of organisms continues to decrease with time, so that by 3 to 4 weeks, only 5% to 15% of adult patients are passing *Salmonella*.
- Some patients may continue to shed *Salmonella* for 1 year or longer. These "chronic carrier" states are rare for serotypes other than *S. typhi*.
- *Salmonella* can produce bacteremia without classic enterocolitis or enteric fever. The clinical syndrome is characterized by persistent bacteremia and prolonged intermittent fever with chills. Stool cultures are frequently negative. Bacteremia is the most common complication of gastroenteritis.

Treatment

- Gastroenteritis is usually self-limiting, and fluid and electrolyte replacement is the primary mode of treatment. Antimotility drugs should be avoided because they increase the risk of mucosal invasion and complications.
- Antibiotics are not indicated. They have no effect on the duration of fever or diarrhea, and their frequent use increases the likelihood of resistance and the duration of fecal shedding. Antibiotics should be used in (1) neonates or infants younger than 1 year of age, (2) persons older than 50 years, (3) patients with primary or secondary immunodeficiency such as acquired immunodeficiency syndrome (AIDS) or chemotherapy patients, and (4) patients with vascular abnormalities or those with prosthetic joints.
- For high-risk patients, **ciprofloxacin** for 5 to 7 days is recommended. For chronic carrier states, the choice of antibiotic should be based on susceptibility testing of the isolate.
- For bacteremia, life-threatening treatment should include the combination of a third-generation cephalosporin (**ceftriaxone,** 2 g IV daily) and **ciprofloxacin,** 500 mg orally twice daily. The duration of antibiotic therapy is dictated by the site.

CAMPYLOBACTERIOSIS

- *Campylobacter* species are thought to be a major cause of diarrhea. Transmission of infection occurs primarily by ingestion of contaminated food or water.

- Incubation usually averages 2 to 4 days. The most common symptoms include diarrhea of varying consistency and severity, abdominal pain, and fever. Nausea, vomiting, headache, myalgias, and malaise may also occur. Bowel movements may be numerous, bloody (dysentery-like), foul smelling, and melenic and range from loose to watery.
- The disease is self-limiting, and signs and symptoms usually resolve in ~1 week but may persist longer in 10% to 20% of patients.
- As with other acute diarrheal illnesses, fluid and electrolyte support is a mainstay of therapy, mainly with ORS.
- Antibiotics are not useful unless initiated within 4 days of the start of illness, as they do not shorten the duration or severity of diarrhea.
- Antibiotics are warranted in patients who present with high fevers, severe bloody diarrhea, prolonged illness (>1 wk), pregnancy, and immunocompromised states, including human immunodeficiency virus infection.
- Erythromycin is considered the drug of choice for treatment. Clarithromycin or azithromycin is equally effective. Antimotility drugs are contraindicated.

YERSINIOSIS

- *Yersinia enterocolitica* and *Y. pseudotuberculosis* are associated with intestinal infection. The organisms have been isolated from a variety of food sources, including raw goat and cow milk.
- These bacteria cause a wide spectrum of clinical syndromes. The majority of cases present with enterocolitis that is mild and self-limiting. Symptoms, generally lasting 1 to 3 weeks, include vomiting, abdominal pain, diarrhea, and fever. A clinical syndrome seen in older children may resemble appendicitis.
- These diseases are generally self-limiting and are easily managed with ORS. Many patients develop a reactive arthritis 1 to 2 weeks after recovery from enteritis.
- Antibiotics should be used in high-risk patients who develop bacteremia (i.e., infants younger than 3 months and patients with cirrhosis or iron overload) or in patients with bone and joint infections.
- Drugs of choice are not yet identified. *Y. enterocolitica* is generally susceptible to **fluoroquinolones,** alone or in combination with **third-generation cephalosporins** or **aminoglycosides**. Alternative agents include **chloramphenicol, tetracycline,** and **trimethoprim–sulfamethoxazole**.
- Suggested antibiotics of choice are given in **Table 39–3**.

ACUTE VIRAL GASTROENTERITIS

ROTAVIRUSES

- The highest frequency of rotavirus-associated diarrhea appears in children younger than 5 years of age. The incubation period is typically 1 to 3 days.
- Clinical manifestations of rotavirus infections vary from asymptomatic (which is common in adults) to severe nausea, vomiting, and diarrhea

with dehydration. Symptoms are characterized initially by nausea and vomiting. The symptoms begin abruptly, with vomiting often preceding the onset of diarrhea. Other signs and symptoms are fever, respiratory symptoms, irritability, lethargy, pharyngeal erythema, rhinitis, red tympanic membranes, and palpable cervical lymph nodes. Dehydration and electrolyte disturbances occur more frequently in children.

- Oral fluid and electrolyte replacement is the cornerstone of treatment. Rotavirus vaccines are available.
- Antimotility agents are not recommended.

CALICIVIRUSES

- Caliciviruses include *Norovirus* (including Norwalk virus) and *Sapovirus*. Calicivirus gastroenteritis is characterized by sudden onset of abdominal cramps with nausea and/or vomiting. Although adults frequently experience nonbloody diarrhea, children experience vomiting more often. Other frequent complaints are myalgias, headache, and malaise, which are accompanied by fever in ~50% of cases. Signs and symptoms generally last only 12 to 48 hours.
- The disease is generally self-limiting and does not require therapy. On occasion, oral rehydration may be required. Rarely is parenteral hydration necessary.

See Chapter 122, Gastrointestinal Infections and Enterotoxigenic Poisonings, authored by Steven Martin and Rose Jung, for a more detailed discussion of this topic.

INTRODUCTION

- **Tables 40–1** and **40–2** present the revised classification systems for adult and child human immunodeficiency virus (HIV) infection.

PATHOGENESIS

TRANSMISSION OF HUMAN IMMUNODEFICIENCY VIRUS

- Infection with HIV occurs through three primary modes: sexual, parenteral, and perinatal. Sexual intercourse, primarily anal and vaginal intercourse, is the most common vehicle for transmission. The probability of HIV transmission from receptive anorectal intercourse is 0.5% to 3% per sexual contact and lower for receptive vaginal intercourse. Condom use reduces the risk of transmission by ~20-fold. Individuals with genital ulcers or sexually transmitted diseases, such as syphilis, chancroid, herpes, gonorrhea, *Chlamydia*, and trichomoniasis, are at great risk for contracting HIV.
- The use of contaminated needles or other injection-related paraphernalia by drug abusers has been the main cause of parenteral transmissions of HIV.
- Healthcare workers have a small risk of occupationally acquiring HIV, mostly through accidental injury, most often percutaneous needlestick injury.
- Perinatal infection, or vertical transmission, is the most common cause of pediatric HIV infection. The risk of mother-to-child transmission is ~25% in the absence of breast-feeding or antiretroviral therapy. Breast-feeding can also transmit HIV.

CLINICAL PRESENTATION

- Persons with HIV infection are categorized as those living with HIV and those with acquired immunodeficiency syndrome (AIDS) diagnosis. An AIDS diagnosis is made when the presence of HIV is confirmed and the CD4 count drops below 200 cells/mm^3 or after an AIDS indicator condition is diagnosed.
- Clinical presentations of primary HIV infection vary, but patients often have a viral syndrome or mononucleosis-like illness with fever, pharyngitis, and adenopathy (**Table 40–3**). Symptoms may last for 2 weeks.
- The probability of progression to AIDS is related to RNA viral load; in one study, 5-year mortality rates were 5% for those with a viral load <4,530 and 49% for those >36,270.
- Most children born with HIV are asymptomatic. On physical examination, they often present with unexplained physical signs such as

TABLE 40–1 Surveillance Case Definition for HIV Infection among Adults and Adolescents (≥13 years) – United States, 2008

Stage	Laboratory evidence (laboratory-confirmed HIV infection *plus*)	Clinical evidence
Stage 1	CD4⁺ cell count ≥500 cells/mm³ or CD4⁺ percentage ≥29	None required (but no AIDS-defining condition)
Stage 2	CD4⁺ cell count 200-499 cells/mm³ or CD4⁺ percentage 14–28	None required (but no AIDS-defining condition)
Stage 3 (AIDS)	CD4⁺ cell count <200 cells/mm³ or CD4⁺ percentage <14	or documentation of an AIDS-defining condition (with laboratory-confirmed HIV infection)
Stage unknown	no information on CD4⁺ counts	and no information on presence of AIDS-defining conditions
AIDS indicator conditions		
Candidiasis of bronchi, trachea, or lungs	Lymphoma, Burkitt	
Candidiasis, esophageal	Lymphoma, immunoblastic	
Cervical cancer, invasive	Lymphoma, primary, for brain	
Coccidioidomycosis, disseminated or extrapulmonary	*Mycobacterium avium* complex or *Mycobacterium kansasii*, disseminated or extrapulmonary	
Cryptococcosis, extrapulmonary	*Mycobacterium tuberculosis*, any site (pulmonary or extrapulmonary)	
Cryptosporidiosis, chronic intestinal (duration >1 month)	*Mycobacterium*, other species or unidentified species, disseminated or extrapulmonary	
Cytomegalovirus disease (other than liver, spleen, or nodes)	*Pneumocystis jiroveci* pneumonia	
Cytomegalovirus retinitis (with loss of vision)	Pneumonia, recurrent	
Encephalopathy, HIV related	Progressive multifocal leukoencephalopathy	
Herpes simplex: chronic ulcer(s) (duration >1 month); or bronchitis, pneumonitis, or esophagitis	*Salmonella* septicemia, recurrent	
Histoplasmosis, disseminated or extrapulmonary	Toxoplasmosis of brain	
Isosporiasis, chronic intestinal (duration >1 month)	Wasting syndrome due to HIV	
Kaposi sarcoma		

Data from Schneider E, Whitmore S, Glynn KM, Dominguez K, et al. Revised surveillance case definitions for HIV infection among adults, adolescents, and children aged <18 months and for HIV infection and AIDS among children aged 18 months to <13 years–United States, 2008. MMWR Recomm Rep 2008;57(RR-10):1–12.

TABLE 40–2	Centers for Disease Control and Prevention 1994 Revised Classification System for HIV Infection in Children Younger Than 13 Years		
Immunologic Categories	**12 Months cells/mm³ (%)ᵃ**	**1–5 Years cells/mm³ (%)ᵃ**	**6–12 Years cells/mm³ (%)ᵃ**
1. No evidence of suppression	≥1,500 (≥25%)	≥1,000 (≥25%)	≥500 (≥25%)
2. Evidence of moderate suppression	750–1,499 (15–24%)	500–999 (15–24%)	200–499 (15–24%)
3. Severe suppression	<750 (<15%)	<500 (<15%)	<200 (<15%)

Immunologic Categories	**N: No Signs/ Symptoms**	**A: Mild Signs/ Symptoms**	**B: Moderate Signs/ Symptoms**	**C: Severe Signs/ Symptoms**
1. No evidence of suppression	N1	A1	B1	C1
2. Evidence of moderate suppression	N2	A2	B2	C2
3. Severe suppression	N3	A3	B3	C3

AIDS, acquired immune deficiency syndrome; HIV, human immunodeficiency virus.
ᵃPercentage of total lymphocytes.

lymphadenopathy, hepatomegaly, splenomegaly, failure to thrive, weight loss or unexplained low birth weight, and fever of unknown origin. Laboratory findings include anemia, hypergammaglobulinemia, altered mononuclear cell function, and altered T-cell subset ratios. The normal range for CD4 cell counts in children is much different than for adults (see Table 40–2).

TABLE 40–3	Clinical Presentation of Primary HIV Infection in Adults

Symptoms
Fever, sore throat, fatigue, weight loss, and myalgia
40–80% of patients will also exhibit a morbilliform or maculopapular rash usually involving the trunk
Diarrhea, nausea, and vomiting
Lymphadenopathy, night sweats
Aseptic meningitis (fever, headache, photophobia, and stiff neck) may be present in one fourth of presenting cases

Other
High viral load (may exceed 1 million copies/mL)
Persistent decrease in CD4 lymphocytes

HIV, human immunodeficiency virus.

- Clinical presentations of the opportunistic infections are presented in Infectious Complications of HIV below.

DIAGNOSIS

- The preferred method for diagnosing HIV is an enzyme-linked immunosorbent assay, which detects antibodies against HIV-1 and is both highly sensitive and specific. False-positives can occur in multiparous women; in recent recipients of hepatitis B, HIV, influenza, or rabies vaccine; following multiple blood transfusions; and in those with liver disease or renal failure or undergoing chronic hemodialysis. False-negatives may occur if the patient is newly infected and the test is performed before antibody production is adequate. The minimum time to develop antibodies is 3 to 4 weeks from initial exposure.
- Positive enzyme-linked immunosorbent assays are repeated in duplicate and if one or both tests are reactive, a confirmatory test is performed for final diagnosis. Western blot assay is the most commonly used confirmatory test, although an indirect immunofluorescence assay is available.
- The viral load test quantifies viremia by measuring the amount of viral RNA. There are several methods used for determining the amount of HIV RNA: reverse transcriptase–coupled polymerase chain reaction, branched DNA, and nucleic acid sequence–based assay. Each assay has its own lower limit of sensitivity, and results can vary from one assay method to the other; therefore, it is recommended that the same assay method be used consistently within patients.
- Viral load can be used as a prognostic factor to monitor disease progression and the effects of treatment.
- The number of CD4 lymphocytes in the blood is a surrogate marker of disease progression. The normal adult CD4 lymphocyte count ranges between 500 and 1,600 cells/mm^3, or 40% to 70% of all lymphocytes.

TREATMENT

- The central goal of antiretroviral therapy is to decrease morbidity and mortality, improve quality of life, restore and preserve immune function, and prevent further transmission through maximum suppression of HIV replication (HIV RNA level that is undetectable).

GENERAL APPROACH TO TREATMENT OF HUMAN IMMUNODEFICIENCY VIRUS INFECTION

- Regular, periodic measurement of plasma HIV RNA levels and CD4 cell counts is necessary to determine the risk of disease progression in an HIV-infected individual and to determine when to initiate or modify antiretroviral treatment regimens.
- Treatment decisions should be individualized by the level of risk indicated by plasma HIV RNA levels and CD4 counts.
- The use of potent combination antiretroviral therapy to suppress HIV replication to below the levels of detection of sensitive plasma HIV RNA

assays limits the potential for selection of antiretroviral-resistant HIV variants, the major factor limiting the ability of antiretroviral drugs to inhibit virus replication and delay disease progression.

- The most effective means to accomplish durable suppression of HIV replication is the simultaneous initiation of combinations of effective anti-HIV drugs with which the patient has not been previously treated and that are not cross-resistant with antiretroviral agents with which the patient has been treated previously.
- Each of the antiretroviral drugs used in combination therapy regimens should always be used according to optimum schedules and dosages.
- Women should receive optimal antiretroviral therapy regardless of pregnancy status.
- The same principles of antiretroviral therapy apply to both HIV-infected children and adults, although the treatment of HIV-infected children involves unique pharmacologic, virologic, and immunologic considerations.
- Persons with acute primary HIV infections should be treated with combination antiretroviral therapy to suppress virus replication to levels below the limit of detection of sensitive plasma HIV RNA assays.
- HIV-infected persons, even those with viral loads below detectable limits, should be considered infectious and should be counseled to avoid sexual and drug-use behaviors that are associated with transmission or acquisition of HIV and other infectious pathogens.
- An excellent source for information on treatment guidelines can be found at *http://aidsinfo.nih.gov/*.
- Treatment is recommended for all HIV-infected persons with an AIDS-defining event, symptomatic disease, or CD4 lymphocyte count <350 cells/mm^3. Therapy is also recommended for symptomatic patients with CD4 counts between 350 and 500 cells/mm^3, and some clinicians would also favor therapy in those with >500 cells/mm^3 (**Table 40–4**).

PHARMACOLOGIC THERAPY

Antiretroviral Agents

- Inhibiting viral replication with a combination of potent antiretroviral therapy has been the most clinically successful strategy in the treatment of HIV infection. There have been four primary groups of drugs used: **entry inhibitors, reverse transcriptase inhibitors, integrase strand transfer inhibitors** (InSTIs), and HIV **protease inhibitors** (PIs) (**Table 40–5**).
- Reverse transcriptase inhibitors are of two types: those that are derivatives of purine-and pyrimidine-based nucleosides and nucleotides (NtRTIs) and those that are not nucleoside or nucleotide based (NNRTIs).
- Current recommendations for treating HIV infection advocate a minimum of three antiretroviral agents: **tenofovir disoproxil fumarate** plus **emtricitabine** with either a ritonavir-enhanced PI (**darunavir** or **atazanavir**), the NNTRI **efavirenz,** or the InSTI **raltegravir.** Multiple alternative regimens are also safe and effective. Efavirenz is the recommended NNRTI except for women who plan to become pregnant or who do not have adequate contraception.

TABLE 40–4 Treatment of Human Immunodeficiency Virus Infection: Antiretroviral Regimens Recommended in Antiretroviral-Naïve Persons

	Preferred Regimens	Limitation
NNRTI based	Efavirenz + tenofovir + emtricitabine (AI)ª	Not in first trimester of pregnancy or in women without adequate contraception
PI based	Darunavir + ritonavir + tenofovir + emtricitabine (AI)	Caution in HCV–HBV co-infection, rash
	Atazanavir + ritonavir + tenofovir + emtricitabine (AI)	Not with high doses of proton-pump-inhibitors, rash
	Raltegravir + tenofovir + emtricitabine (AI)	Twice daily (not once daily)
Alternative regimens (some potential disadvantages versus preferred regimens)		
	Efavirenz + (abacavir or zidovudine) + lamivudine (BI)	Possible reduced efficacy for high viral loads (abacavir), more subcutaneous fat loss (zidovudine)
	Nevirapine + zidovudine + lamivudine (BI)	Not in moderate to severe hepatic disease or in women with CD4 >250 cells/mm³ or men with CD4 >450 cells/mm³
PI based	Atazanavir-ritonavir + (abacavir or zidovudine) + lamivudine (BI)	See above
	Lopinavir-ritonavir (once or twice daily) either with (abacavir or zidovudine) + lamivudine or (tenofovir + emtricitabine) (BI)	Gastrointestinal intolerance, lipids
	Fosamprenavir/ritonavir (once or twice daily) either with (abacavir or zidovudine) + lamivudine or (tenofovir + emtricitabine) (BI)	Rash
	Saquinavir-ritonavir (twice daily) + tenofovir + emtricitabine (BI)	High number of pills/complexity

Acceptable regimens (potential additional disadvantages or pending additional data)

Efavirenz + didanosine + (lamivudine or emtricitabine) (CI)	Mitochondrial toxicities with didanosine
Atazanavir + (abacavir or zidovudine) + lamivudine (CI)	Lower atazanavir concentrations compared with atazanavir-ritonavir
Maraviroc + zidovudine + lamivudine (CII)	Lower virologic activity versus efavirenz, need tropism test
Raltegravir + abacavir or zidovudine + lamivudine	See above
(Darunavir-ritonavir or saquinavir-ritonavir) + (abacavir or zidovudine) + lamivudine	See above

Regimens or components that should not be used

Regimen or component	Comment
Any all NRTI regimen (EI)	Inferior virologic efficacy
Abacavir + didanosine or abacavir + tenofovir (DIII)	Insufficient data
Didanosine + tenofovir (EII)	Inferior virologic efficacy, CD4 declines
Stavudine (EI)	Toxicity including subcutaneous fat loss, peripheral neuropathy, and lactic acidosis
Darunavir or tipranavir or saquinavir without ritonavir (EI)	Insufficient plasma concentrations and efficacy or not studied
Delavirdine (EII)	Inferior virologic efficacy and inconvenient dosing

(continued)

TABLE 40–4 Treatment of Human Immunodeficiency Virus Infection: Antiretroviral Regimens Recommended in Antiretroviral-Naïve Persons (Continued)

	Preferred Regimens	Limitation
Regimens or components that should not be used		
Regimen or component		**Comment**
Enfuvirtide (DIII)		Not studied in naïve patients, inconvenient injections
Etravirine (DIII)		Not studied in naïve patients
Indinavir with or without ritonavir (EIII)		Nephrolithiasis, fluid requirements and inconvenient
Nelfinavir (without ritonavir) (EI)		Inferior virologic efficacy
Ritonavir at virologic doses (EIII)		Gastrointestinal intolerance
Tipranavir-ritonavir (EI)		Inferior virologic efficacy

NRTI, nucleoside reverse transcriptase inhibitor.

Evidence-based Rating Definition

Rating Strength of Recommendation:

A: Both strong evidence for efficacy and substantial clinical benefit support recommendation for use; should always be offered.

B: Moderate evidence for efficacy or strong evidence for efficacy but only limited clinical benefit, supports recommendation for use; should usually be offered.

C: Evidence for efficacy is insufficient to support a recommendation for or against use, or evidence for efficacy might not outweigh adverse consequences (e.g., drug toxicity, drug interactions) or cost of treatment under consideration; use is optional.

D: Moderate evidence for lack of efficacy or for adverse outcome supports recommendation against use; should usually not be offered.

E: Good evidence for lack of efficacy or for adverse outcome supports a recommendation against use; should never be offered. Rating Quality of Evidence Supporting the Recommendation:

I: Evidence from at least one correctly randomized, controlled trial with clinical outcomes and/or validated laboratory endpoints.

II: Evidence from at least one well-designed clinical trial without randomization or observational cohorts with long-term clinical outcomes.

III: Evidence from opinions of respected authorities based on clinical experience, descriptive studies, or reports of consulting committees.

^aLamivudine and emtricitabine are considered interchangeable.

Adapted from Department of Health and Human Services (DHHS) Panel on Antiretroviral Guidelines for Adults and Adolescents. Guidelines for the use of antiretroviral agents in HIV-infected adults and adolescents. December 1, 2009. http://AIDSinfo.NIH.gov.

- Significant drug interactions can occur with many antiretroviral agents:
  - ✓ The latest information on drug interactions of antiretroviral drugs should be consulted.
  - ✓ **Ritonavir** is a potent inhibitor of cytochrome P450 enzyme 3A and is used to reduce clearance of other PIs.
  - ✓ Rifampin may substantially reduce the concentrations of PIs and is contraindicated with the use of most PIs.
  - ✓ Saint John's wort is a potent inducer of metabolism and is contraindicated with PIs and NNRTIs.

TREATMENT DURING PREGNANCY

- In general, pregnant women should be treated like nonpregnant adults with some exceptions. Efavirenz should not be used, particularly in the

TABLE 40–5 Selected Pharmacologic Characteristics of Antiretroviral Compounds

Drug	F (%)	$t_{1/2}$ (hours)[a]	Adult Dose[b] (doses/day)	Plasma C_{max}/C_{min} (μM)	Distinguishing Adverse Effect
Integrase inhibitors (InSTI)					
Raltegravir	?	9	400 mg (2)	1.74/0.22	Increased creatine kinase
Nucleoside (Nucleotide) reverse transcriptase inhibitors (NRTIs)					
Abacavir	83	1.5/20	300 mg (2) or 600 mg (1)	5.2/0.03 7.4[c]	Hypersensitivity
Didanosine	42	1.4/24	200 mg (2) or 400 mg (1)	2.8/0.03 5.6[c]	Peripheral neuropathy, pancreatitis
Emtricitabine	93	10/39	200 mg (1)	7.3/0.04	Pigmentation on soles and palms in non-whites
Lamivudine	86	5/22	150 mg (2) or 300 mg (1)	6.3/1.6 10.5/0.5	Headache, pancreatitis (children)
Stavudine	86	1.4/7	40 mg (2)	2.4/0.04	Lipoatrophy, peripheral neuropathy
Tenofovir	40	17/150	300 mg (1)	1.04/0.4	Renal toxicity (proximal tubule)
Zidovudine	85	2/3.5	200 mg (3) or 300 mg (2)	0.2 3[c]	Anemia, neutropenia, myopathy

(continued)

TABLE 40–5 Selected Pharmacologic Characteristics of Antiretroviral Compounds *(Continued)*

Drug	F (%)	$t_{1/2}$ (hours)[a]	Adult Dose[b] (doses/ day)	Plasma C_{max}/C_{min} (μM)	Distinguishing Adverse Effect
Nonnucleoside reverse transcriptase inhibitors (NNRTIs)					
Delavirdine	85	5.8	400 mg (3) *or* 600 mg (2)	35/14	Rash, elevated liver function tests
Efavirenz	43	48	600 mg (1)	12.9/5.6	Central nervous system disturbances and teratogenicity
Etravirine	?	41	200 mg (2)	1.69/0.86	Rash, nausea
Nevirapine	93	25	200 mg (2)[d]	22/14	Potentially serious rash and hepatotoxicity
Protease inhibitors (PIs)					
Amprenavir[e]	? *or*	9	1,400 mg (2)[e] *or*	9.5/0.7	Rash
Forsamprenavir[e]			1,400 mg (1)[e,f]	14.3/2.9	Rash
Atazanavir	68	7	400 mg (1) *or* 300 mg (1)[f]	3.3/0.23 6.2/0.9	Unconjugated hyperbilirubinemia
Darunavir	82	15	800 mg (1) or 600 mg (2)[f]	11.9/6.5	Hepatitis, rash
Indinavir	60	1.5 1.5	800 mg (3) *or* 400–800 mg (2)[f]	13/0.25	Nephrolithiasis
Lopinavir[g]	?	5.5	800 mg (1) or 400 mg (2)	13.6/7.5	Hyperlipidemia/GI intolerance
Nelfinavir	?	2.6	750 mg (3) *or* 1,250 mg (2)	5.3/1.76 7/1.2	Diarrhea
Ritonavir	60	3–5	600 mg (2)[d] *or* "Boosting doses"	16/5	Gastrointestinal intolerance
Saquinavir	4	3	1,000 mg (2)[f]	3.9/0.55	Mild nausea, bloating
Tipranavir	?	6	500 mg (2)[f]	77.6/35.6	Hepatoxocity, intracranial hemorrhage

(continued)

TABLE 40–5	Selected Pharmacologic Characteristics of Antiretroviral Compounds *(Continued)*				
Drug	**F (%)**	**$t_{1/2}$ (hours)[a]**	**Adult Dose[b] (doses/ day)**	**Plasma C_{max}/C_{min} (μM)**	**Distinguishing Adverse Effect**
Fusion inhibitor					
Enfuvirtide	84	3.8	90 mg (2)	1.1/0.73	Injection-site reactions
Co-receptor inhibitor					
Maraviroc	33	15	300 mg (2)	1.2/0.066	Hepatitis, allergic reaction

C_{max}, maximum plasma concentration; C_{min}, minimum plasma concentration; F, bioavailability; $t_{1/2}$, elimination half-life.

[a]NRTIs: Plasma NRTI $t_{1/2}$/intracellular (peripheral blood mononuclear cells) NRTI-triphosphate $t_{1/2}$; plasma $t_{1/2}$ only for other classes.

[b]Dose adjustment may be required for weight, renal or hepatic disease, and drug interactions.

[c]C_{min} concentration typically below the limit of quantification.

[d]Initial dose escalation recommended to minimize side effects.

[e]Fosamprenavir is a tablet phosphate prodrug of amprenavir. Amprenavir is available only as oral solution.

[f]Must be boosted with low doses of ritonavir (100–200 mg).

[g]Available as coformulation 4:1 lopinavir to ritonavir.

Data from Department of Health and Human Services (DHHS) Panel on Antiretroviral Guidelines for Adults and Adolescents. Guidelines for the use of antiretroviral agents in HIV-infected adults and adolescents; December 1, 2009; Anderson PL, Kakuda TN, Lichtenstein KA. The cellular pharmacology of nucleoside- and nucleotide-analogue reverse-transcriptase inhibitors and its relationship to clinical toxicities. Clin Infect Dis 2004;38(5):743–753; Anderson MS, Kakuda TN, Hanley W, Miller J, et al. Minimal pharmacokinetic interaction between the human immunodeficiency virus nonnucleoside reverse transcriptase inhibitor etravirine and the integrase inhibitor raltegravir in healthy subjects. Antimicrob Agents Chemother 2008;52(12): 4228–4232; and product information for agents.

first trimester, because of the risk of teratogenicity. **Zidovudine** prophylaxis is generally recommended as part of treatment regimens to prevent vertical transmission. Infants also receive zidovudine prophylaxis for 6 weeks after birth.

POSTEXPOSURE PROPHYLAXIS

- Postexposure prophylaxis with a triple-drug regimen consisting of two NtRTIs and a boosted PI is recommended for percutaneous blood exposure involving significant risk (i.e., large-bore needle or large volume of blood or blood from patients with advanced AIDS).
- Two NtRTIs may be offered to healthcare workers with lower risk of exposure such as that involving either the mucous membrane or skin. Treatment is not necessary if the source of exposure is urine or saliva.
- The optimal duration of treatment is unknown, but at least 4 weeks of therapy is advocated. Ideally, treatment should be initiated within 1 to 2 hours of exposure, but treatment is recommended for up to 72 hours postexposure.

EVALUATION OF THERAPEUTIC OUTCOMES

- Following the initiation of therapy, patients are usually monitored at 3-month intervals with immunologic (i.e., CD4 count), virologic (HIV RNA), and clinical assessments.
- There are two general indications to change therapy: significant toxicity and treatment failure.
- Specific criteria to indicate treatment failure have not been established through controlled clinical trials. As a general guide, the following events should prompt consideration for changing therapy:
  - ✓ Less than a 1 log10 reduction in HIV RNA 1 to 4 weeks after the initiation of therapy, or a failure to achieve <400 copies/mL by 24 weeks or <50 copies/mL by 48 weeks
  - ✓ After HIV RNA suppression, repeated detection of HIV-RNA
  - ✓ Failure to achieve a rise in CD4 of 25 to 50 cells/mm³ by 48 weeks
  - ✓ Clinical disease progression, usually the development of a new opportunistic infection

THERAPEUTIC FAILURE

- Regimen failure is commonly associated with antiretroviral resistance, and testing for such resistance is a useful clinical tool.
- Therapeutic failure may be the result of nonadherence to medication, development of drug resistance, intolerance to one or more medications, adverse drug–drug interactions, or pharmacokinetic-pharmacodynamic variability.
- In general, patients failing their first regimens should be treated with at least one new drug representing a new class. Patients should be treated with at least two (preferably three) fully active antiretroviral drugs based on medication history, resistance tests, and new mechanistic drug classes.

INFECTIOUS COMPLICATIONS OF HUMAN IMMUNODEFICIENCY VIRUS

- The development of certain opportunistic infections is directly or indirectly related to the level of CD4 lymphocytes. The principle in the management of opportunistic infections (OIs) is treating HIV infection to enable CD4 cells to recover and be maintained above safe levels. Other important principles are
  - ✓ Preventing exposure to opportunistic pathogens
  - ✓ Using vaccinations to prevent first episodes of disease
  - ✓ Initiating primary chemoprophylaxis at certain CD4 thresholds to prevent first episodes of disease
  - ✓ Treating emergent OIs.
  - ✓ Initiating secondary chemoprophylaxis to prevent disease recurrence
  - ✓ Discontinuing prophylaxis with sustained immune recovery
- The spectrum of infectious diseases observed in HIV-infected individuals and recommended first-line therapies are shown in **Table 40–6.**

TABLE 40–6 Therapies for Common Opportunistic Pathogens in HIV-Infected Individuals

Clinical Disease	Preferred Initial Therapies for Acute Infection in Adults (Strength of Recommendation in Parentheses)	Common Drug- or Dose-Limiting Adverse Reactions
Fungi		
Candidiasis, oral	Fluconazole 100 mg orally for 7–14 days (AI)	Elevated liver function tests, hepatotoxicity, nausea and vomiting
	or	
	Nystatin 500,000 units oral swish (~5 mL) 4 times daily for 7–14 days (BII)	Taste, patient acceptance
Candidiasis, esophageal	Fluconazole 100–200 mg orally or IV daily for 14–21 days (AI)	Same as above
	or	
	Itraconazole 200 mg/day orally for 14–21 days (AI)	Elevated liver function tests, hepatotoxicity, nausea and vomiting
Pneumocystis jirovecii pneumonia	Trimethoprim-sulfamethoxazole IV or orally 15–20 mg/kg/day as trimethoprim component in 3–4 divided doses for 21 days[a] (AI) moderate or severe therapy should be started IV	Skin rash, fever, leucopenia, thrombocytopenia
	or	
	Pentamidine IV 4 mg/kg/day for 21 days[a] (AI)	Azotemia, hypoglycemia, hyperglycemia, arrhythmias
	Mild episodes	Rash, elevated liver enzymes, diarrhea
	Atovaquone suspension 750 mg (5 mL) orally twice daily with meals for 21 days[a] (BI)	
Cryptococcal meningitis	Amphotericin B 0.7 mg/kg/day IV for a minimum of 2 weeks with flucytosine 100 mg/kg/day orally in four divided doses (AI) *followed by*	Nephrotoxicity, hypokalemia, anemia, fever, chills, Bone marrow suppression, Elevated liver enzymes
	Fluconazole 400 mg/day, orally for 8 weeks or until CSF cultures are negative (AI)[a]	Same as above
Histoplasmosis	Liposomal amphotericin B 3 mg/kg/day IV for 3–10 days (AI) *followed by* Itraconazole 200 mg orally thrice daily for 3 days, then twice daily for 12 months[a] (AII)	Same as above

(continued)

TABLE 40–6 Therapies for Common Opportunistic Pathogens in HIV-Infected Individuals *(Continued)*

Clinical Disease	Preferred Initial Therapies for Acute Infection in Adults (Strength of Recommendation in Parentheses)	Common Drug- or Dose-Limiting Adverse Reactions
Fungi		
Coccidioidomycosis	Amphotericin B 0.7–1 mg/kg/day IV until clinical improvement (usually after 500–1,000 mg) then switch to azole (AII)[a] *followed by*	Same as above
	Fluconazole 400–800 mg once daily (meningeal disease) (AII)[a]	Same as above
Protozoa		
Toxoplasmic encephalitis	Pyrimethamine 200 mg orally once, then 50–75 mg/day *plus*	Bone marrow suppression
	Sulfadiazine 1–1.5 g orally 4 times daily *and*	Allergy, rash, drug fever
	Leucovorin 10–25 mg orally daily for 6 weeks (AI)[a]	
Isosporiasis	Trimethoprim and sulfamethoxazole: 160 mg trimethoprim and 800 mg sulfamethoxazole orally or IV 4 times daily for 10 days (AII)[a]	Same as above
Bacteria		
Mycobacterium avium complex	Clarithromycin 500 mg orally twice daily, *plus* ethambutol 15 mg/kg/day orally (AI), *and* For advanced disease, rifabutin 300 mg/day (dose may need adjustment with ART) (AI)[a]	Gastrointestinal intolerance, optic neuritis, peripheral neuritis Rash, gastrointestinal intolerance, Neutropenia, discolored urine, uveitis
Salmonella enterocolitis or bacteremia	Ciprofloxacin 500–750 mg orally (or 400 mg IV) twice daily for 14 days (longer duration for bacteremia or advanced HIV) (AIII)	Gastrointestinal intolerance

Campylobacter enterocolitis	Ciprofloxacin 500 mg orally twice daily *or* Azithromycin 500 mg orally daily for 7 days (or 14 days with bacteremia) (BIII)	Same as above
Shigella enterocolitis	Ciprofloxacin 500 mg orally twice daily for 5 days (or 14 days for bacteremia) (AIII)	Same as above
Viruses		
Mucocutaneous herpes simplex	Acyclovir 5 mg/kg IV every 8 hours until lesions regress, then acyclovir 400 mg orally 3 times daily until complete healing (famciclovir or valacyclovir is alternative) (AII)	Gastrointestinal intolerance, crystalluria
Primary varicella-zoster	Acyclovir 10–15 mg/kg every 8 hours IV for 7–10 days, then switch to oral acyclovir 300 mg 5 times daily after defervescence (famciclovir or valacyclovir is alternative) (AIII)	Obstructive nephropathy, central nervous system symptomatology
Cytomegalovirus (retinitis)	Ganciclovir intraocular implant plus valganciclovir 900 mg twice daily for 14–21 days then once daily until immune recovery from ART (AI)[a]	Neutropenia, thrombocytopenia
Cytomegalovirus esophagitis or colitis	Ganciclovir 5 mg/kg IV every 12 hours for 21 to 28 days (BII)	Same as above

ART, antiretroviral therapy; CSF, cerebrospinal fluid; HIV, human immunodeficiency virus.

[a]Maintenance therapy is recommended.

See Table 40–4 for levels of evidence-based recommendations.

Data from Kaplan JE, Benson C, Holmes KH, Brooks JT, et al. Guidelines for prevention and treatment of opportunistic infections in HIV-infected adults and adolescents: recommendations from CDC, the National Institutes of Health, and the HIV Medicine Association of the Infectious Diseases Society of America. MMWR Recomm Rep 2009;58(RR-4):1–207; quiz CE1–4.

Pneumocystis carinii (Pneumocystis jiroveci)

- *P. jiroveci* pneumonia is the most common life-threatening opportunistic infection in patients with AIDS. The taxonomy of the organism is unclear, having been classified as both protozoan and fungal.

CLINICAL PRESENTATION

- Characteristic symptoms include fever and dyspnea; clinical signs are tachypnea, with or without rales or rhonchi, and a nonproductive or mildly productive cough. Chest radiographs may show florid or subtle infiltrates or may occasionally be normal, although infiltrates are usually interstitial and bilateral. Arterial blood gases may show minimal hypoxia (partial pressure of oxygen [PaO_2] 80–95 mm Hg) but in more advanced disease may be markedly abnormal.
- The onset of *P. carinii* pneumonia (PCP) is often insidious, occurring over a period of weeks. Clinical signs are tachypnea with or without rales or rhonchi and a nonproductive or mildly productive cough occurring over a period of weeks, although more fulminant presentations can occur.

TREATMENT

- Treatment with **trimethoprim–sulfamethoxazole** or parenteral pentamidine is associated with a 60% to 100% response rate. Trimethoprim–sulfamethoxazole is the regimen of choice for treatment and subsequent prophylaxis of PCP in patients with and without HIV.
- Trimethoprim–sulfamethoxazole is given in doses of 15 to 20 mg/kg/day (based on the trimethoprim component) as three or four divided doses for the treatment of PCP. Treatment duration is typically 21 days but must be based on clinical response.
- Trimethoprim–sulfamethoxazole is usually initiated by the IV route, although oral therapy (as oral absorption is high) may suffice in mildly ill and reliable patients or to complete a course of therapy after a response has been achieved with IV administration.
- The more common adverse reactions seen with trimethoprim–sulfamethoxazole are rash (including Stevens–Johnson syndrome), fever, leukopenia, elevated serum transaminases, and thrombocytopenia. The incidence of these adverse reactions is higher in HIV-infected individuals than in those not infected with HIV.
- For pentamidine, side effects include hypotension, tachycardia, nausea, vomiting, severe hypoglycemia or hyperglycemia, pancreatitis, irreversible diabetes mellitus, elevated transaminases, nephrotoxicity, leukopenia, and cardiac arrhythmias.
- The early addition of adjunctive glucocorticoid therapy to anti-PCP regimens has been shown to decrease the risk of respiratory failure and improve survival in patients with AIDS and moderate to severe PCP (PaO_2 ≤70 mm Hg or [alveolar–arterial] gradient ≥35 mm Hg).

TABLE 40–7 Therapies for Prophylaxis of First-Episode Opportunistic Diseases in Adults and Adolescents

Pathogen	Indication	First Choice (Strength of Recommendation in Parentheses)
I. Standard of care		
Pneumocystis jiroveci	CD4+ count <200/mm³ *or* oropharyngeal candidiasis	Trimethoprim–sulfamethoxazole, one double-strength tablet orally once daily (AI) or 1 single-strength tablet orally once daily (AI)
Mycobacterium tuberculosis		
Isoniazid sensitive	(Active TB should be ruled out): + test for latent TB infection with no prior TB treatment history *or* - test for latent TB infection, but close contact with case of active tuberculosis *or* history of untreated or inadequately treated healed TB regardless of latent TB infection test results	Isoniazid 300 mg orally plus pyridoxine, 50 mg orally once daily for 9 months (AII) *or* Isoniazid 900 mg orally twice weekly (BII) plus pyridoxine 50 mg orally daily for 9 months (BII)
For exposure to drug resistant TB	Consult public health authorities	
Toxoplasma gondii	Immunoglobulin G antibody to *Toxoplasma* and CD4+ count <100/mm³	Trimethoprim–sulfamethoxazole, one double-strength tablet orally once daily (AII)
Mycobacterium avium complex	CD4+ count <50/mm³	Azithromycin 1,200 mg orally once weekly (AI) or 600 mg orally twice weekly (BIII) or clarithromycin 500 mg orally twice daily (AI)
Varicella zoster virus (VZV)	Pre-exposure: CD4 ≥200/mm², no history of varicella infection, or, if available, negative antibody to VZV	Varicella vaccination; two doses, three months apart (CIII)
	Postexposure: Significant exposure to chicken pox or shingles for patients who have no history of either condition or, if available, negative antibody to VZV	Varicella-zoster immune globulin, 125 IU per 10 kg (maximum of 625 IU) IM, within 96 hours after exposure to a person with active varicella or herpes zoster (AIII)

(continued)

TABLE 40–7 Therapies for Prophylaxis of First-Episode Opportunistic Diseases in Adults and Adolescents *(Continued)*

Pathogen	Indication	First Choice (Strength of Recommendation in Parentheses)
I. Standard of care		
Streptococcus pneumoniae	CD4 count ≥200 cells/mm³ or no receipt of vaccination in past 5 years. Consider for those with CD4 <200/mm³ and those with an CD4 increase to >200/mm³ on ART (CIII)	23-valent polysaccharide vaccine, 0.5 mL intramuscularly (BII) revaccination every 5 years may be considered (CIII)
Hepatitis B virus	All susceptible patients	Hepatitis B vaccine, three doses (AII). Anti-HBs should be obtained one month after the vaccine series completion (BIII)
Influenza virus	All patients (annually, before influenza season)	Inactivated trivalent influenza virus vaccine (annual): 0.5 mL intramuscularly (AIII)
Hepatitis A virus	All susceptible (anti-hepatitis A virus–negative) patients at increased risk for hepatitis A infection (e.g., chronic liver disease, illegal drug users, men who have sex with men)	Hepatitis A vaccine: two doses (AII) antibody response should be assessed 1 month after vaccination; with revaccination as needed (BIII)
Human papillomavirus (HPV) infection	15–26 year old women	HPV quadravalent vaccine months 0, 2, and 6 (CIII)
Bacteria	Neutropenia	Granulocyte colony-stimulating factor (G-CSF), 5–10 mcg/kg subcutaneously once daily for 2–4 weeks; or granulocyte-macrophage colony-stimulating factor (GM-CSF), 250 mcg/m² subcutaneously for 2–4 weeks (CII)
Histoplasma capsulatum	CD4⁺ count <150/mm³, endemic geographic area and high risk for exposures	Itraconazole 100–200 mg orally once daily (CI)

See Table 40–4 for levels of evidence-based recommendations.

Data from Kaplan JE, Benson C, Holmes KH, Brooks JT, et al. Guidelines for prevention and treatment of opportunistic infections in HIV-infected adults and adolescents: recommendations from CDC, the National Institutes of Health, and the HIV Medicine Association of the Infectious Diseases Society of America. MMWR Recomm Rep 2009;58(RR-4):1-207; quiz CE1-4.

PROPHYLAXIS

(Table 40–7)

- Currently, PCP prophylaxis is recommended for all HIV-infected individuals who have already had previous PCP. Prophylaxis is also recommended for all HIV-infected persons who have a CD4 lymphocyte count <200 cells/mm^3 (i.e., their CD4 cells are <14% of total lymphocytes) or a history of oropharyngeal candidiasis.
- Trimethoprim–sulfamethoxazole is the preferred therapy for both primary and secondary prophylaxis of PCP in adults and adolescents. The recommended dose in adults and adolescents is one double-strength tablet daily.

See Chapter 134, Human Immunodeficiency Virus Infection, authored by Peter L. Anderson, Thomas N. Kakuda, and Courtney V. Fletcher, for a more detailed discussion of this topic.

Influenza

DEFINITION

- Influenza is a viral illness associated with high mortality and high hospitalization rates among persons younger than age 65 years. Seasonal influenza epidemics result in 25 million to 50 million influenza cases, ~200,000 hospitalizations, and more than 30,000 deaths each year in the United States. Overall, more people die of influenza than of any other vaccine-preventable illness.
- The route of influenza transmission is person-to-person via inhalation of respiratory droplets, which can occur when an infected person coughs or sneezes. The incubation period for influenza ranges between 1 and 7 days, with an average incubation of 2 days. Adults are considered infectious from the day before their symptoms begin through 7 days after the onset of illness, whereas children can be infectious for longer than 10 days after the onset of illness. Viral shedding can persist for weeks to months in severely immunocompromised people.

CLINICAL PRESENTATION

- The presentation of influenza is similar to a number of other respiratory illnesses.
- The clinical course and outcome are affected by age, immunocompetence, viral characteristics, smoking, comorbidities, pregnancy, and the degree of preexisting immunity.
- Complications of influenza may include exacerbation of underlying comorbidities, primary viral pneumonia, secondary bacterial pneumonia or other respiratory illnesses (e.g., sinusitis, bronchitis, and otitis), encephalopathy, transverse myelitis, myositis, myocarditis, pericarditis, and Reye's syndrome.

SIGNS AND SYMPTOMS

- Classic signs and symptoms of influenza include rapid onset of fever, myalgia, headache, malaise, nonproductive cough, sore throat, and rhinitis.
- Nausea, vomiting, and otitis media are also commonly reported in children.
- Signs and symptoms typically resolve in 3 to 7 days, although cough and malaise may persist for more than 2 weeks.

LABORATORY TESTS

- The gold standard for diagnosis of influenza is viral culture.
- Rapid antigen and point-of-care tests, direct fluorescence antibody test, and the reverse transcription polymerase chain reaction assay may be used for rapid detection of virus.

- Chest radiograph should be obtained if pneumonia is suspected.
- Rapid tests have allowed for prompt diagnosis and initiation of antiviral therapy and decreased inappropriate use of antibiotics.

PREVENTION

- The best means to decrease the morbidity and mortality associated with influenza is to prevent infection through vaccination. Appropriate infection control measures, such as hand hygiene, basic respiratory etiquette (cover your cough and throw tissues away), and contact avoidance, are also important in preventing the spread of influenza.
- Annual vaccination is recommended for all persons age 6 months or older.
- Vaccination is also recommended for those who live with and/or care for people who are at high risk, including household contacts and healthcare workers.
  - ✓ The ideal time for vaccination is October or November to allow for the development and maintenance of immunity during the peak of the influenza season.
  - ✓ The two vaccines currently available for prevention of influenza are the trivalent influenza vaccine (TIV) and the live-attenuated influenza vaccine (LAIV). The specific strains included in the vaccine each year change based on antigenic drift.
  - ✓ TIV is FDA approved for use in people over 6 months of age, regardless of their immune status. Of note, several commercial products are available and are approved for different age groups (Table 41–1).
  - ✓ Adults older than 65 years benefit from influenza vaccination, including prevention of complications and decreased risk of influenza-related hospitalization and death. However, people in this population may not generate a strong antibody response to the vaccine and may remain susceptible to infection.
  - ✓ The most frequent adverse effect associated with TIV is soreness at the injection site that lasts for <48 hours. TIV may cause fever and malaise in those who have not previously been exposed to the viral antigens in the vaccine. Allergic-type reactions (hives and systemic anaphylaxis) rarely occur after influenza vaccination and are likely a result of a reaction to residual egg protein in the vaccine.
  - ✓ Vaccination should be avoided in persons who are not at high risk for influenza complications and who have experienced Guillain–Barré syndrome within 6 weeks of receiving a previous influenza vaccine.
  - ✓ LAIV is made with live, attenuated viruses and is approved for intranasal administration in healthy people between 2 and 49 years of age (Table 41–2). Advantages of LAIV include its ease of administration, intranasal rather than intramuscular administration, and the potential induction of broad mucosal and systemic immune response.
  - ✓ LAIV is only approved for children over the age of 2 years in part because of data showing an increase in asthma or reactive airway disease in those younger than 5 years.

TABLE 41–1 Approved Influenza Vaccines for Different Age Groups–United States, 2010–2011 Season

Vaccine	Trade Name	Manufacturer	Dose/Presentation	Thimerosal Mercury Content (mcg Hg/0.5 mL dose)	Age Group	Number of Doses
TIV	Fluzone	Sanofi Pasteur	0.25 mL prefilled syringe	0	6–35 months	1 or 2[a]
			0.5 mL prefilled syringe	0	≥36 months	1 or 2[a]
			0.5 mL vial	0	≥36 months	1 or 2[a]
			5 mL multidose vial	25	≥6 months	1 or 2[a]
TIV	Fluvirin	Novartis Vaccine	0.5 mL prefilled syringe	<1	≥4 y	1 or 2[a]
			5 mL multidose vial	25	≥4 y	1 or 2[a]
TIV	Fluarix	GlaxoSmith-Kline	0.5 mL prefilled syringe	0	≥3 y	1
TIV	FluLaval	GlaxoSmith-Kline	5 mL multidose vial	25	>18 y	1
TIV	Afluria	CSL limited	0.5 mL prefilled syringe	0	>6 months	1
			5-mL multidose vial	25		
LAIV	FluMist	MedImmune	0.5 mL sprayer	0	5–49 y	1 or 2[b]

LAIV, live-attenuated influenza vaccine; TIV, trivalent influenza vaccine.

[a]Two doses administered at least 1 month apart are recommended for children ages 6 months to less than 9 years who are receiving influenza vaccine for the first time.

[b]Two doses administered at least 6 weeks apart are recommended for children ages 5 to 9 years who are receiving influenza vaccine for the first time.

From Smith NM, Bresee JS, Shay DK, et al. *Prevention and control of influenza: Recommendations of the Advisory Committee on Immunization Practices (ACIP). MMWR Recomm Rep 2006;55(RR-10):1–42.*

TABLE 41–2	Comparison of Trivalent (TIV) and Live-Attenuated Influenza Vaccine (LAIV)	
Characteristic	**TIV**	**LAIV**
Age groups approved for use	>6 months	5 to 49 years
Immune status requirements	Immunocompetent or immunocompromised	Immunocompetent
Viral properties	Inactivated (killed) influenza A (H3N2), A (H1N1), and B viruses	Live-attenuated influenza A (H3N2), A (H1N1), and B viruses
Route of administration	Intramuscular	Intranasal
Immune system response	High serum IgG antibody response	Lower IgG response and high serum IgA mucosal response

Ig, immunoglobulin.

✓ The adverse effects typically associated with LAIV administration include runny nose, congestion, sore throat, and headache.
✓ LAIV should not be given to immunosuppressed patients or given by healthcare workers who are severely immunocompromised.

POSTEXPOSURE PROPHYLAXIS

- Antiviral drugs available for prophylaxis of influenza should be considered adjuncts but are not replacements for annual vaccination.
- The adamantanes amantadine and rimantadine are currently not recommended for prophylaxis or treatment in the United States because of the rapid emergence of resistance.
- The neuraminidase inhibitors oseltamivir and zanamivir are effective prophylactic agents against influenza in terms of preventing laboratory-confirmed influenza when used for seasonal prophylaxis and preventing influenza illness among persons exposed to a household contact who was diagnosed with influenza. Table 41–3 gives dosing recommendations.
- In those patients who did not receive the influenza vaccination and are receiving an antiviral drug for prevention of disease during the influenza season, the medication should optimally be taken for the entire duration of influenza activity in the community.
- Prophylaxis should be considered during influenza season for the following groups of patients:
  ✓ Persons at high risk of serious illness and/or complications who cannot be vaccinated
  ✓ Persons at high risk of serious illness and/or complications who are vaccinated after influenza activity has begun in their community because the development of sufficient antibody titers after vaccination takes ~2 weeks
  ✓ Unvaccinated persons who have frequent contact with those at high risk

TABLE 41–3 Recommended Daily Dosage of Influenza Antiviral Medications for Treatment and Prophylaxis–United States

Drug	Adult Treatment	Adult Prophylaxis[a]	Pediatric Treatment	Pediatric Prophylaxis

Oseltamivir	75-mg capsule twice daily for 5 days	75-mg capsule daily	≤3 months[b]: 12 mg twice daily
			3–5 months[b]: 20 mg twice daily
			6–11 months[b]: 25 mg twice daily
			≥1 year
			   <15 kg: 30 mg twice daily
			   16–23 kg: 45 mg twice daily
			   23–40 kg: 60 mg twice daily
			   >40 kg: 75 mg twice daily
			All for 5 days
				≤3 months Not recommended situation judged critical due to limited data in this group
				3–5 months[b]: 20 mg daily
				6–11 months[b]: 25 mg daily
				≥1 year
				   ≤15 kg: 30 mg daily
				   16–23 kg: 45 mg daily
				   23–40 kg: 60 mg daily
				   >40 kg: 75 mg daily

Zanamivir	2 inhalations twice daily × 5 days	2 inhalations daily	2 inhalations twice daily × 5 days for ≥7 years old	2 inhalations daily for ≥5 years old
Rimantadine[c]	200 mg/day in 1–2 doses × 7 days	200 mg/day in 1–2 doses	1–9 years old or <40 kg: 6.6 mg/kg/day divided twice daily (max 150 mg/day) ≥10 years old: 200 mg/day in 1–2 doses Treat 5–7 days	1–9 years old: 5 mg/kg daily (max 150 mg/day) ≥10 years old: 200 mg/day in 1–2 doses
Amantadine[c]	200 mg/day in 1–2 doses until 24–48 hours after symptom resolution	Same as treatment doses	>12 years old: same as adult 1–9 years old: 5 mg/kg/day in 1–2 doses; max 150 mg/day ≥10–12 years old: 100 mg orally twice daily	Same as treatment doses

[a]If influenza vaccine is administered, prophylaxis can generally be stopped 14 days after vaccination for non-institutionalized persons. When prophylaxis is being administered following an exposure, prophylaxis should be continued for 10 days after the last exposure. In persons at high risk for complications from influenza for whom vaccination is contraindicated or expected to be ineffective, chemoprophylaxis should be continued for the duration that influenza viruses are circulating in the community during influenza season.

[b]Emergency use authorization for pandemic H1N1 virus from the CDC.

[c]Monotherapy not recommended due to rapid emergence of resistance when used alone.

Data from Fiore AE, Shay DK, Broder K, Iskander JK, Uyeki TM, Mootrey G, et al. Prevention and control of influenza: recommendations of the Advisory Committee on Immunization Practices (ACIP), 2009. MMWR 2009;58(RR-8):1–52.

✓ Persons who may have an inadequate response to vaccination (e.g., advanced human immunodeficiency virus disease)

✓ Long-term care facility residents, regardless of vaccination status, when an outbreak has occurred in the institution

✓ Unvaccinated household contacts of someone who was diagnosed with influenza

- LAIV should not be administered until 48 hours after influenza antiviral therapy has stopped, and influenza antiviral drugs should not be administered for 2 weeks after the administration of LAIV because the antiviral drugs inhibit influenza virus replication.

- Pregnant women, regardless of trimester, should receive annual influenza vaccination with TIV but not with LAIV.

- The adamantanes and neuraminidase inhibitors are not recommended during pregnancy because of concerns regarding the effects of the drugs on the fetus.

- Immunocompromised hosts should receive annual influenza vaccination with TIV but not LAIV.

TREATMENT

GOALS OF THERAPY

- The four primary goals of therapy of influenza are as follows:
  1. Control symptoms
  2. Prevent complications
  3. Decrease work and/or school absenteeism
  4. Prevent the spread of infection

- In the era of pandemic preparedness and increasing resistance, early and definitive diagnosis of influenza is crucial. The currently available antiviral drugs are most effective if started within 48 hours of the onset of illness. Adjunct agents, such as acetaminophen for fever or an antihistamine for rhinitis, may be used concomitantly with the antiviral drugs.

- Patients suffering from influenza should get adequate sleep and maintain a low level of activity. They should stay home from work and/or school in order to rest and prevent the spread of infection. Appropriate fluid intake should be maintained. Cough/throat lozenges, warm tea, or soup may help with symptom control (cough and sore throat).

PHARMACOLOGIC THERAPY

- The two classes of antiviral drugs available for treatment of influenza are the same as those available for prophylaxis and include the adamantanes amantadine and rimantadine and the neuraminidase inhibitors oseltamivir and zanamivir. Because of widespread resistance to the adamantanes among influenza A viruses in the United States, amantadine and rimantadine are not recommended for treatment of influenza until susceptibility can be reestablished.

- Oseltamivir and zanamivir are neuraminidase inhibitors that have activity against both influenza A and influenza B viruses, although resistance to oseltamivir among seasonal influenza A H1N1 is on the rise. When administered within 48 hours of the onset of illness, oseltamivir and zanamivir may reduce the duration of illness by ~1 day versus placebo. Benefits are highly dependent on the timing of initiation of treatment, ideally being within 12 hours of illness onset.

- Oseltamivir is approved for treatment in those older than 1 year; zanamivir is approved for treatment in those older than 7 years. The recommended dosages vary by agent and age (see Table 41–3), and the recommended duration of treatment for both agents is 5 days.

- Neuropsychiatric complications consisting of delirium, seizures, hallucinations, and self-injury in pediatric patients have been reported following treatment with oseltamivir.

- Oseltamivir and zanamivir have been used in pregnancy, but solid clinical safety data are lacking. Both the adamantanes and the neuraminidase inhibitors are excreted in breast milk and should be avoided by mothers who are breast-feeding their infants. More studies are needed in these populations who are at high risk for serious disease and complications from influenza.

EVALUATION OF THERAPEUTIC OUTCOMES

- Patients should be monitored daily for resolution of signs and symptoms associated with influenza, such as fever, myalgia, headache, malaise, nonproductive cough, sore throat, and rhinitis. These signs and symptoms will typically resolve within ~1 week. If the patient continues to exhibit signs and symptoms of illness beyond 10 days or a worsening of symptoms after 7 days, a physician visit is warranted, as this may be an indication of a secondary bacterial infection.

See Chapter 118, Influenza, authored by Jessica C. Njoku and Elizabeth D. Hermsen, for a more detailed discussion of this topic.

CHAPTER 42

Intraabdominal Infections

DEFINITION

- Intraabdominal infections are those contained within the peritoneum or retroperitoneal space. Two general types of intraabdominal infections are discussed throughout this chapter: peritonitis and abscess.
- Peritonitis is defined as the acute, inflammatory response of peritoneal lining to microorganisms, chemicals, irradiation, or foreign body injury. It may be classified as either primary or secondary. With primary peritonitis, an intraabdominal focus of disease may not be evident. In secondary peritonitis, a focal disease process is evident within the abdomen.
- An abscess is a purulent collection of fluid separated from surrounding tissue by a wall consisting of inflammatory cells and adjacent organs. It usually contains necrotic debris, bacteria, and inflammatory cells.

PATHOPHYSIOLOGY

- Table 42–1 summarizes many of the potential causes of bacterial peritonitis. The causes of intraabdominal abscess somewhat overlap those of peritonitis, and, in fact, both may occur sequentially or simultaneously. Appendicitis is the most frequent cause of abscess. Intraabdominal infection results from entry of bacteria into the peritoneal or retroperitoneal spaces or from bacterial collections within intraabdominal organs. When peritonitis results from peritoneal dialysis, skin surface flora are introduced via the peritoneal catheter.
- In primary peritonitis, bacteria may enter the abdomen via the bloodstream or the lymphatic system, by transmigration through the bowel wall, through an indwelling peritoneal dialysis catheter, or via the fallopian tubes in female patients.
- In secondary peritonitis, bacteria most often enter the peritoneum or retroperitoneum as a result of disruption of the integrity of the GI tract caused by diseases or traumatic injuries.
- When bacteria become dispersed throughout the peritoneum, the inflammatory process involves the majority of the peritoneal lining. Fluid and protein shift into the abdomen (called "third spacing") may decrease circulating blood volume and cause shock.
- Peritonitis often results in death because of the effects on major organ systems. Fluid shifts and endotoxins may cause hypotension and shock.
- An abscess begins by the combined action of inflammatory cells (e.g., neutrophils), bacteria, fibrin, and other inflammatory components. Within the abscess, oxygen tension is low, and anaerobic bacteria thrive.

TABLE 42–1 Causes of Bacterial Peritonitis

Primary bacterial peritonitis
  Peritoneal dialysis
  Cirrhosis with ascites
  Nephrotic syndrome

Secondary bacterial peritonitis
  Miscellaneous causes
    Diverticulitis
    Appendicitis
    Inflammatory bowel diseases
    Salpingitis
    Biliary tract infections
    Necrotizing pancreatitis
  Neoplasms
    Intestinal obstruction
    Perforation
  Mechanical GI problems
    Any cause of small bowel obstruction (adhesions and hernia)
  Vascular causes
    Mesenteric arterial or venous occlusion (atrial fibrillation)
    Mesenteric ischemia without occlusion
  Trauma
    Blunt abdominal trauma with rupture of intestine
    Penetrating abdominal trauma
  Iatrogenic intestinal perforation (endoscopy)
  Intraoperative events
  Peritoneal contamination during abdominal operation
  Leakage from GI anastomosis

MICROBIOLOGY

- Primary bacterial peritonitis is often caused by a single organism. In children, the pathogen is usually group A *Streptococcus, Streptococcus pneumoniae, Escherichia coli,* or *Bacteroides* species. When peritonitis occurs in association with cirrhotic ascites, *E. coli* is isolated most frequently.

- Peritonitis in patients undergoing peritoneal dialysis is most often caused by common skin organisms: *Staphylococcus epidermidis, Staphylococcus aureus,* streptococci, and diphtheroids. Gram-negative bacteria associated with peritoneal dialysis infections include *E. coli, Klebsiella,* and *Pseudomonas.*

- Secondary intraabdominal infections are often polymicrobial. The mean number of isolates of microorganisms from infected intraabdominal sites has ranged from 2.9 to 3.7, including an average of 1.3 to 1.6 aerobes and 1.7 to 2.1 anaerobes. The frequencies with which specific bacteria were isolated in intraabdominal infections are given in **Table 42–2**.

TABLE 42-2	Pathogens Isolated from Patients with Intraabdominal Infection		
	Secondary Peritonitis	**Community-Acquired Infection**	**Nosocomial Infection**
Gram-negative bacteria			
Escherichia coli	32–61%	29%	22.5%
Enterobacter	8–26%	5.2%	8.0%
Klebsiella	6–26%	2.8%	4.5%
Proteus	4–23%	1.7%	2.4%
Gram-positive bacteria			
Enterococci	18–24%	10.6%	18%
Streptococci	6–55%	13.7%	10%
Staphylococci	6–16%	3.1%	4.8%
Anaerobic bacteria			
Bacteroides	25–80%	13.7%	10.3%
Clostridium	5–18%	3.5%	3.4%
Fungi	2–5%	3%	4%

Datat from Marshall JC, Innes M. Intensive care unit management of intraabdominal infection. Crit Care Med 2003;31:2228–2237; and Montravers P, Lepape A, Dubreuil L, et al. Clinical and microbiological profiles of community-ucquired and nosocomial infections: Results of the French prospective, observational EBIIA study. J Antimicrob Chemother. 2009;63:785–794.

- The combination of aerobic and anaerobic organisms appears to greatly increase pathogenicity. In intraabdominal infections, facultative bacteria may provide an environment conducive to the growth of anaerobic bacteria.
- Aerobic enteric bacteria and anaerobic bacteria are both pathogens in intraabdominal infection. Aerobic bacteria, particularly *E. coli*, appear responsible for the early mortality from peritonitis, whereas anaerobic bacteria are major pathogens in abscesses, with *Bacteroides fragilis* predominating.
- The role of *Enterococcus* as a pathogen is not clear. Enterococcal infection occurs more commonly in postoperative peritonitis, in the presence of specific risk factors indicating failure of the host defenses, or with the use of broad-spectrum antibiotics.

CLINICAL PRESENTATION

- Intraabdominal infections have a wide spectrum of clinical features often depending on the specific disease process, the location and the magnitude of bacterial contamination, and concurrent host factors. Patients with primary and secondary peritonitis present quite differently (**Table 42–3**).
- If peritonitis continues untreated, the patient may experience hypovolemic shock from fluid loss into the peritoneum, bowel wall, and lumen. This

TABLE 42–3 Clinical Presentation of Peritonitis

Primary Peritonitis

The patient may not be in acute distress, particularly with peritoneal dialysis.

Signs and symptoms

The patient may complain of nausea, vomiting (sometimes with diarrhea), and abdominal tenderness.

Temperature may be only mildly elevated or not elevated in patients undergoing peritoneal dialysis.

Bowel sounds are hypoactive.

The cirrhotic patient may have worsening encephalopathy.

Cloudy dialysate fluid with peritoneal dialysis

Laboratory tests

The patient's WBC count may be only mildly elevated.

Ascitic fluid usually contains >300 leukocytes/mm³, and bacteria may be evident on Gram stain of a centrifuged specimen.

In 60% to 80% of patients with cirrhotic ascites, the Gram stain is negative.

Other diagnostic tests

Culture of peritoneal dialysate or ascitic fluid should be positive.

Secondary Peritonitis

Signs and symptoms

Generalized abdominal pain

Tachypnea

Tachycardia

Nausea and vomiting

Temperature is normal initially, then increases to 37.7 to 38.8°C (100–102°F) within the first few hours; it may continue to rise for the next several hours.

Hypotension and shock if volume is not restored

Decreased urine output due to dehydration

Physical examination

Voluntary abdominal guarding changing to involuntary guarding and a "board-like" abdomen

Abdominal tenderness and distention

Faint bowel sounds that cease over time

Laboratory tests

Leukocytosis (15,000–20,000 WBC/mm³), with neutrophils predominating and an elevated percentage of immature neutrophils (bands)

Elevated hematocrit and BUN because of dehydration

Patient progresses from early alkalosis because of hyperventilation and vomiting to acidosis and lactic acidemia.

Other diagnostic tests

Abdominal radiographs may be useful because free air in the abdomen (indicating intestinal perforation) or distention of the small or large bowel is often evident.

BUN, blood urea nitrogen; WBC, white blood cell.

may be accompanied by generalized sepsis. Intraabdominal abscess may pose a diagnostic challenge, as the symptoms are neither specific nor dramatic.

- The overall outcome from intraabdominal infection depends on five key factors: inoculum size, virulence of the organisms, the presence of adjuvants within the peritoneal cavity that facilitate infection, the adequacy of host defenses, and the adequacy of initial treatment.

TREATMENT

- The goals of treatment are the correction of intraabdominal disease processes or injuries that have caused infection and the drainage of collections of purulent material (e.g., abscess). A secondary objective is to achieve resolution of infection without major organ system complications or adverse treatment effects.
- The three major modalities for the treatment of intraabdominal infection are prompt surgical drainage of the infected site, hemodynamic resuscitation and support of vital functions, and early administration of appropriate antimicrobial therapy to treat infection not removed by surgery.
- Antimicrobials are an important adjunct to drainage procedures in the treatment of intraabdominal infections; however, the use of antimicrobial agents without surgical intervention is usually inadequate. For some specific situations (e.g., most cases of primary peritonitis), drainage procedures may not be required, and antimicrobial agents become the mainstay of therapy.
- In the early phase of serious intraabdominal infections, attention should be given to the maintenance of organ system functions. With generalized peritonitis, large volumes of IV fluids are required to restore vascular volume, to improve cardiovascular function, and to maintain adequate tissue perfusion and oxygenation.

NONPHARMACOLOGIC TREATMENT

- Secondary peritonitis is treated surgically; this is called "source control," which refers to the physical measures undertaken to eradicate the focus of infection. Abdominal laparotomy may be used to correct the cause of peritonitis.
- Aggressive fluid repletion and management are required for the purposes of achieving or maintaining proper intravascular volume to ensure adequate cardiac output, tissue perfusion, and correction of acidosis.
- In the initial hour of treatment, a large volume of IV solution (lactated Ringer solution) may need to be administered to restore intravascular volume. This may be followed by up to 1 L/hour until fluid balance is restored in a few hours.
- In patients with significant blood loss (hematocrit $\leq 25\%$), blood should be given. This is generally in the form of packed red blood cells.
- Enteral or parenteral nutrition facilitates improved immune function and wound healing to ensure recovery.

TABLE 42–4	Agents Recommended for the Treatment of Community-acquired, Complicated Intraabdominal Infections
Agents Recommended for Mild to Moderate Infections	**Agents Recommended for High-Severity Infections**
β-Lactamase inhibitor combinations	
Ampicillin–sulbactam	Piperacillin–tazobactam
Ticarcillin–clavulanate	
Carbapenems	
Ertapenem	Imipenem–cilastatin
	Meropenem
Combination regimens	
Cefazolin or cefuroxime plus metronidazole	Third- or fourth-generation cephalosporins (cefotaxime, ceftriaxone, ceftizoxime, ceftazidime, and cefepime) plus metronidazole
Ciprofloxacin, levofloxacin, moxifloxacin, or gatifloxacin in combination with metronidazole	Ciprofloxacin in combination with metronidazole
	Aztreonam plus metronidazole

Data from Solomkin JS, Mazuski JE, Baron EJ, et al. Guidelines for the selection of anti-infective agents for complicated intraabdominal infections. Clin Infect Dis 2003;37:997–1005; Mazuski JE, Sawyer RG, Nathens AB, et al. The Surgical Infection Society guidelines on antimicrobial therapy for intraabdominal infections: An executive summary. Surg Infect (Larchmt) 2002;3:161–174; and Mazuski JE, Sawyer RG, Nathens AB, et al. The Surgical Infection Society guidelines on antimicrobial therapy for intraabdominal infections: Evidence for recommendations. Surg Infect (Larchmt) 2002;3:175–234.

PHARMACOLOGIC THERAPY

- The goals of antimicrobial therapy are to control bacteremia and to establish the metastatic foci of infection, to reduce suppurative complications after bacterial contamination, and to prevent local spread of existing infection.
- An empiric antimicrobial regimen should be started as soon as the presence of intraabdominal infection is suspected on the basis of likely pathogens.

Recommendations

- Table 42–4 presents recommended and alternative regimens for selected situations. These are general guidelines, not rules, because there are many factors that cannot be incorporated into such a table. Guidelines for initial antimicrobial treatment of specific intraabdominal infections are presented in Table 42–5.
- Evidence-based treatment principles for complicated intraabdominal infections are given in Table 42–6.
- The selection of a specific agent or combination should be based on culture and susceptibility data for peritonitis that occurs from chronic

TABLE 42-5 Guidelines for Initial Antimicrobial Agents for Intraabdominal Infections

	Primary Agents	Alternatives
Primary bacterial peritonitis		
Cirrhosis	Cefotaxime	1. Add clindamycin or metronidazole if anaerobes are suspected
		2. Other third-generation cephalosporins, extended-spectrum penicillins, aztreonam, and imipenem as alternatives
		3. Piperacillin–tazobactam
Peritoneal dialysis	Initial empiric regimens	1. An aminoglycoside may be used in place of ceftazidime or cefepime
	Cefazolin or cephalothin plus ceftazidime or cefepime	2. Imipenem/cilastin or cefepime may be used alone
		3. Quinolones may be used in place of ceftazidime or cefepime if local susceptibilities allow
	1. *Staphylococcus*: penicillinase-resistant penicillin or first-generation cephalosporin	1. Alternative for methicillin resistant staphylococci is vancomycin
		2. For vancomycin-resistant *Staphylococcus aureus*, linezolid, daptomycin, or quinupristin-dalfopristin must be used
	2. *Streptococcus* or *Enterococcus*: ampicillin	1. An aminoglycoside may be added for enterococcal peritonitis
		2. Linezolid or quinupristin-dalfopristin should be used to treat vancomycin-resistant enterococcus not susceptible to ampicillin
	3. Aerobic gram-negative bacilli: ceftazidime or cefepime	1. The regimen should be based on in vitro sensitivity tests
	4. *Pseudomonas aeruginosa*: two agents with differing mechanisms of action, such as an oral quinolone plus ceftazidime, cefepime, tobramycin, or piperacillin	
Secondary bacterial peritonitis		
Perforated peptic ulcer	First-generation cephalosporins	1. Antianaerobic cephalosporins[a]
		2. Possibly add aminoglycoside if patient condition is poor
		3. Aminoglycoside with clindamycin or metronidazole; add ampicillin if patient is immunocompromised or if biliary tract origin of infection

(continued)

TABLE 42-5 Guidelines for Initial Antimicrobial Agents for Intraabdominal Infections (*Continued*)

	Primary Agents	Alternatives
Secondary bacterial peritonitis		
Other	Imipenem-cilastatin, meropenem, ertapenem, or extended-spectrum penicillins with β-lactamase inhibitor	1. Ciprofloxacin with metronidazole 2. Aztreonam with clindamycin or metronidazole 3. Antianaerobic cephalosporins[a]
Abscess		
General	Imipenem-cilastatin, meropenem, ertapenem, or extended-spectrum penicillins with β-lactamase inhibitor	1. Aztreonam with clindamycin or metronidazole 2. Ciprofloxacin with metronidazole 3. Aminoglycoside with clindamycin or metronidazole;
Liver	As above but add a first-generation cephalosporin	Use metronidazole if amoebic liver abscess is suspected
Spleen	Aminoglycoside plus penicillinase-resistant penicillin	Alternatives for penicillinase-resistant penicillin are first-generation cephalosporins or vancomycin
Appendicitis		
Normal or inflamed	Antianaerobic cephalosporins[a] (discontinued immediately postoperation)	1. Ampicillin–sulbactam
Gangrenous or perforated	Imipenem-cilastatin, meropenem, ertapenem, antianaerobic cephalosporins, or extended-spectrum penicillins with β-lactamase inhibitor	1. Aztreonam with clindamycin or metronidazole 2. Ciprofloxacin with metronidazole 3. Aminoglycoside with clindamycin or metronidazole
Acute cholecystitis	First-generation cephalosporin	Aminoglycoside plus ampicillin if severe infection
Cholangitis	Aminoglycoside with ampicillin with or without clindamycin or metronidazole	Use vancomycin instead of ampicillin if patient is allergic to penicillin
Acute contamination from abdominal trauma	Antianaerobic cephalosporins[a] or ampicillin–sulbactam	1. A carbapenem 2. Ciprofloxacin plus metronidazole
Pelvic inflammatory disease	Cefotetan or cefoxitin with doxycycline	1. Clindamycin with gentamicin 2. Ciprofloxacin with doxycycline and metronidazole

Cefoxitin, cefotetan, and ceftizoxime.

TABLE 42–6	Evidence-based Recommendations for Treatment of Complicated Intraabdominal Infections

	Grade of Recommendation*a*
Acute contamination as a result of trauma	
Bowel injuries caused by penetrating, blunt, or iatrogenic trauma that are repaired within 12 hours and intraoperative contamination of the operative field by enteric contents under other circumstances should be treated with antibiotics ≤24 hours.	A-1
Acute appendicitis	
Acute appendicitis without evidence of gangrene, perforation, abscess, or peritonitis requires only prophylactic administration of inexpensive regimens active against facultative and obligate anaerobes.	A-1
Community-acquired infections	
Antibiotics used for empirical treatment of community-acquired intraabdominal infections should be active against empiric gram-negative aerobic and facultative bacilli and β-lactam–susceptible gram-positive cocci.	A-1
For patients with mild-to-moderate community-acquired infections, agents that have a narrower spectrum of activity, such as ampicillin–sulbactam, cefazolin, or cefuroxime–metronidazole, ticarcillin–clavulanate, and ertapenem are preferable to more costly agents that have broader coverage against gram-negative organisms and/or greater risk of toxicity.	A-1
Anaerobic coverage	A-1
Coverage against obligate anaerobic bacilli should be provided for distal small bowel and colon-derived infections and for more proximal GI perforations when obstruction is present.	
Nosocomial infections	
Agents used to treat nosocomial infections in the intensive care unit (e.g., expanded gram-negative bacterial spectrum) should not be routinely used to treat community-acquired infections.	B-2
If a patient with diagnosed infection has previously been treated with an antibiotic, that patient should be treated as if he or she has had a healthcare-associated (nosocomial) infection.	B-3
Aminoglycosides	
Aminoglycosides are not recommended for routine use in community-acquired intraabdominal infections.	A-1
Oral completion therapy	
Completion of the antimicrobial course with oral forms of a quinolone plus metronidazole	A-1
or	
with amoxicillin–clavulanic acid is acceptable for patients who are able to tolerate an oral diet.	B-3

(continued)

TABLE 42–6	Evidence-based Recommendations for Treatment of Complicated Intraabdominal Infections *(Continued)*	
		Grade of Recommendation[a]
Suspected fungal infection		
Antiinfective therapy for *Candida* should be withheld until the infecting species is identified.		C-3
Enterococcal infection		
Routine coverage against *Enterococcus* is not necessary for patients with community-acquired intraabdominal infections.		A-1

[a]Strength of recommendations: A, B, C = good, moderate, and poor evidence to support recommendation, respectively. Quality of evidence: 1 = Evidence from >1 properly randomized, controlled trial. 2 = Evidence from >1 well-designed clinical trial with randomization, from cohort or case-controlled analytic studies; from multiple time series, or from dramatic results from uncontrolled experiments. 3 = Evidence from opinions of respected authorities, based on clinical experience, descriptive studies, or reports of expert communities.

Data from Solomkin JS, Mazuski JE, Baron EJ, et al. Guidelines for the selection of anti-infective agents for complicated intraabdominal infections. Clin Infect Dis 2003;37:997–1005; Mazuski JE, Sawyer RG, Nathens AB, et al. The Surgical Infection Society guidelines on antimicrobial therapy for intraabdominal infections: An executive summary. Surg Infect (Larchmt) 2002;3:161–174; and Mazuski JE, Sawyer RG, Nathens AB, et al. The Surgical Infection Society guidelines on antimicrobial therapy for intraabdominal infections: Evidence for recommendations. Surg Infect (Larchmt) 2002;3:175–234.

peritoneal dialysis. If microbiologic data are unavailable, empiric therapy should be initiated.

- For established intraabdominal infections, most patients are adequately treated with 5 to 7 days of antimicrobial therapy.
- Intraperitoneal administration of antibiotics is preferred over IV therapy in the treatment of peritonitis that occurs in patients undergoing continuous ambulatory peritoneal dialysis. Initial antibiotic regimens should be effective against both gram-positive and gram-negative organisms.
- Suitable antibiotics for initial empiric treatment of continuous ambulatory peritoneal dialysis–associated peritonitis are cefazolin (loading dose 500 mg/L, maintenance dose 125 mg/L in the dialysis solution) plus ceftazidime (loading dose 500 mg/L, maintenance dose 125 mg/L) or cefepime (500 mg/L loading dose and 125 mg/L maintenance dose) or an aminoglycoside (gentamicin/tobramycin, 8 mg/L loading dose and 4 mg/L maintenance dose). If the patient is allergic to cephalosporins, vancomycin (1 g/L loading dose and 25 mg/L maintenance dose) or an aminoglycoside should be substituted.
- Antimicrobial therapy should be continued for at least 1 week after the dialysate fluid is clear and for a total of at least 14 days.
- Antianaerobic cephalosporins or extended-spectrum penicillins are effective in preventing most infectious complications after acute bacterial contamination, such as with abdominal trauma where GI contents enter the peritoneum, and when the patient is seen soon after injury (within 2 hours) and surgical measures are instituted promptly.

- Acute intraabdominal contamination, such as after a traumatic injury, may be treated with a short course (24 hours). For established infections (peritonitis or intraabdominal abscess), an antimicrobial course of at least 7 days is justified.

EVALUATION OF THERAPEUTIC OUTCOMES

- The patient should be continually reassessed to determine the success or failure of therapies.
- Once antimicrobials are initiated and other important therapies described earlier in the Treatment section are used, most patients should show improvement within 2 to 3 days. Usually, temperature will return to near normal, vital signs should stabilize, and the patient should not appear in distress, with the exception of recognized discomfort and pain from incisions, drains, and nasogastric tube.
- At 24 to 48 hours, aerobic bacterial culture results should return. If a suspected pathogen is not sensitive to the antimicrobial agents being given, the regimen should be changed if the patient has not shown sufficient improvement.
- If the isolated pathogen is extremely sensitive to one antimicrobial, and the patient is progressing well, concurrent antimicrobial therapy may often be discontinued.
- With present anaerobic culturing techniques and the slow growth of these organisms, anaerobes are often not identified until 4 to 7 days after culture, and sensitivity information is difficult to obtain. For this reason, there are usually few data with which to alter the antianaerobic component of the antimicrobial regimen.
- Superinfection in patients being treated for intraabdominal infection is often due to *Candida*; however, enterococci or opportunistic gram-negative bacilli such as *Pseudomonas* or *Serratia* may be involved.
- Treatment regimens for intraabdominal infection can be judged successful if the patient recovers from the infection without recurrent peritonitis or intraabdominal abscess and without the need for additional antimicrobials. A regimen can be considered unsuccessful if a significant adverse drug reaction occurs, if reoperation is necessary, or if patient improvement is delayed beyond 1 or 2 weeks.

See Chapter 123, Intraabdominal Infections, authored by Joseph T. DiPiro and Thomas R. Howdieshell, for a more detailed discussion of this topic.

Respiratory Tract Infections, Lower

DEFINITION

- Lower respiratory tract infections include infectious processes of the lungs and bronchi, pneumonia, bronchitis, bronchiolitis, and lung abscess.

BRONCHITIS

ACUTE BRONCHITIS

- *Bronchitis* refers to an inflammatory condition of the large elements of the tracheobronchial tree that is usually associated with a generalized respiratory infection. The inflammatory process does not extend to include the alveoli. The disease entity is frequently classified as either acute or chronic. Acute bronchitis occurs in all ages, whereas chronic bronchitis primarily affects adults.
- Acute bronchitis most commonly occurs during the winter months. Cold, damp climates and/or the presence of high concentrations of irritating substances such as air pollution or cigarette smoke may precipitate attacks.

Pathophysiology

- Respiratory viruses are by far the most common infectious agents associated with acute bronchitis. The common cold viruses rhinovirus and coronavirus and lower respiratory tract pathogens, including influenza virus, adenovirus, and respiratory syncytial virus, account for the majority of cases. *Mycoplasma pneumoniae* also appears to be a frequent cause of acute bronchitis. Other bacterial causes are *Chlamydia pneumoniae* and *Bordetella pertussis*.
- Infection of the trachea and bronchi causes hyperemic and edematous mucous membranes and an increase in bronchial secretions. Destruction of respiratory epithelium can range from mild to extensive and may affect bronchial mucociliary function. In addition, the increase in bronchial secretions, which can become thick and tenacious, further impairs mucociliary activity. Recurrent acute respiratory infections may be associated with increased airway hyperreactivity and possibly the pathogenesis of chronic obstructive lung disease.

Clinical Presentation

- Bronchitis is primarily a self-limiting illness and rarely a cause of death. Acute bronchitis usually begins as an upper respiratory infection. The patient typically has nonspecific complaints, such as malaise and headache, coryza, and sore throat.
- Cough is the hallmark of acute bronchitis. It occurs early and will persist despite the resolution of nasal or nasopharyngeal complaints. Frequently,

the cough is initially nonproductive but progresses, yielding mucopurulent sputum.

- Chest examination may reveal rhonchi and coarse, moist rales bilaterally. Chest radiographs, when performed, are usually normal.
- Bacterial cultures of expectorated sputum are generally of limited utility because of the inability to avoid normal nasopharyngeal flora by the sampling technique. Viral antigen detection tests can be used when a specific diagnosis is necessary. Cultures or serologic diagnosis of *M. pneumoniae* and culture or direct fluorescent antibody detection for *B. pertussis* should be obtained in prolonged or severe cases when epidemiologic considerations would suggest their involvement.

Treatment

- The goals of therapy are to provide comfort to the patient and, in the unusually severe case, to treat associated dehydration and respiratory compromise.
- The treatment of acute bronchitis is symptomatic and supportive in nature. Reassurance and antipyretics alone are often sufficient. Bed rest and mild analgesic-antipyretic therapy are often helpful in relieving the associated lethargy, malaise, and fever. Patients should be encouraged to drink fluids to prevent dehydration and possibly decrease the viscosity of respiratory secretions.
- **Aspirin** or **acetaminophen** (650 mg in adults or 10–15 mg/kg per dose in children with a maximum daily adult dose of 4 g and 60 mg/kg for children) or **ibuprofen** (200–800 mg in adults or 10 mg/kg per dose in children with a maximum daily dose of 3.2 g for adults and 40 mg/kg for children) is administered every 4 to 6 hours.
- In children, aspirin should be avoided and acetaminophen used as the preferred agent because of the possible association between aspirin use and the development of Reye's syndrome.
- Mist therapy and/or the use of a vaporizer may further promote the thinning and loosening of respiratory secretions.
- Persistent, mild cough, which may be bothersome, may be treated with **dextromethorphan**; more severe coughs may require intermittent **codeine** or other similar agents.
- Routine use of antibiotics in the treatment of acute bronchitis is discouraged; however, in patients who exhibit persistent fever or respiratory symptomatology for more than 4 to 6 days, the possibility of a concurrent bacterial infection should be suspected.
- When possible, antibiotic therapy is directed toward anticipated respiratory pathogen(s) (i.e., *Streptococcus pneumoniae* and *Haemophilus influenzae*) and/or those demonstrating a predominant growth upon throat culture.
- *M. pneumoniae,* if suspected by history or positive cold agglutinins (titers ≥1:32) or if confirmed by culture or serology, may be treated with **azithromycin.** Also, a fluoroquinolone with activity against these pathogens (**levofloxacin**) may be used in adults.
- During known epidemics involving the influenza A virus, **amantadine** or **rimantadine** may be effective in minimizing associated symptomatology if administered early in the course of the disease.

CHRONIC BRONCHITIS

Pathophysiology

- Chronic bronchitis is a result of several contributing factors, including cigarette smoking; exposure to occupational dusts, fumes, and environmental pollution; host factors [e.g., genetic factors]; and bacterial or viral infections.
- In chronic bronchitis, the bronchial wall is thickened, and the number of mucus-secreting goblet cells in the surface epithelium of both larger and smaller bronchi is markedly increased. Hypertrophy of the mucous glands and dilation of the mucous gland ducts are also observed. As a result of these changes, patients with chronic bronchitis have substantially more mucus in their peripheral airways, further impairing normal lung defenses and causing mucus plugging of the smaller airways. Continued progression of this pathology can result in residual scarring of small bronchi, augmenting airway obstruction and the weakening of bronchial walls.

Clinical Presentation

- The hallmark of chronic bronchitis is a cough that may range from a mild "smoker's cough" to severe incessant coughing productive of purulent sputum. Expectoration of the largest quantity of sputum usually occurs upon arising in the morning, although many patients expectorate sputum throughout the day. The expectorated sputum is usually tenacious and can vary in color from white to yellow-green.
- The diagnosis of chronic bronchitis is based primarily on clinical assessment and history. By definition, any patient who reports coughing up sputum on most days for at least 3 consecutive months each year for 2 consecutive years suffers from chronic bronchitis. Fig. 43–1 presents a diagnosis and treatment scheme for chronic bronchitis.
- An increased number of polymorphonuclear granulocytes in sputum often suggests continual bronchial irritation, whereas an increased number of eosinophils may suggest an allergic component. The most common bacterial isolates (expressed in percentages of total cultures) identified from sputum culture in patients experiencing an acute exacerbation of chronic bronchitis are given in Table 43–1.
- With the exception of pulmonary findings, the physical examination of patients with mild to moderate chronic bronchitis is usually unremarkable (Table 43–2).

Treatment

- The goals of therapy for chronic bronchitis are to reduce the severity of symptoms, to ameliorate acute exacerbations, and to achieve prolonged infection-free intervals.
- A complete occupational/environmental history for the determination of exposure to noxious, irritating gases, as well as cigarette smoking, must be assessed. Exposure to bronchial irritants should be reduced.
- Attempts should be made with the patient to reduce or eliminate cigarette smoking.

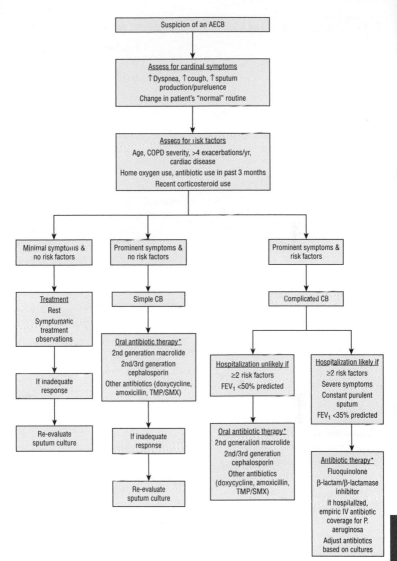

FIGURE 43–1. Clinical algorithm for the diagnosis and treatment of chronic bronchitic patients with an acute exacerbation incorporating the principles of the clinical classification system (AECB, acute exacerbation of chronic bronchitis; COPD, chronic obstructive pulmonary disease; CB, chronic bronchitis; TMP/SMX, trimethoprim/sulfamethoxazole). *See Table 43–4 for commonly used antibiotics and doses.

TABLE 43–1 Common Bacterial Isolates in Chronic Bronchitis

Bacteria	Percentage of Total Cultures
Haemophilus influenzae[a]	45%
Moraxella catarrhalis[a]	30%
Streptococcus pneumoniae[b]	20%
Escherichia coli, Enterobacter species, *Klebsiella,* and *Pseudomonas aeruginosa*	5%

[a]Often β-lactamase positive.
[b]Up to 25% of strains may have intermediate or high resistance to penicillin.

- Humidification of inspired air may promote the hydration (liquefaction) of tenacious secretions, allowing for more effective sputum production. The use of mucolytic aerosols (e.g., *N*-acetylcysteine and deoxyribonuclease) is of questionable therapeutic value. Mucolytics may have the greatest benefit in patients with moderate or severe chronic obstructive pulmonary disease who are not receiving inhaled corticosteroids.
- Postural drainage may assist in promoting clearance of pulmonary secretions.

PHARMACOLOGIC THERAPY

- Oral or aerosolized bronchodilators (e.g., **albuterol** aerosol) may be of benefit to some patients during acute pulmonary exacerbations. For patients who consistently demonstrate limitations in airflow, a therapeutic change of bronchodilators should be considered.

TABLE 43–2 Clinical Presentation of Chronic Bronchitis

Signs and symptoms
Excessive sputum expectoration
Cyanosis (advanced disease)
Obesity

Physical examination
Chest auscultation usually reveals inspiratory and expiratory rales, rhonchi, and mild wheezing with an expiratory phase that is frequently prolonged. There is hyperresonance on percussion with obliteration of the area of cardiac dullness.
Normal vesicular breathing sounds are diminished.
Clubbing of digits (advanced disease)

Chest radiograph
Increase in the anteroposterior diameter of the thoracic cage (observed as a barrel chest)
Depressed diaphragm with limited mobility

Laboratory tests
Erythrocytosis (advanced disease)

Pulmonary function tests
Decreased vital capacity
Prolonged expiratory flow

- Long-term inhalation of **ipratropium** (or **tiotropium**) decreases the frequency of cough, severity of cough, and volume of expectorated sputum.
- The use of antimicrobials has been controversial, although antibiotics are an important component of treatment. Agents should be selected that are effective against likely pathogens, have the lowest risk of drug interactions, and can be administered in a manner that promotes compliance (see **Fig. 43–1**).
- The Anthonisen criteria can be used to determine if antibiotic therapy is indicated. The patient will most likely benefit from antibiotic therapy if two or three of the following are present: (1) increase of shortness of breath, (2) increase in sputum volume, or (3) production of purulent sputum.
- Selection of antibiotics should consider that up to 30% to 40% of *H. influenzae* and 95% to 100% of *M. pneumoniae* are β-lactamase producers; up to 40% of *S. pneumoniae* demonstrate penicillin resistance, with 20% being highly resistant.
- Antibiotics commonly used in the treatment of these patients and their respective adult starting doses are outlined in **Table 43–3**. Duration of symptom-free periods may be enhanced by antibiotic regimens using the upper limit of the recommended daily dose for 5 to 7 days.
- In patients whose history suggests recurrent exacerbations of their disease that might be attributable to certain specific events (i.e., seasonal, winter months), a trial of prophylactic antibiotics might be beneficial. If no

TABLE 43–3	Oral Antibiotics Commonly Used for the Treatment of Acute Respiratory Exacerbations in Chronic Bronchitis	
Antibiotic	**Usual Adult Dose (g)**	**Dose Schedule (doses/day)**
Preferred drugs		
Ampicillin	0.25–0.5	4
Amoxicillin	0.5–0.875	3/2
Amoxicillin–clavulanate	0.5–0.875	3/2
Ciprofloxacin	0.5–0.75	2
Levofloxacin	0.5–0.75	1
Moxifloxacin	0.4	1
Doxycycline	0.1	2
Minocycline	0.1	2
Tetracycline HCl	0.5	4
Trimethoprim–sulfamethoxazole	1 DS[a]	2
Supplemental drugs		
Azithromycin	0.25–0.5	1
Erythromycin	0.5	4
Clarithromycin	0.25–0.5	2
Cephalexin	0.5	4

[a]DS, double-strength tablet (160 mg trimethoprim/800 mg sulfamethoxazole).

TABLE 43–4	Clinical Presentation of Bronchiolitis

Signs and symptoms
Prodrome with irritability, restlessness, and mild fever
Cough and coryza
Vomiting, diarrhea, noisy breathing, and an increase in respiratory rate as symptoms progress
Labored breathing with retractions of the chest wall, nasal flaring, and grunting

Physical examination
Tachycardia and respiratory rate of 40–80/min in hospitalized infants
Wheezing and inspiratory rales
Mild conjunctivitis in one third of patients
Otitis media in 5% to 10% of patients

Laboratory examinations
Peripheral white blood cell count normal or slightly elevated
Abnormal arterial blood gases (hypoxemia and, rarely, hypercarbia)

clinical improvement is noted over an appropriate period (e.g., 2–3 months per year for 2–3 y), prophylactic therapy could be discontinued.

BRONCHIOLITIS

- Bronchiolitis is an acute viral infection of the lower respiratory tract of infants that affects ~50% of children during the first year of life and 100% by 3 years.
- Respiratory syncytial virus is the most common cause of bronchiolitis, accounting for up to 70% of all cases. Parainfluenza viruses are the second most common cause. Bacteria serve as secondary pathogens in only a small minority of cases.

Clinical Presentation

- The most common clinical signs of bronchiolitis are found in Table 43–4. A prodrome suggesting an upper respiratory tract infection, usually lasting from 2 to 8 days, precedes the onset of clinical symptoms.
- As a result of limited oral intake due to coughing combined with fever, vomiting, and diarrhea, infants are frequently dehydrated.
- The diagnosis of bronchiolitis is based primarily on history and clinical findings. The isolation of a viral pathogen in the respiratory secretions of a wheezing child establishes a presumptive diagnosis of infectious bronchiolitis.

Treatment

- Bronchiolitis is a self-limiting illness and usually requires no therapy (other than reassurance, antipyretics, and adequate fluid intake) unless the infant is hypoxic or dehydrated. Otherwise healthy infants can be treated for fever, provided generous amounts of oral fluids, and observed closely.
- In severely affected children, the mainstays of therapy for bronchiolitis are oxygen therapy and IV fluids.

- Aerosolized β-adrenergic therapy appears to offer little benefit for the majority of patients but may be useful in the child with a predisposition toward bronchospasm.
- Because bacteria do not represent primary pathogens in the etiology of bronchiolitis, antibiotics should not be routinely administered. However, many clinicians frequently administer antibiotics initially while awaiting culture results because the clinical and radiographic findings in bronchiolitis are often suggestive of a possible bacterial pneumonia.
- **Ribavirin** may be considered for bronchiolitis caused by respiratory syncytial virus in a subset of patients (those with underlying pulmonary or cardiac disease or with severe acute infection). Use of the drug requires special equipment (small-particle aerosol generator) and specifically trained personnel for administration via oxygen hood or mist tent.

PNEUMONIA

- Pneumonia is the most common infectious cause of death in the United States. It occurs in persons of all ages, although the clinical manifestations are most severe in the very young, the elderly, and the chronically ill.

PATHOPHYSIOLOGY

- Microorganisms gain access to the lower respiratory tract by three routes: they may be inhaled as aerosolized particles, they may enter the lung via the bloodstream from an extrapulmonary site of infection, or aspiration of oropharyngeal contents may occur.
- Lung infections with viruses suppress the bacterial clearing activity of the lung by impairing alveolar macrophage function and mucociliary clearance, thus setting the stage for secondary bacterial pneumonia.
- The vast majority of pneumonia cases acquired in the community by otherwise healthy adults are due to *S. pneumoniae* (pneumococcus) (up to 75% of all acute bacterial pneumonias in the United States). Other common bacterial causes are *M. pneumoniae*, *Legionella*, and *C. pneumoniae*, which are referred to as "atypical" pathogens. Community-acquired pneumonias caused by *Staphylococcus aureus* and gram-negative rods are observed primarily in the elderly, especially those residing in nursing homes, and in association with alcoholism and other debilitating conditions.
- Gram-negative aerobic bacilli and *S. aureus* are also the leading causative agents in hospital-acquired pneumonia.
- Anaerobic bacteria are the most common etiologic agents in pneumonia that follows the gross aspiration of gastric or oropharyngeal contents.
- In the pediatric age group, most pneumonias are due to viruses, especially respiratory syncytial virus, parainfluenza, and adenovirus. Pneumococcus

Hospital-acquired Pneumonia

- The strongest predisposing factor for hospital-acquired pneumonia (HAP) is mechanical ventilation. Factors predisposing patients to HAP include severe illness, long duration of hospitalization, supine positioning, witnessed aspiration, coma, acute respiratory distress syndrome, patient transport, and prior antibiotic exposure.
- The diagnosis of nosocomial pneumonia is usually established by the presence of a new infiltrate on chest radiograph, fever, worsening respiratory status, and the appearance of thick, neutrophil-laden respiratory secretions.

TREATMENT

- Eradication of the offending organism and complete clinical cure are the primary objectives. Associated morbidity should be minimized (e.g., renal, pulmonary, or hepatic dysfunction).
- The first priority on assessing the patient with pneumonia is to evaluate the adequacy of respiratory function and to determine whether there are signs of systemic illness, specifically dehydration, or sepsis with resulting circulatory collapse.
- The supportive care of the patient with pneumonia includes the use of humidified oxygen for hypoxemia, fluid resuscitation, administration of bronchodilators (albuterol) when bronchospasm is present, and chest physiotherapy with postural drainage if there is evidence of retained secretions.
- Important therapeutic adjuncts include adequate hydration (by IV route if necessary), optimal nutritional support, and fever control.
- The treatment of bacterial pneumonia initially involves the empiric use of a relatively broad-spectrum antibiotic (or antibiotics) effective against probable pathogens after appropriate cultures and specimens for laboratory evaluation have been obtained. Therapy should be narrowed to cover specific pathogens once the results of cultures are known.
- Appropriate empiric choices for the treatment of bacterial pneumonias relative to a patient's underlying disease are shown in Table 43–6 for adults and Table 43–7 for children. Dosages for antibiotics to treat pneumonia are provided in Table 43–8.
- Antibiotic concentrations in respiratory secretions in excess of the pathogen minimum inhibitory concentration (MIC) are necessary for successful treatment of pulmonary infections.
- The benefit of antibiotic aerosols or direct endotracheal instillation has not been consistently demonstrated.

EVALUATION OF THERAPEUTIC OUTCOMES

- With community-acquired pneumonia, time for resolution of cough, sputum production, and presence of constitutional symptoms (e.g., malaise, nausea or vomiting, and lethargy) should be assessed.

TABLE 43–6 Evidence-Based Empiric Antimicrobial Therapy for Pneumonia in Adults[a]

Clinical Setting	Usual Pathogens	Empiric Therapy
Outpatient/community acquired		
• Previously healthy	S. pneumoniae, M. pneumoniae, H. influenza, C. pneumoniae, M. catarrhalis	Macrolide/azalide[b], or tetracycline[c]
• Comorbidities (diabetes, heart/lung/liver/renal disease, alcohol'sm		Fluoroquinolone[d] or β-lactam + macrolide[b]
• Elderly	S. pneumoniae, Gram-negative bacilli	Piperacillin/tazobactam or cephalosporin[e] or carbapenem[f]
Inpatient/community acquired		
• Non-ICU	S. pneumoniae, H. influenza, M. pneumoniae, C. pneumoniae, Legionella sp.	Fluoroquinolone[d] or β-lactam + macrolide[b]
• ICU	S. pneumoniae, S. aureus, Legionella sp, gram-negative bacilli, H. influenza	β-lactam + macrolide[b] or fluoroquinolone[d] piperacillin/ taxobactam or meropenem or cefepime + fluoroquinolone[d], or β-lactam + AMG + azithromycin or β-lactam + AMG + respiratory fluoroquinolone[d]
	If MRSA suspected	Above + vancomycin or linezolid
Hospital acquired, ventilator associated, or healthcare associated		
• No risk factors for MDR pathogens	S. pneumoniae, H. influenzae, MSSA enteric Gram-negative bacilli	Ceftriaxone or fluoroquinolone[d] or ampicillin/ sulbactam or ertapenem or doripenem
• Risk factors for MDR pathogen	P. aeruginosa, K. pneumoniae (ESBL), Acinetobacter sp.	Antipseudomonal cephalosporin[e] or antipseudomonal carbapenem or β-lactam/β-lactamase + antipseudomonal fluoroquinolone[d] or AMG[g]
	If MRSA or Legionella sp. suspected	Above + vancomycin or linezolid

(continued)

TABLE 43–6 Evidence-Based Empiric Antimicrobial Therapy for Pneumonia in Adults[a] *(Continued)*

Clinical Setting	Usual Pathogens	Empiric Therapy
Hospital acquired, ventilator associated, or healthcare associated		
• Aspiration	Mouth anaerobes, *S. aureus*, enteric Gram-negative bacilli	Penicillin or clindamycin or piperacillin/tazobactum + AMG[g]
Atypical pneumonia[h]		
• *Legionella pneumophilia*		Fluoroquinolone[d] or doxycycline
• *Mycoplasma pneumonia*		Fluoroquinolone[d] or doxycycline
• *Chlamydophila pneumonia*		Fluoroquinolone[d] or doxycycline
• SARS		Fluoroquinolone[d] or macrolides[b]
• Avian Influenza		Oseltamivir
• H1N1 Influenza		Oseltamivir

MRSA, methicillin resistance staphylococcus aureus; AMG, aminoglycoside; SARS, severe acute respiratory syndrome; ESBL, extended-spectrum β-lactamases.

[a]See section on treatment of bacterial pneumonia

[b]Macrolide/azalide: erythromycin, clarithromycin, azithromycin

[c]Tetracycline: tetracycline, HCl, doxycycline

[d]Fluoroquinolone: ciprofloxacin, levofloxacin, moxifloxacin

[e]Antipseudomonal cephalosporin: cefepime, ceftazidime

[f]Antipseudomonal carbapenem: imipenem, meropenem

[g]Aminoglycoside: amikacin, gentamicin, tobramycin

[h]For tuberculosis, see Chap. 49.

Data from Mandell LA, Wunderink RG, Anzueto A, et al. *Infectious Diseases Society of America/American Thoracic Society consensus guidelines on the management of community-acquired pneumonia in adults. Clin Infect Dis 2007;44 (suppl 2):S27–S72; and Guidelines for the management of adults with hospital-acquired, ventilator- associated, and healthcare-associated pneumonia. Am J Respir Crit Care Med 2005;171:388–416.*

TABLE 43–7	Empirical Antimicrobial Therapy for Pneumonia in Pediatric Patients[a]	
Age	**Usual Pathogen(s)**	**Presumptive Therapy**
1 month	Group B *Streptococcus*, *Haemophilus influenzae* (nontypable), *Escherichia coli*, *Staphylococcus aureus*, Listeria, CMV, RSV, adenovirus	Ampicillin–sulbactam, cephalosporin,[b] carbapenem,[c] ribavirin for RSV
1–3 months	*C. pneumoniae*, possibly *Ureaplasma*, CMV, *Pneumocystis carinii* (afebrile pneumonia syndrome)	Macrolide–azalide,[d] trimethoprim–sulfamethoxazole
	RSV	Ribavirin
	Pneumococcus, S. aureus	Semisynthetic penicillin[e] or cephalosporin[f]
3 months–6 years	*S. pneumoniae, H. influenzae*, RSV, adenovirus, parainfluenza	Amoxicillin or cephalosporin,[f] ampicillin–sulbactam, amoxicillin–clavulanate, ribavirin for RSV
>6 years	*S. pneumoniae, Mycoplasma pneumoniae*, adenovirus	Macrolide–azalide,[d] cephalosporin,[f] amoxicillin–clavulanate

CMV, cytomegalovirus; RSV, respiratory syncytial virus.
[a]See section on treatment of bacterial pneumonia.
[b]Third-generation cephalosporin: ceftriaxone, cefotaxime, or cefepime. Note that cephalosporins are not active against *Listeria*.
[c]Carbapenem: imipenem–cilastatin or meropenem.
[d]Macrolide–azalide: erythromycin or clarithromycin–azithromycin.
[e]Semisynthetic penicillin: nafcillin or oxacillin.
[f]Second generation cephalosporin: cefuroxime or cefprozil.

TABLE 43–8	Antibiotic Doses for the Treatment of Bacterial Pneumonia		
		Daily Antibiotic Dose	
Antibiotic Class	**Antibiotic**	**Pediatric (mg/kg/day)**	**Adult (total dose/day)**
Macrolide	Clarithromycin	15	0.5–1 g
	Erythromycin	30–50	1–2 g
Azalide	Azithromycin	10 mg/kg for 1 day, then 5 mg/kg/day for 4 days	500 mg day 1, then 250 mg/day for 4 days
Tetracycline[a]	Doxycycline	2–5	100–200 mg
	Tetracycline HCl	25–50	1–2 g
Penicillin	Ampicillin	100–200	2–6 g
	Amoxicillin/ amoxicillin–clavulanate[b]	40–90	0.75–1 g

(continued)

519

TABLE 43–8 Antibiotic Doses for the Treatment of Bacterial Pneumonia *(Continued)*

Antibiotic Class	Antibiotic	Daily Antibiotic Dose	
		Pediatric (mg/kg/day)	*Adult (total dose/day)*
	Piperacillin-tazobactam	200–300	12 g
	Ampicillin-sulbactam	100–200	4–8 g
Extended-spectrum Cephalosporins	Ceftriaxone	50–75	1–2 g
	Ceftazidime	150	2–6 g
	Cefepime	100–150	2–4 g
Fluoroquinolones	Moxifloxacin		0.4 g
	Gemifloxacin	20–30	1.2 g
	Levofloxacin	10–15	0.5–0.75 g
	Ciprofloxacin	20–30	0.5–1.5 g
Aminoglycosides	Gentamicin	7.5	3–6 mg/kg
	Tobramycin	7.5	3–6 mg/kg
Carbapenems	Imipenem	60–100	2–4 g
	Meropenem	30–60	1–3 g
Other	Vancomycin	45–60	2–3 g
	Linezolid	20–30	1.2 g

Note: Doses may be increased for more severe disease and may require modification in patients with organ dysfunction.

*a*Tetracyclines are rarely used in pediatric patients, particularly in those younger than 8 years because of tetracycline-induced permanent tooth discoloration.

*b*Higher dose amoxicillin, amoxicillin–clavulanate (e.g., 90 mg/kg/day) is used for penicillin-resistant *Streptococcus pneumoniae*.

*c*Fluoroquinolones are avoided in pediatric patients because of the potential for cartilage damage; however, their use in pediatrics is emerging. Doses shown are extrapolated from adults and will require further study.

Progress should be noted in the first 2 days, with complete resolution in 5 to 7 days.

- With nosocomial pneumonia, the above parameters should be assessed along with white blood cell counts, chest radiograph, and blood gas determinations.

See Chapter 116, Lower Respiratory Tract Infections, authored by Martha G. Blackford, Mark L. Glover, and Michael D. Reed, for a more detailed discussion of this topic.

CHAPTER 44

Respiratory Tract Infections, Upper

OTITIS MEDIA

DEFINITION

- Otitis media is an inflammation of the middle ear. Acute otitis media involves the rapid onset of signs and symptoms of inflammation in the middle ear that manifests clinically as one or more of the following: otalgia (denoted by pulling of the ear in some infants), hearing loss, fever, and irritability. Otitis media with effusion (accumulation of liquid in the middle ear cavity) differs from acute otitis media in that signs and symptoms of an acute infection are absent.
- Otitis media is most common in infants and children. The risk factors for amoxicillin-resistant bacteria in acute otitis media include attendance at a child care center, recent receipt of antibiotic treatment (past 30 days), and age younger than 2 years.

PATHOPHYSIOLOGY

- Approximately 40% to 75% of acute otitis media cases are caused by viral pathogens. *Streptococcus pneumoniae* is the most common bacterial cause of acute otitis media (20–50%). Nontypable strains of *Haemophilus influenzae* and *Moraxella catarrhalis* are each responsible for 15% to 30% and 3% to 20% of cases, respectively.
- Acute bacterial otitis media usually follows a viral upper respiratory tract infection that causes eustachian tube dysfunction and mucosal swelling in the middle ear.
- Between 1% and 50% of *S. pneumoniae* isolates are not susceptible to penicillin, and up to half possess high-level penicillin resistance. Half of *H. influenzae* and 100% of *M. catarrhalis* isolates from the upper respiratory tract produce β-lactamases.

CLINICAL PRESENTATION

- Irritability and tugging on the ear are often the first clues that a child has acute otitis media.
- A diagnosis of acute otitis media requires that three criteria be met: acute onset of signs and symptoms, middle ear effusion, and middle ear inflammation. Middle ear effusion is indicated by any of the following: bulging of the tympanic membrane, limited or absent mobility of the tympanic membrane, air–fluid level behind the tympanic membrane, and otorrhea (Table 44–1).
- Resolution of acute otitis media occurs over 1 week. Pain and fever tend to resolve over 2 to 3 days, with most children becoming asymptomatic at 7 days. Effusions resolve slowly; 90% disappear by 3 months.

TABLE 44–1	Clinical Presentation of Acute Bacterial Otitis Media

General

The acute onset of signs and symptoms of middle ear infection following cold symptoms of runny nose, nasal congestion, or cough

Signs and symptoms

Pain that can be severe (>75% of patients)

Children may be irritable, tug on the involved ear, and have difficulty sleeping.

Fever is present in <25% of patients and, when present, is more often in younger children.

Examination shows a discolored, thickened, bulging eardrum.

Pneumatic otoscopy or tympanometry demonstrates an immobile eardrum; 50% of cases are bilateral.

Draining middle ear fluid occurs (<3% of patients) that usually reveals a bacterial etiology.

Laboratory tests

Gram stain, culture, and sensitivities of draining fluid or aspirated fluid if tympanocentesis is performed

TREATMENT

- The goals of treatment are pain management, prudent antibiotic use, and secondary disease prevention. Acute otitis media should first be differentiated from otitis media with effusion or chronic otitis media.

- Primary prevention of acute otitis media with vaccines should be considered. The seven-valent pneumococcal conjugate vaccine reduced the occurrence of acute otitis media by 6% to 7% during infancy. The vaccine did not benefit older children with a history of acute otitis media.

- Pain of otitis media should be addressed with oral analgesics. **Acetaminophen** or a nonsteroidal antiinflammatory agent, such as **ibuprofen**, should be offered early to relieve pain of acute otitis media. Decongestants or antihistamines should not be recommended for acute otitis media because they provide minimal benefit.

- A brief observation period should be considered to determine whether the patient requires immediate antibiotic therapy because of disease severity or patient characteristics.

- Antimicrobial therapy is used to treat otitis media; however, a high percentage of children will be cured with symptomatic treatment alone.

- Delayed antibiotic treatment (48–72 hours) may be considered in children 6 months to 2 years of age if symptoms are not severe and the diagnosis is uncertain, and in children 2 years of age or older with an uncertain diagnosis. Delayed treatment decreases antibiotic adverse effects and minimizes bacterial resistance.

- High-dose amoxicillin (80–90 mg/kg/day) is the drug of choice for acute otitis media. If β-lactamase-producing pathogens are suspected or known, amoxicillin should be given with **clavulanate** (90 mg/kg/day of amoxicillin with 6.4 mg/kg/day of clavulanate in two divided doses). Treatment recommendations for acute otitis media are found in Table 44–2.

TABLE 44–2	Acute Otitis Media Antibiotic Recommendations			
	Initial Diagnosis		**Failure at 48–72 Hours**	
	Nonsevere	**Severe**[a]	**Nonsevere**	**Severe**[a]
First line	Amoxicillin, high-dose; 80–90 mg/kg/ day divided twice daily	Amoxicillin-clavulanate, high-dose;[b] 90 mg/kg/day of amoxicillin plus 6.4 mg/kg/ day of clavulnate divided twice daily	Amoxicillin-clavulanate, high-dose;[b] 90 mg/kg/ day of amoxicillin plus 6.4 mg/kg/ day of clavulanate divided twice daily	Ceftriaxone (1–3 days)
Non–type 1 allergy	Cefdinir, cefuroxime, cefpodoxime	Ceftriaxone (1–3 days)	Ceftriaxone (1–3 days)	Clindamycin
Type 1 allergy	Azithromycin, clarithromycin		Clindamycin	Clindamycin

[a]Severe = temperature ≥39°C (102°F) and/or severe otalgia.
[b]Amoxicillin-clavulanate 90:6.4 or 14:1 ratio is available in the United States; 7:1 ratio is available in Canada (use amoxicillin 45 mg/kg for one dose, amoxicillin 45 mg/kg with clavulanate 6.4 mg/kg for second dose).
Adapted from McCaig LF, Nawar EW. National Hospital Ambulatory Medical Care Survey: 2004 emergency department summary. Adv Data 2006(372):1–29.

- If treatment failure occurs with amoxicillin, an agent should be chosen with activity against β-lactamase-producing *H. influenzae* and *M. catarrhalis*, as well as drug-resistant *S. pneumoniae*, such as high-dose amoxicillin–clavulanate (recommended) or cefuroxime, cefdinir, cefpodoxime, cefprozil, or intramuscular ceftriaxone.
- Five days of therapy may be used in acute otitis media.
- Surgical insertion of tympanostomy tubes (T tubes) is an effective method for the prevention of recurrent otitis media. Patients with acute otitis media should be reassessed after 3 days, with most children being asymptomatic at 7 days.

Antibiotic Prophylaxis of Recurrent Infections

- Recurrent otitis media is defined as at least three episodes in 6 months or at least four episodes in 12 months. Recurrent infections are of concern because patients younger than 3 years are at high risk for hearing loss and language and learning disabilities. Data from studies generally do not favor prophylaxis.

PHARYNGITIS

- Pharyngitis is an acute infection of the oropharynx or nasopharynx that results in 1% to 2% of all outpatient visits. Although viral causes are most common, group A β-hemolytic *Streptococcus* (GABHS), or *Streptococcus pyogenes*, is the primary bacterial cause.

TABLE 44–3	Clinical Presentation and Diagnosis of Group A Streptococcal Pharyngitis

General
A sore throat of sudden onset that is mostly self-limited
Fever and constitutional symptoms resolving in 3 to 5 days
Clinical signs and symptoms are similar for viral and nonstreptococcal bacterial causes.

Signs and symptoms
Sore throat
Pain on swallowing
Fever
Headache, nausea, vomiting, and abdominal pain (especially in children)
Erythema/inflammation of the tonsils and pharynx with or without patchy exudates
Enlarged, tender lymph nodes
Swollen red uvula, petechiae on the soft palate, and a scarlatiniform rash
Several symptoms that are not suggestive of group A *Streptococcus* are cough, conjunctivitis, coryza, and diarrhea.

Signs suggestive of viral origin for pharyngitis
Conjunctivitis, coryza, cough, and diarrhea

Laboratory tests
Throat swab and culture
Rapid antigen detection testing

- Viruses (e.g., rhinovirus, coronavirus, and adenovirus) cause most of the cases of acute pharyngitis. A bacterial etiology for acute pharyngitis is far less likely. Of all of the bacterial causes, GABHS is the most common (15–30% of cases in pediatric patients and 5–15% in adults).
- Nonsuppurative complications such as acute rheumatic fever, acute glomerulonephritis, and reactive arthritis may occur as a result of pharyngitis with GABHS.

CLINICAL PRESENTATION

- The most common symptom of pharyngitis is sore throat. The clinical presentation of group A streptococcal pharyngitis is presented in **Table 44–3**. Centor criteria are used to predict GABHS pharyngitis (**Table 44–4**).
- Guidelines from the Infectious Disease Society of America, American Academy of Pediatrics, and American Heart Association suggest that testing for group A *Streptococcus* be done in all patients with signs and symptoms. Only those with a positive test for group A *Streptococcus* require antibiotic treatment. Readers are referred to Chap. 117 of *Pharmacotherapy: A Pathophysiologic Approach* for a full discussion of laboratory testing for GABHS.

TREATMENT

- The goals of treatment of pharyngitis are to improve clinical signs and symptoms, minimize adverse drug reactions, prevent transmission to

TABLE 44–4 Modified Centor Criteria for Clinical Prediction of Group A β-Hemolytic Streptococcal Pharyngitis[a]

Criteria	Points
Temperature >38°C (101°F)	1
Absence of cough	1
Swollen, tender anterior cervical nodes	1
Tonsillar swelling or exudate	1
Age	
3–14 years	1
15–44 years	0
45 years or older	−1

Score	Risk of streptococcal infection
≤0	1%–2.5%
1	5%–10%
2	11%–17%
3	28%–35%
≥4	51%–53%

[a]The original Centor score applies to adults only. This modified version allows for age.

From McIsaac WJ, Kellner JD, Aufricht P, et al. Empirical validation of guidelines for the management of pharyngitis in children and adults. JAMA 2004;291(13):1587–1595.

close contacts, and prevent acute rheumatic fever and suppurative complications such as peritonsillar abscess, cervical lymphadenitis, and mastoiditis.

- Antimicrobial therapy should be limited to those who have clinical and epidemiologic features of GABHS pharyngitis, preferably with a positive laboratory test.
- Because pain is often the primary reason for visiting a physician, emphasis on analgesics such as **acetaminophen** and nonsteroidal antiinflammatory drugs (NSAIDs) to aid in pain relief is strongly recommended. However, acetaminophen is a better option because there is some concern that NSAIDs may increase the risk for necrotizing fasciitis or toxic shock syndrome.
- Antimicrobial treatment should be limited to those who have clinical and epidemiologic features of GABHS pharyngitis with a positive laboratory test. **Penicillin** is the drug of choice in the treatment of GABHS pharyngitis (Table 44–5). Table 44–6 presents dosing guidelines for recurrent infections. Table 44–7 presents evidence-based principles for diagnosis of group A *Streptococcus* pharyngitis.
- In patients allergic to penicillin, a macrolide such as **erythromycin** or a first-generation cephalosporin such as **cephalexin** (if the reaction is non-immunoglobulin E–mediated hypersensitivity) can be used. Newer macrolides such as azithromycin and clarithromycin are as effective as erythromycin and cause fewer adverse GI effects.
- If patients are unable to take oral medications, intramuscular **benzathine penicillin** can be given, although it is painful and no longer available in Canada.

TABLE 44-5 Dosing Guidelines for Pharyngitis

Medication	Adult Dosage	Pediatric Dosage	Duration	Rating
Preferred antibiotics				
Penicillin V	250 mg three or four times daily or 500 mg twice daily	50 mg/kg/day divided in three doses	10 days	IB
Penicillin benzathine	1.2 million units intramuscularly	0.6 million units for weight ≤27 kg (50,000 units/kg)	One dose	IB
Penicillin G procaine and benzathine mixture	Not recommended in adolescents and adults	1.2 million units (benzathine 0.9 million units, procaine 0.3 million units)	One dose	IB
Additional effective antibiotics				
Amoxicillin	500 mg three times daily	40-50 mg/kg/day divided in three doses	10 days	IB
Amoxicillin, extended release	775 mg daily	775 mg daily [b]	10 days	IIaB
Cephalexin[a]	250-500 mg orally four times daily	25-50 mg/kg/day divided in four doses	10 days	IB
Clindamycin[a]	20 mg/kg per day divided into 3 doses (maximum 1.8 g/day)		10 days	IIaB
Azithromycin[a]	12 mg/kg once daily (maximum 500 mg)		5 days	IIaB
Clarithromycin[a]	15 mg/kg per day divided in two doses (maximum 250 mg twice daily)		10 days	IIaB
Erythromycin[a]	Variable depending on formulation	Variable depending on formulation	10 days	IIaB

[a]To be prescribed as an alternative to penicillin in penicillin-allergic patients.
[b]Children ages 12 years and older.
Classification of recommendations:
  Class I: Conditions for which there is evidence and/or general agreement that a given procedure or treatment is beneficial, useful, and effective.
  Class II: Conditions for which there is conflicting evidence and/or a divergence of opinion about the usefulness/efficacy of a procedure or treatment.
  Class IIa: Weight of evidence/opinion is in favor of usefulness/efficacy.
  Class IIb: Usefulness/efficacy is less well established by evidence/opinion.
  Class III: Conditions for which there is evidence and/or general agreement that a procedure/treatment is not useful/effective and in some cases may be harmful.
Level of evidence:
  Level of evidence A: Data derived from multiple randomized clinical trials or meta-analyses.
  Level of evidence B: Data derived from a single randomized trial or nonrandomized studies.
  Level of evidence C: Only consensus opinion of experts, cases studies, or standard of care.

From Bisno AL, Gerber MA, Gwaltney JM, Jr., et al. Practice guidelines for the diagnosis and management of group A streptococcal pharyngitis: Infectious Diseases Society of America. Clin Infect Dis 2002;35(2):113–125; Bisno AL. Acute pharyngitis. N Engl J Med 2001;344(3):205–211; American Academy of Pediatrics. Group A streptococcal infections. In: Pickering LK, ed. Red Book 2003: Report of the Committee on Infectious Diseases. 26th ed. Elk Grove Village, IL: American Academy of Pediatrics; 2003:526–536; and Gerber MA, Baltimore RS, Eaton CB, et al. Prevention of rheumatic fever and diagnosis and treatment of acute streptococcal pharyngitis: A scientific statement from the American Heart Association Rheumatic Fever, Endocarditis, and Kawasaki Disease Committee of the Council on Cardiovascular Disease in the Young, the Interdisciplinary Council on Functional Genomics and Translational Biology, and the Interdisciplinary Council on Quality of Care and Outcomes Research; endorsed by the American Academy of Pediatrics. Circulation 2009;119(11):1541–1551.

TABLE 44–6	Antibiotics and Dosing for Recurrent Episodes of Pharyngitis	
Drug	**Adult Dosage**	**Pediatric Dosage**
Clindamycin	600 mg orally divided in two to four doses	20 mg/kg/day orally in three divided doses (maximum 1.8 g/day)
Amoxicillin-clavulanate	500 mg orally twice daily	40 mg/kg/day orally in three divided doses
Penicillin benzathine	1.2 million units intramuscularly for one dose	0.6 million units intramuscularly for weight <27 kg (50,000 units/kg)
Penicillin benzathine with rifampin	As above Rifampin 20 mg/kg/day orally in two divided doses during last 4 days of treatment with penicillin (maximum daily dose 600 mg)	As above Rifampin dose same as adults

From Bisno AL, Gerber MA, Gwaltney JM, Jr., et al. Practice guidelines for the diagnosis and management of group A streptococcal pharyngitis: Infectious Diseases Society of America. Clin Infect Dis 2002;35(2):113–125 by permission of Oxford University Press.

TABLE 44–7	Evidence-based Principles for Diagnosis of Group A *Streptococcus*	
Recommendations		**Level**
Selective use of diagnostic testing in only those with clinical features suggestive of group A *Streptococcus* will increase the proportion of positive tests, as well as results of those truly infected, not carriers.		A-II
Clinical diagnosis cannot be made with certainty even by the most experienced clinician; bacteriologic confirmation is required.		A-II
Throat culture remains the diagnostic standard, with a sensitivity of 90% to 95% for detection of group A *Streptococcus* if done correctly.		A-II
Rapid identification and treatment of patients with disease can reduce transmission, allow patients to return to work or school earlier, and reduce the acute morbidity of the disease.		A-II
The majority of rapid antigen detection tests available have a specificity >95% (minimizes overprescription to those without disease) and a sensitivity of 80% to 90% compared with culture.		A-II
Early initiation of antimicrobial therapy results in faster resolution of signs and symptoms. Delays in therapy (if awaiting cultures) can be made safely for up to 9 days after symptom onset and still prevent major complications such as rheumatic fever.		A-I

Rating:
   Strength of recommendation–A to E
   Evidence to support use: A, good; B, moderate; C, poor
   Evidence against use: D, moderate; E, good
   Quality of evidence–I, II, or III
      I: At least one randomized controlled trial
      II: At least one well-designed clinical trial, not randomized, or a cohort or case-controlled analytical study, or from multiple time series, or from dramatic results of an uncontrolled trial
      III: Opinions of respected authorities
Data from Bisno AL, Gerber MA, Gwaltney JM, et al. Practice guidelines for the diagnosis and management of group A streptococcal pharyngitis (IDSA guidelines). Clin Infect Dis 2002;35:113–125.

- The duration of therapy for group A streptococcal pharyngitis is 10 days to maximize bacterial eradication.

EVALUATION OF THERAPEUTIC OUTCOMES

- Most cases of pharyngitis are self-limited; however, antimicrobial therapy will hasten resolution when given early to proven cases of GABHS. Symptoms generally resolve by 3 or 4 days even without therapy. Follow-up testing is generally not necessary for index cases or in asymptomatic contacts of the index patient.

SINUSITIS

- Sinusitis is an inflammation and/or infection of the paranasal sinus mucosa. The term *rhinosinusitis* is used by some specialists, because sinusitis typically also involves the nasal mucosa. The majority of these infections are viral in origin. It is important to differentiate between viral and bacterial sinusitis to aid in optimizing treatment decisions.
- Acute bacterial sinusitis is most often caused by the same bacteria implicated in acute otitis media: *S. pneumoniae* and *H. influenzae*. These organ-

TABLE 44–8	Clinical Presentation and Diagnosis of Bacterial Sinusitis

General

A nonspecific upper respiratory tract infection that persists beyond 7 to 14 days

Signs and symptoms

Acute
> *Adults:*
>> Nasal discharge/congestion
>> Maxillary tooth pain, facial or sinus pain that may radiate (unilateral in particular), and deterioration after initial improvement
>> Severe or persistent (beyond 7 days) signs and symptoms are most likely bacterial and should be treated with antimicrobials.
>
> *Children:*
>> Nasal discharge and cough for more than 10 to 14 days or severe signs and symptoms such as temperature 39°C (102.2°F) or facial swelling or pain are indications for antimicrobial therapy.

Chronic
> Symptoms are similar to those of acute sinusitis but more nonspecific.
> Rhinorrhea is associated with acute exacerbations.
> Chronic unproductive cough, laryngitis, and headache may occur.
> Chronic/recurrent infections occur three or four times a year and are unresponsive to steam and decongestants.

Laboratory tests

Gram stain, culture, and sensitivities of draining fluid or aspirated fluid if sinus puncture is performed

TABLE 44–9	Acute Bacterial Sinusitis Antibiotic Recommendations[a,b]		
	Uncomplicated	**Treatment Failure or Prior Antibiotic Therapy in Past 4 to 6 Weeks**	**High Suspicion of Penicillin-resistant *Streptococcus pneumoniae***
First line	Amoxicillin	Amoxicillin-clavulanate (high-dose) or cephalosporin	Amoxicillin (high-dose) or clindamycin
Second line	–	Respiratory fluoroquinolone	Respiratory fluoroquinolone
Non–type 1 allergy	Cephalosporin	Cephalosporin	Clindamycin or respiratory fluoroquinolone
Type 1 allergy	Clarithromycin, azithromycin, trimethoprim-sulfamethoxazole, doxycycline, or a respiratory fluoroquinolone	Respiratory fluoroquinolone	Clindamycin or respiratory fluoroquinolone

[a]See Table 44–10 for dosing guidelines in children and adults.
[b]From Anon JB, Jacobs MR, Poole MD, et al. Antimicrobial treatment guidelines for acute bacterial rhinosinusitis. Otolaryngol Head Neck Surg 2004;130(1 Suppl):1–45; Subcommittee on Management of Sinusitis and Committee on Quality Improvement. Clinical practice guideline: Management of sinusitis. Pediatrics 2001;108(3):798–808; and Ip S, Fu L, Balk E, et al. Update on Acute Bacterial Rhinosinusitis: Evidence Report/Technology Assessment No. 124 (Prepared by Tufts-New England Medical Center Evidence-based Practice Center under Contract No. 290-02-0022). AHRQ Pub. No. 05-E020-2. Rockville, MD: Agency for Healthcare Research and Quality; 2005.

isms are responsible for ~70% of bacterial causes of acute sinusitis in both adults and children.

CLINICAL PRESENTATION

- The typical clinical presentation of bacterial sinusitis is presented in Table 44–8.

TREATMENT

- The goals of treatment of acute sinusitis are reducing signs and symptoms, achieving and maintaining patency of the ostia, limiting antimicrobial treatment to those who may benefit, eradicating bacterial infection with appropriate antimicrobial therapy, minimizing the duration of illness, preventing complications, and preventing progression from acute disease to chronic disease.
- Nasal decongestant sprays such as **phenylephrine** and **oxymetazoline** that reduce inflammation by vasoconstriction are often used in sinusitis. Use should be limited to the recommended duration of the product (no

TABLE 44–10	Dosing Guidelines for Acute Bacterial Sinusitis	
Medication	**Adult Dosage**	**Pediatric Dosage**
Amoxicillin	Low dose: 500 mg three times daily High dose: 2 g twice daily	Low dose: 45 mg/kg/day divided in three doses High dose: 90 mg/kg/day divided in two doses
Amoxicillin-clavulanate	Low dose: 500/125 mg three times daily High dose: 2 g/125 mg twice daily	Low dose: 45 mg/kg/day of amoxicillin and 3.2 mg/kg/day of clavulanate divided in three doses High dose: 90 mg/kg/day of amoxicillin and 6.4 mg/kg/day of clavulanate divided in two doses
Cefuroxime	250–500 mg twice daily	15 mg/kg/day divided in two doses
Cefaclor	250–500 mg three times daily	20 mg/kg/day divided in three doses
Cefixime	200–400 mg twice daily	8 mg/kg/day in one dose or divided in two doses
Cefdinir	600 mg daily or divided in two doses	14 mg/kg/day in one dose or divided in two doses
Cefpodoxime	200 mg twice daily	10 mg/kg/day in two divided doses (maximum 400 mg daily)
Cefprozil	250–500 mg twice daily	15–30 mg/kg/day divided in two doses
Doxycycline	100 mg every 12 hours	–
Trimethoprim-sulfamethoxazole	160/800 mg every 12 hours	6–8 mg/kg/day trimethoprim, 30–40 mg/kg/day sulfamethoxazole divided in two doses
Clindamycin	150–450 mg every 6 hours	30–40 mg/kg/day divided in three doses
Clarithromycin	250–500 mg twice daily	15 mg/kg/day divided in two doses
Azithromycin	500 mg day 1, then 250 mg/day × days 2–5	10 mg/kg day 1, then 5 mg/kg/day × days 2–5
Levofloxacin	500 mg daily	–

From Piccirillo JF. Clinical practice: Acute bacterial sinusitis. N Engl J Med 2004;351(9):902–910; Scheid DC, Hamm RM. Acute bacterial rhinosinusitis in adults: 2. Treatment. Am Fam Physician 2004;70(9):1697–1704; and Subcommittee on Management of Sinusitis and Committee on Quality Improvement. Clinical practice guideline: Management of sinusitis. Pediatrics 2001;108(3):798–808.

more than 3 days) to prevent rebound congestion. Oral decongestants may also aid in nasal or sinus patency. Irrigation of the nasal cavity with saline and steam inhalation may be used to increase mucosal moisture, and mucolytics (e.g., guaifenesin) may be used to decrease the viscosity of nasal secretions. Antihistamines should not be used for acute bacterial sinusitis in view of their anticholinergic effects that can dry mucosa and disturb clearance of mucosal secretions.

- Antimicrobial therapy is superior to placebo in reducing or eliminating symptoms, although the benefit is small.
- **Amoxicillin** is first-line treatment for acute bacterial sinusitis. It is cost effective in acute uncomplicated disease, and initial use of newer broad-spectrum agents is not justified. The approach to treating acute bacterial sinusitis is given in Table 44–9. Dosing guidelines are given in Table 44–10.
- The current recommendations are 10 to 14 days, or at least 7 days, of antimicrobial therapy after signs and symptoms are under control.

See Chapter 117, Upper Respiratory Tract Infections, authored by Christopher Frei, Bradi Frei, and George Zhanel, for a more detailed discussion of this topic.

Sepsis and Septic Shock

DEFINITION

- The definitions of terms related to sepsis are given in **Table 45–1**. Physiologically similar systemic inflammatory response syndrome can be seen even in the absence of identifiable infection.

PATHOPHYSIOLOGY

- The sites of infections that most frequently lead to sepsis are the respiratory tract (21–68%), urinary tract (14–18%), and intraabdominal space (14–22%). Sepsis may be caused by gram-negative (38% of sepsis) or gram-positive bacteria (40%), as well as by fungi (17%) or other microorganisms.

- *Escherichia coli* and *Pseudomonas aeruginosa* are the most commonly isolated gram-negative pathogens in sepsis. Other common gram-negative pathogens are *Klebsiella* spp., *Serratia* spp., *Enterobacter* spp., and *Proteus* spp. *P. aeruginosa* is the most frequent cause of sepsis fatality. Common gram-positive pathogens are *Staphylococcus aureus, Streptococcus pneumoniae,* coagulase-negative staphylococci, and *Enterococcus* species.

- *Candida* species (particularly *Candida albicans*) are a common cause of sepsis in hospitalized patients.

- The pathophysiologic focus of gram-negative sepsis has been on the lipopolysaccharide (endotoxin) component of the gram-negative cell wall. Lipid A is a part of the endotoxin molecule from the gram-negative bacterial cell wall that is highly immunoreactive and is responsible for most of the toxic effects. Endotoxin first associates with a protein called lipopolysaccharide-binding protein in plasma. This complex then engages a specific receptor (CD14) on the surface of the macrophage, which activates it and causes release of inflammatory mediators.

- Sepsis involves a complex interaction of proinflammatory (e.g., tumor necrosis factor-α [TNF-α]; interleukin [IL]-1, IL-6) and antiinflammatory mediators (e.g., IL-1 receptor antagonist, IL-4, and IL-10). IL-8, platelet-activating factor, and a variety of prostaglandins, leukotrienes, and thromboxane A_2 are also important.

- TNF-α is considered the primary mediator of sepsis. Concentrations are elevated early in the inflammatory response during sepsis, and there is a correlation with the severity of sepsis. TNF-α release leads to activation of other cytokines associated with cellular damage, and it stimulates release of arachidonic acid metabolites that contribute to endothelial cell damage. IL-6 is a more consistent predictor of sepsis, as it remains elevated for longer periods of time than does TNF-α.

- Antiinflammatory mediators including IL-1 receptor antagonist, IL-4, and IL-10 are also produced in sepsis and inhibit production of

TABLE 45-1	Definitions Related to Sepsis
Condition	**Definition**
Bacteremia (fungemia)	Presence of viable bacteria (fungi) in the bloodstream
Infection	Inflammatory response to invasion of normally sterile host tissue by the microorganisms
Systemic inflammatory response syndrome	Systemic inflammatory response to a variety of clinical insults that can be infection but can also be noninfectious etiology. The response is manifested by two or more of the following conditions: temperature >38°C (100.4°F) or <36°C (96.8°F); heart rate >90 beats/min; respiratory rate >20 breaths/min or $Paco_2$ <32 torr; WBC >12,000 cells/mm³, <4,000 cells/mm³, or >10% immature (band) forms.
Sepsis	Systemic inflammatory response syndrome secondary to infection
Severe sepsis	Sepsis associated with organ dysfunction, hypoperfusion, or hypotension. Hypoperfusion and perfusion abnormalities may include, but are not limited to, lactic acidosis, oliguria, or acute alteration in mental status.
Septic shock	Sepsis with hypotension, despite fluid resuscitation, along with the presence of perfusion abnormalities. Patients who are on inotropic or vasopressor agents may not be hypotensive at the time perfusion abnormalities are measured.
Multiple-organ dysfunction syndrome	Presence of altered organ function requiring intervention to maintain homeostasis
Compensatory antiinflammatory response syndrome	Compensatory physiologic response to systemic inflammatory response syndrome that is considered secondary to the actions of antiinflammatory cytokine mediators

$Paco_2$, partial pressure of carbon dioxide; WBC, white blood cell (count)

proinflammatory cytokines. The net effect can vary depending on the state of activation of the target cell, and the ability of the target cell to release can augment or inhibit the primary mediator. An excess of proinflammatory mediators can cause a systemic inflammatory response syndrome, followed by a compensatory antiinflammatory response syndrome.

- A primary mechanism of injury with sepsis is through endothelial cells. With inflammation, endothelial cells allow circulating cells (e.g., granulocytes) and plasma constituents to enter inflamed tissues, which may result in organ damage.
- Endotoxin activates complement, which then augments the inflammatory response through stimulation of leukocyte chemotaxis, phagocytosis and

lysosomal enzyme release, increased platelet adhesion and aggregation, and production of toxic superoxide radicals.

- Proinflammatory mechanisms in sepsis are also procoagulant and antifibrinolytic. Levels of activated protein C, a fibrinolytic and antiinflammatory substance, are decreased in sepsis.

- Shock is the most ominous complication associated with gram-negative sepsis and causes death in about one half of patients. Another complication is disseminated intravascular coagulation (DIC), which occurs in up to 50% of patients with gram-negative sepsis. DIC is the inappropriate activation of the clotting cascade that causes formation of microthrombi, resulting in consumption of coagulation factors, organ dysfunction, and bleeding. Acute respiratory distress syndrome (ARDS) is another common complication of sepsis.

- The hallmark of the hemodynamic effect of sepsis is the hyperdynamic state characterized by high cardiac output and an abnormally low systemic vascular resistance.

CLINICAL PRESENTATION

- The signs and symptoms of early sepsis are variable and include fever, chills, and a change in mental status with lethargy and malaise. Hypothermia may occur instead of fever. Tachypnea and tachycardia are also evident. White blood cell count is usually elevated, as may be blood sugar. The patient may be hypoxic. Signs and symptoms of early and late sepsis are found in **Table 45–2**.

TABLE 45–2 Signs and Symptoms Associated with Sepsis

Early Sepsis	Late Sepsis
Fever or hypothermia	Lactic acidosis
Rigors, chills	Oliguria
Tachycardia	Leukopenia
Tachypnea	DIC
Nausea, vomiting	Myocardial depression
Hyperglycemia	Pulmonary edema
Myalgias	Hypotension (shock)
Lethargy, malaise	Hypoglycemia
Proteinuria	Azotemia
Hypoxia	Thrombocytopenia
Leukocytosis	ARDS
Hyperbilirubinemia	GI hemorrhage
	Coma

ARDS, acute respiratory distress syndrome; DIC, disseminated intravascular coagulation.

- Progression of uncontrolled sepsis leads to evidence of organ dysfunction, which may include oliguria, hemodynamic instability with hypotension or shock, lactic acidosis, hyperglycemia or hypoglycemia, possibly leukopenia, DIC, thrombocytopenia, ARDS, GI hemorrhage, or coma.

TREATMENT

- The primary goals for treatment of sepsis are as follows:
  1. Timely diagnosis and identification of the pathogen
  2. Rapid elimination of the source of infection
  3. Early initiation of aggressive antimicrobial therapy
  4. Interruption of the pathogenic sequence leading to septic shock
  5. Avoidance of organ failure
- Mortality can be reduced by early placement and use of a central venous catheter, increased fluid volume administration, dobutamine therapy if needed, and red blood cell transfusion, to achieve specific physiologic goals in the first 6 hours. Evidence-based treatment recommendations for sepsis and septic shock from the *Surviving Sepsis* campaign are presented in Table 45–3.

ANTIMICROBIAL THERAPY

- Aggressive, early antimicrobial therapy is critical in the management of septic patients. The regimen selected should be based on the suspected site of infection, likely pathogens and the local antibiotic susceptibility patterns, whether the organism was acquired from the community or a hospital, and the patient's immune status.
- The antibiotics that may be used for empiric treatment of sepsis are listed in Table 45–4. In the nonneutropenic patient with urinary tract infection, fluoroquinolones are generally recommended.
- If *P. aeruginosa* is suspected, or with sepsis from hospital-acquired infections, an antipseudomonal cephalosporin (**ceftazidime** or **cefepime**), antipseudomonal fluoroquinolone (**ciprofloxacin** or **levofloxacin**), or an aminoglycoside should be included in the regimen.
- The antimicrobial regimen should be reassessed after 48 to 72 hours based on microbiologic and clinical data.
- **Vancomycin, daptomycin,** or **linezolid** should be added whenever the risk of methicillin resistant staphylococci is significant.
- The average duration of antimicrobial therapy in the normal host with sepsis is 7 to 10 days, and fungal infections can require 10 to 14 days.
- Suspected systemic mycotic infection leading to sepsis in neutropenic and critically ill patients should be empirically treated with parenteral **fluconazole, caspofungin, anidulafungin,** or **micafungin.** In neutropenic patients, a lipid formulation of **amphotericin B, caspofungin,** or **voriconazole** is recommended.

TABLE 45–3 Evidence-based Treatment Recommendations for Sepsis and Septic Shock

Recommendations	Recommendation Grades[a]
Initial resuscitation (first 6 hours)	
Early goal-directed goals, including CVP 8–12 mm Hg, MAP ≥ 65 mm Hg, central venous oxygen saturation ≥70%	1C
Antibiotic therapy	
IV broad-spectrum antibiotic within 1 hour of diagnosis of septic shock and severe sepsis against likely bacterial/fungal pathogens	1B
Reassess antibiotic therapy daily with microbiology and clinical data to narrow coverage	1C
Fluid therapy	
No clinical outcome difference between colloids and crystalloids	1B
Fluid challenges of 1000 mL of crystalloids or 300–500 mL of colloids over 30 minutes	1D
Vasopressors	
Norepinephrine and dopamine are the initial choices	1C
Maintain MAP ≥ 65 mm Hg	1C
Inotropic therapy	
Use dobutamine when cardiac output remains low despite fluid resuscitation and combined inotropic/vasopressor therapy	1C
Glucose control	
Use IV insulin to keep blood glucose ≤150 mg/dL	2C
Steroids	
IV hydrocortisone for septic shock when hypotension remains poorly responsive to adequate fluid resuscitation and vasopressors	2C
Hydrocortisone dose should be < 300 mg/day	1A
Recombinant human activated protein C (drotrecogin)	
Consider in sepsis-induced organ dysfunction with high risk of death (typically APACHE II ≥25 or multiple organ failure) in the absence of contraindications	2B
Deep vein thrombosis prophylaxis	
Use either low-molecular-weight heparin or low-dose unfractionated heparin in preventing deep vein thrombosis	1A
Stress ulcer prophylaxis	
H2 receptor blocker or proton pump inhibitor is effective	1A, 1B

CVP, central venous pressure; MAP, mean arterial pressure.

[a]Grades of Recommendation, Assessment, Development, and Evaluation (GRADE) system: a structured system for rating quality of evidence and grading strength of recommendation in clinical practice. Quality of evidence: high (grade A), moderate (grade B), low (grade C), or very low (grade D). Strength of recommendation: strong (grade 1) or weak (grade 2).

Adapted from Dellinger RP, Levy MM, Carlet JM, et al. Surviving sepsis campaign: International guidelines for management of severe sepsis and septic shock: 2008. Crit Care Med 2008;36:296–327.

TABLE 45–4 Empiric Antimicrobial Regimens in Sepsis		
	Antimicrobial Regimen	
Infection (Site or Type)	**Community-acquired**	**Hospital-acquired**
Urinary tract	ceftriaxone or ciprofloxacin/ levofloxacin	ciprofloxacin/ levofloxacin or ceftriaxone or ceftazidime
Respiratory tract	levofloxacin[a]/ moxifloxacin or ceftriaxone + clarithromycin/ azithromycin	piperacillin/tazobactam or ceftazidime or cefipime + levofloxacin/ ciprofloxacin or aminoglycoside
Intraabdominal	piperacillin/tazobactam or ciprofloxacin + metronidazole	piperacillin/ tazobactam or carbapenem[b]
Skin/soft tissue	vancomycin or linezolid or daptomycin	vancomycin + ampicillin/sulbactam or piperacillin/ tazobactam
Catheter-related		vancomycin
Unknown		piperacillin/ tazobactam or ceftazidime/ cefipime or imipenem/ meropenem +/– vancomycin not gentamicin.

[a]750 mg orally once daily.
[b]Imipenem, meropenem, doripenem.

HEMODYNAMIC SUPPORT

- Maintenance of adequate tissue oxygenation is important in the treatment of sepsis and is dependent on adequate perfusion and adequate oxygenation of the blood.
- Rapid fluid resuscitation is the best initial therapeutic intervention for treatment of hypotension in sepsis. The goal is to maximize cardiac output by increasing the left ventricular preload, which will ultimately restore tissue perfusion.
- Fluid administration should be titrated to clinical end points such as heart rate, urine output, blood pressure (BP), and mental status. Isotonic crystalloids, such as 0.9% sodium chloride or lactated Ringer solution, are commonly used for fluid resuscitation.

TABLE 45–5	Receptor Activity of Cardiovascular Agents Commonly Used in Septic Shock				
Agent	α_1	α_2	β_1	β_2	**Dopaminergic**
Dopamine	++/+++	?	++++	++	++++
Dobutamine	+	+	++++	++	0
Norepinephrine	+++	+++	+++	+/++	0
Phenylephrine	++/+++	+	?	0	0
Epinephrine	++++	++++	++++	+++	0

α_1, α_1-adrenergic receptor; α_2, α_2-adrenergic receptor; β_1, β_1-adrenergic receptor; β_2, β_2-adrenergic receptor; 0, no activity; ++++, maximal activity; ?, unknown activity.

- Iso-oncotic colloid solutions (plasma and plasma protein fractions), such as 5% albumin and 6% hetastarch, offer the advantage of more rapid restoration of intravascular volume with less volume infused, but there is no significant clinical outcome differences compared with crystalloids. Clinical outcome differences with the use of crystalloids or colloids have not been demonstrated, so crystalloids are generally recommended.

INOTROPE AND VASOACTIVE DRUG SUPPORT

- When fluid resuscitation is insufficient to maintain tissue perfusion, the use of inotropes and vasoactive drugs is necessary. Selection and dosage are based on the pharmacologic properties of various catecholamines and how they influence hemodynamic parameters (Table 45–5).

Suggested Protocol for the Use of Inotropes and Vasoactive Agents

- **Norepinephrine** is a potent α-adrenergic agent (0.01–3 mcg/kg/min) that is useful as a vasopressor to restore adequate BP after failure to restore adequate BP and organ perfusion with appropriate fluid resuscitation.
- **Dopamine** in doses >5 mcg/kg/min is used to support BP and to increase cardiac index (CI). Low-dose dopamine (1–5 mcg/kg/min) is not effective to increase renal and mesenteric perfusion.
- **Dobutamine** (2–20 mcg/kg/min) is an α-adrenergic inotropic agent that many clinicians prefer for improving cardiac output and oxygen delivery. Dobutamine should be considered in severely septic patients with adequate filling pressures and BP but low CI.
- **Epinephrine** (0.1–0.5 mcg/kg/min) increases CI and produces peripheral vasoconstriction. It is reserved for patients who fail to respond to traditional therapies.
- Before administering vasoactive agents, aggressive appropriate fluid resuscitation should occur. Vasoactive agents should not be considered an acceptable alternative to volume resuscitation.

- Administration of activated protein C (**drotrecogin**) to promote fibrinolysis and associated antiinflammatory mechanisms may be beneficial in patients with an **APACHE II** (Acute Physiology and Chronic Health Evaluation II) score >25. This agent reduced mortality in severe sepsis but poses an increased risk of serious bleeding.

See Chapter 128, Severe Sepsis and Septic Shock, authored by S. Lena Kang-Birken and Karla Killgore-Smith, for a more detailed discussion of this topic.

Sexually Transmitted Diseases

The spectrum of sexually transmitted diseases (STDs) includes the classic venereal diseases—gonorrhea, syphilis, chancroid, lymphogranuloma venereum, and granuloma inguinale—as well as a variety of other pathogens known to be spread by sexual contact (Table 46–1). Common clinical syndromes associated with STDs are listed in Table 46–2. The most current information on epidemiology, diagnosis, and treatment of STDs provided by the Centers for Disease Control and Prevention (CDC) can be found at http://www.cdc.gov.

GONORRHEA

- *Neisseria gonorrhoeae* is a gram-negative diplococcus estimated to cause up to 600,000 infections per year in the United States. Humans are the only known host of this intracellular parasite.

CLINICAL PRESENTATION

- Infected individuals may be symptomatic or asymptomatic, have complicated or uncomplicated infections, and have infections involving several anatomical sites.
- The most common clinical features of gonococcal infections are presented in Table 46–3. Approximately 15% of women with gonorrhea develop pelvic inflammatory disease. Left untreated, pelvic inflammatory disease can be an indirect cause of infertility and ectopic pregnancies.
- In 0.5% to 3% of patients with gonorrhea, the gonococci invade the bloodstream and produce disseminated disease. The usual clinical manifestations of disseminated gonococcal infection are tender necrotic skin lesions, tenosynovitis, and monoarticular arthritis.

DIAGNOSIS

- Diagnosis of gonococcal infections can be made by gram-stained smears, culture (the most reliable method), or newer methods based on the detection of cellular components of the gonococcus (e.g., enzymes, antigens, DNA, or lipopolysaccharide) in clinical specimens.
- Although culture of infected fluids is not the most sensitive of diagnostic tests for gonorrhea, it is still the diagnostic test of choice because of the high specificity.
- Alternative methods of diagnosis include enzyme immunoassay, DNA probes, and nucleic acid amplification techniques.

TREATMENT

- **Ceftriaxone** and **cefixime** are the only agents recommended for gonorrhea treatment. Fluoroquinolones are no longer considered a preferred treatment because of increasing resistance (Table 46–4).

TABLE 46–1	Sexually Transmitted Diseases
Disease	**Associated Pathogens**
Bacterial	
Gonorrhea	*Neisseria gonorrhoeae*
Syphilis	*Treponema pallidum*
Chancroid	*Haemophilus ducreyi*
Granuloma inguinale	*Calymmatobacterium granulomatis*
Enteric disease	*Salmonella* spp., *Shigella* spp., *Campylobacter fetus*
Campylobacter infection	*C. jejuni*
Bacterial vaginosis	*Gardnerella vaginalis, Mycoplasma hominis, Bacteroides* spp., *Mobiluncus* spp.
Group B streptococcal infections	Group B *Streptococcus*
Chlamydial	
Nongonococcal urethritis	*Chlamydia trachomatis*
Lymphogranuloma venereum	*C. trachomatis*, type L
Viral	
Acquired immunodeficiency syndrome	Human immunodeficiency virus
Herpes genitalis	Herpes simplex virus, types I and II
Viral hepatitis	Hepatitis A, B, C, and D viruses
Condylomata acuminata	Human papillomavirus
Molluscum contagiosum	Poxvirus
Cytomegalovirus infection	Cytomegalovirus
Mycoplasmal	
Nongonococcal urethritis	*Ureaplasma urealyticum*
Protozoal	
Trichomoniasis	*Trichomonas vaginalis*
Amebiasis	*Entamoeba histolytica*
Giardiasis	*Giardia lamblia*
Fungal	
Vaginal candidiasis	*Candida albicans*
Parasitic	
Scabies	*Sarcoptes scabiei*
Pediculosis pubis	*Phthirus pubis*
Enterobiasis	*Enterobius vermicularis*

- Coexisting chlamydial infection, which is documented in up to 50% of women and 20% of men with gonorrhea, constitutes the major cause of postgonococcal urethritis, cervicitis, and salpingitis in patients treated for gonorrhea. As a result, concomitant treatment with **doxycycline** or **azithromycin** is recommended in all patients treated for gonorrhea. A single dose of azithromycin (2 g) is highly effective against chlamydia.

TABLE 46–2 Selected Syndromes Associated with Common Sexually Transmitted Pathogens

Syndrome	Commonly Implicated Pathogens	Common Clinical Manifestations[a]
Urethritis	*Chlamydia trachomatis*, herpes simplex virus, *Neisseria gonorrhoeae*, *Trichomonas vaginalis*, *Ureaplasma urealyticum*	Urethral discharge, dysuria
Epididymitis	*C. trachomatis*, *N. gonorrhoeae*	Scrotal pain, inguinal pain, flank pain, urethral discharge
Cervicitis/vulvovaginitis	*C. trachomatis*, *Gardnerella vaginalis*, herpes simplex virus, human papillomavirus, *N. gonorrhoeae*, *T. vaginalis*	Abnormal vaginal discharge, vulvar itching/irritation, dysuria, dyspareunia
Genital ulcers (painful)	*Haemophilus ducreyi*, herpes simplex virus	Usually multiple vesicular/pustular (herpes) or papular/pustular (*H. ducreyi*) lesions that may coalesce; painful, tender lymphadenopathy[b]
Genital ulcers (painless)	*Treponema pallidum*	Usually single papular lesion
Genital/anal warts	Human papillomavirus	Multiple lesions ranging in size from small papular warts to large exophytic condylomas
Pharyngitis	*C. trachomatis* (?), herpes simplex virus, *N. gonorrhoeae*	Symptoms of acute pharyngitis, cervical lymphadenopathy, fever[c]
Proctitis	*C. trachomatis*, herpes simplex virus, *N. gonorrhoeae*, *T. pallidum*	Constipation, anorectal discomfort, tenesmus, mucopurulent rectal discharge
Salpingitis	*C. trachomatis*, *N. gonorrhoeae*	Lower abdominal pain, purulent cervical or vaginal discharge, adnexal swelling, fever[d]

[a]For some syndromes, clinical manifestations may be minimal or absent.
[b]Recurrent herpes infection may manifest as a single lesion.
[c]Most cases of pharyngeal gonococcal infection are asymptomatic.
[d]Salpingitis increases the risk of subsequent ectopic pregnancy and infertility.

TABLE 46–3 Presentation of Gonorrhea Infections

	Men	Women
General	Incubation period 1 to 14 days	Incubation period 1 to 14 days
	Symptom onset in 2 to 8 days	Symptom onset in 10 days
Site of infection	Most common—urethra	Most common—endocervical canal
	Others—rectum (usually due to rectal intercourse in men who have sex with men), oropharynx, eye	Others—urethra, rectum (usually due to perineal contamination), oropharynx, eye
Symptoms	May be asymptomatic or minimally symptomatic	May be asymptomatic or minimally symptomatic
	Urethral infection—dysuria and urinary frequency	Endocervical infection—usually asymptomatic or mildly symptomatic
	Anorectal infection—asymptomatic to severe rectal pain	Urethral infection—dysuria, urinary frequency
	Pharyngeal infection asymptomatic to mild pharyngitis	Anorectal and pharyngeal infection—symptoms same as for men
Signs	Purulent urethral or rectal discharge can be scant to profuse	Abnormal vaginal discharge or uterine bleeding; purulent urethral or rectal discharge can be scant to profuse
	Anorectal—pruritus, mucopurulent discharge, bleeding	
Complications	Rare (epididymitis, prostatitis, inguinal lymphadenopathy, urethral stricture)	Pelvic inflammatory disease and associated complications (i.e., ectopic pregnancy, infertility)
	Disseminated gonorrhea	Disseminated gonorrhea (three times more common than in men)

- Pregnant women infected with *N. gonorrhoeae* should be treated with either a **cephalosporin** or **spectinomycin**. **Azithromycin** or **amoxicillin** is the preferred treatment for presumed *Chlamydia trachomatis* infection.
- Treatment of gonorrhea during pregnancy is essential to prevent ophthalmia neonatorum. The CDC recommends that either **tetracycline** (1%) ophthalmic ointment or **erythromycin** (0.5%) ophthalmic ointment be instilled in each conjunctival sac immediately postpartum to prevent ophthalmia neonatorum.

TABLE 46–4 Treatment of Gonorrhea

Type of Infection	Recommended Regimens[a]	Alternative Regimens[b]
Uncomplicated infections of the cervix, urethra, and rectum in adults[c,d]	Ceftriaxone 125 mg IM once,[e] or cefixime 400 mg PO once (tablet or suspension) plus A treatment regimen for presumptive C. trachomatis coinfection if chlamydial infection has not been ruled out (see Table 46–8)	Spectinomycin 2 g IM once,[f] or ceftizoxime 500 mg IM once, or cefotaxime 500 mg IM once, or cefoxitin 2 g IM once with probenecid 1 g PO once plus A treatment regimen for presumptive C. trachomatis coinfection if chlamydial infection has not been ruled out (see Table 46–8)
Gonococcal infections in pregnancy	Ceftriaxone 125 mg IM once,[g,h] or cefixime 400 mg PO once (tablet or suspension) plus A recommended treatment regimen for presumptive C. trachomatis infection during pregnancy,[h] if chlamydial infection has not been ruled out (see Table 46–8)	Spectinomycin 2 g IM once,[f] or ceftizoxime 500 mg IM once, or cefotaxime 500 mg IM once, or cefoxitin 2 g IM once with probenecid 1 g PO once plus A recommended treatment regimen for presumptive C. trachomatis infection during pregnancy,[h] if chlamydial infection has not been ruled out (see Table 46–8)
Disseminated gonococcal infection in adults (>45 kg)[h,i,j,k]	Ceftriaxone 1 g IM or IV every 24 hours[k]	Cefotaxime 1 g IV every 8 hours[k] or ceftizoxime 1 g IV every 8 hours,[k] or spectinomycin 2 g IM every 12 hours[f,k]
Uncomplicated infections of the cervix, urethra, and rectum in children (<45 kg)	Ceftriaxone 125 mg IM once[l]	Spectinomycin 40 mg/kg IM once (not to exceed 2 g)[l]
Gonococcal conjunctivitis in adults	Ceftriaxone 1 g IM once[m]	

Ophthalmic neonatorum	Ceftriaxone 25–50 mg/kg IV or IM once (not to exceed 125 mg)
Infants born to mothers with gonococcal infection (prophylaxis)	Erythromycin (0.5%) ophthalmic ointment in a single application[n]; or Tetracycline (1%) ophthalmic ointment in a single application[o]

CDC, Centers for Disease Control and Prevention; C. trachomatis, Chlamydia trachomatis; PO, orally.

[a]Recommendations are those of the CDC.

[b]A number of other antimicrobials have demonstrated efficacy in treating uncomplicated gonorrhea but are not included in the CDC guidelines.

[c]Treatment failures are usually caused by reinfection and necessitate patient education and sex-partner referral; additional treatment regimens for gonorrhea and chlamydia infections should be administered. Epididymitis should be treated for 10 days (see Table 46–9).

[d]Patients allergic to β-lactams should receive a quinolone. Persons unable to tolerate a β-lactam (penicillin or cephalosporin) or a quinolone should receive spectinomycin.

[e]Also recommended for the treatment of uncomplicated infections of the pharynx in combination with a treatment regimen for presumptive C. trachomatis infection, if chlamydial infection has not been ruled out.

[f]Spectinomycin is currently not available in the United States (January 9, 2010).

[g]Another recommended IM or PO cephalosporin also can be used.

[h]Tetracyclines are contraindicated during pregnancy.

[i]Patients treated with one of the recommended regimens should be treated with doxycycline or azithromycin for possible coexistent chlamydial infection.

[j]Patients with gonococcal meningitis should be treated for 10 to 14 days and those with endocarditis for at least 4 weeks with ceftriaxone 1–2 g IV every 12 hours.

[k]All treatment regimens should be continued for 24–48 hours after improvement begins; at this time therapy can be switched to one of the following oral regimens to complete a 7-day course of treatment: cefixime 400 mg PO twice daily (tablet or suspension) or spectinomycin 2 g IM every 12 hours; fluoroquinolones may be an acceptable alternative if susceptibility can be documented by culture.

[l]Patients with bacteremia or arthritis should receive ceftriaxone 50 mg/kg (max. 1 g) IM or IV once daily for 7 days.

[m]A single lavage of the infected eye should be considered.

[n]Efficacy in preventing chlamydial ophthalmia is unclear.

[o]Tetracycline ophthalmic ointment (1%) is currently not available in the United States (January 9, 2010).

SYPHILIS

- The causative organism of syphilis is *Treponema pallidum,* a spirochete.
- Syphilis is usually acquired by sexual contact with infected mucous membranes or cutaneous lesions, although on rare occasions it can be acquired by nonsexual personal contact, accidental inoculation, or blood transfusion.

CLINICAL PRESENTATION

- The clinical presentation of syphilis is varied, with progression through multiple stages possible in untreated or inadequately treat patients (Table 46–5).

Primary Syphilis

- Primary syphilis is characterized by the appearance of a chancre on cutaneous or mucocutaneous tissue. Chancres persist only for 1 to 8 weeks before spontaneously disappearing.

TABLE 46–5	Presentation of Syphilis Infections
General	
Primary	Incubation period 10 to 90 days (mean 21 days)
Secondary	Develops 2 to 8 weeks after initial infection in untreated or inadequately treated individuals
Latent	Develops 4 to 10 weeks after secondary stage in untreated or inadequately treated individuals
Tertiary	Develops in ~30% of untreated or inadequately treated individuals 10 to 30 years after initial infection
Site of infection	
Primary	External genitalia, perianal region, mouth, and throat
Secondary	Multisystem involvement secondary to hematogenous and lymphatic spread
Latent	Potentially multisystem involvement (dormant)
Tertiary	CNS, heart, eyes, bones, and joints
Signs and symptoms	
Primary	Single, painless, indurated lesion (chancre) that erodes, ulcerates, and eventually heals (typical); regional lymphadenopathy is common; multiple, painful, purulent lesions possible but uncommon
Secondary	Pruritic or nonpruritic rash, mucocutaneous lesions, flu-like symptoms, lymphadenopathy
Latent	Asymptomatic
Tertiary	Cardiovascular syphilis (aortitis or aortic insufficiency), neurosyphilis (meningitis, general paresis, dementia, tabes dorsalis, eighth cranial nerve deafness, blindness), gummatous lesions involving any organ or tissue

Secondary Syphilis

- The secondary stage of syphilis is characterized by a variety of mucocutaneous eruptions, resulting from widespread hematogenous and lymphatic spread of *T. pallidum.*
- Signs and symptoms of secondary syphilis disappear in 4 to 10 weeks; however, in untreated patients, lesions may recur at any time within 4 years.

Latent Syphilis

- Persons with a positive serologic test for syphilis but with no other evidence of disease have latent syphilis.
- Most untreated patients with latent syphilis have no further sequelae; however, ~25% to 30% progress to either neurosyphilis or late syphilis with clinical manifestations other than neurosyphilis.

Tertiary Syphilis and Neurosyphilis

- Forty percent of patients with primary or secondary syphilis exhibit CNS infection.

DIAGNOSIS

- Because *T. pallidum* is difficult to culture in vitro, diagnosis is based primarily on dark-field or direct fluorescent antibody microscopic examination of serous material from a suspected syphilitic lesion or on results from serologic testing.
- Serologic tests are the mainstay in the diagnosis of syphilis and are categorized as nontreponemal or treponemal. Commonly used nontreponemal tests include the Venereal Disease Research Laboratory slide test, the rapid plasma reagin card test, the unheated serum reagin test, and the toluidine red unheated serum test.
- Treponemal tests are more sensitive than nontreponemal tests and are used to confirm the diagnosis (i.e., the fluorescent treponemal antibody absorption).

TREATMENT

- Treatment recommendations from the CDC for syphilis are presented in **Table 46–6.** Parenteral **penicillin G** is the treatment of choice for all stages of syphilis. Benzathine penicillin G is the only penicillin effective for single-dose therapy.
- Patients with abnormal cerebrospinal fluid findings should be treated as having neurosyphilis.
- For pregnant patients, penicillin is the treatment of choice at the dosage recommended for that particular stage of syphilis. To ensure treatment success and prevent transmission to the fetus, some experts advocate an additional intramuscular dose of benzathine penicillin G, 2.4 million units, 1 week after completion of the recommended regimen.
- The majority of patients treated for primary and secondary syphilis experience the Jarisch–Herxheimer reaction after treatment, characterized

TABLE 46–6	Drug Therapy and Follow-up of Syphilis	
Stage/Type of Syphilis	Recommended Regimens[a,b]	Follow-up Serology
Primary, secondary, or early latent syphilis (<1 year's duration)	Benzathine penicillin G 2.4 million units IM in a single dose[c]	Quantitative nontreponemal tests at 6 and 12 months for primary and secondary syphilis; at 6, 12, and 24 months for early latent syphilis[d]
Late latent syphilis (>1 year's duration) or latent syphilis of unknown duration	Benzathine penicillin G 2.4 million units IM once a week for 3 successive weeks (7.2 million units total)	Quantitative nontreponemal tests at 6, 12, and 24 months[e]
Neurosyphilis	Aqueous crystalline penicillin G 18–24 million units IV (3–4 million units every 4 hours or by continuous infusion) for 10–14 days[f] *or* Aqueous procaine penicillin G 2.4 million units IM daily plus probenecid 500 mg PO four times daily, both for 10–14 days[f]	CSF examination every 6 months until the cell count is normal; if it has not decreased at 6 months or is not normal by 2 years, retreatment should be considered
Congenital syphilis (infants with proven or highly probable disease)	Aqueous crystalline penicillin G 50,000 units/kg IV every 12 hours during the first 7 days of life and every 8 hours thereafter for a total of 10 days *or* Procaine penicillin G 50,000 units/kg IM daily for 10 days	Serologic follow-up only recommended if antimicrobials other than penicillin are used
Penicillin-allergic patients[g]		
Primary, secondary, or early latent syphilis	Doxycycline 100 mg PO 2 times daily for 14 days[a,h] *or* Tetracycline 500 mg PO 4 times daily for 14 days[h]	Same as for non–penicillin-allergic patients

(continued)

TABLE 46–6	Drug Therapy and Follow-up of Syphilis *(Continued)*	
Stage/Type of Syphilis	**Recommended Regimens**[a,b]	**Follow-up Serology**
Late latent syphilis (>1 year's duration) or syphilis of unknown duration	Ceftriaxone 1 g IM or IV daily for 8–10 days Doxycycline 100 mg PO twice a day for 28 days[h,i] *or* Tetracycline 500 mg PO 4 times daily for 28 days[h,i]	Same as for non–penicillin-allergic patients

CDC, Centers for Disease Control and Prevention; CSF, cerebrospinal fluid; PO, orally.

[a]Recommendations are those of the CDC.

[b]The CDC recommends that all patients diagnosed with syphilis be tested for HIV infection.

[c]Some experts recommend multiple doses of benzathine penicillin G or other supplemental antibiotics in addition to benzathine penicillin G in HIV-infected patients with primary or secondary syphilis; HIV-infected patients with early latent syphilis should be treated with the recommended regimen for latent syphilis of more than 1 year's duration.

[d]More frequent follow-up (i.e., 3, 6, 9, 12, and 24 months) recommended for HIV-infected patients.

[e]More frequent follow-up (i.e., 6, 12, 18, and 24 months) recommended for HIV-infected patients.

[f]Some experts administer benzathine penicillin G 2.4 million units IM once per week for up to 3 weeks after completion of the neurosyphilis regimens to provide a total duration of therapy comparable to that used for late syphilis in the absence of neurosyphilis.

[g]For nonpregnant patients; pregnant patients should be treated with penicillin after desensitization.

[h]Pregnant patients allergic to penicillin should be desensitized and treated with penicillin.

[i]Limited data suggest that ceftriaxone my be effective, although the optimal dosage and treatment duration are unclear.

by flu-like symptoms such as transient headache, fever, chills, malaise, arthralgia, myalgia, tachypnea, peripheral vasodilation, and aggravation of syphilitic lesions.

- The Jarisch–Herxheimer reaction should not be confused with penicillin allergy. Most reactions can be managed symptomatically with analgesics, antipyretics, and rest.
- CDC recommendations for serologic follow-up of patients treated for syphilis are given in **Table 46–6**. Quantitative nontreponemal tests should be performed at 6 and 12 months in all patients treated for primary and secondary syphilis and at 6, 12, and 24 months for early and late latent disease.
- For women treated during pregnancy, monthly, quantitative, nontreponemal tests are recommended in those at high risk of reinfection.

CHLAMYDIA

- Infections caused by *C. trachomatis* are believed to be the most common STD in the United States that has more than doubled in the past 10 years. *C. trachomatis* is an obligate intracellular parasite that has some similarities to viruses and bacteria.

TABLE 46-7	Presentation of *Chlamydia* Infections	
	Men	**Women**
General	Incubation period–35 days Symptom onset–7 to 21 days	Incubation period–7 to 35 days Usual symptom onset–7 to 21 days
Site of infection	Most common–urethra Others–rectum (receptive anal intercourse), oropharynx, eye	Most common–endocervical canal Others–urethra, rectum (usually due to perineal contamination), oropharynx, eye
Symptoms	More than 50% of urethral and rectal infections are asymptomatic Urethral infection–mild dysuria, discharge Pharyngeal infection–asymptomatic to mild pharyngitis	More than 66% of cervical infections are asymptomatic Urethral infection–usually subclinical; dysuria and frequency uncommon Rectal and pharyngeal infection–symptoms same as for men
Signs	Scant to profuse, mucoid to purulent urethral or rectal discharge Rectal infection–pain, discharge, bleeding	Abnormal vaginal discharge or uterine bleeding; purulent urethral or rectal discharge can be scant to profuse
Complications	Epididymitis, Reiter's syndrome (rare)	Pelvic inflammatory disease and associated complications (i.e., ectopic pregnancy, infertility) Reiter's syndrome (rare)

CLINICAL PRESENTATION

- In comparison with gonorrhea, chlamydial genital infections are more frequently asymptomatic, and when present, symptoms tend to be less noticeable. Table 46-7 summarizes the usual clinical presentation of chlamydial infections.
- Similar to gonorrhea, chlamydia may be transmitted to an infant during contact with infected cervicovaginal secretions. Nearly two thirds of infants acquire chlamydial infection after endocervical exposure, with the primary morbidity associated with seeding of the infant's eyes, nasopharynx, rectum, or vagina.

DIAGNOSIS

- Culture of endocervical or urethral epithelial cell scrapings is the most specific method (close to 100%) for detection of chlamydia, but sensitivity is as low as 70%. Between 3 and 7 days are required for results.
- Tests that allow rapid identification of chlamydial antigens and nucleic acid provide more rapid results, are technically less demanding, are less costly, and in some situations have greater sensitivity than culture.

TABLE 46–8	Treatment of Chlamydial Infections	
Infection	**Recommended Regimens***a*	**Alternative Regimen**
Uncomplicated urethral, endocervical, or rectal infection in adults	Azithromycin 1 g orally once *or* doxycycline 100 mg orally twice daily for 7 days	Ofloxacin 300 mg orally twice daily for 7 days, *or* levofloxacin 500 mg orally once daily for 7 days, *or* erythromycin base 500 mg orally four times daily for 7 days, *or* erythromycin ethyl succinate 800 mg orally four times daily for 7 days
Urogenital infections during pregnancy	Azithromycin 1 g orally as a single dose *or* amoxicillin 500 mg orally three times daily for 7 days	Erythromycin base 500 mg orally four times daily for 7 days, *or* erythromycin base 250 mg orally four times daily for 14 days, *or* erythromycin ethyl succinate 800 mg orally four times daily for 7 days (*or* 400 mg orally four times daily for 14 days)
Conjunctivitis of the newborn or pneumonia in infants	Erythromycin base 50 mg/kg/day orally in four divided doses for 14 days*b*	–

*a*Recommendations are those of the Centers for Disease Control and Prevention.
*b*Topical therapy alone is inadequate and is unnecessary when systemic therapy is administered.

TREATMENT

- Recommended regimens for treatment of chlamydial infections are given in Table 46–8. Single-dose **azithromycin** and 7-day **doxycycline** are the agents of choice.
- Treatment of chlamydial infections with the recommended regimens is highly effective; therefore, posttreatment cultures are not routinely recommended.
- Infants with pneumonitis should receive follow-up testing because erythromycin is only 80% effective.

GENITAL HERPES

- The term *herpes* is used to describe two distinct but antigenically related serotypes of herpes simplex virus (HSV). HSV type 1 (HSV-1) is most commonly associated with oropharyngeal disease; type 2 (HSV-2) is most closely associated with genital disease.

CLINICAL PRESENTATION

- A summary of the clinical presentation of genital herpes is provided in Table 46–9.
- A presumptive diagnosis of genital herpes commonly is made on the basis of the presence of dark-field-negative, vesicular, or ulcerative genital

TABLE 46–9 | Presentation of Genital Herpes Infections

General	Incubation period 2 to 14 days (mean 4 days)
	Can be caused by either HSV-1 or HSV-2

Classification of infection

First-episode primary	Initial genital infection in individuals lacking antibody to either HSV-1 or HSV-2
First-episode nonprimary	Initial genital infection in individuals with clinical or serologic evidence of prior HSV (usually HSV-1) infection
Recurrent	Appearance of genital lesions at some time following healing of first-episode infection

Signs and symptoms

First-episode infections	Most primary infections are asymptomatic or minimally symptomatic
	Multiple painful pustular or ulcerative lesions on external genitalia developing over a period of 7 to 10 days; lesions heal in 2 to 4 weeks (mean, 21 days)
	Flu-like symptoms (e.g., fever, headache, malaise) during first few days after appearance of lesions
	Others—local itching, pain, or discomfort; vaginal or urethral discharge, tender inguinal adenopathy, paresthesias, urinary retention
	Severity of symptoms greater in women than in men
	Symptoms are less severe (e.g., fewer lesions, more rapid lesion healing, fewer or milder systemic symptoms) with nonprimary infections
	Symptoms more severe and prolonged in the immunocompromised
	On average, viral shedding lasts ~11 or 12 days for primary infections and 7 days for nonprimary infections
Recurrent	Prodrome seen in ~50% of patients prior to appearance of recurrent lesions; mild burning, itching, and tingling are typical prodromal symptoms
	Compared with primary infections, recurrent infections associated with (1) fewer lesions that are more localized, (2) shorter duration of active infection (lesions heal within 7 days), and (3) milder symptoms
	Severity of symptoms greater in women than in men
	Symptoms more severe and prolonged in the immunocompromised
	On average, viral shedding lasts ~4 days
	Asymptomatic viral shedding is more frequent during the first year after infection with HSV

(continued)

TABLE 46–9	Presentation of Genital Herpes Infections *(Continued)*
Therapeutic implications of HSV-1 versus HSV-2 genital infection	Primary infections due to HSV-1 and HSV-2 virtually indistinguishable Recurrence rate is greater after primary infection with HSV-1 Recurrent infections with HSV-2 tend to be more severe
Complications	Secondary infection of lesions; extragenital infection due to autoinoculation; disseminated infection (primarily in immunocompromised patients); meningitis or encephalitis; neonatal transmission

HSV, herpes simplex virus.

lesions. A history of similar lesions or recent sexual contact with an individual with similar lesions also is useful in making the diagnosis.
- Tissue culture is the most specific (100%) and sensitive method (80–90%) of confirming the diagnosis of first-episode genital herpes.

TREATMENT

- The goals of therapy in genital herpes infection are to shorten the clinical course, prevent complications, prevent the development of latency and/or subsequent recurrences, decrease disease transmission, and eliminate established latency.
- Palliative and supportive measures are the cornerstone of therapy for patients with genital herpes. Pain and discomfort usually respond to warm saline baths or the use of analgesics, antipyretics, or antipruritics.
- Specific treatment recommendations are given in **Table 46–10**.
- Oral acyclovir, valacyclovir, and famciclovir are the treatments of choice for outpatients with first-episode genital herpes. Treatment does not prevent latency or alter the subsequent frequency and severity of recurrences.
- Continuous oral antiviral therapy reduces the frequency and the severity of recurrences in 70% to 80% of patients experiencing frequent recurrences.
- Acyclovir, valacyclovir, and famciclovir have been used to prevent reactivation of infection in patients seropositive for HSV who undergo transplantation procedures or induction chemotherapy for acute leukemia.
- The safety of **acyclovir** therapy during pregnancy is not established, although there is no evidence of teratogenic effects in humans.

TRICHOMONIASIS

- Trichomoniasis is caused by *Trichomonas vaginalis,* a flagellated, motile protozoan that is responsible for 3 million to 5 million cases per year in the United States.
- Coinfection with other STDs (e.g., gonorrhea) is common in patients diagnosed with trichomoniasis.

TABLE 46–10	Treatment of Genital Herpes	
Type of Infection	**Recommended Regimens**[a,b]	**Alternative Regimen**
First clinical episode of genital herpes[c]	Acyclovir 400 mg po three times daily for 7 to 10 days,[d] *or* Acyclovir 200 mg po five times daily for 7 to 10 days,[d] *or* Famciclovir 250 mg po three times daily for 7 to 10 days,[d] *or* Valacyclovir 1 g po twice daily for 7 to 10 days[d]	Acyclovir 5–10 mg/kg IV every 8 hours for 2 to 7 days or until clinical improvement occurs, followed by oral therapy to complete at least 10 days of total therapy[e]
Recurrent infection		
Episodic therapy	Acyclovir 400 mg po three times daily for 5 days,[f] *or* Acyclovir 800 mg po twice daily for 5 days,[f] *or* Acyclovir 800 mg po three times daily for 2 days,[f] *or* Famciclovir 125 mg po twice daily for 5 days,[f] *or* Valacyclovir 500 mg po twice daily for 3 to 5 days,[f] *or* Valacyclovir 1 g po once daily for 1 day	
Suppressive therapy	Acyclovir 400 mg po twice daily, *or* Famciclovir 250 mg po twice daily, *or* Valacyclovir 500 mg or 1,000 mg po once daily[g]	

CDC, Centers for Disease Control and Prevention; HIV, human immunodeficiency virus.
[a]Recommendations are those of the CDC.
[b]HIV-infected patients can require more aggressive therapy.
[c]Primary or nonprimary first episode.
[d]Treatment duration can be extended if healing is incomplete after 10 days.
[e]Only for patients with severe symptoms or complications that necessitate hospitalization.
[f]Requires initiation of therapy within 24 hours of lesion onset or during the prodrome that precedes some outbreaks.
[g]Valacyclovir 500 mg appears less effective than valacyclovir 1,000 mg in patients with ~10 recurrences per year.

CLINICAL PRESENTATION

- The typical presentation of trichomoniasis in men and women is presented in **Table 46–11**.
- *T. vaginalis* produces nonspecific symptoms also consistent with bacterial vaginosis; thus, laboratory diagnosis is required.
- The simplest and most reliable means of diagnosis is a wet-mount examination of the vaginal discharge. Trichomoniasis is confirmed if characteristic pear-shaped, flagellating organisms are observed. Newer

TABLE 46–11 Presentation of *Trichomonas* Infections

	Men	Women
General	Incubation period 3 to 28 days	Incubation period 3 to 28 days
	Organism may be detectable within 48 hours after exposure to infected partner	
Site of infection	Most common—urethra	Most common—endocervical canal
	Others—rectum (usually due to rectal intercourse in men who have sex with men), oropharynx, eye	Others—urethra, rectum (usually due to perineal contamination), oropharynx, eye
Symptoms	May be asymptomatic (more common in men than women) or minimally symptomatic	May be asymptomatic or minimally symptomatic
	Urethral discharge (clear to mucopurulent)	Scant to copious, typically malodorous vaginal discharge (50–75%) and pruritus (worsen during menses)
	Dysuria, pruritus	Dysuria, dyspareunia
Signs	Urethral discharge	Vaginal discharge
		Vaginal pH 4.5–6
		Inflammation/erythema of vulva, vagina, and/or cervix
		Urethritis
Complications	Epididymitis and chronic prostatitis (uncommon)	Pelvic inflammatory disease and associated complications (i.e., ectopic pregnancy, infertility)
	Male infertility (decreased sperm motility and viability)	Premature labor, premature rupture of membranes, and low-birth-weight infants (risk of neonatal infections is low)
		Cervical neoplasia

diagnostic tests such as monoclonal antibody or DNA probe techniques, as well as polymerase chain reaction tests, are highly sensitive and specific.

TREATMENT

- **Metronidazole** and **tinidazole** are the only antimicrobial agents available in the United States that are consistently effective in *T. vaginalis* infections.
- Treatment recommendations for *Trichomonas* infections are given in **Table 46–12**.
- GI complaints (e.g., anorexia, nausea, vomiting, and diarrhea) are the most common adverse effects with the single 2 g dose of metronidazole

TABLE 46–12 Treatment of Trichomoniasis

Type	Recommended Regimen[a]	Alternative Regimen
Symptomatic and asymptomatic infections	Metronidazole 2 g po in a single dose[b] or Tinidazole 2 g po in a single dose	Metronidazole 500 mg po two times daily for 7 days[c] or Tinidazole 2 g po in a single dose[d]
Treatment in pregnancy	Metronidazole 2 g po in a single dose[e]	

CDC, Centers for Disease Control and Prevention.

[a]Recommendations are those of the CDC.

[b]Treatment failures should be treated with metronidazole 500 mg po twice daily for 7 days. Persistent failures should be managed in consultation with an expert. Metronidazole or tinidazole 2 g po daily for 5 days has been effective in patients infected with *Trichomonas vaginalis* strains mildly resistant to metronidazole, but experience is limited; higher doses also have been used.

[c]Metronidazole labeling approved by the FDA does not include this regimen. Dosage regimens for treatment of trichomoniasis included in the product labeling are the single 2 g dose, 250 mg three times daily for 7 days, and 375 mg twice daily for 7 days. The 250 mg and 375 mg dosage regimens are currently not included in the CDC recommendations.

[d]For treatment failures with metronidazole 2 g as a single dose.

[e]Metronidazole is pregnancy category B, and tinidazole is pregnancy category C; both drugs are contraindicated in the first trimester of pregnancy. Some clinicians recommend deferring metronidazole treatment in asymptomatic pregnant women until after 37 weeks' gestation.

or tinidazole, occurring in 5% to 10% of treated patients. Some patients complain of a bitter, metallic taste in the mouth.

- Patients intolerant of the single 2 g dose because of GI adverse effects usually tolerate the multidose regimen.
- To achieve maximal cure rates and prevent relapse with the single 2 g dose of metronidazole, simultaneous treatment of infected sexual partners is necessary.
- Patients who fail to respond to an initial course usually respond to a second course of metronidazole or tinidazole therapy.
- Patients taking metronidazole should be instructed to avoid alcohol ingestion during therapy and for 1 or 2 days after completion of therapy because of a possible disulfiram-like effect.
- At present, no satisfactory treatment is available for pregnant women with *Trichomonas* infections. Metronidazole and tinidazole are contraindicated during the first trimester of pregnancy.
- Follow-up is considered unnecessary in patients who become asymptomatic after treatment with metronidazole.
- When patients remain symptomatic, it is important to determine if reinfection has occurred. In these cases, a repeat course of therapy, as well as identification and treatment or retreatment of infected sexual partners, is recommended.

TABLE 46–13 Treatment Regimens for Miscellaneous Sexually Transmitted Diseases

Infection	Recommended Regimen[a]	Alternative Regimen
Chancroid (*Haemophilus ducreyi*)	Azithromycin 1 g orally in a single dose *or* Ceftriaxone 250 mg intramuscularly in a single dose *or* Ciprofloxacin 500 mg orally twice daily for 3 days[b] *or* Erythromycin base 500 mg orally four times daily for 7 days	—
Lymphogranuloma venereum	Doxycycline 100 mg orally twice daily for 21 days[c]	Erythromycin base 500 mg orally four times daily for 7 days
Human papillomavirus infection	*Provider-administered therapies:*	
External genital warts	Cryotherapy (e.g., liquid nitrogen or cryoprobe) *or* Podophyllin resin10–25% in compound tincture of benzoin applied to lesions; repeat weekly if necessary,[d,e] *or* Trichloroacetic acid 80–90% or bichloracetic acid 80–90% applied to warts; repeat weekly if necessary *or* Surgical removal (tangential scissor excision, tangential shave excision, curettage, or electrosurgery) *Patient-applied therapies:* Podofilox 0.5% solution or gel applied twice daily for 3 days, followed by 4 days of no therapy; cycle is repeated as necessary for a total of four cycles[e] *or* Imiquimod 5% cream applied at bedtime three times weekly for up to 16 weeks[e]	Intralesional interferon or laser surgery

(continued)

TABLE 46–13	Treatment Regimens for Miscellaneous Sexually Transmitted Diseases *(Continued)*	
Infection	**Recommended Regimen**^{a}	**Alternative Regimen**
Vaginal, urethral meatus, and anal warts	Cryotherapy with liquid nitrogen, or trichloroacetic acid or bichloracetic acid 80–90% as for external human papillomavirus warts; repeat weekly as necessary^f Surgical removal (not for vaginal or urethral meatus warts)	–
Urethral meatus warts	Cryotherapy with liquid nitrogen, or podophyllin resin 10–25% in compound tincture of benzoin applied at weekly intervals^{e,g}	–

^{a}Recommendations are those of the Centers for Disease Control and Prevention.
^{b}Ciprofloxacin is contraindicated for pregnant and lactating women and for persons age <18 years.
^{c}Azithromycin 1 g orally once weekly for 3 weeks can be effective.
^{d}Some experts recommended washing podophyllin off after 1 to 4 hours to minimize local irritation.
^{e}Safety during pregnancy is not established.
^{f}Surgical removal of anal warts is also a recommended treatment.
^{g}Some specialists recommend the use of podofilox and imiquimod for treating distal meatal warts.

OTHER SEXUALLY TRANSMITTED DISEASES

- Several STDs other than those previously discussed occur with varying frequency in the United States and throughout the world. Although an in-depth discussion of these diseases is beyond the scope of this chapter, recommended treatment regimens are given in **Table 46–13**.

See Chapter 126, Sexually Transmitted Diseases, authored by Leroy C. Knodel, for a more detailed discussion of this topic.

CHAPTER 47

Skin and Soft-Tissue Infections

DEFINITION

- Bacterial infections of the skin can be classified as primary or secondary (Table 47–1). Primary bacterial infections are usually caused by a single bacterial species and involve areas of generally healthy skin (e.g., impetigo and erysipelas). Secondary infections, however, develop in areas of previously damaged skin and are frequently polymicrobic.
- The conditions that may predispose a patient to the development of skin and soft-tissue infections (SSTIs) include (1) a high concentration of bacteria; (2) excessive moisture of the skin; (3) inadequate blood supply; (4) availability of bacterial nutrients; and (5) damage to the corneal layer, allowing for bacterial penetration.
- The majority of SSTIs are caused by gram-positive organisms and, less commonly, gram-negative bacteria present on the skin surface. *Staphylococcus aureus* and *Streptococcus pyogenes* account for the majority of SSTIs. Community-associated methicillin-resistant *S. aureus* (CA-MRSA) has recently emerged and is often isolated in otherwise healthy patients.

ERYSIPELAS

- Erysipelas (Saint Anthony's fire) is an infection of the superficial layers of the skin and cutaneous lymphatics. The infection is almost always caused by β-hemolytic streptococci, with *S. pyogenes* (group A streptococci) responsible for most infections.
- The lower extremities are the most common sites for erysipelas. Patients often experience flu-like symptoms (fever and malaise) prior to the appearance of the lesions. The infected area is painful, often a burning pain. Erysipelas lesions are bright red and edematous with lymphatic streaking and clearly demarcated raised margins. Leukocytosis is common, and C-reactive protein is generally elevated.
- Mild to moderate cases of erysipelas in adults are treated with intramuscular **procaine penicillin G** or **penicillin VK**. For more serious infections, aqueous penicillin G, 2 million to 8 million units daily, should be administered IV. Penicillin-allergic patients can be treated with clindamycin or erythromycin.
- Evidence-based recommendations for treatment of SSTIs are found in Table 47–2, and recommended drugs and dosing regimens for outpatient treatment of mild to moderate SSTIs are found in Table 47–3.

IMPETIGO

- Impetigo is a superficial skin infection that is seen most commonly in children. It is highly communicable and spreads through close contact. Most cases are caused by *S. pyogenes*, but *S. aureus* either alone

TABLE 47–1	Bacterial Classification of Important Skin and Soft-Tissue Infections
Primary infections	
Erysipelas	Group A streptococci
Impetigo	*Staphylococcus aureus,* group A streptococci
Lymphangitis	Group A streptococci; occasionally *S. aureus*
Cellulitis	Group A streptococci, *S. aureus*; occasionally other gram-positive cocci, gram-negative bacilli, and/or anaerobes
Necrotizing fasciitis	
Type I	Anaerobes (*Bacteroides* spp., *Peptostreptococcus* spp.) and facultative bacteria (streptococci, Enterobacteriaceae)
Type II	Group A streptococci
Secondary infections	
Diabetic foot infections	*S. aureus,* streptococci, Enterobacteriaceae, *Bacteroides* spp., *Peptostreptococcus* spp., *Pseudomonas aeruginosa*
Pressure sores	*S. aureus,* streptococci, Enterobacteriaceae, *Bacteroides* spp., *Peptostreptococcus* spp., *P. aeruginosa*
Bite wounds	
Animal	*Pasteurella multocida, S. aureus,* streptococci, *Bacteroides* spp.
Human	*Eikenella corrodens, S. aureus,* streptococci, *Corynebacterium* spp., *Bacteroides* spp., *Peptostreptococcus* spp.
Burn wounds	*P. aeruginosa,* Enterobacteriaceae, *S. aureus,* streptococci

or in combination with *S. pyogenes* has emerged as a principal cause of impetigo.

CLINICAL PRESENTATION

- Exposed skin, especially the face, is the most common site for impetigo.
- Pruritus is common, and scratching of the lesions may further spread infection through excoriation of the skin. Other systemic signs of infection are minimal.
- Weakness, fever, and diarrhea are sometimes seen with bullous impetigo.
- Nonbullous impetigo manifests initially as small, fluid-filled vesicles. These lesions rapidly develop into pus-filled blisters that readily rupture. Purulent discharge from the lesions dries to form golden yellow crusts that are characteristic of impetigo.
- In the bullous form of impetigo, the lesions begin as vesicles and turn into bullae containing clear yellow fluid. Bullae soon rupture, forming thin, light brown crusts.
- Regional lymph nodes may be enlarged.

TABLE 47–2 Evidence-based Recommendations for Treatment of Skin and Soft-Tissue Infections

Recommendations	Recommendation Grade
Folliculitis, furuncles, carbuncles	
Folliculitis and small furuncles can be treated with moist heat; large furuncles and carbuncles require incision and drainage. Antimicrobial therapy is unnecessary unless extensive lesions or fever are present.	E-III
Erysipelas	
Most infections are caused by *Streptococcus pyogenes*. Penicillin (oral or IV depending on clinical severity) is the drug of choice.	A-I
If *Staphylococcus aureus* is suspected, a penicillinase-resistant penicillin or first-generation cephalosporin should be used.	A-I
Impetigo	
S. aureus accounts for the majority of infections; consequently, a penicillin-resistant penicillin or first-generation cephalosporin is recommended.	A-I
Topical therapy with mupirocin is equivalent to oral therapy.	A-I
Cellulitis	
Mild to moderate infections can generally be treated with oral agents (dicloxacillin, cephalexin, and clindamycin) unless resistance is high in the community.	A-I
Serious infections should be treated IV with a penicillinase-resistant penicillin (nafcillin) or first-generation cephalosporin (cefazolin). Patients with penicillin allergies should be treated with vancomycin or clindamycin.	A-I
Vancomycin, linezolid, and daptomycin should be used to treat serious infections caused by methicillin-resistant *S. aureus*.	A-I
Necrotizing fasciitis	
Early and aggressive surgical debridement of all necrotic tissue is essential.	A-III
Necrotizing fasciitis caused by *S. pyogenes* should be treated with the combination of clindamycin and penicillin.	A-II
Clostridial gas gangrene (myonecrosis) should be treated with clindamycin and penicillin.	B-III
Diabetic foot infections	
Many mild to moderate infections can be treated with oral agents that possess high bioavailability.	A-II
All severe infections should be treated with IV therapy. After initial response, step-down therapy to oral agents can be used.	C-III
Broad-spectrum antimicrobial therapy is not generally required, except for some severe cases.	B-III

(continued)

TABLE 47–2	Evidence-based Recommendations for Treatment of Skin and Soft-Tissue Infections *(Continued)*

Recommendations	Recommendation Grade
Diabetic foot infections	
Definitive therapy should be based on results of appropriately collected cultures and sensitivities, as well as clinical response to empiric antimicrobial agents.	C-III
Optimal wound care, in addition to appropriate antimicrobial therapy, is essential for wound healing.	A-I
Animal bites	
Many bite wounds can be treated on an outpatient basis with amoxicillin–clavulanic acid.	B-II
Serious infections requiring IV antimicrobial therapy can be treated with a β-lactam/β-lactamase inhibitor combination or second-generation cephalosporin with activity against anaerobes (cefoxitin).	B-II
Animal bites	
Penicillinase-resistant penicillins, first-generation cephalosporins, macrolides, and clindamycin should not be used for treatment because of their poor activity against *Pasteurella multocida.*	D-III
Human bites	
Antimicrobial therapy should provide coverage against *Eikenella corrodens, S. aureus,* and β-lactamase-producing anaerobes.	B-III

Strength of recommendation: A, good evidence for use; B, moderate evidence for use; C, poor evidence for use, optional; D, moderate evidence to support not using; E, good evidence to support not using.

Quality of evidence: I, evidence from one or more properly randomized, controlled trials; II, evidence from one or more well-designed clinical trials without randomization, case-controlled analytic studies, multiple time series, or dramatic results from uncontrolled experiments; III, evidence from expert opinion, clinical experience, descriptive studies, or reports of expert committees.

TREATMENT

- Penicillinase-resistant penicillins (e.g., **dicloxacillin**) are the agents of first choice because of the increased isolation of *S. aureus*. First-generation cephalosporins (e.g., cephalexin) are also effective (see Table 47–3). **Penicillin** may be used for impetigo caused by *S. pyogenes*. It may be administered as either a single intramuscular dose of benzathine penicillin G (300,000–600,000 units in children, 1.2 million units in adults) or as oral penicillin VK given for 7 to 10 days. Penicillin-allergic patients can be treated with oral **clindamycin**.
- The duration of therapy is 7 to 10 days.
- **Mupirocin ointment** is also effective.

TABLE 47–3 Recommended Drugs and Dosing Regimens for Outpatient Treatment of Mild to Moderate Skin and Soft-Tissue Infections

Infection	Oral Adult Dose	Oral Pediatric Dose
Folliculitis	None; warm saline compresses usually sufficient	
Furuncles and carbuncles	Dicloxacillin 250–500 mg every 6 hours Cephalexin 250–500 mg every 6 hours Clindamycin 300–600 mg every 6 to 8 hours[a]	Dicloxacillin 25–50 mg/kg in four divided doses Cephalexin 25–50 mg/kg in four divided doses Clindamycin 10–30 mg/kg/day in three or four divided doses[a]
Erysipelas	Procaine penicillin G 600,000 units intramuscularly every 12 hours Penicillin VK 250–500 mg every 6 hours Clindamycin 150–300 mg every 6 to 8 hours[a] Erythromycin 250–500 mg every 6 hours[a]	Penicillin VK 25,000–90,000 units/kg in four divided doses Clindamycin 10–30 mg/kg in three or four doses[a] Erythromycin 30–50 mg/kg in four divided doses[a]
Impetigo	Dicloxacillin 250–500 mg every 6 hours Cephalexin 250–500 mg every 6 hours Cefadroxil 500 mg every 12 hours Clindamycin 150–300 mg every 6 to 8 hours[a] Mupirocin ointment every 8 hours[a] Retapamulin ointment every 12 hours[a]	Dicloxacillin 25–50 mg/kg in four divided doses Cephalexin 25–50 mg/kg in two to four divided doses Cefadroxil 30 mg/kg in two divided doses Clindamycin 10–30 mg/kg/day in three or four divided doses[a] Mupirocin ointment every 8 hours[a] Retapamulin ointment every 12 hours[a]
Lymphangitis	Initial IV therapy, followed by penicillin VK 250–500 mg every 6 hours Clindamycin 150–300 mg every 6 to 8 hours[a]	Initial IV therapy, followed by penicillin VK 25,000–90,000 units/kg in four divided doses Clindamycin 10–30 mg/kg/day in three or four divided doses[a]
Diabetic foot infections	Amoxicillin–clavulanic acid 875 mg/125 mg every 12 hours Fluoroquinolone (levofloxacin 750 mg every 24 hours **or** moxifloxacin 400 mg every 24 hours) + metronidazole 250–500 mg every 8 hours **or** clindamycin 300–600 mg every 6 to 8 hours[a]	

(continued)

TABLE 47-3 Recommended Drugs and Dosing Regimens for Outpatient Treatment of Mild to Moderate Skin and Soft-Tissue Infections (*Continued*)

Infection	Oral Adult Dose	Oral Pediatric Dose
Animal bite	Amoxicillin–clavulanic acid 875 mg/125 mg every 12 hours Doxycycline 100–200 mg every 12 hours[a] Dicloxacillin 250–500 mg every 6 hours + penicillin VK 250–500 mg every 6 hours Cefuroxime axetil 500 mg every 12 hours + metronidazole 250–500 mg every 8 hours **or** clindamycin 300–600 mg every 6 to 8 hours Fluoroquinolone (levofloxacin 500–750 mg every 24 hours or moxifloxacin 400 mg every 24 hours) **or** clindamycin 300–600 mg every 6 to 8 hours[a] Erythromycin 500 mg every 6 hours + metronidazole 250–500 mg every 8 hours **or** clindamycin 300–600 mg every 6 to 8 hours[a]	Amoxicillin–clavulanic acid 40 mg/kg (of the amoxicillin component) in two divided doses Dicloxacillin 25–50 mg/kg in four divided doses + penicillin VK 40,000–90,000 units/kg in four divided doses Cefuroxime axetil 20–30 mg/kg in two divided doses + metronidazole 30 mg/kg in three or four divided doses **or** clindamycin 10–30 mg/kg/day in three or four divided doses Trimethoprim–sulfamethoxazole 4–6 mg/kg (of the trimethoprim component) every 12 hours + metronidazole 30 mg/kg in three or four divided doses **or** clindamycin 10–30 mg/kg/day in three or four divided doses[a] Erythromycin 30–50 mg/kg in four divided doses + every 12 hours + metronidazole 30 mg/kg in three or four divided doses **or** clindamycin 10–30 mg/kg/day in three or four divided doses[a]
Human bite	Amoxicillin–clavulanic acid 875 mg/125 mg every 12 hours Doxycycline 100–200 mg every 12 hours[a] Dicloxacillin 250–500 mg every 6 hours + penicillin VK 250–500 mg every 6 hours Cefuroxime axetil 500 mg every 12 hours + metronidazole 250–500 mg every 8 hours **or** clindamycin 300–600 mg every 6 to 8 hours Fluoroquinolone (levofloxacin 500–750 mg every 24 hours **or** moxifloxacin 400 mg every 24 hours) + metronidazole 250–500 mg every 8 hours **or** clindamycin 300–600 mg every 6 to 8 hours[a]	Amoxicillin–clavulanic acid 40 mg/kg (of the amoxicillin component) in two divided doses Dicloxacillin 25–50 mg/kg in four divided doses + penicillin VK 40,000–90,000 units/kg in four divided doses Cefuroxime axetil 20–30 mg/kg in two divided doses + metronidazole 30 mg/kg in three or four divided doses **or** clindamycin 10–30 mg/kg/day in three or four divided doses Trimethoprim–sulfamethoxazole 4–6 mg/kg (of the trimethoprim component) every 12 hours + metronidazole 30 mg/kg in three or four divided doses **or** clindamycin 10–30 mg/kg/day in three or four divided doses[a]

[a]Recommended for patients with penicillin allergy.

CELLULITIS

- Cellulitis is an acute, spreading infectious process that initially affects the epidermis and dermis and may subsequently spread within the superficial fascia. This process is characterized by inflammation but with little or no necrosis or suppuration of soft tissue.
- Cellulitis is most often caused by *S. pyogenes* or *S. aureus* (see **Table 47–1**).
- Acute cellulitis with mixed aerobic-anaerobic flora generally occurs in diabetes, where the skin is near a traumatic site or surgical incision, at sites of surgical incisions to the abdomen or perineum, or when host defenses are compromised.

CLINICAL PRESENTATION

- Cellulitis is characterized by erythema and edema of the skin. The lesion, which may be extensive, is painful and nonelevated and has poorly defined margins. Tender lymphadenopathy associated with lymphatic involvement is common. Malaise, fever, and chills are also commonly present. There is usually a history of an antecedent wound from minor trauma, an ulcer, or surgery.
- A Gram stain of a smear obtained by injection and aspiration of 0.5 mL of saline (using a small-gauge needle) into the advancing edge of the erythematous lesion may help in making the microbiologic diagnosis but often yields negative results. Blood cultures are useful, as bacteremia may be present in 30% of cases.

TREATMENT

- The goal of therapy of acute bacterial cellulitis is rapid eradication of the infection and prevention of further complications.
- Antimicrobial therapy of bacterial cellulitis is directed toward the type of bacteria either documented to be present or suspected.
- Local care of cellulitis includes elevation and immobilization of the involved area to decrease local swelling.
- As streptococcal cellulitis is indistinguishable clinically from staphylococcal cellulitis, administration of a semisynthetic penicillin (**nafcillin** or **oxacillin**) or first-generation cephalosporin (**cefazolin**) is recommended until a definitive diagnosis, by skin or blood cultures, can be made (**Table 47–4**). Mild to moderate infections not associated with systemic symptoms may be treated orally with **dicloxacillin** or **cephalexin.** If documented to be a mild cellulitis secondary to streptococci, oral **penicillin VK** or intramuscular **procaine penicillin** may be administered. More severe streptococcal infections should be treated with IV antibiotics (e.g., **ceftriaxone,** 50 to 100 mg/kg as a single dose).
- The usual duration of therapy for cellulitis is 5 to 10 days.
- In penicillin-allergic patients, oral or parenteral **clindamycin** may be used. Alternatively, a first-generation cephalosporin such as cefazolin (1–2 g IV every 6–8 hours) may be used cautiously for patients who have not experienced immediate or anaphylactic penicillin reactions and are penicillin skin test negative. In severe cases in which cephalosporins

TABLE 47–4 Initial Treatment Regimens for Cellulitis Caused by Various Pathogens

Antibiotic	Adult Dose and Route	Pediatric Dose and Route
Staphylococcal or unknown gram-positive infection		
Mild infection	Dicloxacillin 0.25–0.5 g orally every 6 hours[a,b]	Dicloxacillin 25–50 mg/kg/day orally in four divided doses[a,b]
Mild infection suspected CA-MRSA	Trimethoprim–sulfamethoxazole 80 mg/160 mg orally every 8 to 12 hours Doxycycline 100 mg orally every 12 hours	Trimethoprim–sulfamethoxazole 4 mg/kg (trimethoprim component) orally every 8 to 12 hours
Moderate to severe infection	Nafcillin or oxacillin 1–2 g IV every 4 to 6 hours[a,b]	Nafcillin or oxacillin 150–200 mg/kg/day (not to exceed 12 g/24 hours) IV in four to six equally divided doses[a,b]
Streptococcal (documented)		
Mild infection	Penicillin VK 0.5 g orally every 6 hours[a] or procaine penicillin G 600,000 units IM every 8 to 12 hours[a]	Penicillin VK 125–250 mg orally every 6 to 8 h **or** procaine penicillin G 25,000–50,000 units/kg (not to exceed 600,000 units) IM every 8 to 12 hours[a]
Moderate to severe infection	Aqueous penicillin G 1 million–2 million units IV every 4 to 6 hours[a,c]	Aqueous penicillin G 100,000–200,000 units/kg/day IV in four divided doses[a]
Gram-negative bacilli		
Mild infection	Cefaclor 0.5 g orally every 8 h[d] **or** cefuroxime axetil 0.5 g orally every 12 hours[d]	Cefaclor 20–40 mg/kg/day (not to exceed 1 g) orally in three divided doses **or** cefuroxime axetil 0.125–0.25 g (tablets) orally every 12 hours
Moderate to severe infection	Aminoglycoside[e] **or** IV cephalosporin (first- or second-generation, depending on severity of infection or susceptibility pattern)[d]	Aminoglycoside[e] **or** IV cephalosporin (first- or second-generation, depending on severity of infection or susceptibility pattern)
Polymicrobic infection without anaerobes		
	Aminoglycoside[e] + penicillin G 1 million–2 million units every 4 to 6 hours **or** a semisynthetic penicillin (nafcillin 1–2 g every 4–6 hours), depending on isolation of staphylococci or streptococci[b]	Aminoglycoside[e] + penicillin G 100,000–200,000 units/kg/day IV in four divided doses **or** a semisynthetic penicillin (nafcillin 150–200 mg/kg/day [not to exceed 12 g/24 hours] IV in four to six equally divided doses), depending on isolation of staphylococci or streptococci[b]

Mild infection	Amoxicillin–clavulanate 0.875 g orally every 12 hours *or* A fluoroquinolone (ciprofloxacin 0.4 g orally every 12 hours *or* levofloxacin 0.5–0.75 g orally every 24 hours) + clindamycin 0.3–0.6 g orally every 8 hours *or* metronidazole 0.5 g orally every 8 hours	Amoxicillin–clavulanic acid 20 mg/kg/day orally in three divided doses
Moderate to severe infection	Aminoglycoside[e] + clindamycin 0.6–0.9 g IV every 8 hours *or* metronidazole 0.5 g IV every 8 hours *or* Monotherapy with second- or third-generation cephalosporin (cefoxitin 1–2 g IV every 6 hours *or* ceftizoxime 1–2 g IV every 8 hours) *or* Monotherapy with imipenem 0.5 g IV every 6–8 hours, meropenem 1 g IV every 8 hours, ertapenem 1 g IV every 24 hours, doripenem 0.5 g every 8 hours, extended-spectrum penicillins with a β-lactamase inhibitor (piperacillin/tazobactam 4.5 g IV every 6 hours), *or* tigecycline 100 mg IV as loading dose, then 50 mg IV every 12 hours	Aminoglycoside[e] + clindamycin 15 mg/kg/day IV in three divided doses *or* metronidazole 30–50 mg/kg/day IV in three divided doses

CA-MRSA, community-associated methicillin-resistant *Staphylococcus aureus*.

[a] For penicillin-allergic patients, use clindamycin 150–300 mg orally every 6 to 8 hours (pediatric dosing: 10–30 mg/kg/day in three or four divided doses).

[b] For methicillin-resistant staphylococci, use vancomycin 0.5–1 g every 6 to 12 hours (pediatric dosing 40 mg/kg/day in divided doses) with dosage adjustments made for renal dysfunction.

[c] For type II necrotizing fasciitis, use clindamycin 0.6–0.9 g IV every 8 hours (in children, clindamycin 15 mg/kg/day IV in three divided doses).

[d] For penicillin-allergic adults, use a fluoroquinolone (ciprofloxacin 0.5–0.75 g orally every 12 hours or 0.4 g IV every 12 hours; levofloxacin 0.5–0.75 g orally or IV every 24 hours; or moxifloxacin 0.4 g orally or IV every 24 hours).

[e] Gentamicin or tobramycin, 2 mg/kg loading dose, then maintenance dose as determined by serum concentrations.

[f] A fluoroquinolone or aztreonam 1 g IV every 6 hours may be used in place of the aminoglycoside in patients with severe renal dysfunction or other relative contraindications to aminoglycoside use.

cannot be used because of documented methicillin resistance or severe allergic reactions to β-lactam antibiotics, IV **vancomycin** should be administered.

- Initial therapy with trimethoprim–sulfamethoxazole, doxycycline, or clindamycin appears to be effective for CA-MRSA and should be considered in geographic areas in which cases of CA-MRSA are commonly encountered. Alternative agents for documented infections with resistant gram-positive bacteria such as methicillin-resistant staphylococci and vancomycin-resistant enterococci include linezolid, quinupristin/dalfopristin, daptomycin, tigecycline, and telavancin.

- For cellulitis caused by gram-negative bacilli or a mixture of microorganisms, immediate antimicrobial chemotherapy as determined by Gram stain is essential, along with appropriate surgical excision of necrotic tissue and drainage. Gram-negative cellulitis may be treated appropriately with an aminoglycoside or first- or second-generation cephalosporin. If gram-positive aerobic bacteria are also present, penicillin G or a penicillinase-resistant penicillin should be added to the regimen. Therapy should be 10 to 14 days in duration.

DIABETIC FOOT INFECTIONS

- Three key factors are involved in the causation of diabetic foot problems: neuropathy, ischemia, and immunologic defects. Any of these disorders can occur in isolation; however, they frequently occur together.

- There are three major types of diabetic foot infections: deep abscesses, cellulitis of the dorsum, and mal perforans ulcers of the sole of the foot. Osteomyelitis may occur in 30% to 40% of infections.

- Diabetic foot infections are typically polymicrobic (an average of 2.3–5.8 isolates per culture). Staphylococci (especially *S. aureus*) and streptococci are the most common pathogens, although gram-negative bacilli and anaerobes occur in 50% of cases. Common isolates include *Escherichia coli, Klebsiella* spp., *Proteus* spp., *Pseudomonas aeruginosa, Bacteroides fragilis,* and *Peptostreptococcus* spp.

- Patients with peripheral neuropathy often do not experience pain but seek medical attention for swelling or erythema. Lesions vary in size and clinical features. A foul-smelling odor suggests anaerobic organisms. Temperature may be mildly elevated or normal.

TREATMENT

- The goal of therapy is preservation of as much normal limb function as possible while preventing infectious complications. Most infections can be successfully treated on an outpatient basis with wound care and antibiotics.

- Necrotic tissue must be thoroughly debrided, with wound drainage and amputation as required.

- Diabetic glycemic control should be maximized to ensure optimal healing.

- The patient should initially be restricted to bed rest, leg elevation, and control of edema, if present.

- **Amoxicillin–clavulanate** is the agent of choice for oral outpatient treatment; however, this agent does not cover *P. aeruginosa*. Fluoroquinolones with metronidazole or clindamycin are reasonable alternatives.
- Serious polymicrobic infections may be treated with agents used for anaerobic cellulitis (see **Table 47–3**).
- Monotherapy with broad-spectrum parenteral antimicrobials, along with appropriate medical and/or surgical management, is often effective in treating moderate to severe infections (including those in which osteomyelitis is present).
- In penicillin-allergic patients, metronidazole or clindamycin plus either a fluoroquinolone, aztreonam, or, possibly, a third-generation cephalosporin is appropriate.
- Vancomycin is used frequently in severe infections with gram-positive pathogens. With increasing staphylococcal resistance, linezolid, quinupristin/dalfopristin, daptomycin, and tigecycline are alternatives.
- Treatment of soft-tissue infections in diabetic patients should generally be at least 7 to 14 days in duration, although some infections may require an additional 1 to 2 weeks of therapy. However, in cases of underlying osteomyelitis, treatment should continue for 6 to 12 weeks.

INFECTED PRESSURE ULCERS

- A pressure sore is also called a "decubitus ulcer" or "bed sore." A classification system for pressure sores is presented in **Table 47–5**. Many factors are thought to predispose patients to the formation of pressure ulcers: paralysis, paresis, immobilization, malnutrition, anemia, infection, and advanced age. Four factors thought to be most critical to their formation are pressure, shearing forces, friction, and moisture; however, there is still debate as to the exact pathophysiology of pressure sore formation. The areas of highest pressure are generated over the bony prominences.
- Most pressure sores are colonized by bacteria; however, bacteria frequently infect healthy tissue. A large variety of aerobic gram-positive and gram-negative bacteria, as well as anaerobes, are frequently isolated.

CLINICAL PRESENTATION

- More than 95% of all pressure sores are located on the lower part of the body. The most common sites are the sacral and coccygeal areas, ischial tuberosities, and greater trochanter.
- Clinical infection is recognized by the presence of redness, heat, and pain. Purulent discharge, foul odor, and systemic signs (fever and leukocytosis) may be present.
- Pressure sores vary greatly in their severity, ranging from an abrasion to large lesions that can penetrate into the deep fascia involving both bone and muscle.
- Without treatment, an initial, small, localized area of ulceration can rapidly progress to 5 to 6 cm within days.

TABLE 47–5	Pressure Sore Classification
Suspected deep tissue injury	Area of discolored intact skin or blood-filled blister due to damage of underlying soft tissue from pressure and/or shear. Area may be preceded by tissue that is painful, firm, mushy, boggy, warmer, or cooler as compared with adjacent tissue.
Stage 1	Pressure sore is generally reversible, is limited to the epidermis, and resembles an abrasion. Intact skin with nonblanchable redness of a localized area, usually over a bony prominence. The area may be painful, firm, soft, warmer, or cooler as compared with adjacent tissue.
Stage 2	A stage 2 sore also may be reversible; partial thickness loss of dermis presenting as a shallow open ulcer with a red pink wound bed. May also present as an intact or open/ruptured serum-filled blister or as a shiny or dry shallow ulcer.
Stage 3[a]	Full thickness tissue loss. Subcutaneous fat may be visible, but bone, tendon, or muscles are not exposed. May include undermining and tunneling. Depth of the ulcer varies by anatomical location; may range from shallow to extremely deep over areas of significant adiposity.
Stage 4[a]	Full thickness tissue loss with exposed bone, tendon, or muscle; can extend into muscle and/or supporting structures (e.g., fascia, tendon, or joint capsule) making osteomyelitis possible. Often include undermining and tunneling; depth of the ulcer varies by anatomical location.
Unstageable[a]	Full thickness tissue loss in which the base of the ulcer is covered by slough (yellow, tan, gray, green, or brown) and/or eschar (tan, brown, or black) in the wound bed. True depth, and therefore stage, cannot be determined.

[a]Stage 3, Stage 4, and unstageable lesions are unlikely to resolve on their own and often require surgical intervention.

Data from Black J, Baharestani M, Cuddigan J, et al. National Pressure Ulcer Advisory Panel's updated pressure ulcer staging system. Derm Nursing 2007;19:343–349.

PREVENTION AND TREATMENT

- The goal of therapy is to clean and decontaminate the ulcer to promote wound healing by permitting the formation of healthy granulation tissue or to prepare the wound for an operative procedure. The main factors to be considered for successful wound care are (1) relief of pressure; (2) debridement of necrotic tissue; (3) wound cleansing; (4) dressing selection; and (5) prevention, diagnosis, and treatment of infection.
- Prevention is the single most important aspect in the management of pressure sores. Friction and shearing forces can be minimized by proper positioning. Skin care and prevention of soilage are important, with the intent being to keep the surface relatively free from moisture. Relief of pressure (even for 5 min once every 2 hours) is probably the single most important factor in preventing pressure sore formation.
- Medical management is generally indicated for lesions that are of moderate size and of relatively shallow depth (stage 1 or 2 lesions) and are not located over a bony prominence.

- Debridement can be accomplished by surgical or mechanical means (wet-to-dry dressing changes). Other effective therapies are hydrotherapy, wound irrigation, and dextranomers. Pressure sores should be cleaned with normal saline.
- A number of agents have been used to disinfect pressure sores (e.g., povidone–iodine, iodophor, **sodium hypochlorite, hydrogen peroxide,** and **acetic acid**) and other types of open wounds; however, these agents should be avoided, as they impair healing.
- See Table 47–4 for systemic treatment of an infected pressure sore. A short, 2-week trial of topical antibiotic (**silver sulfadiazine** or **triple antibiotic**) is recommended for a clean ulcer that is not healing or is producing a moderate amount of exudate despite appropriate care.

INFECTED BITE WOUNDS

DOG BITES

- Patients at risk of acquiring an infection after a bite have had a puncture wound, have not sought medical attention within 12 hours of injury, and are older than 50 years.
- The infected dog bite is usually characterized by a localized cellulitis and pain at the site of injury. The cellulitis usually spreads proximally from the initial site of injury. If *Pasteurella multocida* is present, a rapidly progressing cellulitis with a gray malodorous discharge may be encountered.
- Most infections are polymicrobial, and the most frequently isolated organisms are *Pasteurella* spp., streptococci, staphylococci, *Moraxella,* and *Neisseria.* The most common anaerobes are *Fusobacterium* spp., *Bacteroides* spp., *Porphyromonas,* and *Prevotella.*
- Wounds should be thoroughly irrigated with a sterile saline solution. Proper irrigation will reduce the bacterial count in the wound.
- The role of antimicrobials for noninfected dog bite wounds remains controversial because only 20% of wounds become infected. Antibiotic recommendations for empiric treatment include a 3- to 5-day course of therapy. Amoxicillin–clavulanic acid is commonly recommended for oral outpatient therapy. Alternative agents include doxycycline and the combination of penicillin VK and dicloxacillin.
- **Trimethoprim–sulfamethoxazole** and **fluoroquinolones** are recommended as alternatives for infections caused by *P. multocida* or those allergic to penicillins (but not in children or pregnant women). **Macrolides** or **azolides** may be considered an alternative in growing children or pregnant women.
- Treatment options for patients requiring IV therapy include β-lactam–β-lactamase inhibitors (**ampicillin–sulbactam** and **piperacillin–tazobactam**), second-generation cephalosporins with antianaerobic activity (**cefoxitin**), and carbapenems.
- If the immunization history of a patient with anything other than a clean minor wound is not known, tetanus/diphtheria toxoids should be administered. Both tetanus/diphtheria toxoids and tetanus immunoglobulin should be administered to patients who have never been immunized.

- If a patient has been exposed to rabies, the treatment objectives consist of thorough irrigation of the wound, tetanus prophylaxis, antibiotic prophylaxis (if indicated), and immunization. Postexposure prophylaxis immunization consists of both passive antibody administration and vaccine administration.

CAT BITES

- Approximately 30% to 50% of cat bites become infected. These infections are frequently caused by *P. multocida,* which has been isolated in the oropharynx of 50% to 70% of healthy cats.
- The management of cat bites is similar to that discussed for dog bites. Antibiotic therapy with penicillin is the mainstay, and therapy is as described for dog bites.

HUMAN BITES

- Infections can occur in 10% to 50% of patients with human bites.
- Infections caused by these injuries are most often caused by the normal oral flora, which includes both aerobic and anaerobic microorganisms. The most frequent aerobic organisms are *Streptococcus* spp., *Staphylococcus* spp., and *Eikenella corrodens.* The most common anaerobic organisms are *Fusobacterium, Prevotella, Porphyromonas,* and *Peptostreptococcus* spp.
- Management of bite wounds consists of aggressive irrigation and topical wound dressing, surgical debridement, and immobilization of the affected area. Primary closure for human bites is not generally recommended. Tetanus toxoid and antitoxin may be indicated.
- If the biter is human immunodeficiency virus (HIV) positive, the victim should have a baseline HIV status determined and then repeated in 3 and 6 months. The bite should be thoroughly irrigated with a virucidal agent such as povidone–iodine. Victims may be offered antiretroviral chemoprophylaxis.
- Patients with noninfected bite injuries should be given prophylactic antibiotic therapy for 3 to 5 days. Amoxicillin–clavulanic acid (500 mg every 8 hours) is commonly recommended. Alternatives for penicillin-allergic patients include fluoroquinolones or trimethoprim–sulfamethoxazole in combination with clindamycin or metronidazole. First-generation cephalosporins, macrolides, clindamycin alone, or aminoglycosides are not recommended, as the sensitivity to *E. corrodens* is variable.
- Patients with serious injuries or clenched-fist injuries should be started on IV antibiotics (cefoxitin 1 g every 6–8 hours), ampicillin–sulbactam (1.5–3 g every 6 hours), or ertapenem (1 g every 24 hours).

See Chapter 119, Skin and Soft-Tissue Infections, authored by Douglas N. Fish, Susan L. Pendland, and Larry H. Danziger, for a more detailed discussion of this topic.

48 Surgical Prophylaxis

DEFINITION

- Antibiotics administered before contamination of previously sterile tissues or fluids are considered prophylactic. The goal of prophylactic antibiotics is to prevent a surgical-site infection (SSI) from developing.
- Presumptive antibiotic therapy is administered when an infection is suspected but not yet proven. Therapeutic antibiotics are required for established infection.
- SSIs are classified as either incisional (e.g., cellulitis of the incision site) or involving an organ or space (e.g., with meningitis). Incisional SSIs may be superficial (skin or subcutaneous tissue) or deep (fascial and muscle layers). Both types, by definition, occur by postoperative day 30. This period extends to 1 year in the case of deep infection associated with prosthesis implantation.

RISK FACTORS FOR SURGICAL WOUND INFECTION

- The traditional classification system developed by the National Research Council (NRC) stratifying surgical procedures by infection risk is reproduced in Table 48–1. The NRC wound classification for a specific procedure is determined intraoperatively and is the primary determinant of whether antibiotic prophylaxis is warranted.
- The Study on the Efficacy of Nosocomial Infection Control (SENIC) analyzed more than 100,000 surgery cases and identified abdominal operations, operations lasting >2 hours, contaminated or dirty procedures, and more than three underlying medical diagnoses as factors associated with an increased incidence of SSI. When the NRC classification described in Table 48–1 was stratified by the number of SENIC risk factors present, the infection rates varied by as much as a factor of 15 within the same operative category.
- The SENIC risk assessment technique has been modified to include the American Society of Anesthesiologists preoperative assessment score (Table 48–2). An American Society of Anesthesiologists score ≥3 was associated with increased SSI risk.

MICROBIOLOGY

- Bacteria involved in SSI are acquired either from the patient's normal flora (endogenous) or from contamination during the surgical procedure (exogenous).
- Loss of protective flora via antibiotics can upset the balance and allow pathogenic bacteria to proliferate and increase infectious risk.
- Normal flora can become pathogenic when translocated to a normally sterile tissue site or fluid during surgical procedures.

TABLE 48–1 National Research Council Wound Classification, Risk of Surgical-Site Infection (SSI), and Indication for Antibiotics

Classification	SSI Rate (%) Preoperative Antibiotics	No Preoperative Antibiotics	Criteria	Antibiotics
Clean	5.1	0.8	No acute inflammation or transection of GI, oropharyngeal, genitourinary, biliary, or respiratory tracts. Elective case, no technique break.	Not indicated unless high-risk procedure[a]
Clean-contaminated	10.1	1.3	Controlled opening of aforementioned tracts with minimal spillage/minor technique break. Clean procedures performed emergently or with major technique breaks.	Prophylactic antibiotics indicated
Contaminated	21.9	10.2	Acute, nonpurulent inflammation present. Major spillage/technique break during clean-contaminated procedure.	Prophylactic antibiotics indicated
Dirty	N/A	N/A	Obvious preexisting infection present (abscess, pus, or necrotic tissue present).	Therapeutic antibiotics required

N/A, not applicable.
[a]High-risk procedures include implantation of prosthetic materials and other procedures in which surgical-site infection is associated with high morbidity.

- According to the National Nosocomial Infections Surveillance System, the five most common pathogens encountered in surgical wounds are *Staphylococcus aureus*, coagulase-negative staphylococci, Enterococci, *Escherichia coli*, and *Pseudomonas aeruginosa*.
- Impaired host defenses, vascular occlusive states, traumatized tissues, and the presence of a foreign body greatly decrease the number of bacteria required to cause an SSI.

TABLE 48–2	American Society of Anesthesiologists Physical Status Classification
Class	**Description**
1	Normal healthy patient
2	Mild systemic disease
3	Severe systemic disease that is not incapacitating
4	Incapacitating systemic disease that is a constant threat to life
5	Not expected to survive 24 hours with or without operation

ANTIBIOTIC ISSUES

SCHEDULING ANTIBIOTIC ADMINISTRATION

- The following principles must be considered when providing antimicrobial surgical prophylaxis:
  - ✓ Antimicrobials should be delivered to the surgical site prior to the initial incision. They should be administered with anesthesia, just prior to initial incision. Antibiotics should not be prescribed to be given "on-call to the OR [operating room]."
  - ✓ Bactericidal antibiotic tissue concentrations should be maintained throughout the surgical procedure.
- Strategies to ensure appropriate antimicrobial prophylaxis use are described in **Table 48–3**.

ANTIMICROBIAL SELECTION

- The choice of the prophylactic antimicrobial depends on the type of surgical procedure, most likely pathogenic organisms, safety and efficacy of the antimicrobial, current literature evidence supporting its use, and cost.
- Typically, gram-positive coverage is included in the choice of surgical prophylaxis, because organisms such as *S. aureus* and *S. epidermidis* are common skin flora.
- Parenteral antibiotic administration is favored because of its reliability in achieving suitable tissue concentrations.
- First-generation cephalosporins (particularly cefazolin) are the preferred choice, particularly for clean surgical procedures. Antianaerobic cephalosporins (e.g., cefoxitin or cefotetan) are appropriate choices when broad-spectrum anaerobic and gram-negative coverage is desired.
- Vancomycin may be considered for prophylactic therapy in surgical procedures involving implantation of a prosthetic device in which the rate of methicillin-resistant *S. aureus* (MRSA) is high. If the risk of MRSA is low and a β-lactam hypersensitivity exists, clindamycin can be used instead of cefazolin in order to limit vancomycin use.

TABLE 48–3	Strategies for Implementing an Institutional Program to Ensure the Appropriate Use of Antimicrobial Prophylaxis in Surgery

1. Educate

Develop an educational program that enforces the importance and rationale of timely antimicrobial prophylaxis.

Make this educational program available to all healthcare practitioners involved in the patient's care.

2. Standardize the ordering process

Establish a protocol (e.g., a preprinted order sheet) that standardizes antibiotic choice according to current published evidence, formulary availability, institutional resistance patterns, and cost.

3. Standardize the delivery and administration process

Use a system that ensures that antibiotics are prepared and delivered to the holding area in a timely fashion.

Standardize the administration time to <1 hour preoperatively.

Designate responsibility and accountability for antibiotic administration.

Provide visible reminders to prescribe or administer prophylactic antibiotics (e.g., checklists).

Develop a system to remind surgeons or nurses to readminister antibiotics intraoperatively during long procedures.

4. Provide feedback

Follow up with regular reports of compliance and infection rates.

RECOMMENDATIONS FOR SPECIFIC TYPES OF SURGERIES

- Specific recommendations are summarized in **Table 48–4.**

GASTRODUODENAL SURGERY

- The risk of infection rises with conditions that increase gastric pH and subsequent bacterial overgrowth, such as obstruction, hemorrhage, malignancy, and acid-suppression therapy (clean-contaminated).
- A single dose of IV **cefazolin** will provide adequate prophylaxis for most cases. Oral **ciprofloxacin** may be used for patients with β-lactam hypersensitivity.
- Postoperative therapeutic antibiotics may be indicated if perforation is detected during surgery, depending on whether an established infection is present.

BILIARY TRACT SURGERY

- Antibiotic prophylaxis has been proven beneficial for surgery involving the biliary tract.
- Most frequently encountered organisms include *E. coli*, *Klebsiella*, and Enterococci. Single-dose prophylaxis with **cefazolin** is currently

TABLE 48–4 Most Likely Pathogens and Specific Recommendations for Surgical Prophylaxis

Type of Operation	Likely Pathogens	Recommended Prophylaxis Regimen[a]	Comments	Grade of Recommendation[b]
GI surgery				
Gastroduodenal	Enteric gram-negative bacilli, gram-positive cocci, oral anaerobes	Cefazolin 1 g × 1 (see text for recommendations for percutaneous endoscopic gastrostomy)	High-risk patients only (obstruction, hemorrhage, malignancy, acid suppression therapy, morbid obesity)	IA
Cholecystectomy	Enteric gram-negative bacilli, anaerobes	Cefazolin 1 g × 1 for high-risk patients Laparoscopic: none	High-risk patients only (acute cholecystitis, common duct stones, previous biliary surgery, jaundice, age >60 years, obesity, diabetes mellitus)	IA
Transjugular intrahepatic portosystemic shunt (TIPS)	Enteric gram-negative bacilli, anaerobes	Ceftriaxone 1 g × 1	Longer-acting cephalosporins preferred	IA
Appendectomy	Enteric gram-negative bacilli, anaerobes	Cefoxitin or cefotetan 1 g × 1	Second intraoperative dose of cefoxitin may be required if procedure lasts longer than 3 hours	IA
Colorectal	Enteric gram-negative bacilli, anaerobes	Orally: neomycin 1 g + erythromycin base 1 at 1 PM, 2 PM, and 11 PM 1 day preoperatively plus mechanical bowel preparation IV: cefoxitin or cefotetan 1 g × 1	Benefits of oral plus IV is controversial except for colostomy reversal and rectal resection	IA

(continued)

TABLE 48–4 Most Likely Pathogens and Specific Recommendations for Surgical Prophylaxis *(Continued)*

Type of Operation	Likely Pathogens	Recommended Prophylaxis Regimen[a]	Comments	Grade of Recommendation[b]
GI endoscopy	Variable, depending on procedure, but typically enteric gram-negative bacilli, gram-positive cocci, oral anaerobes	Orally: amoxicillin 2 g × 1 or IV: ampicillin 2 g × 1 or cefazolin 1 g × 1	Recommended only for high-risk patients undergoing high-risk procedures (see text)	IA
Urologic surgery				
Prostate resection, shock-wave lithotripsy, ureteroscopy	*Escherichia coli*	Ciprofloxacin 500 mg orally or trimethoprim-sulfamethoxazole 1 DS tablet	All patients with positive pre-operative urine cultures should receive a course of antibiotic treatment	IA–IB
removal of external urinary catheters, cystography, urodynamic studies, simple cystourethroscopy	*E. coli*	Ciprofloxacin 500 mg orally or trimethoprim-sulfamethoxazole 1 DS tablet	Should be considered only in patients with risk factors (see text)	IB
Gynecological surgery				
Cesarean section	Enteric gram-negative bacilli, anaerobes, group B streptococci, enterococci	Cefazolin 2 g × 1	Can be given before initial incision or after cord is clamped	IA
Hysterectomy	Enteric gram-negative bacilli, anaerobes, group B streptococci, enterococci	Vaginal: cefazolin 1 g × 1 Abdominal: cefotetan 1 g × 1 or cefazolin 1 g × 1	Metronidazole 1 g IV × 1 is recommended alternative for penicillin allergy	IA
Head and neck surgery				
Maxillofacial surgery	*Staphylococcus aureus*, streptococci oral anaerobes	Cefazolin 2 g or clindamycin 600 mg	Repeat intraoperative dose for operations longer than 4 hours	IA

Head and neck cancer resection	S. aureus, streptococci oral anaerobes	Clindamycin 600 mg at induction and every 8 hours × 2 more doses	Add gentamicin for clean-contaminated procedures	IA
Cardiothoracic surgery				
Cardiac surgery	S. aureus, Staphylococcus epidermidis, Corynebacterium	Cefazolin 1 g every 8 hours × 48 hours	Patients >80 kg (176 lb) should receive 2 g of cefazolin instead; in areas with high prevalence of S. aureus resistance, vancomycin should be considered	IA
Thoracic surgery	S. aureus, S. epidermidis, Corynebacterium, enteric gram-negative bacilli	Cefuroxime 750 mg IV every 8 hours × 48 hours	First-generation cephalosporins are deemed inadequate, and shorter durations of prophylaxis have not been adequately studied	IA
Vascular surgery				
Abdominal aorta and lower extremity vascular surgery	S. aureus, S. epidermidis, enteric gram-negative bacilli	Cefazolin 1 g at induction and every 8 hours × 2 more doses	Although complications from infections may be infrequent, graft infections are associated with significant morbidity	IB
Orthopedic surgery				
Joint replacement	S. aureus, S. epidermidis	Cefazolin 1 g × 1 preoperatively, then every 8 hours × 2 more doses	Vancomycin reserved for penicillin-allergic patients or where institutional prevalence of methicillin-resistant S. aureus warrants use	IA
Hip fracture repair	S. aureus, S. epidermidis	Cefazolin 1 g × 1 preoperatively, then every 8 hours for 48 hours	Compound fractures are treated as if infection is presumed	IA

(continued)

TABLE 48–4 Most Likely Pathogens and Specific Recommendations for Surgical Prophylaxis *(Continued)*

Type of Operation	Likely Pathogens	Recommended Prophylaxis Regimen[a]	Comments	Grade of Recommendation[b]
Open/compound fractures	S. aureus, S. epidermidis, gram-negative bacilli, polymicrobial	Cefazolin 1 g × 1 preoperatively, then every 8 hours for a course of presumed infection	Gram-negative coverage (i.e., gentamicin) often indicated for severe open fractures	IA
Neurosurgery				
CSF shunt procedures	S. aureus, S. epidermidis	Cefazolin 1 g every 8 hours × 3 doses or ceftriaxone 2 g × 1	No agents have been shown to be better than cefazolin in randomized comparative trials.	IA
Spinal surgery	S. aureus, S. epidermidis	Cefazolin 1 g × 1	Limited number of clinical trials comparing different treatment regimens	IB
CSF shunt procedures	S. aureus, S. epidermidis	Cefazolin 1 g every 8 hours × 3 doses or ceftriaxone 2 g × 1	No agents have been shown to be better than cefazolin in randomized comparative trials.	IA
Craniotomy	S. aureus, S. epidermidis	Cefazolin 1 g × 1 or cefotaxime 1 g × 1	IV × 1 can be substituted for patients with penicillin allergy Trimethoprim-sulfamethoxazole (160/800 mg)	IA

[a]One-time doses are optimally infused at induction of anesthesia except as noted. Repeat doses may be required for long procedures. See text for references.
[b]Strength of recommendations:
Category IA: Strongly recommended and supported by well-designed experimental, clinical, or epidemiologic studies.
Category IB: Strongly recommended and supported by some experimental, clinical, or epidemiologic studies and strong theoretical rationale.
Category II: Suggested and supported by suggestive clinical or epidemiologic studies or theoretical rationale.
CSF, cerebrospinal fluid; DS, double strength; GI, gastrointestinal; IV, intravenous(ly).

recommended. **Ciprofloxacin** and **levofloxacin** are alternatives for patients with β-lactam hypersensitivity.

- For low-risk patients undergoing elective laparoscopic cholecystectomy, antibiotic prophylaxis is of no benefit and is not recommended.
- Some surgeons use presumptive antibiotics for cases of acute chole-cystitis or cholangitis and defer surgery until the patient is afebrile, in an attempt to decrease infection rates further, but this practice is controversial.
- Detection of an active infection during surgery (gangrenous gallbladder or suppurative cholangitis) is an indication for therapeutic postoperative antibiotics.

COLORECTAL SURGERY

- Anaerobes and gram-negative aerobes predominate in SSIs (see **Table 48–4**), although gram-positive aerobes are also important. Therefore, the risk of an SSI in the absence of an adequate prophylactic regimen is substantial.
- Reducing bacteria load with a thorough bowel preparation regimen (4 L of polyethylene glycol solution or 90 mL of sodium phosphate solution administered orally the day before surgery) is controversial, even though it is used by most surgeons.
- The combination of 1 g of **neomycin** and 1 g of **erythromycin base** given orally 19, 18, and 9 hours preoperatively is the most commonly used oral regimen in the United States.
- Whether perioperative parenteral antibiotics, in addition to the stan-dard preoperative oral antibiotic regimen, will lower SSI rates further is controversial. Patients who cannot take oral medications should receive parenteral antibiotics.
- Postoperative antibiotics are unnecessary in the absence of any untoward events or findings during surgery.

APPENDECTOMY

- A cephalosporin with antianaerobic activity such as **cefoxitin** or **cefotetan** is currently recommended as a first-line agent. Cefotetan may be superior for longer operations because of its longer duration of action.
- Single-dose therapy with cefotetan is adequate. Intraoperative dosing of cefoxitin may be required if the procedure extends beyond 3 hours.

UROLOGIC PROCEDURES

- As long as the urine is sterile preoperatively, the risk of SSI after uro-logic procedures is low, and the benefit of prophylactic antibiotics in this setting is controversial. *E. coli* is the most frequently encountered organism.
- Antibiotic prophylaxis is warranted for all patients undergoing transure-thral resection of the prostate, or bladder tumors, shock wave lithotripsy, percutaneous renal surgery, or ureteroscopy.

- Specific recommendations are listed in **Table 48–4**.
- Urologic procedures requiring an abdominal approach such as a nephrectomy or cystectomy require prophylaxis appropriate for a clean-contaminated abdominal procedure.

CESAREAN SECTION

- Antibiotics are efficacious to prevent SSIs for women undergoing cesarean section regardless of underlying risk factors.
- **Cefazolin**, 2 g IV, remains the drug of choice. Providing a broader spectrum by using cefoxitin against anaerobes or piperacillin for better coverage against *Pseudomonas* or enterococci, for example, does not lower postoperative infection rates any further in comparative studies.
- The timing of antibiotic administration is controversial, as some advocate administration just after the umbilical cord is clamped, avoiding exposure of the infant to the drug, whereas others advocate administration before the initial incision.

HYSTERECTOMY

- Vaginal hysterectomies are associated with a high rate of postoperative infection when performed without the benefit of prophylactic antibiotics.
- A single preoperative dose of **cefazolin** or **cefoxitin** is recommended for vaginal hysterectomy. For patients with β-lactam hypersensitivity, a single preoperative dose of **metronidazole** or **doxycycline** is effective.
- Abdominal hysterectomy SSI rates are correspondingly lower than vaginal hysterectomy rates. However, prophylactic antibiotics are still recommended regardless of underlying risk factors.
- Both cefazolin and antianaerobic cephalosporins (e.g., **cefoxitin** and **cefotetan**) have been studied extensively for abdominal hysterectomy. Single-dose cefotetan is superior to single-dose cefazolin. The antibiotic course should not exceed 24 hours in duration.

HEAD AND NECK SURGERY

- Use of prophylactic antibiotics during head and neck surgery depends on the procedure type. Clean procedures, such as parotidectomy or a simple tooth extraction, are associated with low rates of SSI. Head and neck procedures involving an incision through a mucosal layer carry a high risk of SSI.
- Specific recommendations for prophylaxis are listed in **Table 48–4**.
- Although typical doses of **cefazolin** are ineffective for anaerobic infections, the recommended 2 g dose produces concentrations high enough to be inhibitory to these organisms. A 24-hour duration has been used in most studies, but single-dose therapy may also be effective.
- For most head and neck cancer resections, 24 hours of clindamycin is appropriate.

CARDIAC SURGERY

- Although most cardiac surgeries are technically clean procedures, prophylactic antibiotics have been shown to lower rates of SSI.

- The usual pathogens are skin flora (see **Table 48–4**) and, rarely, gram-negative enteric organisms.
- Risk factors for developing an SSI after cardiac surgery include obesity, renal insufficiency, connective tissue disease, reexploration for bleeding, and poorly timed administration of antibiotics.
- **Cefazolin** has been extensively studied and is currently considered the drug of choice. Patients weighing > 80 kg should receive 2 g cefazolin rather than 1 g. Doses should be administered no earlier than 60 minutes before the first incision and no later than the beginning of induction of anesthesia.
- Extending antibiotic administration beyond 48 hours does not lower SSI rates.
- **Vancomycin** use may be justified in hospitals with a high incidence of SSI with MRSA or when sternal wounds are to be explored for possible mediastinitis.

NONCARDIAC VASCULAR SURGERY

- Prophylactic antibiotics are beneficial, especially in procedures involving the abdominal aorta and the lower extremities.
- Twenty-four hours of prophylaxis with IV **cefazolin** is adequate. For patients with β-lactam allergy, 24 hours of oral **ciprofloxacin** is effective.

ORTHOPEDIC SURGERY

- Prophylactic antibiotics are beneficial in cases involving implantation of prosthetic material (pins, plates, and artificial joints).
- The most likely pathogens mirror those of other clean procedures and include staphylococci and, infrequently, gram-negative aerobes.
- **Cefazolin** is the best-studied antibiotic and is thus the drug of choice. For hip fracture repairs and joint replacements, it should be administered for 24 hours. **Vancomycin** is not recommended unless a patient has a history of β-lactam hypersensitivity or the propensity for MRSA infection at the institution necessitates its use.

NEUROSURGERY

- The use of prophylactic antibiotics in neurosurgery is controversial.
- Single doses of **cefazolin** or, where required, **vancomycin** appear to lower SSI risk after craniotomy.

MINIMALLY INVASIVE AND LAPAROSCOPIC SURGERY

- The role of prophylactic antimicrobials depends on the type of procedure performed and preexisting risk factors for infection. There are insufficient clinical trials to provide general recommendations.

See Chapter 132, Antimicrobial Prophylaxis in Surgery, authored by Salmaan Kanji, for a more detailed discussion of this topic.

Tuberculosis

DEFINITION

- Tuberculosis (TB) is a communicable infectious disease caused by *Mycobacterium tuberculosis*. It can produce silent, latent infection, as well as progressive, active disease. Globally, 2 billion people are infected and 2 million to 3 million people die from TB each year.
- *M. tuberculosis* is transmitted from person to person by coughing or sneezing. Close contacts of TB patients are most likely to become infected.
- Fifty-nine percent of TB patients in the United States are foreign born, most often from Mexico, the Philippines, Vietnam, India, and China. In the United States, TB disproportionately affects ethnic minorities (African Americans, Hispanics, and Asians).
- Human immunodeficiency virus (HIV) is the most important risk factor for active TB, especially among people 25 to 44 years of age. An HIV-infected individual with TB infection is over 100-fold more likely to develop active disease than an HIV-seronegative patient.

PATHOPHYSIOLOGY

- Primary infection is initiated by the alveolar implantation of organisms in droplet nuclei that are small enough (1–5 mm) to escape the ciliary epithelial cells of the upper respiratory tract and reach the alveolar surface. Once implanted, the organisms multiply and are ingested by pulmonary macrophages, where they are killed, or they continue to multiply. With bacterial multiplication, the macrophages eventually rupture, releasing many bacilli.
- Large numbers of activated macrophages surround the solid caseous (cheese-like) TB foci (the necrotic area) as a part of cell-mediated immunity. Delayed-type hypersensitivity also develops through activation and multiplication of T lymphocytes. Macrophages form granulomas to contain the organisms.
- Successful containment of *M. tuberculosis* requires activation of a subset of CD4 lymphocytes, referred to as TH_1 cells, which activate macrophages through secretion of interferon-γ.
- Approximately 90% of patients who experience primary disease have no further clinical manifestations other than a positive skin test either alone or in combination with radiographic evidence of stable granulomas. Tissue necrosis and calcification of the originally infected site and regional lymph nodes may occur, resulting in the formation of a radiodense area referred to as a *Ghon complex*.
- Approximately 5% of patients (usually children, the elderly, or the immunocompromised) experience progressive primary disease at the site of the primary infection (usually the lower lobes) and frequently by dissemination, leading to meningitis and often to involvement of the upper lobes of the lung as well.

TABLE 49–1	Clinical Presentation of Tuberculosis

Signs and symptoms
Patients typically present with weight loss, fatigue, a productive cough, fever, and night sweats. Frank hemoptysis

Physical examination
Dullness to chest percussion, rales, and increased vocal fremitus are observed frequently on auscultation.

Laboratory tests
Moderate elevations in the white blood cell count with a lymphocyte predominance

Chest radiograph
Patchy or nodular infiltrates in the apical area of the upper lobes or the superior segment of the lower lobes
Cavitation that may show air–fluid levels as the infection progresses

- Approximately 10% of patients develop reactivation disease, which arises subsequent to the hematogenous spread of the organism. In the United States, most cases of TB are believed to result from reactivation.
- Occasionally, a massive inoculum of organisms may be introduced into the bloodstream, causing widely disseminated disease and granuloma formation known as *miliary TB*.

CLINICAL PRESENTATION

- The classic presentation of pulmonary TB is nonspecific, indicative only of a slowly evolving infectious process (Table 49–1). The onset of TB may be gradual. Physical examination is nonspecific but suggestive of progressive pulmonary disease.
- Clinical features associated with extrapulmonary TB vary depending on the organ system(s) involved but typically consist of slowly progressive decline of organ function with low-grade fever and other constitutional symptoms.
- Patients with HIV may have atypical presentation. HIV-positive patients are less likely to have positive skin tests, cavitary lesions, or fever. They have a higher incidence of extrapulmonary TB and are more likely to present with progressive primary disease.
- TB in the elderly is easily confused with other respiratory diseases. It is far less likely to present with positive skin tests, fevers, night sweats, sputum production, or hemoptysis. TB in children may present as typical bacterial pneumonia and is called **progressive primary TB**.

DIAGNOSIS

- The most widely used screening method for tuberculous infection is the tuberculin skin test, which uses purified protein derivative (PPD). Populations most likely to benefit from skin testing are listed in Table 49–2.

TABLE 49–2 Criteria for Tuberculin Skin Test Positivity, by Risk Group

Reaction ≥5 mm of Induration	Reaction ≥10 mm of Induration	Reaction ≥15 mm of Induration
HIV-positive persons	Recent immigrants (i.e., within the last 5 years) from high-prevalence countries	Persons with no risk factors for TB
Recent contacts of TB case patients	Injection drug users	
Fibrotic changes on chest radiograph consistent with prior TB	Residents and employees[a] of the following high-risk congregate settings: prisons and jails, nursing homes and other long-term care facilities for the elderly, hospitals and other healthcare facilities, residential facilities for patients with AIDS, and homeless shelters	
Patients with organ transplants and other immunosuppressed patients (receiving the equivalent of prednisone for ≥1 month)[b]	Mycobacteriology laboratory personnel	
	Persons with the following clinical conditions that place them at high risk: silicosis, diabetes mellitus, chronic renal failure, some hematologic disorders (e.g., leukemias and lymphomas), other specific malignancies (e.g., carcinoma of the head or neck and lung), weight loss ≥10% of ideal body weight, gastrectomy, and jejunoileal bypass	
	Children younger than 4 years or infants, children, and adolescents exposed to adults at high risk	

AIDS, acquired immunodeficiency syndrome; HIV, human immunodeficiency virus; TB, tuberculosis.

[a]For persons who are otherwise at low risk and are tested at the start of employment, a reaction ≥15 mm induration is considered positive.

[b]Risk of TB in patients treated with corticosteroids increases with higher dose and longer duration.

Adapted from Centers for Disease Control and Prevention. Screening for tuberculosis and tuberculosis infection in high-risk populations: Recommendations of the Advisory Council for the Elimination of Tuberculosis. MMWR 1995;44(No. RR-11):19–34.

- The Mantoux method of PPD administration, which is the most reliable technique, consists of the intracutaneous injection of PPD containing 5 tuberculin units. The test is read 48 to 72 hours after injection by measuring the diameter of the zone of induration.
- Some patients may exhibit a positive test 1 week after an initial negative test; this is referred to as a *booster effect*.
- Confirmatory diagnosis of a clinical suspicion of TB must be made via chest radiograph and microbiologic examination of sputum or other infected material to rule out active disease.
- When active TB is suspected, attempts should be made to isolate *M. tuberculosis* from the infected site. Daily sputum collection over 3 consecutive days is recommended.

- Rapid identification tests (e.g., AccuProbe, *M. tuberculosis* direct test, and the strand-displacement amplification test) are now available to detect the bacterium. Also, tests to measure release of interferon-γ in the patient's blood in response to TB antigens can be used to detect latent infection.

DESIRED OUTCOME

- Rapid identification of new cases of TB
- Initiation of specific antituberculosis treatment.
- Prompt resolution of signs and symptoms of disease
- Achievement of a noninfectious state, thus ending isolation
- Adherence to the treatment regimen by the patient
- Cure as quickly as possible (generally with at least 6 months of treatment)

TREATMENT

- Drug treatment is the cornerstone of TB management. A minimum of two drugs, and generally three or four drugs, must be used simultaneously.
- Drug treatment is continued for at least 6 months and up to 2 to 3 years for some cases of multidrug-resistant TB (MDR-TB).
- Measures to assure adherence, such as directly observed therapy, are important.
- Patients with active disease should be isolated to prevent spread of the disease.
- Public health departments are responsible for preventing the spread of TB, finding where TB has already spread using contact investigation.
- Debilitated patients may require therapy for other medical conditions, including substance abuse and HIV infection, and some may need nutritional support.
- Surgery may be needed to remove destroyed lung tissue, space-occupying lesions, and some extrapulmonary lesions.

PHARMACOLOGIC TREATMENT

Latent Infection

- As described in **Table 49–3**, chemoprophylaxis should be initiated in patients to reduce the risk of progression to active disease.
- **Isoniazid**, 300 mg daily in adults, is the preferred treatment for latent TB in the United States, generally given for 9 months.
- Rifampin, 600 mg daily for 4 months, can be used when isoniazid resistance is suspected or when the patient cannot tolerate isoniazid. Rifabutin, 300 mg daily, may be substituted for rifampin for patients at high risk of drug interactions.
- Pregnant women, alcoholics, and patients with poor diets who are treated with isoniazid should receive pyridoxine, 10 to 50 mg daily, to reduce the incidence of CNS effects or peripheral neuropathies.

TABLE 49–3 Recommended Drug Regimens for Treatment of Latent Tuberculosis (TB) Infection in Adults

Drug	Interval and Duration	Comments	Rating[a] (Evidence)[b] HIV–	HIV+
Isoniazid	Daily for 9 months[cd]	In HIV-infected patients, isoniazid may be administered concurrently with nucleoside reverse transcriptase inhibitors, protease inhibitors, or nonnucleoside reverse transcriptase inhibitors	A (II)	A (II)
	Twice weekly for 9 months[cd]	Directly observed therapy must be used with twice-weekly dosing	B (II)	B (II)
Isoniazid	Daily for 6 months[d]	Not indicated for HIV-infected persons, those with fibrotic lesions on chest radiographs, or children	B (I)	C (I)
	Twice weekly for 6 months[d]	Directly observed therapy must be used with twice-weekly dosing	B (II)	B (III)
Rifampin	Daily for 4 months	For persons who are contacts of patients with isoniazid-resistant, rifampin-susceptible TB who cannot tolerate pyrazinamide	B (II)	C (I)

HIV, human immunodeficiency virus; –, negative; +, positive.
[a]Strength of recommendation: A, preferred; B, acceptable alternative; C, offer when A and B cannot be given.
[b]Quality of evidence: I, randomized clinical trial data; II, data from clinical trials that are not randomized or were conducted in other populations; III, expert opinion.
[c]Recommended regimen for children younger than 18 years.
[d]Recommended regimens for pregnant women. Some experts would use rifampin and pyrazinamide for 2 months as an alternative regimen in HIV-infected pregnant women, although pyrazinamide should be avoided during the first trimester.
Adapted from Centers for Disease Control and Prevention. Targeted tuberculin testing and treatment of latent tuberculosis infection. MMWR 2000;49(RR-6):31.

Treating Active Disease

- **Table 49–4** lists options for treatment of culture-positive pulmonary TB caused by drug-susceptible organisms. Doses of antituberculosis drugs are given in **Table 49–5**. The standard TB treatment regimen is isoniazid, rifampin, pyrazinamide, and ethambutol for 2 months, followed by isoniazid and rifampin for 4 months. Ethambutol can be stopped if susceptibility to isoniazid, rifampin, and pyrazinamide is shown.
- Appropriate samples should be sent for culture and susceptibility testing prior to initiating therapy for all patients with active TB. The data should guide the initial drug selection for the new patient. If susceptibility data

TABLE 49–4 Drug Regimens for Culture-Positive Pulmonary Tuberculosis Caused by Drug-Susceptible Organisms

	Initial Phase		Continuation Phase			Range of Total Doses (Minimal Duration)	Rating[a] (Evidence)[b]	
Regimen	Drugs	Interval and Doses[c] (Minimal Duration)	Regimen	Drugs	Interval and Doses[c,d] (Minimal Duration)		HIV−	HIV+
1	Isoniazid, rifampin, pyrazinamide, ethambutol	Seven days per week for 56 doses (8 wk) or 5 days/wk for 40 doses (8 wk)[c]	1a	Isoniazid/ rifampin	Seven days per week for 126 doses (18 wk) or 5 days/wk for 90 doses (18 wk)[c]	182–130 (26 wk)	A (I)	A (II)
			1b	Isoniazid/ rifampin	Twice weekly for 36 doses (18 wk)	92–76 (26 wk)	A (I)	A (II)[f]
			1c[e]	Isoniazid/ rifapentine	Once weekly for 18 doses (18 wk)	74–58 (26 wk)	B (I)	E (I)
2	Isoniazid, rifampin, pyrazinamide, ethambutol	Seven days per week for 14 doses (2 wk), then twice weekly for 12 doses (6 wk) or 5 days/wk for 10 doses (2 wk)[e] then twice weekly for 12 doses (6 weeks)	2a	Isoniazid/ rifampin	Twice weekly for 36 doses (18 wk)	62–58 (26 wk)	A (II)	B (II)[f]
			2b[g]	Isoniazid/ rifapentine	Once weekly for 18 doses (18 wk)	44–40 (26 wk)	B (I)	E (I)

(continued)

TABLE 49–4 Drug Regimens for Culture-Positive Pulmonary Tuberculosis Caused by Drug-Susceptible Organisms *(Continued)*

	Initial Phase		Continuation Phase			Rating[a] (Evidence)[b]	
Regimen	Drugs	Interval and Doses[c] (Minimal Duration)	Regimen	Drugs	Interval and Doses[c,d] (Minimal Duration)	Range of Total Doses (Minimal Duration)	HIV–	HIV+
3	Isoniazid, rifampin, pyrazinamide, ethambutol	Three times weekly for 24 doses (8 wk)	3a	Isoniazid/ rifampin	Three times weekly for 54 doses (18 wk)	78 (26 wk)	B (I)	B (II)
4	Isoniazid, rifampin, ethambutol	Seven days per week for 56 doses (8 wk) or 5 days/wk for 40 doses (8 wk)[c]	4a	Isoniazid/ rifampin	Seven days per week for 217 doses (31 wk) or 5 days/wk for 155 doses (31 wk)[e]	273–195 (39 wk)	C (I)	C (II)
			4b	Isoniazid/ rifampin	Twice weekly for 62 doses (31 wk)	118–102 (39 wk)	C (I)	C (II)

HIV, human immunodeficiency virus.

[a]Ratings: A, preferred; B, acceptable alternative; C, offer when A and B cannot be given; E, should never be given.

[b]Evidence ratings: I, randomized clinical trial; II, data from clinical trials that were not randomized or were conducted in other populations; III, expert opinion.

[c]When directly observed therapy is used, drugs may be given 5 days per week and the necessary number of doses adjusted accordingly. Although there are no studies that compare five with seven daily doses, extensive experience indicates this would be an effective practice.

[d]Patients with cavitation on initial chest radiograph and positive cultures at completion of 2 months of therapy should receive a 7-month (31-wk; either 217 doses [daily] or 62 doses [twice weekly]) continuation phase.

[e]Five-day-a-week administration is always given by directly observed therapy. Rating for 5-day-per-week regimens is A (II).

[f]Not recommended for HIV-infected patients with CD4+ cell counts <100 cells/μL.

[g]Options 1c and 2b should be used only in HIV-negative patients who have negative sputum smears at the time of completion of 2 months of therapy and who do not have cavitation on initial chest radiograph. For patients started on this regimen and found to have a positive culture from the 2-month specimen, treatment should be extended an extra 3 months.

From Centers for Disease Control and Prevention. Treatment of tuberculosis. MMWR 2003;52(RR-11).

TABLE 49-5 Doses[a] of Antituberculosis Drugs for Adults and Children[b]

Drug	Preparation	Adults/Children	Doses			
			Daily	1 × per week	2 × per week	3 × per week
First-line drugs						
Isoniazid	Tablets (50 mg, 100 mg, 300 mg); elixir (50 mg/ 5 mL); aqueous solution (100 mg/mL) for intravenous or intramuscular injection	Adults (max)	5 mg/kg (300 mg)	15 mg/kg (900 mg)	15 mg/kg (900 mg)	15 mg/kg (900 mg)
		Children (max)	10–15 mg/kg (300 mg)	—	20–30 mg/kg (300 mg)	—
Rifampin	Capsule (150 mg, 300 mg); powder may be suspended for oral administration; aqueous solution for intravenous injection	Adults[c] (max)	10 mg/kg (600 mg)	—	10 mg/kg (600 mg)	10 mg/kg (600 mg)
		Children (max)	10–20 mg/kg (600 mg)	—	10–20 mg/kg (600 mg)	—
Rifabutin	Capsule (150 mg)	Adults[c] (max)	5 mg/kg (300 mg)	—	5 mg/kg (300 mg)	5 mg/kg (300 mg)
		Children	Appropriate dosing for children is unknown	Appropriate dosing for children is unknown	Appropriate dosing for children is unknown	Appropriate dosing for children is unknown
Rifapentine	Tablet (150 mg, film coated)	Adults	—	10 mg/kg (continuation phase) (600 mg usual adult dose)	—	—
		Children	The drug is not approved for use in children	The drug is not approved for use in children	The drug is not approved for use in children	The drug is not approved for use in children

(continued)

TABLE 49-5 Doses[a] of Antituberculosis Drugs for Adults and Children[b] *(Continued)*

Drug	Preparation	Adults/Children	Daily	1 × per week	2 × per week	3 × per week
First-line drugs						
Pyrazinamide	Tablet (500 mg, scored)	Adults	1,000 mg (40–55 kg) 1,500 mg (56–75 kg) 2,000 mg (76–90 kg)	— — —	2,000 mg (40–55 kg) 3,000 mg (56–75 kg) 4,000 mg (76–90 kg)[i]	1,500 mg (40–55 kg) 2,500 mg (56–75 kg) 3,000 mg (76–90 kg)[i]
		Children (max)	15–30 mg/kg (2 g)	—	50 mg/kg (2 g)	—
Ethambutol	Tablet (100 mg, 400 mg)	Adults	800 mg (40–55 kg) 1,200 mg (56–75 kg) 1,600 mg (76–90 kg)[i]	— — —	2,000 mg (40–55 kg) 2,800 mg (56–75 kg) 4,000 mg (76–90 kg)[i]	1,200 mg (40–55 kg) 2,000 mg (56–75 kg) 2,400 mg (76–90 kg)[i]
		Children[d] (max)	15–20 mg/kg daily (1 g)	—	50 mg/kg (2.5 g)	—
Second-line drugs						
Cycloserine	Capsule (250 mg)	Adults (max)	10–15 mg/kg/day (1 g in two doses), usually 500–750 mg/day in two doses[e]	There are no data to support intermittent administration	There are no data to support intermittent administration	There are no data to support intermittent administration
		Children (max)	10–15 mg/kg/day (1 g/day)	—	—	—
Ethionamide	Tablet (250 mg)	Adults[f] (max)	15–20 mg/kg/day (1 g/day), usually 500–750 mg/day in a single daily dose or two divided doses[f]	There are no data to support intermittent administration	There are no data to support intermittent administration	There are no data to support intermittent administration

Drug	Preparation		Daily dose	There are no data to support intermittent administration	There are no data to support intermittent administration	There are no data to support intermittent administration
Streptomycin	Aqueous solution (1-g vials) for intravenous or intramuscular administration	Children (max)	15–20 mg/kg/day (1 g/day)	There are no data to support intermittent administration	There are no data to support intermittent administration	There are no data to support intermittent administration
		Adults (max)	20–40 mg/kg/day (1 g)	g –	g, 20 mg/kg	g –
Amikacin/kanamycin	Aqueous solution (500 mg and 1 g vials) for intravenous administration	Children (max)	15–30 mg/kg/day	There are no data to support intermittent administration	There are no data to support intermittent administration	There are no data to support intermittent administration
		Adults (max)	15–30 mg/kg/day (1 g) intravenous or intramuscular as a single daily dose	g –	g, 15–30 mg/kg	g –
Capreomycin	Aqueous solution (1 g vials) for intravenous or intramuscular administration	Adults (max)	15–30 mg/kg/day (1 g) as a single daily dose	There are no data to support intermittent administration	There are no data to support intermittent administration	There are no data to support intermittent administration
		Children (max)		g –	15–30 mg/kg	g –
p-Amino-salicylic acid (PAS)	Granules (4-g packets) can be mixed with food; tablets (500 mg) are still available in some countries, but not in the United States; a solution for intravenous administration is available in Europe	Adults	8–12 g/day in two or three doses	There are no data to support intermittent administration	There are no data to support intermittent administration	There are no data to support intermittent administration

(continued)

TABLE 49-5 Doses*a* of Antituberculosis Drugs for Adults and Children*b* (Continued)

Drug	Preparation	Adults/Children	Daily	1 × per week	2 × per week	3 × per week
					Doses	
Second-line drugs						
		Children (max)	200–300 mg/kg/day in two to four divided doses (10 g)	There are no data to support intermittent administration	There are no data to support intermittent administration	There are no data to support intermittent administration
Moxifloxacin*h*	Tablets (400 mg); aqueous solution (400 mg/250 mL) for intravenous injection	Adults	400 mg daily	There are no data to support intermittent administration	There are no data to support intermittent administration	There are no data to support intermittent administration

*a*Dose per weight is based on ideal body weight. Children weighing more than 40 kg should be dosed as adults.

*b*For purposes of this document, adult dosing begins at age 15 years.

*c*Dose may need to be adjusted when there is concomitant use of protease inhibitors or nonnucleoside reverse transcriptase inhibitors.

*d*The drug can likely be used safely in older children but should be used with caution in children less than 5 years of age, in whom visual acuity can not be monitored. In younger children, ethambutol at the dose of 15 mg/kg per day can be used if there is suspected or proven resistance to isoniazid or rifampin.

*e*It should be noted that although this is the dose recommended generally, most clinicians with experience using cycloserine indicate that it is unusual for patients to be able to tolerate this amount. Serum concentration measurements are often useful in determining the optimal dose for a given patient.

*f*The single daily dose can be given at bedtime or with the main meal.

*g*Dose: 15 mg/kg per day (1 g) but 10 mg/kg in persons older than 59 years of age (750 mg). Usual dose: 750–1,000 mg administered intramuscularly or intravenously, given as a single dose 5–7 days/week and reduced to two or three times per week after the first 2–4 months or after culture conversion, depending on the efficacy of the other drugs in the regimen.

*h*The long-term (more than several weeks) use of moxifloxacin in children and adolescents has not been approved because of concerns about effects on bone and cartilage growth. The optimal dose is not known.

are not available, the drug resistance pattern in the area where the patient likely acquired TB should be used.

- If the patient is being evaluated for the retreatment of TB, it is imperative to know what drugs were used previously and for how long.
- Patients must complete 6 months or more of treatment. HIV-positive patients should be treated for an additional 3 months and at least 6 months from the time that they convert to smear and culture negativity. When isoniazid and rifampin cannot be used, treatment duration becomes 2 years or more, regardless of immune status.
- Patients who are slow to respond, those who remain culture positive at 2 months of treatment, those with cavitary lesions on chest radiograph, and HIV-positive patients should be treated for 9 months and for at least 6 months from the time they convert to smear and culture negativity.

DRUG RESISTANCE

- If the organism is drug resistant, the aim is to introduce two or more active agents that the patient has not received previously. With MDR-TB, no standard regimen can be proposed. It is critical to avoid monotherapy or adding only a single drug to a failing regimen.
- Drug resistance should be suspected in the following situations:
  ✓ Patients who have received prior therapy for TB
  ✓ Patients from geographic areas with a high prevalence of resistance (South Africa, Mexico, Southeast Asia, the Baltic countries, and the former Soviet states)
  ✓ Patients who are homeless, institutionalized, IV drug abusers, and/or infected with HIV
  ✓ Patients who still have acid-fast bacilli–positive sputum smears after 2 months of therapy
  ✓ Patients who still have positive cultures after 2 to 4 months of therapy
  ✓ Patients who fail therapy or relapse after retreatment
  ✓ Patients known to be exposed to MDR-TB cases

SPECIAL POPULATIONS

Tuberculous Meningitis and Extrapulmonary Disease

- In general, **isoniazid, pyrazinamide, ethionamide,** and **cycloserine** penetrate the cerebrospinal fluid readily. Patients with CNS TB are often treated for longer periods (9–12 months). Extrapulmonary TB of the soft tissues can be treated with conventional regimens. TB of the bone is typically treated for 9 months, occasionally with surgical debridement.

Children

- TB in children may be treated with regimens similar to those used in adults, although some physicians still prefer to extend treatment to 9 months. Pediatric doses of drugs should be used.

Pregnant Women

- The usual treatment of pregnant women is isoniazid, rifampin, and ethambutol for 9 months.

- Women with TB should be cautioned against becoming pregnant, as the disease poses a risk to the fetus as well as to the mother. Isoniazid or ethambutol is relatively safe when used during pregnancy. Supplementation with B vitamins is particularly important during pregnancy. **Rifampin** has been rarely associated with birth defects, but those seen are occasionally severe, including limb reduction and CNS lesions. **Pyrazinamide** has not been studied in a large number of pregnant women, but anecdotal information suggests that it may be safe. **Ethionamide** may be associated with premature delivery, congenital deformities, and Down syndrome when used during pregnancy. **Streptomycin** has been associated with hearing impairment in the newborn, including complete deafness. **Cycloserine** is not recommended during pregnancy. Fluoroquinolones should be avoided in pregnancy and during nursing.

Renal Failure

- In nearly all patients, isoniazid and rifampin do not require dose modifications in renal failure. Pyrazinamide and ethambutol typically require a reduction in dosing frequency from daily to three times weekly (**Table 49–6**).

EVALUATION OF THERAPEUTIC OUTCOMES AND PATIENT MONITORING

- The most serious problem with TB therapy is nonadherence to the prescribed regimen. The most effective way to ensure adherence is with directly observed therapy.
- Symptomatic patients should be isolated and have sputum samples sent for acid-fast bacilli stains every 1 to 2 weeks until two consecutive smears are negative. Once on maintenance therapy, patients should have sputum cultures performed monthly until negative, which generally occurs over 2 to 3 months. If sputum cultures continue to be positive after 2 months, drug susceptibility testing should be repeated, and serum drug concentrations should be checked.
- Patients should have blood urea nitrogen, serum creatinine, aspartate transaminase or alanine transaminase, and a complete blood count determined at baseline and periodically, depending on the presence of other factors that may increase the likelihood of toxicity (advanced age, alcohol abuse, and possibly pregnancy). Hepatotoxicity should be suspected in patients whose transaminases exceed five times the upper limit of normal or whose total bilirubin exceeds 3 mg/dL. At this point, the offending agent(s) should be discontinued and alternatives selected.
- Therapy with isoniazid results in a transient elevation in serum transaminases in 12% to 15% of patients and usually occurs within the first 8 to 12 weeks of therapy. Risk factors for hepatotoxicity include patient age, preexisting liver disease, and pregnancy or postpartum state. Isoniazid also may result in neurotoxicity, most frequently presenting as peripheral neuropathy or, in overdose, seizures and coma. Patients with pyridoxine deficiency, such as alcoholics, children, and the malnourished, are at

		Recommended Dose and Frequency for
	Change in	**Patients with Creatinine Clearance <30 mL/min**
Drug	**Frequency?**	**or for Patients Receiving Hemodialysis**

TABLE 49–6 Dosing Recommendations for Adult Patients with Reduced Renal Function and for Adult Patients Receiving Hemodialysis

Drug	Change in Frequency?	Recommended Dose and Frequency for Patients with Creatinine Clearance <30 mL/min or for Patients Receiving Hemodialysis
Isoniazid	No change	300 mg once daily, or 900 mg three times weekly
Rifampin	No change	600 mg once daily, or 600 mg three times weekly
Pyrazinamide	Yes	25–35 mg/kg per dose three times weekly (not daily)
Ethambutol	Yes	15–25 mg/kg per dose three times weekly (not daily)
Levofloxacin	Yes	750–1,000 mg per dose three times weekly (not daily)
Cycloserine	Yes	250 mg once daily, or 500 mg/dose three times weekly[a]
Ethionamide	No change	250–500 mg per dose daily
p-Aminosalicylic acid	No change	4 g per dose twice daily
Streptomycin	Yes	12–15 mg/kg per dose two or three times weekly (not daily)
Capreomycin	Yes	12–15 mg/kg per dose two or three times weekly (not daily)
Kanamycin	Yes	12–15 mg/kg per dose two or three times weekly (not daily)
Amikacin	Yes	12–15 mg/kg per dose two or three times weekly (not daily)

Note: Standard doses are given unless there is intolerance.

The medications should be given after hemodialysis on the day of hemodialysis. Monitoring of serum drug concentrations should be considered to ensure adequate drug absorption, without excessive accumulation, and to assist in avoiding toxicity. Data currently are not available for patients receiving peritoneal dialysis. Until data become available, begin with doses recommended for patients receiving hemodialysis and verify adequacy of dosing using serum concentration monitoring.

[a]The appropriateness of 250 mg daily doses has not been established. There should be careful monitoring for evidence of neurotoxicity.

increased risk, as are patients who are slow acetylators of isoniazid and those predisposed to neuropathy, such as those with diabetes.

- Elevations in hepatic enzymes have been attributed to rifampin in 10% to 15% of patients, with overt hepatotoxicity occurring in <1%. More frequent adverse effects of rifampin include rash, fever, and GI distress.
- Rifampin's induction of hepatic enzymes may enhance the elimination of a number of drugs, most notably protease inhibitors. Women who use oral contraceptives should be advised to use another form of contraception during therapy.
- The red colorizing effects of rifampin on urine, other secretions, and contact lenses should be discussed with the patient.
- Retrobulbar neuritis is the major adverse effect noted in patients treated with ethambutol. Patients usually complain of a change in visual acuity and/or inability to see the color green. Vision testing should be performed on all patients who must receive ethambutol for longer than 2 months.

- Impairment of eighth cranial nerve function is the most important adverse effect of streptomycin. Vestibular function is most frequently affected, but hearing may also be impaired. Audiometric testing should be performed in patients who must receive streptomycin for longer than 2 months. Streptomycin occasionally causes nephrotoxicity.

See Chapter 121, Tuberculosis, authored by Charles A. Peloquin and Rocsanna Namdar, for a more detailed discussion of this topic.

CHAPTER 50

Urinary Tract Infections and Prostatitis

DEFINITION

- Infections of the urinary tract represent a wide variety of clinical syndromes, including urethritis, cystitis, prostatitis, and pyelonephritis.
- A urinary tract infection (UTI) is defined as the presence of microorganisms in the urine that cannot be accounted for by contamination. The organisms have the potential to invade the tissues of the urinary tract and adjacent structures.
- Lower tract infections include cystitis (bladder), urethritis (urethra), prostatitis (prostate gland), and epididymitis. Upper tract infections involve the kidney and are referred to as *pyelonephritis*.
- Uncomplicated UTIs are not associated with structural or neurologic abnormalities that may interfere with the normal flow of urine or the voiding mechanism. Complicated UTIs are the result of a predisposing lesion of the urinary tract, such as a congenital abnormality or distortion of the urinary tract, stone, indwelling catheter, prostatic hypertrophy, obstruction, or neurologic deficit that interferes with the normal flow of urine and urinary tract defenses.
- Recurrent UTIs, three or more UTIs occurring within 1 year, are characterized by multiple symptomatic episodes with asymptomatic periods occurring between these episodes. These infections are due to reinfection or to relapse. Reinfections are caused by a different organism and account for the majority of recurrent UTIs. Relapse represents the development of repeated infections caused by the same initial organism.

PATHOPHYSIOLOGY

- The bacteria causing UTIs usually originate from bowel flora of the host.
- UTIs can be acquired via three possible routes: the ascending, hematogenous, and lymphatic pathways.
- In female patients, the short length of the urethra and proximity to the perirectal area make colonization of the urethra likely. Bacteria are then believed to enter the bladder from the urethra. Once in the bladder, the organisms multiply quickly and can ascend the ureters to the kidney.
- Three factors determine the development of UTI: the size of the inoculum, virulence of the microorganism, and competency of the natural host defense mechanisms.
- Patients who are unable to void urine completely are at greater risk of developing UTIs and frequently have recurrent infections.
- An important virulence factor of bacteria is their ability to adhere to urinary epithelial cells by fimbriae, resulting in colonization of the urinary tract, bladder infections, and pyelonephritis. Other virulence factors are hemolysin, a cytotoxic protein produced by bacteria that lyses a wide

range of cells including erythrocytes, polymorphonuclear leukocytes, and monocytes; and aerobactin, which facilitates the binding and uptake of iron by *Escherichia coli.*

MICROBIOLOGY

- The most common cause of uncomplicated UTIs is *E. coli,* accounting for >80% to 90% of community-acquired infections. Additional causative organisms are *Staphylococcus saprophyticus* (coagulase-negative staphylococcus), *Klebsiella pneumoniae, Proteus* spp., *Pseudomonas aeruginosa,* and *Enterococcus* spp.
- The urinary pathogens in complicated or nosocomial infections may include *E. coli,* which accounts for <50% of these infections, *Proteus* spp., *K. pneumoniae, Enterobacter* spp., *P. aeruginosa,* staphylococci, and enterococci. *Candida* spp. have become common causes of urinary infection in the critically ill and chronically catheterized patient.
- The majority of UTIs are caused by a single organism; however, in patients with stones, indwelling urinary catheters, or chronic renal abscesses, multiple organisms may be isolated.

CLINICAL PRESENTATION

- The typical symptoms of lower and upper UTIs are presented in Table 50-1.
- Symptoms alone are unreliable for the diagnosis of bacterial UTIs. The key to the diagnosis of a UTI is the ability to demonstrate significant numbers of microorganisms present in an appropriate urine specimen to distinguish contamination from infection.

TABLE 50–1	Clinical Presentation of Urinary Tract Infections (UTIs) in Adults

Signs and symptoms

Lower UTI: dysuria, urgency, frequency, nocturia, suprapubic heaviness

Gross hematuria

Upper UTI: flank pain, fever, nausea, vomiting, malaise

Physical examination

Upper UTI: costovertebral tenderness

Laboratory tests

Bacteriuria

Pyuria (WBC >10/mm^3)

Nitrite-positive urine (with nitrite reducers)

Leukocyte esterase-positive urine

Antibody-coated bacteria (upper UTI)

WBC, white blood cell count.

TABLE 50–2	Diagnostic Criteria for Significant Bacteriuria

$\geq 10^2$ CFU coliforms/mL or $\geq 10^5$ CFU noncoliforms/mL in a symptomatic female patient

$\geq 10^3$ CFU bacteria/mL in a symptomatic male patient

$\geq 10^5$ CFU bacteria/mL in asymptomatic individuals on two consecutive specimens

Any growth of bacteria on suprapubic catheterization in a symptomatic patient

$\geq 10^2$ CFU bacteria/mL in a catheterized patient

CFU, colony-forming unit.

- Elderly patients frequently do not experience specific urinary symptoms, but they will present with altered mental status, change in eating habits, or GI symptoms.
- A standard urinalysis should be obtained in the initial assessment of a patient. Microscopic examination of the urine should be performed by preparation of a Gram stain of unspun or centrifuged urine. The presence of at least one organism per oil-immersion field in a properly collected uncentrifuged specimen correlates with >100,000 colony-forming units (CFU)/mL (10^5 CFU/mL) of urine.
- Criteria for defining significant bacteriuria are listed in Table 50–2.
- The presence of pyuria (>10 white blood cells/mm^3) in a symptomatic patient correlates with significant bacteriuria.
- The nitrite test can be used to detect the presence of nitrate-reducing bacteria in the urine (e.g., *E. coli*). The leukocyte esterase test is a rapid dipstick test to detect pyuria.
- The most reliable method of diagnosing UTIs is by quantitative urine culture. Patients with infection usually have >10^5 bacteria/mL of urine, although as many as one third of women with symptomatic infection have <10^5 bacteria/mL.
- A method to detect upper UTI is the antibody-coated bacteria test, an immunofluorescent method that detects bacteria coated with immunoglobulin in freshly voided urine.

TREATMENT

- The goals of treatment for UTIs are to eradicate the invading organisms, prevent or treat systemic consequences of infection, and prevent recurrence of infection.

GENERAL PRINCIPLES

- The management of a patient with a UTI includes initial evaluation, selection of an antibacterial agent and duration of therapy, and follow-up evaluation.
- The initial selection of an antimicrobial agent for the treatment of UTI is primarily based on the severity of the presenting signs and symptoms, the site of infection, and whether the infection is determined to be complicated or uncomplicated.

PHARMACOLOGIC TREATMENT

- The ability to eradicate bacteria from the urinary tract is directly related to the sensitivity of the organism and the achievable concentration of the antimicrobial agent in the urine.
- The therapeutic management of UTIs is best accomplished by first categorizing the type of infection: acute uncomplicated cystitis, symptomatic abacteriuria, asymptomatic bacteriuria, complicated UTIs, recurrent infections, or prostatitis.
- **Table 50–3** lists the most common agents used in the treatment of UTIs, along with comments concerning their general use.
- **Table 50–4** presents an overview of various therapeutic options for outpatient therapy for UTI.
- **Table 50–5** describes empiric treatment regimens for specific clinical situations.

TABLE 50–3	Commonly Used Antimicrobial Agents in the Treatment of Urinary Tract Infections (UTIs)
Agent	**Comments**
Oral therapy	
Trimethoprim–sulfamethoxazole	This combination is highly effective against most aerobic enteric bacteria except *Pseudomonas aeruginosa*. High urinary tract tissue levels and urine levels are achieved, which may be important in complicated infection treatment. Also effective as prophylaxis for recurrent infections.
Penicillins Ampicillin Amoxicillin–clavulanic acid	Ampicillin is the standard penicillin that has broad-spectrum activity. Increasing *Escherichia coli* resistance has limited amoxicillin use in acute cystitis. Drug of choice for enterococci sensitive to penicillin. Amoxicillin–clavulanate is preferred for resistance problems.
Cephalosporins Cephalexin Cefaclor Cefadroxil Cefuroxime Cefixime Cefzil Cefpodoxime	There are no major advantages of these agents over other agents in the treatment of UTIs, and they are more expensive. They may be useful in cases of resistance to amoxicillin and trimethoprim–sulfamethoxazole. These agents are not active against enterococci.
Tetracyclines Tetracycline Doxycycline Minocycline	These agents have been effective for initial episodes of UTIs; however, resistance develops rapidly, and their use is limited. These agents also lead to candidal overgrowth. They are useful primarily for chlamydial infections.
Fluoroquinolones Ciprofloxacin Levofloxacin	The newer quinolones have a greater spectrum of activity, including *P. aeruginosa*. These agents are effective for pyelonephritis and prostatitis. Avoid in pregnancy and with children. Moxifloxacin should not be used because of inadequate urinary concentrations.

(continued)

TABLE 50–3	Commonly Used Antimicrobial Agents in the Treatment of Urinary Tract Infections (UTIs) *(Continued)*
Agent	**Comments**
Oral therapy	
Nitrofurantoin	This agent is effective as both a therapeutic and prophylactic agent in patients with recurrent UTIs. Main advantage is the lack of resistance even after long courses of therapy. Adverse effects may limit use (GI intolerance, neuropathies, and pulmonary reactions).
Azithromycin	Single-dose therapy for chlamydial infections
Fosfomycin	Single-dose therapy for uncomplicated infections
Parenteral therapy	
Aminoglycosides Gentamicin Tobramycin Amikacin	Gentamicin and tobramycin are equally effective; gentamicin is less expensive. Tobramycin has better pseudomonal activity, which may be important in serious systemic infections. Amikacin generally is reserved for multiresistant bacteria.
Penicillins Ampicillin Ampicillin–sulbactam Ticarcillin–clavulanate Piperacillin–tazobactam	These agents generally are equally effective for susceptible bacteria. The extended-spectrum penicillins are more active against *P. aeruginosa* and enterococci and often are preferred over cephalosporins. They are very useful in renally impaired patients or when an aminoglycoside is to be avoided.
Cephalosporins, first-, second-, and third-generation	Second- and third-generation cephalosporins have a broad spectrum of activity against gram-negative bacteria but are not active against enterococci and have limited activity against *P. aeruginosa*. Ceftazidime and cefepime are active against *P. aeruginosa*. They are useful for nosocomial infections and urosepsis due to susceptible pathogens.
Carbapenems/ monobactams Imipenem–cilastatin Meropenem Ertapenem Doripenem	These agents have a broad spectrum of activity, including gram-positive, gram-negative, and anaerobic bacteria. Imipenem, meropenem, and doripenem are active against *P. aeruginosa* and enterococci, but ertapenem is not. All may be associated with candidal superinfections.
Aztreonam	A monobactam that is only active against gram-negative bacteria, including some strains of *P. aeruginosa*. Generally useful for nosocomial infections when aminoglycosides are to be avoided and in penicillin-sensitive patients.
Fluoroquinolones Ciprofloxacin Levofloxacin	These agents have broad-spectrum activity against both gram-negative and gram-positive bacteria. They provide urine and high-tissue concentrations and are actively secreted in reduced renal function.

TABLE 50–4	Overview of Outpatient Antimicrobial Therapy for Lower Tract Infections in Adults			
Indications	**Antibiotic**	**Dose**[a]	**Interval**	**Duration**
Lower tract infections	TMP-SMX	1 DS tablet	Twice daily	3 days
Uncomplicated	Ciprofloxacin	250 mg	Twice daily	3 days
	Levofloxacin	250 mg	Once daily	3 days
	Amoxicillin	500 mg	Twice daily	5–7 days
	Amoxicillin–clavulanate	500 mg	Every 8 hours	5–7 days
	Trimethoprim	100 mg	Twice a day	3–5 days
	Nitrofurantoin macrocrystal	100 mg	Every 6 hours	7 days
	Nitrofurantoin monohydrate	100 mg	Twice daily	5 days
	Fosfomycin	3 g	Single dose	1 day
Complicated	TMP-SMX	1 DS tablet	Twice daily	7–10 days
	Ciprofloxacin	250–500 mg	Twice daily	7–10 days
	Levofloxacin	250 mg	Once daily	10 days
	Levofloxacin	750 mg	Once daily	5 days
	Amoxicillin-clavulanate	500 mg	Every 8 hours	7–10 days
Recurrent infections	Nitrofurantoin	50 mg	Once daily	6 months
	TMP-SMX	½ SS tablet	Once daily	6 months
Acute urethral syndrome	TMP-SMX	1 DS tablet	Twice daily	3 days
Failure of TMP-SMX	Azithromycin	1 g	Single dose	
	Doxycycline	100 mg	Twice daily	7 days
Acute pyelonephritis	TMP-SMX	1 DS tablet	Twice daily	14 days
	Ciprofloxacin	500 mg	Twice daily	14 days
	Levofloxacin	250 mg	Once daily	10 days
	Levofloxacin	750 mg	Once daily	5 days
	Amoxicillin-clavulanate	500 mg	Every 8 hours	14 days

DS, double strength; SS, single strength; TMP-SMX, trimethoprim–sulfamethoxazole.
[a]Dosing intervals for normal renal function.

Acute Uncomplicated Cystitis

- These infections are predominantly caused by *E. coli*, and antimicrobial therapy should be directed against this organism initially. Because the causative organisms and their susceptibilities are generally known, a cost-effective approach to management is recommended that includes a urinalysis and initiation of empiric therapy without a urine culture (**Fig. 50–1**).
- Short-course therapy (3-day therapy) with **trimethoprim–sulfamethoxazole** or a **fluoroquinolone** (e.g., **ciprofloxacin** or **levofloxacin**) is superior to single-dose therapy for uncomplicated infection and should be the treatment of choice. Amoxicillin or sulfonamides are not recommended because of the high incidence of resistant *E. coli*. Follow-up urine cultures are not necessary in patients who respond.

TABLE 50-5 Empirical Treatment of Urinary Tract Infections and Prostatitis

Diagnosis	Pathogens	Treatment Recommendation	Comments
Acute uncomplicated cystitis	Escherichia coli	1. Trimethoprim–sulfamethoxazole for 3 days (A, I)[a]	Short-course therapy more effective than single dose
	Staphylococcus saprophyticus	2. Fluoroquinolone for 3 days (A, II)[a]	β-Lactams as a group are not as effective in acute cystitis than trimethoprim–sulfamethoxazole or the fluoroquinolones[a]
		3. Nitrofurantoin for 5 days (B, I)[a]	
		4. β-Lactams for 3 days (E, III)[a]	
Pregnancy	As above	1. Amoxicillin–clavulanate for 7 days	Avoid trimethoprim–sulfamethoxazole during third trimester
		2. Cephalosporin for 7 days	
		3. Trimethoprim–sulfamethoxazole for 7 days	
Acute pyelonephritis			
Uncomplicated	E. coli	1. Quinolone for 14 days (A, II)[a]	Can be managed as outpatient
		2. Trimethoprim–sulfamethoxazole (if susceptible) for 14 days (B, II)[a]	
	Gram-positive bacteria	1. Amoxicillin or amoxicillin–clavulanic acid for 14 days (B, III)[a]	

(continued)

TABLE 50–5 Empirical Treatment of Urinary Tract Infections and Prostatitis *(Continued)*

Diagnosis	Pathogens	Treatment Recommendation	Comments
Complicated	E. coli Proteus mirabilis Klebisella pneumoniae Pseudomonas aeruginosa Enterococcus faecalis	1. Quinolone for 14 days (B, III)[a] 2. Extended-spectrum penicillin + aminoglycoside (B, III)[a]	Severity of illness will determine duration of IV therapy; culture results should direct therapy Oral therapy may complete 14 days of therapy
Prostatitis	E. coli K. pneumoniae Proteus spp. P. aeruginosa	1. Trimethoprim–sulfamethoxazole for 4 to 6 weeks 2. Quinolone for 4 to 6 weeks	Acute prostatitis may require IV therapy initially Chronic prostatitis may require longer treatment periods or surgery

[a]Strength of recommendations: A, good evidence for; B, moderate evidence for; C, poor evidence for and against; D, moderate against; E, good evidence against. Quality of evidence: I, at least one proper randomized, controlled study; II, one well-designed clinical trial; III, evidence from opinions, clinical experience, and expert committees.

Data from Warren JW, Abrutyn E, Hebel JR, et al. Surviving sepsis campaign guidelines for management of severe sepsis and septic shock. Crit Care Med 2004;32:858–873.

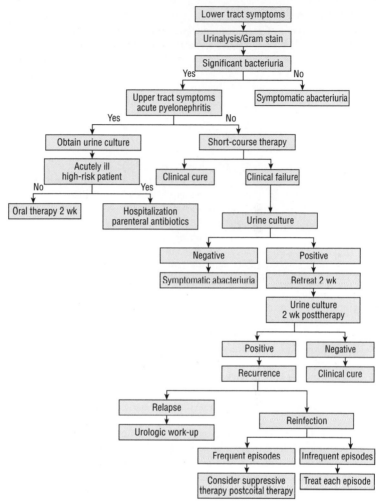

FIGURE 50–1. Management of urinary tract infections in women.

Symptomatic Abacteriuria

- Single-dose or short-course therapy with **trimethoprim–sulfamethoxazole** has been used effectively, and prolonged courses of therapy are not necessary for the majority of patients. If single-dose or short-course therapy is ineffective, a culture should be obtained.
- If the patient reports recent sexual activity, therapy for *Chlamydia trachomatis* should be considered (azithromycin 1 g as a single dose or doxycycline 100 mg twice daily for 7 days).

Asymptomatic Bacteriuria

- The management of asymptomatic bacteriuria depends on the age of the patient and, if female, whether she is pregnant. In children, treatment should consist of conventional courses of therapy, as described for symptomatic infections.
- In the nonpregnant female, therapy is controversial; however, it appears that treatment has little effect on the natural course of infections.

Complicated Urinary Tract Infections

ACUTE PYELONEPHRITIS

- The presentation of high-grade fever (>38.3°C [100.9°F]) and severe flank pain should be treated as acute pyelonephritis, and aggressive management is warranted. Severely ill patients with pyelonephritis should be hospitalized and IV drugs administered initially. Milder cases may be managed with oral antibiotics in an outpatient setting.
- At the time of presentation, a Gram stain of the urine should be performed, along with urinalysis, culture, and sensitivities.
- In the mild to moderately symptomatic patient for whom oral therapy is considered, an effective agent should be administered for at least a 2-week period, although use of highly active agents for 7 to 10 days may be sufficient. Oral antibiotics that have shown efficacy in this setting include **trimethoprim–sulfamethoxazole** and **fluoroquinolones**. If a Gram stain reveals gram-positive cocci, *Streptococcus faecalis* should be considered and treatment directed against this pathogen (**ampicillin**).
- In the seriously ill patient, the traditional initial therapy is an IV **fluoroquinolone**, an **aminoglycoside** with or without **ampicillin**, or an extended-spectrum **cephalosporin** with or without an aminoglycoside.
- If the patient has been hospitalized in the last 6 months, has a urinary catheter, or is in a nursing home, the possibility of *P. aeruginosa* and *enterococci* infection, as well as multiple-resistant organisms, should be considered. In this setting, **ceftazidime, ticarcillin–clavulanic acid, piperacillin, aztreonam, meropenem,** or **imipenem,** in combination with an **aminoglycoside**, is recommended. If the patient responds to initial combination therapy, the aminoglycoside may be discontinued after 3 days.
- Follow-up urine cultures should be obtained 2 weeks after the completion of therapy to ensure a satisfactory response and to detect possible relapse.

URINARY TRACT INFECTIONS IN MEN

- The conventional view is that therapy in men requires prolonged treatment (Fig. 50–2).
- A urine culture should be obtained before treatment, because the cause of infection in men is not as predictable as in women.
- If gram-negative bacteria are presumed, **trimethoprim–sulfamethoxazole** or a **fluoroquinolone** is a preferred agent. Initial therapy is for 10 to 14 days. For recurrent infections in men, cure rates are much higher with a 6-week regimen of **trimethoprim–sulfamethoxazole**.

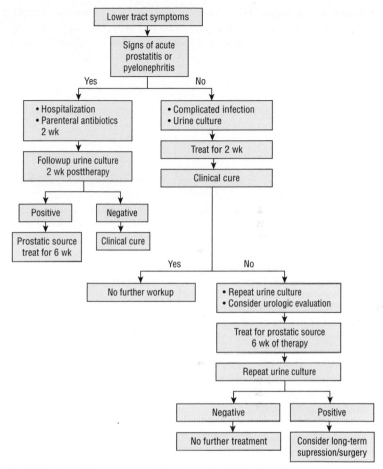

FIGURE 50–2. Management of urinary tract infections in men.

Recurrent Infections

- Recurrent episodes of UTI (reinfections and relapses) account for a significant portion of all UTIs. These patients are most commonly women and can be divided into two groups: those with fewer than two or three episodes per year and those who develop more frequent infections.
- In patients with infrequent infections (i.e., fewer than three infections per year), each episode should be treated as a separately occurring infection. Short-course therapy should be used in symptomatic female patients with lower tract infection.
- In patients who have frequent symptomatic infections, long-term prophylactic antimicrobial therapy may be instituted (see **Table 50–4**). Therapy is generally given for 6 months, with urine cultures followed periodically.

- In women who experience symptomatic reinfections in association with sexual activity, voiding after intercourse may help prevent infection. Also, self-administered, single-dose prophylactic therapy with **trimethoprim–sulfamethoxazole** taken after intercourse has been found to significantly reduce the incidence of recurrent infection in these patients.
- Women who relapse after short-course therapy should receive a 2-week course of therapy. In patients who relapse after 2 weeks, therapy should be continued for another 2 to 4 weeks. If relapse occurs after 6 weeks of treatment, urologic examination should be performed, and therapy for 6 months or even longer may be considered.

SPECIAL CONDITIONS

Urinary Tract Infection in Pregnancy

- In patients with significant bacteriuria, symptomatic or asymptomatic, treatment is recommended to avoid possible complications during the pregnancy. Therapy should consist of an agent with a relatively low adverse-effect potential (**cephalexin, amoxicillin, or amoxicillin/clavulanate**) administered for 7 days.
- Tetracyclines should be avoided because of teratogenic effects, and sulfonamides should not be administered during the third trimester because of the possible development of kernicterus and hyperbilirubinemia. Also, the fluoroquinolones should not be given because of their potential to inhibit cartilage and bone development in the newborn.

Catheterized Patients

- When bacteriuria occurs in the asymptomatic, short-term catheterized patient (<30 days), the use of systemic antibiotic therapy should be withheld and the catheter removed as soon as possible. If the patient becomes symptomatic, the catheter should again be removed, and treatment as described for complicated infections should be started.
- The use of prophylactic systemic antibiotics in patients with short-term catheterization reduces the incidence of infection over the first 4 to 7 days. In long-term catheterized patients, however, antibiotics only postpone the development of bacteriuria and lead to emergence of resistant organisms.

PROSTATITIS

- Prostatitis is an inflammation of the prostate gland and surrounding tissue as a result of infection. It can be either acute or chronic. The acute form is characterized by a severe illness characterized by a sudden onset of fever and urinary and constitutional symptoms. Chronic bacterial prostatitis (CBP) represents a recurring infection with the same organism (relapse). Pathogenic bacteria and significant inflammatory cells must be present in prostatic secretions and urine to make the diagnosis of bacterial prostatitis.
- The exact mechanism of bacterial infection of the prostate is not well understood. The possible routes of infection include ascending infection

TABLE 50–6	Clinical Presentation of Bacterial Prostatitis

Signs and symptoms

Acute bacterial prostatitis: high fever, chills, malaise, myalgia, localized pain (perineal, rectal, sacrococcygeal), frequency, urgency, dysuria, nocturia, and retention

Chronic bacterial prostatitis: voiding difficulties (frequency, urgency, dysuria), low back pain, and perineal and suprapubic discomfort

Physical examination

Acute bacterial prostatitis: swollen, tender, tense, or indurated gland

Chronic bacterial prostatitis: boggy, indurated (enlarged) prostate in most patients

Laboratory tests

Bacteriuria

Bacteria in expressed prostatic secretions

of the urethra, reflux of infected urine into prostatic ducts, invasion by rectal bacteria through direct extension or lymphatic spread, and by hematogenous spread.

- Gram-negative enteric organisms are the most frequent pathogens in acute bacterial prostatitis. *E. coli* is the predominant organism, occurring in 75% of cases.
- CBP is most commonly caused by *E. coli,* with other gram-negative organisms isolated much less often.

CLINICAL PRESENTATION AND DIAGNOSIS

- The clinical presentation of bacterial prostatitis is given in Table 50–6.
- Digital palpation of the prostate via the rectum may reveal a swollen, tender, warm, tense, or indurated prostate. Massage of the prostate will express a purulent discharge, which will readily grow the pathogenic organism. However, prostatic massage is contraindicated in acute bacterial prostatitis because of a risk of inducing bacteremia and associated pain.
- CBP is characterized by recurrent UTIs with the same pathogen.
- Urinary tract localization studies are critical to the diagnosis of CBP.

TREATMENT

- The majority of patients can be managed with oral antimicrobial agents, such as **trimethoprim–sulfamethoxazole** or the fluoroquinolones (**ciprofloxacin** or **levofloxacin**). When IV treatment is necessary, IV to oral sequential therapy with **trimethoprim–sulfamethoxazole** or a fluoroquinolone, such as ciprofloxacin or **ofloxacin**, would be appropriate.
- The total course of therapy should be 4 weeks, which may be prolonged to 6 to 12 weeks with chronic prostatitis.
- Parenteral therapy should be maintained until the patient is afebrile and less symptomatic. The conversion to an oral antibiotic can be considered if the patient has been afebrile for 48 hours or after 3 to 5 days of IV therapy.

- The choice of antibiotics in CBP should include those agents that are capable of crossing the prostatic epithelium into the prostatic fluid in therapeutic concentrations and that also possess the spectrum of activity to be effective.
- The fluoroquinolones (given for 4–6 weeks) appear to provide the best therapeutic option in the management of CBP.

See Chapter 125, Urinary Tract Infections and Prostatitis, authored by Elizabeth A. Coyle and Randall A. Prince, for a more detailed discussion of this topic.

CHAPTER 51

Vaccines, Toxoids, and Other Immunobiologics

DEFINITIONS

- Immunization is the process of introducing an antigen into the body to induce protection against an infectious agent without causing disease.
- Vaccines are substances administered to generate a protective immune response. They can be live attenuated or killed.
- Toxoids are inactivated bacterial toxins. They retain the ability to stimulate the formation of antitoxins, which are antibodies directed against the bacterial toxin.
- Adjuvants are inert substances, such as aluminum salts (i.e., alum), which enhance vaccine antigenicity by prolonging antigen absorption.
- Immune sera are sterile solutions containing antibody derived from human (immunoglobulin [IG]) or equine (antitoxin) sources.

VACCINE AND TOXOID RECOMMENDATIONS

- The recommended schedules for routine immunization of children and adults are shown in **Tables 51–1** and **51–2**, respectively.
- In general, killed vaccines can be administered simultaneously at separate sites. Killed and live attenuated vaccines may be administered simultaneously at separate sites. If they cannot be administered simultaneously, they can be administered at any interval between doses with the exception of cholera (killed) and yellow fever (live) vaccines, which should be given at least 3 weeks apart. If live vaccines are not administered simultaneously, their administration should be separated by at least 4 weeks.
- Vaccination of pregnant women generally is deferred until after delivery because of concern over potential risk to the fetus. Administration of live attenuated vaccines should not be done during pregnancy, and inactivated vaccines may be administered to pregnant women when the benefits outweigh the risks. Hepatitis A, hepatitis B, meningococcal, inactivated polio, and pneumococcal polysaccharide vaccines should be administered to pregnant women who are at risk for contracting these infections. Universal influenza immunization is recommended for women who will be or are pregnant during influenza season.
- In general, severely immunocompromised individuals should not receive live vaccines.
- Patients with chronic conditions that cause limited immunodeficiency (e.g., renal disease, diabetes, liver disease, and asplenia) and who are not receiving immunosuppressants may receive live attenuated and killed vaccines, as well as toxoids.
- Patients with active malignant disease may receive killed vaccines or toxoids but should not be given live vaccines. Live virus vaccines may be administered to persons with leukemia who have not received chemotherapy for at least 3 months.

TABLE 51-1 2010 Childhood and Adolescent Immunization Schedule (Continued)

Catch-up Immunization Schedule for Persons Aged 4 Months Through 18 Years Who Start Late or Who Are More Than 1 Month Behind—United States • 2010
The table below provides catch-up schedules and minimum intervals between doses for children whose vaccinations have been delayed. A vaccine series does not need to be restarted, regardless of the time that has elapsed between doses. Use the section appropriate for the child's age.

Vaccine	Minimum age for dose 1	Persons aged 4 months through 6 years				
		Dose 1 to dose 2	Minimum interval between doses			
			Dose 2 to dose 3	Dose 3 to dose 4	Dose 4 to dose 5	
Hepatitis B[1]	Birth	**4 weeks**	**8 weeks** (and at least 16 weeks after first dose)			
Rotavirus[2]	6 wks	**4 weeks**	**4 weeks**[2]			
Diphtheria, tetanus, pertussis[3]	6 wks	**4 weeks**	**4 weeks**	**6 months**	**6 months**[3]	
Haemophilus influenzae type b[4]	6 wks	**4 weeks** if first dose administered at younger than age 12 months **8 weeks (as final dose)** if first dose administered at age 12–14 months **No further doses needed** if first dose administered at age 15 months or older	**4 weeks**[4] if current age is younger than 12 months **8 weeks (as final dose)**[4] if current age is 12 months or older and first dose administered at younger than age 12 months and second dose administered at younger than 15 months **No further doses needed** if previous dose administered at age 15 months or older	**8 weeks (as final dose)** This dose only necessary for children aged 12 months through 59 months who received 3 doses before age 12 months		
Pneumococcal[5]	6 wks	**4 weeks** if first dose administered at younger than age 12 months **8 weeks (as final dose for healthy children)** if first dose administered at younger than age 12 months or current age 24 through 59 months **No further doses needed** if first dose administered at age 12–14 months administered at age 24 months or older	**4 weeks** if current age is younger than 12 months **8 weeks (as final dose for healthy children)** if current age is 12 months or older **No further doses needed** for healthy children if previous dose administered at age 24 months or older	**8 weeks (as final dose)** This dose only necessary for children aged 12 months through 59 months who received 3 doses before age 12 months or for high-risk children who received 3 doses at any age		

Vaccine	Minimum age for dose 1	Minimum interval between doses			
		Dose 1 to dose 2	Dose 2 to dose 3	Dose 3 to dose 4	Dose 4 to dose 5
Persons aged 4 months through 6 years					
Inactivated poliovirus[5]	6 wks	4 weeks	4 weeks	6 months	
Measles, mumps, rubella[7]	12 mos	4 weeks			
Varicella[8]	12 mos	3 months			
Hepatitis A[9]	12 mos	6 months			
Persons aged 7 through 18 years					
Tetanus, diphtheria/tetanus, diphtheria, pertussis[10]	7 yrs[10]	4 weeks	4 weeks if first dose administered at younger than age 12 months 6 months if first dose administered at 12 months or older	6 months if first dose administered at age younger than age 12 months	
Human papillomavirus[11]	9 yrs	Routine dosing intervals are recommended[11]			
Hepatitis A[9]	12 mos	6 months			
Hepatitis B[1]	Birth	4 weeks	8 weeks (and at least 16 weeks after first dose)		
Inactivated poliovirus[6]	6 wks	4 weeks	4 weeks	6 months	
Measles, mumps, rubella[7]	12 mos	4 weeks			
Varicella[8]	12 mos	3 months if person is younger than age 13 years 4 weeks if person is aged 13 years or older			

(continued)

TABLE 51-1 2010 Childhood and Adolescent Immunization Schedule (Continued)

1. **Hepatitis B vaccine (HepB).**
- administer the 3-dose series to those not previously vaccinated.
- 2-dose series (separated by at least 4 months) of adult formulation Recombivax HB is licensed for children aged 11 through 15 years.

2. **Rotavirus vaccine (RV).**
- The maximum age for the first dose is 14 weeks 6 days. Vaccination should not be initiated for infants aged 15 weeks 0 days or older.
- The maximum age for the final dose in the series is 8 months 0 days.
- If Rotarix was administered for the first and second doses, a third dose is not indicated.

3. **Diphtheria and tetanus toxoids and acellular pertussis vaccine (DTaP).**
- The fifth dose is not necessary if the fourth dose was administered at age 4 years or older.

4. **Haemophilus influenzae type b conjugate vaccine (Hib).**
- Hib vaccine is not generally recommended for persons aged 5 years or older. No efficacy data are available on which to base a recommendation concerning use of Hib vaccine for older children and adults. However, studies suggest good immunogenicity in persons who have sickle cell disease, leukemia, or HIV infection, or who have had a splenectomy; administering 1 dose of Hib vaccine to these persons who have not previously received Hib vaccine is not contraindicated.
- If the first 2 doses were PRP-OMP (PedvaxHIB or Comvax), and administered at age 11 months or younger, the third (and final) dose should be administered at age 12 through 15 months and at least 8 weeks after the second dose.
- If the first dose was administered at age 7 through 11 months, administer the second dose at least 4 weeks later and a final dose at age 12 through 15 months.

5. **Pneumococcal vaccine.**
- Administer 1 dose of pneumococcal conjugate vaccine (PCV) to all healthy children aged 24 through 59 months who have not received at least 1 dose of PCV on or after age 12 months.
- For children aged 24 through 59 months with underlying medical conditions, administer 1 dose of PCV if 3 doses were received previously or administer 2 doses of PCV at least 8 weeks apart if fewer than 3 doses were received previously.
- Administer pneumococcal polysaccharide vaccine (PPSV) to children aged 2 years or older with certain underlying medical conditions, including a cochlear implant, at least 8 weeks after the last dose of PCV. See MMWR 1997;46(No. RR-8).

6. **Inactivated poliovirus vaccine (IPV).**
- The final dose in the series should be administered on or after the fourth birthday and at least 6 months following the previous dose.
- A fourth dose is not necessary if the third dose was administered at age 4 years or older and at least 6 months following the previous dose.
- In the first 6 months of life, minimum age and minimum intervals are only recommended if the person is at risk for imminent exposure to circulating poliovirus (i.e., travel to a polio-endemic region or during an outbreak).

7. **Measles, mumps, and rubella vaccine (MMR).**
- Administer the second dose routinely at age 4 through 6 years. However, the second dose may be administered before age 4, provided at least 28 days have elapsed since the first dose.
- If not previously vaccinated, administer 2 doses with at least 28 days between doses.

8. **Varicella vaccine.**
- Administer the second dose routinely at age 4 through 6 years. However, the second dose may be administered before age 4, provided at least 3 months have elapsed since the first dose.
- For persons aged 12 months through 12 years, the minimum interval between doses is 3 months. However, if the second dose was administered at least 28 days after the first dose, it can be accepted as valid.
- For persons aged 13 years and older, the minimum interval between doses is 28 days.

9. **Hepatitis A vaccine (HepA).**
- HepA is recommended for children aged older than 23 months who live in areas where vaccination programs target older children, who are at increased risk for infection, or for whom immunity against hepatitis A is desired.

10. **Tetanus and diphtheria toxoids vaccine (Td) and tetanus and diphtheria toxoids and acellular pertussis vaccine (Tdap).**
- Doses of DTaP are counted as part of the Td/Tdap series
- Tdap should be substituted for a single dose of Td in the catch-up series or as a booster for children aged 10 through 18 years; use Td for other doses.

11. **Human papillomavirus vaccine (HPV).**
- Administer the series to females at age 13 through 18 years if not previously vaccinated.
- Use recommended routine dosing intervals for series catch-up (i.e., the second and third doses should be administered at 1 to 2 and 6 months after the first dose). The minimum interval between the first and second doses is 4 weeks. The minimum interval between the second and third doses is 12 weeks, and the third dose should be administered at least 24 weeks after the first dose.

Information about reporting reactions after immunization is available online at **http://www.vaers.hhs.gov** or by telephone, **800-822-7967**. Suspected cases of vaccine-preventable diseases should be reported to the state or local health department. Additional information, including precautions and contraindications for immunization, is available from the National Center for Immunization and Respiratory Diseases at **http://www.cdc.gov/vaccines** or telephone, **800-CDC-INFO** (800-232-4636).

Department of Health and Human Services • Centers for Disease Control and Prevention

CS207330-A

TABLE 51–2 2010 Adult Immunization Schedule

Figure 2. Vaccines that might be indicated for adults based on medical and other indications

Indication ▶ / Vaccine ▼	Pregnancy	Immuno-compromising conditions (excluding human immunodeficiency virus [HIV])3-5,13	HIV infection3-5,12,13 CD4+ T lymphocyte count < 200 cells/µL	HIV infection ≥ 200 cells/µL	Diabetes, heart disease, chronic lung disease, chronic alcoholism	Asplenia12 (including elective splenectomy and persistent complement component deficiencies)	Chronic liver disease	Kidney failure, end-stage renal disease, receipt of hemodialysis	Healthcare personnel
Tetanus, diphtheria, pertussis (Td/Tdap)1,*	Td	Substitute 1-time dose of Tdap for Td booster; then boost with Td every 10 yrs							
Human papillomavirus (HPV)2,*		3 doses for females through age 26 yrs							
Varicella3,*	Contraindicated	Contraindicated	Contraindicated		2 doses				
Zoster4	Contraindicated	Contraindicated	Contraindicated			1 dose			
Measles, mumps, rubella (MMR)5,*	Contraindicated	Contraindicated	Contraindicated				1 or 2 doses		
Influenza6,*					1 dose TIV annually				1 dose TIV or LAIV annually
Pneumococcal (polysaccharide)7,8					1 or 2 doses				
Hepatitis A9,*					2 doses				

(continued)

TABLE 51–2 2010 Adult Immunization Schedule (*Continued*)

Figure 2. Vaccines that might be indicated for adults based on medical and other indications

Indication ▶ / Vaccine ▼	Pregnancy	Immuno-compromising conditions (excluding human immunodeficiency virus [HIV])3–5,13	HIV infection3–5,12,13 CD4+ T lymphocyte count <200 cells/µL	HIV infection3–5,12,13 CD4+ T lymphocyte count ≥200 cells/µL	Diabetes, heart disease, chronic lung disease, chronic alcoholism	Asplenia12 (including elective splenectomy and persistent complement component deficiencies)	Chronic liver disease	Kidney failure, end-stage renal disease, receipt of hemodialysis	Healthcare personnel
Hepatitis B10,*				3 doses					
Meningococcal11,*				1 or more doses					

*Covered by the Vaccine Injury Compensation Program.

■ For all persons in this category who meet the age requirements and who lack evidence of immunity (e.g., lack documentation of vaccination or have no evidence of prior infection)

■ Recommended if some other risk factor is present (e.g., on the basis of medical, occupational, lifestyle, or other indications)

□ No recommendation

DEPARTMENT OF HEALTH AND HUMAN SERVICES
CENTERS FOR DISEASE CONTROL AND PREVENTION

These schedules indicate the recommended age groups and medical indications for which administration of currently licensed vaccines is commonly indicated for adults ages 19 years and older, as of January 1, 2010. Licensed combination vaccines may be used whenever any components of the combination are indicated and when the vaccine's other components are not contraindicated. For detailed recommendations on all vaccines, including those used primarily for travelers or that are issued during the year, consult the manufacturers' package inserts and the complete statements from the Advisory Committee on Immunization Practices (www.cdc.gov/vaccines/pubs/acip-list.htm).

The recommendations in this schedule were approved by the Centers for Disease Control and Prevention's (CDC) Advisory Committee on Immunization Practices (ACIP), the American Academy of Family Physicians (AAFP), the American College of Obstetricians and Gynecologists (ACOG), and the American College of Physicians (ACP).

Footnotes

Recommended Adult Immunization Schedule—UNITED STATES · 2010

For complete statements by the Advisory Committee on Immunization Practices (ACIP), visit www.cdc.gov/vaccines/pubs/ACIP-list.htm.

1. Tetanus, diphtheria, and acellular pertussis (Td/Tdap) vaccination

Tdap should replace a single dose of Td for adults aged 19 through 64 years who have not received a dose of Tdap previously.

Adults with uncertain or incomplete history of primary vaccination series with tetanus and diphtheria toxoid-containing vaccines should begin or complete a primary vaccination series. A primary series for adults is 3 doses of tetanus and diphtheria toxoid-containing vaccines; administer the first 2 doses at least 4 weeks apart and the third dose 6–12 months after the second; Tdap can substitute for any one of the doses of Td in the 3-dose primary series. The booster dose of tetanus and diphtheria toxoid-containing vaccine should be administered to adults who have completed a primary series and if the last vaccination was received <10 years previously. Tdap or Td vaccine may be used, as indicated.

If a woman is pregnant and received the last Td vaccination ≥10 years previously, administer Td during the second or third trimester. If the woman received the last Td vaccination <10 years previously, administer Tdap during the immediate postpartum period. A dose of Tdap is recommended for postpartum women, close contacts of infants aged <12 months, and all healthcare personnel with direct patient contact if they have not previously received Tdap. An interval as short as 2 years from the last Td is suggested; shorter intervals can be used. Tdap may be deferred during pregnancy, and Td substituted in the immediate postpartum period, or Tdap can be administered instead of Td to a pregnant woman.

Consult the ACIP statement for recommendations for giving Td as prophylaxis in wound management.

2. Human papillomavirus (HPV) vaccination

HPV vaccination is recommended at age 11 or 12 years with catch-up vaccination at ages 13 through 26 years.

Ideally, vaccine should be administered before potential exposure to HPV through sexual activity; however, females who are sexually active should still be vaccinated consistent with age-based recommendations. Sexually active females who have not been infected with any of the four HPV vaccine types (types 6, 11, 16, 18 all of which HPV4 prevents) or of the two HPV vaccine types (types 16 and 18 both of which HPV2 prevents) receive the full benefit of the vaccination. Vaccination is less beneficial for females who have already been infected with one or more of the HPV vaccine types. HPV4 or HPV2 can be administered to persons with a history of genital warts, abnormal Papanicolaou test, or positive HPV DNA test, because these conditions are not evidence of prior infection with all vaccine HPV types.

HPV4 may be administered to males aged 9 through 26 years to reduce their likelihood of acquiring genital warts. HPV4 would be most effective when administered before exposure to HPV through sexual contact.

A complete series for either HPV4 or HPV2 consists of 3 doses. The second dose should be administered 1–2 months after the first dose; the third dose should be administered 6 months after the first dose. Although HPV vaccination is not specifically recommended for persons with the medical indications described in Figure 2, "Vaccines that might be indicated for adults based on medical and other indications," it may be administered to these persons because the HPV vaccine is not a live-virus vaccine. However, the immune response and vaccine efficacy might be less for persons with the medical indications described in Figure 2 than in persons who do not have the medical indications described or who are immunocompetent. Healthcare personnel are not at increased risk because of occupational exposure, and should be vaccinated consistent with age-based recommendations.

3. Varicella vaccination

All adults without evidence of immunity to varicella should receive 2 doses of single-antigen varicella vaccine if not previously vaccinated or the second dose if they have received only 1 dose, unless they have a medical contraindication. Special consideration should be given to those who (1) have close contact with persons at high risk for severe disease (e.g., healthcare personnel and family contacts of persons with immunocompromising conditions) or (2) are at high risk for exposure or transmission (e.g., teachers; child-care employees; residents and staff members of institutional settings, including correctional institutions; college students; military personnel; adolescents and adults living in households with children; nonpregnant women of childbearing age; and international travelers).

Evidence of immunity to varicella in adults includes any of the following: (1) documentation of 2 doses of varicella vaccine at least 4 weeks apart; (2) U.S.-born before 1980 (although for healthcare personnel and pregnant women, birth before 1980 should not be considered evidence of immunity); (3) history of varicella based on diagnosis or verification of varicella by a healthcare provider (for a patient reporting a history of or presenting with an atypical case, a mild case, or both, healthcare providers should seek either an epidemiologic link with a typical varicella case or to a laboratory-confirmed case or evidence of laboratory confirmation, if it was performed at the time of acute disease); (4) history of herpes zoster based on diagnosis or verification of herpes zoster by a healthcare provider; or (5) laboratory evidence of immunity or laboratory confirmation of disease.

Pregnant women should be assessed for evidence of varicella immunity. Women who do not have evidence of immunity should receive the first dose of varicella vaccine upon completion or termination of pregnancy and before discharge from the healthcare facility. The second dose should be administered 4–8 weeks after the first dose.

4. Herpes zoster vaccination

A single dose of zoster vaccine is recommended for adults aged ≥60 years regardless of whether they report a prior episode of herpes zoster. Persons with chronic medical conditions may be vaccinated unless their condition constitutes a contraindication.

5. Measles, mumps, rubella (MMR) vaccination

Adults born before 1957 generally are considered immune to measles and mumps.

Measles component: Adults born during or after 1957 should receive 1 or more doses of MMR vaccine unless they have (1) a medical contraindication; (2) documentation of vaccination with 1 or more doses of MMR vaccine; (3) laboratory evidence of immunity; or (4) documentation of physician-diagnosed measles.

A second dose of MMR vaccine, administered 4 weeks after the first dose, is recommended for adults who (1) have been recently exposed to measles or are in an outbreak setting; (2) have been vaccinated previously with killed measles vaccine; (3) have been vaccinated with an unknown type of measles vaccine during 1963–1967; (4) are students in postsecondary educational institutions; (5) work in a healthcare facility; or (6) plan to travel internationally.

Mumps component: Adults born during or after 1957 should receive 1 dose of MMR vaccine unless they have (1) a medical contraindication; (2) documentation of vaccination with 1 or more doses of MMR vaccine; (3) laboratory evidence of immunity; or (4) documentation of physician-diagnosed mumps.

A second dose of MMR vaccine, administered 4 weeks after the first dose, is recommended for adults who (1) live in a community experiencing a mumps outbreak and are in an affected age group; (2) are students in postsecondary educational institutions; (3) work in a healthcare facility; or (4) plan to travel internationally.

(continued)

TABLE 51-2 2010 Adult Immunization Schedule (*Continued*)

Rubella component: 1 dose of MMR vaccine is recommended for women who do not have documentation of rubella vaccination, or who lack laboratory evidence of immunity. For women of childbearing age, regardless of birth year, rubella immunity should be determined and women should be counseled regarding congenital rubella syndrome. Women who do not have evidence of immunity should receive MMR vaccine upon completion or termination of pregnancy and before discharge from the healthcare facility.

Healthcare personnel born before 1957: For unvaccinated healthcare personnel born before 1957 who lack laboratory evidence of measles, mumps, and/or rubella immunity or laboratory confirmation of disease, healthcare facilities should consider vaccinating personnel with 2 doses of MMR vaccine at the appropriate interval (for measles and mumps) and 1 dose of MMR vaccine (for rubella), respectively. During outbreaks, healthcare facilities should recommend that 1 unvaccinated healthcare personnel born before 1957 who lack laboratory evidence of measles, mumps, and/or rubella immunity or laboratory confirmation of disease, receive 2 doses of MMR vaccine during an outbreak of measles or mumps, and 1 dose during an outbreak of rubella. Complete information about evidence of immunity is available at www.cdc.gov/vaccines/recs/provisional/default.htm.

6. Seasonal Influenza vaccination

Vaccinate all persons aged ≥50 years and any younger persons who would like to decrease their risk of getting influenza. Vaccinate persons aged 19 through 49 years with any of the following indications.

Medical: Chronic disorders of the cardiovascular or pulmonary systems, including asthma; chronic metabolic diseases, including diabetes mellitus; renal or hepatic dysfunction, hemoglobinopathies, or immunocompromising conditions (including immunocompromising conditions caused by medications or HIV); cognitive, neurologic or neuromuscular disorders; and pregnancy during the influenza season. No data exist on the risk for severe or complicated influenza disease among persons with asplenia; however, influenza is a risk factor for secondary bacterial infections that can cause severe disease among persons with asplenia.

Occupational: All healthcare personnel, including those employed by long-term care and assisted-living facilities, and caregivers of children aged <5 years.

Other: Residents of nursing homes and other long-term care and assisted-living facilities; persons likely to transmit influenza to persons at high risk (e.g., in-home household contacts and caregivers of children aged <5 years, persons aged ≥50 years, and persons of all ages with high-risk conditions). Healthy, nonpregnant adults aged <50 years without high-risk medical conditions who are not contacts of severely immunocompromised persons in special-care units may receive either intranasally administered live, attenuated influenza vaccine (FluMist) or inactivated vaccine. Other persons should receive the inactivated vaccine.

7. Pneumococcal polysaccharide (PPSV) vaccination

Vaccinate all persons with the following indications.

Medical: Chronic lung disease (including asthma); chronic cardiovascular diseases; diabetes mellitus; chronic liver diseases cirrhosis; chronic alcoholism; functional or anatomic asplenia (e.g., sickle cell disease or splenectomy [if elective splenectomy is planned, vaccinate at least 2 weeks before surgery]); immunocompromising conditions including chronic renal failure or nephrotic syndrome; and cochlear implants and cerebrospinal fluid leaks. Vaccinate as close to HIV diagnosis as possible.

Other: Residents of nursing homes or long-term care facilities and persons who smoke cigarettes. Routine use of PPSV is not recommended for American Indians/Alaska Natives or persons aged <65 years unless they have underlying medical conditions that are PPSV indications. However, public health authorities may consider recommending PPSV for American Indians/Alaska Natives and persons aged 50 through 64 years who are living in areas where the risk for invasive pneumococcal disease is increased.

8. Revaccination with PPSV

One-time revaccination after 5 years is recommended for persons with chronic renal failure or nephrotic syndrome; functional or anatomic asplenia (e.g., sickle cell disease or splenectomy); and for persons with immunocompromising conditions. For persons aged ≥65 years, one-time revaccination is recommended if they were vaccinated ≥5 years previously and were younger than aged <65 years at the time of primary vaccination.

9. Hepatitis A vaccination

Vaccinate persons with any of the following indications and any person seeking protection from hepatitis A virus (HAV) infection.

Behavioral: Men who have sex with men and persons who use injection drugs.

Occupational: Persons working with HAV–infected primates or with HAV in a research laboratory setting.

Medical: Persons with chronic liver disease and persons who receive clotting factor concentrates.

Other: Persons traveling to or working in countries that have high or intermediate endemicity of hepatitis A (a list of countries is available at wwwn.cdc.gov/travel/contentdiseases.aspx).

Unvaccinated persons who anticipate close personal contact (e.g., household contact or regular babysitting) with an international adoptee from a country of high or intermediate endemicity during the first 60 days after arrival of the adoptee in the United States should consider vaccination. The first dose of the 2-dose hepatitis A vaccine series should be administered as soon as adoption is planned, ideally ≥2 weeks before the arrival of the adoptee.

Single-antigen vaccine formulations should be administered in a 2-dose schedule at either 0 and 6–12 months (Havrix), or 0 and 6–18 months (Vaqta). If the combined hepatitis A and hepatitis B vaccine (Twinrix) is used, administer 3 doses at 0, 1, and 6 months; alternatively, a 4-dose schedule, administered on days 0, 7, and 21–30 followed by a booster dose at month 12 may be used.

10. Hepatitis B vaccination

Vaccinate persons with any of the following indications and any person seeking protection from hepatitis B virus (HBV) infection.

Behavioral: Sexually active persons who are not in a long-term, mutually monogamous relationship (e.g., persons with more than one sex partner during the previous 6 months); persons seeking evaluation or treatment for a sexually transmitted disease (STD); current or recent injection-drug users; and men who have sex with men.

Occupational: Healthcare personnel and public-safety workers who are exposed to blood or other potentially infectious body fluids.

Medical: Persons with end-stage renal disease, including patients receiving hemodialysis; persons with HIV infection; and persons with chronic liver disease.

Other: Household contacts and sex partners of persons with chronic HBV infection; clients and staff members of institutions for persons with developmental disabilities; and international travelers to countries with high or intermediate prevalence of chronic HBV infection (a list of countries is available at wwwn.cdc.gov/travel/contentdiseases.aspx).

Hepatitis B vaccination is recommended for all adults in the following settings: STD treatment facilities; HIV testing and treatment facilities; facilities providing drug-abuse treatment and prevention services; healthcare settings targeting services to injection-drug users or men who have sex with men; correctional facilities; end-stage renal disease programs and facilities for chronic hemodialysis patients; and institutions and nonresidential daycare facilities for persons with developmental disabilities.

Administer or complete a 3-dose series of HepB to those persons not previously vaccinated. The second dose should be administered 1 month after the first dose; the third dose should be administered at least 2 months after the second dose (and at least 4 months after the first dose). If the combined hepatitis A and hepatitis B vaccine (Twinrix) is used, administer 3 doses at 0, 1, and 6 months; alternatively, a 4-dose schedule, administered on days 0, 7, and 21–30 followed by a booster dose at month 12 may be used.

Adult patients receiving hemodialysis or with other immunocompromising conditions should receive 1 dose of 40 μg/mL (Recombivax HB) administered on a 3-dose schedule or 2 doses of 20 μg/mL (Engerix-B) administered simultaneously on a 4-dose schedule at 0, 1, 2 and 6 months.

11. Meningococcal vaccination

Meningococcal vaccine should be administered to persons with the following indications.

Medical: Adults with anatomic or functional asplenia, or persistent complement component deficiencies.

Other: First-year college students living in dormitories; microbiologists routinely exposed to isolates of *Neisseria meningitides*; military recruits; and persons who travel to or live in countries in which meningococcal disease is hyperendemic or epidemic (e.g., the "meningitis belt" of sub-Saharan Africa during the dry season [December through June]), particularly if their contact with local populations will be prolonged. Vaccination is required by the government of Saudi Arabia for all travelers to Mecca during the annual Hajj.

Meningococcal conjugate vaccine (MCV4) is preferred for adults with any of the preceding indications who are aged ≤55 years; meningococcal polysaccharide vaccine (MPSV4) is preferred for adults aged ≥56 years. Revaccination with MCV4 after 5 years is recommended for adults previously vaccinated with MCV4 or MPSV4 who remain at increased risk for infection (e.g., adults with anatomic or functional asplenia). Persons whose only risk factor is living in on-campus housing are not recommended to receive an additional dose.

12. Selected conditions for which *Haemophilus influenzae* type b (Hib) vaccine may be used

Hib vaccine generally is not recommended for persons aged ≥5 years. No efficacy data are available on which to base a recommendation concerning use of Hib vaccine for older children and adults. However, studies suggest good immunogenicity in patients who have sickle cell disease, leukemia, or HIV infection or who have had a splenectomy. Administering 1 dose of Hib vaccine to these high-risk persons who have not previously received Hib vaccine is not contraindicated.

13. Immunocompromising conditions

Inactivated vaccines generally are acceptable (e.g., pneumococcal, meningococcal, influenza [inactivated influenza vaccine]) and live vaccines generally are avoided in persons with immune deficiencies or immunocompromising conditions. Information on specific conditions is available at www.cdc.gov/vaccines/pubs/acip-list.htm.

- If a person has been receiving high-dose corticosteroids or has had a course lasting longer than 2 weeks, then at least 1 month should pass before immunization with live virus vaccines.
- Responses to live and killed vaccines generally are suboptimal for human immunodeficiency virus (HIV)–infected patients and decrease as the disease progresses.
- General contraindications to vaccine administration include a history of anaphylactic reaction to a previous dose or an unexplained encephalopathy occurring within 7 days of a dose of pertussis vaccine. Immunosuppression and pregnancy are temporary contraindications to live vaccines.
- Whenever possible, transplant patients should be immunized before transplantation. Live vaccines generally are not given after transplantation.

DIPHTHERIA TOXOID ADSORBED AND DIPHTHERIA ANTITOXIN

- Two strengths of diphtheria toxoid are available: pediatric (D) and adult, which contains less antigen. Primary immunization with D is indicated for children younger than 6 weeks of age. Generally, D is given along with tetanus and acellular pertussis (DTaP) vaccines at 2, 4, and 6 months of age, and then at 15 to 18 months and 4 to 6 years of age.
- For nonimmunized adults, a complete three-dose series of diphtheria toxoid should be administered, with the first two doses given at least 4 weeks apart and the third dose 6 to 12 months after the second. The combined preparation, tetanus–diphtheria (Td), is recommended in adults because it contains less diphtheria toxoid than DTaP, with fewer reactions seen from the diphtheria preparation. Booster doses are given every 10 years.
- Adverse effects to diphtheria toxoid include mild to moderate tenderness, erythema, and induration at the injection site.

TETANUS TOXOID, TETANUS TOXOID ADSORBED, AND TETANUS IMMUNOGLOBULIN

- In children, primary immunization against tetanus is usually done in conjunction with diphtheria and pertussis vaccination using DTaP or a combination vaccine that includes other antigens. A 0.5 mL dose is recommended at 2, 4, 6, and 15 to 18 months of age.
- In children 7 years and older and in adults who have not been previously immunized, a series of three 0.5 mL doses of Td are administered intramuscularly (IM) initially. The first two doses are given 1 to 2 months apart and the third dose 6 to 12 months later. Boosters are recommended every 10 years.
- Tetanus toxoid may be given to immunosuppressed patients if indicated.
- Tetanus IG is used to provide passive tetanus immunization after the occurrence of traumatic wounds in nonimmunized or suboptimally immunized persons (see **Table 51–3**). A dose of 250 to 500 units is administered IM. When administered with tetanus toxoid, separate sites for administration should be used.

TABLE 51–3 Tetanus Prophylaxis				
	Clean, Minor		**All Other**	
Vaccination History	**Td**	**TIG**	**Td[a]**	**TIG**
Unknown or fewer than three doses	Yes	No	Yes	Yes
Greater than or equal to three doses	No[a,b]	No	No[a,c]	No

Td, tetanus–diphtheria; TIG, tetanus immunoglobulin.

[a]A single dose of diphtheria, tetanus toxoids, and acellular pertussis should be used for the next dose of Td toxoid.

[b]Yes if >10 years since last dose.

[c]Yes if >5 years since last dose.

- Tetanus IG is also used for the treatment of tetanus. In this setting, a single dose of 3,000 to 6,000 units is administered IM.

HAEMOPHILUS INFLUENZAE TYPE B VACCINES

- *Haemophilus influenzae* type b (Hib) vaccines currently in use are conjugate products, consisting of either a polysaccharide or oligosaccharide of polyribosylribitol phosphate (PRP) covalently linked to a protein carrier.
- Hib conjugate vaccines are indicated for routine use in all infants and children younger than 5 years of age.
- The primary series of Hib vaccination consists of 0.5 mL IM doses at 2, 4, and 6 months of age (for HibTITER [HbOC] and ActHIB [PRP-T]) or doses at 2 and 4 months if PRP-OMP (PRP conjugated to an outer membrane protein) is used (Table 51–4). A booster dose is recommended at age 12 to 15 months.
- For infants ages 7 to 11 months who have not been vaccinated, three doses of HbOC PRP-OMP, or PRP-T should be given: two doses, spaced 4 weeks apart, and then a booster dose at age 12 to 15 months (but at least 8 weeks since dose 2). For unvaccinated children ages 12 to 14 months, two doses should be given, with an interval of 2 months between them. In a child older than 15 months, a single dose of any of the four conjugate vaccines is indicated.

HEPATITIS VACCINES

- Information on hepatitis vaccines can be found in Chap. 24.

TABLE 51–4 *Haemophilus influenzae* Type B Conjugate Vaccine Products		
Vaccine	**Trade Name**	**Protein Carrier**
PRP-T	ActHIB (Sanofi Pasteur)	Tetanus toxoid
PRP-OMP	PedvaxHIB (Merck)	*Neisseria meningitidis* serogroup B outer membrane protein

Note: The polysaccharide is polyribosylribitol phosphate (PRP).

HUMAN PAPILLOMAVIRUS VACCINE

- Bivalent (Cervarix) and quadrivalent (Gardisil) vaccines are available. Both vaccines are recommended as a three-dose series (0, 2, and 6 months) for all female patients 11 to 12 years old and ages 13 to 26 years. The quadrivalent vaccine is licensed for prevention of genital warts in females 9 to 26 years of age.
- The vaccine is well tolerated, with injection site reactions and headache and fatigue occurring as commonly as in placebo groups.

INFLUENZA VIRUS VACCINE

- See Chap. 41 for information regarding influenza vaccination.

MEASLES VACCINE

- Measles vaccine is a live attenuated vaccine that is administered for primary immunization to persons 12 to 15 months of age or older, usually as a combination of measles, mumps, and rubella (MMR). A second dose is recommended at 4 to 6 years of age.
- The vaccine should not be given to immunosuppressed patients (except those infected with HIV) or pregnant women. HIV-infected persons who have never had measles or have never been vaccinated should be given measles-containing vaccine unless there is evidence of severe immunosuppression.
- The vaccine should not be given within 1 month of any other live vaccine unless the vaccine is given on the same day (as with the MMR vaccine).
- Measles vaccine is indicated in all persons born after 1956 or in those who lack documentation of wild virus infection by either history or antibody titers.

MENINGOCOCCAL POLYSACCHARIDE VACCINE

- There are two meningococcal conjugate vaccines; Menactra is licensed for individuals 2 to 55 years old and Menveo for those 11 to 55 years old. They are recommended for all children 11 to 12 years old and others at high risk for invasive meningococcal infection, including high school students and college freshmen who live in dormitories. The polysaccharide vaccine is indicated in high-risk populations such as those exposed to the disease, those in the midst of uncontrolled outbreaks, travelers to an area with epidemic hyperendemic meningococcal disease, and individuals who have terminal complement deficiencies or asplenia.
- The vaccine should be made available to students starting college who wish to decrease their risk for meningococcal disease.
- The polysaccharide vaccine is administered subcutaneously as a single 0.5 mL dose, and the conjugate vaccine is administered by IM injection.

MUMPS VACCINE

- The vaccine (usually given in conjunction with measles and rubella, MMR) is given beginning at age 12 to 15 months, with a second dose prior to entry into elementary school.
- Two doses of mumps vaccine are recommended for school-age children, international travelers, college students, and healthcare workers born after 1956.
- Postexposure vaccination is of no benefit.
- Mumps vaccine should not be given to pregnant women or immuno-suppressed patients. The vaccine should not be given within 6 weeks (preferably 3 months) of administration of IG.

PERTUSSIS VACCINE

- Acellular pertussis vaccine is usually administered in combination with diphtheria and tetanus toxoids (as DTaP).
- The primary immunization series for pertussis vaccine consists of four doses given at ages 2, 4, 6, and 15 to 18 months. A booster dose is recommended at age 4 to 6 years. Adults up to age 64 should receive a pertussis-containing vaccine with their next tetanus vaccine.
- Systemic reactions, such as moderate fever, occur in 3% to 5% of those receiving vaccines. Very rarely, high fever, febrile seizures, persistent crying spells, and hypotonic hyporesponsive episodes occur after vaccination.
- There are only two absolute contraindications to pertussis administration: (1) an immediate anaphylactic reaction to a previous dose and (2) encephalopathy within 7 days of a previous dose, with no evidence of other cause.

PNEUMOCOCCAL VACCINES

- Pneumococcal polysaccharide vaccine is a mixture of capsular polysaccharides from 23 of the 83 most prevalent types of *Streptococcus pneumoniae* seen in the United States.
- Pneumococcal vaccine is recommended for the following immunocompetent persons:
  - ✓ Persons 65 or more years of age. If an individual received vaccine more than 5 years earlier and was under age 65 at the time of administration, revaccination should be given.
  - ✓ Persons ages 2 to 64 years with chronic illness
  - ✓ Persons ages 2 to 64 years with functional or anatomical asplenia. When splenectomy is planned, pneumococcal vaccine should be given at least 2 weeks before surgery.
  - ✓ Persons ages 2 to 64 years living in environments where the risk of invasive pneumococcal disease or its complications is increased. This does not include daycare center employees and children.
- Pneumococcal vaccination is recommended for immunocompromised persons 2 years of age or older with
  - ✓ HIV infection

   ✓ Leukemia, lymphoma, Hodgkin disease, or multiple myeloma
   ✓ Generalized malignancy
   ✓ Chronic renal failure of nephritic syndrome
   ✓ Patients receiving immunosuppressive therapy
   ✓ Organ or bone marrow transplant recipients

- Because children younger than 2 years of age do not respond adequately to the pneumococcal polysaccharide vaccine, a heptavalent pneumococcal conjugate vaccine was created that can be administered at 2, 4, and 6 months of age and between 12 and 15 months of age.

POLIOVIRUS VACCINES

- Two types of trivalent poliovirus vaccines are currently licensed for distribution in the United States: an enhanced inactivated poliovirus vaccine (IPV) and a live attenuated, oral poliovirus vaccine (OPV). IPV is the recommended vaccine for the primary series and booster dose for children in the United States, whereas OPV is recommended in areas of the world that have circulating poliovirus.
- IPV is given to children ages 2, 4, and 6 to 18 months and 4 to 6 years. Primary poliomyelitis immunization is recommended for all children and young adults up to age 18 years. Allergies to any component of IPV, including streptomycin, polymyxin B, and neomycin, are contraindications to vaccine use.
- The routine use of OPV in the United States has been discontinued. OPV is not recommended for persons who are immunodeficient or for normal individuals who reside in a household where another person is immunodeficient. It should not be given during pregnancy because of the small but theoretical risk to the fetus.

RUBELLA VACCINE

- The vaccine is given with measles and mumps vaccines (MMR) at 12 to 15 months of age, then at 4 to 6 years.
- The vaccine should not be given to immunosuppressed individuals, although MMR vaccine should be administered to young children with HIV without severe immunosuppression as soon as possible after their first birthday. The vaccine should not be given to individuals with anaphylactic reaction to neomycin.
- Although the vaccine has not been associated with congenital rubella syndrome, its use in pregnancy is contraindicated. Women should be counseled not to become pregnant for 4 weeks after vaccination.

VARICELLA VACCINE

- Varicella virus vaccine is recommended for all children 12 to 18 months of age, with a second dose prior to entering school between 4 and 6 years of age. It is also recommended for persons above this age if they have not had chickenpox. Persons ages 13 years and older should receive two doses separated by 4 to 8 weeks.

TABLE 51–5	Indications and Dosage of Intramuscular Immunoglobulin in Infectious Diseases
Primary immunodeficiency states	1.2 mL/kg IM, then 0.6 mL/kg every 2–4 weeks
Hepatitis A exposure	0.02 mL/kg IM within 2 weeks if < 1 year or >39 years of age
Hepatitis A prophylaxis	0.02 mL/kg IM for exposure <3 months' duration 0.06 mL/kg IM for exposure up to 5 months' duration
Hepatitis B exposure	0.06 mL/kg (hepatitis B immunoglobulin preferred in known exposures)
Measles exposure	0.25 mL/kg (maximum dose 15 mL) as soon as possible 0.5 mL/kg (maximum dose 15 mL) as soon as possible for immunocompromised individuals
Varicella exposure	0.6–1.2 mL/kg as soon as possible when varicella zoster immunoglobulin is not available

- The vaccine is contraindicated in immunosuppressed or pregnant patients.
- Children with asymptomatic or mildly symptomatic HIV should receive two doses of varicella vaccine 3 months apart.

VARICELLA ZOSTER VACCINE

- The zoster vaccine is recommended for immunocompetent individuals older than 60 years. It should not be used in immunocompromised individuals, including those with HIV or malignancies or in pregnant women.
- Administration of varicella zoster IG is by the IM route (never IV).

IMMUNOGLOBULIN

- IG is available as both IM (IGIM) and IV (IGIV) preparations.
- Table 51–5 lists the suggested dosages for IGIM in various disease states.
- The uses for IGIV are as follows:
  ✓ Primary immunodeficiency states, including both antibody deficiencies and combined deficiencies
  ✓ Idiopathic thrombocytopenic purpura
  ✓ Chronic lymphocytic leukemia in patients who have had a serious bacterial infection
  ✓ Kawasaki disease (mucocutaneous lymph node syndrome)
  ✓ Bone marrow transplant
  ✓ Varicella zoster

RHO(D) IMMUNOGLOBULIN

- Rho(D) IG (RDIg) suppresses the antibody response and formation of anti-Rho(D) in Rho(D)-negative, D^u-negative women exposed to Rho(D)-positive blood and prevents the future chance of erythroblastosis fetalis in subsequent pregnancies with a Rho(D)-positive fetus.

- RDIg, when administered within 72 hours of delivery of a full-term infant, reduces active antibody formation from 12% to between 1% and 2%.
- RDIg is also used in the case of a premenopausal woman who is Rho(D) negative and has inadvertently received Rho(D)-positive blood or blood products.
- RDIg may be used after abortion, miscarriage, amniocentesis, or abdominal trauma.
- RDIg is administered IM only.

See Chapter 133, Vaccines, Toxoids, and Other Immunobiologics, authored by Mary S. Hayney, for a more detailed discussion of this topic.

CHAPTER 52 · Alzheimer's Disease

DEFINITION

- *Alzheimer's disease (AD)* is a progressive dementia affecting cognition, behavior, and functional status with no known cause or cure. Patients eventually lose cognitive, analytical, and physical functioning, and the disease is ultimately fatal.

PATHOPHYSIOLOGY

- The signature findings are intracellular neurofibrillary tangles (NFTs), extracellular neuritic plaques, degeneration of neurons and synapses, and cortical atrophy.
- Mechanisms proposed for these changes are:
  - ✓ β-Amyloid protein aggregation, leading to formation of plaques
  - ✓ Hyperphosphorylation of tau protein, leading to intracellular NFT development and collapse of microtubules
  - ✓ Inflammatory processes
  - ✓ Vasculature injury
  - ✓ Depletion of neurotrophin and neurotransmitters
  - ✓ Oxidative stress
  - ✓ Defective cholesterol metabolism
  - ✓ Mitochondrial dysfunction
  - ✓ Loss of calcium regulation
- Neuritic plaques are lesions found in brain and cerebral vasculature.
- Whether genetic variations promote a primary β-amyloidosis in the majority of patients with AD is unresolved.
- Density of NFTs correlates with severity of dementia.
- Although there is a variety of neurotransmitter deficits, loss of cholinergic activity is most prominent and correlates with AD severity.
- It is clear that replacement of acetylcholine activity cannot compensate for all the changes that take place in AD.
- Deficits that exist in other pathways are
  - ✓ Serotonergic neurons of the raphe nuclei and noradrenergic cells of the locus ceruleus are lost.
  - ✓ Monoamine oxidase type B activity is increased.
  - ✓ Glutamate pathways of the cortex and limbic structures are abnormal.
- Excitatory neurotransmitters, including glutamate, have been implicated as potential neurotoxins in AD.

TABLE 52–1	Stages of Alzheimer's Disease
Mild (MMSE score 26–18)	Patient has difficulty remembering recent events. Ability to manage finances, prepare food, and carry out other household activities declines. May get lost while driving. Begins to withdraw from difficult tasks and to give up hobbies. May deny memory problems.
Moderate (MMSE score 17–10)	Patient requires assistance with activities of daily living. Frequently disoriented with regard to time (date, year, and season). Recall for recent events is severely impaired. May forget some details of past life and names of family and friends. Functioning may fluctuate from day to day. Patient generally denies problems. May become suspicious or tearful. Loses ability to drive safely. Agitation, paranoia, and delusions are common.
Severe (MMSE score 9–0)	Patient loses ability to speak, walk, and feed self. Incontinent of urine and feces. Requires care 24 hours a day, 7 days a week.

MMSE, Mini-Mental State Examination.

Data from Alzheimer's Association. http://www.alz.org/; Rubin CD. The primary care of Alzheimer's disease. Am J Med Sci 2006;332:314–333; and Burns A, Iliffe S. Alzheimer's disease. BMJ 2009;339:b158.

- Risk factors for AD are hypertension, elevated low-density lipoprotein cholesterol, low high-density lipoprotein cholesterol, and diabetes.

CLINICAL PRESENTATION

- The onset of AD is almost imperceptible, but deficits progress over time. Cognitive decline is gradual, and behavioral disturbances may be present in moderate stages. **Table 52–1** shows the stages of AD.

SYMPTOMS

- **Table 52–2** shows the clinical presentation of AD and recommended laboratory and diagnostic tests.

DIAGNOSIS

- The definitive diagnosis of AD is made by examining brain tissue. Useful diagnostic criteria and guidelines are provided by
  - ✓ *Diagnostic and Statistical Manual of Mental Disorders*, 4th ed., text revision
  - ✓ Agency for Healthcare Research and Quality
  - ✓ American Academy of Neurology
  - ✓ National Institute of Neurological and Communicative Disorders and Stroke
  - ✓ Alzheimer's Disease and Related Disorders Association
- Patients with suspected AD should have a history and physical examination with appropriate laboratory and other diagnostic tests, neurologic and psychiatric examinations, standardized rating assessments, functional evaluation, and a caregiver interview.

| **TABLE 52–2** | Clinical Presentation of Alzheimer's Disease |

General
- The patient may have vague memory complaints initially, or the patient's significant other may report that the patient is "forgetful." Cognitive decline is gradual over the course of illness. Behavioral disturbances may be present in moderate stages. Loss of daily function is common in advanced stages.

Symptoms
Cognitive
- Memory loss (poor recall and losing items)
- Aphasia (circumlocution and anomia)
- Apraxia
- Agnosia
- Disorientation (impaired perception of time and unable to recognize familiar people)
- Impaired executive function
Noncognitive
- Depression, psychotic symptoms (hallucinations and delusions)
- Behavioral disturbances (physical and verbal aggression, motor hyperactivity, uncooperativeness, wandering, repetitive mannerisms and activities, and combativeness)
Functional
- Inability to care for self (dressing, bathing, toileting, and eating)

Laboratory tests
- Rule out vitamin B_{12} and folate deficiency
- Rule out hypothyroidism with thyroid function tests
- Blood cell counts, serum electrolytes, liver function tests

Other diagnostic tests
- CT or MRI scans may aid diagnosis.

CT, computed tomography; MRI, magnetic resonance imaging.

- Information about prescription drug use; alcohol or other substance use; family medical history; and history of trauma, depression, or head injury should be obtained. It is important to rule out medication use as a contributor or cause of symptoms (e.g., anticholinergics, sedatives, hypnotics, opioids, antipsychotics, and anticonvulsants) as contributors to dementia symptoms. Other medications may contribute to delirium(e.g., digoxin, nonsteroidal antiinflammatory drugs (NSAIDs), histamine$_2$ receptor antagonists, amiodarone, antihypertensives, and corticosteroids).
- The Folstein Mini-Mental State Examination (MMSE) can help to establish a history of deficits in two or more areas of cognition and establish a baseline against which to evaluate change in severity. The average expected decline in an untreated patient is 2 to 4 points per year.

DESIRED OUTCOME

- The primary goal of treatment in AD is to maintain patient functioning as long as possible. Secondary goals are to treat the psychiatric and behavioral sequelae.

TREATMENT

NONPHARMACOLOGIC THERAPY

- Sleep disturbances, wandering, urinary incontinence, agitation, and aggression should be managed with behavioral interventions whenever possible.
- On initial diagnosis, the patient and caregiver should be educated on the course of illness, available treatments, legal decisions, changes in lifestyle that will be necessary with disease progression, and other quality of life issues.
- The Alzheimer's Association recommends staying physically, mentally, and socially active, adopting a low-fat/low-cholesterol diet rich in dark vegetables and fruit, and managing body weight.

PHARMACOTHERAPY OF COGNITIVE SYMPTOMS

- Managing blood pressure, cholesterol, and blood sugar may reduce the risk of developing AD and may prevent the worsening of dementia in patients with AD.
- Current pharmacotherapeutic interventions are primarily symptomatic attempts to improve or maintain cognition. **Table 52–3** may be used as an algorithm for managing cognitive symptoms in AD.
- Successful treatment reflects a decline of <2 points each year on the MMSE score.

Cholinesterase Inhibitors

- **Table 52–4** summarizes the clinical pharmacology of the cholinesterase inhibitors and **memantine**.
- No direct comparative trials have assessed the effectiveness of one agent over another. **Donepezil, rivastigmine,** and **galantamine** are indicated in mild to moderate AD; donepezil is also indicated in severe AD.

TABLE 52–3	Treatment Options for Cognitive Symptoms in Alzheimer's Disease

- In mild to moderate disease, consider therapy with a cholinesterase inhibitor.
  - Donepezil, *or*
  - Rivastigmine, *or*
  - Galantamine
- Titrate to recommended maintenance dose as tolerated.
- In moderate to severe disease, consider adding antiglutamatergic therapy:
  - Memantine
- Titrate to recommended maintenance dose as tolerated.
- Alternatively, consider memantine or cholinesterase inhibitor therapy alone.
- Behavioral symptoms may require additional pharmacologic approaches.

Data from Burns A, Iliffe S. Alzheimer's disease. N Engl J Med 2010;362:329–344; Lyketsos CG, Colenda CC, Beck C, et al. Position statement of the American Association for Geriatric Psychiatry regarding principles of care for patients with dementia resulting from Alzheimer's disease. Am J Geriatr Psychiatry 2006;14: 561–573; and Lleó A, Greenberg SM, Growdon JH. Current pharmacotherapy for Alzheimer's disease. Annu Rev Med 2006;57:513–533.

TABLE 52–4 Clinical Pharmacology of Cognitive Enhancing Medications

	Donepezil	Rivastigmine	Galantamine	Memantine
Brand Name	Aricept	Exelon	Razadyne	Namenda
Dosage Forms	Tablet Orally disintegrating tablet	Capsule Oral solution Patch	Tablet Oral solution Extended-release (ER) capsule	Tablet Oral solution (Extended-release formulation in development)
Starting Dose	5 mg daily in the evening	1.5 mg twice a day 4.6 mg/day (patch)	4 mg twice a day 8 mg daily for (ER)	5 mg once daily
Maintenance Dose	5–10 mg daily 23 mg daily in moderate to severe AD	3–6 mg twice a day 9.5 mg/day (patch)	8–12 mg twice a day (16–24 mg daily for ER)	10 mg twice a day
Meals	Can be taken with or without food	Take with meals	Take with meals	Can be taken with or without food
Mechanism of Action	Reversible inhibition of acetylcholinesterase	Reversible inhibition of acetylcholinesterase and butyrylcholinesterase	Reversible inhibition of acetylcholinesterase and modulation of nicotinic receptors	Antagonism of N-methyl-D-aspartate (NMDA) receptors
Half-Life	70 hours	1.5 hours	7 hours	60–80 hours
Protein Binding	96%	40%	18%	45%
Metabolism	Substrate (minor) of CYP2D6 and 3A34 glucuronidation	Cholinesterase-mediated hydrolysis	Substrate (minor) of CYP2D6 and 3A34 glucuronidation	Glucuronidation
Renal Elimination	Yes	Major pathway	Yes	Yes

CYP, cytochrome P450.

Data from Namenda (memantine hydrochloride) package insert. St. Louis, MO: Forest Laboratories, 2007; Aricept (donepezil hydrochloride) package insert. Teaneck, NJ: Eisai Co, Ltd, 2006; Exelon (rivastigmine tartrate) package insert. East Hanover, NJ: Novartis Pharmaceuticals, 2006; Razadyne (galantamine hydrobromide) package insert. Titusville, NJ: Ortho-McNeil-Janssen Pharmaceuticals; 2008; and Exelon (rivastigmine) Patch package insert. East Hanover, NJ: Novartis Pharmaceutical, 2009.

- If the decline in MMSE score is >2 to 4 points after treatment for 1 year with the initial agent, it is reasonable to change to a different cholinesterase inhibitor. Otherwise, treatment should be continued with the initial medication throughout the course of the illness.
- The most frequent adverse effects are mild to moderate GI symptoms (nausea, vomiting, and diarrhea), urinary incontinence, dizziness, headache, syncope, bradycardia, muscle weakness, salivation, and sweating. Abrupt discontinuation can cause worsening of cognition and behavior in some patients.
- **Donepezil** (Aricept) is a piperidine derivative with specificity for inhibition of acetylcholinesterase rather than butyrylcholinesterase.
- **Rivastigmine** has central activity at acetylcholinesterase and butyrylcholinesterase sites but low activity at these sites in the periphery.
- **Galantamine** is an acetylcholinesterase inhibitor that also has activity as a nicotinic receptor agonist.
- **Tacrine** was the first cholinesterase inhibitor approved for the treatment of AD, but it has been replaced by safer drugs that are better tolerated.

Other Drugs

- **Memantine** (Namenda) blocks glutamatergic neurotransmission by antagonizing *N*-methyl-d-aspartate receptors, which may prevent excitotoxic reactions. It is used as monotherapy, and data suggest that when it is combined with a cholinesterase inhibitor, there is improvement in cognition and activities of daily living.
  ✓ It is indicated for treatment of moderate to severe AD.
  ✓ It is not metabolized by the liver, but is primarily excreted unchanged in the urine.
  ✓ It is usually well tolerated; side effects include constipation, confusion, dizziness, hallucinations, headache, cough, and hypertension.
  ✓ It is initiated at 5 mg/day and increased weekly by 5 mg/day to the effective dose of 10 mg twice daily. Dosing must be adjusted in patients with renal impairment.
- Guidelines recommend low-dose **aspirin** therapy in patients with AD with significant brain vascular disease.
- Recent trials do not support the use of **estrogen** to prevent or treat cognitive decline.
- Evidence related to the role of **vitamin E** in preventing AD is mixed, and conclusions cannot be drawn at this time. It is not recommended for treatment of AD.
- Because of a significant incidence of side effects and a lack of compelling supporting evidence, neither **NSAIDs** nor **prednisone** is recommended for treatment or prevention of AD.
- There is interest in the use of lipid-lowering agents, especially the 3-hydroxy-3-methylglutaryl coenzyme A–reductase inhibitors, to prevent AD. Thus far, trials of *statin* drugs have not shown significant benefit in prevention or treatment of AD.
- A meta-analysis indicated that EGb 761 (an extract of **ginkgo biloba**) may have some therapeutic effect at doses of 120 to 240 mg of the standard

leaf extract twice daily. However, a large trial using these doses failed to reduce the incidence of dementia or AD. Because of limited efficacy data, the potential for adverse effects (e.g., nausea, vomiting, diarrhea, headache, dizziness, restlessness, weakness, and hemorrhage), and the poor standardization of herbal products, ginkgo biloba is not recommended for prevention or treatment of AD.

✓ Ginkgo biloba should not be used in individuals taking anticoagulants or antiplatelet drugs and should be used cautiously in those taking **NSAIDs.**

• Although initial studies suggest the potential effectiveness of **huperzine A,** it has not been adequately evaluated and is not currently recommended for treatment of AD.

PHARMACOTHERAPY OF NONCOGNITIVE SYMPTOMS

• Pharmacotherapy is aimed at treating psychotic symptoms, inappropriate or disruptive behavior, and depression. Medications and recommended doses for noncognitive symptoms are shown in Table 52–5.

TABLE 52–5	Medications Used for Noncognitive Symptoms of Dementia		
Drugs	**Starting Dose (mg)**	**Maintenance Dose in Dementia (mg/day)**	**Target Symptoms**
Antipsychotics			Psychosis: hallucinations, delusions, suspiciousness
Haloperidol	0.25	1–3	
Olanzapine	2.5	5–10	
Quetiapine	25	100–300	Disruptive behaviors: agitation, aggression
Risperidone	0.25	0.75–2	
Ziprasidone	20	40–160	
Antidepressants			Depression: poor appetite, insomnia, hopelessness, anhedonia, withdrawal, suicidal thoughts, agitation, anxiety
Citalopram	10	10–20	
Escitalopram	5	20–40	
Fluoxetine	5	10–40	
Paroxetine	10	10–40	
Sertraline	25	75–100	
Venlafaxine	25	75–225	
Trazodone	25	75–150	
Anticonvulsants			Agitation or aggression
Carbamazepine	100	200–600	
Valproic acid	125	500–1,000	

Data from Lleó A, Greenberg SM, Growdon JH. Current pharmacotherapy for Alzheimer's disease. Annu Rev Med 2006;57:513–533; Benoit M, Arbus C, Blanchard F, et al. Professional consensus on the treatment of agitation, aggressive behavior, oppositional behavior and psychotic disturbances in dementia. J Nutr Health Aging 2006;10:410–415; and Grossberg GT, Desai AK. Management of Alzheimer's disease. J Gerontol A Biol Sci Med Sci 2003;58A:331–353.

- General guidelines are as follows: (1) use reduced doses, (2) monitor closely, (3) titrate the dosage slowly, (4) document carefully, and (5) periodically attempt to reduce medication in minimally symptomatic patients.
- Psychotropic medications with anticholinergic effects should be avoided because they may worsen cognition.

Cholinesterase Inhibitors and Memantine

- **Cholinesterase inhibitors** and **memantine** have consistently shown modest benefit for management of behavioral symptoms over time but may not significantly reduce acute agitation.

Antipsychotics

- Antipsychotic medications have traditionally been used to treat disruptive behaviors and psychosis in patients with AD, but the risks and benefits must be carefully weighed.
- A meta-analysis found that only 17% to 18% of dementia patients showed a modest treatment response to atypical antipsychotics. Adverse events included somnolence, extrapyramidal symptoms, abnormal gait, worsening cognition, cerebrovascular events, and increased risk of death.
- Typical antipsychotics may also be associated with a small increased risk of death, as well as more severe extrapyramidal effects and hypotension.

Antidepressants

- Depression and dementia have many symptoms in common, and the diagnosis of depression can be difficult, especially later in the course of AD.
- Treatment with a **selective serotonin reuptake inhibitor** (SSRI) is usually initiated in depressed patients with AD, and the best evidence is for **sertraline** and **citalopram.**
- **Buproprion, venlafaxine,** and **mirtazapine** may also be used, but the **tricyclic antidepressants** are usually avoided.

Miscellaneous Therapies

- Use of **benzodiazepines is** not advised except on an "as needed" basis for infrequent episodes of agitation.
- **Carbamazepine, valproic acid,** and **gabapentin** may be alternatives, but evidence is conflicting.

EVALUATION OF THERAPEUTIC OUTCOMES

- Baseline assessment should define therapeutic goals and document cognitive status, physical status, functional performance, mood, thought processes, and behavior. Both the patient and caregiver should be interviewed.
- Because target symptoms of psychiatric disorders may respond differently in demented patients, a detailed list of symptoms to be treated should be documented to aid in monitoring.
- Objective assessments, such as the MMSE for cognition and the Functional Activities Questionnaire for activities of daily living, should be used to quantify changes in symptoms and functioning.

- The patient should be observed carefully for potential side effects of drug therapy. The specific side effects to be monitored and the method and frequency of monitoring should be documented.
- Assessments for drug effectiveness, side effects, compliance, need for dosage adjustment, or change in treatment should occur at least monthly.
- A treatment period of several months to 1 year may be required to determine whether therapy is beneficial.

See Chapter 63, Alzheimer's Disease, authored by Patricia W. Slattum, Russell H. Swerdlow, and Angela Massey Hill, for a more detailed discussion of this topic.

DEFINITIONS

- Epilepsy is defined by the occurrence of at least two unprovoked seizures with or without convulsions separated by at least 24 hours. A seizure results from an excessive discharge of cortical neurons and is characterized by changes in electrical activity as measured by the electroencephalogram (EEG). A convulsion implies violent, involuntary contraction(s) of the voluntary muscles.

PATHOPHYSIOLOGY

- Seizures result from excessive excitation or from disordered inhibition of a population of neurons. Initially, a small number of neurons fire abnormally. Normal membrane conductances and inhibitory synaptic currents then break down, and excitability spreads locally (focal seizure) or more widely (generalized seizure).
- Mechanisms that may contribute to synchronous hyperexcitability include:
  - ✓ Alterations of ion channels in neuronal membranes
  - ✓ Biochemical modifications of receptors
  - ✓ Modulation of second messaging systems and gene expression
  - ✓ Changes in extracellular ion concentrations
  - ✓ Alterations in neurotransmitter uptake and metabolism in glial cells
  - ✓ Modification in the ratio and function of inhibitory circuits
  - ✓ Local imbalances between the main neurotransmitters (e.g., glutamate, γ-aminobutyric acid [GABA]) and neuromodulators (e.g., acetylcholine, norepinephrine, and serotonin)
- Prolonged seizures and continued exposure to glutamate may result in neuronal injury with functional deficits and rewiring of neuronal circuitry.

CLINICAL PRESENTATION

GENERAL

- In most cases, the healthcare provider will not be in a position to witness a seizure. Many patients, particularly those with complex partial (CP) or generalized tonic-clonic (GTC) seizures, are amnestic to the actual seizure event. Obtaining an accurate history and description of the ictal event (including time course) from a third party is important.

SYMPTOMS

- Symptoms of a specific seizure depend on seizure type. Although seizures can vary between patients, they tend to be stereotyped within an individual.

- CP seizures may include somatosensory or focal motor features. They are associated with altered consciousness.
- Absence seizures have only very brief (seconds) periods of altered consciousness.
- GTC seizures are major convulsive episodes and are always associated with a loss of consciousness.

SIGNS

- Interictally (between seizure episodes), there are typically no objective, pathognomonic signs of epilepsy.

LABORATORY TESTS

- There are currently no diagnostic laboratory tests for epilepsy. In some cases, particularly following GTC (or perhaps CP) seizures, serum prolactin levels may be transiently elevated. Laboratory tests may be done to rule out treatable causes of seizures (hypoglycemia, altered serum electrolyte concentrations, infections, etc.) that do not represent epilepsy.

OTHER DIAGNOSTIC TESTS

- EEG is very useful in the diagnosis of various seizure disorders, but the EEG may be normal in some patients who still have the clinical diagnosis of epilepsy.
- A serum prolactin level obtained within 10 to 20 minutes of a tonic-clonic seizure can help differentiate seizure activity from pseudoseizure activity but not from syncope.
- Although magnetic resonance imaging is very useful (especially imaging of the temporal lobes), computed tomography typically is not helpful except in the initial evaluation for a brain tumor or cerebral bleeding.
- The International Classification of Epileptic Seizures (Table 53–1) classifies epilepsy on the basis of clinical description and electrophysiologic findings.
- Partial (focal) seizures begin in one hemisphere of the brain and, unless they become secondarily generalized, result in an asymmetric seizure. Partial seizures manifest as alterations in motor functions, sensory or somatosensory symptoms, or automatisms. If there is no loss of consciousness, the seizures are called *simple partial.* If there is loss of consciousness, they are termed *complex partial,* and the patients may have automatisms, memory loss, or aberrations of behavior. A partial seizure that becomes generalized is termed a *secondarily generalized seizure.*
- Absence seizures generally occur in young children or adolescents and exhibit a sudden onset, interruption of ongoing activities, a blank stare, and possibly a brief upward rotation of the eyes. Absence seizures have a characteristic 2 to 4 cycle/sec spike and slow-wave EEG pattern.
- In generalized seizures, motor symptoms are bilateral, and there is altered consciousness.
- GTC seizures may be preceded by premonitory symptoms (i.e., an aura). A tonic-clonic seizure that is preceded by an aura is likely a partial seizure

TABLE 53–1	International Classification of Epileptic Seizures

I. Partial seizures (seizures begin locally)
  A. Simple (without impairment of consciousness)
    1. With motor symptoms
    2. With special sensory or somatosensory symptoms
    3. With psychic symptoms
  B. Complex (with impairment of consciousness)
    1. Simple partial onset followed by impairment of consciousness—with or without automatisms
    2. Impaired consciousness at onset—with or without automatisms
  C. Secondarily generalized (partial onset evolving to generalized tonic-clonic seizures)
II. Generalized seizures (bilaterally symmetrical and without local onset)
  A. Absence
  B. Myoclonic
  C. Clonic
  D. Tonic
  E. Tonic-clonic
  F. Atonic
  G. Infantile spasms
III. Unclassified seizures
IV. Status epilepticus

Data from Commission on Classification and Terminology of the International League Against Epilepsy. Proposal for revised clinical and electroencephalographic classification of epileptic seizures. Epilepsia 1981;22:489–501; and Commission on Classification and Terminology of the International League Against Epilepsy. Proposal for revised classification of epilepsies and epileptic syndromes. Epilepsia 1989;30:389–399.

that is secondarily generalized. Tonic-clonic seizures begin with a short tonic contraction of muscles followed by a period of rigidity and clonic movements. The patient may lose sphincter control, bite the tongue, or become cyanotic. The episode may be followed by unconsciousness, and frequently the patient goes into a deep sleep.

- Myoclonic jerks are brief shock-like muscular contractions of the face, trunk, and extremities. They may be isolated events or rapidly repetitive.
- In atonic seizures, there is a sudden loss of muscle tone that may be described as a head drop, dropping of a limb, or slumping to the ground.

DIAGNOSIS

- The patient and family should be asked to characterize the seizure for frequency, duration, precipitating factors, time of occurrence, presence of an aura, ictal activity, and postictal state.
- Physical, neurologic, and laboratory examination (SMA-20 [sequential multichannel analysis], complete blood cell count, urinalysis, and special blood chemistries) may identify an etiology. A lumbar puncture may be indicated if there is fever.

DESIRED OUTCOME

- The goal of treatment is to control or reduce the frequency of seizures, minimize side effects, and ensure compliance, allowing the patient to live as normal a life as possible. Complete suppression of seizures must be balanced against tolerability of side effects, and the patient should be involved in defining the balance.

TREATMENT

GENERAL APPROACH

- The treatment of choice depends on the type of epilepsy (Table 53–2) and on drug-specific adverse effects and patient preferences. Fig. 53–1 is a suggested algorithm for treatment of epilepsy.
- Begin with monotherapy; ~50% to 70% of patients can be maintained on one antiepileptic drug (AED), but all are not seizure free.
- About 65% of patients can be maintained on one AED and be well controlled, although not necessarily seizure free.
- Up to 60% of patients with epilepsy are noncompliant; this is the most common reason for treatment failure.
- Drug therapy may not be indicated in patients who have had only one seizure or those whose seizures have minimal impact on their lives. Patients who have had two or more seizures should generally be started on AEDs.
- Factors favoring successful withdrawal of AEDs include a seizure-free period of 2 to 4 years, complete seizure control within 1 year of onset, an onset of seizures after age 2 years and before age 35 years, and a normal EEG and neurologic examination. Poor prognostic factors include a history of a high frequency of seizures, repeated episodes of status epilepticus, a combination of seizure types, and development of abnormal mental functioning. A 2-year, seizure-free period is suggested for absence and rolandic epilepsy, whereas a 4-year, seizure-free period is suggested for simple partial, CP, and absence associated with tonic-clonic seizures. According to the American Academy of Neurology guidelines, discontinuation of AEDs may be considered if the patient is seizure free for 2 to 5 years, if there is a single type of partial seizure or primary GTC seizures, if the neurologic examination and IQ are normal, and if the EEG normalized with treatment. AED withdrawal should always be done gradually.

MECHANISM OF ACTION

- The mechanism of action of most AEDs includes effects on ion channel (sodium and Ca) kinetics, augmentation of inhibitory neurotransmission (increasing CNS GABA), and modulation of excitatory neurotransmission (decreasing or antagonizing glutamate and aspartate). AEDs that are effective against GTC and partial seizures probably work by delaying recovery of sodium channels from activation. Drugs that reduce corticothalamic T-type Ca currents are effective against generalized absence seizures.

TABLE 53–2 Drugs of Choice for Specific Seizure Disorders

Seizure Type	First-Line Drugs	Alternative Drugs[a]	Comments
Partial seizures (newly diagnosed)			
U.S. guidelines	*Adults & adolescents:* Carbamazepine Gabapentin Oxcarbazepine Phenobarbital Phenytoin Topiramate Valproic acid		*FDA approved:* Carbamazepine Lacosamide Phenobarbital Phenytoin Topiramate Valproic acid
U.K. guidelines	Carbamazepine Lamotrigine Oxcarbazepine Topiramate Valproic acid		
ILAE guidelines	*Adults:* Carbamazepine Phenytoin Valproic acid	*Adults:* Gabapentin Lamotrigine Oxcarbazepine Phenobarbital Topiramate	
	Children: Oxcarbazepine	*Children:* Phenobarbital Phenytoin Topiramate Valproic acid	
	Elderly: Gabapentin Lamotrigine	*Elderly:* Carbamazepine	
U.S. Expert Panel 2005	Carbamazepine Lamotrigine Oxcarbazepine	Levetiracetam	
Partial seizures (refractory monotherapy)			
U.S. guidelines	Lamotrigine Oxcarbazepine Topiramate		*FDA approved:* Carbamazepine Lamotrigine Oxcarbazepine Phenobarbital Phenytoin Topiramate Valproic acid
U.K. guidelines	Lamotrigine Oxcarbazepine Topiramate		

(continued)

TABLE 53-2	Drugs of Choice for Specific Seizure Disorders *(Continued)*		
Seizure Type	**First-Line Drugs**	**Alternative Drugs**[a]	**Comments**
Partial seizures (refractory adjunct)			
U.S. guidelines	*Adults:* Gabapentin Lamotrigine Levetiracetam Oxcarbazepine Tiagabine Topiramate Zonisamide *Children:* Gabapentin Lamotrigine Oxcarbazepine Topiramate		*FDA approved:* Carbamazepine Gabapentin Lamotrigine Levetiracetam Oxcarbazepine Phenobarbital Phenytoin Pregabalin Tiagabine Valproic acid Vigabatrin Zonisamide
U.K. guidelines	Gabapentin Lamotrigine Levetiracetam Oxcarbazepine Tiagabine		
Generalized seizures absence (newly diagnosed)			
U.S. guidelines	Lamotrigine		*FDA approved:* Ethosuximide Valproic acid
U.K. guidelines	Lamotrigine		
ILAE guidelines	None	Ethosuximide Lamotrigine Valproic acid	
U.S. Expert Panel 2005	Ethosuximide Valproic acid	Lamotrigine	
Primary generalized (tonic-clonic)			
U.S. guidelines	Topiramate		*FDA approved:* Lamotrigine Levetiracetam Topiramate
U.K. guidelines	Lamotrigine Topiramate		
ILAE guidelines	None	*Adults:* Carbamazepine Lamotrigine Oxcarbazepine Phenobarbital Phenytoin Topiramate Valproic acid	

(continued)

TABLE 53–2	Drugs of Choice for Specific Seizure Disorders *(Continued)*		
Seizure Type	**First-Line Drugs**	**Alternative Drugs[a]**	**Comments**
Primary generalized (tonic-clonic)			
		Children: Carbamazepine Phenobarbital Phenytoin Topiramate Valproic acid	
U.S. Expert Panel 2005	Valproic acid	Lamotrigine Topiramate	
Juvenile myoclonic epilepsy			*FDA approved:* Levetiracetam (myoclonic seizures)
ILAE[28]	None	Clonazepam Lamotrigine Levetiracetam Topiramate Valproic acid Zonisamide	
U.S. Expert Panel 2005	Valproic acid	Levetiracetam Topiramate Zonisamide	

ILAE, International League Against Epilepsy.
[a]Includes possibly effective drugs.
Data from French JA, Kanner AM, Bautista J, et al. Efficacy and tolerability of the new antiepileptic drugs:
   I. Treatment of new onset epilepsy. Neurology 2004;62:1252–1260; French JA, Kanner AM, Bautista J,
   et al. Efficacy and tolerability of the new antiepileptic drugs: II. Treatment of refractory epilepsy. Neurology
   2004;62:1261–1273; National Institute for Clinical Excellence. Newer Drugs for Epilepsy in Adults; 2006.
   http://www.nice.org.uk; National Institute for Clinical Excellence. Newer Drugs for Epilepsy in Children;
   2006. http://www.nice.org.uk; Glauser T, Ben-Menachem E, Bourgeois B, et al. ILAE treatment guidelines:
   Evidenced-based analysis of antiepileptic drug efficacy and effectiveness as initial monotherapy for epileptic
   seizures and syndromes. Epilepsia 2006;47:1094–1120; and Karceski S, Morrell MJ, Carpenter D. Treatment
   of epilepsy in adults: Expert opinion. Epilepsy Behav 2005;7:S1–S64.

SPECIAL CONSIDERATIONS IN THE FEMALE PATIENT

- Estrogen has a seizure-activating effect, whereas progesterone has a seizure-protective effect. Enzyme-inducing AEDs, including topiramate and oxcarbazepine, may cause treatment failures in women taking **oral contraceptives**; a supplemental form of birth control is advised if breakthrough bleeding occurs.
- For catamenial epilepsy (seizures just before or during menses) or seizures that occur at the time of ovulation, conventional AEDs should be tried first, but intermittent supplementation with higher dose AEDs or benzodiazepines should be considered. **Acetazolamide** has been used with limited success. Hormonal therapy (**progestational agents**) may also be effective.

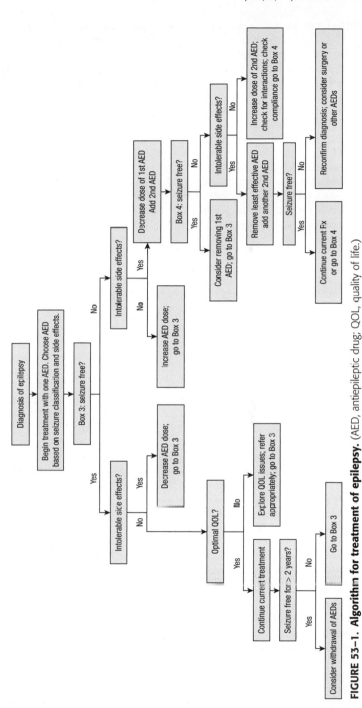

FIGURE 53-1. Algorithm for treatment of epilepsy. (AED, antiepileptic drug; QOL, quality of life.)

651

- About 25% to 30% of women have increased seizure frequency during pregnancy, and a similar percentage have decreased frequency.
- AED monotherapy is preferred in pregnancy. Clearance of **phenytoin, carbamazepine, phenobarbital, ethosuximide, lamotrigine, oxcarbazepine, levetiracetam, topiramate,** and **clorazepate** increases during pregnancy, and protein binding may be reduced. There is a higher incidence of adverse pregnancy outcomes in women with epilepsy, and the risk of congenital malformations is 4% to 6% (twice as high as in nonepileptic women). **Barbiturates** and **phenytoin** are associated with congenital heart malformations and facial clefts. **Valproic acid** and **carbamazepine** are associated with spina bifida (0.5–1%) and hypospadias. Other adverse outcomes are growth, psychomotor, and mental retardation. Valproic acid is associated with a higher rate of fetal malformations compared with the other AEDs, especially at doses >1400 mg/day. Some teratogenic events can be prevented by adequate **folate** intake; **prenatal vitamins with folic acid** (~0.4–5 mg/day) should be given to women of child-bearing potential who are taking AEDs. Higher folate doses should be used in women with a history of a previous pregnancy with a neural tube defect or taking valproic acid. **Vitamin K,** 10 mg/day orally, given to the mother during the last month before delivery can prevent neonatal hemorrhagic disorder. Alternatively, parenteral vitamin K can be given to the newborn at delivery.

PHARMACOKINETICS

- AED pharmacokinetic data are summarized in **Table 53–3.** For populations known to have altered plasma protein binding, free rather than total serum concentrations should be measured if the AED is highly protein bound. Conditions altering AED protein binding include chronic renal failure, liver disease, hypoalbuminemia, burns, pregnancy, malnutrition, displacing drugs, and age (neonates and the elderly). Unbound concentration monitoring is especially useful for **phenytoin.**
- Neonates and infants display decreased efficiency in renal elimination and may metabolize drugs more slowly, but children by age 2 or 3 years may metabolize drugs more rapidly than adults. Thus, neonates and infants require lower doses of AED, but children require higher doses of many AEDs than adults. Lower doses of AEDs are often required in the elderly. Some elderly patients have increased receptor sensitivity to CNS drugs, making the accepted therapeutic range invalid.

THE ROLE OF SERUM CONCENTRATION MONITORING

- Seizure control may occur before the "minimum" of the accepted therapeutic serum range is reached, and some patients may need serum concentrations beyond the "maximum." The therapeutic range for AEDs may be different for different seizure types (e.g., higher for CP seizures than for GTC seizures). Clinicians should determine the optimal serum concentration for each patient. Serum concentrations can be useful to document lack of or loss of efficacy, to establish noncompliance, and to guide therapy in patients with renal and/or hepatic disease and patients

TABLE 53-3 Antiepileptic Drug Pharmacokinetic Data

AED	$t_{1/2}$ (hours)	Time to Steady State (days)	Unchanged (%)	V_D (L/kg)	Clinically Important Metabolite	Protein Binding (%)
Carbamazepine	12 M; 5–14 Co	21–28 for completion of auto-induction	<1	1–2	10,11-epoxide	40–90
Ethosuximide	A 60; C 30	6–12	10–20	0.67	No	0
Felbamate	16–22	5–7	50	0.73–0.82	No	~25
Gabapentin[c]	5–40[b]	1–2	100	0.65–1.04	No	0
Lacosamide	13	3	40	0.6	No	<15
Lamotrigine	25.4 M	3–15	0	1.28	No	40–50
Levetiracetam	7–10	2		0.7	No	<10
Oxcarbazepine	3–13	2		0.7	10-hydroxy-carbazepine	40
Phenobarbital	A 46–136; C 37–73	14–21	20–40	0.6	No	50
Phenytoin	A 10–34; C 5–14	7–28	<5	0.6–8.0	No	90
Pregabalin	A6–7[b]	1–2	90	0.5	No	0
Primidone	A 3.3–19; C 4.5–11	1–4	40	0.43–1.1	PB	80
Rufinamide	6–10	2	4	0.8–1.2	No	26–35

(continued)

TABLE 53–4	Antiepileptic Drug Side Effects *(Continued)*		
	Acute Side Effects		
Antiepileptic Drug	**Concentration Dependent**	**Idiosyncratic**	**Chronic Side Effects**
Valproic acid	GI upset Sedation Unsteadiness Tremor Thrombocytopenia	Acute hepatic failure Acute pancreatitis Alopecia	Polycystic ovary–like syndrome Weight gain Hyperammonemia Menstual cycle irregularities
Vigabatrin	Permanent vision loss Fatigue Somnolence Weight gain Tremor Blurred vision	Abnormal MRI brain signal changes (infants with infantile spasms) Peripheral neuropathy Anemia	Permanent vision loss
Zonisamide	Sedation Dizziness Cognitive impairment Nausea	Rash Metabolic acidosis Oligohydrosis	Kidney stones Weight loss

Data from French JA, Kanner AM, Bautista J, et al. Efficacy and tolerability of the new antiepileptic drugs: I. Treatment of new onset epilepsy. Neurology 2004;62:1252–1260; French JA, Kanner AM, Bautista J, et al. Efficacy and tolerability of the new antiepileptic drugs: II. Treatment of refractory epilepsy. Neurology 2004;62:1261–1273; Leppik IE. Contemporary Diagnosis and Management of the Patient with Epilepsy, 6th ed. Newton, PA: Handbooks in Health Care, 2006:92–149; Halford JJ, Lapointe M. Clinical perspectives on lacosamide. Epilepsy Curr 2009;9:1–9; Cada DJ, Levien TL, Baker DE. Rufinamide. Hosp Pharm 2009;44:412–422; and Sabril [package insert]. Deerfield, IL: Lundbeck Inc; August 2009.

asymptomatic high-turnover bone disease with normal bone mineral density (BMD) or decreased (BMD) and osteoporosis. Laboratory tests may reveal elevated bone-specific alkaline phosphatase and decreased serum Ca and 25-OH vitamin D, as well as intact parathyroid hormone.

DRUG–DRUG INTERACTIONS

- Drug interactions involving AEDs are shown in **Table 53–5.**
- **Phenobarbital, phenytoin, primidone,** and **carbamazepine** are potent inducers of cytochrome P450 (CYP450), epoxide hydrolase, and uridine diphosphate glucuronosyltransferase enzyme systems. **Valproic acid** inhibits many hepatic enzyme systems and displaces some drugs from plasma albumin.
- **Felbamate** and **topiramate** can act as inducers with some isoforms and inhibitors with others.
- Except for **levetiracetam** and **gabapentin,** which are eliminated mostly unchanged by the renal route, AEDs are metabolized wholly or in part by hepatic enzymes.

TABLE 53–5 Interactions Between Antiepileptic Drugs

Antiepileptic Drug	Added Drug	Effect[a]
Carbamazepine (CBZ)	Felbamate	Incr. 10,11 epoxide
		Decr. CBZ
	Oxcarbazepine	Decr. CBZ
	Phenobarbital	Decr. CBZ
	Phenytoin	Decr. CBZ
	Valproic acid	Incr. 10,11 epoxide
Ethosuximide	Carbamazepine	Decr. ethosuximide
	Phenobarbital	Decr. ethosuximide
	Phenytoin	Decr. ethosuximide
Felbamate (FBM)	Carbamazepine	Decr. FBM
	Phenytoin	Decr. FBM
	Valproic acid	Incr. FRM
Gabapentin	No known interactions	
Lacosamide (LAC)	Carbamazepine	Decr. LAC
	Phenobarbital	Decr. LAC
	Phenytoin	Decr. LAC
Lamotrigine (LTG)	Carbamazepine	Decr. LTG
	Phenobarbital	Decr. LTG
	Phenytoin	Decr. LTG
	Primidone	Decr. LTG
	Valproic acid	Incr. LTG
Levetiracetam (LEV)	Carbamazepine	Decr. LEV
	Phenobarbital	Decr. LEV
	Phenytoin	Decr. LEV
Oxcarbazepine	Carbamazepine	Decr. MHD[b]
	Phenobarbital	Decr. MHD[b]
	Phenytoin	Decr. MHD[b]
Phenobarbital (PB)	Felbamate	Incr. PB
	Oxcarbazepine	Incr. PB
	Phenytoin	Incr. PB
	Valproic acid	Incr. PB
Phenytoin (PHT)	Carbamazepine	Incr. or decr. PHT
	Felbamate	Incr. PHT
	Methsuximide	Incr. PHT
	Oxcarbazepine (>1,200 mg/d)	Incr. PHT
	Phenobarbital	Incr. or decr. PHT
	Topiramate	Incr. PHT
	Valproic acid	Decr. Total PHT, then may incr. total PHT
	Vigabatrin	Decr. PHT
Pregabalin	No known interactions	

(continued)

TABLE 53–5	Interactions Between Antiepileptic Drugs *(Continued)*

Antiepileptic Drug	Added Drug	Effect[a]
Primidone (PRM)	Carbamazepine	Decr. PRM
		Incr. PB
	Phenytoin	Decr. PRM
		Incr. PB
	Valproic acid	Incr. PRM
		Incr. PB
Rufinamide (RUF)	Carbamazepine	Decr. RUF
	Phenobarbital	Decr. RUF
	Phenytoin	Decr. RUF
	Primidone	Decr. RUF
	Valproic acid	Incr. RUF
Tiagabine (TGB)	Carbamazepine	Decr. TGB
	Phenobarbital	Decr. TGB
	Phenytoin	Decr. TGB
	Primidone	Decr. TGB
Topiramate (TPM)	Carbamazepine	Decr. TPM
	Phenobarbital	Decr. TPM
	Phenytoin	Decr. TPM
	Primdione	Decr. TPM
	Valproic acid	Decr. TPM
Valproic acid (VPA)	Carbamazepine	Decr. VPA
	Felbamate	Incr. VPA
	Lamotrigine	Decr. VPA (slight)
	Phenobarbital	Decr. VPA
	Phenytoin	Decr. VPA
	Primidone	Decr. VPA
	Topiramate	Decr. VPA
Vigabatrin	No known interactions	
Zonisamide (ZON)	Carbamazepine	Decr. ZON
	Phenobarbital	Decr. ZON
	Phenytoin	Decr. ZON
	Primidone	Decr. ZON

[a]Incr., increased; Decr., decreased.
[b]MHD, 10-mono-hydroxy-derivative.
Data from Patsalos PN, Berry DJ, Bourgeois BFD, et al. Antiepileptic drugs-best practice guidelines for therapeutic drug monitoring: A position paper by the subcommission on therapeutic drug monitoring, ILAE Commission on Therapeutic Strategies. Epilepsia 2008;49:1239–1276; Halford JJ, Lapointe M. Clinical perspectives on lacosamide. Epilepsy Curr 2009;9:1–9; and Cada DJ, Levien TL, Baker DE. Rufinamide. Hosp Pharm 2009;44:412–22.

DOSAGE AND ADMINISTRATION

- Initial and maximal daily doses and target serum concentration ranges are shown in **Table 53–6.** Usually therapy is initiated at one fourth to one third of the anticipated maintenance dose and gradually increased over 3 or 4 weeks to an effective dose. Serum concentrations may be useful, but the therapeutic range must be correlated with clinical outcome.

TABLE 53-6 Antiepileptic Drug Dosing and Target Serum Concentration Ranges

	Trade Name	Usual Initial Dose	Usual Maximum Daily Dose	Target Serum Concentration Range
Barbiturates				
Phenobarbital	Various	1–3 mg/kg/day (10–20 mg/kg LD)	180–300 mg	10–40 mcg/mL (43–172 μmol/L)
Primidone	Mysoline	100–125 mg/day	750–2,000 mg	5–10 mcg/mL (23–46 μmol/L)
Benzodiazepines				
Clonazepam	Klonopin	1.5 mg/day	20 mg	20–70 ng/mL (0.06–0.22 μmol/L)
Diazepam	Valium	PO: 4–40 mg IV: 5–10 mg	PO: 4–40 mg IV: 5–30 mg	100–1,000 ng/mL (0.4–3.5 μmol/L)
Lorazepam	Ativan	PO: 2–6 mg IV: 0.05 mg/kg IM: 0.05 mg/kg	PO: 10 mg IV: 0.05 mg/kg	10–30 ng/mL (31–93 μmol/L)
Hydantoin				
Phenytoin	Dilantin	PO: 3–5 mg/kg (200–400 mg) (15–20 mg/kg LD)	PO: 500–600 mg	Total: 10–20 mcg/mL (40–79 μmol/L) Unbound: 0.5–3 mcg/mL (2–12 μmol/L)
Succinimide				
Ethosuximide	Zarontin	500 mg/day	500–2,000 mg	40–100 mcg/mL (282–708 μmol/L)
Other				
Carbamazepine	Tegretol	400 mg/day	400–2,400 mg	4–12 mcg/mL (17–51 μmol/L)
Felbamate	Felbatol	1,200 mg/day	3,600 mg	30–60 mcg/mL (126–252 μmol/L)

(continued)

TABLE 53–6 Antiepileptic Drug Dosing and Target Serum Concentration Ranges *(Continued)*

	Trade Name	Usual Initial Dose	Usual Maximum Daily Dose	Target Serum Concentration Range
Other				
Gabapentin	Neurontin	900 mg/day	4,800 mg	2–20 mcg/mL (12–117 μmol/L)
Lacosamide	Vimpat	100 mg/day	400 mg	Not defined
Lamotrigine	Lamictal	25 mg every other day if on VPA; 25–50 mg/day if not on VPA	100–150 mg if on VPA; 300–500 mg if not on VPA	4–20 mcg/mL (16–78 μmol/L)
Levetiracetam	Keppra Keppra XR	500–1,000 mg/day	3,000–4,000 mg	12–46 mcg/mL (70–270 μmol/L)
Oxcarbazepine	Trileptal	300–600 mg/day	2,400–3,000 mg	3–35 mcg/mL (MHD) (12–139 μmol/L)
Pregabalin	Lyrica	150 mg/day	600 mg	Not defined
Rufinamide	Banzel	400–800 mg/day	3,200 mg	Not defined
Tiagabine	Gabitril	4–8 mg/day	80 mg	0.02–0.2 mcg/mL (0.05–0.5 μmol/L)
Topiramate	Topamax	25–50 mg/day	200–1,000 mg	5–20 mcg/mL (15–59 μmol/L)
Valproic acid	Depakene Depakene SR Depakote Depakote ER Depacon	15 mg/kg (500–1,000 mg)	60 mg/kg (3,000–5,000 mg)	50–100 mcg/mL (347–693 μmol/L)
Vigabatrin	Sabril	1,000 mg/day	3,000 mg	0.8–36 mcg/mL (6–279 μmol/L)
Zonisamide	Zonegran	100–200 mg/day	600 mg	10–40 mcg/mL (47–188 μmol/L)

IM, intramuscular; LD, loading dões; MHD, 10-monohydroxy- derivative; PO, orally; VPA, valproic acid.

Data from Patsalos PN, Berry DJ, Bourgeois BFD, et al. Antiepileptic drugs-best practice guidelines for therapeutic drug monitoring: A position paper by the subcommission on therapeutic drug monitoring, ILAE Commission on Therapeutic Strategies. Epilepsia 2008;49:1239–1276; Halford JJ, Lapointe M. Clinical perspectives on lacosamide. Epilepsy Curr 2009;9:1–9; Cada DJ, Levien TL, Baker DE. Rufiramide. Hosp Pharm 2009;44:412–422; and Sabril [package insert]. Deerfield, IL: Lundbeck Inc; August 2009.

SPECIFIC ANTIEPILEPTIC DRUGS

Carbamazepine

- Food may enhance the bioavailability of **carbamazepine**.
- Controlled- and sustained-release preparations dosed every 12 hours are bioequivalent to immediate-release preparations dosed every 6 hours. These dosage forms, compared with immediate-release preparations, have lower peaks and higher troughs.
- The liver metabolizes carbamazepine (mostly by CYP3A4), and the major metabolite is carbamazepine-10,11-epoxide, which is active.
- Carbamazepine can induce its own metabolism (autoinduction); this effect begins within 3 to 5 days of dosing initiation and takes 21 to 28 days to become complete.
- Carbamazepine is considered an AED of first choice for newly diagnosed partial seizures and for primary GTC seizures that are not considered an emergency.
- Neurosensory side effects (e.g., diplopia, blurred vision, nystagmus, ataxia, dizziness, and headache) are the most common, occurring in 35% to 50% of patients initially. Carbamazepine may induce hyponatremia, and the incidence may increase with age. Hyponatremia occurs less frequently than with oxcarbazepine.
- Leukopenia is the most common hematologic side effect (up to 10%) but is usually transient. It may be persistent in 2% of patients. Carbamazepine may be continued unless the white blood cell count drops to <2,500/mm³ (2.5×10^9/L) and the absolute neutrophil count drops to <1,000/mm³ (1×10^9/L).
- Rashes may occur in 10% of patients. Other side effects are nausea, hepatitis, osteomalacia, cardiac conduction defects, and lupus-like reactions.
- Carbamazepine may interact with other drugs by inducing their metabolism. **Valproic acid** increases concentrations of the 10,11-epoxide metabolite without affecting the concentration of carbamazepine. The interaction of **erythromycin** and **clarithromycin** (CYP3A4 inhibition) with carbamazepine is particularly significant.
- Loading doses are used only in critically ill patients.
- Although some patients, especially those on monotherapy, may be maintained on twice-a-day dosing, most patients will require dosing two to four times daily, especially children. Larger doses can be given at bedtime. Dose increases can be made every 2 to 3 weeks.
- The sustained- and controlled-release dosage forms allow for twice-a-day dosing. The sustained-release capsule can be opened and sprinkled on food.

Ethosuximide

- **Ethosuximide** is a first-line treatment for absence seizures.
- There is some evidence for nonlinear metabolism at higher serum concentrations. Metabolites are believed to be inactive.
- A loading dose is not required. Titration over 1 to 2 weeks to maintenance doses of 20 mg/kg/day (divided into two doses) usually results in therapeutic serum concentrations.

Felbamate

- **Felbamate** appears to act by blocking *N*-methyl-D-aspartate responses and by modulating GABA$_A$ receptors.
- It is approved for treating atonic seizures in patients with Lennox–Gastaut syndrome and is effective for partial seizures as well.
- Because of the reports of aplastic anemia (1 in 3,000 patients) and hepatitis (1 in 10,000 patients), felbamate is now recommended only for patients refractory to other AEDs. Risk factors for aplastic anemia may be a history of cytopenia, AED allergy or toxicity, viral infection, and/or immunologic problems.

Gabapentin

- **Gabapentin** inhibits high-voltage activated Ca channels and elevates human brain GABA levels. It is a second-line agent for patients with partial seizures who have failed initial treatment. It may also have a role in patients with less severe seizure disorders, such as new-onset partial epilepsy, especially in elderly patients.
- Bioavailability decreases with increasing doses (i.e., is a saturable process). It is eliminated exclusively renally, and dosage adjustment is necessary in patients with impaired renal function.
- Dosing is initiated at 300 mg at bedtime and increased to 300 mg twice daily on the second day and 300 mg three times daily on the third day. Further titrations are then made. The manufacturer recommends usual maintenance doses from 1,800 to 2,400 mg/day.

Lacosamide

- **Lacosamide** is a schedule V controlled substance.
- There is a linear relationship between daily doses and serum concentrations up to 800 mg/day.
- Moderate hepatic and renal impairment have both been shown to increase systemic drug exposure by up to 40%.
- Lacosamide can cause a small increase in the median PR interval.
- The starting dose is 100 mg/day in two divided doses, with dose increase by 100 mg/day every week until a daily dose of 200 mg to 400 mg has been reached.

Lamotrigine

- **Lamotrigine** is useful as both adjunctive therapy for partial seizures and as monotherapy. It may also be a useful alternative for primary generalized seizures, such as absence and as adjunctive therapy for primary GTC seizures.
- The most frequent side effects are diplopia, drowsiness, ataxia, and headache. Rashes are usually generalized, erythematous, and morbilliform, but Stevens–Johnson reaction has also occurred. The incidence of the more serious rashes appears to be increased in patients who are also receiving **valproic acid** and who have rapid dosage titration. Valproic acid substantially inhibits the metabolism of lamotrigine.

Levetiracetam

- Levetiracetam's renal elimination of unchanged drug accounts for 66% of drug clearance, and the dose should be adjusted for impaired renal function. The role of therapeutic drug monitoring is unknown. It has linear pharmacokinetics and is metabolized in blood by nonhepatic enzymatic hydrolysis.
- It is effective in the adjunctive treatment of partial seizures in adults who have failed initial therapy.
- Adverse effects include sedation, fatigue, coordination difficulties, agitation, irritability, and lethargy. A slight decline in red and white blood cells was noted in clinical trials.
- It is believed to have a low potential for pharmacokinetic drug interactions.
- The recommended initial dose is 500 mg orally twice daily. In some intractable seizure patients, the oral dose has been titrated rapidly over 3 days up to 3,000 mg/day (1,500 mg twice daily).

Oxcarbazepine

- **Oxcarbazepine** (a prodrug) is structurally related to **carbamazepine,** but it is converted to a monohydrate derivative, which is the active component.
- It undergoes glucuronide conjugation and is eliminated by the kidneys. Patients with significant renal impairment may require a dose adjustment. The half-life (9.3 ± 1.8 hours) is shorter in patients taking enzyme-inducing drugs. The relationship between dose and serum concentration is linear. It does not autoinduce its own metabolism.
- It is indicated for use as monotherapy or adjunctive therapy for partial seizures in adults and children as young as 4 years of age. It is also a potential first-line drug for patients with primary, generalized convulsive seizures.
- The most frequently reported side effects are dizziness, nausea, headache, diarrhea, vomiting, upper respiratory tract infections, constipation, dyspepsia, ataxia, and nervousness. It generally has fewer side effects than **phenytoin, valproic acid,** or **carbamazepine**. Hyponatremia has been reported in up to 25% of patients and is more likely in the elderly. About 25% to 30% of patients who have had a rash with carbamazepine will have a cross-reaction with oxcarbazepine.
- Concurrent use of oxcarbazepine with **ethinyl estradiol** and **levonorgestrel**-containing contraceptives may render these agents less effective. Oxcarbazepine may increase serum concentrations of **phenytoin** and decrease serum concentrations of **lamotrigine** (induction of uridine diphosphate glucuronosyltransferase).
- In adults, the starting dose of oxcarbazepine as monotherapy is 300 mg once or twice daily. This can be increased by 600 mg/day each week to a maximum dose of 2,400 mg/day. This is titrated to the target dose over 2 weeks. See manufacturer's recommendations for dosing by weight.
- In patients converted from carbamazepine, the typical maintenance doses of oxcarbazepine are 1.5 times the carbamazepine dose or less if patients are on larger carbamazepine doses.

Phenobarbital

- **Phenobarbital** is the drug of choice for neonatal seizures, but in other situations it is reserved for patients who have failed other AEDs.
- Phenobarbital is a potent enzyme inducer and interacts with many drugs. The amount of phenobarbital excreted renally can be increased by giving diuretics and urinary alkalinizers.
- The most common side effects are fatigue, drowsiness, and depression. Phenobarbital impairs cognitive performance. In children, paradoxical hyperactivity can occur.
- **Ethanol** increases phenobarbital metabolism, but **valproic acid, cimetidine,** and **chloramphenicol** inhibit its metabolism.
- Phenobarbital can usually be dosed once daily, and bedtime dosing may minimize daytime sedation.

Phenytoin

- **Phenytoin** is a first-line AED for primary generalized convulsive seizures and for partial seizures. Its place in therapy will be reevaluated as more experience is gained with the newer AEDs.
- Absorption may be saturable at higher doses. Absorption is affected by particle size, and the brand should not be changed without careful monitoring. Food may slow absorption. The intramuscular route is best avoided, as absorption is erratic. Fosphenytoin can safely be administered IV and intramuscularly. Equations are available to normalize the phenytoin concentration in patients with hypoalbuminemia or renal failure.
- Phenytoin is metabolized in the liver mainly by CYP2C9, but CYP2C19 is also involved. Zero-order kinetics occurs within the usual therapeutic range, so any change in dose may produce disproportional changes in serum concentrations.
- In nonacute situations, phenytoin may be initiated in adults at oral doses of 5 mg/kg/day and titrated upward. Subsequent dosage adjustments should be done cautiously because of nonlinearity in elimination. Most adult patients can be maintained on a single daily dose, but children often require more frequent administration. Only extended-release preparations should be used for single daily dosing.
- One author suggested that if the phenytoin serum concentration is less than 7 mcg/mL (28 μmol/L), the daily dose should be increased by 100 mg; if the concentration is 7 to 12 mcg/mL (28 and 48 μmol/L), the daily dose can be increased by 50 mg; and if the concentration is greater than 12 mcg/mL (48 μmol/L), the daily dose can be increased by 30 mg or less.
- Common but usually transient side effects are lethargy, incoordination, blurred vision, higher cortical dysfunction, and drowsiness. At concentrations greater than 50 mcg/mL (200 μmol/L), phenytoin can exacerbate seizures. Chronic side effects include gingival hyperplasia, impaired cognition, hirsutism, vitamin D deficiency, osteomalacia, folic acid deficiency, carbohydrate intolerance, hypothyroidism, and peripheral neuropathy.
- Phenytoin is prone to many drug interactions (see **Table 53–5**). If protein-binding interactions are suspected, free rather than total phenytoin concentrations are a better therapeutic guide.

- Phenytoin decreases **folic acid** absorption, but folic acid replacement enhances phenytoin clearance and can result in loss of efficacy. Phenytoin tablets and suspension contain phenytoin acid, whereas the capsules and parenteral solution are phenytoin sodium. One hundred mg of phenytoin acid is equal to 92 mg of phenytoin sodium. Clinicians should remember that there are two different strengths of phenytoin suspension and capsules.

Pregabalin

- **Pregabalin** is a second-line agent for partial seizures that have failed initial treatment.
- It is eliminated primarily by renal excretion as unchanged drug; dosage adjustment is required in patients with renal dysfunction.
- The most frequent side effects are dizziness, somnolence, ataxia, blurred vision, and weight gain.
- Drug interactions are unlikely to occur. It is a schedule V controlled substance.

Rufinamide

- **Rufinamide** is an adjunctive agent used for Lennox–Gastaut syndrome in patients who have failed valproic acid, topiramate, and lamotrigine.
- It is a triazole derivative, structurally unlike other AEDs.
- It is extensively metabolized with no active metabolites. Children may have a higher clearance of rufinamide than adults.
- It is dosed twice daily because of slow absorption and a short half-life (6–10 hours).
- Common side effects include headache, dizziness fatigue, somnolence, and nausea. Multiorgan hypersensitivity has occurred within 4 weeks of dose initiation in children younger than 12 years.
- Rufinamide is a weak inhibitor of CYP2E1 and a weak inducer of CYP3A4, and it may be involved in several drug interactions with other AEDs.
- Dosing is initiated at 400 to 800 mg/day divided into two doses, with an increase of 400 to 800 mg/day every other day up to 3,200 mg/day (divided into two doses).

Tiagabine

- **Tiagabine** is considered second-line therapy for patients with partial seizures who have failed initial therapy.
- The most frequently reported side effects are dizziness, asthenia, nervousness, tremor, diarrhea, and depression. These side effects are usually transient and can be diminished by taking it with food.
- It is oxidized by CYP3A4 enzymes, and other drugs may alter its clearance.
- Tiagabine is displaced from protein by **naproxen, salicylates,** and **valproate**.
- The minimal effective adult dose level is considered to be 30 mg/day.

Topiramate

- **Topiramate** is a first-line AED for patients with partial seizures as an adjunct or for monotherapy. It is also approved for tonic-clonic seizures in primary generalized epilepsy.

- Approximately 50% of the dose is excreted renally, and tubular reabsorption may be prominently involved.
- The most common side effects are ataxia, impaired concentration, confusion, memory difficulties, dizziness, fatigue, paresthesias, and somnolence. Nephrolithiasis occurs in 1.5% of patients. It has also been associated with acute narrow-angle glaucoma, oligohidrosis, and metabolic acidosis.
- Enzyme inducers may decrease topiramate serum levels.
- Dose increments may occur every 1 or 2 weeks. For patients on other AEDs, doses >600 mg/day do not appear to lead to improved efficacy and may increase side effects.

Valproic Acid and Divalproex Sodium

- **Valproic acid** may potentiate postsynaptic GABA responses, may have a direct membrane-stabilizing effect, and may affect potassium channels.
- The free fraction may increase as the total concentration increases, and free concentrations may be more useful in monitoring than total concentrations, especially at higher concentrations or in patients with hypoalbuminemia. Protein binding is decreased in patients with head trauma.
- At least 10 metabolites have been identified, and some may be active. One may account for hepatotoxicity (4-*ene*-valproic acid), and it is increased by concurrent dosing with enzyme-inducing drugs. At least 67 cases of hepatotoxicity have been reported, and most deaths were in mentally retarded children younger than 2 years who were receiving multiple drug therapy.
- The extended-release formulation (Depakote ER) is 15% less bioavailable than the enteric-coated preparation (Depakote).
- It is first-line therapy for primary generalized seizures, such as absence, myoclonic, and atonic seizures, and is approved for adjunctive and monotherapy treatment of partial seizures. It can also be useful in mixed seizure disorders.
- Side effects are usually mild and include GI complaints, weight gain, drowsiness, ataxia, and tremor. GI complaints may be minimized with the enteric-coated formulation or by giving with food. Thrombocytopenia is common but is responsive to a decrease in dose. Pancreatitis is rare.
- Although **carnitine** administration may partially ameliorate hyperammonemia, it is expensive, and there are only limited data to support routine supplemental use in patients taking valproic acid.
- Valproic acid is an enzyme inhibitor that increases serum concentrations of concurrently administered **phenobarbital** and may increase concentrations of **carbamazepine 10,11-epoxide** without affecting concentrations of the parent drug. It also inhibits the metabolism of **lamotrigine**. Carbapenems and combination oral contraceptives may lower serum levels of valproic acid.
- Twice-daily dosing is reasonable, but children and patients taking enzyme inducers may require three- or four-times-daily dosing.
- The enteric-coated tablet **divalproex sodium** causes fewer GI side effects. It is metabolized in the gut to valproic acid. When switching from Depakote to Depakote-ER, the dose should be increased by 14% to 20%. Depakote ER may be given once daily.

Vigabatrin

- **Vigabatrin** is a first-line agent for infantile spasms and a third-line adjunctive agent for refractory partial epilepsy.
- It undergoes virtually no metabolism and is excreted unchanged in the urine; dosage adjustment is necessary in renally impaired patients.
- Side effects include permanent bilateral concentric visual field constriction, headache, somnolence, fatigue, dizziness, convulsion, hyperactivity in children, nasopharyngitis, and weight gain.
- Vigabatrin induces CYP2C and decreases phenytoin plasma levels by ~20%.

Zonisamide

- **Zonisamide** is a broad-spectrum **sulfonamide** AED that is approved as adjunctive therapy for partial seizures, but it is potentially effective in a variety of partial and primary generalized seizure types.
- It is metabolized primarily by CYP3A4, and ~30% is excreted unchanged.
- The most common side effects are somnolence, dizziness, anorexia, headache, nausea, word-finding difficulties, oligohidrosis, modest weight loss, and irritability. Symptomatic kidney stones may occur in 2.6% of patients. Hypersensitivity reactions may occur in 0.02% of patients, and it should be used with caution if at all in patients with a history of allergy to sulfonamides. Monitoring of renal function may be advisable in some patients.
- The initial dose in adults is 100 mg/day, and daily doses are increased by 100 mg every 2 weeks until a response is seen. The dosage range in adults is 100 to 600 mg/day. It is suitable for once or twice-daily dosing, but once-daily dosing may cause more side effects.

EVALUATION OF THERAPEUTIC OUTCOMES

- Patients should be chronically monitored for seizure control, side effects, social adjustment including quality of life, drug interactions, compliance, and toxicity.
- Screening for neuropsychiatric disorders is also important. Clinical response is more important than serum drug concentrations.
- Patients should be asked to record severity and frequency of seizures in a seizure diary. Patients and family can provide useful input regarding frequency of seizures.

See Chapter 65, Epilepsy, authored by Susan J. Rogers and Jose E. Cavazos, for a more detailed discussion of this topic.

Headache: Migraine and Tension-Type

MIGRAINE HEADACHE

DEFINITION

- Migraine is a common, recurrent, primary headache of moderate to severe intensity that interferes with normal functioning and is associated with gastrointestinal (GI), neurologic, and autonomic symptoms. In migraine with aura, a complex of focal neurologic symptoms precedes or accompanies the attack.

PATHOPHYSIOLOGY

- Replacing previous neuronal and vascular theories of migraine pathophysiology, a combined theory has emerged. Activity in the trigeminovascular system may be regulated partly by serotonergic neurons within the brainstem. Pathogenesis may be related to a defect in the activity of neuronal calcium channels mediating neurotransmitter release in brainstem areas that modulate cerebrovascular tone and nociception. The result may be vasodilation of intracranial extracerebral blood vessels with activation of the trigeminovascular system.
- Twin studies suggest 50% heritability of migraine, with a multifactorial polygenic basis. Migraine triggers may be modulators of the genetic set point that predisposes to migraine headache.
- Specific populations of serotonin (5-hydroxytryptamine [5-HT]) receptors may be involved in the pathophysiology and treatment of migraine headache. Acute antimigraine drugs such as ergot alkaloids and triptan derivatives are agonists of vascular and neuronal $5HT_1$ receptor subtypes, resulting in vasoconstriction and inhibition of vasoactive neuropeptide release and pain signal transmission.

CLINICAL PRESENTATION

Symptoms

- Migraine headache is characterized by recurring episodes of throbbing head pain, frequently unilateral. Migraine headaches can be severe and associated with nausea, vomiting, and sensitivity to light, sound, and/or movement.
- Approximately 20% to 60% of migraineurs experience premonitory symptoms (not to be confused with aura) in the hours or days before the onset of headache. Neurologic symptoms (phonophobia, photophobia, hyperosmia, and difficulty concentrating) are most common, but psychological (anxiety, depression, euphoria, irritability, drowsiness, hyperactivity, and restlessness), autonomic (e.g., polyuria, diarrhea, and constipation), and constitutional (e.g., stiff neck, yawning, thirst, food cravings, and anorexia) symptoms may also occur.

- A migraine aura is experienced by ~31% of migraineurs. The aura typically evolves over 5 to 20 minutes and lasts <60 minutes. Headache usually occurs within 60 minutes of the end of the aura. Visual auras can include both positive features (e.g., scintillations, photopsia, teichopsia, and fortification spectrum) and negative features (e.g., scotoma and hemianopsia). Sensory and motor symptoms such as paresthesias or numbness of the arms and face, dysphasia or aphasia, weakness, and hemiparesis may also occur.
- The migraine headache may occur at any time of day or night but usually occurs in the early morning hours on awakening. Pain is usually gradual in onset, peaking in intensity over minutes to hours and lasting between 4 and 72 hours untreated. Pain is typically reported as moderate to severe and most often involves the frontotemporal region. The headache is usually unilateral and throbbing in nature. GI symptoms (e.g., nausea and vomiting) almost invariably accompany the headache. Other systemic symptoms are anorexia, constipation, diarrhea, abdominal cramps, nasal stuffiness, blurred vision, diaphoresis, facial pallor, and localized facial, scalp, or periorbital edema. Sensory hyperacuity (photophobia, phonophobia, or osmophobia) is frequently reported. Many patients seek a dark, quiet place for rest and relief.
- Once the headache pain wanes, a resolution phase characterized by exhaustion, malaise, and irritability ensues.

DIAGNOSIS

- A comprehensive headache history is the most important element in establishing the diagnosis of migraine.
- In the headache evaluation, diagnostic alarms should be identified. These include acute onset of the "first" or "worst" headache ever, accelerating pattern of headache following subacute onset, onset of headache after age 50 years, headache associated with systemic illness (e.g., fever, nausea, vomiting, stiff neck, and rash), headache with focal neurologic symptoms or papilledema, and new-onset headache in a patient with cancer or human immunodeficiency virus infection.
- A stable pattern of headaches, absence of daily headache, positive family history for migraine, normal neurologic examination, presence of food triggers, menstrual association, long-standing history, improvement with sleep, and subacute evolution are signs suggestive of migraine headache. Aura may signal the migraine headache but is not required for diagnosis.
- Perform a general medical and neurologic physical examination. Check for abnormalities: vital signs (fever and hypertension), funduscopy (papilledema, hemorrhage, and exudates), palpation and auscultation of the head and neck (sinus tenderness, hardened or tender temporal arteries, trigger points, temporomandibular joint tenderness, bruits, nuchal rigidity, and cervical spine tenderness), and neurologic examination (identify abnormalities or deficits in mental status, cranial nerves, deep tendon reflexes, motor strength, coordination, gait, and cerebellar function).
- Diagnostic and laboratory testing may be warranted if there are suspicious headache features or abnormal examination findings. Neuroimaging (computed tomography or magnetic resonance imaging) should be

considered in patients with unexplained findings on the neurologic exam or those with an atypical headache history.

- In selected circumstances and secondary headache presentation, serum chemistries, urine toxicology profiles, thyroid function tests, lyme studies, and other blood tests, such as a complete blood count, antinuclear antibody titer, erythrocyte sedimentation rate, and antiphospholipid antibody titer, may be considered.

DESIRED OUTCOME

- Acute therapy should provide consistent, rapid headache relief with minimal adverse effects and symptom recurrence, as well as minimal disability and emotional distress, thereby enabling the patient to resume normal daily activities. Ideally, patients should be able to manage their headaches effectively without emergency department or physician office visits.

TREATMENT

Nonpharmacologic Treatment

- Application of ice to the head and periods of rest or sleep, usually in a dark, quiet environment, may be beneficial.
- Preventive management should begin with identification and avoidance of factors that provoke migraine attacks (Table 54–1).
- Behavioral interventions (relaxation therapy, biofeedback, and cognitive therapy) are preventive options for patients who prefer nondrug therapy or when drug therapy is ineffective or not tolerated.

Pharmacologic Treatment of Acute Migraine

- A treatment algorithm for migraine headache is shown in Fig. 54–1. Acute migraine therapies (Table 54–2) are most effective when administered at the onset of migraine.
- Pretreatment with an antiemetic (e.g., **metoclopramide, chlorpromazine,** or **prochlorperazine**) 15 to 30 minutes prior to administering oral acute migraine therapy or use of nonoral treatments (rectal suppositories, nasal spray, or injections) may be advisable when nausea and vomiting are severe. In addition to its antiemetic effects, the prokinetic agent metoclopramide helps reverse gastroparesis and enhances absorption of oral medications.
- The frequent or excessive use of acute migraine medications can result in a pattern of increasing headache frequency and drug consumption known as medication-overuse headache. This occurs commonly with overuse of simple or combination analgesics, opiates, ergotamine tartrate, and triptans. This may be avoided by limiting use of acute migraine therapies to 2 or 3 days per week.

ANALGESICS AND NONSTEROIDAL ANTIINFLAMMATORY DRUGS

- **Simple analgesics** and **nonsteroidal antiinflammatory drugs (NSAIDs)** are effective as first-line treatment for mild to moderate migraine attacks. **Aspirin, ibuprofen, naproxen sodium, tolfenamic acid,** and the combination of **acetaminophen** plus **aspirin** and **caffeine** are effective. Some severe attacks are also responsive.

TABLE 54–1	Commonly Reported Triggers of Migraine

Food triggers
Alcohol
Caffeine/caffeine withdrawal
Chocolate
Fermented and pickled foods
Monosodium glutamate (e.g., in Chinese food, seasoned salt, and instant foods)
Nitrate-containing foods (e.g., processed meats)
Saccharin/aspartame (e.g., diet foods or diet sodas)
Tyramine-containing foods

Environmental triggers
Glare or flickering lights
High altitude
Loud noises
Strong smells and fumes
Tobacco smoke
Weather changes

Behavioral–physiologic triggers
Excess or insufficient sleep
Fatigue
Menstruation, menopause
Sexual activity
Skipped meals
Strenuous physical activity (e.g., prolonged overexertion)
Stress or post-stress

Data from Diamond M, Cady R. Initiating and optimizing acute therapy for migraine: The role of patient-centered stratified care. Am J Med 2005;118(Suppl 1):S18–S27; Buse DC, Rupnow FT, Lipton RB. Assessing and managing all aspects of migraine: migraine attacks, migraine-related functional impairment, common comorbidities, and quality of life. Mayo Clin Proc 2009;84(5):422–435; and Kelman L. The triggers or precipitants of the acute migraine attack. Cephalalgia 2007;27(5):394–402.

- NSAIDs appear to prevent neurogenically mediated inflammation in the trigeminovascular system by inhibiting prostaglandin synthesis.
- In general, NSAIDs with a long half-life are preferred, as less frequent dosing is needed. Rectal suppositories and intramuscular (IM) **ketorolac** are options for patients with severe nausea and vomiting.
- The combination of **acetaminophen, aspirin,** and **caffeine** is approved in the United States for relieving migraine pain and associated symptoms.
- Aspirin and acetaminophen are also available by prescription in combination with a short-acting barbiturate (**butalbital**). No randomized, placebo-controlled studies support the efficacy of butalbital-containing formulations for migraine.
- **Midrin** is a **proprietary** combination of **acetaminophen, isometheptene mucate** (a sympathomimetic amine), and **dichloralphenazone** (a chloral hydrate derivative) that has shown modest benefits in placebo-controlled trials. It may be an alternative for patients with mild to moderate migraine attacks.

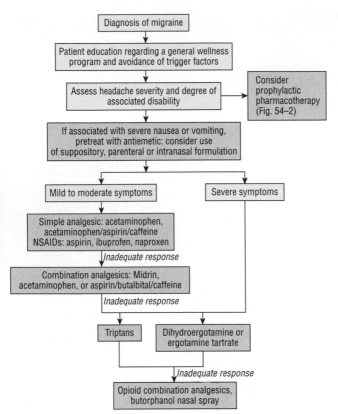

FIGURE 54–1. Treatment algorithm for migraine headaches. (NSAIDs, nonsteroidal antiinflammatory drugs.)

ERGOT ALKALOIDS AND DERIVATIVES

- **Ergot alkaloids** are useful for moderate to severe migraine attacks. They are nonselective $5HT_1$ receptor agonists that constrict intracranial blood vessels and inhibit the development of neurogenic inflammation in the trigeminovascular system. Venous and arterial constriction occurs. They also have activity at dopaminergic receptors.
- **Ergotamine tartrate** is available for oral, sublingual, and rectal administration. Oral and rectal preparations contain caffeine to enhance absorption and potentiate analgesia. Some patients respond preferentially to rectal administration. Dosage should be titrated to produce an effective but subnauseating dose.
- **Dihydroergotamine (DHE)** is available for intranasal and parenteral (IM, IV, or subcutaneous [SC]) administration. Patients can be trained to self-administer DHE by the IM or SC routes.

TABLE 54–2 Acute Migraine Therapies[a]

Medication	Dosage	Comments
Analgesics		
Acetaminophen	1,000 mg at onset; repeat every 4–6 hours as needed	Max. daily dose is 4 g
Acetaminophen 250 mg/aspirin 250 mg/caffeine 65 mg	2 tablets at onset and every 6 hours	Available over-the-counter as Excedrin Migraine
Aspirin or acetaminophen with butalbital, caffeine	1–2 tablets every 4–6 hours	Limit dose to 4 tablets/day and usage to 2 days/week
Isometheptene 65 mg/dichloralphenazone 100 mg/acetaminophen 325 mg (Midrin)	2 capsules at onset; repeat 1 capsule every hour as needed	Max. of 6 capsules/day and 20 capsules/month
Nonsteroidal antiinflammatory drugs		
Aspirin	500–1,000 mg every 4–6 hours	Max. daily dose is 4 g
Ibuprofen	200–800 mg every 6 hours	Avoid doses >2.4 g/day
Naproxen sodium	550–825 mg at onset; can repeat 220 mg in 3–4 hours	Avoid doses >1.375 g/day
Diclofenac potassium	50–100 mg at onset; can repeat 50 mg in 8 hours	Avoid doses >150 mg/day
Ergotamine tartrate		
Oral tablet (1 mg) with caffeine 100 mg	2 mg at onset; then 1–2 mg every 30 minutes as needed	Max. dose is 6 mg/day or 10 mg/week; consider pretreatment with an antiemetic
Sublingual tablet (2 mg)	–	–
Rectal suppository (2 mg) with caffeine 100 mg	Insert ½ to 1 suppository at onset; repeat after 1 hour as needed	Max. dose is 4 mg/day or 10 mg/week; consider pretreatment with an antiemetic
Dihydroergotamine		
Injection 1 mg/mL	0.25–1 mg at onset IM, IV or subcutaneous; repeat every hour as needed	Max. dose is 3 mg/day or 6 mg/week

(continued)

TABLE 54–2 Acute Migraine Therapies[a] *(Continued)*

Medication	Dosage	Comments
Dihydroergotamine		
Nasal spray	One spray (0.5 mg) in each nostril at onset; repeat sequence 15 minutes later (total dose is 2 mg or 4 sprays)	Max. dose is 3 mg/day; prime sprayer 4 times before using; do not tilt head back or inhale through nose while spraying; discard open ampules after 8 hours
Serotonin agonists (triptans)		
Sumatriptan		
Injection	6 mg subcutaneous at onset; can repeat after 1 hour if needed	Max. daily dose is 12 mg
Oral tablets	25, 50, 85 or 100 mg at onset; can repeat after 2 hours if needed	Optimal dose is 50–100 mg; max. daily dose is 200 mg; combination product with naproxen, 85 mg/500 mg
Nasal spray	5, 10, or 20 mg at onset; can repeat after 2 hours if needed	Optimal dose is 20 mg; max. daily dose is 40 mg; single-dose device delivering 5 or 20 mg; administer one spray in one nostril
Zolmitriptan		
Oral tablets	2.5 or 5 mg at onset as regular or orally disintegrating tablet; can repeat after 2 hours if needed	Optimal dose is 2.5 mg; max. dose is 10 mg/day Do not divide ODT dosage form
Nasal spray	5 mg (one spray) at onset; can repeat after 2 hours if needed	Max. daily dose is 10 mg/day
Naratriptan	1 or 2.5 mg at onset; can repeat after 4 hours if needed	Optimal dose is 2.5 mg; max. daily dose is 5 mg

Rizatriptan	5 or 10 mg at onset as regular or orally disintegrating tablet; can repeat after 2 hours if needed	Optimal dose is 10 mg; max. daily dose is 30 mg; onset of effect is similar with standard and orally disintegrating tablets; use 5-mg dose (15 mg/day max.) in patients receiving propranolol
Almotriptan	6.25 or 12.5 mg at onset; can repeat after 2 hours if needed	Optimal dose is 12.5 mg; max. daily dose is 25 mg
Frovatriptan	2.5 or 5 mg at onset; can repeat in 2 hours if needed	Optimal dose 2.5–5 mg; max. daily dose is 7.5 mg (3 tablets)
Eletriptan	20 or 40 mg at onset; can repeat after 2 hours if needed	Max. single dose is 40 mg; max. daily dose is 80 mg
Miscellaneous		
Butorphanol nasal spray	1 spray in 1 nostril (1 mg) at onset; repeat in 1 hour if needed	Limit to 4 sprays/day; consider use only when nonopioid therapies are ineffective or not tolerated
Metoclopramide	10 mg IV at onset	Useful for acute relief in the office or emergency department setting
Prochlorperazine	10 mg IV or IM at onset	Useful for acute relief in the office or emergency department setting

ODT, orally disintegrating tablet.

[a]Limit use of symptomatic medications to 2 or 3 days/week when possible to avoid medication-misuse headache.

Data from Silberstein SD. Migraine. Lancet 2004;363:381–391; Matchar DB, Young WB, Rosenberg JA, et al. Evidence-Based Guidelines for Migraine Headache in the Primary Care Setting: Pharmacological Management of Acute Attacks. The U.S. Headache Consortium; 2000. www.aan.com/professionals/practice/guidelines; Smith TR. The pharmacologic treatment of the acute migraine attack. Clin Fam Pract 2005;7(3):423–444; and Bigal ME, Lipton RB, Krymchantowski AV. The medical management of migraine. Am J Ther 2004;11(2):130–140.

- Nausea and vomiting are common adverse effects of ergotamine derivatives. Pretreatment with an antiemetic should be considered with ergotamine and IV DHE therapy. Other common side effects are abdominal pain, weakness, fatigue, paresthesias, muscle pain, diarrhea, and chest tightness. Symptoms of severe peripheral ischemia (ergotism) include cold, numb, painful extremities; continuous paresthesias; diminished peripheral pulses; and claudication. Gangrenous extremities, myocardial infarction (MI), hepatic necrosis, and bowel and brain ischemia have been reported rarely with ergotamine. Ergotamine derivatives and triptans should not be used within 24 hours of each other.
- Contraindications include renal and hepatic failure; coronary, cerebral, or peripheral vascular disease; uncontrolled hypertension; sepsis; and women who are pregnant or nursing.
- DHE does not appear to cause rebound headache, but dosage restrictions for ergotamine tartrate should be strictly observed to prevent this complication.

SEROTONIN RECEPTOR AGONISTS (TRIPTANS)

- **Sumatriptan, zolmitriptan, naratriptan, rizatriptan, almotriptan, frovatriptan,** and **eletriptan** are appropriate first-line therapies for patients with mild to severe migraine or as rescue therapy when nonspecific medications are ineffective.
- These drugs are selective agonists of the $5HT_{1B}$ and $5HT_{1D}$ receptors. Relief of migraine headache results from (1) normalization of dilated intracranial arteries, (2) peripheral neuronal inhibition, and (3) inhibition of transmission through second-order neurons of the trigeminocervical complex. They also display varying affinity for $5HT_{1A}$, $5HT_{1E}$, and $5HT_{1F}$ receptors.
- **Sumatriptan** is available for oral, intranasal, and SC administration. The SC injection is packaged as an autoinjector device for self-administration by patients. When compared with the oral formulation, SC administration offers enhanced efficacy and a more rapid onset of action. Intranasal sumatriptan also has a faster onset of effect than the oral formulation and produces similar rates of response.
- Second-generation triptans (all except sumatriptan) have higher oral bioavailability and longer half-lives than oral sumatriptan, which could theoretically improve within-patient treatment consistency and reduce headache recurrence. However, comparative clinical trials are necessary to determine their relative efficacy.
- Pharmacokinetic characteristics of the triptans are shown in **Table 54–3**.
- Clinical response to triptans varies among individual patients, and lack of response to one agent does not preclude effective therapy with another member of the class.
- Side effects of triptans include paresthesias, fatigue, dizziness, flushing, warm sensations, and somnolence. Minor injection site reactions are reported with SC use, and taste perversion and nasal discomfort may occur with intranasal administration. Up to 15% of patients report chest tightness, pressure, heaviness, or pain in the chest, neck, or throat. Although the mechanism of these symptoms is unknown, a cardiac source is unlikely

TABLE 54–3	Pharmacokinetic Characteristics of Triptans			
Drug	**Half-Life (Hours)**	**Time to Maximal Concentration (t_{max})**	**Bioavail-ability (%)**	**Elimination**
Almotriptan	3–4	1–3 hours	70	MAO-A, CYP3A4, CYP2D6
Eletriptan	5	1–1.25 hours	50	CYP3A4
Frovatriptan	25	2–4 hours	24–30	Mostly unchanged, CYP1A2
Naratriptan	5–6	2–3 hours	63–74	Largely unchanged, CYP450 (various isoenzymes)
Rizatriptan	2–3		40–45	MAO-A
Oral tablets		1–1.5 hours		
Disintegrating		1.6–2.5 hours		
Sumatriptan	2			MAO-A
SC injection		12–15 minutes	96	
Oral tablets		2.5 hours	14	
Nasal spray		1–2.5 hours	16	
Zolmitriptan	3			CYP1A2, MAO-A
Oral		2–2.5 hours	40	
Disintegrating		3 hours		
Nasal		4 hours		

CYP, cytochrome P450; MAO-A, monoamine oxidase type A.

Data from Silberstein SD. Migraine. Lancet 2004;363:381–391; Smith TR. The pharmacologic treatment of the acute migraine attack. Clin Fam Pract 2005;7(3):423–444; and Matthew NT, Loder EW. Evaluating the triptans. Am J Med 2005;118(Suppl 1):S28–S35.

in most patients. Isolated cases of MI and coronary vasospasm with ischemia have been reported.

- Contraindications include ischemic heart disease, uncontrolled hypertension, cerebrovascular disease, and hemiplegic and basilar migraine. Triptans should not be given within 24 hours of ergotamine derivative administration. Administration within 2 weeks of therapy with monoamine oxidase inhibitors is not recommended. Concomitant use of the triptans with selective serotonin reuptake inhibitors (SSRIs) or the serotonin–norepinephrine reuptake inhibitors can cause serotonin syndrome, a potentially life-threatening condition.

OPIOIDS

- Opioids and derivatives (e.g., **meperidine, butorphanol, oxycodone,** and **hydromorphone**) provide effective relief of intractable migraine but should be reserved for patients with moderate to severe infrequent headaches in whom conventional therapies are contraindicated or as rescue medication after failure to respond to conventional therapies. Opioid therapy should be closely supervised.

TABLE 54–4	Prophylactic Migraine Therapies
Medication	**Dose**
β-Adrenergic antagonists	
Atenolol	25–100 mg/day
Metoprolol[a]	50–200 mg/day in divided doses
Nadolol	80–160 mg/day
Propranolol[a,b]	80–240 mg/day in divided doses
Timolol[b]	20–60 mg/day in divided doses
Antidepressants	
Amitriptyline	25–150 mg at bedtime
Doxepin	10–300 mg at bedtime
Nortriptyline	10–150 mg at bedtime
Protriptyline	5–60 mg at bedtime
Fluoxetine	10–80 mg/day
Venlafaxine[a]	75–225 mg/day
Gapapentin	900–2,400 mg/day in divided doses
Topiramate[b]	100 mg/day in divided doses
Valproic acid/divalproex sodium[b]	500–1,500 mg/day in divided doses
Verapamil[a]	240–480 mg/day in divided doses
Nonsteroidal antiinflammatory drugs[c]	
Ketoprofen[a]	150 mg/day in divided doses
Naproxen sodium[a]	550–1,100 mg/day in divided doses
Coenzyme Q10	300 mg/day in divided doses
Feverfew	10–100 mg/day in divided doses
Magesium gluconate	400–600 mg/day in divided doses
Petasites	150 mg/day in divided doses
Vitamin B$_2$	400 mg/day

[a]Sustained-release formulation available.
[b]FDA approved for prevention of migraine.
[c]Daily or prolonged use limited by potential toxicity.
Data from Silberstein SD. Migraine. Lancet 2004;363:381–391; Bigal ME, Lipton RB. The preventive treatment of migraine. Neurologist 2006;12(4):204–213; Evans RW, Bigal ME, Grosberg B, Lipton RB. Target doses and titration schedules for migraine preventive medications. Headache 2006;46:160–164; and Rapoport AM, Bigal ME. Preventive migraine therapy: What is new. Neurol Sci 2004;25(Suppl 1):S177–S185.

- **Intranasal butorphanol** may provide an alternative to frequent office or emergency department visits for injectable migraine therapies. Onset of analgesia occurs within 15 minutes of administration. Adverse effects include dizziness, nausea, vomiting, drowsiness, and taste perversion. It also a has the potential for dependence and addiction.

Pharmacologic Prophylaxis of Migraine

- Prophylactic therapies (Table 54–4) are administered on a daily basis to reduce the frequency, severity, and duration of attacks, as well as to increase responsiveness to acute symptomatic therapies. A treatment algorithm for prophylactic management of migraine headache is shown in Fig. 54–2.

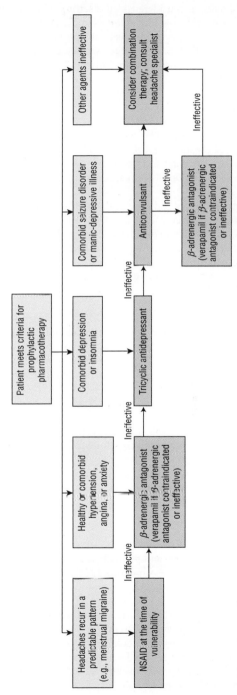

FIGURE 54–2. **Treatment algorithm for prophylactic management of migraine headaches.** (NSAID, nonsteroidal antiinflammatory drug.)

- Prophylaxis should be considered in the setting of recurring migraines that produce significant disability; frequent attacks requiring symptomatic medication more than twice per week; symptomatic therapies that are ineffective, contraindicated, or produce serious side effects; uncommon migraine variants that cause profound disruption and/or risk of neurologic injury; and patient preference to limit the number of attacks.
- Preventive therapy may also be administered intermittently when headaches recur in a predictable pattern (e.g., exercise-induced or menstrual migraine).
- Because efficacy of various prophylactic agents appears to be similar, drug selection is based on side effect profiles and comorbid conditions of the patient. Individual response to a particular agent is unpredictable, and a trial of 2 to 6 months' duration is necessary to judge the efficacy of each medication.
- Only propranolol, timolol, valproic acid, and topiramate are approved by the FDA for migraine prevention.
- Prophylaxis should be initiated with low doses and advanced slowly until a therapeutic effect is achieved or side effects become intolerable.
- Prophylaxis is usually continued for at least 3 to 6 months after headache frequency and severity have diminished, then gradually tapered and discontinued, if possible.

β-ADRENERGIC ANTAGONISTS

- β-Blockers (**propranolol, nadolol, timolol, atenolol,** and **metoprolol**) are the most widely used treatment for prevention of migraine. They are reported to reduce the frequency of attacks by 50% in 60% to 80% of patients. β-Blockers with intrinsic sympathomimetic activity are ineffective.
- Bronchoconstrictive and hyperglycemic effects can be minimized with β_1-selective β-blockers.
- Side effects include drowsiness, fatigue, sleep disturbances, vivid dreams, memory disturbance, depression, GI intolerance, sexual dysfunction, bradycardia, and hypotension.
- β-Blockers should be used with caution in patients with heart failure, peripheral vascular disease, atrioventricular conduction disturbances, asthma, depression, and diabetes.

ANTIDEPRESSANTS

- **Amitriptyline** appears to be the tricyclic antidepressant (TCA) of choice, but **doxepin, nortriptyline,** and **protriptyline** have also been used.
- Their beneficial effects in migraine prophylaxis are independent of antidepressant activity and may be related to downregulation of central $5HT_2$ and adrenergic receptors.
- TCAs are usually well tolerated at the lower doses used for migraine prophylaxis, but anticholinergic effects may limit use, especially in elderly patients or those with benign prostatic hyperplasia or glaucoma. Evening doses are preferred because of sedation. Increased appetite and weight gain can occur. Orthostatic hypotension and slowed atrioventricular conduction are occasionally reported.

- Data for **fluoxetine** are inconsistent, and prospective data evaluating **sertraline, paroxetine, fluvoxamine,** and **citalopram** are lacking.
- SSRIs are considered to be less effective than TCAs for migraine prophylaxis and should not be considered first- or second-line therapy. However, they may be beneficial when depression is a significant contributor to headache combined with an anticonvulsant. Preliminary data suggest a possible benefit with **venlafaxine.**

ANTICONVULSANTS

- **Valproic acid** and **divalproex sodium** (a 1:1 molar combination of valproate sodium and valproic acid) can reduce the frequency, severity, and duration of headaches.
- Side effects of valproic acid and divalproex sodium include nausea (less common with divalproex sodium and gradual dosing titration), tremor, somnolence, weight gain, hair loss, and hepatotoxicity (the risk appears to be low in patients older than 10 years on monotherapy). The extended-release formulation of divalproex sodium is administered once daily and is better tolerated than the enteric-coated formulation.
- Serum levels less than 50 mcg/mL (346 μmol/L) may be equal in efficacy to higher serum concentrations.
- **Topiramate** was recently approved by the FDA for migraine prophylaxis. The dose is initiated at 25 mg/day and increased slowly to minimize side effects, which may include paresthesias, fatigue, anorexia, diarrhea, weight loss, difficulty with memory, and nausea. Kidney stones, acute myopia, acute angle-closure glaucoma, and oligohidrosis have been infrequently reported.
- **Gabapentin** may also have a role in migraine prophylaxis.

CALCIUM CHANNEL BLOCKERS

- **Verapamil** provided only modest benefit in decreasing the frequency of attacks in two placebo-controlled studies. It has little effect on the severity of migraine attacks. It is generally considered a second- or third-line prophylactic agent.

NONSTEROIDAL ANTIINFLAMMATORY DRUGS

- NSAIDs are modestly effective for reducing the frequency, severity, and duration of migraine attacks, but potential GI and renal toxicity can limit daily or prolonged use.
- They may be used intermittently to prevent headaches that recur in a predictable pattern (e.g., menstrual migraine). Treatment should be initiated 1 or 2 days before the time of headache vulnerability and continued until vulnerability is passed.

TENSION-TYPE HEADACHE

DEFINITION

- Tension-type headache is the most common type of primary headache and is more common in women than men. Pain is usually mild to moderate and nonpulsatile. Episodic headaches may become chronic.

PATHOPHYSIOLOGY

- Pain is thought to originate from myofascial factors and peripheral sensitization of nociceptors. Central mechanisms are also involved. Mental stress, nonphysiologic motor stress, a local myofascial release of irritants, or a combination of these may be the initiating stimulus. In predisposed individuals, chronic, tension-type headache can evolve from episodic tension-type headache.
- After activation of supraspinal pain perception structures, a headache occurs because of central modulation of incoming peripheral stimuli.

CLINICAL PRESENTATION

- Premonitory symptoms and aura are absent, and pain is usually mild to moderate, bilateral, nonpulsatile, and in the frontal and temporal areas, but occipital and parietal areas can also be affected.
- Mild photophobia or phonophobia may occur. Pericranial or cervical muscles may have tender spots or localized nodules in some patients.

TREATMENT

- **Simple analgesics** (alone or in combination with caffeine) and **NSAIDs** are the mainstay of acute therapy.
- Nonpharmacologic therapies include reassurance and counseling, stress management, relaxation training, and biofeedback. Physical therapeutic options (e.g., heat or cold packs, ultrasound, electrical nerve stimulation, massage, acupuncture, trigger point injections, and occipital nerve blocks) have performed inconsistently.
- **Acetaminophen, aspirin, ibuprofen, naproxen, ketoprofen, indomethacin,** and **ketorolac** are effective.
- High-dose NSAIDs and the combination of aspirin or acetaminophen with butalbital or, rarely, codeine are effective options. The use of butalbital and codeine combinations should be avoided when possible.
- Acute medication for episodic headache should be taken no more often than 9 days/month to prevent the development of chronic tension-type headache.
- There is no evidence to support the efficacy of muscle relaxants for tension-type headache.
- Preventive treatment should be considered if headache frequency is more than two per week, duration is longer than 3 to 4 hours, or severity results in medication overuse or substantial disability.
- The TCAs are used most often for prophylaxis of tension headache, but **venlafaxine** and **mirtazapine** may also be effective. Injection of botulinum toxin into pericranial muscles has demonstrated inconsistent efficacy and is not recommended.

EVALUATION OF THERAPEUTIC OUTCOMES

- Patients should be monitored for frequency, intensity, and duration of headaches and for any change in the headache pattern. They should be encouraged to keep a headache diary to document frequency, duration, and severity of headaches, headache response, and potential triggers of migraine headaches.

- Patients taking abortive therapy should be monitored for frequency of use of prescription and nonprescription medications and for side effects of medications.
- Patterns of abortive medication use can be documented to establish the need for prophylactic therapy. Prophylactic therapies should also be monitored closely for adverse reactions, abortive therapy needs, adequate dosing, and compliance.

See Chapter 70, Headache Disorders, authored by Deborah S. Minor, for a more detailed discussion of this topic.

CHAPTER 55

Pain Management

DEFINITION

- Pain is an unpleasant, subjective, sensory, and emotional experience associated with actual or potential tissue damage or described in terms of such damage.

PATHOPHYSIOLOGY

NOCICEPTIVE PAIN

- Nociceptive (acute) pain is either somatic (arising from skin, bone, joint, muscle, or connective tissue) or visceral (arising from internal organs, e.g., the large intestine and pancreas).
- Stimulation of free nerve endings known as *nociceptors* is the first step leading to the sensation of pain. These receptors are found in both somatic and visceral structures and are activated by mechanical, thermal, and chemical impulses. Release of bradykinins, hydrogen and potassium ions, prostaglandins, histamine, interleukins, tumor necrosis factor-α, serotonin, and substance P may sensitize and/or activate nociceptors. Receptor activation leads to action potentials that are transmitted along afferent nerve fibers to the spinal cord.
- Action potentials continue from the site of noxious stimuli to the dorsal horn of the spinal cord and then ascend to higher centers. The thalamus may act as a relay station and pass the impulses to central structures where pain is processed further.
- The body modulates pain through several processes. The endogenous opiate system consists of neurotransmitters (e.g., enkephalins, dynorphins, and β-endorphins) and receptors (e.g., μ, δ, and κ) that are found throughout the central nervous system (CNS). Endogenous opioids bind to opioid receptors and modulate the transmission of pain impulses.
- The CNS also contains a descending system for control of pain transmission. This system originates in the brain and can inhibit synaptic pain transmission at the dorsal horn. Important neurotransmitters here include endogenous opioids, serotonin, norepinephrine, and γ-aminobutyric acid.

NEUROPATHIC PAIN AND FUNCTIONAL PAIN

- Neuropathic and functional pain is often described in terms of chronic pain. Neuropathic pain (e.g., postherpetic neuralgia and diabetic neuropathy) is a result of nerve damage, but functional pain (e.g., fibromyalgia, irritable bowel syndrome, and tension-type headache) refers to abnormal operation of the nervous system. Pain circuits may rewire themselves and produce spontaneous nerve stimulation.

- Acute pain (e.g., surgery, trauma, labor, and medical procedures) usually is nociceptive, but it can be neuropathic.
- Chronic pain can be nociceptive, neuropathic/functional, or both (e.g., pain that persists after the healing of the acute injury, pain related to a chronic disease, pain without an identifiable cause, and pain associated with cancer).

CLINICAL PRESENTATION

GENERAL

- Patients may be in obvious acute distress (trauma pain) or appear to have no noticeable suffering.

SYMPTOMS

- Acute pain can be described as sharp or dull, burning, shock-like, tingling, shooting, radiating, fluctuating in intensity, varying in location, and occurring in a timely relationship with an obvious noxious stimulus. Chronic pain can present similarly and often occurs without a timely relationship with a noxious stimulus.
- Over time, the chronic pain presentation may change (e.g., sharp to dull, obvious to vague).

SIGNS

- Acute pain can cause hypertension, tachycardia, diaphoresis, mydriasis, and pallor, but these signs are not diagnostic. These signs are seldom present in chronic pain.
- In acute pain, comorbid conditions are usually not present, and outcomes of treatment are generally predictable. In chronic pain, comorbid conditions are often present, and outcomes of treatment are often unpredictable.
- Pain is always subjective; thus, pain is best diagnosed based on patient description, history, and physical exam. A baseline description of pain can be obtained by assessing PQRST characteristics (palliative and provocative factors, quality, radiation, severity, and temporal factors). Attention should be given to mental factors that may lower the pain threshold (e.g., anxiety, depression, fatigue, anger, and fear). Behavioral, cognitive, social, and cultural factors may also affect the pain experience.
- Neuropathic pain is often chronic, not well described, and not easily treated with conventional analgesics. There may be exaggerated painful responses to normally noxious stimuli (hyperalgesia) or painful responses to normally nonnoxious stimuli (allodynia).

DESIRED OUTCOMES

- The goals of therapy are to minimize pain and provide reasonable comfort and quality of life at the lowest effective analgesic dose. With chronic pain, goals may include rehabilitation and resolution of psychosocial issues.

TREATMENT

- The elderly and the young are at a higher risk for undertreatment of pain because of misunderstanding about the pathophysiology of their pain. **Figs. 55–1** and **55–2** are algorithms for management of acute pain and pain in oncology patients.

NONOPIOID AGENTS

- Analgesia should be initiated with the most effective analgesic with the fewest side effects. Adult dosage, half-life, and selected pharmacodynamics of FDA-approved nonopioid analgesics are shown in **Tables 55–1** and **55–2**.
- The nonopioids are often preferred over the opioids for mild to moderate pain (see **Table 55–1**). The salicylates and nonsteroidal antiinflammatory drugs (NSAIDs) reduce prostaglandins produced by the arachidonic acid cascade, thereby decreasing the number of pain impulses received by the CNS.
- **NSAIDs** may be particularly useful for management of cancer-related bone pain.
- **The salicylate salts** cause fewer GI side effects than aspirin and do not inhibit platelet aggregation.
- Aspirin-like compounds should not be given to children or teenagers with viral illnesses (e.g., influenza or chickenpox), as Reye's syndrome may result.
- **Acetaminophen** has analgesic and antipyretic activity but little antiinflammatory action. It is highly hepatotoxic on overdose.

OPIOID AGENTS

- With oral opioids, the onset of action usually takes about 45 minutes, and peak effect usually is seen in about 1 to 2 hours.
- Equianalgesic doses, dosing guidelines, histamine-releasing characteristics, major adverse effects, and pharmacokinetics of opioids are shown in **Tables 55–2**, **55–3**, and **55–4**. The equianalgesic doses are only a guide, and doses must be individualized.
- Partial agonists and antagonists (e.g., **pentazocine**) compete with agonists for opioid receptor sites and exhibit mixed agonist–antagonist activity. They may have selectivity for analgesic receptor sites and cause fewer side effects.
- In the initial stages of acute pain treatment, analgesics should be given around the clock. As the painful state subsides, as-needed schedules can be used. Around-the-clock administration is also useful for management of chronic pain.
- Patients with severe pain may receive very high doses of opioids with no unwanted side effects, but as pain subsides, patients may not tolerate even low doses.
- Most of the itching or rash reported with the opioids is due to histamine release and mast cell degranulation, not to a true allergic response.

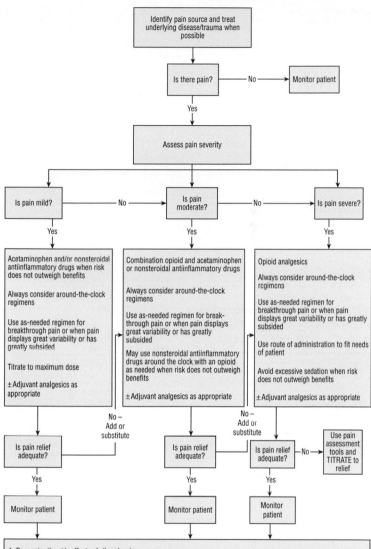

FIGURE 55–1. Algorithm for management of acute pain. *(Data modified from Omnicare, Inc., Acute Pain Pathway.)*

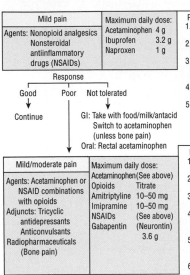

Mild pain	Maximum daily dose:	
Agents: Nonopioid analgesics Nonsteroidal antiinflammatory drugs (NSAIDs)	Acetaminophen	4 g
	Ibuprofen	3.2 g
	Naproxen	1 g

Response

Good → Continue

Poor

Not tolerated → GI: Take with food/milk/antacid
Switch to acetaminophen (unless bone pain)
Oral: Rectal acetaminophen

Principles of therapy
1. Assess the frequency/duration/occurrence/etiology of the pain on a routine basis.
2. If bone pain is present, consideration of an NSAID should be routine.
3. Always dose a medication to its maximum before reverting to the next step, unless pain is totally out of control.
4. If pain is constant or recurring, always dose around-the-clock (ATC).
5. Some authors suggest a lower maximum dose of acetaminophen.

Mild/moderate pain	Maximum daily dose:	
Agents: Acetaminophen or NSAID combinations with opioids Adjuncts: Tricyclic antidepressants Anticonvulsants Radiopharmaceuticals (Bone pain)	Acetaminophen	(See above)
	Opioids	Titrate
	Amitriptyline	10–50 mg
	Imipramine	10–50 mg
	NSAIDs	(See above)
	Gabapentin	(Neurontin) 3.6 g

Principles of therapy
1. Assess the frequency/duration/occurrence/etiology of the pain on a routine basis.
2. Whenever bone pain is present, consideration of an NSAID with opioid should be routine.
3. Pain management needs to take precedence over other therapies.
4. Fulminating sites of pain, especially in bone, need to be evaluated quickly for alternate therapy such as radiation/radiopharmaceuticals.
5. Accurate assessment and history of reported opiate allergies are important. A differentiation between allergy, sensitivity, and side effect needs to be made.
6. Always dose to the maximum of each agent when possible.
7. If pain is constant or recurring, always dose ATC.
8. Consider adjunct therapy when appropriate.
9. When using opioids, prevent constipation with a GI stimulant.

Response

Good → Continue

Poor

Not tolerated → GI: Take with food/milk/antacid
Delete NSAID (unless bone pain)
Oral: See Below

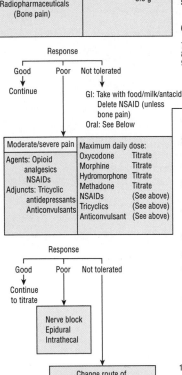

Moderate/severe pain	Maximum daily dose:	
Agents: Opioid analgesics NSAIDs Adjuncts: Tricyclic antidepressants Anticonvulsants	Oxycodone	Titrate
	Morphine	Titrate
	Hydromorphone	Titrate
	Methadone	Titrate
	NSAIDs	(See above)
	Tricyclics	(See above)
	Anticonvulsant	(See above)

Principles of therapy
1. Assess the frequency/duration/occurrence/etiology of the pain on a routine basis.
2. Morphine is often the choice in this category: (1) multiple products available; (2) multiple route of administration options, such as oral, rectal, IM, SC, IV, epidural, and intrathecal; and (3) a known equipotency between these routes that allows a much easier transition.
3. No real practical dosage limits with opioids mentioned; can be titrated to patient response. If myoclonic jerking occurs, consider switching to alternative opioid.
4. Management should be ATC dosing, with sustained-release product and an immediate-release product as for breakthrough pain.
5. Utilize all possible adjuncts to minimize increases in dose.
6. Initial control may require doses higher than those needed in maintenance.
7. A fentanyl patch placed every 72 hours may provide a more convenient dosing regimen when patients are on a stable oral dosing program.
8. Special situations of sudden-onset/sudden-resolution pain, especially along a nerve track, or neuralgias, may require an adjunct of an anticonvulsant and/or tricyclic antidepressant.
9. Any time nonpharmacologic options of radiation, chemotherapy, surgical debulking, or neurologic interventions are used, a total reevaluation of all drug treatment needs to be made.
10. When using opioids, prevent constipation with a GI stimulant.
11. Any new report of pain requires reevaluation.
12. If patient does not tolerate an opioid, consider switching to another opioid.

Response

Good → Continue to titrate

Poor → Nerve block
Epidural
Intrathecal

Not tolerated → Change route of administration (see note 2)
Change opioid (see note 12)

FIGURE 55–2. Algorithm for pain management in oncology patients. *(Data modified from the Kaiser Permanente Algorithm for Pain Management in Patients with Advanced Malignant Disease and Pain (PDQ) Health Professional Version. (Modified in 4/20/10). http://www.cancer.gov/cancertopics/pdq/supportivecare/pain/HealthProfessional.*

TABLE 55-1 FDA-Approved Nonopioid Analgesics for Pain in Adults

Class and Generic Name (Brand Name)	Approximate Half-Life (hour)	Usual Dosage Range (mg)	Maximal Dose (mg/day)
Salicylates			
Acetylsalicylic acid[a]–aspirin (various)	0.25	325–1,000 every 4–6 hour	4,000
Choline and magnesium trisalicylate (various)	9–17	1,000–1,500 every 12 hour 750 every 8 hour (elderly)	3,000
Diflunisal (Dolobid, various)	8–12	500–1,000 initial 250–500 every 8–12 hour	1,500
Salsalate (various)	1	1,000 every 12 hour or 500 every 6 hour	3,000
Para-aminophenol			
Acetaminophen[a] (Tylenol, various)	2–3	325–1,000 every 4–6 hour	4,000[b]
Fenamates			
Meclofenamate (various)	0.8–3.3	50–100 every 4–6 hour	400
Mefenamic acid (Ponstel)	2	Initial 500 250 every 6 hour (max. 7 days)	1,000[c]
Pyranocarboxylic acid			
Etodolac (various) (immediate release)	7.3	200–400 every 6–8 hour	1,000 1,200 with extended-release product
Acetic acid			
Diclofenac potassium [Cataflam, various, Flector (patch)]	1.9	In some patients, initial 100, 50 three times per day Patch available–to be applied twice daily to painful area (intact skin only)	150[d]
Propionic acids			
Ibuprofen[a] (Motrin, Caldolor, various)	2–2.5	200–400 every 4–6 hour Injectable, 400–800 every 6 hour (infused over 30 min)	3,200[e] 2,400[e] 1,200[f]
Fenoprofen (Nalfon, various)	3	200 every 4–6 hour	3,200
Ketoprofen (various)	2	25–50 every 6–8 hour	300 200 with extended-release product
Naproxen (Naprosyn, Anaprox, various)	12–17	500 initial 500 every 12 hour or 250 every 6–8 hour	1,000[c]

(continued)

TABLE 55–1 FDA-Approved Nonopioid Analgesics for Pain in Adults *(Continued)*

Class and Generic Name (Brand Name)	Approximate Half-Life (hours)	Usual Dosage Range (mg)	Maximal Dose (mg/day)
Propionic acids			
Naproxen sodium*a* (Aleve, various)	12–17	In some patients, 440 initial*f* 220 every 8–12 hour*f*	660*f*
Pyrrolizine carboxylic acid			
Ketorolac–parenteral (various)	5–6	30*g*–60 (single IM dose only) 15*g*–30 (single IV dose only) 15*g*–30 every 6 hour (IV dose) (max. 5 days)	30*g* –60 15*g*–30 60*g*–120
Ketorolac–oral, indicated for continuation with parenteral only (various)	5–6	10 every 4–6 hour (max. 5 days, which includes parenteral doses) In non-elderly patients, initial oral dose of 20	40
Pyrazols			
Celecoxib (Celebrex)	11	Initial 400 followed by another 200 on first day, then 200 twice daily	400

FDA, Food and Drug Administration; IM, intramuscular; IV, intravenous; Nd, no data.

*a*Available both as an over-the-counter preparation and as a prescription drug.

*b*Some experts believe 4,000 mg may be too high.

*c*Up to 1,250 mg on the first day.

*d*Up to 200 mg on the first day.

*e*Some individuals may respond better to 3,200 mg as opposed to 2,400 mg, although well-controlled trials show no better response; consider risk versus benefits when using 3,200 mg/day.

*f*Over-the-counter dose.

*g*Dose for elderly and those under 50 kg (110 lbs).

Data from American Pain Society. Principles of Analgesic Use in the Treatment of Acute Pain and Chronic Cancer Pain, 5th ed. Glenview, IL: American Pain Society, 2003; Anonymous. American Hospital Formulary Service. In: McVoy GK, ed. Drug Information. Bethesda, MD: American Society of Health-System Pharmacists, 2009; Anonymous. Facts and Comparisons. Philadelphia, PA. Wolters Kluwer Health. Accessed August 2010. Watkins PB, Kaplowitz N, Slattery TJ, et al. Aminotransferase elevations in healthy adults receiving 4 grams of acetaminophen daily: A randomized controlled trial. JAMA 2006;296:87–93; and Caldolor [package insert]. Nashville, TN: Cumberland Pharmaceuticals Inc.; 2009.

- When allergies occur with one opioid, a drug from a different structural class of opioids may be tried with caution. For these purposes, the mixed agonist–antagonist class behaves most like the morphine-like agonists.
- With patient-controlled analgesia, patients self-administer preset amounts of IV opioids via a syringe pump electronically interfaced with a timing device; thus, patients can balance pain control with sedation.

TABLE 55-2 Adult Dosing Guidelines for Opioids and Nonopioids

Agent(s)	Doses (Use Lowest Effective Dose, Titrate Up or Down Based on Patient Response, Opioid Tolerant Patients May Need Dose Modification)	Notes
NSAIDs/acetaminophen/ aspirin	Dose to maximum before switching to another agent (see Table 55-1)	Used in mild-to-moderate pain May use in conjunction with opioid agents to decrease doses of each Regular alcohol use and of acetaminophen may result in liver toxicity Care must be exercised to avoid overdose when combination products containing these agents are used
Morphine	PO 5–30 mg every 4 hour^a *[PO 5–30 mg every 4 hour^a]* IM 5–20 mg every 4 hour^a IV 5–15 mg every 4 hour^a SR 15–30 mg every 12 hour (may need to be every 8 hour in some patients) Rectal 10–20 mg every 4 hour^a	Drug of choice in severe pain Use immediate-release product with SR product to control breakthrough pain in cancer patients Typical patient controlled analgesia IV dose is 1 mg with a 10 minute lock out interval Every-24-hour products available (Avinza should not exceed doses of 1,600 mg/day)
Hydromorphone	PO 2–4 mg every 4–6 hour^a IM 1–2 mg every 4–6 hour^a IV 0.5–2 mg every 4 hour^a Rectal 3 mg every 6–8 hour^a	Use in severe pain More potent than morphine; otherwise, no advantages Typical patient controlled analgesia IV dose is 0.2 mg with a 10 minute lock out interval Every-24-hour product (Exalgo) available

(continued)

TABLE 55-2 Adult Dosing Guidelines for Opioids and Nonopioids (*Continued*)

Agent(s)	Doses (Use Lowest Effective Dose, Titrate Up or Down Based on Patient Response, Opioid Tolerant Patients May Need Dose Modification)	Notes
Oxymorphone	IM 1–1.5 mg every 4–6 hour[a] IV 0.5 mg every 4–6 hour[a] PO immediate-release 5–10 mg every 4–6 hour[a] PO extended-release 5–10 mg every 12 hour[a]	Use in severe pain No advantages over morphine Use immediate-release product with controlled-release product to control breakthrough pain in cancer or chronic pain patients
Levorphanol	PO 2–3 mg every 6–8 hour[a] (Levo-Dromoran) PO 2 mg every 3–6 hour[a] (Levorphanol Tartrate) IM 1–2 mg every 6–8 hour[a] IV 1 mg every 3–6 hour[a]	Use in severe pain Extended half-life useful in cancer patients In chronic pain, wait 3 days between dosage adjustments
Codeine	PO 15–60 mg every 4–6 hour[a] IM 15–60 mg every 4–6 hour[a]	Use in mild to moderate pain Weak analgesic; use with NSAIDs, aspirin, or acetaminophen, analgesic prodrug
Hydrocodone	PO 5–10 mg every 4–6 hour[a]	Use in moderate/severe pain Most effective when used with NSAIDs, aspirin, or acetaminophen Only available as combination product with other ingredients for pain and/or cough
Oxycodone	PO 5–15 mg every 4–6 hour[a] Controlled release 10–20 mg every 12 hour	Use in moderate/severe pain Most effective when used with NSAIDs, aspirin, or acetaminophen Use immediate-release product with controlled-release product to control breakthrough pain in cancer or chronic pain patients

Meperidine	IM 50–150 mg every 3–4 hour[a] IV 5–10 mg every 5 min prn[a]	Use in severe pain Oral not recommended Do not use in renal failure May precipitate tremors, myoclonus, and seizures Monoamine oxidase inhibitors can induce hyperpyrexia and/or seizures or opioid overdose symptoms
Fentanyl	IV 25–50 mcg/hour IM 50–100 mcg every 1–2 hour[a] Transdermal 25 mcg/hour every 72 hour Transmucosal (Actiq Lozenge) 200 mcg may repeat × 1, 30 min after first dose is started, then titrate Transmucosal (Fentora Buccal Tablet) 100 mcg, may repeat × 1, 30 min after first dose is started, then titrate	Used in severe pain Do not use transdermal in acute pain Transmucosal for breakthrough cancer pain in patients already receiving or tolerant to opioids. Always start with lowest dose despite daily opioid intake
Methadone	PO 2.5–10 mg every 8–12 hour[a] IM 2.5–10 mg every 8–12 hour[a]	Effective in severe chronic pain Sedation can be major problem Some chronic pain patients can be dosed every 12 hours Equianalgesic dose of methadone when compared with other opioids will decrease progressively the higher the previous opioid dose. Avoid dose titrations more frequently than weekly in chronic pain maintenance
Propoxyphene	PO 100 mg every 4 hour[c] (napsylate) PO 65 mg every 4 hour[c] (HCl) (maximum 600 mg daily of napsylate, 390 mg HCl)	Use in moderate pain Weak analgesic; most effective when used with NSAIDs, aspirin, or acetaminophen This drug is not recommended in the elderly Will cause carbamazepine levels to increase 100 mg of napsylate salt = 65 mg of HCl salt

(continued)

TABLE 55–2 Adult Dosing Guidelines for Opioids and Nonopioids (*Continued*)

Agent(s)	Doses (Use Lowest Effective Dose, Titrate Up or Down Based on Patient Response, Opioid Tolerant Patients May Need Dose Modification)	Notes
Pentazocine	PO 50–100 mg every 3–4 hour[b] (max. 600 mg daily, for those 50 mg tablet containing 0.5 mg of naloxone) PO 25 mg every 4 hour[b] (max. 150 mg daily, for those 25 mg tablet containing 325 mg of acetaminophen)	Second-line agent for moderate-to-severe pain May precipitate withdrawal in opiate-dependent patients Parenteral doses not recommended
Butorphanol	IM 1–4 mg every 3–4 hour[b] IV 0.5–2 mg every 3–4 hour[b] Intranasal 1 mg (1 spray) every 3–4 hour[b] If inadequate relief after initial spray, may repeat in other nostril × 1 in 60–90 min Max. 2 sprays (one per nostril) every 3–4 hour[b]	Second-line agent for moderate-to-severe pain May precipitate withdrawal in opiate-dependent patients
Nalbuphine	IM/IV 10 mg every 3–6 hour[b] (max. 20 mg dose, 160 mg daily)	Second-line agent for moderate-to-severe pain May precipitate withdrawal in opiate-dependent patients
Buprenorphine	IM 0.3 mg every 6 hour[b] Slow IV 0.3 mg every 6 hour[b] May repeat × 1, 30–60 min after initial dose	Second-line agent for moderate-to-severe pain May precipitate withdrawal in opiate-dependent patients Transdermal delivery systems (5, 10, 20 micrograms/hour) available for every 7 day administration Naloxone may not be effective in reversing respiratory depression

Naloxone	IV 0.4–2 mg	When reversing opiate side effects in patients needing analgesia, dilute and titrate (0.1–0.2 mg every 2–3 min) so as not to reverse analgesia
Tramadol	PO 50–100 mg every 4–6 hour[b] If rapid onset not required, start 25 mg/day and titrate over several days Extended release PO 100 mg every 24 hour	Maximum dose for nonextended-release, 400 mg/24 hours; maximum for extended release, 300 mg/24 hours Decrease dose in patient with renal impairment and in the elderly
Tapentadol	PO 50–100 mg every 4–6 hour[b]	First day of therapy may administer second dose after the first within 1 hour Maximum dose first day 700 mg, max. dose thereafter 600 mg

IM, intramuscular; IV, intravenous; NSAID, nonsteroidal antiinflammatory drug; PO, oral; prn, as needed; SR, sustained release; HCL, hydrochloride

[a]May start with an around-the-clock regimen and switch to prn if/when the painful signal subsides or is episodic.

[b]May reach a ceiling analgesic effect.

Data from American Pain Society: *Principles of Analgesic Use in the Treatment of Acute Pain and Chronic Cancer Pain, 5th ed.* Glenview, IL: American Pain Society, 2003; *Tapentadol [package insert].* Raritan NJ: PriCara, Division of Ortho-McNeil-Janssen Pharmaceuticals, Inc; 2009; Anonymous. American Hospital Formulary Service. In: McEvoy GK, ed. Drug Information. Bethesda, MD: American Society of Health-System Pharmacists, 2009; Anonymous. *Facts and Comparisons.* Philadelphia, PA: Wolters Kluwer Health. Accessed August 2010; and Anonymous. Micromedex 2.0. Thomson Reuters. Accessed August 2010.

TABLE 55–3 Opioid Analgesics, Central Analgesics, and Opioid Antagonists

Class and Generic Name (Brand Name)	Chemical Source	Relative Histamine Release	Route	Equianalgesic Dose in Adults (mg)	Approximate Onset (min)/ Half-Life (hour)
Phenanthrenes (morphine-like agonists)					
Morphine (various)	Naturally occurring	+++	IM PO	10 30	10–20/2
Hydromorphone (Dilaudid, various)	Semisynthetic	+	IM PO	1.5 7.5	10–20/2–3
Oxymorphone (Numorphan, Opana)	Semisynthetic	+	IM PO	1 10	10–20/2–3
Levorphanol (various)	Semisynthetic	+	IM PO	Variable Variable	10–20/12–16
Codeine (various)	Naturally occurring	+++	IM PO	15–30ª 15–30ª	10–30/3
Hydrocodone (available as combination)	Semisynthetic	N/A	PO	5–10ª	30–60/4
Oxycodone (various)	Semisynthetic	+	PO	15–30ᵇ	30–60/2–3

Phenylpiperidines (meperidine-like agonists)					
Meperidine (Demerol, various)	Synthetic	+++	IM PO	75 300^b, not recommended	10–20/3–5
Fentanyl (Sublimaze, Duragesic, various)	Synthetic	+	IM Transdermal Buccal, transmucosal	0.1 25^c Variable^d Variable^d	7–15/3–4
Diphenylheptanes (methadone-like agonists)					
Methadone (Dolophine, various)	Synthetic	+	IM PO IM PO	Variable^e (acute) Variable^e (acute) Variable^e (chronic) Variable^e (chronic)	30–60/12–190
Propoxyphene (Darvon, various)	Synthetic	N/A	PO	65^a	30–60/6–12
Agonist–antagonist derivatives					
Pentazocine (Talwin, various)	Synthetic	N/A	IM PO	Not recommended 50^a	15–30/2–3
Butorphanol (Stadol, various)	Synthetic	N/A	IM Intranasal	2 1^a (one spray)	10–20/3–4
Nalbuphine (Nubain, various)	Synthetic	N/A	IM	10	<15/5
Buprenorphine (Buprenex, various)	Synthetic	N/A	IM	0.3	10–20/2–3

(continued)

TABLE 55-3 Opioid Analgesics, Central Analgesics, and Opioid Antagonists *(Continued)*

Class and Generic Name (Brand Name)	Chemical Source	Relative Histamine Release	Route	Equianalgesic Dose in Adults (mg)	Approximate Onset (min)/ Half-Life (hour)
Antagonist					
Naloxone (Narcan, various)	Synthetic	N/A	IV	0.4–2[f]	1–2 (IV), 2–5 (IM)/ 0.5–1.3
Central analgesics					
Tramadol (Ultram, various)	Synthetic	N/A	PO	50–100[a,g]	<60/5–7
Tapentadol (Nucynta)	Synthetic	N/A	PO	50–100[a,g]	Within 60/4

IM, intramuscular; IV, intravenous; PO, oral.

[a]Starting dose only (equianalgesia not shown).

[b]Starting doses lower (oxycodone 5–10 mg, meperidine 50–150 mg).

[c]Equivalent PO morphine dose = variable.

[d]For breakthrough pain only.

[e]The equianalgesic dose of methadone when compared with other opioids will decrease progressively the higher the previous opioid dose.

[f]Starting doses to be used in cases of opioid overdose.

[g]First day of dosing may administer second dose 1 hour after first dose.

Data from American Pain Society. Principles of Analgesic Use in the Treatment of Acute Pain and Chronic Cancer Pain, 5th ed. Glenview, IL: American Pain Society, 2003; Gutstein HB, Akil H. Opioid analgesics. In: Brunton LL, Lazo AS, Parker KL, eds. The Pharmacological Basis of Therapeutics, 11th ed. New York: McGraw-Hill, 2006:547–590; McPherson ML. Demystifying Opioid Conversion Calculations. A Guide For Effective Dosing. Bethesda, MD: American Society of Health-System Pharmacists, 2010; Pasero C, Portenoy RK, McCaffery M. Opioid analgesics. In: McCaffery M, Pasero C, eds. Pain. St. Louis, MO: Mosby, 1999:161–299; Anonymous. American Hospital Formulary Service. In: McVoy GK, ed. Drug Information. Bethesda, MD: American Society of Health-System Pharmacists, 2009; Anonymous. Facts and Comparisons. Philadelphia, PA: Wolters Kluwer Health. Accessed August 2010; Tapentadol [package insert]. Raritan NJ: PriCara, Division of Ortho-McNeil-Janssen Pharmaceuticals, Inc; 2009; and Li F. Pharmacologically induced histamine release: sorting out hypersensitivity reactions to opioids. Drug Therapy topics 2006:35 http://depts.washington.edu/druginfo/DTT/2006_Vol35_FilesN35N4.pdf.

TABLE 55-4	Major Adverse Effects of the Opioid Analgesics
Effect	**Manifestation**
Mood changes	Dysphoria, euphoria
Somnolence	Sedation, inability to concentrate
Stimulation of chemoreceptor trigger zone	Nausea, vomiting
Respiratory depression	Decreased respiratory rate
Decreased gastrointestinal motility	Constipation
Increase in sphincter tone	Biliary spasm, urinary retention (varies among agents)
Histamine release	Urticaria, pruritus, rarely exacerbation of asthma (varies among agents)
Tolerance	Larger doses for same effect
Dependence	Withdrawal symptoms upon abrupt discontinuation

Data from Stimmel B. Pain, Analgesia and Addiction: The Pharmacology of Pain. New York: Raven Press, 1983:1, 2, 63, 241–245, 259, 266; and Gutstein HB, Akil H. Opioid analgesics. In: Brunton LL, Lazo AS, Parker KL, eds. The Pharmacological Basis of Therapeutics, 11th ed. New York: McGraw-Hill, 2006:547–590.

- Administration of opioids directly into the CNS (**Table 55–5**; epidural and intrathecal/subarachnoid routes) is becoming prominent for acute pain, chronic noncancer pain, and cancer pain. These methods require careful monitoring because of reports of marked sedation, respiratory depression, pruritus, nausea, vomiting, urinary retention, and hypotension. **Naloxone** is used to reverse respiratory depression, but continuous infusion may be required.

TABLE 55-5	Intraspinal Opioids			
Agent	**Single Dose (mg)**	**Onset of Pain Relief (minute)**	**Duration of Pain Relief (hour)**	**Continual Infusion Dose (mg/ hour)**
Epidural route				
Morphine	1–6	30	6–24	0.1–1
Hydromorphone	0.8–1.5	5–8	4–8	0.1–0.3
Fentanyl	0.025–0.1	5	2–8	0.025–0.1
Sufentanil	0.01–0.06	5	2–4	0.01–0.05
Subarachnoid route				
Morphine	0.1–0.3	15	8–34	–
Fentanyl	0.005–0.025	5	3–6	–

Data from American Pain Society. Principles of Analgesic Use in the Treatment of Acute Pain and Chronic Cancer Pain, 5th ed. Glenview, IL: American Pain Society, 2003; and Gutstein HB, Akil H. Opioid analgesics. In: Brunton LL, Lazo AS, Parker KL, eds. The Pharmacological Basis of Therapeutics, 11th ed. New York: McGraw-Hill, 2006:547–590.

- Intrathecal and epidural opioids are often administered by continuous infusion or patient-controlled analgesia. They are safe and effective when given simultaneously with intrathecal or epidural local anesthetics such as **bupivacaine**. All agents administered directly into the CNS should be preservative-free.

Morphine and Congeners (Phenanthrenes)

- **Morphine** is considered by many clinicians to be the first-line agent for moderate to severe pain. Nausea and vomiting are more likely in ambulatory patients and with the initial dose.
- Respiratory depression increases progressively as doses are increased. It often manifests as a decrease in respiratory rate, and the cough reflex is also depressed. Patients with underlying pulmonary dysfunction are at risk for increased respiratory compromise. Respiratory depression can be reversed by **naloxone.**
- The combination of opioid analgesics with alcohol or other CNS depressants amplifies CNS depression and is potentially harmful and possibly lethal.
- **Morphine** produces venous and arteriolar dilation, which may result in orthostatic hypotension. Hypovolemic patients are more susceptible to morphine-induced hypotension. Morphine is often considered the opioid of choice to treat pain associated with myocardial infarction, as it decreases myocardial oxygen demand.
- Morphine can cause constipation, spasms of the sphincter of Oddi, urinary retention, and pruritus (secondary to histamine release) (see **Table 55–4**). In patients with head trauma who are not ventilated, morphine-induced respiratory depression can increase intracranial pressure and cloud the neurologic examination results.

Meperidine and Congeners (Phenylpiperidines)

- **Meperidine** is less potent and has a shorter duration of action than morphine.
- With high doses or in patients with renal failure, the metabolite normeperidine accumulates, causing tremor, muscle twitching, and possibly seizures. In most settings, it offers no advantages over morphine, and it should not be used long term. It should be avoided in the elderly and those with renal dysfunction.
- Meperidine should not be combined with monoamine oxidase inhibitors because of the possibility of severe respiratory depression or excitation, delirium, hyperpyrexia, and convulsions.
- **Fentanyl** is a synthetic opioid structurally related to meperidine. It is often used in anesthesiology as an adjunct to general anesthesia. It is more potent and shorter acting than meperidine. Transdermal fentanyl can be used for treatment of chronic pain requiring opioid analgesics. After a patch is applied, it takes 12 to 24 hours to obtain optimal analgesic effect, and analgesia may last 72 hours. It may take 6 days after increasing a dose before new steady-state levels are achieved. Thus, the fentanyl patch should not be used for acute pain. A fentanyl lozenge and a buccal dosage form are available for treatment of breakthrough cancer pain.

Methadone and Congeners (Diphenylheptanes)

- **Methadone** has oral efficacy, extended duration of action, and ability to suppress withdrawal symptoms in heroin addicts. With repeated doses, the analgesic duration of action of methadone is prolonged, but excessive sedation may also result. Although effective for acute pain, it is used for chronic cancer pain and increasingly for chronic noncancer pain.
- There is a growing number of methadone-related deaths. Cardiac arrhythmias may occur, especially with higher doses. The equinalgesic dose of methadone may decrease with higher doses of the previous opioid.

Opioid Agonist–Antagonist Derivatives

- This class produces analgesia and has a ceiling effect on respiratory depression and lower abuse potential than morphine. However, psychotomimetic responses (e.g., hallucinations and dysphoria with **pentazocine**), a ceiling analgesic effect, and the propensity to initiate withdrawal in opioid-dependent patients have limited their widespread use.

Opioid Antagonists

- **Naloxone** is a pure opioid antagonist that binds competitively to opioid receptors but does not produce an analgesic response. It is used to reverse the toxic effects of agonist and agonist–antagonist opioids.

Central Analgesic

- **Tramadol** and **tapentadol** are centrally acting analgesics. Tramadol, which is indicated for moderate to moderately severe pain, binds to μ opiate receptors and weakly inhibits norepinephrine and serotonin reuptake. Tapentadol, for moderate to severe pain, binds to the same receptor and inhibits norepinephrine.
- They have side effect profiles similar to that of other opioid analgesics. They may also increase the risk of seizures. Tramadol may be useful for treating chronic pain, especially neuropathic pain, but it has little advantage over other opioid analgesics for acute pain. Tapentadol, a schedule II controlled substance, may be useful for acute pain.

Combination Therapy

- The combination of an opioid and nonopioid oral analgesic often results in analgesia superior to monotherapy and may allow for lower doses of each agent.

REGIONAL ANALGESIA

- Regional analgesia with local anesthetics (**Table 55–6**) can provide relief of both acute and chronic pain. Anesthetics can be positioned by injection (i.e., in joints, in the epidural or intrathecal space, or along nerve roots) or applied topically.

TABLE 55–6 Local Anesthetics[a]

Agent (Brand Name)	Onset (minute)	Duration (hour)
Esters		
Procaine (Novocain, various)	2–5	0.25–1
Chloroprocaine (Nesacaine, various)	6–12	0.5
Tetracaine (Pontocaine)	≤15	2–3
Amides		
Mepivacaine (Polocaine, various)	3–5	0.75–1.5
Bupivacaine (Marcaine, various)	5	2–4
Lidocaine (Xylocaine, various)	<2	0.5–1
Prilocaine (Citanest)	<2	1–2
Ropivacaine[b] (Naropin)	10–30	0.5–6

[a]Unless otherwise indicated, values are for infiltrative anesthesia.
[b]Epidural administration.
Data from Anonymous. American Hospital Formulary Service. In: McVoy GK, ed. Drug Information. Bethesda, MD: American Society of Health-System Pharmacists, 2009; and Anonymous. Facts and Comparisons. Philadelphia, PA. Wolters Kluwer Health. Accessed August 2010.

- High plasma concentrations can cause CNS excitation and depression (dizziness, tinnitus, drowsiness, disorientation, muscle twitching, seizures, and respiratory arrest). Cardiovascular effects include myocardial depression. Skillful technical application, frequent administration, and specialized follow-up procedures are required.

SPECIAL CONSIDERATIONS IN CANCER PAIN

- An algorithm for pain management in oncology patients is shown in **Fig. 55–2**. Pharmacologic therapies should be coupled with psychological, surgical, and supportive therapies using an interdisciplinary approach.
- Individualization of therapy is essential, and continuous assessment of pain response, side effects, and behavior is required.
- **NSAIDs** are especially effective for bone pain. **Strontium 89** and **samarium 153 lexidronam** are also effective.
- Around-the-clock schedules in conjunction with as-needed doses are employed when patients experience breakthrough pain.
- **Methadone** has regained prominence in treating cancer pain. It has a prolonged mechanism of action, N-methyl-D-aspartate receptor antagonist activity (d-isomer), and is inexpensive. However, it can be difficult to titrate.

SPECIAL CONSIDERATIOINS IN CHRONIC NONCANCER PAIN

- As pain becomes more chronic, hypertension, tachycardia, and diaphoresis become less evident, and depression, sleep disturbances, anxiety, irritability, work problems, and family instability tend to dominate.

- An integrated, interdisciplinary, systematic approach (e.g., pain clinic) is preferred. Placebos should not be used. Maximal benefit may take months to years.

EVALUATION OF THERAPEUTIC OUTCOMES

- Pain intensity, pain relief, and medication side effects must be assessed on a regular basis. The timing and regularity of assessment depend on the type of pain, medications administered, route of administration, and other therapies being used. Postoperative pain and acute exacerbations of cancer pain may require hourly assessment, whereas chronic nonmalignant pain may need only daily (or less frequent) monitoring.
- With chronic pain, a monitoring tool such as the Brief Pain Inventory, Initial Pain Assessment Inventory, or McGill Pain Questionnaire may be useful. Quality of life must also be assessed on a regular basis in all patients.
- The best management of opioid-induced constipation is prevention. Patients should be counseled on proper intake of fluids and fiber, and a laxative should be added with chronic opioid use.

See Chapter 69, Pain Management, authored by Terry J. Baumann, Jennifer M. Strickland, and Chris M. Herndon, for a more detailed discussion of this topic.

DEFINITION

- Parkinson's disease (PD) has highly characteristic neuropathologic findings and a clinical presentation, including motor deficits and, in some cases, mental deterioration.

PATHOPHYSIOLOGY

- The two hallmark features in the substantia nigra pars compacta are loss of neurons and the presence of Lewy bodies. There is a positive correlation between the degree of nigrostriatal dopamine loss and severity of motor symptoms. PD is relatively asymptomatic until profound depletion (70–80%) of substantia nigra pars compacta neurons has occurred.
- Reduced activation of dopamine-1 and dopamine-2 receptors results in greater inhibition of the thalamus. Clinical improvement may be more tied to restoring activity at the dopamine-2 receptor than at the dopamine-1 receptor. Loss of presynaptic nigrostriatal dopamine neurons results in inhibition of thalamic activity and reduced activation of the motor cortex.

CLINICAL PRESENTATION

- PD develops insidiously and progresses slowly. Clinical features are summarized in Table 56–1. Initial symptoms may be sensory, but as the disease progresses, one or more classic primary features presents (e.g., resting tremor, rigidity, bradykinesia, and postural instability that may lead to falls).
- Resting tremor is often the sole presenting complaint. However, only two thirds of PD patients have tremor on diagnosis, and some never develop this sign. Tremor is present most commonly in the hands, often begins unilaterally, and sometimes has a characteristic "pill-rolling" quality. Resting tremor is usually abolished by volitional movement and is absent during sleep.
- Muscular rigidity involves increased muscular resistance to passive range of motion and can be cogwheel in nature. It commonly affects both upper and lower extremities, and facial muscles may be affected.
- Intellectual deterioration is not inevitable, but some patients deteriorate in a manner indistinguishable from Alzheimer's disease.

DIAGNOSIS

- Clinically, PD is diagnosed when at least two of the following are present: limb muscle rigidity, resting tremor (at 3–6 Hz and abolished by movement), or bradykinesia. A diagnosis of PD can be made with a high level of confidence when there is resting tremor, bradykinesia or rigidity, prominent asymmetry, and a positive response to dopaminergic medication.

TABLE 56–1	Presentation of Parkinson's Disease (PD)

General features
- For clinically probable IPD, the patient exhibits at least two of the following: resting tremor, rigidity, or bradykinesia. Asymmetric onset and severity of these features is typical.
- Postural instability (difficulty with maintaining balance) is more common in advanced PD.

Motor symptoms
- The patient experiences decreased manual dexterity, difficulty arising from a seated position, diminished arm swing during ambulation, dysarthria (slurred speech), dysphagia (difficulty with swallowing), festinating gait (tendency to pass from a walking to a running pace), flexed posture (axial, upper/lower extremities), "freezing" at initiation of movement, hypomimia (reduced facial animation), hypophonia (reduced voice volume), and micrographia (diminution of handwritten letters/ symbols).

Autonomic and sensory symptoms
- The patient experiences bladder and anal sphincter disturbances, constipation, diaphoresis, fatigue, olfactory disturbance, orthostatic blood pressure changes, pain, paresthesia, paroxysmal vascular flushing, seborrhea, sexual dysfunction, and sialorrhea (drooling).

Mental status changes
- The patient experiences anxiety, apathy, bradyphrenia (slowness of thought processes), confusional state, dementia, depression, hallucinosis/psychosis (typically drug induced), and sleep disorders (excessive daytime sleepiness, insomnia, obstructive sleep apnea, and rapid eye movement sleep behavior disorder).

Laboratory tests
- No laboratory tests are available to diagnose PD.

Other diagnostic tests
- Genetic testing is not routinely helpful.
- Neuroimaging may be useful for excluding other diagnoses.
- Medication history should be obtained to rule out drug-induced parkinsonism.

- A number of other conditions must also be excluded, such as medication-induced parkinsonism (e.g., induced by antipsychotics, phenothiazine antiemetics, or metoclopramide). Other neurologic conditions (e.g., essential tremor, corticobasal ganglionic degeneration, multiple system atrophy, and progressive supranuclear palsy) must be ruled out.

DESIRED OUTCOME

- The goals of treatment are to minimize symptoms, disability, and side effects while maintaining quality of life. Education of patients and caregivers is critical, and exercise and proper nutrition are essential.

TREATMENT

PHARMACOLOGIC THERAPY

- An algorithm for management of early and late PD is shown in **Fig. 56–1**.
- A summary of available antiparkinsonian medications is listed in **Table 56–2**.

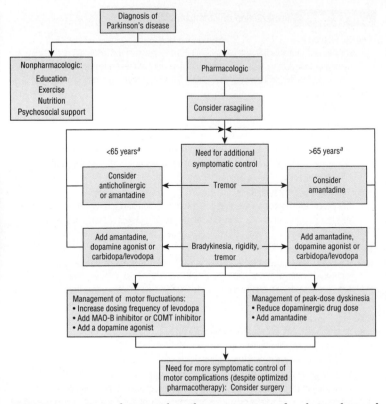

FIGURE 56–1. General approach to the management of early to advanced Parkinson's disease. *ᵃAge is not the sole determinant for drug choice. Others factors such as cognitive function and overall safety and tolerability of drug (especially in the elderly) should be considered.*

- Monotherapy usually begins with a monoamine oxidase-B (MAO-B) inhibitor, or if the patient is physiologically young, a dopamine agonist. For patients who are older, cognitively impaired, or having moderately severe functional impairment, L-dopa (e.g., **carbidopa/levodopa**) is preferred.
- With the development of motor fluctuations, addition of a catechol-*O*-methyltransferase (COMT) inhibitor should be considered to extend L-dopa duration of activity. Alternatively, addition of an MAO-B inhibitor or dopamine agonist should be considered.
- For management of L-dopa-induced peak-dose dyskinesias, the addition of **amantadine** should be considered.

Anticholinergic Medications

- Anticholinergic drugs can be effective for tremor and sometimes dystonic features in some patients but rarely show substantial benefit for

TABLE 56–2 Drugs Used in Parkinson's Disease[a]

Generic Name	Trade Name	Dosage Range[b] (mg/day)	Dosage Forms (mg)
Anticholinergic drugs			
Benztropine	Cogentin	0.5–4	0.5, 1, 2
Trihexyphenidyl	Artane	1–6	2, 5, 2/5mL
Carbidopa/levodopa products			
Carbidopa/L-dopa	Sinemet	300–1,000[c]	10/100, 25/100, 25/250
Carbidopa/L-dopa ODT	Parcopa	300–1,000[c]	10/100, 25/100, 25/250
Carbidopa/L-dopa CR	Sinemet CR	400–1,000[c]	25/100, 50/200
Carbidopa/L-dopa/ entacapone	Stalevo	600–1,600[d]	12.5/50/200, 18.75/75/200, 25/100/200, 31.25/125/200, 37.5/150/200, 50/200/200
Carbidopa	Lodosyn	25–75	25
Dopamine agonists			
Apomorphine	Apokyn	3–12	30/3 mL
Bromocriptine	Parlodel	15–40	2.5, 5
Pramipexole	Mirapex	1.5–4.5	0.125, 0.25, 0.5, 1, 1.5
Pramipexole ER	Mirapex ER	1.5–4.5	0.375, 0.75, 1.5, 3, 4.5
Ropinirole	Requip	9–24	0.25, 0.5; 1, 2, 3, 4, 5
Ropinirole XL	Requip XL	8–24	2, 4, 6, 8, 12
COMT inhibitors			
Entacapone	Comtan	200–1,600	200
Tolcapone	Tasmar	300–600	100, 200
MAO-B inhibitors			
Rasagiline	Azilect	0.5–1	0.5, 1
Selegiline	Eldepryl	5–10	5
Selegiline ODT	Zelapar	1.25–2.5	1.25, 2.5
Miscellaneous			
Amantadine	Symmetrel	200–300	100, 50/5 mL

COMT, catechol-O-methyltransferase; CR, controlled release; MAO, monoamine oxidase; ODT, orally disintegrating tablet.
[a]Marketed in the United States for idiopathic Parkinson's disease.
[b]Dosages may vary beyond stated range.
[c]Dosages expressed as L-dopa component.
[d]Dosages expressed as entacapone component.

bradykinesia or other disabilities. They can be used as monotherapy or in conjunction with other antiparkinsonian drugs. They differ little from each other in therapeutic potential or adverse effects.

- Anticholinergic side effects include dry mouth, blurred vision, constipation, and urinary retention. More serious reactions include forgetfulness, confusion, sedation, depression, and anxiety. Patients with preexisting cognitive deficits and the elderly are at greater risk for central anticholinergic side effects.

Amantadine

- Amantadine often provides modest benefit for tremor, rigidity, and bradykinesia. It may also decrease dyskinesia at relatively high doses (400 mg/day).
- Adverse effects include sedation, vivid dreams, dry mouth, depression, hallucinations, anxiety, dizziness, psychosis, and confusion. Livedo reticularis (a diffuse mottling of the skin in the upper or lower extremities) is a common but reversible side effect.
- Doses should be reduced in patients with renal dysfunction (100 mg/day with creatinine clearances of 30–50 mL/min [0.5–0.84 mL/s], 100 mg every other day for creatinine clearances of 15–29 mL/min [0.25–0.49 mL/s], and 200 mg every 7 days for creatinine clearances less than 15 mL/min [0.25 mL/s]) and those on hemodialysis.

Levodopa and Carbidopa/Levodopa

- L-dopa, the most effective drug available, is the immediate precursor of dopamine. It crosses the blood–brain barrier, whereas dopamine, **carbidopa**, and **benserazide** do not. Ultimately, all PD patients will require L-dopa.
- The decision whether to start L-dopa as soon as the diagnosis is made or only when symptoms compromise social, occupational, or psychological well-being has generated controversy.
- In the CNS and elsewhere, L-dopa is converted by L-amino acid decarboxylase (L-AAD) to dopamine. In the periphery, L-AAD can be blocked by administering carbidopa or benserazide. Carbidopa therefore increases the CNS penetration of exogenously administered L-dopa and decreases adverse effects (e.g., nausea, vomiting, cardiac arrhythmias, postural hypotension, and vivid dreams) from peripheral L-dopa metabolism to dopamine. Benserazide is unavailable in the United States.
- Starting L-dopa at 300 mg/day (in divided doses) in combination with carbidopa often achieves adequate relief of disability. The usual maximal dose of L-dopa is 800 to 1,000 mg/day.
- About 75 mg of carbidopa is required to effectively block peripheral L-AAD, but some patients may need more. Carbidopa/L-dopa is most widely used in a 25/100 mg tablet, but 25/250 mg and 10/100 mg dosage forms are also available. Controlled-release preparations of carbidopa/L-dopa are available in 50/200 mg and 25/100 mg strengths. For patients with difficulty swallowing, an orally disintegrating tablet is available. If peripheral adverse effects are prominent, 25 mg carbidopa (Lodosyn) tablets are available.

TABLE 56–3	Common Motor Complications and Possible Initial Treatments
Effect	**Possible Treatments**
End-of-dose "wearing off" (motor fluctuation)	Increase frequency of carbidopa/ʟ-dopa doses; add either COMT inhibitor or MAO-B inhibitor or dopamine agonist
"Delayed on" or "no on" response	Give carbidopa/ʟ-dopa on empty stomach; use carbidopa/ʟ-dopa ODT; avoid carbidopa/ʟ-dopa CR; use apomorphine subcutaneous
Start hesitation ("freezing")	Increase carbidopa/ʟ-dopa dose; add a dopamine agonist or MAO-B inhibitor; utilize physical therapy along with assistive walking devices or sensory cues (e.g., rhythmic commands, stepping over objects)
Peak-dose dyskinesia	Provide smaller doses of carbidopa/ʟ-dopa; add amantadine

COMT, catechol-*O*-methyltransferase; CR, controlled release; MAO, monoamine oxidase; ODT, orally disintegrating tablet.

- There is marked intra- and intersubject variability in time to peak plasma concentrations after oral ʟ-dopa. Meals delay gastric emptying, but antacids promote gastric emptying. ʟ-dopa is absorbed primarily in the proximal duodenum by a saturable large neutral amino acid transport system. Large neutral amino acids (including high-protein meals) can interfere with bioavailability.

- ʟ-dopa is not bound to plasma proteins, and the elimination half-life is ~1 hour. The addition of carbidopa or benserazide can extend the half-life to 1.5 hours, and the addition of a COMT inhibitor (e.g., **entacapone**) can extend it to ~2 to 2.5 hours.

- Long-term ʟ-dopa-associated motor complications can be disabling. The most common of these are end-of-dose "wearing off" and "peak-dose dyskinesias." The risk of developing motor fluctuations or dyskinesias is felt to be ~10% per year of ʟ-dopa therapy. However, motor complications can occur as early as 5 to 6 months after starting ʟ-dopa, especially when excessive doses are used initially. Table 56–3 shows the motor complications associated with long-term treatment with carbidopa/ʟ-dopa and suggested management strategies.

- "End-of-dose wearing off" is common and related to the increasing loss of neuronal storage capability for dopamine and the short half-life of ʟ-dopa. Bedtime administration of a dopamine agonist or a sustained-release formulation product (e.g., carbidopa/ʟ-dopa CR, ropinirole XL, or pramipexole ER) can help reduce nocturnal off episodes and improve functioning upon awakening.

- "Delayed-on" or "no-on" can result from delayed gastric emptying or decreased absorption in the duodenum. Crushing the tablet of carbidopa/ʟ-dopa and taking with a glass of water or using the orally disintegrating tablet formulation on an empty stomach can help. Subcutaneous apomorphine may also be used as rescue therapy.

- "Freezing," a sudden, episodic inhibition of lower extremity motor function, may be worsened by anxiety and may increase the risk of falls.

- Dyskinesias are involuntary choreiform movements, usually involving the neck, trunk, and extremities. They are usually associated with peak striatal dopamine levels. Less commonly, dyskinesias also can develop during the rise and fall of L-dopa effects (the dyskinesias-improvement-dyskinesias or diphasic pattern of response).
- "Off-period dystonia," sustained muscle contractions that occur more commonly in distal lower extremities (e.g., feet or toes), occur often in the early morning hours. They may be treated with bedtime administration of sustained-release products, use of baclofen, or selective denervation with botulinum toxin.

Monoamine Oxidase B Inhibitors

- At therapeutic doses, **selegiline** and **rasagiline**, selective inhibitors of MAO-B, are unlikely to induce a "cheese reaction" (hypertension, headache) unless excessive amounts of dietary tyramine ($\geq$400 mg) are ingested. However, concomitant MAO-B inhibitors with meperidine and other selected analgesics is contraindicated because of a small risk of serotonin syndrome. Selegiline and rasagiline may be neuroprotective.
- Selegiline (deprenyl; Eldepryl) is an irreversible MAO-B inhibitor that blocks dopamine breakdown and can modestly extend the duration of action of L-dopa (up to 1 hour). It often permits reduction of the L-dopa dose by as much as one half.
- Selegiline also increases the peak effects of L-dopa and can worsen preexisting dyskinesias or psychiatric symptoms, such as delusions and hallucinations. Other adverse effects include insomnia and jitteriness. The oral disintegrating tablet may provide improved response and fewer side effects compared with the conventional formulation.
- Metabolites of selegiline are l-methamphetamine and L-amphetamine.
- Studies evaluating its neuroprotective properties suggest that selegiline can delay the need for L-dopa by ~9 months and has symptomatic effects, but there is no firm evidence that it can slow neurodegeneration.
- Rasagiline, another MAO-B inhibitor, has similar effects as selegiline in enhancing L-dopa effects and modest beneficial effect as monotherapy. Early initiation is associated with better long-term outcomes.
- When an adjunctive agent is required for managing motor fluctuations, rasagiline may provide 1 hour of extra "on" time during the day. It is considered a first-line agent (as is entacapone) for managing motor fluctuations.

Catechol-*O*-Methyltransferase Inhibitors

- **Tolcapone** (Tasmar) and **entacapone** (Comtan) are used only in conjunction with carbidopa/L-dopa to prevent the peripheral conversion of L-dopa to dopamine (increasing the area under the curve of L-dopa by ~35%). Thus, "on" time is increased by ~1 to 2 hours. These agents significantly decrease "off" time and decrease L-dopa dosage requirements. Concomitant use of nonselective MAO inhibitors should be avoided to prevent inhibition of the pathways for normal catecholamine metabolism.
- COMT inhibition is more effective than controlled-release carbidopa/L-dopa in providing consistent extension of effect.

- The starting and recommended dose of tolcapone is 100 mg three times daily as an adjunct to carbidopa/L-dopa. Its use is limited by the potential for fatal liver toxicity. Strict monitoring of liver function is required, and tolcapone should be discontinued if liver function tests are above the upper limit of normal or any signs or symptoms suggestive of hepatic failure exist. It should be reserved for patients with fluctuations that have not responded to other therapies.
- Because entacapone has a shorter half-life, 200 mg is given with each dose of carbidopa/L-dopa up to eight times a day. Dopaminergic adverse effects may occur and are managed easily by reducing the carbidopa/L-dopa dose. Brownish orange urine discoloration may occur (as with tolcapone), but there is no evidence of hepatotoxicity from entacapone.

Dopamine Agonists

- The ergot derivative **bromocriptine** (Parlodel) and the nonergots **pramipexole** (Mirapex) and **ropinirole** (Requip) are beneficial adjuncts in patients with deteriorating response to L-dopa, those experiencing fluctuation in response to L-dopa, and those with limited clinical response to L-dopa due to inability to tolerate higher doses. They decrease the frequency of "off" periods and provide an L-dopa-sparing effect.
- The dose of dopamine agonists is best determined by slow titration to enhance tolerance and to find the least dose that provides optimal benefit.
- The nonergots are safer and are effective as monotherapy in mild to moderate PD as well as adjuncts to L-dopa in patients with motor fluctuations.
- Bromocriptine is not commonly used because of an increased risk of pulmonary fibrosis and reduced efficacy compared with the other agonists.
- There is less risk of developing motor complications from monotherapy with dopamine agonists than from L-dopa. Because younger patients are more likely to develop motor fluctuations, dopamine agonists are preferred in this population. Older patients are more likely to experience psychosis and orthostatic hypotension from dopamine agonists; therefore, carbidopa/L-dopa may be the best initial medication in elderly patients, particularly if cognitive problems or dementia is present.
- Common side effects of dopamine agonists are nausea, confusion, hallucinations, lightheadedness, lower extremity edema, postural hypotension, sedation, and vivid dreams. Less common are compulsive behaviors, psychosis, and sleep attacks. Hallucinations and delusions can be managed using a stepwise approach (**Table 56–4**). When added to L-dopa, dopamine agonists may worsen dyskinesias.
- **Pramipexole** is initiated at a dose of 0.125 mg three times daily and increased every 5 to 7 days as tolerated to a maximum of 1.5 mg 3 times a day. It is primarily renally excreted, and the initial dose must be adjusted in renal insufficiency. A once-daily extended-release formulation is available.
- **Ropinirole** is initiated at 0.25 mg three times daily and increased by 0.25 mg three times daily on a weekly basis to a maximum of 24 mg/day. It is metabolized by cytochrome P450 1A2; fluoroquinolones and smoking may alter ropinirole clearance. A once-daily formulation is available.

TABLE 56–4 Stepwise Approach to Management of Drug-induced Hallucinosis and Psychosis in Parkinson's Disease

1. General measures such as evaluating for electrolyte disturbance (especially hypercalcemia or hyponatremia), hypoxemia, or infection (especially encephalitis, sepsis, or urinary tract infection).
2. Simplify the antiparkinsonian regimen as much as possible by discontinuing or reducing the dosage of medications with the highest risk-to-benefit ratio first.[a]
   a. Discontinue anticholinergics, including other nonparkinsonian medications with anticholinergic activity such as antihistamines or tricyclic antidepressants.
   b. Taper and discontinue amantadine.
   c. Discontinue monoamine oxidase-B inhibitor.
   d. Taper and discontinue dopamine agonist.
   e. Consider reduction of L-dopa (especially evening doses) and discontinuation of catechol-O-methyltransferase inhibitors.
3. Consider atypical antipsychotic medication if disruptive hallucinosis or psychosis persists.
   a. Quetiapine 12.5–25 mg at bedtime; gradually increase by 25 mg each week if necessary, until hallucinosis or psychosis improved or
   b. Clozapine 12.5–50 mg at bedtime; gradually increase by 25 mg each week if necessary until hallucinosis or psychosis improved (requires frequent monitoring for leukopenia).

[a]If dosage reduction or medication discontinuation is either infeasible or undesirable, go to step 3.

- **Apomorphine** is a nonergot dopamine agonist given as a subcutaneous "rescue" injection. For patients with advanced PD with intermittent "off" episodes despite optimized therapy, subcutaneous apomorphine triggers an "on" response within 20 minutes, and duration of effect is up to 100 minutes. Most patients require 0.06 mg/kg. Prior to injection, patients should be premedicated with the antiemetic trimethobenzamide. It is contraindicated with the serotonin-3-receptor blockers (e.g., ondansetron).

EVALUATION OF THERAPEUTIC OUTCOMES

- Patients and caregivers should be educated so that they can participate in treatment by recording medication administration times and duration of "on" and "off" periods.
- Symptoms, side effects, and activities of daily living must be scrupulously monitored and therapy individualized. Concomitant medications that may worsen motor symptoms, memory, falls, or behavioral symptoms should be discontinued if possible.

See Chapter 68, Parkinson's Disease, authored by Jack J. Chen, Merlin V. Nelson, and David M. Swope, for a more detailed discussion of this topic.

CHAPTER 57

Status Epilepticus

DEFINITION

- Status epilepticus (SE) is any seizure lasting longer than 30 minutes, whether or not consciousness is impaired, or recurrent seizures without an intervening period of consciousness between seizures. SE is a medical emergency with significant morbidity and mortality, and aggressive treatment of seizures that last 5 minutes or more is strongly recommended. **Table 57–1** shows the classification of SE. This chapter focuses on generalized convulsive status epilepticus (GCSE), the most common and severe form of SE.

PATHOPHYSIOLOGY

- Seizure initiation is likely caused by an imbalance between excitatory (e.g., glutamate, calcium, sodium, substance P, and neurokinin B) neurotransmission and inhibitory (γ-aminobutyric acid [GABA], adenosine, potassium, neuropeptide Y, opioid peptides, and galanin) neurotransmission.
- Seizure maintenance is largely caused by glutamate acting on postsynaptic N-methyl-D-aspartate [NMDA] and α-amino-3-hydroxy-5-methyl-isoxazole-4-propionate [AMPA]/akinate receptors. Sustained depolarization can result in neuronal death.
- There is evidence that $GABA_A$ receptors may be modified during SE and become less responsive to endogenous agonists and antagonists.
- Two phases of GCSE have been identified. During phase I, each seizure produces marked increases in plasma epinephrine, norepinephrine, and steroid concentrations that may cause hypertension, tachycardia, and cardiac arrhythmias. Muscle contractions and hypoxia can cause acidosis, hypotension, shock, rhabdomyolysis, and secondary hyperkalemia, and acute tubular necrosis may ensue.
- Phase II begins 30 minutes into the seizure, and the patient begins to decompensate. The patient may become hypotensive, and cerebral blood flow may be compromised. Serum glucose may be normal or decreased, and hyperthermia, respiratory deterioration, hypoxia, and ventilatory failure may develop.
- In prolonged seizures, motor activity may cease, but electrical seizures may persist.

MORBIDITY AND MORTALITY

- Younger children, the elderly, and those with preexisting epilepsy have a higher propensity for sequelae.
- Recent estimates suggest a mortality rate of up to 16% in children, 20% in adults, and 38% in the elderly.
- Variables affecting outcome are (1) the time between onset of GCSE and the initiation of treatment and (2) the duration of the seizure. The

TABLE 57–1	International Classification of Status Epilepticus		
Convulsive		**Nonconvulsive**	
International	*Traditional Terminology*	*International*	*Traditional Terminology*
Primary generalized SE • Tonic-clonic[a,b] • Tonic[c] • Clonic[c] • Myoclonic[b] • Erratic[d]	Grand mal, epilepticus convulsivus	Absence[c]	Petit mal, spike-and-wave stupor, spike-and-slow-wave or 3/s spike-and-wave, epileptic fugue, epilepsia minora continua, epileptic twilight, minor SE
Secondary generalized SE[a,b] • Tonic • Partial seizures with secondary generalization		Partial SE[a,b] Simple partial Somatomotor Dysphasic Other types Complex partial	Focal motor, focal sensory, epilepsia partialis continua, adversive SE Elementary Temporal lobe, psychomotor, epileptic fugue state, prolonged epileptic stupor, prolonged epileptic confusional state, continuous epileptic twilight state

SE, status epilepticus.
[a]Most common in older children.
[b]Most common in adolescents and adults.
[c]Most common in infants and young children.
[d]Most common in neonates.

mortality rate is 2.6% for those with seizures lasting 10 to 29 minutes and 19% for those with seizures lasting longer than 30 minutes. Another report showed that those with seizures lasting longer than 60 minutes had a mortality rate of 32%.

CLINICAL PRESENTATION AND DIAGNOSIS

SYMPTOMS

- Impaired consciousness (e.g., ranging from lethargy to coma)
- Disorientation (once GCSE is controlled)
- Pain associated with injuries (e.g., tongue lacerations, shoulder dislocations, and head and facial trauma)

SIGNS

Early

- Generalized convulsions
- Acute injuries or CNS insults that cause extensor or flexor posturing
- Hypothermia or fever suggestive of intercurrent illnesses (e.g., sepsis or meningitis)
- Incontinence
- Normal blood pressure or hypotension
- Respiratory compromise

Late

- Clinical seizures may or may not be apparent
- Pulmonary edema with respiratory failure
- Cardiac failure (dysrhythmias, arrest, or cardiogenic shock)
- Hypotension or hypertension
- Disseminated intravascular coagulation or multiorgan failure
- Rhabdomyolysis
- Hyperpyremia

DIAGNOSIS

Initial Laboratory Tests

- Complete blood count (CBC) with differential
- Serum chemistry profile (e.g., electrolytes, calcium, magnesium, glucose, serum creatinine, alanine aminotransferase [ALT], and aspartate aminotransferase [AST])
- Urine drug/alcohol screen
- Blood cultures
- Arterial blood gases (ABG) to assess for metabolic and respiratory acidosis
- Serum drug concentrations if previous anticonvulsant use is suspected or known

Other Diagnostic Tests

- Spinal tap if CNS infection suspected
- Electroencephalograph (EEG) should be obtained immediately and once clinical seizures are controlled
- Computed tomography (CT) with and without contrast
- Magnetic resonance imaging (MRI)
- Radiograph if indicated to diagnose fractures
- Electrocardiogram (ECG)

DESIRED OUTCOME

- The goals of treatment are (1) terminate clinical and electrical seizure activity, (2) minimize side effects, (3) prevent recurrent seizures, and (4) avoid pharmacoresistent epilepsy and/or neurologic sequelae.

TREATMENT

- For any tonic-clonic seizure that does not stop automatically or when doubt exists regarding the diagnosis, treatment of GCSE should begin during the diagnostic workup. An algorithm for treatment of GCSE is shown in **Fig. 57–1**. Loading and maintenance doses used in the pharmacologic management of GCSE are shown in **Table 57–2**.
- Normal to high blood pressure should be maintained.
- All patients should receive IV glucose, and **thiamine** (100 mg IV) should be given prior to glucose in adults.
- Metabolic and/or respiratory acidosis should be assessed by ABG measurements to determine pH, partial pressure of oxygen (Pao_2), partial pressure of carbon dioxide ($Paco_2$), and HCO_3. If pH is <7.2, secondary to metabolic acidosis, sodium bicarbonate should be given.

BENZODIAZEPINES

- A **benzodiazepine** should be administered as soon as possible if the patient is actively seizing. Generally, one or two IV doses will stop seizures within 2 to 3 minutes. Diazepam, lorazepam, and midazolam are equally effective. If seizures have stopped, a longer-acting anticonvulsant should be given.
- **Diazepam** is extremely lipophilic and quickly distributed into the brain, but it redistributes rapidly into body fat, causing a very short duration of effect (0.25–0.5 hours). Therefore, a longer-acting anticonvulsant (e.g., **phenytoin** or **phenobarbital**) should be given immediately after the diazepam. The initial dose of diazepam can be repeated if the patient does not respond within 5 minutes.
- **Lorazepam** is currently considered the benzodiazepine of choice by most practitioners. It takes longer to reach peak brain levels than diazepam but has a longer duration of action (12–24 hours). Patients chronically on benzodiazepines may require larger doses. The administration rate of diazepam and lorazepam should not exceed 5 and 2 mg/min, respectively, because the propylene glycol in the vehicle can cause dysrhythmia and hypotension.
- **Midazolam** is water soluble and diffuses rapidly into the CNS but has a very short half-life. It must be given by continuous infusion. There is increasing interest in using it buccally and intramuscularly when IV access cannot be obtained readily.
- With benzodiazepine administration, a brief period of cardiorespiratory depression (<1 min) may occur and can necessitate assisted ventilation or require intubation, especially if the benzodiazepine is used with a barbiturate. Hypotension may occur with high doses of benzodiazepines.

PHENYTOIN

- **Phenytoin** has a long half-life (20–36 hours), but it cannot be delivered fast enough to be considered a first-line agent. It takes longer to control seizures than do the benzodiazepines because it enters the brain more slowly. It causes less respiratory depression and sedation than the

PREHOSPITAL CARE
- Monitor vital signs (HR, RR)
- Consider PR diazepam (0.5 mg/kg/dose up to 10–20 mg) or IM midazolam (0.1–0.2 mg/kg)
- Transport to hospital if seizures persist

INITIAL HOSPITAL CARE
- Assess and control airway and cardiac function; pulse oximetry
- 100% oxygen
- Place IV catheter
- Intraosseous if unable to place IV and patient is older than 6 y
- Begin IV fluids
- Thiamine 100 mg (adult)
- Pyridoxine 50–100 mg (infant)
- Glucose (adult: 50 mL of 50%; children: 1 mL/kg of 25%)
- Naloxone 0.1 mg/kg for suspected narcotic overdose
- Antibiotics if suspected infection

LABORATORY STUDIES
- CBC with differential
- Serum chemistry profile (e.g., electrolytes, glucose, renal/hepatic function, calcium, magnesium)
- Arterial blood gas
- Blood cultures
- Serum anticonvulsant concentration
- Urine drug/alcohol screen

EARLY STATUS
0–10 min
- IV lorazepam (4 mg adults; 0.03–0.1 mg/kg at 2 mg/min pediatrics) may repeat if no response in 5 min
- Additional therapy may not be required if seizures stop and cause identified 10–30 min
- IV phenytoin or fosphenytoin PE[a] adults: 10–20 mg/kg at rate of 50 mg/min or 150 mg/min PE, respectively; infants/children: 15–20 mg/kg at a rate of 1–3 mg/kg/min

ESTABLISHED STATUS (30–60 min)
Seizures continue:
- Additional IV 5 mg/kg dose of either phenytoin or fosphenytoin PE[a] may be given in unresponsive patients[b]
- IV phenobarbital[a] 20 mg/kg at a rate of 100 mg/min in adults and 30 mg/min in infants/children[b]

REFRACTORY STATUS (>60 min)
Clinical or electrical seizures continue.
- IV phenobarbital[a] additional 10 mg/kg; 10 mg/kg may be given every hour until seizures stop or
- IV valproate 15–25 mg/kg followed by 1–4 mg/kg/hours[b] or
- General anesthesia with either
  IV midazolam 2 mg/kg bolus followed by 50–500 mcg/kg/hours
  IV pentobarbital 15–20 mg/kg bolus over 1 hour then 1–3 mg/kg/hours to burst suppression on EEG. If hypotension occurs slow rate of infusion or begin dopamine or
  IV propofol 1–2 mg/kg bolus followed by ≤4 mg/kg/hours
Once seizures controlled, taper midazolam, pentobarbital, propofol over 12 hours. If seizures recur start infusion and titrate to effective dose over 12 hours.

FIGURE 57–1. Algorithm for the management of generalized convulsive status epilepticus (GCSE). (CBC, complete blood cell count; EEG, electroencephalogram; HR, heart rate; PE, phenytoin sodium equivalents; PR, per rectum; RR, respiratory rate.) [a]Because variability exists in dosing, monitor serum concentration. [b]If seizure is controlled, begin maintenance dose, and optimize using serum concentration monitoring.

TABLE 57–2 Medications Used in the Initial Treatment of Generalized Convulsive Status Epilepticus

Anticonvulsant (Route)	Loading Dose (Maximum Dose)		Rate of Infusion		Maintenance Dose	
	Adult	Pediatric	Adult	Pediatric	Adult	Pediatric
Diazepam (IV bolus)	0.25 mg/kg[a,b,c] (40 mg)	0.25–0.5 mg/kg[a,c] (0.75 mg/kg)	<5 mg/min	<5 mg/min	Not used	Not used
Fosphenytoin IV	15–20 mg PE/kg	15–20 mg PE/kg	150 mg PE/min	3 mg PE/kg/min	4–5 mg PE/kg/day	5–10 mg PE/kg/day
Lorazepam (IV bolus)	4 mg[a,b,c] (8 mg)	0.1 mg/kg[a,c] (4 mg)	2 mg/min	2 mg/min	Not used	Not used
Midazolam IV	200 mcg/kg[a,d]	150 mcg/kg[a,d]	0.5–1 mg/min	2–3 min	50–500 mcg/kg/hour[e]	60–120 mcg/kg/hour[e]
Phenobarbital IV	10–20 mg/kg[e]	15–20 mg/kg[e]	100 mg/min	30 mg/min	1–4 mg/kg/day[e]	3–5 mg/kg/day[e]
Phenytoin IV	10–20 mg/kg[f]	10–20 mg/kg[f]	50 mg/min[g]	1–3 mg/kg/min	4–5 mg/kg/day[e]	5–10 mg/kg/day[e]

GCSE, generalized convulsive status epilepticus; PE, phenytoin equivalents.

[a]Doses can be repeated every 10 to 15 minutes until the maximum dosage is given.

[b]Initial doses in the elderly are 2 to 5 mg.

[c]Larger doses can be required if patients chronically on a benzodiazepine (e.g., clonazepam).

[d]Can be given by the intramuscular, rectal, or buccal routes.

[e]Titrate dose as needed.

[f]Administer additional loading dose based on serum concentration.

[g]The rate should not exceed 25 mg/min in elderly patients and those with known atherosclerotic cardiovascular disease.

benzodiazepines or **phenobarbital**, but it is associated with administration-related cardiovascular toxicity (the vehicle is 40% propylene glycol). These administration-related problems are more likely to occur with large loading doses or in critically ill patients with marginal blood pressure.

- Phenytoin should be diluted to ≤5 mg/mL in normal saline. The maximum rate of infusion is 50 mg/min in adults (25 mg/min in the elderly) and 3 mg/kg/min in children <50 kg. Vital signs and ECG should be obtained during administration. If arrhythmias or hypotension occurs or if the QT interval widens, the rate should be slowed. Maintenance doses should be started within 12 to 24 hours of the loading dose.
- If the patient has been on phenytoin prior to admission and the phenytoin concentration is known, this should be considered in determining a loading dose.
- A reduction in the loading dose is recommended for elderly patients, and a larger loading dose is required in obese patients.
- For seizures continuing after the initial loading dose, some practitioners have recommended an additional loading dose of 5 mg/kg (after waiting 60 min for response), but additional phenytoin may result in toxicity and exacerbation of seizures. There is no evidence that a total loading dose >20 mg/kg will be of benefit in these patients.
- Phenytoin is associated with pain and burning during infusion. Phlebitis may occur with chronic infusion, and tissue necrosis is likely on infiltration. Intramuscular administration is not recommended.

FOSPHENYTOIN

- **Fosphenytoin,** the water-soluble phosphate ester of phenytoin, is a phenytoin prodrug.
- The dose of fosphenytoin sodium is expressed as phenytoin sodium equivalents (PE).
- Adverse reactions include nystagmus, dizziness, and ataxia. Paresthesias and pruritus typically disappear within 5 to 10 minutes after the infusion.
- Continuous ECG, blood pressure, and respiratory status monitoring is recommended for all loading doses of fosphenytoin. Serum phenytoin concentrations should not be obtained for at least 2 hours after IV and 4 hours after intramuscular administration of fosphenytoin.

PHENOBARBITAL

- The Working Group on Status Epilepticus recommends that **phenobarbital** be given after a benzodiazepine plus phenytoin has failed. Most practitioners agree that phenobarbital is the long-acting anticonvulsant of choice in patients with hypersensitivity to the hydantoins or in those with cardiac conduction abnormalities.
- To avoid overdosing, estimated lean body mass should be used in obese patients.
- Peak brain concentrations occur 12 to 60 minutes after IV dosing. On average, seizures are controlled within minutes of the loading dose.
- If the initial loading dose does not stop the seizures within 20 to 30 minutes, an additional 10 to 20 mg/kg dose may be given. If seizures continue,

a third 10 mg/kg load may be given. There is no maximum dose beyond which further doses are likely to be ineffective. Once seizures are controlled, the maintenance dose should be started within 12 to 24 hours.

- The risk of apnea and hypopnea can be more profound in patients already treated with benzodiazepines. If significant hypotension develops, the infusion should be slowed or stopped.

REFRACTORY GENERALIZED CONVULSIVE STATUS EPILEPTICUS

- When adequate doses of a benzodiazepine, phenytoin, or phenobarbital have failed, the condition is termed refractory. Failure to aggressively treat early increases the likelihood of nonresponse. Doses of agents used to treat refractory GCSE are given in Table 57–3.
- A meta-analysis showed that among patients refractory to GCSE, pentobarbital had a 92% response rate, compared with midazolam (80%) and propofol (73%). Breakthrough seizures were least common with pentobarbital (12%, compared with propofol [15%] and midazolam [51%]). Hypotension was more common with midazolam.

Benzodiazepines

- **Midazolam** has been suggested by some practitioners as the first-line treatment for refractory GCSE. Most patients respond within 1 hour, but the infusion rate should be increased every 15 minutes in those who do not. Tachyphylaxis can develop, and dosing should be guided by EEG response.
- Once seizures are terminated, dosages can be decreased by 1 mcg/kg/min every 2 hours. Successful discontinuation is enhanced by maintaining serum **phenytoin** concentrations >20 mg/L (79 μmol/L) and **phenobarbital** concentrations >40 mg/L (172 μmol/L).
- Hypotension and poikilothermia can occur and may require supportive therapies.
- Refractory GCSE has also been treated with large-dose, continuous infusion **lorazepam**. Lorazepam contains propylene glycol, which can accumulate and cause marked osmolar gap, metabolic acidosis, and renal toxicity.

Medically Induced Coma

- If there is inadequate response to high doses of **midazolam**, anesthetizing is recommended. Intubation and respiratory support are mandatory during **barbiturate** coma, and continuous monitoring of vital signs is essential. A short-acting barbiturate (e.g., **pentobarbital** or **thiopental**) is generally preferred (see Fig. 57–1).
- **Pentobarbital** should be initiated with a loading dose in accordance with the guidelines given in Table 57–3. Serum concentration of 40 mg/L (177 μmol/L) is necessary to induce an isoelectric EEG. If hypotension occurs, the rate of administration should be slowed, or dopamine should be administered. The loading dose should be followed immediately by an infusion according to Table 57–3, increasing gradually until there is burst suppression on the EEG or adverse effects occur. Twelve hours after a

TABLE 57-3 Medications Used to Treat Refractory Generalized Convulsive Status Epilepticus

Anticonvulsant (Route)	Loading Dose		Infusion Duration		Maintenance Dose	
	Adult	Pediatric	Adult	Pediatric	Adult	Pediatric
Lacosamide	200–300 mg	NA	3–5 min	NA	200 mg/day	NA
Levetiracetam IV	500–2,000 mg	15–70 mg/kg	33–66 mg/min	2–5 mg/kg/min	750–9,000 mg/day	20–60 mg/kg/day
Lidocaine IV	55–100 mg	1 mg/kg (max. dose = 3–5 mg/kg in first hour)	≤2 min	≤2 min	1.5–3.5 mg/kg/hour	1.2–3 mg/kg/hour
Midazolam IV	200 mcg/kg[a]	150 mcg/kg[c]	0.5–1 mg/min	0.5–1 mg/min	50–500 mcg/kg/hour[b]	60–120 mcg/kg/hour[b]
Pentobarbital IV	10–20 mg/kg	15–20 mg/kg	Over 1–2 hours	Over 1–2 hours	1–5 mg/kg/hour[b]	1–5 mg/kg/hour[b]
Propofol IV	2 mg/kg	3 mg/kg	Over 10 sec	Over 20–30 sec	5–10 mg/kg/hour[b]	2–18 mg/kg/hour[c]
Topiramate PO	300–1,600 mg	5–10 mg/kg	NA	NA	400–1,600 mg/day	5–10 mg/kg/day
Valproate IV	15–45 mg/kg	20–25 mg/kg	3 mg/kg/min	3 mg/kg/min	1–4 mg/kg/hour[b]	1–4 mg/kg/hour[b]

GCSE, generalized convulsive status epilepticus; NA, not available; PO, orally.

[a]Doses can be repeated twice every 10 to 15 minutes until the maximum dosage is given.

[b]Titrate dose as needed.

[c]Generally recommended not to exceed a dose of 4 mg/kg/hour and a duration of 48 hours.

burst suppression pattern is obtained, the rate of pentobarbital infusion should be titrated downward every 2 to 4 hours to determine if GCSE is in remission.

Valproate

- Refer to **Table 57–3** for dosing guidelines for adults and children. The manufacturer recommends that IV **valproate** be given no faster than 3 mg/kg/min.
- Some have suggested that the maintenance infusion rate should be adjusted as follows: (1) if no metabolic enzyme inducers are present, the continuous infusion rate is 1 mg/kg/hour; (2) if one or more inducers are present (e.g., phenobarbital or phenytoin), the rate is 2 mg/kg/hour; and (3) if inducers and pentobarbital coma are present, the rate is 4 mg/kg/hour.
- There are no reports of respiratory depression; hemodynamic instability is rare, but vital signs should be monitored closely during the loading dose.

Propofol

- **Propofol** is very lipid soluble, has a large volume of distribution, and has a rapid onset of action. It has comparable efficacy to midazolam for refractory GCSE. It has been associated with metabolic acidosis, hemodynamic instability, and bradyarrhythmias that are refractory to treatment.
- An adult dose can provide greater than 1,000 cal/day as lipid and cost over $800/day.

Other Agents

- **Topiramate** tablets can be crushed and dissolved in a small amount of water. Response tends to be delayed hours to days. It may induce metabolic acidosis and kidney stones.
- Levetiracetam is not hepatically metabolized and is minimally protein bound.
- Lidocaine is not recommended unless other agents have failed. **Table 57–3** shows the recommended dosing guidelines. It has a rapid onset of action. Fasciculations, visual disturbances, and tinnitus may occur at serum concentrations between 6 and 8 mg/L (25.6–34.2 μmol/L). Seizures and obtundation may develop when serum concentrations exceed 8 mg/L (34.2 μmol/L).

EVALUATION OF THERAPEUTIC OUTCOMES

- An EEG is a key tool that allows practitioners to determine when abnormal electrical activity has been aborted and may assist in determining which anticonvulsant was effective. Vital signs must be monitored during the infusion. The infusion site must be assessed for any evidence of infiltration before and during administration of phenytoin.

See Chapter 66, Status Epilepticus, authored by Stephanie J. Phelps, Collin A. Hovinga, and James W. Wheless, for a more detailed discussion of this topic.

CHAPTER 58

Assessment of Nutrition Status and Nutrition Requirements

DEFINITIONS

- Nutrition assessment allows identification of individuals at risk for under- and overnutrition.
- Undernutrition is the result of inadequate nutrition intake, impaired absorption of nutrients, or inappropriate use of ingested nutrients. Changes in subcellular, cellular, and/or organ function can occur and increase the risk of morbidity and mortality.

CLASSIFICATION OF NUTRITIONAL DISEASES

- Undernutrition can result from a deficiency in protein and calories or from a single nutrient (e.g., vitamins or trace elements).
- Types of protein-energy malnutrition are marasmus (deficiency in total intake or nutrient utilization), kwashiorkor (relative protein deficiency), and mixed marasmus-kwashiorkor.
- Single-nutrient deficiencies can occur, usually in combination with any protein-energy malnutrition.
- For information on overnutrition or obesity, see Chap. 60.

NUTRITION SCREENING

- Nutrition screening provides a systematic way to identify individuals at risk for undernutrition and should be a rapid and simple process done in any care environment.
- Risk factors for undernutrition include any disease state, complicating condition, treatment, or socioeconomic condition that results in decreased nutrient intake, altered metabolism, and/or malabsorption. The presence of three or four risk factors puts a person at risk for undernutrition.
- The Joint Commission on Accreditation of Healthcare Organizations standards require a nutrition screening typically within 24 hours of hospital admission. Patients determined to be at "nutrition risk" need a nutrition assessment and care plan.

NUTRITION ASSESSMENT

- Nutrition assessment is the first step in developing a nutrition care plan. The goals of nutrition assessment are to identify the presence (or risk) of developing undernutrition and complications, estimate nutrition needs, and establish baseline parameters for assessing the outcome of therapy.

- This assessment should include a nutrition-focused history, a physical exam including anthropometrics, and laboratory measurements.

CLINICAL EVALUATION

- Medical and dietary history should include weight changes within 6 months, dietary intake changes, GI symptoms, functional capacity, and disease states.
- Physical examination should focus on assessment of lean body mass (LBM) and physical findings of vitamin, trace element, and essential fatty acid deficiencies.

ANTHROPOMETRIC MEASUREMENTS

- Anthropometric measurements are physical measurements of the size, weight, and proportions of the human body used to compare an individual with normative standards for a population. The most common measurements are weight, stature, head circumference (for children younger than 3 years of age) waist circumference, and measurements of limb size (e.g., skinfold thickness and midarm muscle and wrist circumferences), along with bioelectrical impedance analysis (BIA).
- Interpretation of actual body weight should consider ideal weight for height, usual body weight, fluid status, and age. Change over time can be calculated as the percentage of usual body weight. Unintentional weight loss >10% in less than 6 months correlates with poor clinical outcome in adults.
- Ideal body weight provides a population reference standard against which the actual body weight can be compared to detect both under- and overnutrition (Table 58–1). See Table 58–2 for body weight equations.
- The best indicator of adequate nutrition in children is the appropriate rate of growth. Weight, stature, and head circumference should be plotted on the appropriate growth curve and compared with usual growth velocities (Table 58–3). Additionally, the average weight gain for infants is 24 to 35 g/day for term infants and 10 to 25 g/day for preterm infants.
- Body mass index (BMI) is another index of weight-for-height that is highly correlated with body fat. Interpretation of BMI should include consideration of gender, frame size, and age. BMI values >25 kg/m^2 are indicative of overweight, and values <18.5 kg/m^2 are indicative of undernutrition. BMI is calculated as follows:

$$\text{Body weight (kg)}/[\text{height (m)}]^2$$

- Measurements of skinfold thickness estimate subcutaneous fat, midarm muscle circumference estimates skeletal muscle mass, and waist circumference estimates abdominal fat content.
- BIA is a simple, noninvasive, and relatively inexpensive way to measure LBM. It is based on differences between fat tissue and lean tissue's resistance to conductivity. Fluid status should be considered in interpretation of BIA results.

TABLE 58-1	Evaluation of Body Weight
Actual body weight (ABW) compared with ideal body weight (IBW)	
ABW <69% IBW	Severe malnutrition
ABW 70–79% IBW	Moderate malnutrition
ABW 80–89% IBW	Mild malnutrition
ABW 90–120% IBW	Normal
ABW >120% IBW	Overweight
ABW ≥150% IBW	Obese
ABW ≥200% IBW	Morbidly obese
Actual body weight (ABW) compared with usual body weight (UBW)	
ABW 85–95% UBW	Mild malnutrition
ABW 75–84% UBW	Moderate malnutrition
ABW <75% UBW	Severe malnutrition
Body mass index (BMI) (kg/m^2) or (lb/in^2)	**Interpretation**
Adults	
<16	Severe malnutrition
16–16.9	Moderate malnutrition
17–18.9	Mild malnutrition
19–24.9	Healthy
25–29.9	Overweight
30–40	Moderate obesity
>40	Severe or morbid obesity
Children	
BMI-for-age <5th percentile	Underweight
BMI-for-age 5th–84th percentile	Healthy
BMI-for-age 85th–94th percentile	Overweight
BMI-for-age ≥95th percentile	Obese

BIOCHEMICAL AND IMMUNE FUNCTION STUDIES

- LBM can be assessed by measuring serum visceral proteins (Table 58-4). They are best for assessing uncomplicated semistarvation and recovery, and poor for assessing status during acute stress. Visceral proteins must be interpreted relative to overall clinical status because they are affected by factors other than nutrition.

TABLE 58-2	Body Weight Equations
Ideal body weight (IBW)	
Adult males:	IBW (kg) = 48 + (2.7 × inches over 5 ft)
Adult females:	IBW (kg) = 45 + (2.3 × inches over 5 ft)
Children (1–18 yr):	IBW (kg) = ([height in cm]^2 × 1.65)/1,000
Adjusted body weight for obesity	
Adjusted IBW = {[Actual body weight (kg) − IBW (kg)] × 0.25} + IBW	

TABLE 58–3	Expected Growth Velocities in Term Infants and Children	
Age	**Weight (g/day)**	**Height (cm/month)**[a]
0–3 months	24–35	2.8–3.4
4–6 months	15–21	1.7–2.4
7–12 months	10–13	1.3–1.6
1–3 years	5–9	0.6–1
4–6 years	5–6	0.5–0.6
7–10 years	7–11	0.4–0.5

Example of growth assessment:
Age: 2 months; weight: 3.9 kg; weight at 1 month of age, 3.1 kg; days since last wt: 30
Growth velocity = [(3.9 kg – 3.1 kg) × 1,000 g/kg]/30 days = 26.7 g/day
Interpretation: normal growth

[a]Growth velocity of 1 cm/month is equivalent to 0.4 in/month.

- Nutrition affects immune status both directly and indirectly. Total lymphocyte count and delayed cutaneous hypersensitivity reactions are immune function tests useful in nutrition assessment, but their lack of specificity limits their usefulness as nutrition status markers.
- Total lymphocyte count is obtained from a complete blood count with differential (% lymphocyte × total number of white blood cells). Values <1,500 cells/mm³ (1.5×10^9 cells/L) have been associated with nutrition depletion.
- Delayed cutaneous hypersensitivity is commonly assessed using antigens to which the patient has been previously sensitized. The recall antigens used most frequently are mumps, *Candida albicans,* and *Trichophyton.* Anergy is associated with severe malnutrition, and immune response may be restored with nutrition repletion.

SPECIFIC NUTRIENT DEFICIENCIES

- Biochemical assessment of trace element, vitamin, and essential fatty acid deficiencies should be based on the nutrient's function, but few practical methods are available. Therefore, most assays measure serum concentrations of the individual nutrient.
- Clinical syndromes are associated with deficiencies of the following trace elements: zinc, copper, manganese, selenium, chromium, iodine, fluoride, molybdenum, and iron.
- Single vitamin deficiencies are uncommon; multiple vitamin deficiencies more commonly occur with undernutrition. For information on iron deficiency and other anemias, see Chap. 33.
- Essential fatty acid deficiency is rare but can occur with prolonged lipid-free parenteral nutrition, very-low-fat enteral formulas or diets, severe fat malabsorption, or severe malnutrition. The body can synthesize all fatty acids except for linoleic and linolenic acid, which should constitute ~5% of total calorie intake.

TABLE 58–4 Visceral Proteins Used for Assessment of Lean Body Mass

Serum Protein	Half-Life (days)	Function	Factors Resulting in Increased Values	Factors Resulting in Decreased Values
Albumin	18–20	Maintains plasma oncotic pressure; transports small molecules	Dehydration, anabolic steroids, insulin, infection	Overhydration, edema, kidney dysfunction, nephrotic syndrome, poor dietary intake, impaired digestion, burns, congestive heart failure, cirrhosis, thyroid/adrenal/pituitary hormones, trauma, sepsis
Transferrin	8–9	Binds Fe in plasma and transports Fe to bone	Fe deficiency, pregnancy, hypoxia, chronic blood loss, estrogens	Chronic infection, cirrhosis, burns, enteropathies, nephrotic syndrome, cortisone, testosterone
Prealbumin (transthyretin)	2–3	Binds T_3 and to a lesser extent T_4; carrier for retinol-binding protein	Kidney dysfunction	Cirrhosis, hepatitis, stress, inflammation, surgery, hyperthyroidism, cystic fibrosis, burns, kidney dysfunction, zinc deficiency

Fe, iron; T_3, triiodothyronine, T_4, thyroxine.

- Carnitine can be synthesized from lysine and methionine, but synthesis is decreased in premature infants. Low carnitine levels can occur in premature infants receiving parenteral nutrition or carnitine-free diets.

ASSESSMENT OF NUTRIENT REQUIREMENTS

- Assessment of nutrient requirements must be made in the context of patient-specific factors (e.g., age, gender, size, disease state, clinical condition, nutrition status, and physical activity).

expenditure (MREE, kcal/day) is then calculated using the abbreviated Weir equation:

$$MREE = (3.94\ Vo_2 + 1.11\ Vco_2) \times 1.44$$

- Data from indirect calorimetry can also be used to determine a respiratory quotient. Values >1 suggest overfeeding, whereas values <0.7 suggest a ketogenic diet, fat gluconeogenesis, or ethanol oxidation. Respiratory quotient (RQ) is calculated as follows:

$$RQ = Vco_2/Vo_2$$

- Limitations of indirect calorimetry include limited availability, calibration errors, and other errors.

PROTEIN, FLUID, AND MICRONUTRIENT REQUIREMENTS
Protein

- Protein requirements are based on age, nutrition status, disease state, and clinical condition. The usual recommended daily protein allowances are 0.8 g/kg for adults, 1 to 1.5 g/kg for adults over 60 years of age, 1.5 to 2 g/kg for patients with metabolic stress (e.g., infection, trauma, and surgery), and 2.5 to 3 g/kg for patients with burns. See Table 58–5 for recommendations for children.
- Daily protein requirements can be individualized by measuring the nitrogen in a 24-hour urine collection (UUN), because nitrogen is found only in protein and at a relatively constant ratio of 1 g/6.25 g protein. Nitrogen output is then compared with nitrogen intake. Nitrogen output is approximated by the following:

$$\text{Nitrogen output (g/day)} = UUN + 4$$

Fluid

- Daily adult fluid requirements are ~30 to 35 mL/kg, 1 mL/kcal (or per every 4.19 kJ) ingested, or 1,500 mL/m^2.
- Daily fluid requirements for children and preterm infants who weigh <10 kg are at least 100 mL/kg. An additional 50 mL/kg should be provided for each kilogram of body weight between 11 and 20 kg, and 20 mL/kg for each kilogram >20 kg.
- Examples of factors that result in increased fluid requirements include GI losses, fever, sweating, and increased metabolism, whereas kidney or cardiac failure and hypoalbuminemia with starvation are examples of factors that result in decreased fluid requirements.
- Fluid status is assessed by monitoring urine output and specific gravity, serum electrolytes, and weight changes. An hourly urine output of at least 1 mL/kg for children and 40 to 50 mL for adults is needed to ensure tissue perfusion.

Micronutrients

- Requirements for micronutrients (i.e., electrolytes, trace elements, and vitamins) vary with age, gender, route of administration, and underlying clinical conditions.

- Sodium, potassium, magnesium, and phosphorus requirements are typically decreased in patients with kidney failure, whereas calcium requirements are increased (see Chaps. 77 and 79).

DRUG–NUTRIENT INTERACTIONS

- Concomitant drug therapy can alter serum concentrations of vitamins (Table 58–7), minerals, and electrolytes.
- Some drug delivery systems contain nutrients. For example, the vehicle for propofol is 10% lipid emulsion, and most IV therapies include dextrose or sodium.

EVALUATION OF THERAPEUTIC OUTCOMES

- Most markers of nutrition status are not ideal. They were first used in epidemiologic studies of large populations and, when applied to individuals, lack specificity and sensitivity.

TABLE 58–7 Drug and Vitamin Interactions

Drug	Effect
Antacids	Thiamine deficiency
Antibiotics	Vitamin K deficiency
Cathartics	Increased requirements for vitamins D, C, and B_6
Cholestyramine	Vitamins A, D, E, and K, β-carotene malabsorption
Colestipol	Vitamins A, D, E, and K, β-carotene malabsorption
Corticosteroids	Decreased vitamins A, D, and C
Diuretics (loop)	Thiamine deficiency
Histamine$_2$-antagonists	Vitamin B_{12} deficiency
Isoniazid	Vitamin B_6 and niacin deficiency
Isotretinoin	Vitamin A increases toxicity
Mercaptopurine	Niacin deficiency
Methotrexate	Folic acid inhibits effect
Orlistat	Vitamins A, D, E, and K malabsorption
Pentamidine	Folic acid deficiency
Phenobarbital	Vitamin D malabsorption; vitamin C affects protein binding
Phenytoin	Vitamin D malabsorption; altered vitamin C binding; effect reversed by folic acid
Primidone	Folic acid deficiency
Proton pump inhibitors	Vitamin B_{12} deficiency
Sulfasalazine	Folic acid malabsorption
Trimethoprim	Folic acid depletion
Warfarin	Vitamin K inhibits effect; vitamins A, C, and E may affect prothrombin time
Zidovudine	Folic acid and B_{12} deficiencies increase myelosuppression

- Weight and serum albumin concentration have the best correlation with clinical outcome; the cost-effectiveness of other biochemical parameters is not known.
- Anthropometric measures are probably most useful with long-term nutrition support.
- Continuous reassessment is required because nutrition requirements are dynamic.

See Chapter 149, Assessment of Nutrition Status and Nutrition Requirements, authored by Katherine Hammond Chessman and Vanessa J. Kumpf, for a more detailed discussion of this topic.

CHAPTER 59

Enteral Nutrition

DEFINITION

- Enteral nutrition (EN) is the delivery of nutrients by tube or mouth into the GI tract. This chapter focuses on delivery through a feeding tube.

PATHOPHYSIOLOGY

- Digestion and absorption are the GI processes that generate usable fuels for the body. Understanding the mechanisms of these processes can enhance rational use of EN support.
- Digestion is the stepwise conversion of complex chemical and physical nutrients via mechanical, enzymatic, and physicochemical processes into molecular forms that can be absorbed from the GI tract.
- Nutrients are absorbed across the intestinal cell membrane and reach the systemic circulation through the portal venous or splanchnic lymphatic systems, provided the GI or biliary tract does not excrete them.
- Many factors can alter these stepwise processes and interfere with digestion and absorption, such as functional immaturity of the neonatal gut.

CLINICAL PRESENTATION AND INDICATIONS

- Clinical presentation of protein-energy malnutrition and nutrition assessment are discussed in Chap. 58.
- EN is indicated for the patient who cannot or will not eat enough to meet nutritional requirements and who has a functioning GI tract. Additionally, a method of enteral access must be possible. Potential indications include neoplastic disease, organ failure, hypermetabolic states, GI disease, and neurologic impairment.
- The only absolute contraindications are mechanical obstruction and necrotizing enterocolitis. Conditions that challenge the success of EN include severe diarrhea, protracted vomiting, enteric fistulas, severe GI hemorrhage, and intestinal dysmotility.
- EN has replaced parenteral nutrition (PN) (see Chap. 61) as the preferred method for the feeding of critically ill patients requiring specialized nutrition support. Advantages of EN over PN include maintaining GI tract structure and function; fewer metabolic, infectious, and technical complications; and lower costs.
- The optimal time to initiate EN is controversial. Early initiation within 24 to 48 hours of hospitalization is recommended for critically ill patients because this approach appears to decrease infectious complications and reduce mortality. If patients are only mildly to moderately stressed and well nourished, EN initiation can be delayed until oral intake is inadequate for 7 to 14 days.

DESIRED OUTCOME

- The goal of EN is to provide calories, macronutrients, and micronutrients to patients who are unable to achieve these requirements from an oral diet.

TREATMENT

ENTERAL ACCESS

- EN can be administered through four routes, which have different indications, tube placement options, advantages, and disadvantages (Table 59–1). The choice depends on the anticipated duration of use and the feeding site (i.e., stomach vs small bowel).
- Short-term access is generally easier to initiate, less invasive, and less costly than long-term access. Feeding tubes used for short-term access are not suitable for long-term use owing to patient discomfort, long-term complications, and mechanical failure.
- The most frequently used short-term routes are accessed by inserting a tube through the nose and threading it into the stomach (nasogastric), duodenum (nasoduodenal), or jejunum (nasojejunal).
- The stomach is generally the least expensive and least labor-intensive access site; however, patients who have impaired gastric emptying are at risk for aspiration and pneumonia.
- Long-term access should be considered when EN is anticipated for more than 4 to 6 weeks. The most popular option is gastrostomy followed by jejunostomy.
- The gastrostomy exit site requires general stoma care to prevent inflammation and infection. Jejunostomy may be appropriate in patients at high risk of gastroesophageal reflux disease and aspiration, and with impaired gastric motility or delayed gastric emptying.

ADMINISTRATION METHODS

- EN can be administered by continuous, cyclic, bolus, and intermittent methods. The choice depends on the feeding tube location, patient's clinical condition, intestinal function, residence environment, and tolerance to tube feeding.
- Continuous EN is preferred for initiation and has the advantage of being well tolerated. It has the disadvantages of cost and inconvenience because of pump and administration sets.
- Cyclic EN has the advantage of allowing breaks from the infusion system, thereby increasing mobility, especially if EN is administered nocturnally.
- Bolus EN is most commonly used in long-term care residents who have a gastrostomy. This method has the advantage of requiring little administration time (e.g., 5–10 min) and minimal equipment (e.g., a syringe). Bolus EN has the potential disadvantages of causing cramping, nausea, vomiting, aspiration, and diarrhea.

TABLE 59-1 Options and Considerations in the Selection of Enteral Access

Access	EN Duration/Patient Characteristics	Tube Placement Options	Advantages	Disadvantages
Nasogastric or orogastric	Short term Intact gag reflex Normal gastric emptying	Manually at bedside	Ease of placement Allows for all methods of administration Inexpensive Multiple commercially available tubes and sizes	Potential tube displacement Potential increased aspiration risk
Nasoduodenal or nasojejunal	Short term Impaired gastric motility or emptying High risk of GER or aspiration	Manually at bedside Fluoroscopically Endoscopically	Potential reduced aspiration risk Allows for early postinjury or postoperative feeding Multiple commercially available tubes and sizes	Manual transpyloric passage requires greater skill Potential tube displacement or clogging Bolus or intermittent feeding not tolerated
Gastrostomy	Long term Normal gastric emptying	Surgically Endoscopically Radiologically Laparoscopically	Allows for all methods of administration Large-bore tubes less likely to clog Multiple commercially available tubes and sizes Low-profile buttons available	Attendant risks associated with each type of procedure Potential increased aspiration risk Risk of stoma site complications
Jejunostomy	Long term Impaired gastric motility or gastric emptying High risk of GER or aspiration	Surgically Endoscopically Radiologically Laparoscopically	Allows for early postinjury or postoperative feeding Potential reduced aspiration risk Multiple commercially available tubes and sizes Low-profile buttons available	Attendant risks associated with each type of procedure Bolus or intermittent feeding not tolerated Risk of stoma site complications

EN, enteral nutrition; GER, gastroesophageal reflux.

- Intermittent EN is similar to bolus EN except that the feeding is administered over 20 to 60 minutes, which improves tolerability but requires more equipment (e.g., reservoir bag and infusion pump). Like bolus EN, intermittent EN mimics normal eating patterns. As compared with continuous EN, bolus or intermittent EN minimizes the development of cholestatic liver disease.

INITIATION AND ADVANCEMENT PROTOCOL

- Protocols outlining initiation and advancement criteria are a useful strategy to optimize achievement of nutrient goals based on GI tolerance. Clinical signs of intolerance include abdominal distention or cramping, high gastric residual volumes, aspiration, and diarrhea.
- Continuous EN feedings are typically started in adults at 20 to 50 mL/hour and advanced by 10 to 25 mL/hour every 4 to 8 hours until the goal is achieved. Intermittent EN feedings are started at 120 mL every 4 hours and advanced by 30 to 60 mL every 8 to 12 hours.
- EN feedings are typically started in children at 1 to 2 mL/kg/hour for continuous feeding or 2 to 4 mL/kg per bolus with advancement by similar amounts every 4 to 24 hours. Feedings are started at lower rates or volumes in premature infants, usually 10 to 20 mL/kg/day.
- The practice of diluting hyperosmolar EN formulations should be avoided unless necessary to increase fluid intake.

FORMULATIONS

- Historically, EN formulations were created to provide essential nutrients, including macronutrients (e.g., carbohydrates, fats, and proteins) and micronutrients (e.g., electrolytes, trace elements, vitamins, and water).
- Over time, formulations have been enhanced to improve tolerance and meet specific patient needs. For example, nutraceuticals or pharmaconutrients are added to modify the disease process or improve clinical outcome; however, these health claims are not regulated by the FDA.
- The molecular form of the protein source determines the amount of digestion required for absorption within the small bowel. The carbohydrate component usually provides the major source of calories; polymeric entities are preferred over elemental sugars. Vegetable oils are the most common sources of fat in EN formulations.
- Fiber, in the form of soy polysaccharides, has been added to several EN formulations. In addition to providing an excellent energy source, potential benefits include trophic effects on colonic mucosa, promotion of sodium and water absorption, and regulation of bowel function.
- Osmolality is a function of the size and quantity of ionic and molecular particles primarily related to protein, carbohydrate, electrolyte, and mineral content. The osmolality of EN formulations for adults ranges from 300 to 900 mOsm/kg (300–900 mmol/kg), and an osmolality <450 mOsm/kg (450 mmol/kg) is recommended for children. Osmolality is commonly thought to affect GI tolerability, but there is a lack of supporting evidence.

CLASSIFICATION OF ENTERAL FEEDING FORMULATIONS

- EN formulations are classified by their composition and intended patient population (**Table 59–2**). Formularies should focus on clinically significant characteristics of available products, avoid duplicate formulations, and include only specialty formulations with evidence-based indications.

TABLE 59–2	Adult Enteral Feeding Formulation Classification System	
Category	**Features**	**Indications**
Standard polymeric	Isotonic 1–1.2 kcal/mL (4.2–5 kJ/mL) NPC:N 125:1 to 150:1 May contain fiber	Designed to meet the needs of the majority of patients Patients with functional GI tract Not suitable for oral use
High protein	NPC:N <125:1 May contain fiber	Patients with protein requirements >1.5 g/kg/day, such as trauma, burns, pressure sores, or wounds Patients receiving propofol
High caloric density	1.5–2 kcal/mL (6.3–8.4 kJ/mL) Lower electrolyte content per calorie Hypertonic	Patients requiring fluid and/or electrolyte restriction, such as kidney insufficiency
Elemental	High proportion of free amino acids Low in fat	Patients who require low fat Use has generally been replaced by peptide-based formulations
Peptide-based	Contains dipeptides and tripeptides Contains MCTs	Indications/benefits not clearly established. Trial may be warranted in patients who do not tolerate intact protein due to malabsorption.
Disease-specific		
Kidney	Caloric dense Protein content varies Low electrolyte content	Alternative to high caloric density formulations, but generally more expensive
Liver	Increased branched-chain and decreased aromatic amino acids	Patients with hepatic encephalopathy
Lung	High fat, low carbohydrate Antiinflammatory lipid profile and antioxidants	Patients with ARDS and severe ALI
Diabetes mellitus	High fat, low carbohydrate	Alternative to standard, fiber-containing formulation in patients with uncontrolled hyperglycemia

(continued)

TABLE 59–2	Adult Enteral Feeding Formulation Classification System *(Continued)*	
Category	**Features**	**Indications**
Immune-modulating	Supplemented with glutamine, arginine, nucleotides, and/or omega-3 fatty acids	Patients undergoing major elective GI surgery, trauma, burns, head and neck cancer, and critically ill patients on mechanical ventilation. Use with caution in patients with sepsis. Select nutrients may be beneficial or harmful in subgroups of critically ill patients.
Oral supplement	Sweetened for taste Hypertonic	Patients who require supplementation to an oral diet

ALI, acute lung injury; ARDS, acute respiratory distress syndrome; GI, gastrointestinal; MCT, medium-chain triglyceride; NPC:N, nonprotein calorie-to-nitrogen ratio.

- Most EN products are ready-to-use prepackaged liquids, which have the advantages of convenience and lower susceptibility to microbiologic contamination. The major disadvantage is storage space. Closed-system containers provide a prefilled, sterile 1 to 1.5 L supply of EN formula that does not require refrigeration and has a longer hang time than ready-to-use products.

- Polymeric formulations contain a well-proportioned mix of macronutrients, with or without fiber, and are best suited for tube feeding due to lack of sweetening to maintain isotonicity. Standard formulations have a nonprotein calorie:nitrogen ratio of 125:1 to 150:1.

- High-protein formulations have a nonprotein calorie:nitrogen ratio <125:1. Candidates for these formulations require >1.5 g of protein/kg/day and are generally critically ill because of trauma, burns, pressure sores, surgical wounds, or high fistula output.

- High caloric density formulations are indicated for patients requiring restriction of fluids, electrolytes, or both, such as patients with kidney insufficiency or congestive heart failure.

- Elemental or peptide-based formulations have partially hydrolyzed protein or fat components. Peptide-based formulations replace some of the protein with dipeptides and tripeptides, thereby optimizing absorption in patients with impaired digestive or absorptive capacity.

- Disease state–specific formulations are designed to meet unique nutrient requirements and to manage metabolic abnormalities. Use of low-carbohydrate formulations supplemented with specific fatty acids and antioxidants have resulted in improved outcomes for patients with acute respiratory distress syndrome. Immune-modulating formulations benefit some critically ill patients but should be used cautiously, if at all, in patients with preexisting severe sepsis.

TABLE 59–3	Suggested Monitoring for Patients on Enteral Nutrition	
Parameter	During Initiation of EN Therapy	During Stable EN Therapy
Vital signs	Every 4–6 hours	As needed with suspected change (i.e., fever)
Clinical assessment		
Weight	Daily	Weekly
Length/height (children)	Weekly–monthly	Monthly
Head circumference (<3 y of age)	Weekly–monthly	Monthly
Total intake/output	Daily	As needed with suspected change in intake/output
Tube-feeding intake	Daily	Daily
Enterostomy tube site assessment	Daily	Daily
GI tolerance		
Stool frequency/volume	Daily	Daily
Abdomen assessment	Daily	Daily
Nausea or vomiting	Daily	Daily
Gastric residual volumes	Every 4–8 hours (varies)	As needed when delayed gastric emptying suspected
Tube placement	Prior to starting, then ongoing	Ongoing
Laboratory		
Electrolytes, BUN/serum creatinine, glucose	Daily	Every 1–3 months
Calcium, magnesium, phosphorus	Three to seven times/week	Every 1–3 months
Liver function tests	Weekly	Every 1–3 months
Trace elements, vitamins	If deficiency/ toxicity suspected	If deficiency/ toxicity suspected

BUN, blood urea nitrogen; EN, enteral nutrition; GI, gastrointestinal.

- Oral supplements are not intended for tube feeding. They are sweetened to improve taste and are therefore hypertonic.
- A *module* is a powder or liquid that can be added to a commercially available product. Alternatively, a modular product can be mixed to concentrate nutrients in less volume.
- Oral rehydration formulations are used to maintain hydration or treat dehydration. They can be administered by mouth or feeding tube. The glucose content of these formulations can decrease fecal water loss and generate a positive electrolyte balance.

COMPLICATIONS

- Patients should be monitored for metabolic, GI, and mechanical complications (Table 59–3).
- Metabolic complications associated with EN are analogous to those of PN (see Chap. 61), but the occurrence is lower.

- GI complications include nausea, vomiting, abdominal distention, cramping, aspiration, diarrhea, and constipation. Gastric residual volume is thought to increase the risk of vomiting and aspiration. Although the definition is controversial, residual is probably excessive if it is >200 to 500 mL in adults, or if it is 2 to 3 times the bolus volume or twice the hourly infusion rate in children. The determination should be based on a trend rather than an isolated finding and should be made in conjunction with the presence of symptoms.

- The stepwise approach for managing excessive gastric residual volume with GI symptoms is slowing, not stopping, the tube feeding; initiating metoclopramide or erythromycin; considering a transpyloric feeding tube; trying a proton pump inhibitor or histamine$_2$-receptor antagonist to decrease gastric secretion volume; and minimizing use of narcotics, sedatives, and other agents that delay gastric emptying.

- In addition to avoiding excessive gastric residuals, methods for preventing aspiration pneumonia include keeping the head of the bed at 30° to 45° during feeding and for 30 to 60 minutes after intermittent infusions and changing from bolus to intermittent or continuous administration.

- Management of diarrhea should be directed at identifying and correcting the cause. The most common causes are sorbitol contained in many liquid medications, drug therapy, infection, malabsorption, and factors related to tube feeding (e.g., rapid delivery or advancement, intolerance to composition, large volume administered into small bowel, and formula contamination). Switching to a fiber-containing, lower fat, peptide-based, or lactose-free formulation can be beneficial. After excluding infectious etiologies, pharmacologic intervention (e.g., opiates, **diphenoxylate,** or **loperamide**) can be used to control severe diarrhea.

- Mechanical complications include tube occlusion or malposition and nasopulmonary intubation. Techniques for clearing occluded tubes include pancreatic enzymes in sodium bicarbonate and using a declogging device. Techniques for maintaining patency include flushing with at least 30 mL of water before and after medication administration and intermittent feedings and at least every 8 hours during continuous feeding.

DRUG DELIVERY VIA FEEDING TUBE

- Administering drugs via tube feeding is a common practice, but drug dissolution or therapeutic effect can be altered if the tube tip is placed in the small bowel. If the drug is a solid that can be crushed (e.g., *not* a sublingual, sustained-release, or enteric-coated formulation) or is a capsule, the powder can be mixed with 15 to 30 mL of solvent and administered. Otherwise, a liquid dosage preparation should be used. Multiple medications should be administered separately, each followed by flushing the tube with 5 mL or more of water.

- Mixing of liquid medications with EN formulations can cause physical incompatibilities that inhibit drug absorption and clog small-bore feeding tubes. Incompatibility is more common with formulations containing

TABLE 59–4	Medications with Special Considerations for Enteral Feeding Tube Administration	
Drug	**Interaction**	**Comments**
Phenytoin	Reduced bioavailability in the presence of tube feedings. Possible binding of phenytoin to calcium caseinates or protein hydrolysates in enteral feeding	A suggestion to minimize interaction is to hold tube feeding 1–2 hours before and after phenytoin, but this has no proven benefit. Adjust tube feeding rate to account for time held for phenytoin administration. Monitor phenytoin serum concentrations and clinical response closely. Consider switching to IV phenytoin route if unable to reach therapeutic serum concentration.
Fluoroquinolones Tetracycline	Potential for reduced bioavailability because of complexation of drug with divalent and trivalent cations found in enteral feeding	Consider holding tube feeding 1 hour before and after administration. Avoid jejunal administration of ciprofloxacin. Monitor clinical response.
Warfarin	Decreased absorption of warfarin because of enteral feeding; therapeutic effect antagonized by vitamin K in enteral formulations	Adjust warfarin dose based on INR. Anticipate need to increase warfarin dose when enteral feedings are started and decrease dose when enteral feedings are stopped.
Omeprazole Lansoprazole	Administration via feeding tube complicated by acid-labile medication within delayed-release, base-labile granules	Granules become sticky when moistened with water and may occlude small-bore tubes. Suggested that granules be mixed with acidic liquid when given via a gastric feeding tube. An oral liquid suspension can be extemporaneously prepared for administration via a feeding tube.

INR, international normalized ratio.

intact (vs hydrolyzed) protein and medications formulated as acidic syrups. Mixing of liquid medications and EN formulations should be avoided whenever possible.

- The most significant drug–nutrient interactions result in reduced bioavailability and suboptimal pharmacologic effect (Table 59–4). Continuous feeding requires interruption for drug administration, and medications should be spaced between bolus feedings.

EVALUATION OF THERAPEUTIC OUTCOMES

- Assessing the outcome of EN includes monitoring objective measures of body composition, protein and energy balance, and subjective outcome for physiologic muscle function and wound healing.
- Measures of disease-related morbidity include length of hospital stay, infectious complications, and patient's sense of well-being. Ultimately, the successful use of EN avoids the need for PN.

See Chapter 152, Enteral Nutrition, authored by Vanessa J. Kumpf and Katherine Hammond Chessman, for a more detailed discussion of this topic.

60   Obesity

DEFINITION

- Obesity occurs when there is an imbalance between energy intake and energy expenditure over time, resulting in increased energy storage.

ETIOLOGY

- The etiology of obesity is usually unknown, but it is likely multifactorial and related to varying contributions from genetic, environmental, and physiologic factors.
- Genetic factors appear to be the primary determinants of obesity in some individuals, whereas environmental factors are more important in others. Identification of the total number and identity of contributing genes is an area of extensive research.
- Environmental factors include reduced physical activity or work, abundant food supply, relatively sedentary lifestyles, increased availability of high-fat foods, and cultural factors and religious beliefs.
- Medical conditions including Cushing disease and growth hormone deficiency or genetic syndromes such as Prader–Willi syndrome can be associated with weight gain.
- Medications associated with weight gain include insulin, corticosteroids, some antidepressants, antipsychotics, and several anticonvulsants.

PATHOPHYSIOLOGY

- Many neurotransmitters and neuropeptides stimulate or depress the brain's appetite network, impacting total calorie intake.
- The degree of obesity is determined by the net balance of energy ingested relative to energy expended over time. The single largest determinant of energy expenditure is metabolic rate, which is expressed as *resting energy expenditure* or *basal metabolic rate*. Physical activity is the other major factor that affects total energy expenditure.
- The major types of adipose tissue are (1) white adipose tissue, which manufactures, stores, and releases lipid; and (2) brown adipose tissue, which dissipates energy via uncoupled mitochondrial respiration. Adrenergic stimulation activates lipolysis in fat cells and increases energy expenditure in adipose tissue and skeletal muscle.

CLINICAL PRESENTATION

- Obesity is associated with serious health risks and increased mortality. Central obesity reflects high levels of intraabdominal or visceral fat that is associated with the development of hypertension, dyslipidemia, type 2

TABLE 60–1	Classification of Overweight and Obesity by Body Mass Index (BMI), Waist Circumference, and Associated Disease Risk		
			Disease Risk^a (Relative to Normal Weight and Waist Circumference)
	BMI (kg/m²)	**Obesity Class**	**Men ≤40 in (≤102 cm) Women ≤35 in (≤89 cm)**	**>40 in (>102 cm) >35 in (>89 cm)**
Underweight	<18.5		–	–
Normal weight^b	18.5–24.9		–	–
Overweight	25–29.9		Increased	High
Obesity	30–34.9	I	High	Very high
	35–39.9	II	Very high	Very high
Extreme obesity	≥40	III	Extremely high	Extremely high

^{a}Disease risk for type 2 diabetes, hypertension, and cardiovascular disease.
^{b}Increased waist circumference can also be a marker for increased risk even in persons of normal weight.
Adapted from Preventing and Managing the Global Epidemic of Obesity: Report of the World Health Organization Consultation on Obesity. Geneva: World Health Organization; 1997. National Institutes of Health, National Heart, Lung and Blood Institute, http://www.nhlbi.nih.gov/guidelines/obesity/ob_home.htm.

diabetes, and cardiovascular disease. Other obesity comorbidities are osteoarthritis and changes in the female reproductive system.

- Excess body fat can be determined by skinfold thickness, body density using underwater body weight, bioelectrical impedance and conductivity, dual-energy x-ray absorptiometry, computed axial tomography scan, and magnetic resonance imaging. Unfortunately, many of these methods are too expensive and time consuming for routine use.
- Body mass index (BMI) and waist circumference (WC) are recognized, acceptable markers of excess body fat that independently predict disease risk (**Table 60–1**).
- BMI is calculated as weight (kg) divided by the square of the height (m²).
- WC, the most practical method of characterizing central adiposity, is the narrowest circumference between the last rib and the top of the iliac crest.

DESIRED OUTCOME

- Weight management is considered successful when goals are achieved. Goals may include losing a predefined amount of weight, decreasing the rate of weight gain, or maintaining a weight-neutral status, depending on the clinical situation.

TREATMENT

GENERAL APPROACH

- Successful obesity treatment plans incorporate diet, exercise, behavior modification with or without pharmacologic therapy, and/or surgery (**Fig. 60–1**). Weight loss of 5% to 10% of initial weight is a reasonable goal

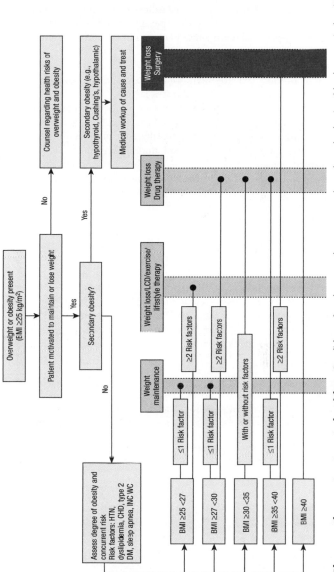

FIGURE 60–1. Pharmacotherapy treatment algorithm. Candidates for pharmacotherapy are selected on the basis of body mass index (BMI) and waist circumference (WC) criteria, along with consideration of concurrent risk factors. Medication therapy is always used as an adjunct to a comprehensive weight loss program that includes diet, exercise, and behavioral modification. CHD, coronary heart disease; DM, diabetes mellitus; HTN, hypertension; WC, ≥40 in [≥102 cm] for men and ≥35 in [≥89 cm] for women; LCD, low-calorie diet.

for most obese patients. Measures of success not only include pounds lost but also improvement in comorbid conditions, including blood pressure, blood glucose, and lipids.

- Many diets exist to aid weight loss. Regardless of the program, energy consumption must be less than energy expenditure. A reasonable goal is loss of 0.5 to 1 kg per week with a diet balanced in fat, carbohydrate, and protein intake.

- Increased physical activity combined with reduced calorie intake and behavior modification can augment weight loss and improve obesity-related comorbidities and cardiovascular risk factors.

- The primary aim of behavior modification is to help patients choose lifestyles conducive to safe and sustained weight loss. Behavioral therapy is based on principles of human learning, which use stimulus control and reinforcement to substitute desirable behaviors for learned, undesirable habits.

- Bariatric surgery, which reduces the stomach volume or absorptive surface of the alimentary tract, remains the most effective intervention for obesity. Surgery should be reserved for those with BMI >35 or 40 kg/m² and significant comorbidities due to the morbidity and mortality associated with the surgical procedures.

PHARMACOLOGIC THERAPY

(Table 60–2)

- The debate regarding the role of pharmacotherapy remains heated, fueled by the need to treat a growing epidemic and by the fallout from the removal of several agents from the market because of adverse reactions.

- Long-term pharmacotherapy may have a role for patients who have no contraindications to approved drug therapy. The National Institutes

TABLE 60–2	Pharmacotherapeutic Agents for Weight Loss		
Class	**Availability**	**Status**	**Daily Dosages (mg)**
Gastrointestinal lipase inhibitor			
Orlistat (Xenical)	Rx	Long-term use	360 (3 divided doses)
Orlistat (Alli)	OTC	Long-term use	180 (3 divided doses)
Noradrenergic/serotonergic agent			
Sibutramine (Meridia, Reductil)[a]	Rx	Long-term use	5–15
Noradrenergic agents			
Phendimetrazine (Prelu-2, Bontril, Plegine, Obezine, Statobex, X-trozine)	Rx	Short-term use	70–105
Phentermine (Fastin, Adipex-P, Ionamin)	Rx	Short-term use	15–37.5
Diethylpropion (Tenuate, Tenuate Dospan)	Rx	Short-term use	75

OTC, over-the-counter; Rx, prescription.
[a]Sibutramine was withdrawn from the U.S. market in October of 2010.

of Health guidelines recommend consideration of pharmacotherapy in adults with BMI ≥30 kg/m² and/or WC ≥40 in (102 cm) for men or 35 in (89 cm) for women, or BMI of 27 to 30 kg/m² with at least two concurrent risk factors if 6 months of diet, exercise, and behavioral modification failed to achieve weight loss.

- **Orlistat** (180 or 360 mg in three divided doses/day) induces weight loss by lowering dietary fat absorption; it also improves lipid profiles, glucose control, and other metabolic markers. Soft stools, abdominal pain or colic, flatulence, fecal urgency, and/or incontinence occur in 80% of individuals using prescription strength, are mild to moderate in severity, and improve after 1 to 2 months of therapy. Orlistat is approved for long-term use. It interferes with the absorption of fat-soluble vitamins, **cyclosporine,** and **levothyroxine**. A nonprescription formulation is also available.
- **Phentermine** (30 mg in the morning or 8 mg before meals) has less powerful stimulant activity and lower abuse potential than amphetamines and was an effective adjunct in placebo-controlled studies. Adverse effects (e.g., increased blood pressure, palpitations, arrhythmias, mydriasis, and altered insulin or oral hypoglycemic requirements) and interactions with monoamine oxidase inhibitors have implications for patient selection. It is labeled for short-term use.
- **Diethylpropion** (25 mg before meals or 75 mg of extended-release formulation every morning) is more effective than placebo in achieving short-term weight loss. Diethylpropion should not be used in patients with severe hypertension or significant cardiovascular disease. Diabetic patients may experience decreased insulin or oral hypoglycemic dosage requirements soon after beginning therapy and prior to substantial weight loss.
- **Amphetamines** should generally be avoided because of their powerful stimulant effects and addictive potential.
- Herbal, natural, and food-supplement products are often used to promote weight loss (**Table 60–3**). The FDA does not strictly regulate these products, so the ingredients may be inactive and present in variable concentrations. After more than 800 reports of serious adverse events (e.g.,

TABLE 60–3	Common Herbal/Natural Products and Food Supplements Used for Weight Loss[a]	
Herbal/Natural/Food Supplements	**Active Moiety**	**Proposed Mechanism**
Bitter orange	M-synephrine	Noradrenergic
Calcium pyruvate	Pyruvate	Unknown
Chromium picolinate	Chromium	Unknown
Chitosan	Cationic polysaccharide	Block fat absorption
Garcinia cambogia extract (citrin)	Hydroxycitric acid	Unknown
Guarana extract	Caffeine	Noradrenergic
Hoodia	P57	Unknown
Various tea extracts	Caffeine	Noradrenergic

[a]Safety and efficacy not documented.

seizures, stroke, and death) were attributed to ephedrine alkaloids, the FDA decided to exclude them from dietary supplements.

EVALUATION OF THERAPEUTIC OUTCOMES

- Evaluation requires careful clinical, biochemical, and, if necessary, psychological evaluation. Progress should be assessed in a healthcare setting once or twice monthly for 1 to 2 months, then monthly. Each encounter should document weight, WC, BMI, blood pressure, medical history, and tolerability of drug therapy.
- Medication therapy should be discontinued after 3 to 4 months if the patient has failed to demonstrate weight loss or maintenance of prior weight.
- Diabetic patients require more intense medical monitoring and self-monitoring of blood glucose. Weekly healthcare visits for 1 to 2 months may be necessary until the effects of diet, exercise, and weight loss medication become more predictable.
- Patients with hyperlipidemia or hypertension should be monitored to assess the effects of weight loss on appropriate end points.

See Chapter 154, Obesity, authored by Judy T. Chen, Amy Heck Sheehan, Jack A. Yanovski, and Karim Anton Calis, for a more detailed discussion of this topic.

61 Parenteral Nutrition

DEFINITION

- Parenteral nutrition (PN) provides macro- and micronutrients by central or peripheral venous access to meet specific nutritional requirements of the patient.

INDICATIONS

- Identifying candidates and deciding when to initiate PN are difficult decisions because data are conflicting, and published guidelines are not consistent.
- In general, PN should be considered when a patient cannot meet nutritional requirements through use of the GI tract. Consensus guidelines are based on clinical experience and investigations in specific populations (Table 61–1).
- PN should be considered after suboptimal nutritional intake for 1 day in preterm infants, 2 to 3 days in term infants, 3 to 5 days in critically injured children, 5 to 7 days in other children, and 7 to 14 days in older children and adults. The route and type of PN depend on the patient's clinical state and expected length of PN therapy (Fig. 61–1).

DESIRED OUTCOME

- Optimal nutrition therapy requires defining the patient's nutrition goals, determining the nutrient requirements to achieve those goals, delivering the required nutrients, and assessing the nutrition regimen.
- Goals of nutrition support include correcting caloric and nitrogen imbalances, fluid or electrolyte abnormalities, and vitamin or trace element abnormalities, without causing or worsening other metabolic complications.
- Specific caloric goals include adequate energy intake to promote growth and development in children, energy equilibrium and preservation of fat stores in well-nourished adults, and positive energy balance in malnourished patients with depleted fat stores.
- Specific nitrogen goals are positive nitrogen balance or nitrogen equilibrium and improvement in serum concentration of protein markers (e.g., transferrin or prealbumin).

COMPONENTS OF PARENTERAL NUTRITION

MACRONUTRIENTS

- Macronutrients (i.e., water, protein, dextrose, and IV fat emulsion [IVFE]) are used for energy (dextrose, fat) and as structural substrates (protein and fats).

TABLE 61–1 Indications for Adult Parenteral Nutrition

1. Inability to absorb nutrients via the GI tract because of one or more of the following:
   a. Massive small bowel resection: usually patients with <100 cm (39 in)of small bowel distal to the ligament of Treitz without a colon, or <50 cm (20 in) of small bowel with an intact colon
   b. Intractable vomiting when adequate EN is not expected for 7–14 days
   c. Severe diarrhea
   d. Bowel obstruction
   e. GI fistulas: PN is indicated in patients with prolonged inadequate nutritional intake longer than 5 to 7 days who are not candidates for EN.

2. Cancer: antineoplastic therapy, radiation therapy, or HSCT
   a. PN may be used in moderately to severely malnourished patients receiving active anticancer treatment who are not candidates for EN.
   b. PN is not routinely indicated for well-nourished or mildly malnourished patients undergoing surgery, chemotherapy, or radiation therapy.
   c. PN is unlikely to benefit patients with advanced cancer whose malignancy is unresponsive to treatment. However, use may be appropriate for carefully selected patients who have failed trials of less-invasive medical therapies and have good performance status, an estimated life expectancy of longer than 40 to 60 days, and strong social and financial support.
   d. PN is appropriate for patients undergoing HSCT who are malnourished and who are anticipated to be unable to ingest and/or absorb adequate nutrients for 7 to 14 days. PN should be discontinued as soon as toxicities have resolved after stem cell engraftment.

3. Pancreatitis: PN may be used in patients with severe pancreatitis with prolonged inadequate nutritional intake longer than 5 to 7 days who are not candidates for EN. PN should be used when EN exacerbates abdominal pain, ascites, or fistula output.

4. Critical care
   a. PN should be used in those patients in whom EN is contraindicated or is unlikely to provide adequate nutritional requirements within 5 to 10 days.
   b. Organ failure (liver, renal, or respiratory): PN should be used in patients with moderate to severe catabolism when EN is contraindicated.
   c. Burns: PN should be used in those patients in whom EN is contraindicated or is unlikely to provide adequate nutritional requirements within 4 or 5 days.

5. Perioperative PN
   a. Preoperative: for 7 to 14 days for patients with moderate to severe malnutrition who are undergoing major GI surgery, if the operation can be safely postponed
   b. Postoperative: PN should be used in patients in whom EN is contraindicated or is unlikely to provide adequate nutritional requirements within 7 to 10 days.

6. Hyperemesis gravidarum: when EN is not tolerated

7. Eating disorders: PN should be considered for patients with anorexia nervosa and severe malnutrition who are unable or unwilling to ingest adequate nutrition.

EN, enteral nutrition; GI, gastrointestinal; HSCT, hematopoietic stem cell transplantation; PN, parenteral nutrition.
Data from ASPEN Board of Directors and the Clinical Guidelines Taskforce. Administration of specialized nutrition support. JPEN J Parenter Enteral Nutr 2002;26:18SA–21SA; McClave SA, Martindale R, Vanek VW, et al. Guidelines for the provision and assessment of nutrition support therapy in the adult critically ill patient: Society of Critical Care Medicine (SCCM) and American Society for Parenteral and Enteral Nutrition (A.S.P.E.N.). JPEN J Parenter Enteral Nutr 2009;33:277–316; August DA, Huhmann MB. American Society for Parenteral and Enteral Nutrition (A.S.P.E.N.) Board of Directors. A.S.P.E.N. clinical guidelines: Nutrition support therapy during adult anticancer treatment and in hematopoietic cell transplantation. JPEN J Parenter Enteral Nutr 2009;33:472-500; and ASPEN Board of Directors and the Clinical Guidelines Taskforce. Specific guidelines for disease–Adults. JPEN J Parenter Enteral Nutr 2002;26:61SA–96SA.

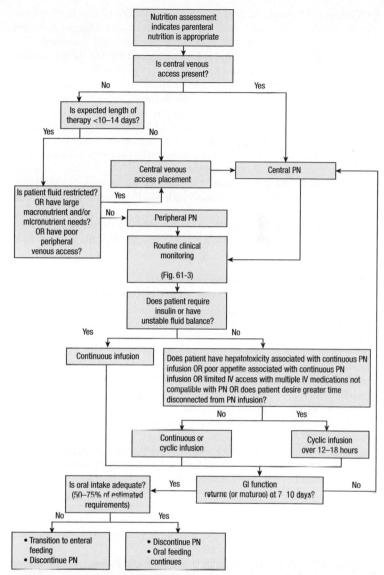

FIGURE 61–1. The route of parenteral nutrition (PN) and the infusion type depend on the patient's clinical status and the expected length of therapy.

Amino Acids

- Protein is provided as crystalline amino acids (CAAs). When oxidized, 1 g of protein yields 4 calories (~ 17 J). Including the caloric contribution from protein in calorie calculations is controversial; therefore, PN calories can be calculated as either total or nonprotein calories.

- Standard CAA products contain a balanced profile of essential, semiessential, and nonessential L-amino acids and are designed for patients with "normal" organ function and nutritional requirements. Standard CAA products differ in amino acid, total nitrogen, and electrolyte content but have similar effects on protein markers.
- Modified amino acid solutions are designed for patients with altered protein requirements associated with hepatic encephalopathy, renal failure, and metabolic stress or trauma. However, these solutions are expensive, and their role in disease-specific PN regimens is controversial.
- Conditionally essential amino acids such as taurine, aspartic acid, and glutamic acid are available in some commercially available CAA solutions. Other conditionally essential amino acids, such as cysteine, carnitine, and glutamine, are not included because they are unstable or insoluble. Cysteine and carnitine are commonly added to PN solutions compounded for newborns.
- More concentrated CAA solutions (i.e., 15–20%) are attractive for patients who have large protein needs, such as the critically ill, but are fluid restricted.

Dextrose

- The primary energy source in PN solutions is carbohydrate, usually as dextrose monohydrate. Available concentrations range from 5% to 70%. When oxidized, 1 g of hydrated dextrose provides 3.4 kcal (14.2 kJ).
- Recommended doses for routine clinical care rarely exceed 5 mg/kg/min in older critically ill children (1–11 yr old) and adults. Minimum requirements for neonates are 6 to 10 mg/kg/min. Higher infusion rates contribute to the development of hyperglycemia, excess carbon dioxide production, and increased biochemical markers for liver function.
- Glycerol is a non-insulin-dependent source of carbohydrate that can be used to improve glycemic control for patients with impaired insulin secretion or activity. A major disadvantage of the available glycerol solution is the dilute concentration of carbohydrate and amino acids (3% of each). Most adult patients require 3 to 4 L/day of glycerol solution and supplemental IVFE to meet minimal energy requirements.

Intravenous Fat Emulsion

- Commercially available IVFEs provide calories and essential fatty acids. These products differ in triglyceride source, fatty acid content, and essential fatty acid concentration.
- When oxidized, 1 g of fat yields 9 kcal (38 kJ). Because of the caloric contribution from egg phospholipid and glycerol, caloric content of IVFE is 1.1 kcal/mL (4.6 kJ/mL) for the 10%, 2 kcal/mL (8.4 kJ/mL) for the 20%, and 3 kcal/mL (12.6 kJ/mL) for the 30% emulsions.
- Essential fatty acid deficiency can be prevented by giving IVFE, 0.5 to 1 g/kg/day for neonates and infants and 100 g/wk for adults.
- IVFE 10% and 20% products can be administered by a central or peripheral vein, added directly to PN solution as a total nutrient admixture (TNA) or three-in-one system (lipids, protein, glucose, and additives), or piggybacked with a CAA and dextrose solution, commonly

referred to as a two-in-one solution. IVFE 30% is approved only for TNA preparation.

- IVFE is contraindicated in patients with an impaired ability to clear fat emulsion and should be administered cautiously to patients with egg allergy.
- The caloric contribution from **propofol** infusions can require adjustment of a patient's nutrition regimen. The caloric contribution from **amphotericin** liposomal and lipid complex formulations is not clinically relevant.

MICRONUTRIENTS

- Micronutrients (i.e., vitamins, trace elements, and electrolytes) are required to support metabolic activities for cellular homeostasis such as enzyme reactions, fluid balance, and regulation of electrophysiologic processes.
- Multivitamin products have been formulated to comply with guidelines for adults, children, and infants. These products contain 13 essential vitamins, including vitamin K.
- Requirements for trace elements depend on the patient's age and clinical condition. Examples include using higher doses of zinc in patients with high-output ostomies or diarrhea; restricting or withholding manganese and copper in patients with cholestatic liver disease; and restricting or withholding chromium, molybdenum, andselenium in patients with renal failure.
- Chromium, copper, manganese, selenium, and zinc are considered essential and available as single- or multiple-entity products for addition to PN solutions.
- Sodium, potassium, calcium, magnesium, phosphorus, chloride, and acetate are necessary components of PN for maintenance of numerous cellular functions.
- Patients with normal organ function and serum electrolyte concentrations should receive daily maintenance doses of electrolytes during PN.
- Electrolyte requirements depend on the patient's age, disease state, organ function, drug therapy, nutrition status, and extrarenal losses.

DESIGNING A PARENTERAL NUTRITION REGIMEN

ROUTES OF PARENTERAL NUTRITION ADMINISTRATION

- The patient's clinical condition determines the appropriate route of administration (see **Fig. 61–1**).
- Peripheral parenteral nutrition (PPN) candidates do not have large nutritional requirements, are not fluid restricted, and are expected to regain GI tract function within 10 to 14 days. Solutions for PPN have lower final concentrations of amino acid (3–5%), dextrose (5–10%), and micronutrients as compared with central parenteral nutrition (CPN).
- Primary advantages of PPN include a lower risk of infectious, metabolic, and technical complications.

TABLE 61–2	Osmolarities of Select Parenteral Nutrients
Nutrient	**Osmolarity**
Amino acid	100 mOsm/%
Dextrose	50 mOsm/%
Lipid emulsion (20%)	1.3–1.5 mOsm/g
Sodium (acetate, chloride)	2 mOsm/mEq
Sodium phosphate	3 mOsm/mEq sodium
Potassium (acetate, chloride)	2 mOsm/mEq
Potassium phosphate	1.7–2.7 mOsm/mEq potassium
Magnesium sulfate	1 mOsm/mEq
Calcium gluconate	1.4 mOsm/mEq

- PPN use is limited by relatively poor peripheral vein tolerance to hypertonic solutions. Thrombophlebitis is a common complication; this risk is greater with solution osmolarities >600 to 900 mOsm/L (600–900 mmol/L) (**Table 61–2**).
- CPN is useful in patients who require PN for more than 7 to 14 days and who have large nutrient requirements, poor peripheral venous access, or fluctuating fluid requirements.
- CPN solutions are highly concentrated hypertonic solutions that must be administered through a large central vein. The choice of venous access site depends on factors including patient age and anatomy. Peripherally inserted central catheters (PICCs) are often used for both short- and long-term central venous access in acute or home care settings.
- Disadvantages include risks associated with catheter insertion, use, and care. Central venous access has a greater potential for infection.

CONSTRUCTING THE PARENTERAL NUTRITION REGIMEN

- PN regimens for adults can be based on formulas (**Fig. 61–2**), computer programs, or standardized order forms. Order forms are popular because they help educate practitioners and foster cost-efficient nutrition support by minimizing errors in ordering, compounding, and administering.
- Pediatric PN regimens typically require an individualized approach because practice guidelines often recommend nutrient intake based on weight. Labeling should reflect "amount per day" and also "amount per kilogram per day."

INITIATING AND ADVANCING THE PARENTERAL NUTRITION INFUSION

- PN solutions should be administered with an infusion pump.
- A 0.22 μm filter is recommended for CAA and dextrose solutions to remove particulate matter, air, and microorganisms. Because IVFE

Calculation of an Adult Parenteral Nutrition Regimen

Patient case: A patient's daily nutritional requirements have been estimated to be 100 g protein and 2,000 total kcal. The patient has a central venous access and reports no history of hyperlipidemia or egg allergy. The patient is not fluid restricted. The PN solution will be compounded as an individualized regimen using a single-bag, 24-hour infusion of a 2-in-1 solution with intravenous fat emulsion (IVFE) piggybacked into the PN infusion line. Determine the total PN volume and administration rate by calculating the macronutrient stock solution volumes required to provide the desired daily nutrients. The stock solutions used to compound this regimen are 10% crystalline amino acids (CAA), 70% dextrose, and 20% IVFE.

1. Determine the daily IVFE calories and volume

    *   2,000 kcal/day × 30–40% of total calories as fat = 600–800 kcal/day
        Choose IVFE 20% 250 mL/day × 2 kcal/mL = 500 kcal/day

2. Determine the 70% dextrose stock solution volume

    *   Determine dextrose calories
        Dextrose calories = TOTAL – IVFE – Protein
        2,000 kcal – 500 kcal IVFE – (4 kcal/g × 100 g CAA) = 1,100 kcal

    *   Calculate required dextrose (grams)
        1,100 kcal ÷ 3.4 kcal/g dextrose = 324 g dextrose

    *   Determine 70% dextrose volume
        70 g/100 mL = 324 g/X mL 70% dextrose;   X = 463 mL 70% dextrose

3. Calculate the 10% CAA stock solution volume

    *   10 g/100 mL = 100 g/X mL 10% CAA;   X = 1,000 mL 10% CAA

4. Determine the 2-in-1 PN volume and administration rate

    *   Calculate CAA/dextrose volume
        463 mL 70% dextrose + 1,000 mL 10% CAA = 1,463 mL CAA–dextrose

    *   Add 100–200 mL for additives
        Total 2-in-1 volume = approximately 1,600–1,700 mL/day

    *   Calculate the administration rate
        1,600–1,700 mL/day ÷ 24 hours = 67–71 mL/hour; round to 65–70 mL/hour

5. Choose final 2-in-1 PN regimen and determine provided nutrient amounts:

    *   Final 2-in-1 regimen
        100 g CAA/324 gm dextrose in 1,680 mL/day to infuse at 70 mL/hour
        + 20% IVFE 250 mL to infuse at 2 mL/hour

    *   Calculate macronutrient calories

20% IVFE calories:	250 mL × 2 kcal/mL =	500 kcal
Dextrose calories:	324 g × 3.4 kcal/g =	1,102 kcal
Protein calories:	100 g × 4 kcal/g =	400 kcal
Total kcal:		2,002 kcal
Nonprotein kcal:		1,002 kcal

FIGURE 61–2. Calculation of an adult PN regimen. To convert to energy units of kilojoules (kJ), multiply valus with kilocalories as the numerator (kcal, kcal/mL, kcal/kg, kcal/g) by 4.18 to give the corresponding value in kilojoules (kJ, kJ/mL, kJ/kg, kJ/g).

particles measure ~0.5 μm, IVFE should be administered separately and piggybacked into the PN line beyond the in-line filter. Use of a 1.2 μm filter with TNA solutions is recommended by the FDA to prevent catheter occlusion caused by precipitates or lipid aggregates and to remove *Candida albicans*.

- Although protocols for initiating adult PN differ, the rate is typically increased gradually over 12 to 24 hours to prevent hyperglycemia. When discontinuing PN, the infusion rate is gradually decreased to prevent hypoglycemia.

- The dose of IVFE in adults ranges from 1 to 2.5 g/kg/day, not to exceed 30% to 60% of total calories. Administering IVFE over 12 to 24 hours appears to promote IVFE clearance and minimize the risk of negative effects on pulmonary and immune function and also eliminates the need for a test dose.

- Pediatric PN solutions are initiated with a volume calculated to meet daily maintenance fluid requirements. Individual substrates are advanced daily as tolerated with the goal protein dose achieved by day 3 of therapy; institutional practices vary. Transition from PN to EN is recommended over a period of days to weeks.

- The starting dose of IVFE is 0.5 g/kg/day in neonates and 0.5 to 1 g/kg/day in older children. This dose is increased by 0.5 to 1 g/kg/day to a maximum of 3 g/kg/day. Another strategy is to infuse IVFE over 20 to 24 hours or at a rate of 0.15 g/kg/hour.

- Cyclic PN (e.g., 12–18 hours/day) is useful in hospitalized patients who have limited venous access and require other medications necessitating interruption of PN infusion, to prevent or treat hepatotoxicities associated with continuous PN therapy, and to allow home patients to resume normal lifestyles. Patients with severe glucose intolerance or unstable fluid balance may not tolerate cyclic PN.

EVALUATION OF THERAPEUTIC OUTCOMES

- Routine evaluation should include assessment of the clinical condition of the patient, with a focus on nutritional and metabolic effects of the PN regimen.

- Biochemical and clinical parameters should be monitored routinely in patients receiving PN (**Fig. 61–3**).

COMPOUNDING, STORAGE, AND INFECTION CONTROL

- The United States Pharmacopeia (USP) chapter 797 details procedures and requirements for compounding sterile preparations, including PN formulations. In general, the type of solution being prepared dictates the methods of compounding, storage, and infusion. The two most common types of PN solutions are two-in-one solutions, with or without IVFE piggybacked into the PN line, and TNAs.

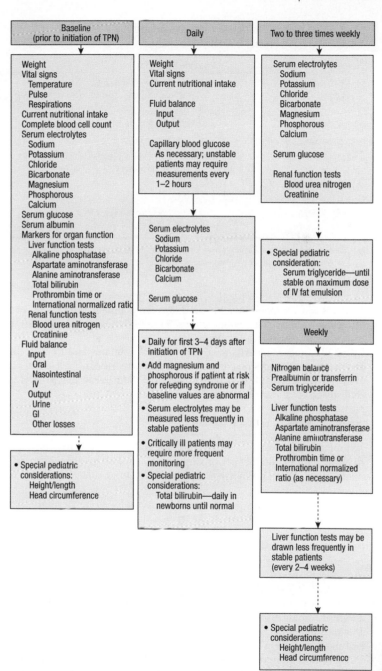

FIGURE 61-3. Monitoring strategy for parenteral nutrition. (TPN, total parenteral nutrition.)

TABLE 61–3 Metabolic Abnormalities Associated with Parenteral Nutrition Macronutrients

Abnormality	Possible Etiologies
Hyperglycemia	Metabolic stress, infection, corticosteroids, pancreatitis, diabetes mellitus, peritoneal dialysis, excessive dextrose administration
Hypoglycemia	Abrupt dextrose withdrawal, excessive insulin
Excess carbon dioxide production	Excess dextrose administration
Hypertriglyceridemia	Metabolic stress, familial hyperlipidemia, pancreatitis, excess IVFE dose; rapid IVFE infusion rate
Abnormal liver function tests (elevated ALT, AST, Alk Phos, Bili)	Metabolic stress, infection, excess carbohydrate intake, excess caloric intake, EFAD; long-term PN therapy

Alk Phos, alkaline phosphatase; ALT, alanine aminotransferase; AST, aspartate aminotransferase; Bili, bilirubin; EFAD, essential fatty acid deficiency; IVFE, intravenous fat emulsion; PN, parenteral nutrition.

- Methods for compounding PN solutions vary among institutions and often involve automated compounders. Sterility should be ensured during compounding, storage, and administration.
- USP 797 storage standards for CAA–dextrose solutions and Centers for Disease Control and Prevention (CDC) infusion recommendations for IVFE should be followed. Compliance with IVFE recommendations is challenging for pediatric patients.

STABILITY AND COMPATIBILITY

- Appropriate resources should be consulted for current compatibility and stability information before mixing components (e.g., manufacturer's information, *Trissel's Handbook on Injectable Drugs*, and *King Guide to Parenteral Admixtures*).
- In general, preparation of an unstable TNA formulation can be minimized by maintaining the final concentrations of CAA >4%, dextrose >10%, and IVFE >2%.
- Precipitation of calcium and phosphorus is a common interaction that is potentially life-threatening.
- Bicarbonate should not be added to acidic PN solutions; a bicarbonate precursor salt (e.g., acetate) is preferred.
- Vitamins can be adversely affected by changes in solution pH, other additives, storage time, solution temperature, and exposure to light. Vitamins should be added to the PN solution near the time of administration and should not be in the PN solution for more than 24 hours.
- Using the PN admixture as a drug vehicle consolidates dosage units and has other advantages; however, compatibility and stability data are not available for many PN solutions. Medications frequently added to PN solutions include regular insulin and histamine$_2$ antagonists.

COMPLICATIONS OF PARENTERAL NUTRITION

- PN can cause mechanical or technical (e.g., malfunctions in delivery system and catheter-related complications), infectious (e.g., colonization of the catheter or direct microbial invasion of the skin), metabolic (Table 61–3), and nutritional complications.

See Chapter 151, Parenteral Nutrition, authored by Todd W. Mattox and Catherine M. Crill, for a more detailed discussion of this topic.

CHAPTER 62

Breast Cancer

DEFINITION

- Breast cancer is a malignancy originating from breast tissue. This chapter distinguishes between early stages, which are potentially curable, and metastatic breast cancer (MBC), which is usually incurable.

EPIDEMIOLOGY

- The strongest risk factors for breast cancer are female gender and increasing age. Additional risk factors include endocrine factors (e.g., early menarche, nulliparity, late age at first birth, and hormone replacement therapy), genetic factors (e.g., personal and family history, mutations of tumor suppresser genes [*BRCA1* and *BRCA2*]), and environmental and lifestyle factors (e.g., radiation exposure).
- Breast cancer cells often spread undetected by contiguity, lymph channels, and through the blood early in the course of the disease, resulting in metastatic disease after local therapy. The most common metastatic sites are lymph nodes, skin, bone, liver, lungs, and brain.

CLINICAL PRESENTATION

- The initial sign in most women with breast cancer is a painless lump that is typically solitary, unilateral, solid, hard, irregular, and nonmobile. Less common initial signs are pain and nipple changes. More advanced cases present with prominent skin edema, redness, warmth, and induration.
- Symptoms of MBC depend on the site of metastases but may include bone pain, difficulty breathing, abdominal pain or enlargement, jaundice, and mental status changes.
- Many women first detect some breast abnormalities themselves, but it is increasingly common for breast cancer to be detected during routine screening mammography in asymptomatic women.

DIAGNOSIS

- Initial workup for a woman presenting with a localized lesion or suggestive symptoms should include a careful history, physical examination of the breast, three-dimensional mammography, and, possibly, other breast imaging techniques, such as ultrasound and magnetic resonance imaging (MRI).

- Breast biopsy is indicated for a mammographic abnormality that suggests malignancy or for a palpable mass on physical examination.

STAGING

- Stage (anatomical extent of disease) is based on the size of the primary tumor extent and size (T_{1-4}), presence and extent of lymph node involvement (N_{1-3}), and presence or absence of distant metastases (M_{0-1}). The staging system determines prognosis and assists with treatment decisions. Simplistically stated, these stages may be represented as follows:
  ✓ *Early Breast Cancer*
    - Stage 0: Carcinoma in situ or disease that has not invaded the basement membrane
    - Stage I: Small primary tumor without lymph node involvement
    - Stage II: Involvement of regional lymph nodes
  ✓ *Locally Advanced Breast Cancer*
    - Stage III: Usually a large tumor with extensive nodal involvement in which the node or tumor is fixed to the chest wall; also includes inflammatory breast cancer, which is rapidly progressive
  ✓ *Advanced or Metastatic Breast Cancer*
    - Stage IV: Metastases in organs distant from the primary tumor

PATHOLOGIC EVALUATION

- The development of malignancy is a multistep process with preinvasive (or noninvasive) and invasive phases. The goal of treatment for noninvasive carcinomas is to prevent the development of invasive disease.
- The pathologic evaluation of breast lesions establishes the histologic diagnosis and the presence or absence of prognostic factors.
- Most breast carcinomas are adenocarcinomas and are classified as ductal or lobular.

PROGNOSTIC FACTORS

- The ability to predict prognosis is used to design treatment recommendations to maximize quantity and quality of life.
- Tumor size and the presence and number of involved axillary lymph nodes are primary factors in assessing the risk for breast cancer recurrence and subsequent metastatic disease. Other disease characteristics that provide prognostic information are histologic subtype, nuclear or histologic grade, lymphatic and vascular invasion, and proliferation indices.
- The estrogen receptor (ER) and progesterone receptor (PR) are two hormone receptors used as indicators of breast cancer prognosis and to predict response to hormone therapy.
- HER2/*neu* (HER2) overexpression is associated with transmission of growth signals that control aspects of normal cell growth and division. Overexpression of HER2 is associated with increased tumor aggressiveness, rates of recurrence, and mortality.
- Genetic profiling tools provide additional prognostic information to aid in treatment decisions for subgroups of patients with otherwise favorable prognostic features.

DESIRED OUTCOME

- The goal of therapy with early and locally advanced breast cancer is cure. The goals of therapy with MBC are to improve symptoms, improve quality of life, and prolong survival.

TREATMENT

- The treatment of breast cancer is rapidly evolving. Specific information regarding the most promising interventions can be found only in the primary literature.
- Treatment can cause substantial toxicity, which differs depending on the individual agent, administration method, and combination regimen. Because a comprehensive review of toxicities is beyond the scope of this chapter, appropriate references should be consulted.

EARLY BREAST CANCER

Local-Regional Therapy

- Surgery alone can cure most patients with in situ cancers and approximately one half of those with stage II cancers.
- Breast-conserving therapy (BCT) is appropriate primary therapy for most women with stage I and II disease; it is preferable to modified radical mastectomy because it produces equivalent survival rates with cosmetically superior results. BCT consists of lumpectomy (i.e., excision of the primary tumor and adjacent breast tissue) followed by radiation therapy (RT) to prevent local recurrence.
- RT is administered to the entire breast over 4 to 6 weeks to eradicate residual disease after BCT. Reddening and erythema of the breast tissue with subsequent shrinkage of total breast mass are minor complications associated with RT.
- Simple or total mastectomy involves removal of the entire breast without dissection of underlying muscle or axillary nodes. This procedure is used for carcinoma in situ where the incidence of axillary node involvement is only 1% or with local recurrence following BCT.
- Axillary lymph nodes should be sampled for staging and prognostic information. Lymphatic mapping with sentinel lymph node biopsy is a new, less invasive alternative to axillary dissection; however, the procedure is controversial because of the lack of long-term data.

Systemic Adjuvant Therapy

- Systemic adjuvant therapy is the administration of systemic therapy following definitive local therapy (surgery, radiation, or both) when there is no evidence of metastatic disease but a high likelihood of disease recurrence. The goal of such therapy is cure.
- Chemotherapy, hormonal therapy, or both result in improved disease-free survival and/or overall survival (OS) for all treated patients.
- The National Comprehensive Cancer Network practice guidelines reflect the trend toward the use of chemotherapy in all women regardless of

menopausal status, along with the addition of hormonal therapy in all women with receptor-positive disease regardless of age or menopausal status.

- Genetic tests are being prospectively validated as decision-support tools for adjuvant chemotherapy in ER-positive, node-negative breast cancer to identify characteristics of the primary tumor that may predict for the likelihood of distant recurrence and/or death.

ADJUVANT CHEMOTHERAPY

- Early administration of effective combination chemotherapy at a time of low tumor burden should increase the likelihood of cure and minimize emergence of drug-resistant tumor cell clones. Combination regimens have historically been more effective than single-agent chemotherapy (**Table 62–1**).

TABLE 62–1 Selected Adjuvant Chemotherapy Regimens for Breast Cancer	
AC[a,b]	**TC[a,c]**
Doxorubicin 60 mg/m² IV, day 1 Cyclophosphamide 600 mg/m² IV, day 1 Repeat cycles every 21 days for 4 cycles	Docetaxel 75 mg/m² IV, day 1 Cyclophosphamide 600 mg/m² IV, day 1 Repeat cycles every 21 days for 4 cycles
FAC[d,m]	**TAC[a,e]**
Fluorouracil 500 mg/m² IV, days 1 and 4 Doxorubicin 50 mg/m² IV continuous infusion over 72 hours Cyclophosphamide 500 mg/m² IV, day 1 Repeat cycles every 21–28 days for 6 cycles	Docetaxel 75 mg/m² IV, day 1 Doxorubicin 50 mg/m² IV bolus, day 1 Cyclophosphamide 500 mg/m² IV, day 1 (Doxorubicin should be given first) Repeat cycles every 21 days for 6 cycles (must be given with growth factor support)
AC → Paclitaxel[a,f]	**Paclitaxel → FAC[g,m]**
Doxorubicin 60 mg/m² IV, day 1 Cyclophosphamide 600 mg/m² IV, day 1 Repeat cycles every 21 days for 4 cycles Followed by: Paclitaxel 80 mg/m² IV weekly Repeat cycles every 7 days for 12 cycles	Paclitaxel 80 mg/m² per week IV over 1 hour every week for 12 weeks Followed by: Fluorouracil 500 mg/m² IV, days 1 and 4 Doxorubicin 50 mg/m² IV continuous infusion over 72 hours Cyclophosphamide 500 mg/m² IV, day 1 Repeat cycles every 21–28 days for 4 cycles[g]
FEC[h]	**CEF[i]**
Fluorouracil 500 mg/m² IV, day 1 Epirubicin 100 mg/m² IV bolus, day 1 Cyclophosphamide 500 mg/m² IV, day 1 Repeat cycle every 21 days for 6 cycles	Cyclophosphamide 75 mg/m² per day orally on days 1–14 Epirubicin 60 mg/m² IV, days 1 and 8 Fluorouracil 600 mg/m² IV, days 1 and 8 Repeat cycles every 21 days for 6 cycles (requires prophylactic antibiotics or growth factor support)

(continued)

| **TABLE 62–1** | Selected Adjuvant Chemotherapy Regimens for Breast Cancer *(Continued)* |

CMF[j,k]	**Dose-Dense AC → Paclitaxel**[a,l,n]
Cyclophosphamide 100 mg/m^2 per day orally, days 1–14	Doxorubicin 60 mg/m^2 IV bolus, day 1
Methotrexate 40 mg/m^2 IV, days 1 and 8	Cyclophosphamide 600 mg/m^2 IV, day 1
Fluorouracil 600 mg/m^2 IV, days 1 and 8	Repeat cycles every 14 days for 4 cycles
Repeat cycles every 28 days for 6 cycles	(must be given with growth factor support)
or	Followed by:
Cyclophosphamide 600 mg/m^2 IV, day 1	Paclitaxel 175 mg/m^2 IV over 3 hours
Methotrexate 40 mg/m^2 IV, day 1	Repeat cycles every 14 days for 4 cycles
Fluorouracil 600 mg/m^2 IV, days 1 and 8	(must be given with growth factor support)
Repeat cycles every 21 days for 6 cycles	

AC, Adriamycin (doxorubicin), Cytoxan (cyclophosphamide); CAF, Cytoxan (cyclophosphamide), Adriamycin (doxorubicin), 5 fluorouracil; CEF, cyclophosphamide, epirubicin, 5-fluorouracil; CMF, cyclophosphamide, methotrexate, 5-flourouracil; FAC, 5-fluorouracil, Adriamycin (doxorubicin), cyclophosphamide; FEC, 5-fluorouracil, epirubicin, cyclophosphamide; TAC, Taxotere (docetaxel), Adriamycin (doxorubicin) cyclophosphamide; TC, Taxotere (docetaxel), cyclophosphamide.

[a]Designated as a preferred regimen in the NCCN Breast Cancer Guidelines.
[b]From Fisher B, Brown AM, Dimitrov NV, et al. J Clin Oncol 1990;8:1483.
[c]From Jones SE, Savin MA, Holmes FA, et al. J Clin Oncol 2006;24.5381.
[d]From Buzdar AU, Hortobagyi GN, Singletary SE, et al. In: Salmon S, ed. Adjuvant Therapy of Cancer, VIII. Philadelphia, PA: Lippincott-Raven, 1997:93–100.
[e]From Martin M, Dienkowski T, Mackey J, et al. N Engl J Med 2005;352:2302.
[f]From Sparano JA, Wang M, Martino S, et al. N Engl J Med 2008;358:1663–1671.
[g]From Green MC, Buzdar AU, Smith T, et al. J Clin Oncol 2005;23:5983.
[h]From French Adjuvant Study Group. J Clin Oncol 2001;19:602.
[i]From Levine MN, Bramwell VH, Pritchard KI, et al. J Clin Oncol 1998;16:2651.
[j]From Bonadonna G, Brusamolino E, Valagussa P, et al. N Engl J Med 1976;294:405.
[k]From Fisher B, Redmond C, Dimitrov NV, et al. N Engl J Med 1989;320:473.
[l]From Citron ML, Berry DA, Cirrincione C, et al. J Clin Oncol 2003;21:1431–1439.
[m]FAC may also be given with bolus doxorubicin administration, and the fluorouracil dose is then given on days 1 and 8.
[n]Another way to give these agents in a dose-dense manner is A → P → C as sequential single agents, in the same doses indicated above, every 14 days for 4 cycles each with growth factor support.

- Anthracycline-containing regimens (e.g., **doxorubicin** and **epirubicin**) significantly reduce the rate of recurrence and improve OS 5 and 10 years after treatment as compared with regimens that contain **cyclophosphamide, methotrexate,** and **fluorouracil**. Both node-negative and node-positive patients benefit from anthracycline-containing regimens.
- The addition of taxanes, **docetaxel** and **paclitaxel,** a newer class of agents, to adjuvant regimens comprised of the drugs listed above resulted in consistently and significantly improved disease-free survival and OS in node-positive breast cancer patients. The use of taxane-containing regimens in node-negative patients remains controversial.
- Chemotherapy should be initiated within 12 weeks of surgical removal of the primary tumor. The optimal duration of adjuvant treatment is unknown but appears to be on the order of 12 to 24 weeks, depending on the regimen used.

- *Dose intensity* refers to the amount of drug administered per unit of time, which can be achieved by increasing dose, decreasing time between doses, or both. *Dose density* is one way of achieving dose intensity by decreasing time between treatment cycles.
- Dose-dense regimens may be considered as options for adjuvant therapy for node-positive breast cancer.
- Increasing doses in standard regimens appears to not be beneficial and may be harmful.
- Decreasing doses in standard regimens should be avoided unless necessitated by severe toxicity.
- Short-term toxicities of adjuvant chemotherapy are generally well tolerated, especially with the availability of serotonin-antagonist and substance P/neurokinin 1–antagonist antiemetics and colony-stimulating factors.
- Survival benefit for adjuvant chemotherapy in stage I and II breast cancer is modest. The absolute reduction in mortality at 10 years is 5% in node-negative and 10% in node-positive disease.

ADJUVANT BIOLOGIC THERAPY

- Trastuzumab in combination with adjuvant chemotherapy is indicated in patients with early stage, HER2-positive breast cancer. The risk of recurrence was reduced up to 50% in clinical trials.
- Unanswered questions with the use of adjuvant trastuzumab include optimal concurrent chemotherapy, optimal dose, schedule and duration of therapy, and use of other concurrent therapeutic modalities.

ADJUVANT ENDOCRINE THERAPY

- **Tamoxifen, toremifene,** oophorectomy, ovarian irradiation, luteinizing hormone–releasing hormone (LHRH) agonists, and aromatase inhibitors are hormonal therapies used in the treatment of primary or early-stage breast cancer. Tamoxifen was the gold standard adjuvant hormonal therapy for 3 decades and is generally considered the adjuvant hormonal therapy of choice for premenopausal women. It has both estrogenic and antiestrogenic properties, depending on the tissue and gene in question.
- Tamoxifen 20 mg daily, beginning soon after completing chemotherapy and continuing for 5 years, reduces the risk of recurrence and mortality. Tamoxifen is usually well tolerated. Symptoms of estrogen withdrawal (hot flashes and vaginal bleeding) may occur but decrease in frequency and intensity over time. Tamoxifen reduces the risk of hip radius and spine fractures. It increases the risks of stroke, pulmonary embolism, deep vein thrombosis, and endometrial cancer, particularly in women age 50 years or older.
- Premenopausal women benefit from ovarian ablation with LHRH agonists (e.g., **goserelin**) in the adjuvant setting, either with or without concurrent tamoxifen. Trials are ongoing to further define the role of LHRH agonists.
- Guidelines recommend incorporation of aromatase inhibitors into adjuvant hormonal therapy for postmenopausal, hormone-sensitive breast cancer. The following options are currently recommended: (1) an aromatase inhibitor for 5 years; (2) tamoxifen for 2 to 3 years, followed

by an aromatase inhibitor for a total of 5 years of endocrine therapy; or (3) tamoxifen for 5 years, followed by an aromatase inhibitor for another 5 years. Experts believe that the three available aromatase inhibitors—**anastrozole, letrozole,** and **exemestane**—have similar antitumor efficacy and toxicity profiles. Adverse effects with aromatase inhibitors include bone loss/osteoporosis, hot flashes, myalgia/arthralgia, vaginal dryness/atrophy, mild headaches, and diarrhea.

- The optimal drug, dose, sequence, and duration of administration of aromatase inhibitors in the adjuvant setting are not known.

LOCALLY ADVANCED BREAST CANCER (STAGE III)

- Neoadjuvant or primary chemotherapy is the initial treatment of choice. Benefits include rendering inoperable tumors resectable and increasing the rate of BCT.
- Primary chemotherapy with either an anthracycline- or taxane-containing regimen is recommended. The use of trastuzumab with chemotherapy is appropriate for patients with HER2-positive tumors.
- Surgery followed by chemotherapy and adjuvant RT should be administered to minimize local recurrence.
- Cure is the primary goal of therapy for most patients with stage III disease.

METASTATIC BREAST CANCER (STAGE IV)

- MBC is not curable; therefore, the goals of treatment are to improve symptoms and quality of life and to extend survival.
- The choice of therapy for MBC is based on the site of disease involvement and the presence or absence of certain characteristics, as described below.

Endocrine Therapy

- Endocrine therapy is the treatment of choice for patients who have hormone receptor–positive metastases in soft tissue, bone, pleura, or, if asymptomatic, viscera. Compared with chemotherapy, endocrine therapy has an equal probability of response and a better safety profile.
- Patients are sequentially treated with endocrine therapy until their tumors cease to respond, at which time chemotherapy can be given.
- Historically, the choice of an endocrine therapy was based primarily on toxicity and patient preference, but study results have led to changes in MBC treatment (**Table 62–2**).
- Aromatase inhibitors reduce circulating and target organ estrogens by blocking peripheral conversion from an androgenic precursor, the primary source of estrogens in postmenopausal women. The third-generation aromatase inhibitors **anastrozole, letrozole,** and **exemestane** are more selective and potent than the prototype, **aminoglutethimide.** Anastrozole, letrozole, and exemestane are approved as second-line therapy of advanced breast cancer in postmenopausal women; anastrozole and letrozole are also approved for first-line therapy in these patients. When compared with tamoxifen, patients receiving anastrozole and letrozole had similar response rates and longer median time to

TABLE 62–2	Endocrine Therapies Used for Metastatic Breast Cancer		
Class	**Drug**	**Dose**	**Side Effects**
Aromatase inhibitors			
Nonsteroidal	Anastrozole	1 mg orally daily	Hot flashes, bone
	Letrozole	2.5 mg orally daily	loss/osteoporosis,
Steroidal	Exemestane	25 mg orally daily	arthralgias, myalgias, headaches, diarrhea, mild nausea
Antiestrogens			
SERMs	Tamoxifen	20 mg orally daily	Hot flashes, vaginal
	Toremifene	60 mg orally daily	discharge, mild nausea, thromboembolism, endometrial hyperplasia/cancer
SERDs	Fulvestrant	250 mg IM every 28 days	Hot flashes, injection site reactions, possibly thromboembolism
LHRH analogues	Goserelin	3.6 mg SC every 28 days	Hot flashes, amenorrhea, menopausal symptoms, injection site reactions (extended formulations of more than 28 days are not recommended for the treatment of breast cancer)
	Leuprolide	3.75 mg IM every 28 days	
	Triptorelin	3.75 mg IM every 28 days	
Progestins	Megestrol acetate	40 mg orally four times daily	Weight gain, hot flashes, vaginal bleeding, edema, thromboembolism
	Medroxyprogesterone	400–1,000 mg IM every week	
Androgens	Fluoxymesterone	10 mg orally twice daily	Deepening voice, alopecia, hirsutism, facial/truncal acne, fluid retention, menstrual irregularities, cholestatic jaundice
Estrogens	Diethylstilbestrol	5 mg orally three times daily	Nausea/vomiting, fluid retention, anorexia, thromboembolism, hepatic dysfunction, myocardial infarction
	Ethinyl estradiol	1 mg orally three times daily	
	Conjugated estrogens	2.5 mg orally three times daily	

IM, intramuscularly; LHRH, luteinizing hormone–releasing hormone; SC, subcutaneously; SERD, selective estrogen receptor downregulator; SERM, selective estrogen receptor modulator.

progression as well as lower incidence of thromboembolic events and vaginal bleeding.

- **Tamoxifen** is the antiestrogen of choice in premenopausal women whose tumors are hormone receptor positive, unless metastases occur within 1 year of adjuvant tamoxifen. Maximal beneficial effects do not occur for at least 2 months. In addition to the side effects described for adjuvant therapy, tumor flare or hypercalcemia occurs in ~5% of patients with MBC.
- **Toremifene** has similar efficacy and tolerability as tamoxifen and is an alternative to tamoxifen in postmenopausal patients. **Fulvestrant** is a second-line intramuscular agent with similar efficacy and safety when compared with anastrozole in patients who progressed on tamoxifen.
- Ovarian ablation (oophorectomy) is considered by some to be the endocrine therapy of choice in premenopausal women and produces similar overall response rates as tamoxifen. Medical castration with an LHRH analogue (**goserelin, leuprolide,** or **triptorelin**) is a reversible alternative to surgery. If used as first-line therapy for MBC, combination therapy with tamoxifen is recommended.
- Progestins are generally reserved for third-line therapy. They cause weight gain, fluid retention, and thromboembolic events.

Chemotherapy

- Chemotherapy is used as initial therapy for women with hormone receptor–negative tumors and after failure of endocrine therapy.
- The choice of treatment depends on the individual. Agents used previously as adjuvant therapy can be repeated unless the cancer recurred within 1 year. Single agents are associated with lower response rates than combination therapy, but time to progression and OS are similar. Single agents are better tolerated, an important consideration in the palliative metastatic setting (Table 62–3). Treatment with sequential single agents is recommended over combination regimens unless the patient has rapidly progressive disease, life-threatening visceral disease, or the need for rapid symptom control.

TABLE 62–3	Selected Chemotherapy Regimens for Metastatic Breast Cancer
Single-Agent Chemotherapy	
Paclitaxel[a,b]	**Vinorelbine**[c]
Paclitaxel 175 mg/m^2 IV over 3 hours	Vinorelbine 30 mg/m^2 IV, days 1 and 8
Repeat cycles every 21 days	Repeat cycles every 21 days
or	*or*
Paclitaxel 80 mg/m^2/week IV over 1 hour	Vinorelbine 25–30 mg/m^2/week IV
Repeat dose every 7 days	Repeat cycles every 7 days (adjust dose based on absolute neutrophil count; see product information)
	(continued)

| **TABLE 62–3** | Selected Chemotherapy Regimens for Metastatic Breast Cancer *(Continued)* |

Single-Agent Chemotherapy

Docetaxel[d,e]	**Gemcitabine**[f]
Docetaxel 60–100 mg/m² IV over 1 hour Repeat cycles every 21 days *or* Docetaxel 30–35 mg/m²/week IV over 30 minutes Repeat dose every 7 days	Gemcitabine 600–1,000 mg/m²/week IV, days 1, 8, and 15 Repeat cycles every 28 days (may need to hold day 15 dose based on blood counts)[g]
Protein-bound Paclitaxel[g,h]	**Ixabepilone**[i]
Protein-bound Paclitaxel 260 mg/m² IV over 30 minutes Repeat cycles every 21 days *or* Protein-bound Paclitaxel 100–150 mg/m² IV over 30 minutes on days 1, 8, and 15 Repeat cycle every 28 days	Ixabepilone 40 mg/m² IV over 3 hours Repeat cycles every 21 days
Capecitabine[j]	**Liposomal doxorubicin**[k]
Capecitabine 2,000–2,500 mg/m² per day orally, divided twice daily for 14 days Repeat cycles every 21 days	Liposomal doxorubicin 30–50 mg/m² IV over variable duration Repeat cycles every 28 days

Combination Chemotherapy Regimens

Docetaxel + capecitabine[l]	**Paclitaxel + Gemcitabine**[m]
Docetaxel 75 mg/m² IV over 1 hour, day 1 Capecitabine 2,000–2,500 mg/m² per day orally divided twice daily for 14 days Repeat cycles every 21 days	Paclitaxel 175 mg/m² IV over 3 hours, day 1 Gemcitabine 1250 mg/m² IV days 1 and 8 Repeat cycles every 21 days
Ixabepilone + capecitabine[i]	**Paclitaxel + bevacizumab**[n]
Ixabepilone 40 mg/m² IV over 3 hours, day 1 Capecitabine 1,750–2,000 mg/m²/day orally divided twice daily for 14 days Repeat cycles every 21 days	Paclitaxel 90 mg/m² IV over 1 hour, days 1, 8, and 15 Bevacizumab 10 mg/kg IV over 30–90 minutes, days 1 and 15 Repeat cycles every 28 days

[a]From Taxol (paclitaxel) product information. Princeton, NJ: Bristol-Myers Squibb; July 2007.
[b]From Perez EA, Vogelci, Irwin DH, et al. Clin Oncol 2001;19:4216.
[c]From Zelek L, Barthier S, Riofrio M, et al. Cancer 2001;92:2267.
[d]From Taxotere (docetaxel) product information. Bridgewater, NJ: Sanofi-aventis; 2008.
[e]From Hainsworth JD, Burris HA 3rd, Erlaud JB, et al. J Clin Oncol 1998;16:2164.
[f]From Carmichael J, Possinger K, Philip P, et al. J Clin Oncol 1995;13:2731.
[g]From Abraxane (paclitaxel protein-bound particles for injectable suspension) product information. Bridgewater, NJ: Abraxis Bioscience; September 2009.
[h]From Gradishar WJ, Krasnojon D, Cheporov S, et al. J Clin Oncol 2009;27:3611–3619.
[i]From Boehnke Michaud L. J Oncol Pharm Pract 2009;15(2):95–106.
[j]From Gralow, JR. Breast Cancer Res Treat 2005;89 Suppl 1: S9–S15.
[k]From O'Brien ME, Wigler N, Inbar M, et al. Ann Oncol 2004;15(3):440–449.
[l]From O'Shaughnessy J, Miles D, Vukelja S, et al. J Clin Oncol 2002;20(12):2812–2823.
[m]From Gemzar (gemcitabine) product information. Indianapolis, IN: Eli Lilly and Company; May 2007.
[n]From Miller K, Wang M, Gralow J, et al. N Engl J Med 2007;357(26):2666–2676.

- Combination regimens produce objective responses in ~60% of patients previously unexposed to chemotherapy, but complete responses occur in <10% of patients. The median duration of response is 5 to 12 months; the median survival is 14 to 33 months. A specific chemotherapy regimen is continued until there is unequivocal evidence of progressive disease or intolerable side effects.
- **Anthracyclines** and **taxanes** produce response rates of 50% to 60% when used as first-line therapy for MBC. Single-agents **capecitabine, vinorelbine,** and **gemcitabine** have response rates of 20% to 25% when used after an anthracycline and a taxane.
- **Ixabepilone,** a microtubule stabilizing agent, is indicated as monotherapy or in combination with capecitabine in patients with MBC who have progressive disease despite treatment with the above agents. Response rates and time to progression were increased with combination therapy as compared with capecitabine alone.

Biologic or Targeted Therapy

- **Trastuzumab,** a monoclonal antibody that binds to HER2, produces response rates of 15% to 20% when used as a single agent and increases response rates, time to progression, and OS when combined with chemotherapy. It has been studied in doublet (**taxane–trastuzumab** and **vinorelbine–trastuzumab**) and triplet (**trastuzumab–taxane–platinum**) combinations, but the optimum regimen is unknown.
- Trastuzumab is well tolerated, but the risk of cardiotoxicity is 5% with single-agent trastuzumab and unacceptably high in combination with an anthracycline.
- **Lapatinib,** an oral tyrosine kinase inhibitor that targets both HER2 and the epidermal growth factor receptor, improved response rates and time to progression in combination with capecitabine, as compared with capecitabine alone, in patients previously treated with an anthracycline, taxane, and trastuzumab. The most common adverse events were rash and diarrhea.
- The role of **bevacizumab,** a monoclonal antibody targeted against vascular endothelial growth factor, in MBC is currently not clearly defined.

Radiation Therapy

- Radiation is commonly used to treat painful bone metastases or other localized sites of disease, including brain and spinal cord lesions. Pain relief is seen in ~90% of patients who receive RT.

PREVENTION OF BREAST CANCER

- Three classes of agents being studied for pharmacologic risk reduction of breast cancer include retinoids, selective estrogen receptor modulators (SERMs), and aromatase inhibitors.
- The most clinical information is available for the SERMs, **tamoxifen** and **raloxifene,** which reduce the rates of invasive breast cancer in women at high risk for developing the disease. Rates of endometrial cancer and deep

vein thromboses are higher in patients receiving tamoxifen, but the overall quality of life is similar between the two agents.

EVALUATION OF THERAPEUTIC OUTCOMES

EARLY BREAST CANCER

- The goal of adjuvant therapy in early-stage disease is cure. Because there is no clinical evidence of disease when adjuvant therapy is administered, assessment of this goal cannot be fully evaluated for years after initial diagnosis and treatment.
- Adjuvant chemotherapy can cause substantial toxicity. Because maintaining dose intensity is important in the cure of disease, supportive care should be optimized with measures such as antiemetics and growth factors.

LOCALLY ADVANCED BREAST CANCER

- The goal of neoadjuvant chemotherapy in locally advanced breast cancer is cure. Complete pathologic response, determined at the time of surgery, is the desired end point.

METASTATIC BREAST CANCER

- Optimizing quality of life is the therapeutic end point in the treatment of patients with MBC. Many valid and reliable tools are available for objective assessment of quality of life.
- The least toxic therapies are used initially, with increasingly aggressive therapies applied in a sequential manner that does not significantly compromise quality of life.
- Tumor response is measured by clinical chemistry (e.g., liver enzyme elevation in patients with hepatic metastases) or imaging techniques (e.g., bone scans or chest radiographs).
- Assessment of the clinical status and symptom control of the patient is often adequate to evaluate response to therapy.

See Chapter 136, Breast Cancer, authored by Laura Boehnke Michaud, Chad M. Barnett, and Francisco J. Esteva, for a more detailed discussion of this topic.

CHAPTER 63

Colorectal Cancer

DEFINITION

- Colorectal cancer is a malignant neoplasm involving the colon, rectum, and anal canal.

PATHOPHYSIOLOGY

- Development of a colorectal neoplasm is a multistep process of genetic and phenotypic alterations of normal bowel epithelium structure and function leading to unregulated cell growth, proliferation, and tumor development.
- Features of colorectal tumorigenesis include genomic instability, activation of oncogene pathways, mutational inactivation of tumor-suppressor genes, and activation of growth factor pathways.
- Adenocarcinomas account for >90% of tumors of the large intestine.

PREVENTION AND SCREENING

- Primary prevention is aimed at preventing colorectal cancer in an at-risk population. To date, the only strategy shown to reduce the risk is chemoprevention with celecoxib in people with familial adenomatous polyposis.
- Secondary prevention is aimed at preventing malignancy in a population that has already manifested an initial disease process. Secondary prevention includes procedures ranging from colonoscopic removal of precancerous polyps detected during screening colonoscopy to total colectomy for high-risk individuals (e.g., familial adenomatous polyposis).
- Current United States guidelines for average-risk individuals include annual occult fecal blood testing starting at age 50 years and examination of the colon every 5 or 10 years, depending on the procedure.

CLINICAL MANIFESTATIONS

- Signs and symptoms of colorectal cancer can be extremely varied, subtle, and nonspecific. Patients with early-stage colorectal cancer are often asymptomatic, and lesions are usually detected by screening procedures.
- Blood in the stool is the most common sign; however, any change in bowel habits, vague abdominal discomfort, or abdominal distention may be a warning sign. Less common signs and symptoms include nausea, vomiting, and, if anemia is severe, fatigue.
- Approximately 19% of patients with colorectal cancer present with metastatic disease. The most common site of metastasis is the liver, followed by the lungs and bones.

DIAGNOSIS

- When colorectal carcinoma is suspected, a careful personal and family history and physical examination should be performed.
- The entire large bowel should be evaluated by colonoscopy or flexible sigmoidoscopy with double-contrast barium enema.
- Baseline laboratory tests should include complete blood cell count, international normalized ratio (INR), activated partial thromboplastin time, liver and renal function tests, and serum carcinoembryonic antigen (CEA). Serum CEA can serve as a marker for monitoring colorectal cancer response to treatment, but it is too insensitive and nonspecific to be used as a screening test for early-stage colorectal cancer.
- Radiographic imaging studies may include chest radiographs, bone scan, chest and abdominal computed tomography scans, positron emission tomography, ultrasonography, and magnetic resonance imaging.
- Immunodetection of tumors using tumor-directed antibodies is an imaging technique for determining the location and extent of extrahepatic disease. These tests might also be useful for identifying metastatic or recurrent disease in patients with rising CEA levels.
- Stage of colorectal cancer should be determined at diagnosis to predict prognosis and to develop treatment options. Stage is based on the size of the primary tumor (T_{1-4}), presence and extent of lymph node involvement (N_{0-2}), and presence or absence of distant metastases (M).
  - ✓ Stage I disease involves tumor invasion of the submucosa (T_1) or muscularis propria (T_2) and negative lymph nodes.
  - ✓ Stage II disease involves tumor invasion through the muscularis propria into pericolorectal tissues (T_3), or penetration to the surface of the visceral peritoneum (T_{4a}), or directly invades or is adherent to other organs or structures (T_{4b}), and negative lymph nodes.
  - ✓ Stage III disease includes T_{1-4} and positive regional lymph nodes.
  - ✓ Stage IV disease includes any T, any N, and distant metastasis.

PROGNOSIS

- Stage at diagnosis is the most important independent prognostic factor for survival and disease recurrence. Five-year relative survival is ~92% for those with localized tumor at diagnosis as compared with 11% for those with metastatic disease at diagnosis.
- Poor prognostic clinical factors at diagnosis include bowel obstruction or perforation, rectal bleeding, high preoperative CEA level, distant metastases, and location of the primary tumor in the rectum or rectosigmoid area. Studies to determine the prognostic use of genetic factors are ongoing.

DESIRED OUTCOME

- The goal of treatment depends on the stage of disease. Stages I, II, and III are potentially curable; the intent is to eradicate micrometastatic disease. Twenty to thirty percent of patients with metastatic disease may be cured if their metastases are resectable. Most stage IV disease is incurable; palliative treatment is given to reduce symptoms, avoid disease-related complications, and prolong survival.

TREATMENT

GENERAL APPROACH

- Treatment modalities are surgery, radiation therapy (RT), chemotherapy, and biomodulators. Adjuvant therapy for early-stage disease and treatment of metastatic disease will be discussed separately.

OPERABLE DISEASE

Surgery

- Complete surgical resection of the primary tumor is a curative approach for patients with operable colorectal cancer.
- Surgery for colon cancer generally involves complete tumor resection with an appropriate margin of tumor-free bowel and a regional lymphadenectomy.
- Surgery for rectal cancer depends on the area involved. Although <33% of these patients require permanent colostomy, frequent complications include urinary retention, incontinence, impotence, and locoregional recurrence.
- Common complications of surgery for both colon and rectal cancer include infection, anastomotic leakage, obstruction, adhesions, and malabsorption syndromes.

Adjuvant Therapy for Colon Cancer

- Adjuvant therapy is administered after complete tumor resection to eliminate residual local or metastatic microscopic disease. Adjuvant therapy is not indicated for stage I colorectal cancer because >90% of patients are cured by surgical resection alone.
- Results of adjuvant chemotherapy studies in patients with stage II disease are conflicting. Despite a lack of consensus among practitioners, the approach to treatment of high-risk stage II and stage III disease is similar.
- Adjuvant chemotherapy is the standard of care for stage III colon cancer.

Adjuvant Radiation Therapy

- Adjuvant RT has no definitive role in colon cancer because most recurrences are extrapelvic and occur in the abdomen.
- Acute adverse effects associated with RT include hematologic depression, dysuria, diarrhea, abdominal cramping, and proctitis. Chronic symptoms may persist for months after RT and may involve diarrhea, proctitis, enteritis, small bowel obstruction, perineal tenderness, and impaired wound healing.

Adjuvant Chemotherapy

- **Fluorouracil** is the most widely used chemotherapeutic agent for colorectal cancer. **Leucovorin** is usually added to fluorouracil as a biochemical modulator to enhance cytotoxic activity.

- Administration method affects clinical activity and toxicity. Fluorouracil is administered by IV bolus or by continuous IV infusion. Efficacy evaluations favor continuous infusion fluorouracil, but none of the combination regimens with leucovorin has proven superior with regard to overall patient survival.
- Continuous IV infusion of fluorouracil is generally well tolerated but is associated with palmar-plantar erythrodysesthesia (hand–foot syndrome) and stomatitis. IV bolus administration is associated with leukopenia, which is dose limiting and can be life threatening. Both administration methods are associated with a similar incidence of mucositis, diarrhea, nausea and vomiting, and alopecia.
- In rare cases, patients deficient in dihydropyrimidine dehydrogenase, responsible for the catabolism of fluorouracil, develop severe toxicity, including death, after fluorouracil administration.
- **Capecitabine,** an oral prodrug of fluorouracil, has efficacy and safety profiles similar to those of IV infusion of fluorouracil.
- National guidelines recommend **oxaliplatin**-based regimens as the first-line option for patients with stage III colon cancer who can tolerate combination therapy. It is commonly administered with fluorouracil/leucovorin.
- Oxaliplatin is associated with paresthesia, neutropenia, and GI toxicity. *Acute neuropathy* is reversible within 2 weeks, usually occurs peripherally but may occur in the jaw and tongue, and is precipitated by exposure to cold. *Persistent neuropathy* is cumulative and is characterized by paresthesias, dysesthesias, and hypoesthesias that usually resolve with dosage reductions or cessation of oxaliplatin therapy.
- Selection of an adjuvant regimen (**Table 63–1**) is based on patient-specific factors, including performance status, comorbid conditions, and patient preference based on lifestyle factors.
- Fluorouracil/leucovorin regimens currently have limited use but are acceptable options in patients who cannot receive oxaliplatin and are unable to tolerate oral capecitabine.

Adjuvant Therapy for Rectal Cancer

- Rectal cancer is more difficult to resect with wide margins, so local recurrences are more frequent than with colon cancer. Adjuvant RT plus chemotherapy is considered the standard of care for stages II and III rectal cancer.
- RT reduces the risk of local tumor recurrence in patients undergoing surgery for rectal cancer. RT is given prior to surgery to decrease tumor size, making it more resectable. Postoperative RT is used to treat a defined area but is associated with more toxicity.
- Fluorouracil enhances the cytotoxic effects of RT. Compared with surgery alone, the combination of adjuvant fluorouracil and RT for 6 months reduces local and distant tumor recurrences and improves survival in stages II and III rectal cancer.
- Preoperative (neoadjuvant) RT shrinks rectal tumors prior to surgical resection, improving sphincter preservation. Preoperative infusional fluorouracil-based chemotherapy plus RT is the preferred

TABLE 63–1	Chemotherapy Regimens for the Adjuvant Treatment of Colorectal Cancer	
Regimen	**Agents**	**Comment**
FOLFOX4[a]	Oxaliplatin 85 mg/m^2 IV day 1 Leucovorin 200 mg/m^2 per day IV over 2 hours days 1 and 2 Fluorouracil 400 mg/m^2 IV bolus, after leucovorin, then 600 mg/m^2 CIV over 22 hours days 1 and 2 • Repeat every 14 days	Improved OS and DFS as compared with infusional fluorouracil–leucovorin–based regimens.
FLOX[b]	Oxaliplatin 85 mg/m^2 IV administered on weeks 1, 3, and 5 Fluorouracil 500 mg/m^2 IV bolus weekly for 6 weeks Leucovorin 500 mg/m^2 IV weekly for 6 weeks • Each cycle lasts 8 weeks and is repeated for three cycles	Improved DFS as compared with bolus fluorouracil-leucovorin–based regimens. Increased toxicity compared with FOLFOX4.
Capecitabine	Capecitabine 1,250 mg/m^2 PO twice daily on days 1 through 14 every 21 days	Equivalent DFS as compared with the Mayo Clinic regimen with improved tolerability.
Fluorouracil-based regimens		
Roswell Park regimen[c]	Fluorouracil 600 mg/m^2 per day IV, day 1 Leucovorin 500 mg/m^2 per day IV over 2 hours • Repeat weekly for 6 of 8 weeks	
Mayo Clinic regimen[d]	Fluorouracil 425 mg/m^2 per day IV, days 1–5 Leucovorin 20 mg/m^2 per day IV, days 1–5 • Repeat every 4 to 5 weeks	
de Gramont regimen[e]	Fluorouracil 400 mg/m^2 per day IV bolus, followed by 600 mg/m^2 CIV over 22 hours, days 1 and 2 for 2 consecutive days Leucovorin 200 mg/m^2 per day IV over 2 hours days 1 and 2 • Repeat every 2 weeks	Improved safety as compared with the Mayo Clinic regimen.

CIV, continuous intravenous infusion; DFS, disease-free survival; OS, overall survival.
[a]Giantonio BJ, Catalano PJ, Meropol NJ, et al. J Clin Oncol 2007;25:1539–1544.
[b]Kuebler JP, Wieand HS, O'Connell MJ, et al. J Clin Oncol 2007;25:2198–2204.
[c]Wolmark N, Rockette H, Fisher B, et al. J Clin Oncol 1993;11:1879–1887.
[d]O'Connell MJ, Mailliard JA, Kahn MJ, et al. J Clin Oncol 1997;15:246–250.
[e]de Gramont A, Bosset JF, Milan C, et al. J Clin Oncol 1997;15:808–815.

treatment for resectable T_3N_0 or any T, N_{1-2} lesions. Patients should receive adjuvant chemotherapy following surgery to total 6 months of chemotherapy.
- Neoadjuvant fluorouracil or capecitabine chemoradiation followed by surgery should be considered for locally unresectable tumors (T_4).
- All patients who receive preoperative chemotherapy for rectal cancer should receive postoperative chemotherapy, regardless of whether the disease was initially resectable.

METASTATIC DISEASE

Initial Therapy

- Chemotherapy is the primary treatment modality for metastatic colorectal cancer (MCRC). Currently, most MCRCs are incurable. Initial chemotherapy is administered with palliative intent: to reduce symptoms, improve quality –of life, and extend survival. In general, treatment options are similar for metastatic cancer of the colon and rectum.
- Surgical resection of discrete metastases in select patients may extend disease-free survival. Resection of hepatic-limited metastases may result in cure. Adjuvant chemotherapy may be administered, but the optimal regimen remains to be determined.
- Neoadjuvant chemotherapy is administered to patients with liver metastases to increase complete resection rates with resectable or unresectable liver lesions. **Oxaliplatin**-based regimens with or without **bevacizumab** are commonly used. A total of 6 months of chemotherapy (pre- and postoperative) should be administered.
- Symptom control is the primary goal of RT in advanced or metastatic colorectal cancer.

Chemotherapy

- Site(s) of tumor involvement and history of prior chemotherapy help define a management strategy for MCRC. Various chemotherapy regimens are recommended by national guidelines for initial palliative chemotherapy (**Table 63–2**). The results of recent meta-analyses suggest that palliative chemotherapy improves survival in MCRC.
- The most important factor in patient survival is not the initial chemotherapy regimen but ensuring that patients receive all three active drugs (fluorouracil, irinotecan, and oxaliplatin) at some point in their treatment course.
- Either **irinotecan** or **oxaliplatin** plus **fluorouracil** and **leucovorin** is recommended as first-line therapy for MCRC (FOLFOX, FOLFIRI). These regimens result in improved response rates and progression-free survival, as well as improved median survival.
- **Irinotecan** is a topoisomerase I inhibitor. Early- and late-onset diarrhea and neutropenia are dose-limiting toxicities of irinotecan.
- Early-onset diarrhea occurs 2 to 6 hours after administration and is characterized by lacrimation, diaphoresis, abdominal cramping, flushing, and/

TABLE 63–2 Chemotherapeutic Regimens for Metastatic Colorectal Cancer

Regimen		Major Dose-limiting Toxicities/Comments
Initial therapy		
Oxaliplatin plus fluorouracil plus leucovorin		
Oxaliplatin plus bimonthly infusional fluorouracil; FOLFOX4[e]	Oxaliplatin 85 mg/m² IV day 1 plus bolus fluorouracil 400 mg/m² IV plus leucovorin 200 mg/m² IV followed by fluorouracil 600 mg/m² IV in 22-hour infusion on days 1 and 2, every 2 weeks	Sensory neuropathy, neutropenia
mFOLFOX6[f]	Oxaliplatin 85 mg/m² IV day 1 plus leucovorin 400 mg/m² IV on day 1 followed by fluorouracil 400 mg/m² IV bolus on day 1, then 1,200 mg/m²/day for 2 days (total 2,400 mg/m² over 45–48 hours) continuous infusion, repeat every 2 weeks	Sensory neuropathy, neutropenia; easier administration as compared with FOLFOX4
Irinotecan plus fluorouracil plus leucovorin		
Irinotecan plus infusional fluorouracil; FOLFIRI[g]	Irinotecan 180 mg/m² IV plus leucovorin 400 mg/m² IV plus bolus fluorouracil 400 mg/m², followed by fluorouracil 2,400 mg/m² CIV infusion over 46 hours on day 1, repeated every 2 weeks	Nausea, diarrhea, mucositis, neutropenia
Biweekly irinotecan plus infusional fluorouracil[h]	Irinotecan 180 mg/m² IV day 1 plus leucovorin 400 mg/m², then fluorouracil 400 mg/m² IV, followed by fluorouracil 600 mg/m² CIV infusion over 22 hours, days 1 and 2, repeated every 2 weeks	Neutropenia, diarrhea
Bevacizumab		
Bevacizumab plus fluorouracil-based regimens	Bevacizumab 5 mg/kg IV every 2 weeks plus fluorouracil and leucovorin (given in any schedule below) or FOLFOX or CapeOx or FOLFIRI	Hypertension, thrombosis, proteinuria from bevacizumab added to toxicities of regimen chosen

(continued)

TABLE 63-2 Chemotherapeutic Regimens for Metastatic Colorectal Cancer (*Continued*)

	Regimen	Major Dose-limiting Toxicities/Comments
Capecitabine		
Capecitabine monotherapy[j]	See Table 63-1[a]	Diarrhea, hand-foot syndrome
CapeOx[k]	Oxaliplatin 130 mg/m² day 1 plus capecitabine 850 mg/m² twice a day for 14 days, repeat every 3 weeks	Diarrhea, hand-foot syndrome, neuropathies
Fluorouracil plus leucovorin only		
Bolus plus infusional fluorouracil; (LV5FU2); de Gramont regimen[i]	See Table 63-1[a]	Neutropenia, mucositis
Salvage therapy[b]		
Irinotecan		
Weekly irinotecan[k]	Irinotecan 125 mg/m² IV every week for 4 of 6 weeks	Neutropenia, diarrhea
Every-3-weeks irinotecan[l]	Irinotecan 350 mg/m² IV every 3 weeks	Neutropenia, diarrhea (less-than-weekly irinotecan)
Oxaliplatin plus fluorouracil plus leucovorin		
Oxaliplatin plus bimonthly infusional fluorouracil; FOLFOX4[m]	Same as FOLFOX4 above; CapeOx may be used in place of FOLFOX4	Sensory neuropathy, neutropenia
Cetuximab		
Cetuximab plus irinotecan[cn]	Continue irinotecan as previously dosed, plus cetuximab 400 mg/m² IV loading dose, then cetuximab 250 mg/m² IV weekly thereafter; if cetuximab is used for FOLFIRI, the dose is the same	Asthenia, diarrhea, nausea, acneiform rash, vomiting

Cetuximab[d,n]	Cetuximab 400 mg/m² IV loading dose, then cetuximab 250 mg/m² IV weekly thereafter	Papulopustular and follicular rash, asthenia, constipation, diarrhea, allergic reactions, hypomagnesemia
Panitumumab	6 mg/kg IV over 60 minutes every 2 weeks	Rash, hypomagnesemia, rare allergic reactions
Fluorouracil		
Protracted continuous infusion[o]	Fluorouracil 250–300 mg/m² daily CIV infusion until disease progression	Mucositis, hand–foot syndrome

[a]Doses and schedule the same as those in the adjuvant setting.
[b]See Fig. 63-1 for comments or salvage regimens.
[c]If irinotecan-refractory disease.
[d]If patient cannot tolerate irinotecan.
[e]Giantonio BJ, Catalano PJ, Meropol NJ, et al. J Clin Oncol 2007;25:1539–1544.
[f]Hochster HS, Hart LL, Ramanathan RK, et al. J Clin Oncol 2008;26:3523–3529.
[g]Tournigand C, Andre T, Achille E et al. J Clin Oncol 2004;22:229–237.
[h]Douillard J, Cunningham D, Roth A, et al. Lancet 2000;355:1041–1047.
[i]Twelves C. Eur J Cancer 2002;38:15–20.
[j]de Gramont A, Bosset JF, Milan C, et al. J Clin Oncol 1997;15:808–815.
[k]Saltz LB, Cox JV, Blanke C, et al. N Engl J Med 2000;343:905–914.
[l]Cunningham D, Pyrhonen S, James R, et al. Lancet 1998;352:1413–1418.
[m]deGramont A, Figer A, Seymour M, et al. J Clin Oncol 2000;18:2938–2947.
[n]Cunningham D, Humblet Y, Siena S, et al. N Engl J Med 2004;351:337–345.
[o]Rougier P, Van Cutsem E, Bajetta E, et al. Lancet 1998;352:1407–1412.

or diarrhea. These cholinergic symptoms respond to IV or subcutaneous **atropine,** 0.25 to 1 mg.

- Late-onset diarrhea occurs 1 to 12 days after administration, lasts 3 to 5 days, and can be fatal. Late-onset diarrhea requires aggressive, high-dose **loperamide** beginning with 4 mg after the first soft or watery stool, followed by 2 mg every 2 hours until symptom free for 12 hours.

- **Capecitabine** monotherapy is suitable for first-line therapy in patients not likely to tolerate IV chemotherapy. Capecitabine is s suitable replacement for infusional fluorouracil in combination with oxaliplatin (CapeOx).

- **Bevacizumab** is a humanized monoclonal antibody directed against vascular endothelial growth factor. The addition of bevacizumab to fluorouracil-based regimens improves response rates, time to progression, and median survival compared with chemotherapy alone, and the resulting four-drug regimens are considered first-line therapy for MCRC.

- Bevacizumab is associated with hypertension, which is easily managed with oral antihypertensive agents. Other safety concerns are bleeding, thrombocytopenia, and proteinuria. GI perforation is a rare but potentially fatal complication necessitating prompt evaluation of abdominal pain associated with vomiting or constipation.

- **Cetuximab** is a chimeric monoclonal antibody directed against epidermal growth factor receptor. Common adverse events include acne-like skin rash, asthenia, lethargy, malaise, and fatigue.

- Treatment guidelines also include the addition of cetuximab to FOLFIRI, FOLFOX, or CapeOx as initial therapy in patients with wild-type *KRAS* tumors only.

Second-Line Therapy

- The selection of second-line chemotherapy is primarily based on the type of prior therapy received, as well as the response to prior treatments, site and extent of disease, and patient factors and treatment preferences. The optimal sequence of regimens has not been established. **Fig. 63–1** depicts an algorithm for the treatment of refractory metastatic disease.

- If disease progressed on first-line bevacizumab, data do not support continued use.

- Cetuximab, either alone or in combination with irinotecan, can be used in patients with disease progression on irinotecan. Cetuximab monotherapy can also be considered as salvage therapy in patients with irinotecan- or oxaliplatin-refractory disease.

- **Panitumumab** is a human monoclonal antibody directed against epidermal growth factor receptor. Common adverse events are dermatologic toxicities, fatigue, abdominal pain, nausea, and diarrhea. As with cetuximab, the use of panitumumab should be limited to patients with wild-type *KRAS* tumors only.

- Panitumumab is approved for use in MCRC that no longer responds to previous therapy with fluorouracil, irinotecan, or oxaliplatin.

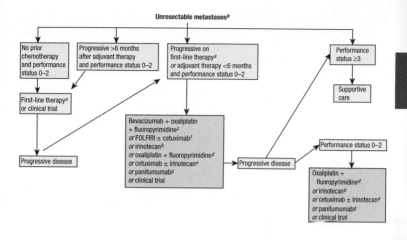

Unresectable metastases[h]

[a] Bevacizumab + oxaliplatin + fluoropyrimidine (e.g., infusional 5-FU/LV (FOLFOX) *or* capecitabine (CapeOx)); *or* bevacizumab + irinotecan + infusional 5-FU/LV (FOLFIRI); *or* bevacizumab + 5FU/LV; *or* capecitabine ± bevacizumab; *or* 5-FU/LV ± bevacizumab.

[b] If no prior irinotecan.

[c] If first-line regimen did not contain bevacizumab or oxaliplatin.

[d] If no prior oxaliplatin.

[e] If irinotecan-refractory or intolerant and no prior cetuximab.

[f] If *KRAS* wild-type and first-line regimen did not contain irinotecan.

[g] If *KRAS* wild-type and no prior cetuximab or panitumumab.

[h] Initial unresectable metastases may be converted to resectable disease in selected patients who exhibit a good tumor response to systemic chemotherapy. Those patients may be candidates for surgical tumor resection followed by adjuvant chemotherapy.

FIGURE 63–1. Algorithm for treatment of unresectable or refractory metastatic colorectal cancer.

- Patients with hepatic-predominant disease whose disease progresses with systemic therapy may be candidates for hepatic-directed therapies such as chemoembolization, cryotherapy, or radiofrequency ablation.

EVALUATION OF THERAPEUTIC OUTCOMES

- The goals of monitoring are to evaluate the benefit of treatment and to detect recurrence.
- Patients who undergo curative surgical resection, with or without adjuvant therapy, require routine follow-up.
- Patients should be evaluated for anticipated side effects such as loose stools or diarrhea, nausea or vomiting, mouth sores, fatigue, and fever.
- Patients should be closely monitored for side effects that require aggressive intervention, such as irinotecan-induced diarrhea and bevacizumab-induced GI perforation. Patients should be evaluated for other treatment-specific side effects, such as oxaliplatin-induced neuropathy, cetuximab and panitumumab-induced skin rash, and bevacizumab-induced hypertension and proteinuria.

785

- Less than one half of patients develop symptoms of recurrence, such as pain syndromes, changes in bowel habits, rectal or vaginal bleeding, pelvic masses, anorexia, and weight loss. CEA levels may help detect recurrences in asymptomatic patients.
- Quality-of-life indices should be monitored, especially in patients with metastatic disease.

See Chapter 138, Colorectal Cancer, authored by Lisa E. Davis, Weijing Sun, and Patrick J. Medina, for a more detailed discussion of this topic.

64 Lung Cancer

DEFINITION

- Lung cancer is a solid tumor originating from bronchial epithelial cells. This chapter distinguishes between non–small cell lung cancer (NSCLC) and small cell lung cancer (SCLC) because they have different natural histories and responses to therapy.

PATHOPHYSIOLOGY

- Lung carcinomas arise from normal bronchial epithelial cells that have acquired multiple genetic lesions and are capable of expressing a variety of phenotypes.
- Activation of protooncogenes, inhibition or mutation of tumor suppressor genes, and production of autocrine growth factors contribute to cellular proliferation and malignant transformation. Molecular changes, such as overexpression of c-KIT in SCLC and epidermal growth factor receptor (EGFR) in NSCLC, also affect disease prognosis and response to therapy.
- Cigarette smoking is responsible for ~80% of lung cancer cases. Other risk factors are exposure to respiratory carcinogens (e.g., asbestos and benzene), genetic risk factors, and history of other lung diseases (e.g., chronic obstructive pulmonary disease [COPD] and asthma).
- The major cell types are SCLC (~15% of all lung cancers), adenocarcinoma (~50%), squamous cell carcinoma (<30%), and large cell carcinoma. The last three types are grouped together and referred to as NSCLC.

CLINICAL PRESENTATION

- The most common initial signs and symptoms are cough, dyspnea, chest pain or discomfort, with or without hemoptysis. Many patients also exhibit systemic symptoms such as anorexia, weight loss, and fatigue.
- Disseminated disease can cause neurologic deficits from CNS metastases, bone pain or pathologic fractures secondary to bone metastases, or liver dysfunction from hepatic involvement.
- Paraneoplastic syndromes commonly associated with lung cancers include cachexia, hypercalcemia, syndrome of inappropriate antidiuretic hormone secretion, and Cushing's syndrome. These syndromes may be the first sign of an underlying malignancy.

DIAGNOSIS

- Chest radiography, endobronchial ultrasound, computed tomography (CT) scan, and positron emission tomography (PET) scan are the most valuable diagnostic tests. Integrated CT–PET technology appears to improve diagnostic accuracy in staging NSCLC over CT or PET alone.

- Pathologic confirmation of lung cancer is established by examination of sputum cytology and/or tumor biopsy by bronchoscopy, mediastinoscopy, percutaneous needle biopsy, or open-lung biopsy.

- All patients must have a thorough history and physical examination to detect signs and symptoms of the primary tumor, regional spread of the tumor, distant metastases, paraneoplastic syndromes, and ability to withstand aggressive surgery or chemotherapy.

STAGING

- The World Health Organization has established a TNM staging classification for lung cancer based on the primary tumor size and extent (T), the regional lymph node involvement (N), and the presence or absence of distant metastases (M).

- A simpler system is commonly used to compare treatments. Stage I includes tumors confined to the lung without lymphatic spread, stage II includes large tumors with ipsilateral peribronchial or hilar lymph node involvement, stage III includes other lymph node and regional involvement, and stage IV includes any tumor with distant metastases.

- A two-stage classification is widely used for SCLC. Limited disease is confined to one hemithorax and can be encompassed by a single radiation port. All other disease is classified as extensive.

TREATMENT

NON–SMALL CELL LUNG CANCER

Desired Outcome

- The stage of NSCLC and the patient's comorbidities and performance status (i.e., the ability to perform activities of daily living) determine which treatment modalities will be used. The intent of treatment—curative or palliative—influences the aggressiveness of therapy.

Recommendations for Chemotherapy, Radiation Therapy, and Surgery

- Local disease (stages IA, IB, and IIA) is associated with a favorable prognosis. Surgery is the mainstay of treatment and may be used with radiation and/or adjuvant (postoperative) chemotherapy (Table 64–1). The adjuvant treatment regimen of choice is not clear.

- Patients with locally advanced disease (stages IIB and IIIA) may undergo surgery. Adjuvant chemotherapy is the standard of care. Some centers use neoadjuvant (preoperative) chemoradiation, but this is not considered the standard of care. Nonresectable locally advanced disease may be treated with both an active **cisplatin**-based regimen and radiotherapy.

- Four to six cycles of doublet chemotherapy with **cisplatin** or **carboplatin** plus **docetaxel, gemcitabine, paclitaxel, pemetrexed,** or **vinorelbine** (see Table 64-1) are recommended as first-line palliative chemotherapy for patients with unresectable stage III or IV disease. Cisplatin-based doublets improve survival and quality of life in this patient population as compared with best supportive care or single-agent chemotherapy. No combination was found to be superior; tolerance of expected toxicities may contribute to the decision.
- Non-platinum-based combination regimens (e.g., **gemcitabine–paclitaxel** and **gemcitabine–docetaxel**) are recommended as first-line therapy of advanced NSCLC in patients with a contraindication to a platinum (cisplatin or carboplatin) agent.

TABLE 64–1	Common Chemotherapy Regimens Used to Treat Lung Cancer
Non–small cell lung carcinoma[a]	
Carboplatin/paclitaxel/bevacizumab	Carboplatin AUC 6 mg/mL/min on day 1
	Paclitaxel 200 mg/m^2 IV on day 1
	Bevacizumab 15 mg/kg IV on day 1
	Repeat cycle every 3 weeks. Continue bevacizumab until progression
Carboplatin/pemetrexed	Carboplatin AUC 5 mg/mL/min on day 1
	Pemetrexed 500 mg/m^2 IV on day 1
	Repeat cycle every 3 weeks
Cetuximab/cisplatin/vinorelbine	Cetuximab 400 mg/m^2 IV first dose on day 1, then 250 mg/m^2 IV weekly
	Cisplatin 80 mg/m^2 IV on day 1
	Vinorelbine 25 mg/m^2 IV on day 1 and day 8
	Repeat cycle every 3 weeks
Cisplatin/paclitaxel (CP)	Cisplatin 75 mg/m^2 IV on day 1
	Paclitaxel 175 mg/m^2 over 24 hours IV on day 1
	Repeat cycle every 21 days[b]
	or
	Cisplatin 80 mg/m^2 IV on day 1
	Paclitaxel 175 mg/m^2 IV over 3 hours on day 1
	Repeat cycle every 21 days[c]
Gemcitabine/cisplatin (GC)	Gemcitabine 1,000 mg/m^2 IV on days 1, 8, and 15
	Cisplatin 100 mg/m^2 IV on day 1
	Repeat cycle every 28 days[b]
Gemcitabine/cisplatin (GCq21)	Gemcitabine 1,200 mg/m^2 on days 1 and 8
	Cisplatin 80 mg/m^2 IV on day 1
	Repeat cycle every 21 days[d]
	or
	Gemcitabine 1,250 mg/m^2 on days 1 and 8
	Cisplatin 80 mg/m^2 IV on day 1
	Repeat cycle every 21 days[c]

(continued)

TABLE 64-1	Common Chemotherapy Regimens Used to Treat Lung Cancer (Continued)

Non–small cell lung carcinoma[a]

Docetaxel/cisplatin (DC)	Docetaxel 75 mg/m^2 IV on day 1 Cisplatin 75 mg/m^2 IV on day 1 Repeat cycle every 21 days[b]
Paclitaxel/carboplatin (PCb)	Paclitaxel 225 mg/m^2 over 3 hours IV on day 1 Carboplatin AUC 6 IV on day 1 Repeat cycle every 21 days[b,e] *or* Paclitaxel 175 mg/m^2 IV over 3 hours on day 1 Carboplatin AUC 6 IV on day 1 Repeat cycle every 21 days for 6 cycles[f]
Vinorelbine/cisplatin (VC)	Vinorelbine 25 mg/m^2 IV weekly Cisplatin 100 mg/m^2 IV on day 1 Repeat cycle every 28 days[e] *or* Vinorelbine 30 mg/m^2 IV on days 1 and 8 Cisplatin 80 mg/m^2 IV on day 1 Repeat cycle every 21 days[d]
Etoposide/cisplatin (EP)	Etoposide 100 mg/m^2 IV on days 1, 2, and 3 Cisplatin 100 mg/m^2 IV on day 1 Repeat cycle every 28 days[b]
Vinorelbine/gemcitabine (VG)	Vinorelbine 25 mg/m^2 IV on days 1 and 8 Gemcitabine 1,000 mg/m^2 on days 1 and 8 Repeat cycle every 21 days[d,g]
Paclitaxel/gemcitabine (PG)	Paclitaxel 175 mg/m^2 IV over 3 hours on day 1 Gemcitabine 1,250 mg/m^2 on days 1 and 8 Repeat cycle every 21 days[c]
Gemcitabine/docetaxel (GD)	Gemcitabine 1,000 mg/m^2 IV on days 1 and 8 Docetaxel 100 mg/m^2 IV on day 8 Repeat cycle every 21 days[h]
Paclitaxel/vinorelbine (PV)	Paclitaxel 135 mg/m^2 IV on day 1 Vinorelbine 25 mg/m^2 IV on day 1 Repeat cycle every 14 days for 9 cycles[f]

Small cell lung carcinoma[i]

Etoposide/cisplatin (EP)	Cisplatin 80 mg/m^2 IV on day 1 Etoposide 100 mg/m^2 IV on days 1, 2, and 3 Repeat cycle every 3 weeks[i,j] *or*
Etoposide/cisplatin (EP)	Cisplatin 60 mg/m^2 IV on day 1 Etoposide 120 mg/m^2 IV on days 1, 2, and 3 Repeat cycle every 3 weeks[k]

(continued)

TABLE 64-1	Common Chemotherapy Regimens Used to Treat Lung Cancer (Continued)

Small cell lung carcinoma[l]

Cisplatin/irinotecan (IP)	Cisplatin 60 mg/m² IV on day 1 Irinotecan 60 mg/m² IV on days 1, 8, and 15 Repeat cycle every 4 weeks[i,j] *or* Cisplatin 30 mg/m² IV on day 1 Irinotecan 65 mg/m² IV on days 1 and 8 Repeat cycle every 3 weeks[k]

AUC, area under the curve.

[a]NCCN Clinical Practice Guidelines in Oncology: Non-Small Cell Lung Cancer. National Comprehensive Cancer Network, 2010. http://www.nccn.org/professionals/physician_gls/PDF/nscl.pdf.

[b]Schiller JH, Harrington D, Belani CP, et al. N Engl J Med 2002;346:92–98.

[c]Smit EF, van Meerbeeck JP, Lianes P, et al. J Clin Oncol 2003;21:3909–3917.

[d]Gridelli C, Gallo C, Shepherd FA, et al. J Clin Oncol 2003;21:3025–3034.

[e]Kelly K, Crowley J, Bunn PA, Jr, et al. J Clin Oncol 2001;19:3210–3218.

[f]Stathopoulos GP, Veslemes M, Georgatou N, et al. Ann Oncol 2004;15:1048–1055.

[g]Lilenbaum RC, Chen CS, Chidiac T, et al. Ann Oncol 2005;16:97–101.

[h]Georgoulias V, Ardavanis A, Tsiafaki X, et al. J Clin Oncol 2005;23:2937–2945.

[i]Noda K, Nishiwaki Y, Kawahara M, et al. N Engl J Med 2002;346:85–91.

[j]Lara PN Jr, Gandara DR, Natale RB. Clin Lung Cancer 2006;7:353–356.

[k]Hanna N, Bunn PA Jr, Langer C, et al. J Clin Oncol 2006;24:2038–2043.

[l]NCCN Clinical Practice Guidelines in Oncology: Small Cell Lung Cancer. National Comprehensive Cancer Network, 2010. http://www.nccn.org/professionals/physician_gls/PDF/sclc.pdf.

- **Docetaxel, pemetrexed,** and an oral EGFR inhibitor, **erlotinib,** are options for unresectable stage III or IV NSCLC patients with good performance status who progress during or after first-line therapy.
- **Cetuximab,** a monoclonal antibody that binds to the extracellular portion of the EGFR receptor, in combination with cisplatin and vinorelbine, prolongs median overall survival by 1 month in patients with advanced NSCLC.
- **Bevacizumab,** a recombinant, humanized monoclonal antibody, neutralizes vascular endothelial growth factor. The addition of bevacizumab to carboplatin–paclitaxel is recommended in advanced NSCLC of nonsquamous cell histology in patients with no history of hemoptysis and no CNS metastasis who are not receiving therapeutic anticoagulation.
- Palliative radiation therapy with chemotherapy may help control local and systemic disease and reduce disease-related symptoms. The optimal delivery method, schedule, and radiation therapy dosages when used with chemotherapy are yet to be determined.

SMALL CELL LUNG CANCER

Desired Outcome

- The goal of treatment is cure or prolonged survival, which requires aggressive combination chemotherapy.

Surgery and Radiation Therapy

- There is no clear role for surgery in SCLC.
- SCLC is very radiosensitive. Radiotherapy has been combined with chemotherapy to treat limited disease SCLC. This combined-modality therapy prevents local tumor recurrences but only modestly improves survival over chemotherapy alone.
- Radiotherapy is used to prevent and treat brain metastases, a frequent occurrence with SCLC. Prophylactic cranial irradiation is used in patients with limited or extensive disease to reduce the risk of brain metastases. Neurologic and intellectual impairment is associated with prophylactic cranial irradiation, although other factors may contribute.
- Radiotherapy followed by combination chemotherapy is recommended for patients with symptomatic brain metastases. **Dexamethasone** and **anticonvulsants** are also administered for symptom control and seizure prevention, respectively.

Chemotherapy

- Chemotherapy with concurrent radiation is recommended for limited- and extensive-disease SCLC. Single-agent chemotherapy is inferior to doublet chemotherapy.
- The most frequently used regimen is **cisplatin** or **carboplatin** combined with **etoposide**. **Irinotecan** in combination with cisplatin has also been shown to be active (see **Table 64–1**). Overall response rates and survival durations are generally superior for patients with limited-stage versus those with extensive-stage disease.
- Recurrent SCLC is usually less sensitive to chemotherapy. If recurrence occurs in >3 months, national guidelines recommend **gemcitabine**, **topotecan**, irinotecan, paclitaxel, docetaxel, CAV (**cyclophosphamide, doxorubicin,** and **vincristine**), and **vinorelbine.**
- Patients with SCLC that recurs within 3 months of first-line chemotherapy are considered refractory to chemotherapy and unlikely to respond to a second-line regimen.

EVALUATION OF THERAPEUTIC OUTCOMES

- Tumor response to chemotherapy for NSCLC should be evaluated at the end of the second or third cycle and at the end of every second cycle thereafter. Patients with stable disease, objective response, or measurable decrease in tumor size should continue treatment until four to six cycles have been administered. Responding patients with nonsquamous histology should be considered for maintenance therapy with pemetrexed.
- Efficacy of first-line therapy for SCLC should be determined after two or three cycles of chemotherapy. If there is no response or progressive disease, therapy can be discontinued or changed to a non-cross-resistant regimen. If responsive to chemotherapy, the induction regimen should be administered for four to six cycles.

- Intensive therapeutic monitoring is required for all patients with lung cancer to avoid drug-related and radiotherapy-related toxicities. These patients frequently have numerous concurrent medical problems requiring close attention.
- References should be consulted for management of common toxicities associated with the aggressive chemotherapy regimens used for lung cancer.

See Chapter 137, Lung Cancer, authored by Deborah A. Frieze and Val R. Adams, for a more detailed discussion of this topic.

DEFINITION

- Lymphomas are a heterogeneous group of malignancies that arise from immune cells residing predominantly in lymphoid tissues. Differences in histology have led to the classification of Hodgkin and non-Hodgkin lymphoma (HL and NHL, respectively), which are addressed separately in this chapter.

HODGKIN LYMPHOMA

PATHOPHYSIOLOGY

- Current hypotheses indicate that B-cell transcriptional processes are disrupted, which prevents expression of B-cell surface markers and production of immunoglobulin messenger RNA. Alterations in the normal apoptotic pathways favor cell survival and proliferation.
- Malignant Reed–Sternberg cells overexpress nuclear factor-κ B, which is associated with cell proliferation and anti-apoptotic signals. Infections with viral and bacterial pathogens upregulate nuclear factor-κ B. Epstein–Barr virus is found in many, but not all, HL tumors.

CLINICAL PRESENTATION

- Most patients with HL present with a painless, rubbery, enlarged lymph node in the supradiaphragmatic area and commonly have mediastinal nodal involvement. Less common asymptomatic adenopathy of the inguinal and axillary regions may be present at diagnosis.
- Constitutional, or "B," symptoms (e.g., fever, drenching night sweats, and weight loss) are present at diagnosis in ~25% of patients with HL.

DIAGNOSIS AND STAGING

- Diagnosis requires the presence of Reed–Sternberg cells in the lymph node biopsy.
- Staging is performed to provide prognostic information and to guide therapy. Clinical staging is based on noninvasive procedures such as history, physical examination, laboratory tests, and radiography, including positron emission tomography (PET). Pathologic staging is based on biopsy findings of strategic sites (e.g., muscle, bone, skin, spleen, and abdominal nodes) using an invasive procedure (e.g., laparoscopy).
- Approximately half of the patients have localized disease (stages I, II, and IIE). The other half have advanced disease at diagnosis, of which 10% to 15% is stage IV.
- Prognosis predominantly depends on age and stage; patients older than 65 to 70 years have a lower cure rate than younger patients. Patients with limited stage disease (stages I and II) have a 90% to 95% cure rate,

whereas those with advanced disease (stages III and IV) have a 60% to 80% cure rate.

TREATMENT SUMMARY

- The treatment goal for HL is to maximize curability while minimizing short- and long-term treatment-related complications.
- Treatment options include radiation therapy, chemotherapy, or both (combined-modality therapy). The therapeutic role of surgery is limited, regardless of stage.
- Combination chemotherapy is the primary treatment modality for most patients with HL.
- Radiation therapy is an integral part of treatment and can be used alone for select patients with early-stage disease, although most patients will receive chemotherapy and radiation. *Involved-field radiation* targets a single field of HL. *Extended-field* or *subtotal nodal radiation* targets the involved field and an uninvolved area. Total nodal radiation targets all areas.
- Long-term complications of radiotherapy, chemotherapy, and chemo-radiotherapy include gonadal dysfunction, secondary malignancies, and cardiac disease. Patients treated for HL are at increased risk of developing secondary malignancies of the lung, breast, GI tract, and connective tissue, as well as leukemia.

Initial Chemotherapy

- Two to eight cycles of chemotherapy should be administered, depending on the stage of disease and the presence of risk factors (Tables 65–1 and 65–2).

Salvage Chemotherapy

- The response to salvage therapy depends on the extent and site of recurrence, previous therapy, and duration of first remission. The choice of salvage therapy should be guided by the response to the initial therapy and a patient's ability to tolerate therapy.
- Patients who relapse after an initial complete response can be treated with the same regimen, a non cross-resistant regimen, radiation therapy, or high-dose chemotherapy and autologous hematopoietic stem cell transplantation (HSCT).
- The lack of complete remission after initial therapy or relapse within 1 year after completing initial therapy is associated with a poor prognosis. Patients with these prognostic factors are candidates for high-dose chemotherapy and HSCT.

NON-HODGKIN LYMPHOMA

PATHOPHYSIOLOGY

- NHLs are derived from monoclonal proliferation of malignant B or, less commonly, T lymphocytes and their precursors. The current classification

TABLE 65–1 General Treatment Recommendations for Hodgkin Lymphoma	
Early-stage disease	
Favorable disease (stage IA or IIA with no risk factors)	Two cycles of Stanford V or four cycles of ABVD followed by involved-field radiation
Unfavorable disease (stage IA or IIA with risk factors [e.g., B symptoms, extranodal disease, bulky disease, three or more sites of nodal involvement, or an ESR >50 mm/h; ≥13.9 μm/s])	Two to four cycles of ABVD plus involved-field radiation; if radiation is omitted, six cycles of ABVD are recommended.
Advanced-stage disease	
Favorable disease (stage III or IV)	Six to eight cycles of ABVD plus radiation to residual disease sites
Unfavorable prognosis (stage III or IV with four or more poor prognostic factors [e.g., low serum albumin, low hemoglobin, male gender, age ≥45 years, high WBC, lymphocytopenia])	Six to eight cycles of escalated-dose BEACOPP plus radiation to residual disease sites
Relapsed disease	
Relapse after radiation	Six to eight cycles of chemotherapy with or without radiation (treat as if this were primary advanced disease)
Relapse after primary chemotherapy[a]	Salvage chemotherapy at conventional doses or high-dose chemotherapy and autologous hematopoietic stem cell transplantation

ABVD, Doxorubicin (Adriamycin), bleomycin, vinblastine, and dacarbazine; BEACOPP, bleomycin, etoposide, doxorubicin (Adriamycin), cyclophosphamide, vincristine (Oncovin), procarbazine, and prednisone; ESR, erythrocyte sedimentation rate; WBC, white blood cell count.
[a]A standard regimen or approach does not exist. See Table 65–2 for details of chemotherapy regimens.

schemes characterize NHLs according to cell of origin, clinical features, and morphologic features.

- The World Health Organization (WHO) classification uses the term *grade* to refer to histologic parameters such as cell and nuclear size, density of chromatin, and proliferation fraction, and the term *aggressiveness* to denote clinical behavior of a tumor.

CLINICAL PRESENTATION

- Patients present with a variety of symptoms, which depend on the site of involvement and whether it is nodal or extranodal.
- Adenopathy can be localized or generalized. Involved nodes are painless, rubbery, and discrete and are usually located in the cervical and supraclavicular regions. Mesenteric or GI involvement can cause nausea, vomiting, obstruction, abdominal pain, palpable abdominal mass, or

TABLE 65–2 Combination Chemotherapy Regimens for Hodgkin Lymphoma

Drug	Dosage (mg/m²)	Route	Days
MOPP			
Mechlorethamine	6	IV	1, 8
Vincristine (Oncovin)	1.4	IV	1, 8
Procarbazine	100	Oral	1–14
Prednisone	40	Oral	1–14
Repeat every 21 days			
ABVD			
Doxorubicin (Adriamycin)	25	IV	1, 15
Bleomycin	10	IV	1, 15
Vinblastine	6	IV	1, 15
Dacarbazine	375	IV	1, 15
Repeat every 28 days			
MOPP/ABVD			
Alternating months of MOPP and ABVD			
MOPP/ABV hybrid			
Mechlorethamine	6	IV	1
Vincristine (Oncovin)	1.4	IV	1
Procarbazine	100	Oral	1–7
Prednisone	40	Oral	1–14
Doxorubicin (Adriamycin)	35	IV	8
Bleomycin	10	IV	8
Vinblastine	6	IV	8
Repeat every 28 days			
Stanford V			
Doxorubicin	25	IV	Weeks 1, 3, 5, 7, 9, 11
Vinblastine	6	IV	Weeks 1, 3, 5, 7, 9, 11
Mechlorethamine	6	IV	Weeks 1, 5, 9
Etoposide	60	IV	Weeks 3, 7, 11
Vincristine	1.4ᵃ	IV	Weeks 2, 4, 6, 8, 10, 12
Bleomycin	5	IV	Weeks 2, 4, 6, 8
Prednisone	40	Oral	Every other day for 12 weeks; begin tapering at week 10
One course (12 weeks)			
Procarbazine	100	Oral	1–7
Repeat every 21 days			

(continued)

TABLE 65–2	Combination Chemotherapy Regimens for Hodgkin Lymphoma *(Continued)*		
Drug	**Dosage (mg/m²)**	**Route**	**Days**
BEACOPP (escalated-dose)			
Bleomycin	10	IV	8
Etoposide	200	IV	1–3
Doxorubicin (Adriamycin)	35	IV	1
Cyclophosphamide	1,250	IV	1
Vincristine (Oncovin)	1.4[a]	IV	8
Procarbazine	100	Oral	1–7
Prednisone	40	Oral	1–14
Granulocyte colony-stimulating factor		Subcutaneously	8+
Repeat every 21 days			

[a]Vincristine dose capped at 2 mg.

GI bleeding. Bone marrow involvement can cause symptoms related to anemia, neutropenia, or thrombocytopenia.

- Forty percent of patients with NHL present with B symptoms—fever, drenching night sweats, and weight loss.

DIAGNOSIS AND STAGING

- Diagnosis is established by biopsy of an involved lymph node.
- Diagnostic workup of NHL is generally similar to that of HL.
- Systems for classifying NHLs continue to evolve. Lymphomas can be classified by degree of aggressiveness. Slow-growing or indolent lymphomas are favorable (untreated survival measured in years), whereas rapid-growing or aggressive lymphomas are unfavorable (untreated survival measured in weeks to months).
- Prognosis depends on histologic subtype and clinical risk factors (e.g., age >60 years, performance status of 2 or more, abnormal lactate dehydrogenase, extranodal involvement, and stage III or IV disease). These risk factors are used to calculate the International Prognostic Index; it is most useful in patients with aggressive lymphomas.
- A newer prognostic index for patients with indolent (follicular) lymphomas uses similar risk factors except that poor performance status is replaced with low hemoglobin (<12 g/dL [<120 g/L; 7.45 mmol/L]). Current research is focused on the prognostic importance of phenotypic and molecular characteristics of NHL.

DESIRED OUTCOME

- The primary treatment goals for NHL are to relieve symptoms and, whenever possible, cure the patient of disease while minimizing the risk of serious toxicity.

TREATMENT

General Principles

- Appropriate therapy for NHL depends on many factors, including patient age, histologic type, stage and site of disease, presence of adverse prognostic factors, and patient preference.
- Treatment is divided into two categories: limited disease (e.g., localized disease; Ann Arbor stages I and II) and advanced disease (e.g., Ann Arbor stage III or IV and stage II patients with poor prognostic features).
- Treatment options include radiation therapy, chemotherapy, and biologic agents.
- Radiation therapy is rarely suitable for remission induction because NHL is rarely localized at diagnosis. It is used more commonly in advanced disease, mainly as a palliative measure.
- Effective chemotherapy ranges from single-agent therapy for indolent lymphomas to aggressive, complex combination regimens for aggressive lymphomas.
- Treatment strategies are summarized for the most common NHLs as examples of how to treat indolent (i.e., follicular) and aggressive (i.e., diffuse large B-cell) lymphomas. Strategies are also summarized for acquired immunodeficiency syndrome (AIDS)–related lymphoma.

Indolent Lymphomas

- Follicular lymphomas occur in older adults, with a majority having advanced disease at diagnosis. At diagnosis, most patients have the chromosomal translocation t(14;18). The clinical course is generally indolent, with median survival of 8 to 10 years. The natural history of follicular lymphoma is unpredictable, with spontaneous regression of objective disease seen in 20% to 30% of patients.

LOCALIZED FOLLICULAR LYMPHOMA

- Options for stage I and II follicular lymphoma include locoregional radiation therapy and immunotherapy (i.e., **rituximab**) with or without chemotherapy or radiation therapy.
- Radiation therapy is the standard treatment and is usually curative. Chemotherapy is not recommended, unless the patient has high-risk, stage II disease.

ADVANCED FOLLICULAR LYMPHOMA

- Management of stages III and IV indolent lymphoma is controversial because standard approaches are not curative. Median time to relapse is only 18 to 36 months. After relapse, response can be reinduced; however, response rates and durations decrease with each retreatment.
- Therapeutic options are diverse and include watchful waiting, radiation therapy, single-agent therapy, combination chemotherapy, biologic therapy, radioimmunotherapy, and combined-modality therapy. Immediate aggressive therapy does not improve survival compared with conservative therapy (i.e., watchful waiting followed by single-agent chemotherapy, **rituximab,** or radiation therapy, when treatment is needed).

- Oral alkylating agents **chlorambucil** or **cyclophosphamide,** used alone or in combination with **prednisone,** are the mainstay of treatment. These single agents are as effective as combination regimens and produce minimal toxicity, but secondary acute leukemia is a concern. **Bendamustine** is an IV alkylating agent approved for relapsed or refractory indolent NHL.

- Two adenosine analogues, **fludarabine** and **cladribine,** produce high response rates in previously untreated and relapsed advanced follicular lymphoma. Their use is associated with prolonged myelosuppression and profound immunosuppression, increasing the risk of opportunistic infections.

- **Rituximab,** a chimeric monoclonal antibody directed at the CD20 molecule on B cells, has become one of the most widely used therapies for follicular lymphoma. Rituximab is approved for first-line therapy either alone or combined with chemotherapy and as maintenance therapy for patients with stable disease or with partial or complete response following induction chemotherapy.

- The most common chemotherapy regimen used with rituximab is the CHOP regimen (Table 65–3). Several different maintenance rituximab schedules have been studied. No consistent overall survival benefit has been observed with maintenance rituximab. Practice guidelines list rituximab maintenance as an option in both first- and second-line therapy, but the strength of the recommendation depends on the treatment setting.

- Adverse effects are usually infusion related, especially after the first infusion of rituximab, and consist of fever, chills, respiratory symptoms, fatigue, headache, pruritus, and angioedema. Patients should receive oral **acetaminophen,** 650 mg, and **diphenhydramine,** 50 mg, 30 minutes before the infusion.

- Anti-CD20 radioimmunoconjugates are mouse antibodies linked to radioisotopes (e.g., [131]I-**tositumomab** and [90]Y-**ibritumomab tiuxetan**). They have the advantage of delivering radiation to tumor cells expressing the CD20 antigen and to adjacent tumor cells that do not express it. They have the disadvantage of damaging adjacent normal tissue (e.g., bone marrow).

- Radioimmunotherapy was initially used as salvage therapy and is being evaluated as first-line therapy in combination with CHOP.

TABLE 65–3 Combination Chemotherapy for Non-Hodgkin Lymphoma (CHOP)[a,b]

Drug	Dose (mg/m²)	Route	Days
Cyclophosphamide	750	IV	1
Doxorubicin	50	IV	1
Vincristine	1.4	IV	1
Prednisone	100	Oral	1–5

[a]Cycle should be repeated every 21 days.
[b]Rituximab 375 mg/m² on day 1 is commonly added (R-CHOP).

- Radioimmunotherapy is generally well tolerated. Toxicities include infusion-related reactions, myelosuppression, and possibly myelodysplastic syndrome or acute myelogenous leukemia. ^{131}I-tositumomab can cause thyroid dysfunction.
- The decision to use radioimmunotherapy requires consideration of the complexity, risks, and cost. The ideal candidate has limited bone marrow involvement and adequate blood cell counts.
- High-dose chemotherapy followed by HSCT is an option for relapsed follicular lymphoma. The recurrence rate is lower after allogeneic than after autologous HSCT, but the benefit is offset by increased treatment-related mortality.

Aggressive Lymphomas

- Diffuse large B-cell lymphomas (DLBCLs) are the most common lymphoma in patients of all ages but most commonly seen in the seventh decade. Extranodal disease is present at diagnosis in 30% to 40% of patients. The International Prognostic Index score correlates with prognosis. Diffuse aggressive lymphomas are sensitive to chemotherapy, with cure achieved in some patients.

TREATMENT OF LOCALIZED DISEASE

- Stage I and nonbulky stage II should be treated with three or four cycles of rituximab and CHOP (R-CHOP) (**Table 65–3**) followed by locoregional radiation therapy.
- Patients with at least one adverse risk factor should receive six to eight cycles of R-CHOP followed by locoregional radiation therapy.

TREATMENT OF ADVANCED DISEASE

- Bulky stage II and stages III and IV lymphoma should be treated with R-CHOP or rituximab and CHOP-like chemotherapy until achieving complete response (usually four cycles). Two or more additional cycles should be given following complete response for a total of six to eight cycles. Maintenance therapy following a complete response does not improve survival.
- High-dose chemotherapy with autologous HSCT should be considered in high risk patients who respond to standard chemotherapy and are candidates for autologous HSCT.
- Although historically, elderly adults have lower complete response and survival rates than younger patients, full dose R-CHOP is recommended as initial treatment for aggressive lymphoma in the elderly.

TREATMENT OF REFRACTORY OR RELAPSED DISEASE

- Approximately one third of patients with aggressive lymphoma will require salvage therapy at some point. Salvage therapy is more likely to induce response if the response to initial chemotherapy was complete (chemosensitivity) than if it was primarily or partially resistant to chemotherapy.
- High-dose chemotherapy with autologous HSCT is the therapy of choice for younger patients with chemosensitive relapse.

- Salvage regimens incorporate drugs not used as initial therapy. Commonly used regimens include DHAP (**dexamethasone, cytarabine,** and **cisplatin**), ESHAP (**etoposide, methylprednisolone,** cytarabine, and cisplatin), and MINE (**mesna, ifosfamide, mitoxantrone,** and **etoposide**). None is clearly superior to the others.
- ICE (ifosfamide, **carboplatin,** and etoposide) appears to be better tolerated than cisplatin-containing regimens, especially in elderly adults.
- Rituximab is being evaluated in combination with many salvage regimens.

NON-HODGKIN LYMPHOMA IN ACQUIRED IMMUNODEFICIENCY SYNDROME

- Patients with AIDS have more than a 100-fold increased risk of developing NHL, which is usually aggressive (e.g., Burkitt or DLBCL).
- Treatment of AIDS-related lymphoma is difficult because underlying immunodeficiency increases the risk of treatment-related myelosuppression.
- Standard combination regimens (e.g., CHOP) yield disappointing results. Newer approaches, including dose-adjusted EPOCH (etoposide, prednisone, vincristine, cyclophosphamide, and doxorubicin), appear promising. The role of rituximab in the treatment of AIDS-related DLBCL is not clear.
- Prophylactic antibiotics should be continued during chemotherapy, but the optimal timing for highly active antiretroviral therapy (HAART) is not clear in patients with AIDS-related lymphoma.

EVALUATION OF THERAPEUTIC OUTCOMES

- The primary outcome to be identified is tumor response, which is based on physical examination, radiologic evidence, PET/computed tomography (CT) scanning, and other baseline findings. Complete response is desirable because it yields the only chance for cure.
- Patients are evaluated for response at the end of four cycles or, if treatment is shorter, at the end of treatment.
- Optimal outcomes for most types of lymphoma may require delivery of full doses on time. Hematopoietic growth factors and other supportive care measures are often needed to achieve this goal.
- To optimize chemotherapy administration, the clinician must identify, monitor, treat, and prevent or minimize treatment-related toxicity. Pertinent laboratory data and other procedures should be reviewed to establish a baseline for monitoring purposes.

See Chapter 140, Lymphomas, authored by Alexandre Chan and Gary C. Yee, for a more detailed discussion of this topic.

66 Prostate Cancer

DEFINITION

- Prostate cancer is a malignant neoplasm that arises from the prostate gland. Prostate cancer has an indolent course; localized prostate cancer is curable by surgery or radiation therapy, but advanced prostate cancer is not yet curable.

PATHOPHYSIOLOGY

- The normal prostate is composed of acinar secretory cells that are altered when invaded by cancer. The major pathologic cell type is adenocarcinoma (>95% of cases).
- Prostate cancer can be graded. Well-differentiated tumors grow slowly, whereas poorly differentiated tumors grow rapidly and have a poor prognosis.
- Metastatic spread can occur by local extension, lymphatic drainage, or hematogenous dissemination. Skeletal metastases from hematogenous spread are the most common sites of distant spread. The lung, liver, brain, and adrenal glands are the most common sites of visceral involvement, but these organs are not usually involved initially.
- The rationale for hormone therapy is based on the effect of androgens on the growth and differentiation of the normal prostate (Fig. 66–1).
- The testes and the adrenal glands are the major sources of androgens, specifically dihydrotestosterone (DHT).
- Luteinizing hormone–releasing hormone (LH-RH) from the hypothalamus stimulates the release of luteinizing hormone (LH) and follicle-stimulating hormone (FSH) from the anterior pituitary gland.
- LH complexes with receptors on the Leydig cell testicular membrane and stimulates the production of testosterone and small amounts of estrogen.
- FSH acts on testicular Sertoli cells to promote maturation of LH receptors and produce an androgen-binding protein.
- Circulating testosterone and estradiol influence the synthesis of LH-RH, LH, and FSH by a negative-feedback loop at the hypothalamic and pituitary level.
- Only 2% of total plasma testosterone is present in the active unbound state that penetrates the prostate cell, where it is converted to DHT by 5-α-reductase. DHT subsequently binds with a cytoplasmic receptor and is transported to the cell nucleus, where transcription and translation of stored genetic material occur.

CHEMOPREVENTION

- The risk of prostate cancer was reduced ~25% in patients taking **finasteride** for treatment of benign prostatic hypertrophy (BPH), but prostate cancer diagnosed in patients on finasteride is more aggressive.

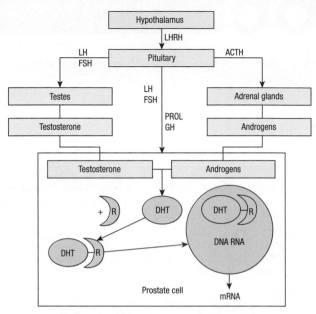

FIGURE 66–1. Hormonal regulation of the prostate gland. (ACTH, adreno-corticotropic hormone; DHT, dihydrotestosterone; FSH, follicle-stimulating hormone; GH, growth hormone; LH, luteinizing hormone; LH-RH, luteinizing hormone–releasing hormone; mRNA, messenger RNA; PROL, prolactin; R, receptor.)

- Current guidelines do not recommend the use of finasteride or **dutaseride** for prostate cancer chemoprevention. Although finasteride reduces the prevalence of prostate cancer, the impact on prostate cancer morbidity or mortality has not been demonstrated.

SCREENING

- Screening for prostate cancer is controversial. The current approach involves offering a baseline prostate-specific antigen (PSA) and digital rectal exam (DRE) at age 40 with annual evaluations beginning at age 50 for men of normal risk. Earlier testing is recommended for men at higher risk for prostate cancer.
- DRE is commonly employed for screening of prostate cancer. It has the advantages of specificity, low cost, safety, and ease of performance. DRE has the disadvantages of relative insensitivity and interobserver variability.
- PSA is a glycoprotein produced and secreted by the epithelial cells of the prostate gland. Acute urinary retention, acute prostatitis, and BPH influence PSA, thereby limiting the usefulness of PSA alone for early detection. PSA is a useful marker for monitoring response to therapy.

CLINICAL PRESENTATION

- Localized prostate cancer is usually asymptomatic.
- Locally invasive prostate cancer is associated with ureteral dysfunction or impingement, such as alterations in micturition (e.g., urinary frequency, hesitancy, and dribbling).
- Patients with advanced disease commonly present with back pain and stiffness due to osseous metastases. Untreated spinal cord lesions can lead to cord compression. Lower extremity edema can occur as a result of lymphatic obstruction. Anemia and weight loss are nonspecific signs of advanced disease.

DESIRED OUTCOME

- In early-stage prostate cancer, the goal is to minimize morbidity and mortality. Surgery and radiation therapy are curative but also associated with significant morbidity and mortality. In advanced prostate cancer, treatment focuses on providing symptom relief and maintaining quality of life.

TREATMENT

GENERAL APPROACH TO TREATMENT

- The initial treatment for prostate cancer depends on the disease stage, Gleason score, presence of symptoms, and patient's life expectancy. The most appropriate therapy for early-stage prostate cancer is unknown. See **Tables 66–1** and **66–2** for management recommendations based on risk of recurrence.
- The major initial treatment modality for advanced prostate cancer is androgen ablation (e.g., orchiectomy or LH-RH agonists with or without antiandrogens). After disease progression, secondary hormonal manipulations, cytotoxic chemotherapy, and supportive care are used.

NONPHARMACOLOGIC THERAPY

Expectant Management

- Expectant management, also known as *observation* or *watchful waiting*, involves monitoring the course of the disease and initiating treatment if disease progresses or the patient becomes symptomatic. PSA and DRE are performed every 6 months.
- Advantages include avoiding adverse effects of definitive therapies and minimizing risk of unnecessary therapies. The major disadvantage is the risk of cancer progression requiring more intense therapy.

Surgery and Radiation Therapy

- Bilateral orchiectomy rapidly reduces circulating androgens to castrate levels. Many patients are not surgical candidates, owing to advanced age or perceived unacceptability. Nonetheless, orchiectomy is the preferred

TABLE 66–1	Management of Prostate Cancer with Low and Intermediate Recurrence Risk	
Recurrence Risk	**Expected Survival**	**Initial Therapy**
Low	Less than 10	Expectant management or radiation therapy
T$_1$–T$_{2a}$ and Gleason 2–6 and PSA less than 10 ng/mL (10 mcg/L) and less than 5% tumor in specimen	Greater than or equal to 10	Expectant management or radical prostatectomy with or without pelvic lymph node dissection or radiation therapy
	Less than 10	Expectant management or radical prostatectomy with or without pelvic lymph node dissection or radiation therapy with or without 4–6 months of androgen deprivation therapy
Intermediate T$_{2b}$–T$_{2c}$ or Gleason 7 or PSA 10–20 ng/mL (10–20 mcg/L)	Greater than or equal to 10	Radical prostatectomy with or without pelvic lymph node dissection or radiation therapy with or without 4–6 months of androgen deprivation therapy

initial treatment for patients with impending spinal cord compression or ureteral obstruction.

- Radical prostatectomy and radiation therapy are generally considered equivalent for localized prostate cancer, and neither has been shown to be superior to observation alone. They are potentially curative therapies but are associated with complications that must be weighed against expected benefit. Consequently, many patients postpone therapy until the onset of symptoms.

TABLE 66–2	Management of Prostate Cancer with High and Very High Recurrence Risk
Recurrence Risk	**Initial Therapy**
High T$_{3a}$, Gleason 8–10, PSA greater than 20 ng/mL (20 mcg/L)	ADT (2–3 years) and radiation therapy, or short-term ADT and radiation therapy for those with a single high risk factor or radical prostatectomy with or without pelvic lymph node dissection
Locally Advanced, Very High T$_{3b}$–T$_4$	ADT (2–3 years) or radiation therapy + ADT (4–6 months) or radical prostatectomy
Very High Any T, N$_1$	ADT (2–3 years) or radiation therapy + ADT (4–6 months)
Very High Any T, Any N, M$_1$	ADT 2–3 years

ADT, androgen deprivation therapy to achieve serum testosterone levels less than 50 ng/dL (1.7 nmol/L)
LHRH agonist (medical castrations or surgical are equivalent)

- Complications of radical prostatectomy include blood loss, stricture formation, incontinence, lymphocele, fistula formation, anesthetic risk, and impotence. Nerve-sparing techniques facilitate return of sexual potency after prostatectomy.
- Acute complications of radiation therapy include cystitis, proctitis, hematuria, urinary retention, penoscrotal edema, and impotence.
- Chronic complications of radiation therapy include proctitis, diarrhea, cystitis, enteritis, impotence, urethral stricture, and incontinence.

PHARMACOLOGIC THERAPY

Drug Treatments of First Choice

LUTEINIZING HORMONE–RELEASING HORMONE AGONISTS

- LH-RH agonists are a reversible method of androgen ablation, providing response rates of ~80%, which is similar to that of orchiectomy.
- There are no comparative trials of LH-RH agonists, so the choice is usually based on cost (**Table 66–3**) and on patient and physician preference. **Leuprolide acetate** is administered daily. **Leuprolide depot** and **goserelin acetate implant** can be administered monthly, or every 12 or 16 weeks.

TABLE 66–3	Comparative Costs of Hormone Therapy for Advanced Prostate Cancer	
Drug	**Dose**	**Average Wholesale Price per Month of Therapy**
Leuprolide depot	7.5 mg/month	$781.90
Leuprolide depot	22.5 mg/12 wk	$781.89
Leuprolide depot	30 mg/16 wk	$781.89
Goserelin implant	3.6 mg every 28 days	$451.19
Goserelin implant	10.8 mg/12 wk	$451.19
Flutamide	750 mg/day	$390.79
Bicalutamide	50 mg/day	$523.92
Nilutamide	300 mg/day for first month, then 150 mg/day	$830.28, then $415.14
Combined Androgen Blockade		**Average Wholesale Price per 3 Months of Therapy**
Leuprolide depot 22.5 mg/12 wk		
+ flutamide	750 mg/day	$3,518.03
+ bicalutamide	50 mg/day	$3,917.42
+ nilutamide	150 mg/day	$3,591.08
Goserelin depot 10.8 mg/12 wk		
+ flutamide	750 mg/day	$2,525.95
+ bicalutamide	50 mg/day	$2,925.34
+ nilutamide	150 mg/day	$2,599.00

Compiled from Drug Topics, Annual Pharmacists' Reference (Red Book). *Montvale, NJ: Thomson Healthcare,* 2008.

Triptorelin LA and **triptorelin depot** are administered every 84 and 28 days, respectively.

- The most common adverse effects of LH-RH agonists are disease flare-up during the first week of therapy (e.g., increased bone pain or urinary symptoms), hot flashes, erectile impotence, decreased libido, and injection-site reactions. Use of an antiandrogen (e.g., **flutamide, bicalutamide,** or **nilutamide**) prior to initiation of LH-RH therapy and for 2 to 4 weeks after is a strategy to minimize initial tumor flare.

- Decreases in bone mineral density complicate androgen deprivation therapy (ADT), resulting in increased risk of osteoporosis, osteopenia, and skeletal fractures. Patients should take calcium and vitamin D supplements and have a baseline bone mineral density.

GONADOTROPIN-RELEASING HORMONE ANTAGONISTS

- The gonadotropin-releasing hormone (GnRH) antagonist **degarelix** binds reversibly to GnRH receptors in the pituitary gland, reducing the production of testosterone to castrate levels in 7 days or less. A major advantage of degarelix over LH-RH agonists is the lack of tumor flare.

- Degarelix is administered as a subcutaneous injection every 28 days. Injection site reactions are the most frequently reported adverse effects and include pain, erythema, swelling, induration and nodules.

ANTIANDROGENS

- Monotherapy with **flutamide, bicalutamide,** and **nilutamide** is no longer recommended due to decreased efficacy as compared with patients treated with LH-RH agonist therapy. Antiandrogens are indicated for advanced prostate cancer only when combined with an LH-RH agonist (flutamide and bicalutamide]) or orchiectomy (nilutamide). In combination, antiandrogens can reduce the LH-RH agonist–induced flare.

- The adverse effects of antiandrogens are gynecomastia, hot flushes, GI disturbances, liver function test abnormalities, and breast tenderness. GI disturbances consist of diarrhea for flutamide and bicalutamide and nausea or constipation for nilutamide. Flutamide is also associated with methemoglobinemia; nilutamide causes visual disturbances (impaired dark adaptation), alcohol intolerance, and interstitial pneumonitis.

COMBINED ANDROGEN BLOCKADE

- The role of combined androgen blockade (CAB), also referred to as maximal androgen deprivation or total androgen blockade, continues to be evaluated. The combination of LH-RH agonists or orchiectomy with antiandrogens is the CAB approach most extensively studied.

- Randomized trial results are mixed when candidates for second-line therapy are treated with combinations of antiandrogens plus either LH-RH agonists or orchiectomy. The most recent meta-analysis showed only a slight survival benefit at 5 years for maximal androgen blockade with flutamide or nilutamide (27.6%) compared with conventional medical or surgical castration alone (24.7%).

- Some investigators consider CAB to be the initial hormone therapy of choice for newly diagnosed patients because the major benefit is seen in patients with minimal disease. Some argue that treatment should not be delayed because combined androgen deprivation trials demonstrate a survival advantage for young patients with good performance status and minimal disease who were initially treated with hormone therapy.
- Until definitive trials are published, it is appropriate to use either LH-RH agonist monotherapy or CAB as initial therapy for metastatic prostate cancer.

Alternative Drug Treatments

- The selection of salvage therapy depends on what was used as initial therapy. Radiotherapy can be used after radical prostatectomy. Androgen ablation can be used after radiation therapy or radical prostatectomy.
- If testosterone levels are not suppressed (i.e., >20 ng/dL [0.7 nmol/L]) after initial LH-RH agonist therapy, an antiandrogen or orchiectomy may be indicated. If testosterone levels are suppressed, the disease is considered androgen independent and should be treated with palliative therapy.
- If initial therapy consisted of an LH-RH agonist and antiandrogen, then androgen withdrawal should be attempted. Mutations of the androgen receptor may allow antiandrogens to become agonists. Withdrawal produces responses lasting 3 to 14 months in up to 35% of patients.
- Androgen synthesis inhibitors provide symptomatic but brief relief in ~50% of patients. **Aminoglutethimide** causes adverse effects in 50% of patients, such as lethargy, ataxia, dizziness, and self-limiting rash. The adverse effects of **ketoconazole** are GI intolerance, transient increases in liver and renal function tests, and hypoadrenalism.
- Bisphosphonates such as **pamidronate** and **zoledronic acid** or **denosumab,** a human monoclonal antibody targeted against receptor activator of nuclear factor κ B ligand (RANKL) may prevent skeletal morbidity, such as pathologic fractures and spinal code compression, when used for hormone-refractory prostate cancer in patients with clinically significant bone loss. Usual dosages are pamidronate, 90 mg every month, and zoledronic acid, 4 mg every 3 to 4 weeks.
- After hormonal options are exhausted, palliation can be achieved with **strontium 89** or **samarium 153 lexidronam** for bone-related pain, analgesics, glucocorticoids, local radiotherapy, or chemotherapy.

CHEMOTHERAPY

- **Docetaxel,** 75 mg/m² every 3 weeks, combined with **prednisone,** 5 mg twice daily, has been shown to prolong survival in hormone-refractory metastatic prostate cancer. The most common adverse events are nausea, alopecia, and myelosuppression. Docetaxel can also cause fluid retention and peripheral neuropathy.
- The combination of **estramustine,** 280 mg by mouth three times daily on days 1 to 5, and docetaxel, 60 mg/m² on day 2 of a 21-day cycle, also improves survival in hormone-refractory metastatic prostate cancer.

Estramustine causes a decrease in testosterone and a corresponding increase in estrogen, which results in an increase in thromboembolic events, gynecomastia, and decreased libido.

EVALUATION OF THERAPEUTIC OUTCOMES

- For definitive, curative therapy, objective parameters to monitor include primary tumor size, involved lymph nodes, and tumor markers such as PSA. PSA level is checked every 6 months for the first 5 years, then annually.
- With metastatic disease, clinical benefit can be documented by evaluating performance status, weight, quality of life, analgesic requirements, and PSA or DRE at 3-month intervals.
- Patients should be monitored for treatment-related adverse events, especially events that are amenable to intervention.

See Chapter 139, Prostate Cancer, authored by LeAnn B. Norris and Jill M. Kolesar, for a more detailed discussion of this topic.

67   Renal Cell Carcinoma

DEFINITION

- Renal cell carcinoma (RCC) is a less common malignancy affecting the parenchyma of the kidney. The most established risk factors for RCC include smoking, obesity, and hypertension.

SUBTYPES AND PATHOPHYSIOLOGY

CLEAR CELL

- Clear cell is the predominant subtype, affecting the proximal tubule as a result of inactivation of the von Hippel–Lindau (VHL) tumor suppressor gene on chromosome 3p25, leading to increased production of growth factors, including vascular endothelial growth factor (VEGF), transforming growth factor (TGF), and platelet-derived growth factor (PDGF), as well as others responsible for angiogenesis and cell growth.
- Inactivation of both copies of the tumor suppressor gene VHL in a healthy kidney is described as sporadic disease, resulting in a single, unilateral tumor, whereas patients with hereditary disease are more likely to present with multicentric, bilateral tumors. This subtype is more likely to metastasize than other subtypes.
- The VHL gene produces the VHL protein (pVHL) and regulates cellular response to oxygen. When VHL is mutated or silenced in clear cell RCC, pVHL is unable to bind and target hypoxia-inducible factor (HIF)-1α for proteasome destruction, resulting in activation of hypoxia-inducible genes such as VEGF, PDGF, and TGF.
- Therapies for RCC target these hypoxia-inducible genes.

PAPILLARY

- Papillary subtypes occur in the proximal tubule, accounting for 5% to 10% of RCC cases. They are associated with multiple genetic abnormalities, commonly diagnosed as localized disease, and have a more favorable prognosis than clear cell.
- Hereditary papillary type 1 cases are associated with mutations in the mesenchymal-epithelial transition (MET) oncogene, located at chromosome 7q31-34.
- Papillary type 2 occurs in patients with a history of skin and uterine leiomyomas in their 20s and 30s.

CHROMOPHORE AND ONCOCYTOMA

- Chromophore and oncocytoma subtypes occur in the intercalated cells of the collecting system, accounting for 5% to 10% of RCC cases. Both are associated with a wide variety of chromosomal abnormalities.
- Oncocytomas are relatively benign and rarely metastasize.

CLINICAL PRESENTATION AND DIAGNOSIS

- Most cases of RCC are diagnosed incidentally following computed tomography (CT) scans done for unrelated reasons.
- Classic triad symptoms of flank pain, hematuria, and palpable abdominal mass are seen in <10% of patients. Other presenting symptoms are fatigue, weight loss, anemia, hypertension, fever, and lower extremity edema. Patients with metastatic disease may present with bone pain, adenopathy, and pulmonary symptoms.
- Sporadic RCC often presents as a single tumor in a patient at least 60 years old. Hereditary RCC more commonly presents as numerous bilateral, cystic tumors in a patient younger than age 50 with other malignancies or a strong family history of RCC or other malignancies.
- Laboratory evaluation should include complete blood count, serum calcium, serum creatinine, liver function tests, lactate dehydrogenase, coagulation profile, and urinalysis. In addition to CT scans, magnetic resonance imaging of the chest, abdomen, and pelvis further characterizes the renal tumor and determines stage.

STAGING AND PROGNOSIS

- Factors associated with prognosis include positive surgical margins, metastatic spread, presence of sarcomatoid architecture, and tumor subtype, grade, and stage, with tumor stage being the most powerful prognostic indicator.
- The Memorial Sloan-Kettering Cancer Center (MSKCC) Prognostic Factors Model was developed for patients with metastatic disease. Patients with none of the poor prognostic risk factors are considered low risk, one or two factors are intermediate risk, and three or more factors are high risk (**Table 67–1**). These criteria are used by clinicians to determine optimal therapy for patients and are included in national guidelines.

TABLE 67–1 MSKCC Poor Prognostic Factors
• Karnofsky Performance Status (KPS) <80%
• Low serum hemoglobin (<13 g/dL [<130 g/L; 8.07 mmol/L] for men and <11.5 g/dL [<115 g/L; 7.14 mmol/L] for women)
• Elevated corrected calcium (>10 mg/dL [2.50 mmol/L])
• Elevated serum LDH (≥300 U/L [≥ 5.00 μkat/L] or 1.5 × ULN)
• Absence of prior nephrectomy (has been shown to be a function of duration of time between diagnosis and start of therapy, with >1 year delay being considered a poor prognostic factor)
Expanded criteria in untreated patients include
• Two or more sites of metastatic disease
• Prior radiotherapy

LDH, lactate dehydrogenase; ULN, upper limit of normal; MSKCC, Memorial Sloan-Kettering Cancer Center.

TREATMENT

- Surgery with curative intent is the initial treatment recommended in patients with localized disease confined to the kidney (stage I, II, or III disease).
- Historically, patients with advanced disease were treated with immunotherapy following nephrectomy, but most patients currently receive a targeted therapy.
- Selection of a specific targeted agent for first-line treatment of metastatic RCC is based on underlying tumor histology and MSKCC risk criteria. The optimal sequencing of targeted agents is currently the subject of ongoing clinical trials.

SURGERY

- The size and location of the renal tumor, the number of tumors present, and whether the patient has a single kidney or a known genetic predisposition are patient-specific factors that determine whether patients undergo a total nephrectomy or nephron-sparing surgery.
- Nephrectomy is preferred for large (4–7 cm), centrally located tumors and is associated with a higher risk of developing chronic kidney disease (CKD).
- Nephron-sparing surgery usually refers to partial nephrectomy, but it also refers to radiofrequency ablation (RFA) and cryoablation. Partial nephrectomy has been shown to have equivalent outcomes to total nephrectomy in appropriately selected patients. Partial nephrectomy candidates include those with smaller (<4 cm) tumors located in the cortical region, bilateral tumors, and those with compromised renal function.
- Extended lymphadenectomy without lymph node involvement is controversial.
- Observation is recommended postsurgery, with imaging of the chest and abdomen every 4 to 6 months. Adjuvant chemotherapy and radiation therapy are not indicated.
- In patients with advanced (stage IV) disease, surgical resection of the tumor and/or metastatic sites is used. Ideal candidates are those with minimal regional lymphadenopathy and a solitary metastatic site in the lung, bone, brain, or soft tissue.

IMMUNOTHERAPY

- Interferon-α (IFN-α) and Interleukin-2 (IL-2) were the standard of care in metastatic RCC until the recent emergence of targeted therapies. Treatment with INF-α and IL-2 is limited by low response rates (6–30% and 5–20%, respectively) and high toxicity. The cytokine INF-α remains the comparator for novel treatments in metastatic RCC, as it is better tolerated than IL-2 and can be self-administered.
- IL-2 toxicities include hypotension, diarrhea, chills, vomiting, dyspnea, and peripheral edema that are related to capillary leak syndrome. Treatment delays and discontinuation are frequently seen.

TABLE 67–2 Comparison of Targeted Agents in Patients with Metastatic Renal Cell Carcinoma

Targeted Agent	Indication (NCCN Guidelines Category of Recommendation)	Dosing	Adverse Effects	Precautions	Drug Interactions
Sunitinib[a]	First-line therapy for metastatic RCC (category 1) and second-line after progression on cytokine therapy (category 1) or tyrosine kinase inhibitor (category 2A)	50 mg orally daily × 4 weeks, then off 2 weeks	Leukopenia, thrombocytopenia, diarrhea, nausea, vomiting, anorexia, constipation, mucositis, hypertension, hand-foot syndrome, hair discoloration, hypothyroidism, decreased LVEF	Discontinue sunitinib if clinical manifestations of CHF occur. Delay or reduce dose if no clinical manifestations of CHF but EF <50% and >20% below baseline	CYP 3A4 inducers may decrease sunitinib exposure CYP 3A4 inhibitors may increase sunitinib exposure
Sorafenib[b]	Second-line therapy for metastatic RCC after progression on cytokine therapy (category 1) or tyrosine kinase therapy (category 2A) and first-line therapy only in select patients (category 2A)	400 mg orally twice daily	Diarrhea, nausea, vomiting, anorexia, fatigue, hand-foot syndrome, desquamating rash, hypertension, fatigue, cardiac ischemia, hemorrhagic events	Consider discontinuing therapy if clinical manifestations of cardiac ischemia or hemorrhagic event occurs	UGT1A1 and UGT1A9 substrates may have increased exposure when coadministered with sorafenib due to inhibition of glucuronidation Docetaxel and doxorubicin exposure may increase when coadministered with sorafenib CYP 3A4 inducers may decrease sorafenib exposure

Pazopanib[c]	First-line therapy for metastatic RCC (category 1) and second-line after progression on cytokine therapy (category 1) or tyrosine kinase inhibitor (category 3)	Initiate at 400 mg orally daily and increase to 800 mg orally daily	ALT elevation, leukopenia, thrombocytopenia, diarrhea, nausea, vomiting, hypertension, hair discoloration, QT prolongation, hemorrhage, thromboembolism, hypothyroidism	Temporarily discontinue therapy in patients undergoing surgery	CYP 3A4 inducers may decrease pazopanib exposure CYP 3A4 inhibitors may increase pazopanib exposure
Bevacizumab[d]	First-line therapy for metastatic RCC in combination with interferon (category 1) and second-line monotherapy after progression on cytokine therapy (category 2B)	10 mg/kg IV every 2 weeks	Epistaxis, hemorrhage, delayed wound healing, hypertension, thromboembolic events, proteinuria, GI perforation, dry skin, rhinitis, taste alteration	Do not administer within 4 weeks of surgery; monitor blood pressure and urine protein	None known
Temsirolimus[e]	First-line therapy for metastatic RCC in patients with poor prognosis (category 1) and an option for patients of other risk groups (category 2B). Second-line therapy after progression on cytokine therapy (category 2B) or tyrosine kinase therapy (category 2B)	25 mg IV once weekly	Anorexia, asthenia, edema, hypersensitivity reactions, infections, interstitial lung disease, mucositis, nausea, rash, wound healing complications Laboratory abnormalities: anemia, hyperglycemia, hyperlipidemia, hypertriglyceridemia, hypophosphatemia, leukopenia, lymphopenia, thrombocytopenia, and elevated alkaline phosphatase, aspartate transaminase, and serum creatinine	Avoid live vaccinations and close contact with those who received live vaccines; monitor blood glucose, serum cholesterol, creatinine, triglycerides, liver function tests, chemistry, and hematologic parameters	CYP3A4 inhibitors may increase exposure CYP3A4 inducers may decrease exposure

(continued)

TABLE 67-2 Comparison of Targeted Agents in Patients with Metastatic Renal Cell Carcinoma (*Continued*)

Targeted Agent	Indication (NCCN Guidelines Category of Recommendation)	Dosing	Adverse Effects	Precautions	Drug Interactions
Everolimus[f]	Second-line therapy following progression on tyrosine kinase therapy (category 1)	10 mg orally daily	Abdominal pain, asthenia, cough, dehydration, diarrhea, dyspnea, fatigue, infections, pneumonitis, and stomatitis Laboratory abnormalities: anemia, hypercholesterolemia, hypertriglyceridemia, hyperglycemia, lymphopenia, and increased serum creatinine	Hepatic impairment (Child-Pugh class B), reduce dose to 5 mg orally daily; avoid live vaccinations and close contact with those who received live vaccines; monitor blood glucose, serum cholesterol, creatinine, triglycerides, liver function tests, chemistry, and hematologic parameters	CYP3A4 and PgP inhibitors may increase exposure CYP3A4 inducers may decrease exposure

ALT, alanine aminotransferase; CHF, congestive heart failure; EF, ejection fraction; GI, gastrointestinal; IV, intravenous(ly); LVEF, left ventricular ejection fraction; NCCN, National Comprehensive Cancer Network; RCC, renal cell carcinoma.

^aSunitinib (Sutent) prescribing information: Pfizer, Inc New York, NY. Revised February 2010.

^bSorafenib (Nexavar) prescribing information: Bayer Healthcare Pharmaceuticals, Inc. Wayne, NJ. Revised February 2009.

^cPazopanib (Votrient) prescribing information: GlaxoSmithKline, Inc. Research Triangle Park, NC. Revised October 2009.

^dBevacizumab (Avastin) prescribing information: Genentech, Inc. San Francisco, CA. Revised July 2009.

^eTemsirolimus (Torisel) prescribing information: Wyeth Pharmaceuticals Inc. Philadelphia, PA. Revised September 2008.

^fEverolimus (Afinitor) prescribing information: Novartis Pharmaceuticals Corp. East Hanover, NJ. Revised March 2009.

Data from The NCCN Clinical Practice Guidelines in Oncology™ Kidney Cancer (Version 1.2010). Available at: NCCN.org. Accessed August 15, 2009. To view the most recent and complete version of the NCCN guidelines, go to NCCN.org; Escudier B, Pluzanska A, Koralewski P, et al. Bevacizumab plus interferon alpha-2a for treatment of metastatic renal cell carcinoma: A randomized, double-blind, phase III trial. Lancet 2007;370:2103–2111; Motzer RJ, Hutson TE, Tomczak P, et al. Sunitinib versus interferon alfa in metastatic renal cell carcinoma. N Eng J Med 2007;356:1115–1124; Escudier B, Eisen T, Stadler WM, et al. Sorafenib in advanced clearcell renal-cell carcinoma. N Eng J Med 2007;356:125–134; Horner MJ, Ries LAG, Krapcho M, et al. (eds). SEER Cancer Statistics Review, 1975–2006. National Cancer Institute. http://seer.cancer.gov/csr/1975_2006/; Sternberg CN, Davis ID, Mardiak J, et al. Pazopanib in locally advanced or metastatic renal cell carcinoma: Results of a randomized phase III trial. J Clin Oncol 2010;28:1061–1068; Escudier BJ, Bellmunt J, Negrier S, et al. Phase III trial of bevacizumab plus interferon alfa-2a in patients with metastatic renal cell carcinoma (AVOREN): final analysis of overall survival. J Clin Oncol 2010;28:2144–2150; Motzer RJ, Escudier B, Oudard S, et al. Efficacy of everolimus in advanced renal cell carcinoma: A double-blind, randomised, placebocontrolled phase III trial. Lancet 2008;372:449–456; and Jemal A, Siegel R, Xu J, Ward E. Cancer Statistics, 2010. CA Cancer J Clin 2010;50:277–300.

- INF-α treatment is associated with chills, fever, asthenia, fatigue, headache, diarrhea, and liver function abnormalities, as well as depression and other neuropsychiatric symptoms.

TARGETED THERAPIES

- Since 2005, six new drugs have been approved either as first- or second-line therapy for metastatic RCC: **sunitinib**, **sorafenib**, **pazopanib**, **bevacizumab** (in combination with INF-α), **temsirolimus**, and **everolimus** (Table 67–2).
- **Sunitinib**, **sorafenib**, and **pazopanib** are orally administered antiangiogenic agents that inhibit multiple tyrosine kinases, including VEGFR and PDGFR. Improved response rates of 30% to 45% were seen with sunitinib as compared with cytokines in clinical trials. It was relatively well tolerated, with most adverse events managed by supportive care or dose modification.
- Sorafenib and pazopanib are generally well tolerated with few grade 3 or 4 adverse events, although ~5% of patients on sorafenib reported cardiac infarct or ischemic events.
- Clinical studies have demonstrated that these three oral agents have different efficacy and toxicity profiles (see **Table 67–2**). Both sunitinib and sorafenib appear to benefit the subgroup of patients with non–clear cell histology.
- **Bevacizumab** is a humanized monoclonal antibody that binds circulating VEGF, inhibiting its effects. The addition of bevacizumab to INF-α improves progression-free survival and objective response rates as compared with single-agent INF-α but not overall survival. Treatment was discontinued more often in the bevacizumab group due to proteinuria, hypertension, and GI perforation.
- IV **temsirolimus** and oral **everolimus** are mTOR (mammalian target of rapamycin) inhibitors. Single-agent temsirolimus improved overall survival as compared with INF-α or combination therapy in patients with poor prognostic features. Patients receiving temsirolimus were more likely to experience hyperlipidemia, hyperglycemia, and hypercholesterolemia, which were not unexpected based on the role of mTOR in the regulation of glucose and lipid metabolism.
- Everolimus is superior to placebo for progression-free survival in patients with clear cell RCC who had disease progression following sorafenib or sunitinib. Adverse events were similar to those seen with temsirolimus.

See Chapter 146, Renal Cell Carcinoma, authored by Christine M. Walko, Ninh M. La-Beck, and Mark D. Walsh, for a more detailed discussion of this topic.

68 Glaucoma

DEFINITION

- Glaucomas are ocular disorders that lead to an optic neuropathy characterized by changes in the optic nerve head (optic disk) that is associated with loss of visual sensitivity and field.

PATHOPHYSIOLOGY

- There are two major types of glaucoma: open-angle glaucoma, which accounts for most cases and is therefore the focus of this chapter, and closed-angle glaucoma. Either type can be a primary inherited disorder, congenital, or secondary to disease, trauma, or drugs.

- In open-angle glaucoma, the specific cause of optic neuropathy is unknown. Increased intraocular pressure (IOP) was historically considered to be the sole cause. Additional contributing factors include increased susceptibility of the optic nerve to ischemia, excitotoxicity, autoimmune reactions, and other abnormal physiologic processes.

- Although IOP is a poor predictor of which patients will have visual field loss, the risk of visual field loss increases with increasing IOP. IOP is not constant; it changes with pulse, blood pressure, forced expiration or coughing, neck compression, and posture. IOP demonstrates diurnal variation with a minimum pressure around 6 P.M. and a maximum pressure upon awakening.

- The balance between the inflow and outflow of aqueous humor determines IOP. Inflow is increased by β-adrenergic agents and decreased by α_2- and β-adrenergic blockers, dopamine blockers, carbonic anhydrase inhibitors (CAIs), and adenylate cyclase stimulators. Outflow is increased by cholinergic agents, which contract the ciliary muscle and open the trabecular meshwork, and by prostaglandin analogues and β- and α_2-adrenergic agonists, which affect uveoscleral outflow.

- Secondary open-angle glaucoma has many causes, including exfoliation syndrome, pigmentary glaucoma, systemic diseases, trauma, surgery, ocular inflammatory diseases, and drugs. Secondary glaucoma can be classified as pretrabecular (normal meshwork is covered and prevents outflow of aqueous humor), trabecular (meshwork is altered or material accumulates in the intertrabecular spaces), or posttrabecular (episcleral venous blood pressure is increased).

- Many drugs can increase IOP (**Table 68–1**). The potential to induce or worsen glaucoma depends on the type of glaucoma and on whether it is adequately controlled.

TABLE 68–1	Drugs That May Induce or Potentiate Increased Intraocular Pressure

Open-angle glaucoma
  Ophthalmic corticosteroids (high risk)
  Systemic corticosteroids
  Nasal/inhaled corticosteroids
  Fenoldopam
  Ophthalmic anticholinergics
  Succinylcholine
  Vasodilators (low risk)
  Cimetidine (low risk)

Closed-angle glaucoma
  Topical anticholinergics
  Topical sympathomimetics
  Systemic anticholinergics
  Heterocyclic antidepressants
  Low-potency phenothiazines
  Antihistamines
  Ipratropium
  Benzodiazepines (low risk)
  Theophylline (low risk)
  Vasodilators (low risk)
  Systemic sympathomimetics (low risk)
  CNS stimulants (low risk)
  Selective serotonin reuptake inhibitors
  Imipramine
  Venlafaxine
  Topiramate
  Tetracyclines (low risk)
  Carbonic anhydrase inhibitors (low risk)
  Monoamine oxidase inhibitors (low risk)
  Topical cholinergics (low risk)

- Closed-angle glaucoma occurs when there is a physical blockage of the trabecular meshwork, resulting in increased IOP.

CLINICAL PRESENTATION

- Open-angle glaucoma is slowly progressive and is usually asymptomatic until the onset of substantial visual field loss. Central visual acuity is maintained, even in late stages.
- In closed-angle glaucoma, patients typically experience intermittent prodromal symptoms (e.g., blurred or hazy vision with halos around

lights and, occasionally, headache). Acute episodes produce symptoms associated with a cloudy, edematous cornea; ocular pain; nausea, vomiting, and abdominal pain; and diaphoresis.

DIAGNOSIS

- The diagnosis of *open-angle glaucoma* is confirmed by the presence of characteristic optic disk changes and visual field loss, with or without increased IOP. *Normal tension glaucoma* refers to disk changes, visual field loss, and IOP <21 mm Hg (2.8 kPa). *Ocular hypertension* refers to IOP >21 mm Hg (2.8 kPa) without disk changes or visual field loss.
- For *closed-angle glaucoma*, the presence of a narrow angle is usually visualized by gonioscopy. IOP is generally markedly elevated (e.g., 40–90 mm Hg [5.3–12 kPa]) when symptoms are present. Additional signs include hyperemic conjunctiva, cloudy cornea, shallow anterior chamber, and occasionally edematous and hyperemic optic disk.

DESIRED OUTCOME

- The goal of drug therapy in patients with glaucoma is to preserve visual function by reducing the IOP to a level at which no further optic nerve damage occurs.

TREATMENT OF OCULAR HYPERTENSION AND OPEN-ANGLE GLAUCOMA

- Treatment is indicated for ocular hypertension if the patient has a significant risk factor such as IOP >25 mm Hg (3.3 kPa), vertical cup:disk ratio >0.5, or central corneal thickness <555 μm. Additional risk factors to be considered are family history of glaucoma, black race, severe myopia, and presence of only one eye. The goal of therapy is to lower the IOP by 20% to 30% from baseline to decrease the risk of optic nerve damage.
- Treatment is indicated for all patients with elevated IOP and characteristic optic disk changes or visual field defects. An initial target IOP reduction of 30% is desired in patients with open-angle glaucoma.
- Drug therapy is the most common initial treatment and is initiated in a stepwise manner (Fig. 68–1), starting with lower concentrations of a single well-tolerated topical agent (Table 68–2). Historically, β-blockers (e.g., **timolol**) were the treatment of choice and continue to be used if there are no contraindications to potential β-blockade caused by systemic absorption. Systemic effects may be reduced by the use of gel-forming liquid or suspension formulations. Beta-blockers have the advantage of low cost owing to generic formulations.
- Newer agents are also suitable for first-line therapy. Prostaglandin analogs (e.g., **latanoprost, bimatoprost,** and **travoprost**) have the advantage of strong potency, unique mechanism suitable for combination therapy, good safety profile, and once-a-day dosing. **Brimonidine**

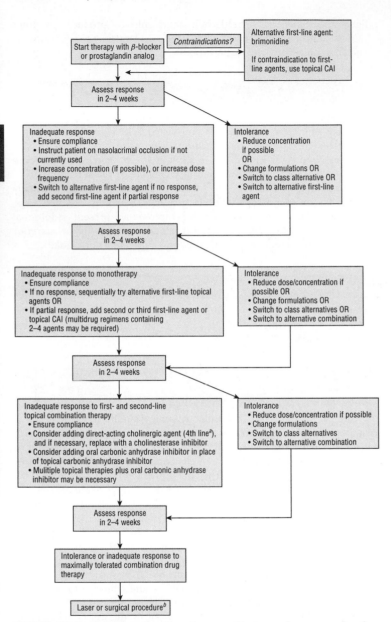

FIGURE 68–1. Algorithm for the pharmacotherapy of open-angle glaucoma. [a]Fourth-line agents not commonly used any longer. [b]Most clinicians believe the laser procedure should be performed earlier (e.g., after three-drug maximum or with a poorly adherent patient). (CAI, carbonic anhydrase inhibitor.)

TABLE 68–2 Topical Drugs Used in the Treatment of Open-Angle Glaucoma

Drug	Pharmacologic Properties	Common Brand Names	Dose Form	Strength (%)	Usual Dose[a]	Mechanism of Action
β-Adrenergic blocking agents						
Betaxolol	Relative β_1-selective	Generic	Solution	0.5	1 drop twice daily	All reduce aqueous production of ciliary body
		Betoptic-S	Suspension	0.25	1 drop twice daily	
Carteolo	Nonselective, intrinsic sympathomimetic activity	Generic	Solution	1	1 drop twice daily	
Levobunolol	Nonselective	Betagan	Solution	0.25, 0.5	1 drop twice daily	
Metipranolol	Nonselective	OptiPranolol	Solution	0.3	1 drop twice daily	
Timolol	Nonselective	Timoptic, Betimol, Istalol	Solution	0.25, 0.5	1 drop once or twice daily	
		Timoptic-XE	Gelling solution	0.25, 0.5	1 drop every day[a]	
Nonspecific adrenergic agonists						
Dipivefrir	Prodrug	Propine	Solution	0.1	1 drop twice daily	Increased aqueous humor outflow
α_2-Adrenergic agonists						
Apraclonidine	Specific α_2-agonists	Iopidine	Solution	0.5, 1	1 drop two or three times daily	Both reduce aqueous humor production; brimonidine known to also increase uveoscleral outflow; only brimonidine has primary indication
Brimonidine		Alphagan P	Solution	0.15, 0.1	1 drop two or three times daily	

(continued)

TABLE 68–2 Topical Drugs Used in the Treatment of Open-Angle Glaucoma (*Continued*)

Drug	Pharmacologic Properties	Common Brand Names	Dose Form	Strength (%)	Usual Dose[a]	Mechanism of Action
Cholinergic agonists, direct acting						
Carbachol	Irreversible	Carboptic, Isopto Carbachol	Solution	1.5, 3	1 drop two or three times daily	All increase aqueous humor outflow through trabecular meshwork
Pilocarpine	Irreversible	Isopto Carpine, Pilocar	Solution	0.25, 0.5, 1, 2, 4, 6, 8, 10	1 drop two or three times daily	
		Pilopine HS	Gel	4	1 drop four times daily Every 24 hours at bedtime	
Cholinesterase inhibitors						
Echothiophate		Phospholine Iodide	Solution	0.125	Once or twice daily	
Carbonic anhydrase inhibitors						
Topical						
Brinzolamide	Carbonic anhydrase type II inhibition	Azopt	Suspension	1	Two or three times daily	All reduce aqueous humor production of ciliary body
Dorzolamide		Trusopt	Solution	2	Two or three times daily	
Systemic						
Acetazolamide		Generic	Tablet	125 mg, 250 mg	125–250 mg two to four times daily	
			Injection	500 mg/vial	250–500 mg	
		Diamox Sequels	Capsule	500 mg	500 mg twice daily	
Methazolamide		Generic	Tablet	25 mg, 50 mg	25–50 mg two or three times daily	

Prostaglandin analogs					
Latanoprost	Prostaglandin $F_{2\alpha}$ analogue	Xalatan	Solution	0.005	1 drop every night	Increases aqueous uveoscleral outflow and to a lesser extent trabecular outflow
Bimatoprost	Prostamide analog	Lumigan	Solution	0.03	1 drop every night
Travoprost		Travatan Z	Solution	0.004	1 drop every night
Combinations					
Timolol-dorzolamide		Cosopt	Solution	Timolol 0.5% dorzolamide 2%	1 drop twice daily
Timolol-brimonidine		Combigan	Solution	Timolol 0.5% brimonidine 0.2%	1 drop twice daily

[a]The use of nasolacrimal occlusion will increase the number of patients successfully treated with longer dosage intervals.

has the theoretical advantage of neuroprotection, which has not yet been demonstrated in humans. Topical CAIs are also suitable for first-line therapy.

- **Pilocarpine** and **dipivefrin**, a prodrug of **epinephrine**, are used as third-line therapies because of adverse events or reduced efficacy as compared with newer agents.
- **Carbachol**, topical cholinesterase inhibitors, and oral CAIs (e.g., **acetazolamide**) are used as last-resort options after failure of less toxic options.
- The optimal timing of laser trabeculoplasty or surgical trabeculectomy is controversial, ranging from initial therapy to after failure of third- or fourth-line drug therapy. Antiproliferative agents such as **fluorouracil** and **mitomycin C** are used to modify the healing process and maintain patency.

TREATMENT OF CLOSED-ANGLE GLAUCOMA

- Acute closed-angle glaucoma with high IOP requires rapid reduction of IOP. Iridectomy is the definitive treatment, which produces a hole in the iris that permits aqueous flow to move directly from the posterior to the anterior chamber.
- Drug therapy of an acute attack typically consists of an osmotic agent and secretory inhibitor (e.g., β-blocker, α_2-agonist, **latanoprost**, or CAI), with or without pilocarpine.
- Osmotic agents are used because they rapidly decrease IOP. Examples include **glycerin**, 1 to 2 g/kg orally, and **mannitol**, 1 to 2 g/kg IV.
- Although traditionally the drug of choice, pilocarpine use is controversial as initial therapy. Once IOP is controlled, pilocarpine should be given every 6 hours until iridectomy is performed.
- Topical corticosteroids can be used to reduce ocular inflammation and synechiae.

EVALUATION OF THERAPEUTIC OUTCOMES

- Successful outcomes require identifying an effective, well-tolerated regimen; closely monitoring therapy; and patient adherence. Whenever possible, therapy for open-angle glaucoma should be started as a single agent in one eye to facilitate evaluation of drug efficacy and tolerance. Many drugs or combinations may need to be tried before the optimal regimen is identified.
- Monitoring therapy for open-angle glaucoma should be individualized. IOP response is assessed every 4 to 6 weeks initially, every 3 to 4 months after IOPs become acceptable, and more frequently after therapy is changed. The visual field and disk changes are monitored annually, unless glaucoma is unstable or worsening.
- Patients should be monitored for loss of control of IOP (tachyphylaxis), especially with β-blockers or **apraclonidine**. Treatment can be temporarily discontinued to monitor its benefit.

- There is no specific target IOP because the correlation between IOP and optic nerve damage is poor. Typically, a 25% to 30% reduction is desired.
- The target IOP also depends on disease severity and is generally <21 mm Hg (2.8 kPa) for early visual field loss or optic disk changes, with progressively lower targets for greater damage. Targets as low as <10 mm Hg (1.3 kPa) are desired for very advanced disease, continued damage at higher IOPs, normal-tension glaucoma, and pretreatment pressures in the low to midteens.
- Using more than one drop per dose increases the risk of adverse events and cost but not efficacy.
- Patients should be educated about possible adverse effects and methods for preventing them.
- Patients should be taught how to administer topical therapy. With a forefinger pulling down the lower eyelid to form a pocket, the patient should place the dropper over the eye, look at the tip of the bottle, and then look up and place a single drop in the eye. To maximize topical activity and minimize systemic absorption, the patient should close the lid for 1 to 3 minutes after instillation and place the index finger over the nasolacrimal drainage system in the inner corner of the eye.
- If more than one topical drug is required, instillation should be separated by 5 to 10 minutes to provide optimal ocular contact.
- Adherence to drug therapy should be monitored because it is commonly inadequate and a cause of therapy failure.

See Chapter 103, Glaucoma, authored by Richard G. Fiscella, Timothy S. Lesar, and Deepak P. Edward, for a more detailed discussion of this topic.

CHAPTER **69** Anxiety Disorders

DEFINITION

- Anxiety disorders include a constellation of disorders in which anxiety and associated symptoms are irrational or experienced at a level of severity that impairs functioning. The characteristic features are anxiety and avoidance.

PATHOPHYSIOLOGY

- *Noradrenergic model.* This model suggests that the autonomic nervous system of anxious patients is hypersensitive and overreacts to various stimuli. The locus ceruleus may have a role in regulating anxiety, as it activates norepinephrine release and stimulates the sympathetic and parasympathetic nervous systems. Chronic noradrenergic overactivity downregulates α_2-adrenoreceptors in patients with generalized anxiety disorder (GAD) and posttraumatic stress disorder (PTSD). Patients with social anxiety disorder (SAD) appear to have a hyperresponsive adrenocortical response to psychological stress.
- *γ-Aminobutyric acid (GABA) receptor model.* GABA is the major inhibitory neurotransmitter in the CNS. Many antianxiety drugs target the $GABA_A$ receptor. **Benzodiazepines** enhance the inhibitory effects of GABA, which has a strong regulatory or inhibitory effect on serotonin 5-hydroxytroptamine, 5-HT), norepinephrine, and dopamine systems. Anxiety symptoms may be linked to underactivity of GABA systems or downregulated central benzodiazepine receptors. In patients with GAD, benzodiazepine binding in the left temporal lobe is reduced. Abnormal sensitivity to antagonism of the benzodiazepine-binding site and decreased binding was demonstrated in panic disorder. Growth hormone response to baclofen in patients with generalized SAD suggests an abnormality of central $GABA_B$ receptor function. Abnormalities of GABA inhibition may lead to increased response to stress in patients with PTSD.
- *5-HT model.* GAD symptoms may reflect excessive 5-HT transmission or overactivity of the stimulatory 5-HT pathways. Patients with SAD have greater prolactin response to **buspirone** challenge, indicating an enhanced central serotonergic response. The role of 5-HT in panic disorder is unclear, but it may have a role in the development of anticipatory anxiety. Preliminary data suggest that the 5-HT and $5\text{-}HT_2$ antagonist *meta*-chlorophenylpiperazine causes increased anxiety in patients with PTSD.
- Patients with PTSD have a hypersecretion of corticotropin-releasing factor but demonstrate subnormal levels of cortisol at the time of trauma and

chronically. Dysregulation of the hypothalamic-pituitary-adrenal axis may be a risk factor for eventual development of PTSD.

- Functional neuroimaging studies suggest that frontal and occipital brain areas are integral to the anxiety response. Patients with panic disorder may have abnormal activation of the parahippocampal region and prefrontal cortex at rest. Panic anxiety is associated with activation of brainstem and basal ganglia regions. Patients with GAD have an abnormal increase in cortical activity and a decrease in basal ganglia activity. In patients with SAD, there may be abnormalities in the amygdala, hippocampus, and various cortical regions. Lower hippocampal volumes in patients with PTSD may be a precursor for subsequent development of PTSD.

CLINICAL PRESENTATION

GENERALIZED ANXIETY DISORDER

- The clinical presentation of GAD is shown in **Table 69–1**. The diagnostic criteria require persistent symptoms most days for at least 6 months. The anxiety or worry must be about a number of matters and is accompanied by at least three psychological or physiologic symptoms. The illness has a gradual onset at an average age of 21 years. The course of illness is chronic, with multiple spontaneous exacerbations and remissions. There is a high percentage of relapse and a low rate of recovery.

PANIC DISORDER

- Symptoms usually begin as a series of unexpected panic attacks. These are followed by at least 1 month of persistent concern about having another panic attack.

TABLE 69–1 Clinical Presentation of Generalized Anxiety Disorder
Psychologic and cognitive symptoms
• Excessive anxiety
• Worries that are difficult to control
• Feeling keyed up or on edge
• Poor concentration or mind going blank
Physical symptoms
• Restlessness
• Fatigue
• Muscle tension
• Sleep disturbance
• Irritability
Impairment
• Social, occupational, or other important functional areas
• Poor coping skills

Data from American Psychiatric Association. Diagnostic and Statistical Manual of Mental Disorders, Fourth Edition, Text Revision. Washington, DC: American Psychiatric Association, 2000:429–484; and Baldwin DS, Anderson IM, Nutt DJ, et al. Evidence-based guidelines for the pharmacological treatment of anxiety disorders: Recommendations from the British Society for Psychopharmacology. J Psychopharmacology 2005;19:567–596.

TABLE 69–2	Clinical Presentation of a Panic Attack

Psychological symptoms
- Depersonalization
- Derealization
- Fear of losing control, going crazy, or dying

Physical symptoms
- Abdominal distress
- Chest pain or discomfort
- Chills
- Dizziness or light-headedness
- Feeling of choking
- Hot flushes
- Palpitations
- Nausea
- Paresthesias
- Shortness of breath
- Sweating
- Tachycardia
- Trembling or shaking

Data from American Psychiatric Association. Diagnostic and Statistical Manual of Mental Disorders, Fourth Edition, Text Revision. Washington, DC: American Psychiatric Association, 2000:429–484; Baldwin DS, Anderson IM, Nutt DJ, et al. Evidence-based guidelines for the pharmacological treatment of anxiety disorders: Recommendations from the British Society for Psychopharmacology. J Psychopharmacology 2005;19:567–596; and Katon WJ. Panic disorder. N Engl J Med 2006;354:2360–2367.

- Symptoms of a panic attack are shown in **Table 69–2**. During an attack, there must be at least four physical symptoms in addition to psychological symptoms. Symptoms reach a peak within 10 minutes and usually last no more than 20 or 30 minutes.
- Up to 70% of patients eventually develop agoraphobia, which is avoidance of specific situations (e.g., being in crowded places or while crossing bridges) where they fear a panic attack might occur. Patients may become homebound.

SOCIAL ANXIETY DISORDER

- The essential feature of SAD is an intense, irrational, and persistent fear of being negatively evaluated in a social or performance situation. Exposure to the feared situation usually provokes a panic attack. Symptoms of SAD are shown in **Table 69–3**. The fear and avoidance of the situation must interfere with daily routine or social/occupational functioning. It is a chronic disorder with a mean age of onset in the mid-teens.
- In the generalized subtype, fear is of many social situations where embarrassment may occur. In the discrete or specific subtype, fear is limited to one or two situations (e.g., performing and public speaking).

POSTTRAUMATIC STRESS DISORDER

- In PTSD, exposure to a traumatic event causes intense fear, helplessness, or horror.

TABLE 69–3	Clinical Presentation of Social Anxiety Disorder

Fears of being
- Scrutinized by others
- Embarrassed
- Humiliated

Some feared situations
- Eating or writing in front of others
- Interacting with authority figures
- Speaking in public
- Talking with strangers
- Use of public toilets

Physical symptoms
- Blushing
- "Butterflies in the stomach"
- Diarrhea
- Sweating
- Tachycardia
- Trembling

Types
- Generalized: fear and avoidance extend to a wide range of social situations
- Nongeneralized: fear limited to one or two situations

Data from American Psychiatric Association. Diagnostic and Statistical Manual of Mental Disorders, Fourth Edition, Text Revision. Washington, DC: American Psychiatric Association, 2000:429–484; Muller JE, Koen LK, Seedat S, et al. Social anxiety disorder: Current treatment recommendations. CNS Drugs 2005;19(5):377–391; and Schneier FR. Social anxiety disorder. N Engl J Med 2006;355(10):1029–1036.

- The clinical presentation of PTSD is shown in **Table 69–4**. Patients must have at least one reexperiencing symptom, three signs or symptoms of persistent avoidance of stimuli, and at least two symptoms of increased arousal. Symptoms from each category must be present longer than 1 month and cause significant distress or impairment. PTSD can occur at any age, and the course is variable.
- Most persons with PTSD meet criteria for another mental disorder; for example, ~80% have concurrent depression, anxiety disorder, or substance abuse or dependence.

DIAGNOSIS

- Evaluation of the anxious patient requires a complete physical and mental status examination; appropriate laboratory tests; and a medical, psychiatric, and drug history.
- Anxiety symptoms may be associated with medical illnesses (**Table 69–5**) or drug therapy (**Table 69–6**).
- Anxiety symptoms may be present in several major psychiatric illnesses (e.g., mood disorders, schizophrenia, organic mental syndromes, and substance withdrawal).

TABLE 69–4	Clinical Presentation of Posttraumatic Stress Disorder

Re-Experiencing symptoms
- Recurrent, intrusive distressing memories of the trauma
- Recurrent, disturbing dreams of the event
- Feeling that the traumatic event is recurring (e.g., dissociative flashbacks)
- Physiologic reaction to reminders of the trauma

Avoidance symptoms
- Avoidance of conversations about the trauma
- Avoidance of thoughts or feelings about the trauma
- Avoidance of activities that are reminders of the event
- Avoidance of people or places that arouse recollections of the trauma
- Inability to recall an important aspect of the trauma
- Anhedonia
- Estrangement from others
- Restricted affect
- Sense of a foreshortened future (e.g., does not expect to have a career, marriage)

Hyperarousal symptoms
- Decreased concentration
- Easily startled
- Hypervigilance
- Insomnia
- Irritability or anger outbursts

Subtypes
- Acute: duration of symptoms is less than 3 months
- Chronic: symptoms last for longer than 3 months
- With delayed onset: onset of symptoms is at least 6 months posttrauma

Data from American Psychiatric Association. Diagnostic and Statistical Manual of Mental Disorders, Fourth Edition, Text Revision. Washington, DC: American Psychiatric Association, 2000:429–484.; and Ballenger JC, Davidson JRT, Lecrubier Y, et al. Consensus statement update on posttraumatic stress disorder from the International Consensus Group on Depression and Anxiety. J Clin Psychiatry 2004;65(Suppl 1):55–62.

DESIRED OUTCOME

- The desired outcomes of treatment of GAD are to reduce severity, duration, and frequency of the symptoms and to improve overall functioning. The long-term goal is minimal or no anxiety or depressive symptoms, no functional impairment, and improved quality of life.
- The goals of therapy of panic disorder include a complete resolution of panic attacks, marked reduction in anticipatory anxiety and phobic fears, elimination of phobic avoidance, and resumption of normal activities. After treatment, 40% to 50% of patients continue to have occasional panic attacks and phobic avoidance.
- The goals of treatment of SAD are to reduce the physiologic symptoms and phobic avoidance, increase participation in desired social activities, and improve quality of life.
- The goals of therapy of PTSD are to decrease core symptoms, disability, and comorbidity and improve quality of life and resilience to stress.

TABLE 69–5	Common Medical Illnesses Associated with Anxiety Symptoms

Cardiovascular
Angina, arrhythmias, cardiomyopathy, congestive heart failure, hypertension, ischemic heart disease, myocardial infarction

Endocrine and metabolic
Cushing's disease, diabetes, hyperparathyroidism, hyperthyroidism, hypothyroidism, hypoglycemia, hyponatremia, hyperkalemia, pheochromocytoma, vitamin B_{12} or folate deficiencies

Neurologic
Migraine, seizures, stroke, neoplasms, poor pain control

Respiratory system
Asthma, chronic obstructive pulmonary disease, pulmonary embolism, pneumonia

Others
Anemias, cancer, systemic lupus erythematosus, vestibular dysfunction

Data from Roy-Byrne PP, Wagner A. Primary care perspectives on generalized anxiety disorder. J Clin Psychiatry 2004;(65 Suppl 13):20–26; Roy-Byrne PP, Davidson KW, Kessler RC, et al. Anxiety disorders and comorbid medical illness. Gen Hosp Psychiatry 2008;30:208–225; and Rogers MP, Wolfe DJ. Anxiety in the medical patient. Psychiatric Times 2007;24(3):1–4.

TREATMENT

GENERALIZED ANXIETY DISORDER

- For patients with GAD, nonpharmacologic modalities include psychotherapy, short-term counseling, stress management, cognitive therapy, meditation, supportive therapy, and exercise. Patients with GAD should be educated to

TABLE 69–6	Drugs Associated with Anxiety Symptoms

Anticonvulsants: carbamazepine, phenytoin
Antidepressants: selective serotonin reuptake inhibitors, serotonin norepinephrine reuptake inhibitors, bupropion
Antihypertensives: clonidine, felodipine
Antibiotics: quinolones, isoniazid
Bronchodilators: albuterol, theophylline
Corticosteroids: prednisone
Dopa agonists: amantadine, levodopa
Herbals: ma huang, ginseng, ephedra
Illicit substances: ecstasy, marijuana
Nonsteroidal antiinflammatory drugs: ibuprofen, indomethacin
Stimulants: amphetamines, methylphenidate, nicotine, caffeine, cocaine
Sympathomimetics: pseudoephedrine, phenylephrine
Thyroid hormones: levothyroxine
Toxicity: anticholinergics, antihistamines, digoxin

Data from American Psychiatric Association. Diagnostic and Statistical Manual of Mental Disorders, Fourth Edition, Text Revision. Washington, DC: American Psychiatric Association, 2000:429–484; and Rogers MP, Wolfe DJ. Anxiety in the medical patient. Psychiatric Times 2007;24(3):1–4.

TABLE 69–7	Drug Choices for Anxiety Disorders		
Anxiety Disorder	**First Line Drugs**	**Second Line Drugs**	**Alternatives**
Generalized anxiety	Duloxetine Escitalopram Paroxetine Sertraline Venlafaxine XR	Benzodiazepines Buspirone Imipramine	Hydroxyzine Pregabalin Quetiapine
Panic disorder	SSRIs Venlafaxine XR	Alprazolam Citalopram Clomipramine Clonazepam Imipramine	Phenelzine
Social anxiety disorder	Escitalopram Fluvoxamine CR Paroxetine Sertraline Venlafaxine XR	Clonazepam Citalopram	Clonazepam Gabapentin Mirtazapine Phenelzine Pregabalin

SSRI, selective serotonin reuptake inhibitor; XR, extended-release; CR, controlled-release.

Data from Bandelow B, Zohar J, Hollander E, et al. World Federation of Societies of Biological Psychiatry (WFSBP) guidelines for the pharmacological treatment of anxiety, obsessive-compulsive and posttraumatic stress disorders - first revision. World J Biol Psychiatry 2008;9(4):248–312; Davidson JR, Zhang W, Connor KM, et al. A psychopharmacological treatment algorithm for generalized anxiety disorder (GAD). J Psychopharmacol 2010;24(1):3–26; Baldwin DS, Anderson IM, Nutt DJ, et al. Evidence-based guidelines for the pharmacological treatment of anxiety disorders: Recommendations from the British Society for Psychopharmacology. J Psychopharmacology 2005;19:567–596; Schneier FR. Social anxiety disorder. N Engl J Med 2006;355(10):1029–1036, and American Psychiatric Association. Practice guideline for the treatment of patients with panic disorder. Arlington, VA: American Psychiatric Association, 2009. http://www.psychiatryonline.com/pracGuide/pracGuideTopic_9.aspx.

avoid caffeine, stimulants, excessive alcohol, and diet pills. Cognitive behavioral therapy (CBT) is the most effective psychological therapy for GAD; ideally, patients with GAD should have psychological therapy, alone or in combination with antianxiety drugs. However, CBT is not widely available.

- Drug choices for anxiety disorders are shown in **Table 69–7**, and nonbenzodiazepine antianxiety agents for GAD are shown in **Table 69–8**.
- Kava kava is not recommended as an anxiolytic because of reports of a lack of efficacy and hepatotoxicity.
- **Hydroxyzine** is often used in primary care settings, but it is considered a second-line agent.
- **Pregabalin** produced anxiolytic effects similar to **lorazepam, alprazolam,** and **venlafaxine** in acute trials. Sedation and dizziness were the most common adverse effects, and the dose should be tapered over 1 week upon discontinuation.
- The FDA has established a link between antidepressant use and suicidality (suicidal thinking and behaviors) in children, adolescents, and young adults 18 to 24 years old. All antidepressants carry a black box warning advising caution in the use of all antidepressants in this population, and the FDA also recommends specific monitoring parameters. The clinician

TABLE 69–8	Nonbenzodiazepine Antianxiety Agents for Generalized Anxiety Disorder		
Generic Name	**Trade Name**	**Starting Dose**	**Dosage Range (mg/day)[a]**
Antidepressants			
Duloxetine[b]	Cymbalta	30 or 60 mg/day	60–120
Escitalopram[b]	Lexapro	10 mg/day	10–20
Imipramine[c]	Tofranil	50 mg/day	75–200
Paroxetine[b,c]	Paxil Pexeva	20 mg/day	20–50
Sertraline[c]	Zoloft	50 mg/day	50–200
Venlafaxine XR[b,c]	Effexor XR	37.5 or 75 mg/day	75–225[d]
Azapirone			
Buspirone[b,c]	BuSpar	7.5 mg twice per day	15–60[d]
Diphenylmethane			
Hydroxyzine[b,c,e]	Vistaril	25 or 50 mg 4 times daily	200–400
Anticonvulsant			
Pregabalin	Lyrica	50 mg 3 times daily	150–600
Atypical Antipsychotic			
Quetiapine XR	Seroquel XR	50 mg at bedtime	150–300

XR, extended-release.

[a]Elderly patients are usually treated with approximately one-half of the dose listed.
[b]FDA approved for generalized anxiety disorder.
[c]Available generically.
[d]No dosage adjustment is required in elderly patients.
[e]FDA approved for anxiety and tension in children in divided daily doses of 50–100 mg.

Data from Bandelow B, Zohar J, Hollander E, et al. World Federation of Societies of Biological Psychiatry (WFSBP) guidelines for the pharmacological treatment of anxiety, obsessive-compulsive and posttraumatic stress disorders - first revision. World J Biol Psychiatry 2008;9(4):248–312; Kavoussi R. Pregabalin: From molecule to medicine. Eur Neuropsychopharmacol 2006;16:S128–S133; Gao K, Sheehan DV, Calabrese JR. Atypical antipsychotics in primary generalized anxiety disorder or comorbid with mood disorders. Expert Rev Neurother 2009;9(8):1147–1158; Paxil [package insert]. Research Triangle Park, NC: GlaxoSmithKline; August 2007; Cymbalta [package insert]. Indianapolis, IN: Eli Lilly and Company; November 2009; Lexapro [package insert]. St. Louis, MO: Forest Pharmaceuticals, Inc.; March 2009; Effexor XR [package insert]. Philadelphia, PA: Wyeth Pharmaceuticals, Inc.; July 2009; and Vistaril [package insert]. New York: Pfizer Labs; December 2009.

should consult the FDA-approved labeling or the FDA website for additional information (see Chap. 71).

Antidepressants

- Antidepressants are efficacious for acute and long-term management of GAD. They are considered the treatment of choice for long-term management of chronic anxiety, especially in the presence of depressive symptoms. Antianxiety response requires 2 to 4 weeks.
- **Selective serotonin reuptake inhibitors (SSRIs)** and **extended-release venlafaxine** and **duloxetine** are effective in acute therapy, with response rates of 60% to 68%. **Imipramine** may be used when patients fail to respond to SSRIs.

TABLE 69–9 Benzodiazepine Antianxiety Agents

Generic Name	Brand Name	Approved Dosage Range (mg/day)[a]	Approximate Equivalent Dose (mg)
Alprazolam[b]	Niravam,[c] Xanax, Xanax XR	0.75–4 1–10[d]	0.5
Chlordiazepoxide[b]	Librium	25–400	10
Clonazepam[b]	Klonopin Klonopin Wafers[c]	1–4[d]	0.25
Clorazepate[b]	Tranxene Tranxene SD	7.5–60	7.5
Diazepam[b]	Valium	2–40	5
Lorazepam[b]	Ativan	0.5–10	1
Oxazepam[b]	Serax	30–120	15

XR, extended-release; SD, sustained-release.

[a]Elderly patients are usually treated with approximately one-half of the dose listed.

[b]Available generically.

[c]Orally disintegrating formulation.

[d]Panic disorder dose.

Equivalent dose data from Chouinard G. Issues in the clinical use of benzodiazepines: Potency, withdrawal and rebound. J Clin Psychiatry 2004;65(Suppl 5):7–12.

- Common side effects of the **SSRIs** are somnolence, nausea, ejaculation disorders, decreased libido, dry mouth, insomnia, and fatigue. Tricyclic anti-depressants (**TCAs**) commonly cause sedation, orthostatic hypotension, anticholinergic effects, and weight gain. TCAs are very toxic on overdose.

Benzodiazepine Therapy

- The benzodiazepines are the most effective, safe, and frequently prescribed drugs for the treatment of acute anxiety (**Table 69–9**). All benzodiazepines are equally effective anxiolytics, and most of the improvement occurs in the first 2 weeks of therapy. They are considered to be more effective for somatic and autonomic symptoms of GAD, whereas antidepressants are considered more effective for the psychic symptoms (e.g., apprehension and worry).
- It is theorized that benzodiazepines ameliorate anxiety through potentiation of GABA activity.
- The dose must be individualized. Some patients require longer treatment.
- The elderly have an enhanced sensitivity to benzodiazepines and may experience falls when on benzodiazepine therapy.

PHARMACOKINETICS

- Benzodiazepine pharmacokinetic properties are shown in **Table 69–10**.
- **Diazepam** and **clorazepate** have high lipophilicity and are rapidly absorbed and distributed into the CNS. They have a shorter duration of effect after a single dose than would be predicted on the basis of half-life, as they are rapidly distributed to the periphery.

TABLE 69–10 Pharmacokinetics of Benzodiazepine Antianxiety Agents

Generic Name	Time to Peak Plasma Level (hours)	Elimination Half-Life, Parent (hours)	Metabolic Pathway	Clinically Significant Metabolites	Protein Binding (%)
Alprazolam	1–2	12–15	Oxidation	–	80
Chlordiazepoxide	1–4	5–30	N-Dealkylation Oxidation	Desmethylchlordiazepoxide Demoxepam DMDZ[a]	96
Clonazepam	1–4	30–40	Nitroreduction	–	85
Clorazepate	1–2	Prodrug	Oxidation	DMDZ	97
Diazepam	0.5–2	20–80	Oxidation	DMDZ Oxazepam	98
Lorazepam	2–4	10–20	Conjugation	–	85
Oxazepam	2–4	5–20	Conjugation	–	97

[a]Desmethyldiazepam (DMDZ) half-life 50–100 hours.

Data from Rosenbaum JF, Arana GW, Hyman SE, et al. Handbook of Psychiatric Therapy, 5th ed. Philadelphia, PA: Lippincott Williams & Wilkins, 2005; Benzodiazepines. Facts and Comparisons 4.0 Online. Wolters Kluwer Health, Inc; 2009. http://online.factsandcomparisons.com.

- **Lorazepam** and **oxazepam** are less lipophilic and have a slower onset but a longer duration of action. They are not recommended for immediate relief of anxiety.
- **Intramuscular (IM) diazepam** and **chlordiazepoxide** should be avoided because of variability in rate and extent of absorption. **IM lorazepam** provides rapid and complete absorption.
- **Clorazepate**, a prodrug, is converted to **desmethyldiazepam** in the stomach through a pH-dependent process that may be impaired by concurrent antacid use. Several other benzodiazepines are also converted to desmethyldiazepam, which has a long half-life and can accumulate, especially in the elderly and those with impaired oxidation.
- Intermediate- or short-acting benzodiazepines are preferred for chronic use in the elderly and those with liver disorders because of minimal accumulation and achievement of steady state within 1 to 3 days.

ADVERSE EVENTS

- The most common side effect of benzodiazepines is CNS depression. Tolerance usually develops to this effect. Other side effects are disorientation, psychomotor impairment, confusion, aggression, excitement, and anterograde amnesia.

ABUSE, DEPENDENCE, WITHDRAWAL, AND TOLERANCE

- Those with a history of drug abuse are at the greatest risk for becoming benzodiazepine abusers.
- Benzodiazepine dependence is defined by the appearance of a predictable withdrawal syndrome (i.e., anxiety, insomnia, agitation, muscle tension, irritability, nausea, malaise, diaphoresis, nightmares, depression, hyperreflexia, tinnitus, delusions, hallucinations, and seizures) upon abrupt discontinuation.

BENZODIAZEPINE DISCONTINUATION

- After benzodiazepines are abruptly discontinued, three events can occur:
  - ✓ Rebound symptoms are an immediate but transient return of original symptoms with an increased intensity compared with baseline.
  - ✓ Recurrence or relapse is the return of original symptoms at the same intensity as before treatment.
  - ✓ Withdrawal is the emergence of new symptoms and a worsening of preexisting symptoms.
- The onset of withdrawal symptoms is within 24 to 48 hours after discontinuation of short-elimination half-life benzodiazepines and 3 to 8 days after discontinuation of long elimination half life drugs.
- Discontinuation strategies include the following:
  - ✓ A 25% per week reduction in dosage until 50% of the dose is reached, then dosage reduction by one eighth every 4 to 7 days. If therapy exceeds 8 weeks, a taper over 2 to 3 weeks is recommended, but if duration of treatment is 6 months, a taper over 4 to 8 weeks should ensue. Longer durations of treatment may require a 2- to 4-month taper.
  - ✓ Adjunctive use of **carbamazepine** can help to reduce withdrawal symptoms during the benzodiazepine taper.

DRUG INTERACTIONS

- Drug interactions with the benzodiazepines are generally pharmacodynamic or pharmacokinetic. The combination of **benzodiazepines** with **alcohol** or other **CNS depressants** may be fatal.
- **Alprazolam** dose should be reduced by 50% if **nefazodone** (Serzone) or **fluvoxamine** is added.

Dosing and Administration

- Initial doses should be low, and dosage adjustments can be made weekly (see **Table 69–9**).
- Treatment of acute anxiety generally should not exceed 4 weeks. Persistent symptoms should be managed with antidepressants.
- Benzodiazepines with a long half-life may be dosed once daily at bedtime and may provide nighttime hypnotic and anxiolytic effects the next day.
- In the elderly, doses should be low, and short-elimination half-life agents chosen. Close monitoring is required for sedation and falls.

Buspirone Therapy

- **Buspirone** is a 5-HT_{1A} partial agonist that lacks anticonvulsant, muscle relaxant, sedative-hypnotic, motor impairment, and dependence-producing properties.
- It is considered a second-line agent for GAD because of inconsistent reports of efficacy, delayed onset of effect, and lack of efficacy for comorbid depressive and anxiety disorders (e.g., panic disorder or SAD). It is the agent of choice in patients who fail other anxiolytic therapies or in patients with a history of alcohol or substance abuse. It is not useful for situations requiring rapid antianxiety effects or as-needed therapy.
- It has a mean $t_{1/2}$ of 2.5 hours, and it is dosed two to three times daily.
- Side effects include dizziness, nausea, and headaches.

DRUG INTERACTIONS

- **Buspirone** may elevate blood pressure in patients taking a monoamine oxidase inhibitor (MAOI).
- **Verapamil, itraconazole,** and **fluvoxamine** can increase buspirone levels, and **rifampin** reduces buspirone blood levels by 10-fold.

DOSING AND ADMINISTRATION

- Buspirone doses can be titrated in increments of 5 mg/day every 2 or 3 days as needed.
- The onset of anxiolytic effects requires 2 weeks or more; maximum benefit may require 4 to 6 weeks.
- When switching from a benzodiazepine to buspirone, the benzodiazepine should be tapered slowly.

Evaluation of Therapeutic Outcomes

- Initially, anxious patients should be monitored once to twice weekly for reduction in anxiety symptoms, improvement in functioning, and side effects. The Hamilton Rating Scale for Anxiety or the Sheehan Disability Scale may assist in the evaluation of drug response.

TABLE 69–11 Drugs Used in the Treatment of Panic Disorder

Class/Generic Name	Brand Name	Starting Dose	Antipanic Dosage Range (mg)
Selective serotonin reuptake inhibitors			
Citalopram[a]	Celexa	10 mg/day	20–60[b]
Escitalopram	Lexapro	5 mg/day	10–20[b]
Fluoxetine[a]	Prozac	5 mg/day	10–30[b]
Fluvoxamine[a]	Luvox	25 mg/day	100–300[b]
Paroxetine[a]	Paxil	10 mg/day	20–60[c]
	Pexeva		
	Paxil CR	12.5 mg/day	25–75[c]
Sertraline[a]	Zoloft	25 mg/day	50–200[c]
Serotonin norepinephrine reuptake inhibitor			
Venlafaxine XR[a]	Effexor XR	37.5 mg/day	75–225[c]
Benzodiazepines			
Alprazolam[a]	Xanax	0.25 mg 3 times a day	4–10[c]
	Xanax XR	0.5–1 mg/day	1–10[c]
Clonazepam[a]	Klonopin	0.25 mg once or twice per day	1–4[c]
Diazepam[a]	Valium	2–5 mg 3 times a day	5–20[b]
Lorazepam[a]	Ativan	0.5–1 mg 3 times a day	2–8[b]
Tricyclic antidepressant			
Imipramine[a]	Tofranil	10 mg/day	75–250[b]
Monoamine oxidase inhibitor			
Phenelzine	Nardil	15 mg/day	45–90[b]

[a]Available generically.
[b]Dosage used in clinical trials but not FDA approved.
[c]Dosage is FDA approved.
Data from Bandelow B, Zohar J, Hollander E, et al. World Federation of Societies of Biological Psychiatry (WFSBP) guidelines for the pharmacological treatment of anxiety, obsessive-compulsive and posttraumatic stress disorders - first revision. World J Biol Psychiatry 2008;9(4):248–312; Katon WJ. Panic disorder. N Engl J Med 2006;354:2360–2367; and American Psychiatric Association. Practice guideline for the treatment of patients with panic disorder. Arlington, VA: American Psychiatric Association, 2009. http://www.psychiatryonline.com/pracGuide/pracGuideTopic_9.aspx.

PANIC DISORDER

General Therapeutic Principles

- Antipanic drugs are shown in **Table 69–11.** An algorithm for drug therapy of panic disorder is shown in **Fig. 69–1.**
- A meta-analysis showed that **SSRIs, TCAs,** and **benzodiazepines** are similarly effective, with 50% to 80% of patients responding. **Alprazolam, clonazepam, sertraline, paroxetine,** and **venlafaxine** are FDA approved for this indication.
- SSRIs are first-line agents, but benzodiazepines are the most commonly used drugs for panic disorder.

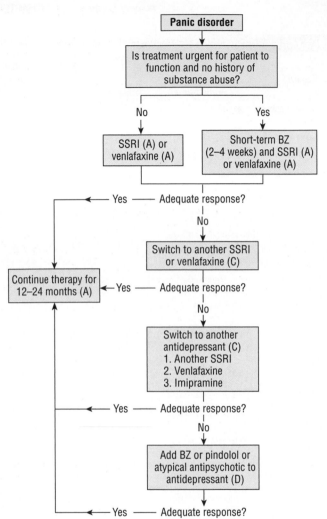

FIGURE 69–1. Algorithm for the pharmacotherapy of panic disorder.
Strength of recommendations: A = directly based on category I evidence (i.e.,
meta-analysis of randomized controlled trials [RCT] or at least one RCT); B =
directly based on category II evidence (i.e., at least one controlled study without
randomization or one other type of quasi-experimental study); C = directly based
on category III evidence (i.e., nonexperimental descriptive studies); D = directly
based on category IV evidence (i.e., expert committee reports or opinions and/
or clinical experience of respected authorities). (BZ, benzodiazepine; SSRI, selective serotonin reuptake inhibitor.) *(Data from American Psychiatric Association.
Practice guideline for the treatment of patients with panic disorder. Arlington,
VA: American Psychiatric Association, 2009. http://www.psychiatryonline.com/
pracGuide/pracGuideTopic_9.aspx; and National Institute for Clinical Excellence.
The Management of Panic Disorder and Generalized Anxiety Disorder in Primary
Care and Secondary Care: Clinical Guideline 22. London: National Collaborating
Centre for Mental Health, December 2004.)*

- Most patients without agoraphobia improve with pharmacotherapy alone, but if agoraphobia is present, CBT typically is initiated concurrently.
- Patients treated with CBT are less likely to relapse than those treated with **imipramine** alone. For patients who cannot or will not take medications, CBT alone is indicated.
- Patients must be educated to avoid **caffeine**, drugs of abuse, and stimulants.
- Antidepressants, especially the SSRIs, are preferred in elderly patients and youth. The benzodiazepines are second line in these patients because of potential problems with disinhibition.

Antidepressants

- Stimulatory side effects (e.g., anxiety, insomnia, jitteriness, and irritability) can occur in **TCA**- and **SSRI**-treated patients. This may affect compliance and hinder dose increases. Low initial doses and gradual dose titration may eliminate these effects (see **Table 69–11**).
- **Imipramine** blocks panic attacks within 4 weeks in 75% of patients, but maximal improvement, including reduced anticipatory anxiety and antiphobic response, requires 8 to 12 weeks.
- About 25% of patients with panic disorder discontinue **TCAs** because of side effects.
- All **SSRIs** eliminate panic attacks in 60% to 80% of patients. The antipanic effect requires 4 weeks, and some patients do not respond until 8 to 12 weeks.
- Low initial doses of **SSRIs** and gradual titration to the antipanic dose are required to avoid stimulatory side effects.
- Approximately 54% to 60% of patients became panic-free on extended-release venlafaxine, 75 mg or 150 mg.

Benzodiazepines

- **Benzodiazepines** are second-line agents except when rapid response is essential. They should not be used as monotherapy in patients with panic disorder with a history of depression or **alcohol** or drug abuse. Benzodiazepines are often used concomitantly with antidepressants in the first 4 to 6 weeks to produce a more rapid onset of antipanic effects.
- Relapse rates of 50% or higher are common despite slow drug tapering.
- **Alprazolam** and **clonazepam** are the most frequently used of the benzodiazepines and are well accepted by patients. Therapeutic response typically occurs in 1 to 2 weeks. With alprazolam, the duration of action may be as little as 4 to 6 hours with breakthrough symptoms between dosing. The use of extended-release alprazolam or clonazepam avoids this problem.

DOSING AND ADMINISTRATION

- The starting dose of **clonazepam** is 0.25 mg twice daily, with a dose increase to 1 mg by the third day. Increases by 0.25 to 0.5 mg every 3 days to 4 mg/day can be made if needed.
- The starting dose of **alprazolam** is 0.25 to 0.5 mg three times daily (or 0.5 mg once daily of extended-release alprazolam), slowly increasing over several weeks to an ideal dose. Most patients require 3 to 6 mg/day.

- Usually patients are treated for 12 to 24 months before discontinuation over 4 to 6 months is attempted. Many patients require long-term therapy. Successful maintenance with single weekly doses of **fluoxetine** has been described.

Evaluation of Therapeutic Outcomes

- Patients with panic disorder should be seen every 2 weeks during the first few weeks to adjust medication doses based on symptom improvement and to monitor side effects. Once stabilized, they can be seen every 2 months. The Panic Disorder Severity Scale (with a remission goal of 3 or less with no or mild agoraphobic avoidance, anxiety, disability, or depressive symptoms) and the Sheehan Disability Scale (with a goal of less than or equal to 1 on each item) can be used to measure for disability. During drug discontinuation, the frequency of appointments should be increased.

SOCIAL ANXIETY DISORDER

- Patients with SAD often respond more slowly and less completely than patients with other anxiety disorders.
- After improvement, at least 1 year of maintenance treatment is recommended to maintain improvement and decrease the rate of relapse. Long-term treatment may be needed for patients with unresolved symptoms, comorbidity, an early onset of disease, or a prior history of relapse.
- CBT (exposure therapy, cognitive restructuring, relaxation training, and social skills training) and pharmacotherapy are considered equally effective in SAD, but CBT can lead to a greater likelihood of maintaining response after treatment termination. Even after response, most patients continue to experience more than minimal residual symptoms.
- CBT and social skills training are effective in children with SAD. Evidence supports the efficacy of SSRIs and serotonin norepinephrine reuptake inhibitors in children 6 to 17 years of age. Individuals up to 24 years of age should be closely monitored for increased risk of suicidality.
- Drugs used in treatment of SAD are shown in **Table 69–12**, and an algorithm for treatment of SAD is shown in **Fig. 69–2**.
- Response rates of SSRIs in SAD ranged from 50% to 80% after 8 to 12 weeks of treatment. **Paroxetine, sertraline, extended-release fluvoxamine, and extended-release venlafaxine** are approved for treatment of generalized SAD and are first-line agents.
- With **SSRI** treatment, the onset of effect is delayed 4 to 8 weeks, and maximum benefit is often not observed until 12 weeks or longer.
- The TCAs are not effective for SAD.
- Limited data suggest that **citalopram** is also effective for SAD, but mixed results have been reported for **fluoxetine**.
- **SSRIs** are initiated at doses similar to those used for depression (see **Table 69–12**). If there is comorbid panic disorder, the **SSRI** dose should be started at one fourth to one half the usual starting dose of antidepressants. The dose should be tapered slowly during discontinuation to decrease the risk of relapse.

TABLE 69–12	Drugs Used in the Treatment of Generalized Social Anxiety Disorder		
Class/Generic Name	**Brand Name**	**Starting Dose**	**Dosage Range (mg/day)**
Selective serotonin reuptake inhibitors			
Citalopram[a]	Celexa	20 mg/day	20–40[b]
Escitalopram	Lexapro	5 mg/day	10–20[b]
Fuvoxamine CR	Luvox CR	100 mg	100–300[c]
Paroxetine[a]	Paxil	10 mg/day	10–60[c]
Paroxetine CR	Paxil CR	12.5 mg/day	12.5–37.5[c]
Sertraline[a]	Zoloft	25–50 mg/day	50–200[c]
Serotonin-norepinephrine reuptake inhibitor			
Venlafaxine XR[a]	Effexor XR	75 mg/day	75–225[c]
Monoamine oxidase inhibitor			
Phenelzine	Nardil	15 mg at bedtime	60–90[b]
Alternative agents			
Buspirone[a,d]	BuSpar	10 mg twice per day	45–60[b]
Clonazepam[a,d]	Klonopin	0.25 mg/day	1–4[b]
Gabapentin[a]	Neurontin	100 mg 3 times a day	900–3,600[b]
Mirtazapine[a]	Remeron	15 mg at bedtime	30[b]
Pregabalin	Lyrica	100 mg 3 times a day	600[b]
Quetiapine	Seroquel	25 mg at bedtime	25–400[b]

XR, extended-release; CR, controlled-release.
[a]Available generically.
[b]Dosage used in clinical trials but not FDA approved.
[c]Dosage is FDA approved.
[d]Used as augmenting agent.
Data from Bandelow B, Zohar J, Hollander E, et al. World Federation of Societies of Biological Psychiatry (WFSBP) guidelines for the pharmacological treatment of anxiety, obsessive-compulsive and posttraumatic stress disorders - first revision. World J Biol Psychiatry 2008;9(4).248–312; Muller JE, Koen LK, Seedat S, et al. Social anxiety disorder: Current treatment recommendations. CNS Drugs 2005;19(5):377–391; Schneier FR. Social anxiety disorder. N Engl J Med 2006;355(10):1029–1036; Stein M, Stein DJ. Social anxiety disorder. Lancet 2008; 371(9618):1115–1125; and Vaishnavi S, Alamy S, Zhang W, et al. Quetiapine as monotherapy for social anxiety disorder: a placebo-controlled study. Prog Neuropsychopharmacol Biol Psychiatry 2007;31(7):1464–1469.

- Some patients unresponsive to **SSRIs** have improved with **extended-release venlafaxine**. Response has been reported by week 3.
- **Benzodiazepines** should be reserved for patients at low risk of substance abuse, those who require rapid relief, or those who have not responded to other therapies.
- **Clonazepam** is the most extensively studied benzodiazepine for treatment of generalized SAD. It improved fear and phobic avoidance, interpersonal sensitivity, fears of negative evaluation, and disability measures. Adverse effects include sexual dysfunction, unsteadiness, dizziness, and poor concentration. Clonazepam should be tapered at a rate not to exceed 0.25 mg every 2 weeks.
- **Gabapentin** was effective for SAD, and the onset of effect was 2 to 4 weeks. **Pregabalin** was superior to placebo at a dose of 600 mg/day.

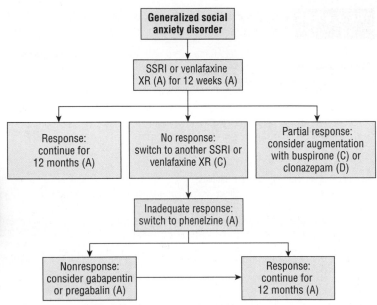

FIGURE 69–2. Algorithm for the pharmacotherapy of generalized social anxiety disorder. Strength of recommendations: A = directly based on category I evidence (i.e., meta-analysis of randomized controlled trials [RCT] or at least one RCT); B = directly based on category II evidence (i.e., at least one controlled study without randomization or one other type of quasi-experimental study); C = directly based on category III evidence (i.e., nonexperimental descriptive studies); D = directly based on category IV evidence (i.e., expert committee reports or opinions and/or clinical experience of respected authorities). (SSRI, selective serotonin reuptake inhibitor.) *(Data from Bandelow B, Zohar J, Hollander E, et al. World Federation of Societies of Biological Psychiatry (WFSBP) guidelines for the pharmacological treatment of anxiety, obsessive-compulsive and posttraumatic stress disorders - first revision. World J Biol Psychiatry 2008;9(4):248–312; and Stein M, Stein DJ. Social anxiety disorder. Lancet 2008;371(9618):1115–1125.)*

- *β*-**Blockers** blunt the peripheral autonomic symptoms of arousal (e.g., rapid heart rate, sweating, blushing, and tremor) and are often used to decrease anxiety in performance-related situations. For specific SAD, 10 to 80 mg of **propranolol** or 25 to 100 mg of **atenolol** can be taken 1 hour before the performance. A test dose should be taken at home on a day before the performance to be sure adverse effects will not be problematic.
- Patients with incomplete response to a first-line agent may benefit from augmentation with **buspirone** or **clonazepam**.
- **Phenelzine**, a monoamine oxidase inhibitor (**MAOI**), is effective but is reserved for treatment-resistant patients because of dietary restrictions, potential drug interactions, and adverse effects.
- Patients with SAD should be monitored for symptom response, adverse effects, and overall functionality and quality of life. Patients should be

TABLE 69–13	Antidepressants Used in the Treatment of Posttraumatic Stress Disorder	
Class/Generic Name	**Starting Dose**	**Dosage Range (mg/day)**
Selective serotonin reuptake inhibitors		
Citalopram[a]	20 mg/day	20–60[b]
Escitalopram	5 or 10 mg/day	10–20[b]
Fluoxetine[a]	10 mg/day	10–60[b]
Fluvoxamine[a]	50 mg/day	100–300[b]
Paroxetine[a]	10–20 mg/day	20–50[c]
Sertraline[a]	25 mg/day	50–200[c]
Other agents		
Amitriptyline[a]	25 or 50 mg/day	50–300[b]
Imipramine[a]	25 or 50 mg/day	50–300[b]
Mirtazapine[a]	15 mg/night	15–60[b]
Phenelzine	15 or 30 mg every night	15–90[b]
Venlafaxine extended-release[a]	37.5 mg/day	37.5–300[b]

[a]Available generically.
[b]Dosage used in clinical trials but not FDA approved.
[c]Dosage is FDA approved.

Data from Ballenger JC, Davidson JRT, Lecrubier Y, et al. Consensus statement update on posttraumatic stress disorder from the International Consensus Group on Depression and Anxiety. J Clin Psychiatry 2004;65(Suppl 1):55–62; International Psychopharmacology Algorithm Project: Post-traumatic Stress Disorder, 2005. http://www.ipap.org/ptsd/index.htp; Paxil [package insert]. Research Triangle Park, NC: GlaxoSmithKline; August 2009; and Zoloft [package insert]. New York, NY: Pfizer, Inc.; January 2009.

seen weekly during dosage titration and monthly once stabilized. Patients should be asked to keep a diary to record symptoms and their severity. The clinician-related Liebowitz Social Anxiety Scale and the patient-rated Social Phobia Inventory can be used to monitor severity of symptoms and symptom change.

POSTTRAUMATIC STRESS DISORDER

- Immediately after the trauma, patients should receive treatment individualized to their presenting symptoms (e.g., **nonbenzodiazepine hypnotic** or short courses of CBT). Brief courses of CBT in close proximity to the trauma resulted in lower rates of PTSD.
- If symptoms (e.g., hyperarousal, avoidance, dissociation, insomnia, and depression) persist for 3 to 4 weeks, and there is social or occupational impairment, patients should receive pharmacotherapy or psychotherapy, or both.
- Psychotherapies for PTSD include anxiety management (e.g., stress-inoculation training, eye movement desensitization and reprocessing, relaxation training, biofeedback, and distraction techniques), CBT, group therapy, hypnosis, psychodynamic therapies, and psychoeducation. Psychotherapy may be used in patients with mild symptoms, those who prefer not to use medications, or in conjunction with drugs in those with severe symptoms to improve response.

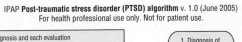

IPAP **Post-traumatic stress disorder (PTSD) algorithm** v. 1.0 (June 2005)
For health professional use only. Not for patient use.

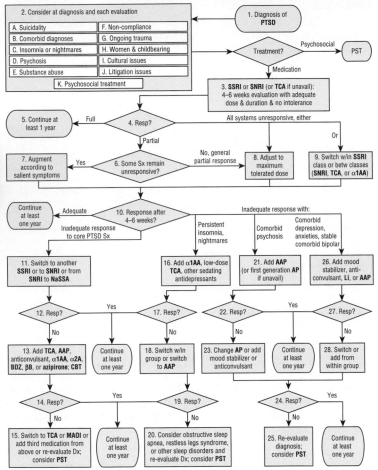

KEY: α1AA, α₁–adrenergic antagonist; α2A, α₂-agonist; AP, Antipsychotic; AAP, Atypical antipsychotic; βB, Beta-blocker; BDZ, Benzodiazepine; CBT, Cognitive behavioral therapy; Dx, Diagnosis; Li, Lithium; MAOI, Monamine oxidase inhibitor; NaSSA, Noradrenergic and selective serotonergic antidepressant; PST, Psychosocial treatment; Resp, Response; SNRI, Serotonin and noradrenaline reuptake inhibitor; SSRI, Selective serotonin reuptake inhibitor; Sx, Symptoms; TCA, Tricyclic antidepressant

FIGURE 69–3. Algorithm for the pharmacotherapy of posttraumatic stress disorder. Levels of evidence (LOE): 1 = more than one adequately powered placebo-controlled trial (i.e., n = 30 per group or greater); 2 = one or more small placebo-controlled trials of monotherapy, combination or augmentation therapy; 3 = case series or open-label trials; 4 = either no published evidence, or presence of clinical consensus. LOE: Node 3 – LOE 1 (sertraline, paroxetine, fluoxetine); LOE 2 (mirtazapine, TCAs, MAOIs); LOE 3 (citalopram); LOE 4 (fluvoxamine); Node 7 – LOE 2 (prazosin, nefazodone, TCAs); LOE 3 (trazodone); Node 9 – LOE 4; Node 13 – Aggression, LOE 2 (prazosin, risperidone, olanzapine), Insomnia/nightmares,

FIGURE 69–3. (continued) LOE 3 (trazodone), Anxiety/agitation, LOE 2 (risperidone), LOE 3 (olanzapine, buspirone), LOE 4 (tiagabine, β-blockers, α_2-agonists); Node 15 – LOE 4; Node 16 – LOE 2, 3 (prazosin); LOE 4 (trazodone, TCAs, olanzapine, mirtazapine, quetiapine, zolpidem); Node 18 – LOE 4; Node 21 – LOE 2 (risperidone), LOE 3 (olanzapine, quetiapine) LOE 4 (SSRIs, anticonvulsants, antiadrenergics); Node 23 – LOE 4; Node 26 – LOE 4; Node 28 – LOE 4 (α1AA, α_1-adrenergic antagonist; α2A, α_2-agonist; AP, antipsychotic; AAP, atypical antipsychotic; βB, beta-blocker; BDZ, benzodiazepine; CBT, cognitive behavioral therapy; Dx, diagnosis; Li, lithium; MAOI, monoamine oxidase inhibitor; NaSSA, noradrenergic and selective serotonergic antidepressant; PST, psychosocial treatment; PTSD, posttraumatic stress disorder; Resp, response; SNRI, serotonin and norepinephrine reuptake inhibitor; SSRI, selective serotonin reuptake inhibitor; Sx, symptoms; TCA, tricyclic antidepressant.) *(Data from International Psychopharmacology Algorithm Project: Post-traumatic Stress Disorder, 2005. http://www.ipap.org/ ptsd/index.htp.)*

- Table 69–13 shows antidepressants used in the treatment of PTSD, and Fig. 69–3 shows an algorithm for the pharmacotherapy of PTSD.
- The **SSRIs** and **venlafaxine** are first-line pharmacotherapy for PTSD. The **TCAs** and **MAOIs** may also be effective, but they have less favorable side effect profiles.
- **Sertraline** and **paroxetine** are approved for acute treatment of PTSD, and sertraline is approved for long-term management of PTSD.
- Antiadrenergics and atypical antipsychotics can be used as augmenting agents.
- The **SSRIs** are believed to be more effective for numbing symptoms than other drugs. About 60% of sertraline-treated patients showed improvement in arousal and avoidance/numbing symptoms. Similar numbers of patients have been shown to improve on **paroxetine** and **venlafaxine**. **Fluoxetine** was effective in a placebo-controlled trial, and **fluvoxamine** and **escitalopram** were effective in an open trial.
- Sertraline and fluoxetine were effective in preventing relapse.
- **Amitriptyline, imipramine,** and **mirtazapine** can be considered second-line drugs. **Phenelzine** is a third-line drug for PTSD after **SSRIs** have failed.
- If there is no improvement in the acute stress response 3 to 4 weeks following trauma, SSRIs should be started in a low dose with slow titration upward toward antidepressant doses. Six to 12 weeks is an adequate duration of treatment to determine response.
- Responders to drug therapy should continue treatment for at least 12 months. When discontinued, drug therapy should be tapered slowly over a period of 1 month or more to reduce the likelihood of relapse.
- Antiadrenergic drugs (**prazosin**) can be useful in some patients with PTSD, and antipsychotics (**risperidone, quetiapine,** and **olanzapine**), α_1-adrenergic antagonists, antidepressants, mood stabilizers, anticonvulsants, β-blockers, and **buspirone** may be used as augmenting agents in partial responders.

- Patients should be seen weekly for the first month, then biweekly through the second month. During months 3 to 6, patients can be seen monthly, then every 1 to 2 months from months 6 to 12. Patients should be monitored for symptom response, side effects, and treatment adherence.

See Chapter 79, Anxiety Disorders I, authored by Sarah T. Melton and Cynthia K. Kirkwood, and Chapter 80, Anxiety Disorders II, authored by Cynthia K. Kirkwood, Lisa B. Phipps, and Barbara G. Wells, for a more detailed discussion of this topic.

CHAPTER 70

Bipolar Disorder

DEFINITION

- Bipolar disorder, previously known as *manic-depressive illness,* is a cyclical, lifelong disorder with recurrent extreme fluctuations in mood, energy, and behavior. Diagnosis requires the occurrence, during the course of the illness, of a manic, hypomanic, or mixed episode (not caused by any other medical condition, substance, or psychiatric disorder).

ETIOLOGY AND PATHOPHYSIOLOGY

- Medical conditions, medications, and somatic treatments that may induce mania are shown in **Table 70–1**.
- See Chap. 71 for medical conditions, substance use disorders, and medications associated with depressive symptoms.
- Etiology and pathophysiology of bipolar disorder are summarized in **Table 70–2**.

CLINICAL PRESENTATION AND DIAGNOSIS

- The *Diagnostic and Statistical Manual of Mental Disorders,* 4th ed., text revision, classifies bipolar disorders as (1) bipolar I, (2) bipolar II, (3) cyclothymic disorder, and (4) bipolar disorder not otherwise specified. **Table 70–3** defines mood disorders by type of episode. **Table 70–4** describes the evaluation and diagnostic criteria for mood disorders.

MAJOR DEPRESSIVE EPISODE

- In bipolar depression, patients often have mood lability, hypersomnia, low energy, psychomotor retardation, cognitive impairments, anhedonia, decreased sexual activity, slowed speech, carbohydrate craving, and weight gain.
- Delusions, hallucinations, and suicide attempts are more common in bipolar depression than in unipolar depression.

MANIC EPISODE

- Acute mania usually begins abruptly, and symptoms increase over several days. The severe stages may include bizarre behavior, hallucinations, and paranoid or grandiose delusions. There is marked impairment in functioning or the need for hospitalization.
- Manic episodes may be precipitated by stressors, sleep deprivation, antidepressants, CNS stimulants, or bright light.

TABLE 70–1	Secondary Causes of Mania

Medical conditions that induce mania

- CNS disorders (brain tumor, strokes, head injuries, subdural hematoma, multiple sclerosis, systemic lupus erythematosus, temporal lobe seizures, Huntington's disease)
- Infections (encephalitis, neurosyphilis, sepsis, human immunodeficiency virus)
- Electrolyte or metabolic abnormalities (calcium or sodium fluctuations, hyper- or hypoglycemia)
- Endocrine or hormonal dysregulation (Addison's disease, Cushing's disease, hyper- or hypothyroidism, menstrual-related or pregnancy-related or perimenopausal mood disorders)

Medications or drugs that induce mania

- Alcohol intoxication
- Drug withdrawal states (alcohol, α_2-adrenergic agonists, antidepressants, barbiturates, benzodiazepines, opiates)
- Antidepressants (MAOIs, TCAs, 5-HT and/or NE and/or DA reuptake inhibitors, 5-HT antagonists)
- DA-augmenting agents (CNS stimulants: amphetamines, cocaine, sympathomimetics; DA agonists, releasers, and reuptake inhibitors)
- Hallucinogens (LSD, PCP)
- Marijuana intoxication precipitates psychosis, paranoid thoughts, anxiety, and restlessness
- NE-augmenting agents (α_2-adrenergic antagonists, β-agonists, NE reuptake inhibitors)
- Steroids (anabolic, adrenocorticotropic hormone, corticosteroids)
- Thyroid preparations
- Xanthines (caffeine, theophylline)
- Over-the-counter weight loss agents and decongestants (ephedra, pseudoephedrine)
- Herbal products (St. John's wort)

Somatic therapies that induce mania

- Bright light therapy
- Sleep deprivation

CNS, central nervous system; DA, dopamine; 5-HT, serotonin; LSD, lysergic acid diethylamide; MAOI, monoamine oxidase inhibitor; NE, norepinephrine; PCP, phencyclidine; TCA, tricyclic antidepressant.

Data from American Psychiatric Association: Diagnostic and Statistical Manual of Mental Disorders, Fourth Edition, Text Revision . Washington, DC: American Psychiatric Association, 2000:345–401; and Kaplan HI, Sadock BJ. Synopsis of Psychiatry: Behavioral Sciences/Clinical Psychiatry, 8th ed. Baltimore, MD: Lippincott Williams & Wilkins, 1998:530.

HYPOMANIC EPISODE

- There is no marked impairment in social or occupational functioning, no delusions, and no hallucinations.
- During a hypomanic episode, some patients may be more productive and creative than usual, but 5% to 15% of patients may rapidly switch to a manic episode.

MIXED EPISODE

- Mixed episodes occur in up to 40% of all episodes, are often difficult to diagnose and treat, and are more common in younger and older patients and women.

TABLE 70–2 Etiologic Theories of Bipolar Disorder

Genetic factors

80%–90% of patients with bipolar disorder have a biologic relative with a mood disorder (e.g., bipolar disorder, major depression, cyclothymia, or dysthymia).

First-degree relatives of bipolar patients have a 15%–35% lifetime risk of developing any mood disorder and a 5%–10% lifetime risk for developing bipolar disorder.

The concordance rate of mood disorders is 60%–80% for monozygotic twins and 14%–20% for dizygotic twins.

Linkage studies suggest that certain loci on genes and the X chromosome may contribute to genetic susceptibility of bipolar disorder.

Nongenetic factors

Perinatal insult

Head trauma

Environmental factors

Desynchronization of circadian or seasonal rhythms cause diurnal variations in mood and sleep patterns and can result in seasonal recurrences of mood episodes.

Changes in the sleep-wake cycle or light-dark cycle can precipitate episodes of mania or depression.

Bright light therapy can be used for the treatment of winter depression and can precipitate hypomania, mania, or mixed episodes.

Psychosocial or physical stressors

Stressful life events often precede mood episodes and can increase recurrence rates and prolong time to recovery from mood episodes.

Nutritional factors

Deficiency of essential amino acid precursors in the diet can cause a dysregulation of neurotransmitter activity (e.g., L-tryptophan deficiency causes a decrease in 5-HT and melatonin synthesis and activity).

Deficiency in essential fatty acids (e.g., omega-3 fatty acids) can cause a dysregulation of neurotransmitter activity.

Neurotransmitter/neuroendocrine/hormonal theories

Dysregulation between excitatory and inhibitory neurotransmitter systems; excitatory: NE, DA, glutamate, and aspartate; inhibitory: 5-HT and GABA.

Monoamine hypothesis

An excess of catecholamines (primarily NE and DA) cause mania.

Agents that decrease catecholamines are used for the treatment of mania (e.g., DA antagonists and α_2-adrenergic agonists).

Deficit of neurotransmitters (primarily NE, DA, and/or 5-HT) cause depression.

Agents that increase neurotransmitter activity are used for the treatment of depression (e.g., 5-HT and NE/DA reuptake inhibitors and MAOIs).

Dysregulation of amino acid neurotransmitters

Deficiency of GABA or excessive glutamate activity causes dysregulation of neurotransmitters (e.g., increased DA and NE activity).

Agents that increase GABA activity or decrease glutamate activity are used for the treatment of mania and for mood stabilization (e.g., benzodiazepines, lamotrigine, lithium, or valproic acid).

Cholinergic hypothesis

Deficiency of acetylcholine causes an imbalance in cholinergic-adrenergic activity and can increase the risk of manic episodes.

(continued)

TABLE 70–2 Etiologic Theories of Bipolar Disorder *(Continued)*

Nongenetic factors

Cholinergic hypothesis

Agents that increase acetylcholine activity can decrease manic symptoms (e.g., use of cholinesterase inhibitors or augmentation of muscarinic cholinergic activity).

Increased central acetylcholine levels can increase the risk of depressive episodes.

Agents that decrease acetylcholine activity can alleviate depressive symptoms (i.e., anticholinergic agents).

Secondary messenger system dysregulation

Abnormal G protein functioning dysregulates adenylate cyclase activity, phosphoinositide responses, sodium/potassium/calcium channel exchange, and activity of phospholipases.

Abnormal cyclic adenosine monophosphate and phosphoinositide secondary messenger system activity.

Abnormal protein kinase C activity and signaling pathways.

Hypothalamic-pituitary-thyroid axis dysregulation

Hyperthyroidism can precipitate manic-like symptoms.

Hypothyroidism can precipitate a depression and be a risk factor for rapid cycling; thyroid supplementation can be used for refractory rapid cycling and augmentation of antidepressants in unipolar depression.

Positive antithyroid antibody titers reported in patients with bipolar disorder.

Hormonal changes during the female life cycle can cause dysregulation of neurotransmitters (e.g., premenstrual, postpartum, and perimenopause).

Membrane and cation theories

Abnormal neuronal calcium and sodium activity and homeostasis cause neurotransmitter dysregulation.

Hypocalcemia has been associated with causing anxiety, mood irritability, mania, psychosis, and delirium.

Hypercalcemia has been associated with causing depression, stupor, and coma.

Extracellular and intracellular calcium concentrations may affect the synthesis and release of NE, DA, and 5-HT, as well as the excitability of neuronal firing.

Sensitization and kindling theories

Recurrences of mood episodes cause behavioral sensitivity and electrophysiologic kindling (similar to the amygdala-kindling models for seizures in animals) and can result in rapid or continuous mood cycling.

DA, dopamine; GABA, γ-aminobutyric acid; 5-HT, serotonin; MAOI, monoamine oxidase inhibitor; NE, norepinephrine.
Data from Goldberg JF, Harrow M, eds. Bipolar Disorders: Clinical Course and Outcome. Washington, DC: American Psychiatric Press, 1999; Kelso JR. Arguments for the genetic basis of the bipolar spectrum. J Affect Disord 2003;73:183–197; Lenox RH, Gould TD, Manji HK. Endophenotypes in bipolar disorder. Am J Med Genet 2002;114:391–406; Baron M. Manic-depressive genes and the new millennium: Poised for discovery. Mol Psychiatry 2002;7:342–358; Bezchlibnyk Y, Young LT. The neurobiology of bipolar disorder: Focus on signal transduction pathways and the regulation of gene expression. Can J Psychiatry 2002;47:135–148; Goodnick PJ, ed. Mania: Clinical and Research Perspectives. Washington, DC: American Psychiatric Press, 1998; Soares JC. Can brain imaging studies provide a "mood stabilizer signature?" Mol Psychiatry 2002;7(Suppl 1):S64–S70; Manji HK, Moore GJ, Chen G. Bipolar disorder: leads from the molecular and cellular mechanisms of action of mood stabilizers. Br J Psychiatry Suppl 2001;41:S107–S119; Gould TD, Manji HK. Signaling networks in the pathophysiology and treatment of mood disorders. J Psychosom Res 2002;53:687–697; Sobczak S, Honig A, van Duinen M, Riedel WJ. Serotonergic dysfunction in bipolar disorders: A literature review of serotonergic challenge studies. Bipolar Disord 2002;4:347–356; Freeman MP, Wosnitzer Smith K, Freeman SA, et al. The impact of reproductive events on the course of bipolar disorder in women. J Clin Psychiatry 2002;63:284–287; Ketter TA, Wang PW. The emerging differential roles of GABAergic and antiglutamatergic agents in bipolar disorders. J Clin Psychiatry 2003;64(Suppl 3):15–20; White HS. Mechanism of action of newer anticonvulsants. J Clin Psychiatry 2003;64(Suppl 8):5–8; Rasgon N, Bauer M, Glenn T, et al. Menstrual cycle related mood changes in women with bipolar disorder. Bipolar Disord 2003;5:48–52; and Mahmood T, Silverstone T. Serotonin and bipolar disorder. J Affect Disord 2001;66:1–11.

TABLE 70-3 Mood Disorders Defined by Episodes

Disorder Subtype	Episode(s)[a]
Major depressive disorder, single episode	Major depressive episode
Major depressive disorder, recurrent	Two or more major depressive episodes
Bipolar disorder, type I[b]	Manic episode ± major depressive or mixed episode
Bipolar disorder, type II[c]	Major depressive episode + hypomanic episode
Dysthymic disorder	Chronic subsyndromal depressive episodes
Cyclothymic disorder[d]	Chronic fluctuations between subsyndromal depressive and hypomanic episodes (2 years for adults and 1 year for children and adolescents)
Bipolar disorder not otherwise specified	Mood states do not meet criteria for any specific bipolar disorder

[a]The length and severity of a mood episode and the interval between episodes varies from patient to patient. Manic episodes are usually briefer and end more abruptly than major depressive episodes. The average length of untreated manic episodes ranges from 4 to 13 months. Episodes can occur regularly (at the same time or season of the year) and often cluster at 12-month intervals. Women have more depressive episodes than manic episodes, whereas men have a more even distribution of episodes.

[b]For bipolar I disorder, 90% of individuals who experience a manic episode later have multiple recurrent major depressive, manic, hypomanic, or mixed episodes alternating with a normal mood state.

[c]Approximately 5%-15% of patients with bipolar II disorder will develop a manic episode over a 5-year period. If a manic or mixed episode develops in a patient with bipolar II disorder, the diagnosis is changed to bipolar I disorder.

[d]Patients with cyclothymic disorder have a 15%-50% risk of later developing a bipolar I or II disorder.

Data from American Psychiatric Association: Diagnostic and Statistical Manual of Mental Disorders, Fourth Edition, Text Revision. Washington, DC: American Psychiatric Association, 2000:345–401; American Psychiatric Association. Practice guideline for the treatment of patients with bipolar disorder (revision). Am J Psychiatry 2002;159:1–50; and Goldberg JF, Harrow M, eds. Bipolar Disorders: Clinical Course and Outcome. Washington, DC: American Psychiatric Press, 1999.

- Patients with mixed states often have comorbid alcohol and substance abuse, severe anxiety symptoms, a higher suicide rate, and a poorer prognosis.

COURSE OF ILLNESS

- The average age of onset of a first manic episode is 21 years. Usually there is normal functioning between episodes.
- Rapid cyclers (10–20% of bipolar patients) have four or more episodes per year (major depressive, manic, mixed, or hypomanic). Rapid-cycling and mixed states are associated with a poorer prognosis and nonresponse to antimanic agents. Risk factors for rapid cycling include biologic rhythm dysregulation; alcohol, antidepressant, or stimulant use; hypothyroidism; and premenstrual and postpartum states.
- Women are more likely to have mixed states, depressive episodes, and rapid cycling than men.

TABLE 70–4 Evaluation and Diagnosis of Mood Episodes

Diagnosis Episode	Impairment of Functioning or Need for Hospitalization[a]	DSM-IV-TR Criteria[b]
Major depressive	Yes	>2-Week period of either depressed mood or loss of interest or pleasure in normal activities, associated with at least five of the following symptoms: • Depressed, sad mood (adults); can be irritable mood in children • Decreased interest and pleasure in normal activities • Decreased appetite, weight loss • Insomnia or hypersomnia • Psychomotor retardation or agitation • Decreased energy or fatigue • Feelings of guilt or worthlessness • Impaired concentration and decision making • Suicidal thoughts or attempts
Manic	Yes	>1-Week period of abnormal and persistent elevated mood (expansive or irritable), associated with at least three of the following symptoms (four if the mood is only irritable): • Inflated self-esteem (grandiosity) • Decreased need for sleep • Increased talking (pressure of speech) • Racing thoughts (flight of ideas) • Distractible (poor attention) • Increased activity (either socially, at work, or sexually) or increased motor activity or agitation • Excessive involvement in activities that are pleasurable but have a high risk for serious consequences (buying sprees, sexual indiscretions, poor judgment in business ventures)
Hypomanic	No	At least 4 days of abnormal and persistent elevated mood (expansive or irritable); associated with at least three of the following symptoms (four if the mood is only irritable): • Inflated self-esteem (grandiosity) • Decreased need for sleep • Increased talking (pressure of speech) • Racing thoughts (flight of ideas) • Increased activity (either socially, at work, or sexually) or increased motor activity or agitation
Hypomanic	No	• Excessive involvement in activities that are pleasurable but have a high risk for serious consequences (buying sprees, sexual indiscretions, poor judgment in business ventures)

(continued)

	TABLE 70–4 Evaluation and Diagnosis of Mood Episodes *(Continued)*	
Diagnosis Episode	**Impairment of Functioning or Need for Hospitalization**[a]	**DSM-IV-TR Criteria**[b]
Mixed	Yes	Criteria for both a major depressive episode and manic episode (except for duration) occur nearly every day for at least a 1-week period
Rapid cycling	Yes	>4 Major depressive or manic episodes (manic, mixed, or hypomanic) in 12 months

[a]Impairment in social or occupational functioning; need for hospitalization because of potential self-harm, harm to others, or psychotic symptoms.

[b]The disorder is not caused by a medical condition (e.g., hypothyroidism) or substance-induced disorder (e.g., antidepressant treatment, medications, electroconvulsive therapy).

Reprinted with permission from American Psychiatric Association: Diagnostic and Statistical Manual of Mental Disorders, 4th ed., Text Revision. Washington, DC: American Psychiatric Association, 2000:345–401.

- Suicide attempts occur in up to 50% of patients with bipolar disorder, and ~10% to 19% of individuals with bipolar I disorder commit suicide. Patients with bipolar II disorder may be more likely than those with bipolar I to attempt suicide.
- Bipolar patients with substance abuse disorders are more likely to have an earlier onset of illness, mixed states, higher relapse rates, poorer response to treatment, higher suicide risk, and more hospitalizations.
- Episodes may become longer in duration and more frequent with aging.

DESIRED OUTCOME

- The goals of treatment are shown in Table 70–5.

TREATMENT

GENERAL APPROACH

- The general approach to treatment is shown in Table 70–5.

NONPHARMACOLOGIC THERAPY

- Psychoeducation for the patient and family includes:
  - ✓ Early signs and symptoms of mania and depression and how to chart mood changes
  - ✓ Importance of compliance with therapy
  - ✓ Psychosocial or physical stressors that may precipitate an episode and strategies for coping with stressful life events
  - ✓ Limiting substances and drugs that can trigger mood episodes
  - ✓ Development of a crisis intervention plan

TABLE 70–5	General Principles for the Management of Bipolar Disorder

Goals of treatment

- Eliminate mood episode with complete remission of symptoms (i.e., acute treatment)
- Prevent recurrences or relapses of mood episodes (i.e., continuation phase treatment)
- Return to complete psychosocial functioning
- Maximize adherence with therapy
- Minimize adverse effects
- Use medications with the best tolerability and fewest drug interactions
- Treat comorbid substance use and abuse
- Eliminate alcohol, marijuana, cocaine, amphetamines, and hallucinogens
- Minimize nicotine use and stop caffeine intake at least 8 hours prior to bedtime
- Avoidance of stressors or substances that precipitate an acute episode

Monitor for

- Mood episodes: document symptoms on a daily mood chart (document life stressors, type of episode, length of episode, and treatment outcome); monthly and yearly life charts are valuable for documenting patterns of mood cycles
- Medication adherence (missing doses of medications is a primary reason for nonresponse and recurrence of episodes)
- Adverse effects, especially sedation and weight gain (manage rapidly and vigorously to avoid noncompliance)
- Suicidal ideation or attempts (suicide completion rates with bipolar I disorder are 10%–15%; suicide attempts are primarily associated with depressive episodes, mixed episodes with severe depression or presence of psychosis)

Data from American Psychiatric Association. Practice guideline for the treatment of patients with bipolar disorder (revision). Am J Psychiatry 2002;159:1–50; Goodnick PJ, ed. Mania: Clinical and Research Perspectives. Washington, DC: American Psychiatric Press, 1998; and Suppes T, Dennehy EB, Hirschfeld RM, et al. The Texas implementation of medication algorithms: update to the algorithms for treatment of bipolar I disorder. J Clin Psychiatry 2005;66:870–886.

- Other nonpharmacologic approaches include:
  - ✓ Psychotherapy (e.g., individual, group, and family), interpersonal therapy, and/or cognitive behavioral therapy
  - ✓ Stress reduction techniques, relaxation therapy, massage, yoga, and so on
  - ✓ Sleep (regular bedtime and awake schedule; avoid alcohol or caffeine intake prior to bedtime)
  - ✓ Nutrition (regular intake of protein-rich foods or drinks and essential fatty acids; supplemental vitamins and minerals)
  - ✓ Exercise (regular aerobic and weight training at least three times a week)
  - ✓ The use of electroconvulsive therapy for severe mania or mixed episodes, psychotic depression, or rapid cycling should be considered for those patients who do not respond to medications.
  - ✓ The role of repetitive transcranial stimulation has yet to be defined.

PHARMACOLOGIC THERAPY

- An example treatment algorithm for the acute treatment of mood episodes in patients with bipolar I disorder is shown in **Table 70–6**.

TABLE 70-6 Algorithm and Guidelines for the Acute Treatment of Mood Episodes in Patients with Bipolar I Disorder

Acute Manic or Mixed Episode		Acute Depressive Episode	

Acute Manic or Mixed Episode

General guidelines

Assess for secondary causes of mania or mixed states (e.g., alcohol or drug use)

Discontinue antidepressants

Taper off stimulants and caffeine if possible

Treat substance abuse

Encourage good nutrition (with regular protein and essential fatty acid intake), exercise, adequate sleep, stress reduction, and psychosocial therapy

Hypomania

First, optimize current mood stabilizer or initiate mood-stabilizing medication: lithium,[a] valproate,[a] carbamazepine,[a] or SGAs

Consider adding a benzodiazepine (lorazepam or clonazepam) for short-term adjunctive treatment of agitation or insomnia if needed

Alternative medication treatment options: oxcarbazepine

Mania

First, two or three drug combinations: lithium,[a] valproate,[a] or SGA **plus** a benzodiazepine (lorazepam or clonazepam) and/or antipsychotic for short-term adjunctive treatment of agitation or insomnia; lorazepam is recommended for catatonia

Do not combine antipsychotics

Alternative medication treatment options: carbamazepine[a]; if patient does not respond or tolerate, consider oxcarbazepine

Acute Depressive Episode

General guidelines

Assess for secondary causes of depression (e.g., alcohol or drug use)

Taper off antipsychotics, benzodiazepines or sedative-hypnotic agents if possible

Treat substance abuse

Encourage good nutrition (with regular protein and essential fatty acid intake), exercise, adequate sleep, stress reduction, and psychosocial therapy

Mild to moderate depressive episode

First, initiate and/or optimize mood stabilizing medication: lithium[a] or quetiapine

Alternative anticonvulsants: lamotrigine[b] valproate[a] antipsychotics: fluoxetine/ olanzapine combination

Severe depressive episode

First, optimize current mood stabilizer or initiate mood-stabilizing medication: lithium[a] or quetiapine

Alternative fluoxetine/olanzapine combination

If psychosis is present, initiate an antipsychotic in combination with above

Do not combine antipsychotics

Alternative anticonvulsants: lamotrigine[b] valproate,[a]

Second, if response is inadequate, consider carbamazepine[a] or adding antidepressant

(continued)

TABLE 70–6 Algorithm and Guidelines for the Acute Treatment of Mood Episodes in Patients with Bipolar I Disorder (Continued)

Acute Manic or Mixed Episode		Acute Depressive Episode	
Hypomania	**Mania**	**Mild to moderate depressive episode**	**Severe depressive episode**
Second, if response is inadequate, consider a two-drug combination: • Lithium[c] **plus** an anticonvulsant or an SGA • Anticonvulsant **plus** an anticonvulsant or SGA	**Second,** if response is inadequate, consider a three-drug combination: • Lithium[a] **plus** an anticonvulsant **plus** an antipsychotic • Anticonvulsant **plus** an anticonvulsant **plus** an antipsychotic **Third,** if response is inadequate, consider ECT for mania with psychosis or catatonia[d], or add clozapine for treatment refractory illness		**Third,** if response is inadequate, consider a three drug combination: • Lithium **plus** lamotrigine[b] **plus** an antidepressant • Lithium **plus** quetiapine **plus** an antidepressant **Fourth,** if response is inadequate, consider ECT for treatment-refractory illness and depression with psychosis or catatonia[d]

ECT, electroconvulsive therapy; MAOI, monoamine oxidase inhibitor; SNRI, serotonin–norepinephrine reuptake inhibitor; SGA, second-generation antipsychotic, SSRI, selective serotonin reuptake inhibitor; TCA, tricyclic antidepressant.

[a]Use standard therapeutic serum concentration ranges if clinically indicated; if partial response or breakthrough episode, adjust dose to achieve higher serum concentrations without causing intolerable adverse effects; valproate is preferred over lithium for mixed episodes and rapid cycling; lithium and/or lamotrigine is preferred over valproate for bipolar depression.

[b]Lamotrigine is not approved for the acute treatment of depression, and the dose must be started low and slowly titrated up to decrease adverse effects if used for maintenance therapy of bipolar I disorder. Lamotrigine may be initiated during acute treatment with plans to transition to this medication for long-term maintenance. A drug interaction and a severe dermatologic rash can occur when lamotrigine is combined with valproate (i.e, lamotrigine doses must be halved from standard dosing titration).

[c]Controversy exists concerning the use of antidepressants, and they are often considered third line in treating acute bipolar depression, except in patients with no recent history of severe acute mania or potentially in bipolar II patients.

[d]ECT is used for severe mania or depression during pregnancy and for mixed episodes; prior to treatment, anticonvulsants, lithium, and benzodiazepines should be tapered off to maximize therapy and minimize adverse effects.

Data from American Psychiatric Association. Practice guideline for the treatment of patients with bipolar disorder (revision). Am J Psychiatry 2002;159:1–50; Canadian Network for Mood and Anxiety Treatments (CANMAT) and International Society for Bipolar Disorders (ISBD) collaborative update of CANMAT guidelines for the management of patients with bipolar disorder: update 2009. Bipolar Disord 2009;11:225–255; and Suppes T, Dennehy EB, Hirschfeld RM, et al. The Texas implementation of medication algorithms: update to the algorithms for treatment of bipolar I disorder. J Clin Psychiatry 2005;66:870–886.

Treatments of First Choice

- **Lithium, divalproex sodium (valproate), extended-release carbamazepine, aripiprazole, olanzapine, quetiapine, risperidone,** and **ziprasidone** are currently approved by the FDA for treatment of acute mania in bipolar disorder. **Lithium, divalproex sodium, aripiprazole, olanzapine,** and **lamotrigine** are approved for maintenance treatment of bipolar disorder. **Quetiapine** is the only monotherapy antipsychotic that is FDA approved for bipolar depression.

- **Lithium** is the drug of choice for bipolar disorder with euphoric mania, whereas valproate has better efficacy for mixed states, irritable/dysphoric mania, and rapid cycling compared with lithium.

- Combination therapies (e.g., lithium plus **valproate** or **carbamazepine**; lithium or valproate plus a second-generation antipsychotic) may provide better acute response and prevention of relapse and recurrence than monotherapy in some bipolar patients, especially those with mixed states or rapid cycling.

- Useful guidelines include the following: Canadian Network for Mood and Anxiety Treatments; International Society for Bipolar Disorders Guidelines; Practice Guideline for the Treatment of Patients with Bipolar Disorder (Revision) published by the American Psychiatric Association; Texas Medication Algorithm Project developed by the Texas Department of Mental Health and Mental Retardation; World Federation of Societies of Biological Psychiatry guideline; Practice Parameters for the Assessment and Treatment of Children and Adolescents with Bipolar Disorder, developed by the American Academy of Child and Adolescent Psychiatry; and the Treatment Guidelines for Children and Adolescents with Bipolar Disorder.

- Lithium was the first established mood stabilizer and is still considered a first-line agent for acute mania and continuation treatment of both bipolar I and II disorders. It may require 6 to 8 weeks for antidepressant response. Long-term use of lithium reduces suicide risk by 6- to 8-fold. Patients with rapid cycling or mixed states may not respond as well to lithium monotherapy as to some anticonvulsants.

- **Divalproex sodium** (**sodium valproate**) is now the most prescribed mood stabilizer in the United States. There are limited data supporting its use for acute depressive episodes.

- **Carbamazepine** is also commonly used for acute and maintenance therapy. Only the extended-release formulation is FDA approved for bipolar disorder. Some data support the efficacy of oxcarbazepine, but it is not FDA approved for bipolar disorder in the United States.

- **Lamotrigine** is approved for the maintenance treatment of bipolar I disorder. It has been used as monotherapy or add-on therapy for refractory bipolar depression.

- First- and second-generation antipsychotics, such as **aripiprazole, haloperidol, olanzapine, quetiapine, risperidone,** and **ziprasidone** are effective as monotherapy or as add-on therapy to lithium or valproate for acute mania. Prophylactic use of antipsychotics can be needed for some patients with recurrent mania or mixed states, but the risks versus

861

benefits must be weighed in view of long-term side effects (e.g., obesity, type 2 diabetes, hyperlipidemia, hyperprolactinemia, cardiac disease, and tardive dyskinesia).

Alternative Treatments

- High-potency benzodiazepines (e.g., **clonazepam** and **lorazepam**) are commonly used alternatives to (or in combination with) antipsychotics for acute mania, agitation, anxiety, panic, and insomnia or in those who cannot take mood stabilizers. **Intramuscular (IM) lorazepam** may be used for acute agitation. A relative contraindication for long-term benzodiazepines is a history of drug or alcohol abuse or dependency.

- Antidepressants are routinely added for the treatment of acute depression, but **tricyclic antidepressants** and venlafaxine are associated with an increased risk of inducing mania in bipolar I disorder. Some guidelines recommend avoiding antidepressants in the treatment of bipolar depression or limiting their use to brief intervals, but evidence suggests that coadministration of therapeutic doses of mood stabilizers can reduce the risk of antidepressant-induced switching. Generally, the antidepressant should be withdrawn 2 to 6 months after remission and the patients maintained on a mood stabilizer.

- **Nimodipine** may be more effective than **verapamil** for rapid-cycling bipolar disorder because of its anticonvulsant properties, high lipid solubility, and good penetration into the brain.

Special Populations

- Approximately 20% to 50% of women with bipolar disorder relapse postpartum; prophylaxis with mood stabilizers (e.g., **lithium** or **valproate**) is recommended immediately postpartum to decrease the risk of relapse.

- Current estimates of the rate of occurrence of Epstein anomaly in infants exposed to lithium during the first trimester is between 1:1,000 and 1:2,000.

- When **lithium** is to be used during pregnancy, it should be given at the lowest effective dose to avoid "floppy" infant syndrome, hypothyroidism, and nontoxic goiter in the infant.

- Serum concentrations in the nursing infant are 10% to 50% of the mother's serum concentration; thus, breast-feeding is usually discouraged for women taking lithium.

- When **valproate** is taken during the first trimester, the risk of neural tube defect is ~5%. For **carbamazepine,** the risk is estimated to be 0.5% to 1%.

- Administration of folic acid can reduce the risk of neural tube defects.

- Women taking valproate may breast-feed, but mother and infant should have identical laboratory monitoring.

Drug Class Information

- Product information, dosing and administration, clinical use, and proposed mechanisms of action for agents used for bipolar disorder are shown in **Table 70–7.**

- Guidelines for baseline and routine laboratory monitoring of mood stabilizers are shown in Table 70–8.

TABLE 70–7 Products, Dosage and Administration, and Clinical Use of Agents Used in the Treatment of Bipolar Disorder

Generic Name	Trade Name	Dosage and Administration	Clinical Use
Lithium salts: FDA approved for bipolar disorder			
Lithium carbonate[a,c]	Eskalith Eskalith CR Lithobid	900–2,400 mg/day in 2–4 divided doses, preferably with meals. There is wide variation in the dosage needed to achieve therapeutic response and trough serum lithium concentration (i.e., 0.6–1.2 mEq/L (mmol/L)) for maintenance therapy and 1.0–1.2 mEq/L (mmol/L) for acute mood episodes taken 8–12 hours after the last dose).	Use alone or in combination with other drugs (e.g., valproate, carbamazepine, antipsychotics) for the acute treatment of mania and for maintenance treatment.
Lithium citrate[a,c]	Cibalith-S		
Anticonvulsants: FDA-approved for bipolar disorder			
Divalproex sodium[a]	Depakote Depakote ER	750–3,000 mg/day (20–60 mg/kg/day) given once daily or in divided doses for delayed-release divalproex or valproic acid.	Use alone or in combination with other drugs (e.g., lithium, carbamazepine, antipsychotics) for the acute treatment of mania and for maintenance treatment.
Valproic acid[a]	Stavzor	A loading dose of divalproex (20–30 mg/kg/day) can be given, then 20 mg/kg per day and titrated to a serum concentration of 50–125 mcg/mL (346–866 μmol/L) or clinical response.	Use caution when combining with lamotrigine because of potential drug interaction.
Lamotrigine[c]	Lamictal	50–400 mg/day in divided doses. Dosage should be slowly increased (e.g., 25 mg/day for 2 wk, then 50 mg/day for wk 3 and 4, then 50-mg/day increments at weekly intervals up to 200 mg/day).	Use alone or in combination with other drugs (e.g., lithium, carbamazepine) for long-term maintenance treatment for bipolar I disorder.
Carbamazepine	Equetro[a]	200–1,800 mg/day in 2–4 divided doses Dosage should be slowly increased according to response and adverse effects (e.g., 100–200 mg twice daily and increase by 200 mg/day at weekly intervals). Dose can be increased rapidly for inpatients. Extended-release tablets should be swallowed whole and not be broken or chewed.	Use alone or in combination with other medications (e.g., lithium, valproate, antipsychotics) for the acute and long-term maintenance treatment of mania or mixed episodes for bipolar I disorder. APA guidelines recommend reserving it for patients unable to tolerate or who have inadequate response to lithium or valproate.

(continued)

TABLE 70–7 Products, Dosage and Administration, and Clinical Use of Agents Used in the Treatment of Bipolar Disorder (*Continued*)

Generic Name	Trade Name	Dosage and Administration	Clinical Use
Anticonvulsants: Not FDA approved for bipolar disorder			
Carbamazepine	Tegretol, Epitol, Tegretol-XR, Carbatrol	200–1,800 mg/day in 2–4 divided doses. Dosage should be slowly increased according to response and adverse effects (e.g., 100–200 mg twice daily and increase by 200 mg/day at weekly intervals). Dose can be increased rapidly for inpatients. Administer conventional tablets and suspension with meals. Extended-release tablets should be swallowed whole and not be broken or chewed. Carbatrol capsules can be opened and contents sprinkled over food.	Use alone or in combination with other medications (e.g., lithium, valproate, anti-psychotics) for the acute and long-term maintenance treatment of mania or mixed episodes for bipolar I disorder. APA guidelines recommend reserving it for patients unable to tolerate or who have inadequate response to lithium or valproate.
Valproic acid Valproate sodium	Depakene Depacon	750–3,000 mg/day (20–60 mg/kg/day) given once daily or in divided doses for delayed-release divalproex or valproic acid. A loading dose of divalproex (20–30 mg/kg/day) can be given, then 20 mg/kg/day and titrated to a serum concentration of 50–125 mcg/mL (346–866 μmol/L) or clinical response.	Use alone or in combination with other drugs (e.g., lithium, carbamazepine, antipsychotics) for the acute treatment of mania and for maintenance treatment. Use caution when combining with lamotrigine because of potential drug interaction.
Oxcarbazepine	Trileptal	300–1,200 mg/day in two divided doses. Dosage should be slowly adjusted up and down according to response and adverse effects (e.g., 150–300 mg twice daily and increase by 300–600 mg/day at weekly intervals). Dose can be increased rapidly for inpatients.	Use after patients have failed treatment with carbamazepine or have intolerable side effects. May have fewer adverse effects and be better tolerated than carbamazepine.

Atypical antipsychotics: FDA-approved for bipolar disorder

Aripiprazole[a,c] Olanzapine[a,c]	Abilify Zyprexa Zyprexa Zydis	10–30 mg/day once daily. 5–20 mg/day once daily or in divided doses.	May be used in combination with lithium, valproate, or carbamazepine for the acute treatment of mania or mixed states (primarily with psychotic features) for bipolar I disorder.
Olanzapine and Fluoxetine[b]	Symbyax	6–12 mg olanzapine and 25–50 mg fluoxetine daily.	
Quetiapine[a,c] Risperidone[a]	Seroquel Risperdal Risperdal M-Tab	50–800 mg/day in divided doses or once daily when stabilized. 0.5–6 mg/day once daily or in divided doses.	
Ziprasidone[a]	Geodon	40–160 mg/day in divided doses. Administer with food.	
Benzodiazepines		Dosage should be slowly adjusted up and down according to response and adverse effects.	Use in combination with other medications (e.g., antipsychotics, lithium, valproate) for the acute treatment of mania or mixed episodes. Use as a short-term adjunctive sedative-hypnotic agent.

FDA approved agents may be used as monotherapy in various phases of the illness as noted by a,b,c

[a] FDA approved for acute mania.
[b] FDA approved for acute bipolar depression.
[c] FDA approved for maintenance.

Data from American Psychiatric Association. Practice guideline for the treatment of patients with bipolar disorder (revision). Am J Psychiatry 2002;159:1–50; Goldberg JF, Harrow M, eds. Bipolar Disorders: Clinical Course and Outcome. Washington, DC: American Psychiatric Press, 1999; Goodnick PJ, ed. Mania: Clinical and Research Perspectives. Washington, DC: American Psychiatric Press, 1998; Manji HK, Bowden CL, Belmaker RH, eds. Bipolar Medications: Mechanisms of Action. Washington, DC: American Psychiatric Press, 2000; White HS. Mechanism of action of newer anticonvulsants. J Clin Psychiatry 2003;64(Suppl 8):5–8; and Canadian Network for Mood and Anxiety Treatments (CANMAT) and International Society for Bipolar Disorders (ISBD) collaborative update of CANMAT guidelines for the management of patients with bipolar disorder: update 2009. Bipolar Disord 2009;11:225–255.

TABLE 70–8 Guidelines for Baseline and Routine Laboratory Tests and Monitoring for Agents Used in the Treatment of Bipolar Disorder

	Baseline: Physical Examination & General Chemistry[a]	Hematologic Tests[b]		Metabolic Tests[c]		Liver Function Tests[d]		Renal Function Tests[e]		Thyroid Function Tests[f]		Serum Electrolytes[g]		Dermatologic[h]	
	Baseline	Baseline	6–12 months	Baseline	6–12 months	Baseline	6–12 months	Baseline	6–12 months	Baseline	6–12 months	Baseline	6–12 months	Baseline	3–6 months
SGAs[i]	X			X	X										
Carbamazepine[j]	X	X	X			X	X	X						X	X
Lamotrigine[k]	X													X	X
Lithium[l]	X	X	X	X	X			X	X	X	X	X		X	X
Oxcarbazepine[m]	X	X	X	X	X							X	X		
Valproate[n]	X	X	X	X	X	X	X							X	X

[a]Screen for drug abuse and serum pregnancy.
[b]Complete blood cell count (CBC) with differential and platelets.
[c]Fasting glucose, serum lipids, weight.
[d]Lactate dehydrogenase, aspartate aminotransferase, alanine aminotransferase, total bilirubin, alkaline phosphatase.
[e]Serum creatinine, blood urea nitrogen, urinalysis, urine osmolality, specific gravity.
[f]Triiodothyronine, total thyroxine, thyroxine uptake, and thyroid-stimulating hormone.
[g]Serum sodium.
[h]Rashes, hair thinning, alopecia.
[i]Second-generation antipsychotics: Monitor for increased appetite with weight gain (primarily in patients with initial low or normal body mass index); monitor closely if rapid or significant weight gain occurs during early therapy; cases of hyperlipidemia and diabetes reported.

[j]Carbamazepine: Manufacturer recommends CBC and platelets (and possibly reticulocyte counts and serum iron) at baseline, and that subsequent monitoring be individualized by the clinician (e.g., CBC, platelet counts, and liver function tests every 2 weeks during the first 2 months of treatment, then every 3 months if normal). Monitor more closely if patient exhibits hematologic or hepatic abnormalities or if the patient is receiving a myelotoxic drug; discontinue if platelets are <100,000/mm³ (<100 × 10⁹/L), if white blood cell (WBC) count is <3,000/mm³ (<3 × 10⁹/L) or if there is evidence of bone marrow suppression or liver dysfunction. Serum electrolyte levels should be monitored in the elderly or those at risk for hyponatremia. Carbamazepine interferes with some pregnancy tests.

[k]Lamotrigine: If renal or hepatic impairment, monitor closely and adjust dosage according to manufacturer's guidelines. Serious dermatologic reactions have occurred within 2–8 weeks of initiating treatment and are more likely to occur in patients receiving concomitant valproate, with rapid dosage escalation, or using doses exceeding the recommended titration schedule.

[l]Lithium: Obtain baseline electrocardiogram for patients older than 40 years or if preexisting cardiac disease (benign, reversible T-wave depression can occur). Renal function tests should be obtained every 2–3 months during the first 6 months, then every 6–12 months; if impaired renal function, monitor 24-hour urine volume and creatinine every 3 months; if urine volume >3 L/day, monitor urinalysis, osmolality, and specific gravity every 3 months. Thyroid function tests should be obtained once or twice during the first 6 months, then every 6–12 months; monitor for signs and symptoms of hypothyroidism; if supplemental thyroid therapy is required, monitor thyroid function tests and adjust thyroid dose every 1–2 months until thyroid function indices are within normal range, then monitor every 3–6 months.

[m]Oxcarbazepine: Hyponatremia (serum sodium concentrations <125 mEq/L [mmol/L]) has been reported and occurs more frequently during the first 3 months of therapy; serum sodium concentrations should be monitored in patients receiving drugs that lower serum sodium concentrations (e.g., diuretics or drugs that cause inappropriate antidiuretic hormone secretion) or in patients with symptoms of hyponatremia (e.g., confusion, headache, lethargy, and malaise). Hypersensitivity reactions have occurred in approximately 25%–30% of patients with a history of carbamazepine hypersensitivity and requires immediate discontinuation.

[n]Valproate: Weight gain reported in patients with low or normal body mass index. Monitor platelets and liver function during first 3–6 months if evidence of increased bruising or bleeding. Monitor closely if patients exhibit hematologic or hepatic abnormalities or in patients receiving drugs that affect coagulation, such as aspirin or warfarin; discontinue if platelets are <100,000/mm³ (<100 × 10⁹/L) or if prolonged bleeding time. Pancreatitis, hyperammonemic encephalopathy, polycystic ovary syndrome, increased testosterone, and menstrual irregularities have been reported; not recommended during first trimester of pregnancy due to risk of neural tube defects.

Data from American Psychiatric Association. Practice guideline for the treatment of patients with bipolar disorder (revision). Am J Psychiatry 2002;159:1–50; Goodnick PJ, ed. Mania: Clinical and Research Perspectives. Washington, DC: American Psychiatric Press, 1998; McEvoy GK, Miller J, Snow EK, et al. Lithium salts. AHFS Drug Information 2007. Bethesda, MD: American Society of Health-System Pharmacists, 2007:2566–2575; McEvoy GK, Miller J, Snow EK, et al. Valproate sodium, valproic acid, divalproex sodium. AHFS Drug Information 2007. Bethesda, MD: American Society of Health-System Pharmacists, 2007:2255–2262; McEvoy GK, Miller J, Snow EK, et al. Carbamazepine. AHFS Drug Information 2007. Bethesda, MD: American Society of Health-System Pharmacists, 2007:2220–2225; McEvoy GK, Miller J, Snow EK, et al. Oxcarbazepine. AHFS Drug Information 2007. Bethesda, MD: American Society of Health-System Pharmacists, 2007:2244–2246; McEvoy GK, Miller J, Snow EK, et al. Lamotrigine. AHFS Drug Information 2007. Bethesda, MD: American Society of Health-System Pharmacists, 2007:2233–2239; and American Diabetes Association, American Psychiatric Association, American Association of Clinical Endocrinologists, et al. Consensus development conference on antipsychotic drugs and obesity and diabetes. Diabetes Care 2004;27:596–601.

- For more information on the side effects, pharmacokinetics, and drug interactions of specific agents, refer to Chap. 72 on schizophrenia, Chap. 71 on major depressive disorder, and Chap. 53 on epilepsy.

ANTIPSYCHOTICS

- Both first- and second-generation antipsychotics are effective in ~70% of patients with acute mania associated with agitation, aggression, and psychosis.
- Depot antipsychotics (e.g., **haloperidol decanoate, fluphenazine decanoate,** and **risperidone long-acting injection**) can be used for maintenance therapy of bipolar disorder with noncompliance or treatment resistance.
- Controlled studies in acute mania suggest that **lithium** or **valproate** plus an antipsychotic is more effective than any of these agents alone.
- Adjunctive second-generation antipsychotics can be beneficial for breakthrough manic episodes or if there is incomplete response to lithium or valproate monotherapy.
- Both **quetiapine** and the combination of **fluoxetine/olanzapine** are effective for acute bipolar depression.
- **Clozapine** monotherapy has acute and long-term mood stabilizing effects in refractory bipolar disorder, including mixed mania and rapid cycling, but requires regular white blood cell monitoring for agranulocytosis.
- Higher initial doses of antipsychotics (e.g., 20 mg/day of **olanzapine**) are required for acute mania, but once mania is controlled (usually 7–28 days), the antipsychotic can be gradually tapered and discontinued and the patient maintained on the mood stabilizer alone.

CARBAMAZEPINE

- **Carbamazepine** is usually reserved for lithium-refractory patients, rapid cyclers, or mixed states. It has acute antimanic effects, but its long-term effectiveness is unclear. It also seems to be effective for bipolar depression.
- The combination of carbamazepine with **lithium, valproate,** and antipsychotics is often used for manic episodes in treatment-resistant patients.
- Carbamazepine induces the hepatic metabolism of antidepressants, anticonvulsants, and antipsychotics; thus, dosage adjustments may be required.
- Acute overdoses of carbamazepine are potentially lethal.
- Women who receive carbamazepine require higher doses of **oral contraceptives** or alternative contraceptive methods.
- Certain medications (e.g., **cimetidine, diltiazem, erythromycin, fluoxetine, fluvoxamine, isoniazid, itraconazole, ketoconazole, nefazodone, propoxyphene,** and **verapamil**) added to carbamazepine therapy may cause carbamazepine toxicity.
- Doses can be started at 400 to 600 mg/day in divided doses and increased by 200 mg/day every 2 to 4 days up to 10 to 15 mg/kg/day. Outpatients should be titrated upward more slowly to avoid side effects. Many patients are able to tolerate once-daily dosing once their mood episode has stabilized.

- During the first month of therapy, serum concentrations can decrease because of autoinduction of metabolizing enzymes, requiring a dose increase.
- Carbamazepine serum levels are usually obtained every 1 or 2 weeks during the first 2 months, then every 3 to 6 months during maintenance therapy. Serum samples are drawn 10 to 12 hours after the dose and at least 4 to 7 days after dosage initiation or change. Most clinicians attempt to maintain levels between 6 and 10 mcg/mL (25–42 mmol/L), but some patients may require 12 to 14 mcg/mL (51–59 mmol/L) (**Table 70–8**).

LAMOTRIGINE

- **Lamotrigine** is effective for the maintenance treatment of bipolar I disorder in adults. It has both antidepressant and mood-stabilizing effects, and it may have augmenting properties when combined with lithium or valproate. It has low rates of switching patients to mania. Although it is less effective for acute mania compared with lithium and valproate, it may be beneficial for the maintenance therapy of treatment-resistant bipolar I and II disorders, rapid cycling, and mixed states. It is often used for bipolar II patients.
- Common adverse effects include headache, nausea, dizziness, ataxia, diplopia, drowsiness, tremor, rash, and pruritus. Although most rashes resolve with continued therapy, some progress to life-threatening conditions, such as Stevens–Johnson syndrome. The incidence of rash appears to be greatest with concomitant administration of **valproate**, rapid dose escalation of lamotrigine, and higher than recommended lamotrigine initial doses. In patients taking valproate, the lamotrigine dose should be about one half the standard dose, and upward titration must be slower than usual.
- For maintenance treatment of bipolar disorder, the usual dosage range of lamotrigine is 50 to 300 mg/day. The target dose is generally 200 mg/day (100 mg/day when combined with valproate, which decreases the clearance of lamotrigine, and 400 mg/day when combined with **carbamazepine**). For patients not taking medications that affect lamotrigine's clearance, the dose is 25 mg/day for the first 2 weeks, then 50 mg/day for 3 to 4 weeks, then 100 mg/day for the next week, then 200 mg/day.

LITHIUM

- Lithium is rapidly absorbed; it is not protein bound, not metabolized, and is excreted unchanged in the urine and other body fluids.
- Lithium is effective for acute mania, but it may require 6 to 8 weeks to show antidepressant efficacy. It may be more effective for elated mania and less effective for mania with psychotic features, mixed episodes, rapid cycling, and when alcohol and drug abuse is present. Maintenance therapy is more effective in patients with fewer episodes, good functioning between episodes, and when there is a family history of good response to lithium. It produces a prophylactic response in up to two thirds of patients and reduces suicide risk by 8- to 10-fold.
- Patients with serum concentrations between 0.8 mEq/L and 1 mEq/L (mmol/L) may have fewer relapses than those with lower serum concentrations.

- Lithium augmentation of antidepressants, carbamazepine, lamotrigine, and valproate can improve response, but it may increase the risk of sedation, weight gain, GI complaints, and tremor.
- Combining lithium with **first-generation antipsychotics** may cause neurotoxicity (e.g., delirium, severe tremors, cerebellar dysfunction, and extrapyramidal symptoms). Lithium should be withdrawn and discontinued at least 2 days before electroconvulsive therapy.
- Combining lithium with **verapamil** or **diltiazem** has been reported to cause neurotoxicity and severe bradycardia.
- Initial side effects are often dose related and are worse at peak serum concentrations (1–2 hours postdose). Lowering the dose, taking smaller doses with food, using extended-release products, and once-daily dosing at bedtime may help.
- GI distress may be minimized by standard approaches or by adding antacids or antidiarrheals.
- Muscle weakness and transient lethargy occur in ~30% of patients. Polydipsia with polyuria and nocturia occurs in up to 70% of patients and is managed by changing to once-daily dosing at bedtime.
- Up to 40% of patients complain of headache, memory impairment, confusion, poor concentration, and impaired motor performance. A fine hand tremor may occur in up to 50% of patients. Hand tremor may be treated with **propranolol**, 20 to 120 mg/day.
- Lithium reduces the kidneys' ability to concentrate urine and may cause a nephrogenic diabetes insipidus with low urine-specific gravity and low osmolality polyuria (urine volume >3 L/day). This may be treated with **loop diuretics, thiazide diuretics,** or **triamterene**. If a thiazide diuretic is used, lithium doses should be decreased by 50% and lithium and potassium levels monitored.
- Long-term lithium therapy is associated with a 10% to 20% risk of morphologic renal changes (e.g., glomerular sclerosis, tubular atrophy, and interstitial nephritis).
- Lithium-induced nephrotoxicity is rare if patients are maintained on the lowest effective dose, if once-daily dosing is used, if good hydration is maintained, and if toxicity is avoided.
- Up to 30% of patients on maintenance lithium therapy develop transiently elevated serum concentrations of thyroid-stimulating hormone, and 5% to 35% of patients develop a goiter and/or hypothyroidism, which is dose-related and more likely to occur in women. This is managed by adding **levothyroxine** to the regimen.
- Lithium may cause cardiac effects, including T-wave flattening or inversion (up to 30% of patients), atrioventricular block, and bradycardia. If a patient has preexisting cardiac disease, a cardiologist should be consulted and an electrocardiogram obtained at baseline and regularly during therapy.
- Other late-appearing lithium side effects are benign reversible leukocytosis, acne, alopecia, exacerbation of psoriasis, pruritic dermatitis, maculo-papular rash, folliculitis, and weight gain.
- Lithium toxicity can occur with serum levels greater than 1.5 mEq/L (mmol/L), but the elderly may have toxic symptoms at therapeutic levels. Severe toxic symptoms may occur with serum concentrations above

2 mEq/L (mmol/L), including vomiting, diarrhea, incontinence, incoordination, impaired cognition, arrhythmias, and seizures. Permanent neurologic impairment and kidney damage may occur as a result of toxicity.

- Several factors predispose to lithium toxicity, including sodium restriction, dehydration, vomiting, diarrhea, drug interactions that decrease lithium clearance, heavy exercise, sauna baths, hot weather, and fever. Patients should be told to maintain adequate sodium and fluid intake and to avoid excessive coffee, tea, cola, and other caffeine-containing beverages and alcohol.

- If lithium toxicity is suspected, the patient should discontinue lithium and go immediately to the emergency room. Hemodialysis is generally required when serum lithium levels are greater than 4 mEq/L (mmol/L) for patients on long-term treatment, or greater than 6 to 8 mEq/L (mmol/L) after acute poisoning.

- Lithium is usually initiated with low to moderate doses (600 mg/day divided into two or three doses) for prophylaxis, and higher doses (900–1,200 mg/day, divided into two or three doses) for acute mania. Immediate-release preparations should be given two or three times daily, whereas extended-release products can be given once or twice daily. After patients are stabilized, many patients can be switched to once-daily dosing.

- Initially, serum lithium concentrations are checked once or twice weekly. After a desired serum concentration is achieved, levels should be drawn in 2 weeks, and if stable, they can be drawn every 3 to 6 months.

- Lithium clearance increases by 50% to 100% during pregnancy. Serum levels should be monitored monthly during pregnancy and weekly the month before delivery. At delivery, a dose reduction to prepregnancy doses and adequate hydration are recommended.

- For bipolar prophylaxis in elderly patients, serum concentrations of 0.4 to 0.6 mEq/L (mmol/L) are recommended.

OXCARBAZEPINE

- **Oxcarbazepine** has mood-stabilizing effects similar to those of carbamazepine, but with milder side effects, no autoinduction of metabolizing enzymes, and potentially fewer drug interactions. There are fewer data supporting its efficacy than there are for carbamazepine's efficacy, but the American Psychiatric Association treatment guidelines recommend oxcarbazepine in any situation where one would use carbamazepine. However, disagreement surrounds its place in therapy.

- Dose-related side effects include dizziness, sedation, headache, ataxia, fatigue, vertigo, abnormal vision, diplopia, nausea, vomiting, and abdominal pain. It causes more hyponatremia than carbamazepine.

- It induces the metabolism of **oral contraceptives**, and alternative contraception measures are required.

VALPROATE SODIUM AND VALPROIC ACID

- **Valproate** is as effective as **lithium** and **olanzapine** for pure mania, and it can be more effective than lithium for rapid cycling, mixed states, and bipolar disorder with substance abuse. It reduces the frequency of recurrent manic, depressive, and mixed episodes.

- **Lithium, carbamazepine, antipsychotics,** or **benzodiazepines** can augment the antimanic effects of valproate. Valproate can be added to lithium or carbamazepine to achieve synergistic effects. Second-generation antipsychotics can be added to valproate for breakthrough mania or if there is partial response to antipsychotic monotherapy.
- The most frequent dose-related side effects of valproate are GI complaints, fine hand tremor, and sedation. A β-blocker may alleviate tremors. Other side effects are ataxia, lethargy, alopecia, pruritus, prolonged bleeding, transient increases in liver enzymes, weight gain, and hyperammonemia.
- For healthy inpatient adults with mania, the starting dose of valproate is typically 20 mg/kg/day in divided doses over 12 hours. The daily dose is adjusted by 250 to 500 mg every 1 to 3 days based on response and tolerability.
- For outpatients who are hypomanic, euthymic, or for elderly patients, the starting dose is generally 5 to 10 mg/kg/day in divided doses. This is gradually increased to the optimal dose. After establishing the optimal dose, the dose can be given twice daily or at bedtime if tolerated.
- Extended-release divalproex can be given once daily, but bioavailability can be 15% lower than that of immediate release.

EVALUATION OF THERAPEUTIC OUTCOMES

- Monitoring parameters are discussed in **Table 70–5.**
- Patients who have a partial response or nonresponse to therapy should be reassessed for an accurate diagnosis, concomitant medical or psychiatric conditions, and medications or substances that exacerbate mood symptoms.
- Patients and family members should be actively involved in treatment to monitor target symptoms, response, and side effects. Standardized rating scales may be useful in monitoring for response.

See Chapter 78, Bipolar Disorder, authored by Shannon J. Drayton, for a more detailed discussion of this topic.

CHAPTER 71

Major Depressive Disorder

DEFINITION

- The essential feature of major depressive disorder is a clinical course that is characterized by one or more major depressive episodes without a history of manic, mixed, or hypomanic episodes.

PATHOPHYSIOLOGY

- *Biogenic amine hypothesis.* Depression may be caused by decreased brain levels of the neurotransmitters norepinephrine, serotonin (5-HT), and dopamine.
- *Postsynaptic changes in receptor sensitivity.* Studies of many antidepressants have demonstrated that desensitization or downregulation of norepinephrine or 5-HT_{1A} receptors may relate to onset of antidepressant effects.
- *Dysregulation hypothesis.* This theory emphasizes a failure of homeostatic regulation of neurotransmitter systems, rather than absolute increases or decreases in their activities. Effective antidepressants are theorized to restore efficient regulation to these systems.
- *5-HT/norepinephrine link hypothesis.* This theory suggests that there is a link between 5-HT and norepinephrine activity, and that both the serotonergic and noradrenergic systems are involved in the antidepressant response.
- *The role of dopamine.* Several reviews suggest that increased dopamine neurotransmission in the mesolimbic pathway may be related to the mechanism of action of antidepressants.

CLINICAL PRESENTATION

- Emotional symptoms may include diminished ability to experience pleasure, loss of interest in usual activities, sadness, pessimistic outlook, crying spells, hopelessness, anxiety (present in ~90% of depressed outpatients), feelings of guilt, and psychotic features (e.g., auditory hallucinations and delusions).
- Physical symptoms may include fatigue, pain (especially headache), sleep disturbance, appetite disturbance (decreased or increased), loss of sexual interest, and GI and cardiovascular complaints (especially palpitations).
- Intellectual or cognitive symptoms may include decreased ability to concentrate or slowed thinking, poor memory for recent events, confusion, and indecisiveness.
- Psychomotor disturbances may include psychomotor retardation (slowed physical movements, thought processes, and speech) or psychomotor agitation.

TABLE 71–1 DSM-IV-TR Criteria for Major Depressive Episode

A. Five (or more) of the following symptoms have been present during the same 2-week period and represent a change from previous functioning; at least one of the symptoms is either (1) depressed mood or (2) loss of interest or pleasure.

Note: Do not include symptoms that are clearly due to a general medical condition or mood-incongruent delusions or hallucinations.

1. Depressed mood most of the day nearly every day
2. Markedly diminished interest or pleasure in all, or almost all, activities most of the day nearly every day
3. Significant weight loss when not dieting or weight gain (e.g., a change of more than 5% of body weight in a month), or decrease or increase in appetite nearly every day
4. Insomnia or hypersomnia nearly every day
5. Psychomotor agitation or retardation nearly every day (observable by others, not merely subjective feelings of restlessness or being slowed down)
6. Fatigue or loss of energy nearly every day
7. Feelings of worthlessness or excessive or inappropriate guilt nearly every day
8. Diminished ability to think or concentrate, or indecisiveness, nearly every day
9. Recurrent thoughts of death (not just fear of dying), recurrent suicidal ideation without a specific plan, or a suicide attempt or a specific plan for committing suicide

B. The symptoms cause clinically significant distress or impairment in social, occupational, or other important areas of functioning.

C. The symptoms are not due to the direct physiological effects of a substance (e.g., a drug of abuse, a medication) or a general medical condition (e.g., hypothyroidism).

D. The symptoms are not better accounted for by bereavement (i.e., after the loss of a loved one), the symptoms persist for longer than 2 months or are characterized by marked functional impairment, morbid preoccupation with worthlessness, suicidal ideation, psychotic symptoms, or psychomotor retardation.

Reprinted with permission from the Diagnostic and Statistical Manual of Mental Disorders, Text Revision, Fourth Edition, (Copyright © 2000). American Psychiatric Association.

DIAGNOSIS

- Major depression is characterized by one or more episodes of major depression, as defined by the *Diagnostic and Statistical Manual of Mental Disorders,* 4th ed., text revision (**Table 71–1**). Symptoms must have been present nearly every day for at least 2 weeks. Patients with major depressive disorder may have one or more recurrent episodes of major depression during their lifetime.

- When a patient presents with depressive symptoms, it is necessary to investigate the possibility of a medical-, psychiatric-, and/or drug-induced cause (**Table 71–2**).

- Depressed patients should have a medication review, physical examination, mental status examination, a complete blood count with differential, thyroid function tests, and electrolyte determinations.

TABLE 71–2 Common Medical Conditions, Substance Use Disorders, and Medications Associated with Depressive Symptoms

General medical conditions

Endocrine diseases
Hypothyroidism
Addison's or Cushing's disease

Deficiency states
Pernicious anemia
Wernicke encephalopathy
Severe anemia

Infections
AIDS
Encephalitis
Human immunodeficiency virus
Mononucleosis
Sexually transmitted diseases
Tuberculosis

Collagen disorder
Systemic lupus erythematosus

Metabolic disorders
Electrolyte imbalance
Hypokalemia
Hyponatremia
Hepatic encephalopathy

Cardiovascular disease
Coronary artery disease
Congestive heart failure
Myocardial infarction

Neurologic disorders
Alzheimer's disease
Epilepsy
Huntington's disease
Multiple sclerosis
Pain
Parkinson's disease
Poststroke

Malignant disease

Substance use disorders (including *intoxication* and *withdrawal*)

Alcoholism
Marijuana abuse and dependence
Nicotine dependence
Opiate abuse and dependence (e.g., heroin)
Psychostimulant abuse and dependence (e.g., cocaine)

Drug therapy

Antihypertensives
Clonidine
Diuretics
Guanethidine sulfate
Hydralazine hydrochloride
Methyldopa
Propranolol
Reserpine

Hormonal therapy
Oral contraceptives
Steroids/adrenocorticotropic hormone

Acne therapy
Isotretinoin

Other
Interferon-β_{1a}

Data from American Psychiatric Association. Diagnostic and Statistical Manual of Mental Disorders, Fourth Edition, Text Revision. Washington, DC: American Psychiatric Association, 2000; Sofuoglu M, Dudish-Poulsen S, Poling J, et al. The effect of individual cocaine withdrawal symptoms on outcomes in cocaine users. Addict Behav 2005;30:1125–1134; and Patten SB, Barbui C. Drug-induced depression: a systematic review to inform clinical practice. Psychother Psychosom 2004;73:207–215.

DESIRED OUTCOME

- The goals of treatment of the acute depressive episode are to eliminate or reduce the symptoms of depression, minimize adverse effects, ensure compliance with the therapeutic regimen, facilitate a return to a premorbid level of functioning, and prevent further episodes of depression.

TREATMENT

NONPHARMACOLOGIC TREATMENT

- If the depressive episode is of mild to moderate severity, psychotherapy may be the first-line therapy. The efficacy of psychotherapy and antidepressants is considered to be additive. Psychotherapy alone is not recommended for the acute treatment of patients with severe and/or psychotic major depressive disorders. For uncomplicated nonchronic major depressive disorder, combined treatment may provide no unique advantage. Cognitive therapy, behavioral therapy, and interpersonal psychotherapy appear to be equal in efficacy.
- Electroconvulsive therapy (ECT) is a safe and effective treatment for major depressive disorder. It is considered when a rapid response is needed, risks of other treatments outweigh potential benefits, there has been a poor response to drugs, and the patient expresses a preference for ECT. A rapid therapeutic response (10–14 days) has been reported. Relative contraindications include increased intracranial pressure, cerebral lesions, recent myocardial infarction, recent intracerebral hemorrhage, bleeding, and otherwise unstable vascular conditions. Adverse effects of ECT include confusion, memory impairment (retrograde and anterograde), prolonged apnea, treatment emergent mania, headache, nausea, muscle aches, and cardiovascular dysfunction. Relapse rates during the year following ECT are high unless maintenance antidepressants are prescribed.
- Bright light therapy (i.e., the patient looks into a 10,000 lux intensity light box for ~30 min/day) may be used for patients with seasonal affective disorder and as adjunctive use for major depression.

PHARMACOLOGIC THERAPY

General Therapeutic Principles

- Table 71–3 shows adult doses of antidepressants.
- In general, antidepressants are equal in efficacy in groups of patients when administered in comparable doses.
- Factors that influence the choice of antidepressant include the patient's history of response, history of familial response, concurrent medical conditions, presenting symptoms, potential for drug–drug interactions, comparative side effect profiles of various drugs, patient preference, and drug cost.
- Between 65% and 70% of patients with major depression improve with drug therapy.
- Psychotically depressed individuals generally require either ECT or combination therapy with an antidepressant and an antipsychotic agent.

TABLE 71-3 Adult Dosages for Currently Available Antidepressant Medications[a]

Generic Name	Trade Name	Suggested Therapeutic Plasma Concentration ng/mL (nmol/L)	Initial Dose (mg/day)	Usual Dosage Range (mg/day)
Serotonin selective reuptake inhibitors				
Citalopram	Celexa		20	20–60
Escitalopram	Lexapro		10	10–20
Fluoxetine	Prozac		20	20–60
Fluvoxamine	Luvox		50	50–300
Paroxetine	Paxil		20	20–60
Sertraline	Zoloft		50	50–200
Serotonin/norepinephrine reuptake inhibitors				
Venlafaxine	Effexor		37.5–75	75–225
Desvenlafaxine	Pristiq		50	50
Duloxetine	Cymbalta		30	30–90
Aminoketone				
Bupropion	Wellbutrin		150	150–300
Triazolopyridines				
Nefazodone	Serzone		100	200–600
Trazodone	Desyrel		50	150–300
Tetracyclic				
Mirtazapine	Remeron		15	15–45
Tricyclics				
Tertiary amines				
Amitriptyline	Elavil	120–250 (433–903)[b]	25	100–300
Clomipramine	Anafranil		25	100–250
Doxepin	Sinequan		25	100–300
Imipramine	Tofranil	200–350 (713–1248)[c]	25	100–300
Secondary amines				
Desipramine	Norpramin	100–300 (375–1126)[c]	25	100–300
Nortriptyline	Pamelor	50–150 (190–570)	25	50–200
Monoamine oxidase inhibitors				
Phenelzine	Nardil		15	30–90
Selegiline (transdermal)	Emsam		6[d]	6–12[d]
Tranylcypromine	Parnate		10	20–60

[a]Doses listed are total daily doses; elderly patients are usually treated with approximately one-half of the dose listed.
[b]Parent drug plus metabolite.
[c]It has been suggested that combined imipramine + desipramine concentrations should fall between 150–240 ng/mL (555–900 nmol/L).
[d]Transdermal delivery system designed to deliver stated dose continuously over a 24-hour period.
Data from American Psychiatric Association. Practice guideline for the treatment of patients with major depressive disorder (revision). Am J Psychiatry 2000;157(Suppl):1–45; Baldessarini RJ. Drugs and the treatment of psychiatric disorders: Depression and anxiety disorders. In: Hardman JG, Limbrid LE, Goodman A, et al, eds. Goodman and Gilman's The Pharmacological Basis of Therapeutics, 10th ed. New York: McGraw-Hill, 2000:447–484; Mann JJ. The medical management of depression. N Engl J Med 2005;353:1819–1834; Patkar AA, Pae C-U, Masand PS. Transdermal selegiline: the new generation of monoamine oxidase inhibitors. CNS Spectrums 2006;11:363–375; and Watanabe MD, Winter ME. Tricyclic antidepressants: amitriptyline, desipramine, imipramine, and nortriptyline. In: Winter ME, ed. Basic Clinical Pharmacokinetics, 4th ed. Baltimore, MD: Lippincott Williams & Wilkins, 2004:423–437.

- The acute phase of treatment lasts 6 to 10 weeks, and the goal is remission (i.e., absence of symptoms).
- The continuation phase lasts 4 to 9 months after remission. The goal is to eliminate residual symptoms or prevent relapse.
- The maintenance phase lasts at least 12 to 36 months, and the goal is to prevent recurrence of a separate episode of depression.
- Some clinicians recommend lifelong maintenance therapy for persons at greatest risk for recurrence (i.e., persons younger than 40 years with two or more prior episodes and persons of any age with three or more prior episodes).
- Educating the patients and their support systems regarding the delay in antidepressant effects (typically 2–4 weeks) and the importance of adherence should occur before therapy is started and throughout treatment.

Drug Classification

- **Table 71-3** shows the commonly accepted classification of available antidepressants.
- **Table 71-4** shows the relative potency and selectivity of the antidepressants for inhibition of norepinephrine and 5-HT reuptake and relative side effect profiles.
- The **selective serotonin reuptake inhibitors** (SSRIs) inhibit the reuptake of 5-HT into the presynaptic neuron. They are generally chosen as first-line antidepressants because of their safety in overdose and improved tolerability compared with earlier agents.
- **Tricyclic antidepressants** (TCAs) are effective for all depressive subtypes, but their use has diminished because of the availability of equally effective therapies that are safer on overdose and better tolerated. In addition to inhibiting the reuptake of norepinephrine and 5-HT, they block adrenergic, cholinergic, and histaminergic receptors.
- The monoamine oxidase inhibitors (MAOIs) **phenelzine** and **tranyl-cypromine** increase the concentrations of norepinephrine, 5-HT, and dopamine within the neuronal synapse through inhibition of the mono-amine oxidase (MAO) enzyme system. Both drugs are nonselective inhibitors of MAO-A and MAO-B. **Selegiline** is available as a transdermal patch for treatment of major depression. It inhibits MAO-A and MAO-B in the brain but has reduced effects on MAO-A in the gut.
- The triazolopyridines **trazodone** and **nefazodone** are antagonists at the 5-HT$_2$ receptor and inhibit the reuptake of 5-HT. They can also enhance 5-HT$_{1A}$ neurotransmission. They have negligible affinity for cholinergic and histaminergic receptors. An extended-release preparation of trazodone was recently approved. Nefazodone carries a black box warning for liver failure.
- **Bupropion's** most potent neurochemical action is blockade of dopamine reuptake; it blocks the reuptake of norepinephrine to a lesser extent.
- The serotonin–norepinephrine reuptake inhibitors include **venlafaxine, desvenlafaxine,** and **duloxetine.**
- **Maprotiline** and **amoxapine** are inhibitors of norepinephrine reuptake, with less effect on 5-HT reuptake.
- **Mirtazapine** enhances central noradrenergic and serotonergic activity through the antagonism of central presynaptic α_2-adrenergic autoreceptors

TABLE 71–4 Relative Potencies of Norepinephrine and Serotonin Reuptake Blockade and Side-Effect Profile of Antidepressant Drugs

	Reuptake Antagonism		Anticholinergic Effects	Sedation	Orthostatic Hypotension	Seizures[a]	Conduction Abnormalities[a]
	Norepinephreine	Serotonin					
Serotonin selective reuptake inhibitors							
Citalopram	0	+++	0	+	0	++	0
Escitalopram	0	+++	0	0	0	0	0
Fluoxetine	0	+++	0	0	0	++	0
Fluvoxamine	0	+++	0	0	0	++	0
Paroxetine	0	+++	+	+	0	++	0
Sertraline	0	+++	0	0	0	++	0
Serotonin/norepinephrine reuptake inhibitors							
Venlafaxine[c] and desvenlafaxine[c]	+++	+++	+	+	0	++	+
Duloxetine[c]	+++	+++	+	0	+	0	0
Aminoketone							
Bupropion[d]	+	0	+	0	0	+++	+
Triazolopyridines							
Nefazodone	0	++	0	++	++	++	+
Trazodone	0	++	0	+++	++	++	++
Tetracyclic							
Mirtazapine	0	0	+	++	++	0	+

(continued)

TABLE 71–4 Relative Potencies of Norepinephrine and Serotonin Reuptake Blockade and Side-Effect Profile of Antidepressant Drugs (Continued)

	Reuptake Antagonism		Anticholinergic Effects	Sedation	Orthostatic Hypotension	Seizures[a]	Conduction Abnormalities[a]
	Norepinephrine[e]	Serotonin					
Tetracyclic							
Tertiary amines							
Amitriptyline	++	++++	++++	++++	+++	+++	+++
Clomipramine	++	+++	++++	++++	++	++++	+++
Doxepin	++	++	+++	++++	++	+++	+++
Imipramine	+++	+++	+++	+++	++++	+++	+++
Secondary amines							
Desipramine	++++	+	++	++	++	++	++
Nortriptyline	+++	++	++	++	+	++	+
Monoamine oxidase inhibitors							
Phenelzine	++	++	+	++	++	+	
Selegiline	0	0	0	+	++	0	0
Tranylcypromine	++	+	+	+	++	+	+

++++, high; +++, moderate; ++, low; +, very low; 0, absent.

[a] These are uncommon side effects of antidepressant drugs, particularly when used at normal therapeutic doses.

[b] Venlafaxine: primarily 5-HT at lower doses, NE at higher doses and DA at very high doses.

[c] Duloxetine: balanced 5-HT and NE reuptake inhibition.

[d] Bupropion: also blocks dopamine reuptake.

Data from Baldessarini RJ. Drugs and the treatment of psychiatric disorders: Depression and anxiety disorders. In: Hardman JG, Limbird LE, Goodman A, et al, eds. Goodman and Gilman's The Pharmacological Basis of Therapeutics, 10th ed. New York: McGraw-Hill, 2000:447–484; Mann JJ. The medical management of depression. N Engl J Med 2005;353:1819–1834; Stahl SM, Grady MM, Moret C, Briley M. SNRIs: Their pharmacology, clinical efficacy, and tolerability in comparison with other classes of antidepressants. CNS Spectrums 2005;10:732–747; Horst WD, Preskorn SH. Mechanism of action and clinical characteristics of three atypical antidepressants: Venlafaxine, nefazodone, bupropion. J Affect Disord 1998;51:237–254; and Patkar AA, Pae C-U, Masand PS. Transdermal selegiline: the new generation of monoamine oxidase inhibitors. CNS Spectrums 2006;11:363–375.

and heteroreceptors. It also antagonizes 5-HT$_2$ and 5-HT$_3$ receptors and blocks histamine receptors.

- **St. John's wort** is an herbal nonprescription medication containing hypericum, which shows mixed results regarding efficacy. It is associated with several drug–drug interactions. Its potency, purity, and manufacture are not regulated by the FDA. Because depression is a potentially life-threatening disease, all antidepressant treatments should be overseen by a trained healthcare professional.

Adverse Effects

- Adverse-effect profiles of the various antidepressants are summarized in Table 71–4.

Tricyclic Antidepressants and Other Heterocyclics

- Anticholinergic side effects (e.g., dry mouth, blurred vision, constipation, urinary retention, tachycardia, memory impairment, and delirium) and sedation are more likely to occur with the tertiary amine **TCAs** than with the secondary amine TCAs.
- **Desipramine** is associated with an increased risk of death in patients with a family history of sudden cardiac death, cardiac dysrhythmias, or cardiac conduction disturbances.
- Orthostatic hypotension and resultant syncope, a common and potentially serious adverse effect of the **TCAs,** occurs as a result of α_1-adrenergic antagonism. Additional side effects include cardiac conduction delays and heart block, especially in patients with preexisting conduction disease.
- Other side effects that may lead to noncompliance are weight gain and sexual dysfunction.
- Abrupt withdrawal of **TCAs** (especially high doses) may result in symptoms of cholinergic rebound (e.g., dizziness, nausea, diarrhea, insomnia, and restlessness).
- **Amoxapine** is a demethylated metabolite of loxapine and, as a result of its postsynaptic receptor DA-blocking effects, may be associated with extrapyramidal side effects.
- **Maprotiline,** a tetracyclic drug, causes seizures at a higher incidence than do standard TCAs and is contraindicated in patients with a history of seizure disorder. The ceiling dose is considered to be 225 mg/day.

Venlafaxine

- **Venlafaxine** may cause a dose-related increase in diastolic blood pressure. Dosage reduction or discontinuation may be necessary if sustained hypertension occurs. Other side effects are similar to those associated with the SSRIs (e.g., nausea and sexual dysfunction).

Duloxetine

- The most common side effects of **duloxetine** are nausea, dry mouth, constipation, decreased appetite, insomnia, and increased sweating.

Selective Serotonin Reuptake Inhibitors

- The SSRIs produce fewer sedative, anticholinergic, and cardiovascular adverse effects than the TCAs and are less likely to cause weight gain than the TCAs. The primary adverse effects are nausea, vomiting, diarrhea, headache, insomnia, fatigue, and sexual dysfunction. A few patients have anxiety symptoms early in treatment.

Triazolopyridines

- **Trazodone** and **nefazodone** cause minimal anticholinergic effects. Sedation, dizziness, and orthostatic hypotension are the most frequent dose-limiting side effects.
- Priapism occurs rarely with trazodone use (1 in 6,000 male patients). Surgical intervention may be required, and impotence may result.
- A black box warning for life-threatening liver failure was added to the prescribing information for nefazodone. Treatment with nefazodone should not be initiated in individuals with active liver disease or with elevated baseline serum transaminases.

Aminoketone

- The occurrence of seizures with **bupropion** is dose related and may be increased by predisposing factors (e.g., history of head trauma or central nervous system [CNS] tumor). At the ceiling dose (450 mg/day), the incidence of seizures is 0.4%. Other side effects are nausea, vomiting, tremor, insomnia, dry mouth, and skin reactions. It is contraindicated in patients with bulimia or anorexia nervosa.

Mirtazapine

- **Mirtazapine**'s most common adverse effects are somnolence, weight gain, dry mouth, and constipation.

Monoamine Oxidase Inhibitors

- The most common adverse effect of MAOIs is postural hypotension (more likely with **phenelzine** than **tranylcypromine**), which can be minimized by divided-daily dosing. Anticholinergic side effects are common but less severe than with the TCAs. Phenelzine causes mild to moderate sedating effects, but tranylcypromine is often stimulating, and the last dose of the day is administered in the early afternoon. Sexual dysfunction in both genders is common. Phenelzine has been associated with hepatocellular damage and weight gain.
- Hypertensive crisis is a potentially fatal adverse reaction that can occur when MAOIs are taken concurrently with certain foods, especially those high in tyramine (**Table 71-5**), and with certain drugs (**Table 71-6**). Symptoms of hypertensive crisis include occipital headache, stiff neck, nausea, vomiting, sweating, and sharply elevated blood pressure. Hypertensive crisis may be treated with agents such as captopril. Education of patients taking MAOIs regarding dietary and medication restrictions is critical.

Pharmacokinetics

- The pharmacokinetics of the antidepressants is summarized in **Table 71-7**.
- The major metabolic pathways of the **TCAs** are demethylation, hydroxylation, and glucuronide conjugation. Metabolism of the TCAs appears to

TABLE 71–5	Dietary Restrictions for Patients Taking Monoamine Oxidase Inhibitors[a]

Aged cheeses[b]
Sour cream[c]
Yogurt[c]
Cottage cheese[c]
American cheese[c]
Mild Swiss cheese[c]
Wine[d] (especially Chianti and sherry)
Beer
Herring (pickled, salted, dry)
Sardines
Snails
Anchovies
Canned, aged, or processed meats
Monosodium glutamate
Liver (chicken or beef, more than 2 days old)
Fermented foods
Canned figs
Raisins
Pods of broad beans (fava beans)
Yeast extract and other yeast products
Meat extract (marmite)
Soy sauce
Chocolate[e]
Coffee[e]
Ripe avocado
Sauerkraut
Licorice

[a]According to the FDA-approved Prescribing Information for the transdermal selegiline patch, patients receiving the 6 mg/24-hour dose are not required to modify their diet. However, patients receiving the 9 or 12 mg/24 hours are still required to follow the dietary restrictions similar to the other MAOIs.
[b]Clearly warrants absolute prohibition (e.g., English Stilton, blue, Camembert, cheddar).
[c]Up to 2 oz (59 mL) daily is acceptable.
[d]3 oz (89 mL) white wine or a single cocktail is acceptable.
[e]Up to 2 oz (59 mL) daily is acceptable; larger amounts of decaffeinated coffee are acceptable.
Data from Anonymous. Lexi-comp online™ interaction analysis. Lexi-Comp Online, Lexi-Comp, Inc. http://online.lexi.com; and Anonymous. Drug interactions. Thomson MICROMEDEX Healthcare Series. https://www.thomsonhc.com.

be linear within the usual dosage range, but dose-related kinetics cannot be ruled out in the elderly.

- The SSRIs, with the possible exception of **citalopram** and **sertraline,** may have a nonlinear pattern of drug accumulation with chronic dosing.
- **Mirtazapine** is primarily eliminated in the urine.
- Factors reported to influence **TCA** plasma concentrations include disease states (e.g., renal or hepatic dysfunction), genetics, age, cigarette smoking, and concurrent drug administration. Similarly, hepatic

TABLE 71–6	Medication Restrictions for Patients Taking Monoamine Oxidase Inhibitors
Amphetamines	Local anesthetics containing sympathomimetic vasoconstrictors
Appetite suppressants	
Asthma inhalants	Meperidine
Buspirone	Methyldopa
Carbamazepine	Methylphenidate
Cocaine	Other antidepressants[a]
Cyclobenzaprine	Other MAOIs
Decongestants (topical and systemic)	Reserpine
Dextromethorphan	Rizatriptan
Dopamine	Stimulants
Ephedrine	Sumatriptan
Epinephrine	Sympathomimetics
Guanethidine	Tryptophan
Levodopa	

[a]Tricyclic antidepressants may be used with caution by experienced clinicians in treatment-resistant populations.
Data from Anonymous. Lexi-comp online™ interaction analysis. Lexi-Comp Online, Lexi-Comp, Inc. http://online.lexi.com; and Anonymous. Drug interactions. Thomson MICROMEDEX Healthcare Series. https://www.thomsonhc.com.

impairment, renal impairment, and age have been reported to influence the pharmacokinetics of **SSRIs**.

- In acutely depressed patients, there is a correlation between antidepressant effect and plasma concentrations for some **TCAs**. Table 71–3 shows suggested therapeutic plasma concentration ranges. The best-established therapeutic range is for **nortriptyline**, and data suggest a therapeutic window.
- Some indications for plasma level monitoring include inadequate response, relapse, serious or persistent adverse effects, use of higher than standard doses, suspected toxicity, elderly patients, children and adolescents, pregnant patients, patients of African or Asian descent (because of slower metabolism), cardiac disease, suspected noncompliance, suspected pharmacokinetic drug interactions, and changing brands.
- Plasma concentrations should be obtained at steady state, usually after a minimum of 1 week at constant dosage. Sampling should be done during the elimination phase, usually in the morning, 12 hours after the last dose. Samples collected in this manner are comparable for patients on once-daily, twice-daily, or thrice-daily regimens.

Drug–Drug Interactions

- Selected drug interactions of the newer-generation antidepressants are summarized in **Table 71–8**.
- The very slow elimination of **fluoxetine** and **norfluoxetine** makes it critical to ensure a 5-week washout after fluoxetine discontinuation before starting an **MAOI**. Potentially fatal reactions may occur when any **SSRI** or **TCA** is coadministered with an MAOI.

TABLE 71–7 Pharmacokinetic Properties of Antidepressants

Generic Name	Elimination Half-Life (hours)[a]	Time of Peak Plasma Concentration (hours)	Plasma Protein Binding (%)	Percentage Bioavailable	Clinically Important Metabolites
Serotonin selective reuptake inhibitors					
Citalopram	33	2–4	80	≥80	None
Escitalopram	27–32	5	56	80	None
Fluoxetine	4–6 days[b]	4–8	94	95	Norfluoxetine
Fluvoxamine	15–26	2–8	77	53	None
Paroxetine	24–31	5–7	95	36[c]	None
Sertraline	27	6–8	99	36[c]	None
Serotonin/norepinephrine reuptake inhibitors					
Venlafaxine	5	2	27–30	45	O-Desmethylvenlafaxine
Desvenlafaxine	11	7.5	30	80	None
Duloxetine	12	6	90	50	None
Aminoketone					
Bupropion	10–21	3	82–88	[d]	Hydroxybupropion Threohydrobupropion Erythrohydrobupropion
Triazolopyridines					
Nefazodone	2–4	1	99	20	Meta-chlorophenylpiperazine
Trazodone	6–11	1–2	92	[d]	Meta-chlorophenylpiperazine

(continued)

TABLE 71–7 Pharmacokinetic Properties of Antidepressants (*Continued*)

Generic Name	Elimination Half-Life (hours)[a]	Time of Peak Plasma Concentration (hours)	Plasma Protein Binding (%)	Percentage Bioavailable	Clinically Important Metabolites
Tetracyclic					
Mirtazapine	20–40	2	85	50	None
Tricyclics					
Tertiary amines					
Amitriptyline	9–46	1–5	90–97	30–60	Nortriptyline
Clomipramine	20–24	2–6	97	36–62	Desmethylclomipramine
Doxepin	8–36	1–4	68–82	13–45	Desmethyldoxepin
Imipramine	6–34	1.5–3	63–96	22–77	Desipramine
Secondary amines					
Desipramine	11–46	3–6	73–92	33–51	2-Hydroxydesipramine
Nortriptyline	16–88	3–12	87–95	46–70	10-Hydroxynortriptyline

[a]Biologic half-life in slowest phase of elimination.

[b]4–6 days with chronic dosing; norfluoxetine, 4–16 days.

[c]Increases 30%–40% when taken with food.

[d]No data available.

Data from Stahl SM, Grady MM, Moret C, Briley M. SNRIs: Their pharmacology, clinical efficacy, and tolerability in comparison with other classes of antidepressants. CNS Spectrums 2005;10:732–747; Hemeryck A, Belpaire FM. Selective serotonin reuptake inhibitors and cytochrome P-450 medicated drug-drug interactions: an update. Curr Drug Metab 2002;3:13–37; Kent JM. SNaRIs, NaSSAs, and NaRIs: new agents for the treatment of depression. Lancet 2000;355:911–918; and DeVane CL. Differential pharmacology of newer antidepressants. J Clin Psychiatry 1998;59(Suppl 20):85–93.

TABLE 71–8 Selected Drug Interactions of Newer-Generation Antidepressants

Antidepressant	Interacting Drug/Drug Class	Effect
Serotonin/norepinephrine reuptake inhibitors		
Venlafaxine and desvenlafaxine	MAOIs	Potential for hypertensive crisis, serotonin syndrome, delirium
	Sibutramine	Serotonin syndrome
	Triptans	Serotonin syndrome
Duloxetine	MAOIs	Potential for hypertensive crisis, serotonin syndrome, delirium
	Sibutramine	Serotonin syndrome
	Thioridazine	Thioridazine C_{max} increased; prolonged QTc interval
	Triptans	Serotonin syndrome
Serotonin selective reuptake inhibitors		
Citalopram and escitalopram	MAOIs	Potential for hypertensive crisis, serotonin syndrome, delirium
	Linezolid (*MAOI effects*)	Serotonin syndrome
	Sibutramine	Serotonin syndrome
	Triptans	Serotonin syndrome
Fluoxetine	Alprazolam	Increased plasma concentrations and half-life of alprazolam; increased psychomotor impairment
	Antipsychotics (e.g., haloperidol and risperidone)	Increased antipsychotic concentrations; increased extrapyramidal side effects
	β-Adrenergic blockers	Increased metoprolol serum concentrations; increased bradycardia; possible heart block
	Carbamazepine	Increased plasma concentrations of carbamazepine; symptoms of carbamazepine toxicity
	Linezolid (*MAOI effects*)	Serotonin syndrome
	MAOIs	Potential for hypertensive crisis, serotonin syndrome, delirium
	Phenytoin	Increased plasma concentrations of phenytoin; symptoms of phenytoin toxicity

(continued)

887

TABLE 71–8 Selected Drug Interactions of Newer-Generation Antidepressants *(Continued)*

Antidepressant	Interacting Drug/Drug Class	Effect
Serotonin selective reuptake inhibitors		
	TCAs	Markedly increased TCA plasma concentrations; symptoms of TCA toxicity
	Sibutramine	Serotonin syndrome
	Triptans	Serotonin syndrome
	Thioridazine	Thioridazine C_{max} increased; prolonged QTc interval
Fluvoxamine	Alosetron	Increased alosetron AUC (6-fold) and half-life (3-fold)
	Alprazolam	Increased AUC of alprazolam by 96%, increased alprazolam half-life by 71%; increased psychomotor impairment
	β-Adrenergic blockers	Fivefold increase in propranolol serum concentration; bradycardia and hypotension
	Carbamazepine	Increased plasma concentrations of carbamazepine; symptoms of carbamazepine toxicity
	Clozapine	Increased clozapine serum concentrations; increased risk for seizures and orthostatic hypotension
	Diltiazem	Bradycardia
	MAOIs	Potential for hypertensive crisis, serotonin syndrome, delirium
	Methadone	Increased methadone plasma concentrations; symptoms of methadone toxicity
	Ramelteon	Increased AUC (190-fold) and C_{max} (70-fold)
	Sibutramine	Serotonin syndrome
	TCAs	Increased TCA plasma concentration; symptoms of TCA toxicity
	Theophylline and caffeine	Increased serum concentrations of theophylline or caffeine; symptoms of theophylline or caffeine toxicity
	Thioridazine	Thioridazine C_{max} increased; prolonged QTc interval
	Warfarin	Increased hypoprothrombinemic response to warfarin
Paroxetine	Antipsychotics (e.g., haloperidol, perphenazine and risperidone)	Increased antipsychotic concentrations; increased central nervous system and extrapyramidal side effects

β-Adrenergic blockers	Increased metoprolol serum concentrations; increased bradycardia; possible heart block
Linezolid (*MAOI effects*)	Serotonin syndrome
MAOIs	Potential for hypertensive crisis, serotonin syndrome, delirium
TCAs	Markedly increased TCA plasma concentrations; symptoms of TCA toxicity
Sibutramine	Serotonin syndrome
Triptans	Serotonin syndrome
Thioridazine	Thioridazine C_{max} increased; prolonged QTc interval
Sertraline	
Linezolid (*MAOI effects*)	Serotonin syndrome
MAOIs	Potential for hypertensive crisis, serotonin syndrome, delirium
Sibutramine	Serotonin syndrome
Triptans	Serotonin syndrome
Tetracyclic	
Mirtazapine	
Carbamazepine	Mirtazapine concentration decrease (60%)
MAOIs	Theoretically central serotonin syndrome could occur
Aminoketone	
Bupropion	
MAOIs	Potential for hypertensive crisis
Medications that lower seizure threshold	Increased incidence of seizures

AUC, area under the curve; C_{max}, maximum concentration; MAOI, monoamine oxidase inhibitor.
Data from Anonymous. Lexi-comp online™ interaction analysis. Lexi-Comp Online, Lexi-Comp, Inc. http://online.lexi.com; and Anonymous. Drug interactions. Thomson MICROMEDEX Healthcare Series. https://www.thomsonhc.com.

TABLE 71–9	Second- and Third-Generation Antidepressants and Cytochrome (CYP) P450 Enzyme Inhibitory Potential			
	CYP Enzyme			
Drug	*1A2*	*2C*	*2D6*	*3A4*
Buproprion	0	0	+	0
Citalopram	0	0	+	NA
Escitalopram	0	0	+	0
Fluoxetine	0	++	++++	++
Fluvoxamine	++++	++	0	+++
Mirtazapine	0	0	0	0
Nefazodone	0	0	0	++++
Paroxetine	0	0	++++	0
Sertraline	0	++	+	+
(des)Venlafaxine	0	0	0/+	0

++++, high; +++, moderate; ++, low; +, very low; 0, absent.

Data from Preskorn SH. Clinically relevant pharmacology of selective serotonin reuptake inhibitors: An overview with emphasis on pharmacokinetics and effects on oxidative drug metabolism. Clin Pharmacokinet 1997;32(Suppl 1):1–21; Hemeryck A, Belpaire FM. Selective serotonin reuptake inhibitors and cytochrome P-450 mediated drug-drug interactions: an update. Curr Drug Metab 2002;3:13–37; Kent JM. SNaRIs, NaSSAs, and NaRIs: new agents for the treatment of depression. Lancet 2000;355:911–918; and DeVane CL. Differential pharmacology of newer antidepressants. J Clin Psychiatry 1998;59(Suppl 20):85–93.

- Increased plasma concentrations of **TCAs** and symptoms of toxicity may occur when **fluoxetine** and **paroxetine** are added to a TCA regimen.
- The combination of an SSRI with another 5-HT augmenting agent can lead to the serotonin syndrome, which is characterized by symptoms such as clonus, hyperthermia, and mental status changes.
- The ability of an SSRI, or any antidepressant, to inhibit or induce the activity of the cytochrome P450 (CYP450) enzymes can be a significant contributory factor in determining its capability to cause a pharmacokinetic drug–drug interaction.
- **Table 71–9** compares second- and third-generation antidepressants for their effects on the enzymes of the CYP450 system.
- The drug interaction literature should be consulted for detailed information concerning any real or potential drug interaction involving any psychotherapeutic agent.

SPECIAL POPULATIONS

Elderly Patients

- Prominent symptoms of depression in the elderly are loss of appetite, cognitive impairment, sleeplessness, anergia, fatigue, physical complaints, and loss of interest in and enjoyment of the normal pursuits of life.
- The **SSRIs** are often selected as first-choice antidepressants in elderly patients.
- **Bupropion** and **venlafaxine** may also be chosen because of their milder anticholinergic and less frequent cardiovascular side effects.

Children and Adolescents

- Symptoms of depression in childhood include boredom, anxiety, failing adjustment, and sleep disturbance.
- Data supporting efficacy of antidepressants in children and adolescents are sparse. **Fluoxetine** is the only antidepressant that is FDA approved for treatment of depression in patients younger than 18 years of age.
- The FDA has established a link between antidepressant use and suicidality (suicidal thinking and behaviors) in children, adolescents, and young adults 18 to 24 years old. All antidepressants carry a black box warning providing cautions in the use of all antidepressants in this population, and the FDA also recommends specific monitoring parameters. The clinician should consult the FDA-approved labeling or the FDA website for additional information. However, several retrospective longitudinal reviews of the use of antidepressants in children found no significant increase in the risk of suicide attempts or deaths.
- Several cases of sudden death have been reported in children and adolescents taking **desipramine**. A baseline electrocardiogram (ECG) is recommended before initiating a TCA in children and adolescents, and an additional ECG is advised when steady-state plasma concentrations are achieved. TCA plasma concentration monitoring is critical to ensure safety.

Pregnancy

- As a general rule, if effective, nondrug approaches are preferred when treating depressed pregnant patients.
- One study showed that pregnant women who discontinued antidepressants were five times more likely to relapse during their pregnancy than were women who continued treatment.
- No major teratogenic effects have been identified with the **SSRIs** or **TCAs**. However, evaluations to date suggest a possible association of **fluoxetine** with low birth weight and respiratory distress. Another study reported a sixfold greater likelihood of the occurrence of persistent pulmonary hypertension of newborn infants exposed to an SSRI after the twentieth week of gestation.
- The risks of untreated depression in pregnancy should be considered. These included low birth weight, maternal suicidality, potential for hospitalization or marital discord, poor prenatal care, and difficulty caring for other children.

Refractory Patients

- Most "treatment-resistant" depressed patients have received inadequate therapy. Issues to be considered in patients who have not responded to treatment include the following: (1) Is the diagnosis correct? (2) Does the patient have a psychotic depression? (3) Has the patient received an adequate dose and duration of treatment? (4) Do adverse effects preclude adequate dosing? (5) Has the patient been compliant with the prescribed regimen? (6) Was treatment outcome measured adequately? (7) Is there a coexisting or preexisting medical or psychiatric disorder? (8) Was a stepwise approach to treatment used? (9) Are there other factors that interfere with treatment?

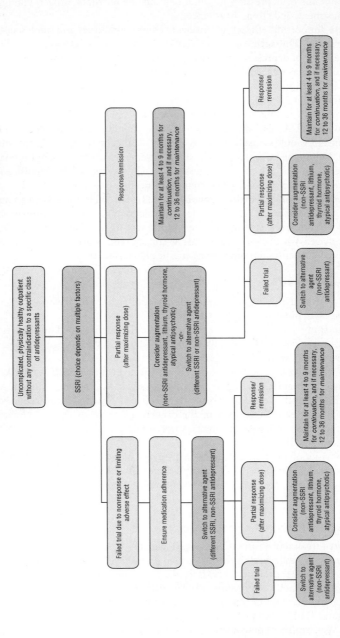

FIGURE 71–1. Algorithm for treatment of uncomplicated major depressive disorder. (SSRI, selective serotonin reuptake inhibitor.)

- The STAR*D study showed that one in three depressed patients who previously did not achieve remission with an antidepressant became symptom-free with the help of an additional medication (e.g., **sustained-release bupropion**), and one in four achieved remission after switching to a different antidepressant (e.g., **extended-release venlafaxine**).
- The current antidepressant may be stopped and a trial initiated with an agent of unrelated chemical structure (e.g., **mirtazapine** or **nortriptyline**).
- Alternatively, the current antidepressant may be augmented (potentiated) by the addition of another agent (e.g., **lithium** or **triiodothyronine [T_3]**), or another antidepressant can be added. An atypical antipsychotic can be used to augment antidepressant response.
- The practice guideline of the American Psychiatric Association recommends that after 6 to 8 weeks of antidepressant treatment, partial responders should consider changing the dose, augmenting the antidepressant, or adding psychotherapy or ECT. For those with no response, options include changing to another antidepressant or the addition of psychotherapy or ECT.
- An algorithm for treatment of depression including refractory patients is shown in **Fig. 71–1**.

Clinical Application

- A 6-week antidepressant trial at a maximum dosage is considered an adequate trial. Patients must be told about the expected lag time of 2 to 4 weeks before the onset of antidepressant effect.
- Elderly patients should receive one half the initial dose given to younger adults, and the dose is increased at a slower rate. The elderly may require 6 to 12 weeks of treatment to achieve the desired antidepressant response.
- To prevent relapse, antidepressants should be continued at full therapeutic doses for 4 to 9 months after remission.

EVALUATION OF THERAPEUTIC OUTCOMES

- Several monitoring parameters, in addition to plasma concentrations, are useful in managing patients. Patients must be monitored for adverse effects, remission of previously documented target symptoms, and changes in social or occupational functioning. Regular monitoring should be assured for several months after antidepressant therapy is discontinued.
- Patients given **venlafaxine** should have blood pressure monitored regularly.
- Patients older than age 40 years should receive a pretreatment ECG before starting TCA therapy, and follow-up ECGs should be performed periodically.
- Patients should be monitored for emergence of suicidal ideation after initiation of any antidepressant, especially in the first few weeks of treatment.
- In addition to the clinical interview, psychometric rating instruments allow for rapid and reliable measurement of the nature and severity of depressive and associated symptoms.

See Chapter 77, Major Depressive Disorder, authored by Christian J. Teter, Judith C. Kando, and Barbara G. Wells, for a more detailed discussion of this topic.

DEFINITION

- Schizophrenia is a chronic heterogeneous syndrome of disorganized and bizarre thoughts, delusions, hallucinations, inappropriate affect, cognitive deficits, and impaired psychosocial functioning.

PATHOPHYSIOLOGY

- Multiple etiologies likely exist.
- Increased ventricular size, decreased brain size, and brain asymmetry have been reported. Lower hippocampal volume may correspond to impairment in neuropsychological testing.
- *Dopaminergic hypothesis.* Psychosis may result from hyper- or hypoactivity of dopaminergic processes in specific brain regions. This may include the presence of a dopamine receptor defect.
- Positive symptoms (see Diagnosis section below) may be more closely associated with dopamine receptor hyperactivity in the mesocaudate, whereas negative symptoms (see Diagnosis section below) and cognitive symptoms (see Diagnosis section below) may be most closely related to dopamine receptor hypofunction in the prefrontal cortex.
- *Glutamatergic dysfunction.* A deficiency of glutamatergic activity produces symptoms similar to those of dopaminergic hyperactivity and possibly symptoms seen in schizophrenia.
- *Serotonin* (5-hydroxytriptamine *[5-HT]*) *abnormalities.* Schizophrenic patients with abnormal brain scans have higher whole blood 5-HT concentrations; these concentrations correlate with increased ventricular size.

CLINICAL PRESENTATION

- Symptoms of the acute episode may include the following: being out of touch with reality; hallucinations (especially hearing voices); delusions (fixed false beliefs); ideas of influence (actions controlled by external influences); disconnected thought processes (loose associations); ambivalence (contradictory thoughts); flat, inappropriate, or labile affect; autism (withdrawn and inwardly directed thinking); uncooperativeness, hostility, and verbal or physical aggression; impaired self-care skills; and disturbed sleep and appetite.
- After the acute psychotic episode has resolved, the patient typically has residual features (e.g., anxiety, suspiciousness, lack of volition, lack of motivation, poor insight, impaired judgment, social withdrawal, difficulty in learning from experience, and poor self-care skills). Patients often have comorbid substance abuse and are nonadherent with medications.

DIAGNOSIS

- The *Diagnostic and Statistical Manual of Mental Disorders*, 4th ed., text revision (*DSM-IV-TR*), specifies the following criteria for the diagnosis of schizophrenia:
  ✓ Persistent dysfunction lasting longer than 6 months
  ✓ Two or more symptoms (present for at least 1 month), including hallucinations, delusions, disorganized speech, grossly disorganized or catatonic behavior, and negative symptoms
  ✓ Significantly impaired functioning (work, interpersonal, or self-care)
- The *DSM-IV-TR* classifies symptoms as positive or negative.
- Positive symptoms (the ones most affected by antipsychotic drugs) include delusions, disorganized speech (association disturbance), hallucinations, behavior disturbance (disorganized or catatonic), and illusions.
- Negative symptoms include alogia (poverty of speech), avolition, affective flattening, anhedonia, and social isolation.
- Cognitive dysfunction is another symptom category that includes impaired attention, working memory, and executive function.

DESIRED OUTCOME

- The goals of treatment include the following: alleviation of target symptoms, avoidance of side effects, improvement in psychosocial functioning and productivity, compliance with the prescribed regimen, and involvement of the patient in treatment planning.

TREATMENT

- A thorough mental status examination, physical and neurologic examination, complete family and social history, psychiatric diagnostic interview, and laboratory workup (complete blood count, electrolytes, hepatic function, renal function, electrocardiogram [ECG], fasting serum glucose, serum lipids, thyroid function, and urine drug screen) should be performed prior to treatment.

GENERAL THERAPEUTIC PRINCIPLES

- Second-generation antipsychotics (SGAs) (also known as *atypical antipsychotics*), except clozapine, are the agents of first choice in the treatment of schizophrenia. SGAs (e.g., **clozapine, olanzapine, risperidone, quetiapine, ziprasidone,** and **aripiprazole**) may have superior efficacy for the treatment of negative symptoms and cognition, but this is controversial.
- SGAs cause few or no acutely occurring extrapyramidal side effects. Other attributes ascribed include minimal or no propensity to cause tardive dyskinesia (TD) and less effect on serum prolactin than the first-generation antipsychotics (FGAs) (also called typical antipsychotics). **Clozapine** is the only SGA that fulfills all these criteria.

- SGAs have an increased risk for metabolic side effects, including weight gain, hyperlipidemia, and diabetes mellitus.
- The Clinical Antipsychotic Trials of Intervention Effectiveness study showed that olanzapine, compared with quetiapine, risperidone, ziprasidone, and perphenazine, has modest superiority in persistence of maintenance therapy but more metabolic side effects.
- Selection of an antipsychotic should be based on (1) the need to avoid certain side effects, (2) concurrent medical or psychiatric disorders, and (3) patient or family history of response. Fig. 72–1 is an algorithm for management of first episode psychosis.

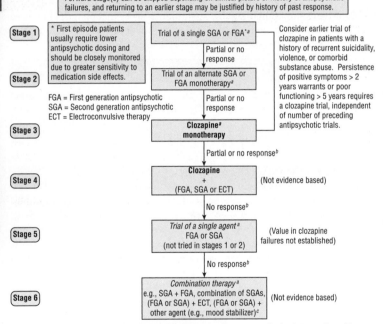

Algorithm for the pharmacotherapy of schizophrenia

Choice of antipsychotic (AP) should be guided by considering the clinical characteristics of the patient and the efficacy and side effect profiles of available medication.

Forward stage(s) can be skipped depending on clinical picture or history of antipsychotic failures, and returning to an earlier stage may be justified by history of past response.

Stage 1 — * First episode patients usually require lower antipsychotic dosing and should be closely monitored due to greater sensitivity to medication side effects.

Trial of a single SGA or FGA*a

Partial or no response

Stage 2 — Trial of an alternate SGA or FGA monotherapy a

FGA = First generation antipsychotic
SGA = Second generation antipsychotic
ECT = Electroconvulsive therapy

Partial or no response

Stage 3 — Clozapine a monotherapy

Consider earlier trial of clozapine in patients with a history of recurrent suicidality, violence, or comorbid substance abuse. Persistence of positive symptoms > 2 years warrants or poor functioning > 5 years requires a clozapine trial, independent of number of preceding antipsychotic trials.

Partial or no response b

Stage 4 — Clozapine + (FGA, SGA or ECT)   (Not evidence based)

No response b

Stage 5 — Trial of a single agent a FGA or SGA (not tried in stages 1 or 2)   (Value in clozapine failures not established)

No response b

Stage 6 — Combination therapy a e.g., SGA + FGA, combination of SGAs, (FGA or SGA) + ECT, (FGA or SGA) + other agent (e.g., mood stabilizer)c   (Not evidence based)

aIf patient is inadequately adherent at any stage, the clinician should assess contributing factors and consider switching to long-acting monotherapy antipsychotic treatment,

bA treatment refractory evaluation should be performed to reexamine diagnosis, substance abuse, medication adherence, and psychosocial stressors. cognitive behavioral therapy and other psychosocial augmentations should be considered.

cWhenever a second medication is added to an antipsychotic (other than clozapine) for the purpose of improving psychotic symptoms, the patient is considered to be in stage 6.

FIGURE 72–1. Patient entry into the algorithm is determined by individual patient history, clinical presentation, and consideration of potential side-effect risk. Either first episode patients or patients who have been off of medications and are reentering treatment with no history of poor response to antipsychotics are entered at stage 1. Algorithm stages can be skipped if clinically

FIGURE 72–1. *(continued)* appropriate, and one can go back stages if indicated. In general, inadequately responding patients should not remain in stages 1 or 2 longer than 12 weeks at therapeutic doses. Stage 3 should be at least 6 months. In stages 4, 5, and 6, a 12-week trial is recommended, and if there is greater than or equal to 20% improvement in positive symptoms at week 12, the medication trial warrants extension for an additional 12 weeks with dose titration as clinically warranted. The levels of evidence for algorithm recommendations are as follows: stage 1, level A for efficacy for both first-generation antipsychotics (FGAs) and second-generation antipsychotics (SGAs); stage 2, level A; stage 3, level A; stage 4, level C; stage 5, level C; stage 6, level C. Level A is supported by one or more randomized controlled trials. Level B is supported by large cohort studies, epidemiologic studies, and so on. Level C is supported only by case series, case reports, or expert opinion.

Data from Moore TA, Buchanan RW, Buckley PF, et al. The Texas Medication Algorithm Project antipsychotic algorithm for schizophrenia: 2006 update. J Clin Psychiatry 2007;68:1751–1762; Buchanan RW, Kreyenbuhl J, Kelly DL, et al. The 2009 schizophrenia PORT psychopharmacological treatment recommendations and summary statements. Schizophr Bull 2010;36:71–93; and Alvarez-Jimenez M, Parker AG, Hetrick SE, et al. Preventing the second episode: a systematic review and meta-analysis of psychosocial and pharmacological trials in first-episode psychosis. Schizophrenia Bulletin 2009 Nov 9. [Epub ahead of print]

- All FGAs are equal in efficacy in groups of patients when used in equipotent doses.
- Dosage equivalents (expressed as chlorpromazine [CPZ]-equivalent dosages—the equipotent dosage of an FGA compared with 100 mg of CPZ) may be useful when switching from one FGA to another (Table 72–1).
- Predictors of good antipsychotic response include a prior good response to the drug selected, absence of alcohol or drug abuse, acute onset and short duration of illness, acute stressors or precipitating factors, later age of onset, affective symptoms, family history of affective illness, compliance with the prescribed regimen, and good premorbid adjustment. Negative symptoms are generally less responsive to antipsychotic therapy.
- An initial dysphoric response, demonstrated by a dislike of the medication or feeling worse, combined with anxiety or akathisia, is associated with a poor drug response, adverse effects, and nonadherence.
- If partial or poor adherence is an issue, a long-acting or depot injectable antipsychotic should be considered (e.g., risperidone microspheres, paliperidone palmitate, extended-release olanzapine, haloperidol decanoate, or fluphenazine decanoate).

PHARMACOKINETICS

- Pharmacokinetic parameters and major metabolic pathways of antipsychotics are summarized in Table 72–2.
- Antipsychotics are highly lipophilic and highly bound to membranes and plasma proteins.

TABLE 72–1 Available Antipsychotics: Doses and Dosage Forms

Generic Name	Trade Name	Traditional Equivalent Dose (mg)	Usual Dosage Range (mg/day)	Manufacturer's Maximum Dose (mg/day)[a]	Dosage Forms[b]
First-generation antipsychotics (traditional or typical antipsychotics)					
Chlorpromazine	Thorazine	100	100–800	2,000	T,L,LC,I,C-ER,S
Fluphenazine	Prolixin	2	2–20	40	T,L,LC,I,LAI
Haloperidol	Haldol	2	2–20	100	T,LC,I,LAI
Loxapine	Loxitane	10	10–80	250	C,LC
Molindone	Moban	10	10–100	225	T,LC
Perphenazine	Trilafon	10	10–64	64	T,LC,I
Thioridazine	Mellaril	100	100–800	800	T,LC
Thiothixene	Navane	4	4–40	60	C,LC
Trifluoperazine	Stelazine	5	5–40	80	T,LC,I
Second-generation antipsychotics (atypical antipsychotics)					
Aripiprazole	Abilify	NA	15–30	30	T,O,L
Asenapine	Saphris	NA	10–20	20	SL
Clozapine	Clozaril	NA	50–500	900	T,O
Iloperidone	Fanapt	NA	2–24	24	T
Olanzapine	Zyprexa	NA	10–20	20	T,I,O
Paliperidone	Invega	NA	3–9	12	ER
Paliperidone palmitate	Invega Sustenna	NA	39–234	234	LAI
Quetiapine	Seroquel	NA	250–500	800	T
Risperidone	Risperdal	NA	2–8	16	T,O,L
Risperidone	Risperdal Consta	NA	25–50 mg every 2 wk	50	LAI
Ziprasidone	Geodon	NA	40–160	200	C,I

[a]NA. This parameter does not apply to atypical antipsychotics.
[b]C, capsule; ER or SR, extended or sustained release; I, injection; L, liquid solution, elixir, or suspension; LC, liquid concentrate; LAI, long-acting injectable; O, orally disintegrating tablets; R, rectal suppositories; SL, sublingual tablet; T, tablet.

- They have large volumes of distribution and are largely metabolized through the cytochrome P450 pathways (except ziprasidone).
- **Risperidone** and its active metabolite 9-OH-resperidone are metabolized by CYP2D6. Polymorphic metabolism should be considered in those with side effects at low doses (~40% of African Americans and Asians can have increased side effects from risperidone and other drugs metabolized through CYP2D6).
- Most antipsychotics have half-lives of elimination in the range of 20 to 40 hours. After dosage stabilization, most antipsychotics (except

TABLE 72–2	Pharmacokinetic Parameters of Selected Antipsychotics			
Drug	**Bioavailability (%)**	**Half-Life (hours)**	**Major Metabolic Pathways**	**Active Metabolites**
Selected first-generation antipsychotics (FGAs)				
Chlorpromazine	10–30	8–35	FMO3, CYP3A4	7-hydroxy, others
Fluphenazine	20–50	14–24	CYP2D6	?
Fluphenazine decanoate		14.2 ± 2.2[a] days	CYP2D6	
Haloperidol	40–70	12–36	CYP1A2, CYP2D6, CYP3A4	Reduced haloperidol
Haloperidol decanoate		21 days	CYP1A2, CYP2D6, CYP3A4	Reduced haloperidol
Perphenazine	20–25	8.1–12.3	CYP2D6	7-OH-perphenazine
Second-generation antipsychotics (SGAs)				
Aripiprazole	87	48–68	CYP3A4, CYP2D6	Dehydroaripiprazole
Asenapine	<2% PO 35% SL Nonlinear	13–39	CYP1A2, UGT1A4	None known
Clozapine	12–81	11–105	CYP1A2, CYP3A4, CYP2C19	Desmethylclozapine
Iloperidone	96	18–33	CYP2D6, CYP3A4	P88
Olanzapine	80	20–70	CYP1A2, CYP3A4, FMO3	N-glucuronide; 2-OH-methyl; 4-N-oxide
Paliperidone ER	28	23	Renal unchanged (59%) Multiple pathways	None known
Paliperidone Palmitate		25–49 days	Renal unchanged (59%) Multiple pathways	None known
Quetiapine	9 ± 4	6.88	CYP3A4	7-OH-quetiapine
Risperidone	68	3–24	CYP2D6	9-OH-risperidone
Risperidone Consta		3–6 days	CYP2D6	9-OH-risperidone
Ziprasidone	59	4–10	Aldehyde oxidase, CYP3A4	None

[a]Based on multiple dose data. Single dose data indicate a β–half-life of 6–10 days.

Data from Citrome L. Paliperidone Palmitate – a review of the efficacy, safety and cost of a new second-generation depot antipsychotic medication. Int J Clin Pract 2010;64:216–239; Citrome L. Iloperidone for schizophrenia: a review of the efficacy and safety profile for this newly commercialized second-generation antipsychotic. Int J Clin Pract 2009;63:1237–1248; Citrome L. Asenapine for schizophrenia and bipolar disorder: a review of the efficacy and safety profile for this newly approved sublingually absorbed second-generation antipsychotic. Int J Clin Pract 2009;63:1762–1784; Harrison TS, Goa KL. Long-acting risperidone: A review of its use in schizophrenia. CNS Drugs 2004;18:113–132; Ereshefsky L, Saklad SR, Jann MW, et al. Future of depot neuroleptic therapy: Pharmacokinetics and pharmacodynamic approaches. J Clin Psychiatry 1984;45(5 pt 2):50–59; Ereshefsky L, Toney G, Saklad SR, Seidel DR. A loading dose strategy for converting from oral to depot haloperidol. Hosp Community Psychiatry 1993;44:1155–1161; De Leon A, Patel NC,

TABLE 72–2 *(continued)*

Crismon ML. Aripiprazole: A comprehensive review of its pharmacology, clinical efficacy, and tolerability. Clin Ther 2004;26:649–666; Mauri MC, Volonteri LS, Colasanti A, et al. Clinical pharmacokinetics of atypical antipsychotics: a critical review of the relationship between plasma concentrations and clinical response. Clin Pharmacokinet 2007;46:359–388; Zhou SF, Liu JP, Chowbay B. Polymorphism of human cytochrome P450 enzymes and its clinical impact. Drug Metabolism Reviews 2009;41:89–295; Spina E, de Leon J. Metabolic drug interactions with newer antipsychotics: a comparative review. Basic Clin Pharmacol Toxicol 2007;100:4–22; and Urichuk L, Prior TI, Dursun, Baker G. Metabolism of atypical antipsychotics: involvement of cytochrome P450 enzymes and relevance for drug-drug interactions. Curr Drug Metabo 2008;9:410–418.

quetiapine and **ziprasidone**) can be dosed once daily. It may be possible to dose SGAs less often than their plasma kinetics would suggest.

- A 12-hour postdose **clozapine** serum concentration of at least 350 ng/mL (1.07 μmol/L) is recommended.
- Serum concentration monitoring of clozapine should be done before exceeding 600 mg daily in patients who develop unusual or severe adverse side effects, in those taking concomitant medications that might cause drug interactions, in those with age or pathophysiologic changes suggesting altered kinetics, and in those suspected of being nonadherent to their regimens.

INITIAL THERAPY

- The goals during the first 7 days are decreased agitation, hostility, anxiety, and aggression and normalization of sleep and eating patterns.
- In general, titrate over the first few days to an average effective dose. After 1 week at a stable dose, a modest dosage increase may be considered. If there is no improvement within 3 to 4 weeks at therapeutic doses, then an alternative antipsychotic should be considered (i.e., move to the next treatment stage in the algorithm; see **Fig. 72–1**).
- In partial responders who are tolerating the antipsychotic well, it may be reasonable to titrate above the usual dose range with close monitoring for response and side effects.
- In general, rapid titration of antipsychotic dose is not recommended.
- Intramuscular (IM) antipsychotic administration (e.g., aripiprazole 5.25–9.75 mg, ziprasidone 10–20 mg, olanzapine 2.5–10 mg, or haloperidol 2–5 mg) can be used to calm agitated patients. However, this approach does not improve the extent of response, time to remission, or length of hospitalization.
- IM **lorazepam**, 2 mg, as needed in combination with the maintenance antipsychotic may actually be more effective in controlling agitation than using additional doses of the antipsychotic. The combination of IM lorazepam and IM **olanzapine** is not recommended because of the risk of hypotension, CNS depression, and respiratory depression.

STABILIZATION THERAPY

- During weeks 2 and 3, the goals should be to improve socialization, self-care habits, and mood. Improvement in formal thought disorder may require an additional 6 to 8 weeks.

- Most patients require a dose of 300 to 1,000 mg of CPZ equivalents (of FGAs) daily or SGAs in usual labeled doses. Dose titration may continue every 1 to 2 weeks as long as the patient has no side effects.
- If symptom improvement is not satisfactory after 8 to 12 weeks, a different strategy (see **Fig. 72–1**) should be tried.

MAINTENANCE THERAPY

- Medication should be continued for at least 12 months after remission of the first psychotic episode. Continuous treatment is necessary in most patients at the lowest effective dose.
- Antipsychotics (especially FGAs and **clozapine**) should be tapered slowly before discontinuation to avoid rebound cholinergic withdrawal symptoms.
- In general, when switching from one antipsychotic to another, the first should be tapered and discontinued over 1 to 2 weeks after the second antipsychotic is initiated.

Depot Antipsychotic Medications

- The principle for conversion from oral antipsychotics to depot formulations is as follows:
  ✓ Stabilize on an oral dosage form of the same agent (or at least a short trial of 3–7 days) to be sure the medication is tolerated adequately.
- **Risperidone Consta** is the first SGA to be available as a long-acting injectable. The recommended starting dose is 25 mg. Usual dosing range is 25 to 50 mg deep IM every 2 weeks. It is a suspension of drug in glycolic acid–lactate copolymer microspheres. Significant risperidone serum concentrations are measurable about 3 weeks after single-dose administration. Thus, oral medication must be administered for at least 3 weeks after beginning injections. Dose adjustments should be made no more often than every 4 weeks.
- **Paliperidone palmitate** is started at a dose of 234 mg on day 1 and 156 mg 1 week later. No overlap of oral dosing is necessary. Monthly IM doses are then titrated between 39 and 234 mg.
- For **fluphenazine decanoate**, an esterified formulation in sesame seed oil, the simplest conversion is the Stimmel method, which uses 1.2 times the oral daily dose for stabilized patients, rounding up to the nearest 12.5 mg interval, administered IM in weekly doses for the first 4 to 6 weeks (1.6 times the oral daily dose for patients who are more acutely ill). Subsequently, fluphenazine decanoate may be administered once every 2 to 3 weeks. Oral fluphenazine may be overlapped for 1 week.
- For **haloperidol decanoate**, an esterified formulation in sesame seed oil, a factor of 10 to 15 times the oral daily dose is commonly recommended, rounding up to the nearest 50-mg interval, administered IM in a once-monthly dose with oral haloperidol overlap for 1 month.
- Haloperidol and fluphenazine decanoate should be administered by a deep, "Z-track" IM method. Long-acting risperidone is injected by deep IM injection in the gluteus maximus, but Z-tracking is not necessary.

- In patients previously unexposed to the drug, an oral test dose of the medication is recommended before long-acting antipsychotics are given.

MANAGEMENT OF TREATMENT-RESISTANT SCHIZOPHRENIA

- Only **clozapine** has shown superiority over other antipsychotics in randomized clinical trials for the management of treatment-resistant schizophrenia.
- Symptomatic improvement with clozapine often occurs slowly in resistant patients; as high as 60% of patients may improve if clozapine is used for up to 6 months.
- Because of the risk of orthostatic hypotension, clozapine is usually titrated more slowly than other antipsychotics. If a 12.5 mg test dose does not produce hypotension, then 25 mg of clozapine at bedtime is recommended, increased to 25 mg twice daily after 3 days, then increased in 25 to 50 mg/day increments every 3 days until a dose of at least 300 mg/day is reached.
- Augmentation therapy involves the addition of a nonantipsychotic drug to an antipsychotic in a poorly responsive patient, whereas combination treatment involves using two antipsychotics simultaneously.
- Responders to augmentation therapy usually improve rapidly. If there is no improvement, the augmenting agent should be discontinued.
- Mood stabilizers (e.g., **lithium, valproic acid,** and **carbamazepine**) used as augmentation agents may improve labile affect and agitated behavior. A placebo-controlled trial supports faster symptom improvement when **divalproex** is combined with either olanzapine or **risperidone**. The 2009 Schizophrenia Patient Outcomes Research Team (PORT) recommendations do not endorse the use of mood stabilizer augmentation in resistant patients.
- **Selective serotonin reuptake inhibitors (SSRIs)** have been used with FGAs with improvement of negative symptoms. SSRIs have been used for obsessive-compulsive symptoms that worsen or arise during **clozapine** treatment.
- Combining an FGA and an SGA and combining different SGAs have been suggested, but no data exist to support or refute these strategies and the 2009 PORT recommendations do not support their use. If a series of antipsychotic monotherapies fails, a time-limited combination trial may be attempted. If there is no improvement within 6 to 12 weeks, one of the drugs should be tapered and discontinued.

ADVERSE EFFECTS

- **Table 72–3** presents the relative incidence of common categories of antipsychotic side effects.

Autonomic Nervous System

- Anticholinergic side effects include impaired memory, dry mouth, constipation, tachycardia, blurred vision, inhibition of ejaculation, and urinary

TABLE 72-3	Relative Side Effect Incidence of Commonly Used Antipsychotics[a,b]					
	Sedation	EPS	Anticholinergic	Orthostasis	Weight Gain	Prolactin
Aripiprazole	+	+	+	+	+	+
Asenapine	+	++	+/−	++	+	+
Chlorpromazine	++++	+++	+++	++++	++	+++
Clozapine	++++	+	++++	++++	++++	+
Fluphenazine	+	++++	+	+	+	++++
Haloperidol	+	++++	+	+	+	++++
Iloperidone	+	+/−	++	+++	++	+
Olanzapine	++	++	++	++	++++	+
Paliperidone	+	++	+	++	++	++++
Perphenazine	++	++++	++	+	+	++++
Quetiapine	++	+	+	++	++	+
Risperidone	+	++	+	++	++	++++
Thioridazine	++++	+++	++++	++++	+	+++
Thiothixene	+	++++	+	+	+	++++
Ziprasidone	++	++	+	+	+	+

EPS, extrapyramidal side effects; Relative side-effect risk: ±, negligible; +, low; ++, moderate; +++, moderately high; ++++, high.

[a]Side effects shown are relative risk based on doses within the recommended therapeutic range.
[b]Individual patient risk varies depending on patient-specific factors.

retention. Elderly patients are especially sensitive to these side effects. Low-potency FGAs, clozapine, and olanzapine are most likely to cause anticholinergic effects.

- Dry mouth can be managed with increased intake of fluids, oral lubricants (Xerolube), ice chips, or the use of sugarless chewing gum or hard candy.
- Constipation can be treated with increases in exercise, fluid, and dietary fiber intake.

Central Nervous System

EXTRAPYRAMIDAL SYSTEM

Dystonia

- Dystonias are prolonged tonic muscle contractions, with rapid onset (usually within 24–96 hours of dosage initiation or dosage increase); they may be life threatening (e.g., pharyngeal-laryngeal dystonias). Other dystonias are trismus, glossospasm, tongue protrusion, blepharospasm, oculogyric crisis, torticollis, and retrocollis. Dystonic reactions occur primarily with FGAs. Risk factors include younger patients (especially male), use of high-potency agents, and high dose.

TABLE 72–4 Agents Used to Treat Extrapyramidal Side Effects

Generic Name	Equivalent Dose (mg)	Daily Dosage Range (mg)
Antimuscarinics		
Benztropine[a]	1	1–8[b]
Biperiden[a]	2	2–8
Trihexyphenidyl	2	2–15
Antihistaminic		
Diphenhydramine[a]	50	50–400
Dopamine agonist		
Amantadine	NA	100–400
Benzodiazepines		
Lorazepam[a]	NA	1–8
Diazepam	NA	2–20
Clonazepam	NA	2–8
β-Blockers		
Propranolol	NA	20–160

NA, not applicable

[a]Injectable dosage form can be given intramuscularly for relief of acute dystonia.

[b]Dosage can be titrated to 12 mg/day with careful monitoring; nonlinear pharmacokinetics have been reported.

- Treatment includes IM or IV anticholinergics (**Table 72–4**) or **benzo-diazepines**. **Benztropine mesylate**, 2 mg, or **diphenhydramine**, 50 mg, may be given IM or IV, or **diazepam**, 5 to 10 mg slow IV push, or **lorazepam**, 1 to 2 mg IM, may be given. Relief usually occurs within 15 to 20 minutes of IM injection or within 5 minutes of IV administration. The dose should be repeated if no response is seen within 15 minutes of IV injection or 30 minutes of IM injection.
- Prophylactic anticholinergic medications (but not amantadine) are reasonable when using high-potency FGAs (e.g., **haloperidol** and **fluphenazine**), in young men and in patients with a history of dystonia.
- Dystonias can be minimized through the use of lower initial doses of FGAs and by using SGAs instead of FGAs.

Akathisia

- Symptoms include subjective complaints (feelings of inner restlessness) and/or objective symptoms (pacing, shuffling, or tapping feet). Akathisia occurs in 20% to 40% of patients taking FGAs.
- Treatment with anticholinergics is disappointing, and reduction in antipsychotic dose may be the best intervention. Another alternative is to switch to an SGA, although akathisia occasionally occurs with the SGAs. **Quetiapine** and **clozapine** appear to have the lowest risk for causing akathisia.
- **Diazepam** may be used (5 mg three times daily), but efficacy data are conflicting.
- **Propranolol** (up to 160 mg/day), **nadolol** (up to 80 mg/day), and **metoprolol** (up to 100 mg/day) are reported to be effective.

Pseudoparkinsonism

- Patients with pseudoparkinsonism may have any of four cardinal symptoms:
  - ✓ Akinesia, bradykinesia, or decreased motor activity, including mask-like facial expression, micrographia, slowed speech, and decreased arm swing
  - ✓ Tremor (predominantly at rest and decreasing with movement)
  - ✓ Rigidity, which may present as stiffness (cogwheel rigidity is seen as the patient's limbs yield in jerky, ratchet-like fashion when moved passively by the examiner)
  - ✓ Postural abnormalities, including stooped, unstable posture and slow, shuffling, or festinating gait
- Risk factors are FGAs (especially in high dose), increasing age, and possibly female gender.
- Accessory symptoms include seborrhea, sialorrhea, hyperhidrosis, fatigue, dysphagia, and dysarthria. A variant is rabbit syndrome, a perioral tremor.
- The onset of symptoms is usually 1 to 2 weeks after initiation of antipsychotic therapy or dose increase. The risk of pseudoparkinsonism with SGAs is low except in the case of **risperidone** in doses greater than 6 mg/day.
- Anticholinergics are an effective treatment (see **Table 72–4**). **Benztropine** has a half-life that allows once- to twice-daily dosing. Dose increases >6 mg/day must be slow because of nonlinear pharmacokinetics. **Trihexyphenidyl, diphenhydramine,** and **biperiden** usually require three-times-daily dosing. Diphenhydramine produces more sedation, but all of the anticholinergics have been abused for euphoriant effects.
- **Amantadine** is as efficacious as anticholinergics and has less effect on memory.
- An attempt should be made to taper and discontinue these agents 6 weeks to 3 months after symptoms resolve.

Tardive Dyskinesia

- TD is sometimes irreversible and is characterized by abnormal involuntary movements occurring with chronic antipsychotic therapy.
- The classic presentation is buccolingual-masticatory (BLM) or orofacial movements. Symptoms may become severe enough to interfere with chewing, wearing dentures, speech, respiration, or swallowing. Facial movements include frequent blinking, brow arching, grimacing, upward deviation of the eyes, and lip smacking. Involvement of the extremities occurs in later stages (restless choreiform and athetotic movements of the limbs). Truncal movements are classically reported in young adults. Movements may worsen with stress, decrease with sedation, and disappear with sleep.
- The Abnormal Involuntary Movement Scale (AIMS) and the Dyskinesia Identification System: Condensed User Scale (DISCUS) should be used to screen (at baseline and at least quarterly) and can facilitate early detection of TD, but neither scale is diagnostic.
- Dosage reduction or discontinuation may have significant effect on outcome, with a complete disappearance of symptoms in some patients (especially if implemented early in the course of TD).

- Prevention of TD is best accomplished by (1) using antipsychotics only when there is a clear indication and at the lowest effective dose for the shortest duration possible; (2) using SGAs as first-line agents; (3) using the DISCUS or other scales to assess for early signs of TD at least quarterly; (4) discontinuing antipsychotics or switching to SGAs (e.g., **risperidone** or **olanzapine**) at the earliest symptoms of TD, if possible; and (5) using antipsychotics only short term to abort aggressive behavior in nonpsychotic patients.
- Risk factors for TD include duration of antipsychotic therapy, higher dose, possibly cumulative dose, increasing age, occurrence of acute extrapyramidal symptoms, poor antipsychotic response, diagnosis of organic mental disorder, diabetes mellitus, mood disorders, and possibly female gender.
- To date, there are no reports of TD with **clozapine** monotherapy. Switching the patient with TD to clozapine is a first-line strategy, especially in patients with moderate to severe dyskinesias.

SEDATION AND COGNITION

- Administration of most or all of the daily dose at bedtime can decrease daytime sedation and may eliminate the need for hypnotics.
- The SGAs as first-line treatment have been shown to improve cognition (attention to tasks and improved working memory) over a 9-month period. However, the schizophrenia-focused Clinical Antipsychotic Trials of Intervention Effectiveness (CATIE) showed no difference in cognitive improvement between SGAs and the FGA perphenazine.

SEIZURES

- There is an increased risk of drug-induced seizures in all patients treated with antipsychotics. The highest risk for antipsychotic-induced seizures is with the use of **CPZ** or **clozapine**. Seizures are more likely with initiation of treatment and with the use of higher doses and rapid dose increases.
- When an isolated seizure occurs, a dosage decrease is recommended, and anticonvulsant therapy is usually not recommended.
- If a change in antipsychotic therapy is required, **risperidone, molindone, thioridazine, haloperidol, pimozide, trifluoperazine,** and **fluphenazine** may be considered.

THERMOREGULATION

- In temperature extremes, patients taking antipsychotics may experience their body temperature adjusting to ambient temperature (poikilothermia). Hyperpyrexia can lead to heat stroke. Hypothermia is also a risk, particularly in elderly patients. These problems are more common with the use of low-potency FGAs and can occur with the more anticholinergic SGAs.

NEUROLEPTIC MALIGNANT SYNDROME

- Neuroleptic malignant syndrome occurs in 0.5% to 1% of patients taking FGAs. It may be more frequent with high-potency FGAs, injectable or depot FGAs, in dehydrated patients, or in those with organic mental disorders. It has been reported with the SGAs, including **clozapine**, but is less frequent than with the FGAs.

- Symptoms develop rapidly over 24 to 72 hours and include body temperature exceeding 38°C (100.4°F), altered level of consciousness, autonomic dysfunction (tachycardia, labile blood pressure, diaphoresis, tachypnea, and urinary or fecal incontinence), and rigidity.
- Laboratory evaluation frequently shows leukocytosis, increases in creatine kinase (CK), aspartate aminotransferase (AST), alanine aminotransferase (ALT), lactate dehydrogenase (LDH), and myoglobinuria.
- Treatment should begin with antipsychotic discontinuation and supportive care.
- **Bromocriptine**, used in theory to reverse dopamine blockade, reduces rigidity, fever, or CK levels in up to 94% of patients. **Amantadine** has been used successfully in up to 63% of patients. **Dantrolene** has been used as a skeletal muscle relaxant, with favorable effects on temperature, respiratory rate, and CK in up to 81% of patients.
- Rechallenge with the lowest effective dose of SGA may be considered only for patients in need of reinstitution of antipsychotics following observation for at least 2 weeks without antipsychotics. There must be careful monitoring and slow-dose titration.

Endocrine System

- Antipsychotic-induced elevations in prolactin levels with associated galactorrhea and menstrual irregularities are common. These effects may be dose related and are more common with the use of FGAs, risperidone, and palperidone.
- Possible management strategies for galactorrhea include switching to an SGA (e.g., **aripiprazole** or **ziprasidone**).
- Weight gain is frequent with antipsychotic therapy involving SGAs, including **olanzapine, clozapine, risperidone,** and **quetiapine,** but ziprasidone and aripiprazole are associated with minimal weight gain.
- Schizophrenics have a higher prevalence of type 2 diabetes than nonschizophrenics. Antipsychotics may adversely affect glucose levels in diabetic patients. New-onset diabetes has been reported with use of the SGAs. Olanzapine has the highest risk of new-onset diabetes, followed by risperidone and quetiapine. The risk with aripiprazole and ziprasidone is somewhat less.
- The 2009 PORT recommends olanzapine as first-line therapy.

Cardiovascular System

- The incidence of orthostatic hypotension (defined as >20 mm Hg drop in systolic pressure upon standing) is greatest with low-potency FGAs and combination antipsychotics. Diabetics with cardiovascular disease and the elderly are predisposed.
- Tolerance to this effect may occur within 2 to 3 months. Reducing the dose or changing to an antipsychotic with less α-adrenergic blockade may also help.
- Low-potency piperidine phenothiazines (e.g., **thioridazine**), **clozapine, iloperodone,** and **ziprasidone** are more likely to cause ECG changes.

- ECG changes include increased heart rate, flattened T waves, ST-segment depression, and prolongation of QT and PR intervals. Torsades de pointes have been reported with **thioridazine**, which may be a cause of cardiac sudden death. A black box warning about this has been added to the labeling of thioridazine.
- Ziprasidone prolonged the QTc interval about one half as much as thioridazine. Ziprasidone's effect on the ECG is probably without clinical sequelae except in patients with baseline risk factors. Iloperidone also prolongs the QTc interval.
- It has been recommended to discontinue a medication associated with QTc prolongation if the interval consistently exceeds 500 msec.
- In patients older than 50 years, pretreatment ECG and serum potassium and magnesium levels are recommended.

Lipid Effects

- Some SGAs and phenothiazines cause elevations in serum triglycerides and cholesterol. The risk for this effect may be less with risperidone, ziprasidone, and aripiprazole.
- Metabolic syndrome consists of raised triglycerides ($\geq$150 mg/dL [170 mmol/L]), low high-density lipoprotein cholesterol ($\leq$40 mg/dL [103 mmol/L] for men, $\leq$50 mg/dL [1.29 mmol/L] for women), elevated fasting glucose ($\geq$100 mg/dL [5.6 mmol/L]), blood pressure elevation ($\geq$130/85 mm Hg), and weight gain (abdominal circumference >102 cm [40 in] for men, >88 cm [34 in] for women).

Psychiatric Side Effects

- Akathisia, akinesia, and dysphoria can result in "behavioral toxicity." Symptoms may include apathy and withdrawal, and patients may appear depressed.
- Chronic confusion and disorientation can occur in the elderly.
- Delirium and psychosis may occur with high doses of FGAs or combinations of FGAs with anticholinergics.

Ophthalmologic Effects

- Impairment in visual accommodation results from paresis of ciliary muscles. Photophobia may also result. If severe, **pilocarpine** ophthalmic solution may be necessary.
- Exacerbation of narrow-angle glaucoma can occur with use of antipsychotics or anticholinergics.
- Opaque deposits in the cornea and lens may occur with chronic phenothiazine treatment, especially with **chlorpromazine**. Although visual acuity is not usually affected, periodic slit-lamp examinations are recommended with use of long-term phenothiazines. Baseline and periodic slit-lamp examinations are also recommended for **quetiapine**-treated patients because of cataract development and lenticular changes in animal studies.
- Retinitis pigmentosa can result from **thioridazine** doses >800 mg daily (the recommended maximum dose) and can cause permanent visual impairment or blindness.

Genitourinary System

- Urinary hesitancy and retention are commonly reported, especially with low-potency FGAs and **clozapine**, and men with benign prostatic hypertrophy are especially prone.
- Urinary incontinence is especially problematic with **clozapine**.
- Risperidone produces at least as much sexual dysfunction as FGAs, but other SGAs (which have a weaker effect of prolactin) are less likely to have this effect.

Hematologic System

- Transient leukopenia may occur with antipsychotic therapy, but it typically does not progress to clinically significant parameters.
- If the white blood cell count (WBC) is <3,000/mm³ (3 × 10⁹/L), or the absolute neutrophil count (ANC) is <1,000/mm³ (1 × 10⁹/L), the antipsychotic should be discontinued, and the WBC monitored closely until it returns to normal, with monitoring for secondary infections.
- Agranulocytosis reportedly occurs in 0.01% of patients receiving FGAs, and it may occur more frequently with **chlorpromazine** and **thioridazine**. The onset is usually within the first 8 weeks of therapy. It may initially manifest as a local infection (e.g., sore throat, leukoplakia, and erythema and ulcerations of the pharynx). These symptoms should trigger an immediate WBC.
- The risk of developing agranulocytosis with **clozapine** is ~0.8%. Increasing age and female gender are associated with greater risk. The greatest risk appears to be between months 1 and 6 of treatment. WBC monitoring is required weekly for the first 6 months, every 2 weeks for months 7 through 12, then monthly if all WBCs are normal (as mandated by the product labeling). If the WBC drops to <2,000/mm³ (2 × 10⁹/L) or the ANC is <1,000/mm³ (1 × 10⁹/L), clozapine should be discontinued. In cases of mild to moderate neutropenia (granulocytes between 2,000 and 3,000/mm³ [2 × 10⁹/L and 3 × 10⁹/L]) or ANC between 1,000 and 1,500/mm³ (1 × 10⁹/L and 1.5 × 10⁹/L), which occurs in up to 2% of patients, clozapine should be discontinued, with daily monitoring of complete blood counts until values return to normal.

Dermatologic System

- Allergic reactions are rare and usually occur within 8 weeks of initiating therapy. They manifest as maculopapular, erythematous, or pruritic rashes. Drug discontinuation and topical steroids are recommended when they occur.
- Contact dermatitis, including on the oral mucosa, may occur. Swallowing of the oral concentrate quickly may decrease problems.
- Both FGAs and SGAs can cause photosensitivity. Erythema and severe sunburns can occur. Patients should be educated to use maximal blocking sunscreens, hats, protective clothing, and sunglasses when in the sun.
- Blue-gray or purplish discoloration of skin exposed to sunlight may occur with higher doses of low-potency phenothiazines (especially **chlorpromazine**) long term. This may occur with concurrent corneal or lens pigmentation.

TABLE 73-3 Pharmacokinetics of Benzodiazepine Receptor Agonists

Generic Name (Brand Name)	t_{max} (Hours)[a]	Half-Life[b] (Hours)	Daily Dose Range (mg)	Metabolic Pathway	Clinically Significant Metabolites
Estazolam (ProSom)	2	12–15	1–2	Oxidation	–
Eszopiclone (Lunesta)	1–1.5	6	2–3	Oxidation Demethylation	–
Flurazepam (Dalmane)	1	8	15–30	Oxidation	Hydroxyethylflurazepam, flurazepam aldehyde
				N-dealkylation	N-desalkylflurazepam[c]
Quazepam (Doral)	2	39	7.5–15	Oxidation, N-dealkylation	2-Oxo-quazepam, N-desalkylflurazepam[c]
Temazepam (Restoril)	1.5	10–15	15–30	Conjugation	–
Triazolam (Halcion)	1	2	0.125–0.25	Oxidation	–
Zaleplon (Sonata)	1	1	5–10	Oxidation	–
Zolpidem (Ambien)	1.6	2–2.6	5–10	Oxidation	–

[a]Time to peak plasma concentration.
[b]Half-life of parent drug.
[c]N-desalkylflurazepam, mean half-life 47 to 100 hours.

- The benzodiazepine receptor agonists are the most commonly used drugs for insomnia. They all carry a caution regarding anaphylaxis, facial angioedema, complex sleep behaviors (e.g., sleep driving, phone calls, and sleep eating). They include the newer nonbenzodiazepine γ-aminobutyric acid$_A$ (GABA$_A$) agonists and the traditional benzodiazepines, which also bind to GABA$_A$ (**Table 73–3**).

Nonbenzodiazepine GABA$_A$ Agonists

- In general, the nonbenzodiazepine hypnotics do not have significant active metabolites, and they are associated with less withdrawal, tolerance, and rebound insomnia than the benzodiazepines.
- Zolpidem, chemically unrelated to benzodiazepines or barbiturates, acts selectively at the GABA$_A$-receptor and has minimal anxiolytic and no muscle relaxant or anticonvulsant effects. It is comparable in effectiveness to benzodiazepine hypnotics, and it has little effect on sleep stages. Its duration is ~6 to 8 hours, and it is metabolized to inactive metabolites. Common side effects are drowsiness, amnesia, dizziness, headache, and GI complaints. Rebound effects when discontinued and tolerance with prolonged use are minimal, but theoretical concerns about abuse exist. It

appears to have minimal effects on next-day psychomotor performance. The usual dose is 10 mg (5 mg in the elderly or those with liver impairment), which can be increased up to 20 mg nightly. Cases of psychotic reactions and sleep eating have been reported. It should be taken on an empty stomach.

- Zaleplon also binds to the GABA$_A$ receptor. It has a rapid onset, a half-life of ~1 hour, and no active metabolites. It does not reduce nighttime awakenings or increase the total sleep time. It may be best used for middle-of-the-night awakenings. It does not appear to cause significant rebound insomnia or next-day psychomotor impairment. The most common side effects are dizziness, headache, and somnolence. The recommended dose is 10 mg (5 mg in the elderly).

- Eszopiclone has a rapid onset and a duration of action of up to 6 hours. The most common adverse effects are somnolence, unpleasant taste, headache, and dry mouth. It may be taken nightly for up to 6 months.

Benzodiazepine Hypnotics

- The pharmacokinetic properties of benzodiazepine hypnotics are summarized in **Table 73–3**.
- Benzodiazepines, which bind to GABA$_A$ receptors, have sedative, anxiolytic, muscle relaxant, and anticonvulsant properties. They increase stage 2 sleep and decrease REM and delta sleep.
- Overdose fatalities are rare unless benzodiazepines are taken with other CNS depressants.
- **Triazolam** is distributed quickly because of its high lipophilicity and thus has a short duration of effect. **Erythromycin, nefazodone, fluvoxamine,** and **ketoconazole** reduce the clearance of triazolam and increase plasma concentrations.
- **Estazolam** and **temazepam** are intermediate in their duration of action.
- The effects of **flurazepam** and **quazepam** are long because of active metabolites.
- With the exception of **temazepam**, which is eliminated by conjugation, benzodiazepine hypnotics are metabolized by microsomal oxidation followed by glucuronide conjugation.
- *N*-desalkylflurazepam accounts for most of **flurazepam's** pharmacologic effects. This metabolite may help when daytime anxiety or early morning awakening is present, but daytime sedation with impaired psychomotor performance may occur.

BENZODIAZEPINE ADVERSE EFFECTS

- Side effects include drowsiness, psychomotor incoordination, decreased concentration, and cognitive deficits.
- Tolerance to the daytime CNS effects (e.g., drowsiness, psychomotor impairment, and decreased concentration) may develop in some individuals.
- Tolerance to hypnotic effects develops after 2 weeks of continuous use of **triazolam**. Efficacy of **flurazepam, quazepam**, and **temazepam** lasts for at least 1 month of continuous nightly use. **Estazolam** reportedly maintains efficacy at maximum dosage (2 mg nightly) for up to 12 weeks.

- Anterograde amnesia has been reported with most benzodiazepines. Using the lowest dose possible minimizes amnesia.
- Rebound insomnia occurs frequently with high doses of **triazolam**, even when used intermittently.
- Rebound insomnia can be minimized by using the lowest effective dose and tapering the dose upon discontinuation.
- There is an association between falls and hip fractures and the use of long-elimination half-life benzodiazepines; thus, **flurazepam** and **quazepam** should be avoided in the elderly.

SLEEP APNEA

- Apnea is repetitive episodes of cessation of breathing during sleep. The goals of therapy are to alleviate sleep-disordered breathing (**Fig. 73–1**).

OBSTRUCTIVE SLEEP APNEA

- Obstructive sleep apnea (OSA) is potentially life threatening and characterized by repeated episodes of nocturnal breathing cessation. It is caused by occlusion of the upper airway, and blood oxygen (O_2) desaturation can occur. In severe episodes, there is heavy snoring, severe gas exchange disturbances, and respiratory failure, causing gasping. These episodes may occur up to 600 times/night.
- Episodes may be caused by obesity or fixed upper airway lesions, enlarged tonsils, amyloidosis, and hypothyroidism. Complications include arrhythmias, hypertension, cor pulmonale, and sudden death.
- The apneic episode is terminated by a reflex action in response to the fall in blood O_2 saturation that causes a brief arousal during which breathing resumes.
- Patients with OSA usually complain of excessive daytime sleepiness. Other symptoms are morning headache, poor memory, and irritability.

Treatment

- Nonpharmacologic approaches are the treatments of choice (e.g., weight loss [which should be implemented for all overweight patients], tonsillectomy, nasal septal repair, and nasal positive airway pressure [PAP], which may be continuous or bilevel). Other surgical therapies, such as uvulopalatopharyngoplasty and tracheostomy, may be necessary in severe cases.
- The most important pharmacologic intervention is avoidance of all CNS depressants and drugs that promote weight gain. Angiotensin-converting enzyme (ACE) inhibitors can also worsen sleep-disordered breathing.
- Modafinil is approved by the FDA to improve wakefulness in those who have residual daytime sleepiness while treated with PAP. It should be used only in patients who are using optimal PAP therapy to alleviate sleep-disordered breathing and in those who are free of cardiovascular disease.

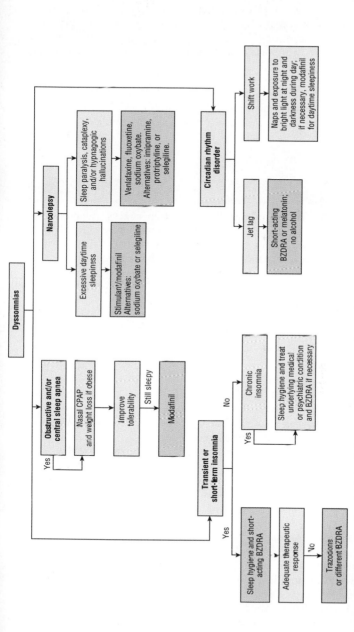

FIGURE 73–1. Algorithm for treatment of dyssomnias. (BZDRA, benzodiazepine receptor agonist; CPAP, continuous positive airway pressure.) (Modified with permission from Jermaine DM. Sleep Disorders. In: Carter BL, Angaran DM, Lake KD, Raebel MA, eds. Pharmacotherapy Self-Assessment Program, 2nd ed. Neurology and Psychiatry. Kansas City: American College of Clinical Pharmacy, 1995;146–147.)

CENTRAL SLEEP APNEA

- Central sleep apnea (CSA), which is less frequent than OSA, is characterized by repeated episodes of apnea caused by temporary loss of respiratory effort during sleep. It may be caused by autonomic nervous system lesions, neurologic diseases, high altitudes, and congestive heart failure.

Treatment

- PAP with or without supplemental O_2 improves CSA.
- **Acetazolamide** causes a metabolic acidosis that stimulates respiratory drive and may be beneficial for high altitude, heart failure, and idiopathic CSA.

NARCOLEPSY

- The essential features of narcolepsy are sleep attacks, cataplexy, hypnagogic hallucinations, and sleep paralysis. Individuals with narcolepsy complain of excessive daytime sleepiness, sleep attacks that last up to 30 minutes, fatigue, impaired performance, and disturbed nighttime sleep. They have multiple arousals during the night.
- Cataplexy is sudden bilateral loss of muscle tone with collapse, which is often precipitated by highly emotional situations.
- The hypocretin/orexin neurotransmitter system may play a central role in narcolepsy. An autoimmune process may cause destruction of hypocretin-producing cells.

TREATMENT

- The goal of therapy is to maximize alertness during waking hours and improve quality of life (see **Fig. 73–1**).
- Good sleep hygiene, as well as two or more brief daytime naps daily (as little as 15 min), should be encouraged.
- Medications used to treat narcolepsy are shown in **Table 73–4**. Pharmacotherapy focuses on excessive daytime sleepiness and cataplexy.
- **Modafinil** is considered the standard for treatment of excessive daytime sleepiness, but armodafinil (the active R-isomer) is also FDA approved for this purpose. Evidence suggests no tolerance or withdrawal after abrupt discontinuation and no risk of abuse.
- Side effects of modafinil include headache, nausea, nervousness, and insomnia.
- **Amphetamines** and **methylphenidate** have a fast onset of effect and durations of 3 to 4 hours and 6 to 10 hours, respectively, for excessive daytime sleepiness. Divided daily doses are recommended, but sustained-release formulations are available. Amphetamines are associated with more likelihood of abuse and tolerance. Side effects include insomnia, hypertension, palpitations, and irritability.
- The most effective treatment for cataplexy is the **tricyclic antidepressants, fluoxetine**, or **venlafaxine. Imipramine, protriptyline, clomipramine,**

TABLE 73–4 Drugs Used to Treat Narcolepsy

Generic Name	Trade Name	Daily Dosage Range (mg)
Excessive daytime somnolence		
Dextroamphetamine	Dexedrine	5–60
Dextroamphetamine/ Amphetamine salts[a]	Adderall	5–60
Methamphetamine[b]	Desoxyn	5–15
Lisdexamfetamine	Vyvanse	20–70
Methylphenidate	Ritalin	30–80
Modafinil	Provigil	200–400
Armodafinil	Nuvigil	150–250
Sodium oxybate[c]	Xyrem	4.5–9 grams per night
Adjunct agents for cataplexy		
Fluoxetine	Prozac	20–80
Imipramine	Tofranil	50–250
Nortriptyline	Aventyl, Pamelor	50–200
Protriptyline	Vivactil	5–30
Venlafaxine	Effexor	37.5–225
Selegiline	Eldepryl	20–40

[a]Dextroamphetamine sulfate, dextroamphetamine saccharate, amphetamine aspartate, and amphetamine sulfate.
[b]Not available in some states.
[c]Also is effective at treating cataplexy.
Data from Morgenthaler TI, Kapur VK, Brown T, et al. Practice parameters for the treatment of narcolepsy and other hypersomnias of central origin. Sleep 2007;30:1705–1711.

fluoxetine, and **nortriptyline** are effective in ~80% of patients. Selegiline improves hypersomnolence and cataplexy.

- **Sodium oxybate** (γ-hydroxybutyrate; a potent sedative-hypnotic) improves excessive daytime sleepiness and decreases episodes of sleep paralysis, cataplexy, and hypnagogic hallucinations. It is taken at bedtime and repeated 2.5 to 4 hours later. Side effects include nausea, somnolence, confusion, dizziness, and incontinence.

EVALUATION OF THERAPEUTIC OUTCOMES

- Patients with short-term or chronic insomnia should be evaluated after 1 week of therapy to assess for drug effectiveness, adverse events, and adherence to nonpharmacologic recommendations. Patients should be instructed to maintain a sleep diary, including a daily recording of awakenings, medications taken, naps, and an index of sleep quality.
- Patients with OSA should be evaluated after 1 to 3 months of treatment for improvement in alertness, daytime symptoms, and weight reduction. The bed partner can report on snoring and gasping.

- Monitoring parameters for pharmacotherapy of narcolepsy include reduction in daytime sleepiness, cataplexy, hypnagogic and hypnopompic hallucinations, and sleep paralysis. Patients should be evaluated regularly during medication titration, then every 6 to 12 months to assess adverse drug events (e.g., mood changes, sleep disturbances, and cardiovascular abnormalities).

See Chapter 81, Sleep Disorders, authored by John M. Dopp and Bradley G. Phillips, for a more detailed discussion of this topic.

CHAPTER 74

Substance-Related Disorders

DEFINITIONS

- The substance-related disorders include disorders of intoxication, dependence, and withdrawal. Substance dependence or addiction can be viewed as a chronic illness that can be successfully controlled with treatment but cannot be cured and is associated with a high relapse rate.
- *Addiction.* A primary chronic neurobiologic disease, with genetic, psychosocial, and environmental factors influencing its development and manifestations. It is characterized by behaviors that include one or more of the following 5Cs: chronicity, impaired control over drug use, compulsive use, continued use despite harm, and craving.
- *Intoxication.* Development of a substance-specific syndrome after recent ingestion and presence in the body of a substance; it is associated with maladaptive behavior during the waking state caused by the effect of the substance on the central nervous system (CNS).
- *Physical dependence.* A state of adaptation that is manifested by a drug class–specific withdrawal syndrome that can be produced by abrupt cessation, rapid dose reduction, decreasing blood level of the drug, and/or administration of an antagonist.
- *Substance abuse.* A maladaptive pattern of substance use characterized by repeated adverse consequences related to the repeated use of the substance.
- *Substance dependence.* The characteristic feature is a continued maladaptive pattern of substance use in spite of repeated adverse consequences related to the repeated use.
- *Tolerance.* A state of adaptation in which exposure to a drug induces changes that result in a diminution of one or more of the drug's effects over time.
- *Withdrawal.* The development of a substance-specific syndrome after cessation of or reduction in intake of a substance that was used regularly.

DIVERSION OF PHARMACEUTICAL CONTROLLED SUBSTANCES

- Between 1995 and 2002 there was a 163% increase in emergency room visits tied to the abuse of prescription drugs.
- CNS agents (primarily pain relievers) were involved in 47% of drug-related suicide attempts presenting to emergency departments in 2005 in the United States.
- In 2006 all incidents of emergency department visits related to illegal drug use or nonmedical use of a legal drug, 28% involved legal pharmaceuticals only.
- Internet-based prescription mills are a major source of diversion of controlled substances.

TABLE 74-2 Dependence on Sedative-Hypnotics

Generic Name	Common Trade Names	Oral Sedating Dose (mg)	Physical Dependence Daily Dose and Time Needed to Produce Dependence	Time Before Onset of Withdrawal (hours)	Peak Withdrawal Symptoms (days)[a]
Benzodiazepines					
Alprazolam	Xanax	0.25–8	8–16 mg × 42 days (est.)	8–24	2–3
Clorazepate	Tranxene	7.5–15	45–180 mg × 42–120 days	12–24	5–8
Diazepam	Valium	5–10	40–100 mg × 42–120 days	12–24	5–8
Flunitrazepam	Rohypnol	1–2	8–10 mg × 42 days (est.)	24–36	2–3
Barbiturates					
Amobarbital	Amytal	65–100	Same	8–12	2–5
Secobarbital	Seconal, Seco-8	100	800–2,200 mg × 35–37 days	6–12	2–3
Equal parts of secobarbital and amobarbital	Tuinal	100	Same	6–12	2–3
Pentobarbital	Nembutal	100	Same	6–12	2–3
Nonbarbiturate sedative-hypnotics					
Chloral hydrate	Noctec	250	Exact dose unknown; 12 g/day chronically has led to delirium upon sudden withdrawal	6–12	2–3
Meprobamate	Equanil, Miltown, Meprotabs	400	1.6–3.2 g × 270 days	8–12	3–8

[a]Withdrawal symptoms are tremor, tachycardia, diaphoresis, nausea, vomiting, elevated blood pressure, delirium, seizures, and hallucinations.

CARISOPRODOL

- Carisoprodol is used in the outpatient setting for muscle spasms and back pain.
- It is structurally and pharmacologically related to meprobamate, and meprobamate is one of its metabolites.
- It can cause drowsiness, dizziness, vertigo, ataxia, tremor, irritability, syncope, insomnia, tachycardia, postural hypotension, nausea, weakness, euphoria, and confusion.
- Overdose can cause shock, stupor, coma, respiratory depression, and death.

OPIATES

- Signs and symptoms of opioid intoxication are euphoria, dysphoria, apathy, sedation, and attention impairment. Signs and symptoms of withdrawal are lacrimation, rhinorrhea, mydriasis, piloerection, diaphoresis, diarrhea, yawning, fever, insomnia, and muscle aches. The onset of withdrawal ranges from a few hours after stopping heroin to 3 to 5 days after stopping methadone. Duration of withdrawal ranges from 3 to 14 days. Occurrence of delirium suggests withdrawal from another drug (e.g., **alcohol**).
- **Heroin** can be snorted, smoked, and given IV. Complications of heroin use include overdoses, anaphylactic reactions to impurities, nephrotic syndrome, septicemia, endocarditis, and acquired immunodeficiency.
- **Oxycodone**, a controlled-release dosage form, is sometimes crushed by abusers to get the full 12-hour effect almost immediately. Snorting or injecting the crushed tablet can lead to overdose and death.
- **Opiates** are commonly combined with stimulants (e.g., cocaine [speedball]) or alcohol.
- Methadone has caused an increased number of deaths in recent years. Converting to methadone from other opioid agonists can be tricky, and death can occur when done improperly.
- Peak respiratory depressant effects occur later and last longer than peak analgesic effects.
- **Dextromethorphan** is an over-the-counter drug that causes depressant and mild hallucinogenic effects in high doses. Excessive doses can cause significant hallucinations and CNS depression.
- Acute overdoses are treated with naloxone.

CENTRAL NERVOUS SYSTEM STIMULANTS

COCAINE

- **Cocaine** may be the most behaviorally reinforcing of all drugs. Ten percent of people who begin to use the drug "recreationally" go on to heavy use.
- It blocks reuptake of catecholamine neurotransmitters and causes a depletion of brain dopamine.
- The hydrochloride salt is inhaled or injected. It can be converted to cocaine base (crack or rock) and smoked to achieve almost instant absorption and intense euphoria. Tolerance to the "high" develops quickly. The

high from snorting can last 15 to 30 minutes; the high from smoking can last 5 to 10 minutes.

- In the presence of alcohol, cocaine is metabolized to cocaethylene, a longer-acting compound than cocaine with a greater risk for causing death.
- The elimination half-life of cocaine is 1 hour.
- Adverse events include ulceration of nasal mucosa and nasal septal collapse, tachycardia, heart failure, hyperthermia, shock, seizures, psychosis (similar to paranoid schizophrenia), and sudden death.
- Signs and symptoms of cocaine intoxication are agitation, elation, euphoria, grandiosity, loquacity, hypervigilance, sweating or chills, nausea, vomiting, tachycardia, arrhythmias, respiratory depression, mydriasis, altered blood pressure, and seizures. Signs and symptoms of withdrawal are fatigue, sleep disturbances, nightmares, depression, changes in appetite, bradyarrhythmias, myocardial infarction (MI), and tremors.
- Withdrawal symptoms begin within hours of discontinuation and last up to several days.

METHAMPHETAMINE

- **Methamphetamine** (known as speed, meth, and crank) can be taken orally, rectally, intranasally, by IV injection, and by smoking. The hydrochloride salt (known as ice, crystal, and glass) is a clear crystal.
- Systemic effects of methamphetamine are similar to those of cocaine. Inhalation or IV injection results in an intense rush that lasts a few minutes. Methamphetamine has a longer duration of effect than cocaine. Pharmacologic effects include increased wakefulness, increased physical activity, decreased appetite, increased respiration, hyperthermia, euphoria, irritability, insomnia, confusion, tremors, anxiety, paranoia, aggressiveness, convulsions, increased heart rate and blood pressure, stroke, and death.
- Methamphetamine intoxication is an acute condition that may result in death; pharmacotherapy may be indicated for seizures.
- Symptoms of withdrawal include depression, altered mental status, drug craving, dyssomnia, and fatigue. Duration of withdrawal from methamphetamine ranges from 3 days to several months, but these individuals are usually not in acute distress. Occurrence of delirium suggests withdrawal from another drug (e.g., **alcohol**).
- **Ephedrine** and **pseudoephedrine** can be extracted from cold and allergy tablets and converted in illegal labs to methamphetamine.
- In the United States, federal law now requires that pseudoephedrine-containing products be kept behind a counter and that identification be shown at the time of purchase.

OTHER DRUGS OF ABUSE

NICOTINE

- Cigarette smoking continues to be the leading cause of preventable morbidity and mortality in the United States. It increases the risks of cardiovascular diseases, lung cancer, other cancers, and nonmalignant respiratory diseases.

- **Nicotine** is a ganglionic cholinergic-receptor agonist with pharmacologic effects that are dose dependent. Effects include CNS and peripheral nervous system stimulation and depression; respiratory stimulation; skeletal muscle relaxation; catecholamine release by the adrenal medulla; peripheral vasoconstriction; and increased blood pressure, heart rate, cardiac output, and oxygen consumption. Low doses of nicotine produce increased alertness and improved cognitive functioning. Higher doses stimulate the "reward" center in the limbic system.
- Abrupt cessation results in onset of withdrawal symptoms usually within 24 hours, which include anxiety, cravings, difficulty concentrating, frustration, irritability, hostility, insomnia, and restlessness.

METHAMPHETAMINE ANALOGUES

- The analogues of current concern include 3,4-methylenedioxyamphetamine (**MDA**) and 3,4-methylenedioxymethamphetamine (**MDMA**; also known as ecstasy, Adam, X, and Stacy).
- MDMA is usually taken by mouth as a tablet, capsule, or powder, but it can also be smoked, snorted, or injected. Taken by mouth, effects last 4 to 6 hours.
- MDMA stimulates the CNS, causes euphoria and relaxation, and produces a mild hallucinogenic effect. It can cause muscle tension, nausea, faintness, chills, sweating, panic, anxiety, depression, hallucinations, and paranoid thinking. It increases heart rate and blood pressure and destroys serotonin (5-HT)-producing neurons in animals. It is considered to be neurotoxic in humans.

MARIJUANA

- **Marijuana** (known as reefer, pot, grass, and weed) is the most commonly used illicit drug. The principal psychoactive component is Δ^9-**tetrahydrocannabinol** (**THC**). **Hashish**, the dried resin of the top of the plant, is more potent than the plant itself. Pharmacologic effects begin immediately and last 1 to 3 hours.
- Chronic exposure is not usually associated with a withdrawal syndrome, but sudden discontinuation by heavy users can cause a withdrawal syndrome.
- Initial effects of marijuana use include increased heart rate, dilated bronchial passages, and bloodshot eyes. Subsequent effects include euphoria, dry mouth, hunger, tremor, sleepiness, anxiety, fear, distrust, panic, incoordination, poor recall, amotivation, and toxic psychosis. Other physiologic effects are sedation, difficulty in performing complex tasks, and disinhibition. Endocrine effects include amenorrhea, decreased testosterone production, and inhibition of spermatogenesis. Signs and symptoms of marijuana intoxication are tachycardia, conjunctival congestion, increased appetite, dry mouth, euphoria, apathy, and hallucinations.
- THC is detectable on toxicologic screening for up to 4 to 5 weeks in chronic users.

- Daily use of one to three joints appears to produce about the same lung damage and potential cancer risk as smoking five times as many tobacco cigarettes.

PHENCYCLIDINE AND KETAMINE

- **Phencyclidine (PCP)** (known as angel dust and crystal) is often misrepresented as **lysergic acid diethylamide (LSD)** or THC. It is commonly smoked with marijuana (crystal joint) but can be taken orally or IV.
  - ✓ Signs and symptoms of PCP intoxication include very unpredictable behavior, increased blood pressure, tachycardia, ataxia, slurred speech, euphoria, agitation, anxiety, hostility, and psychosis. At toxic doses, coma, seizures, and respiratory and cardiac arrest may occur.
- **Ketamine** (known as special K, jet, and green), chemically related to PCP, is a veterinary anesthetic that can cause hallucinations, delirium, and vivid dreams.
  - ✓ It is usually injected but can be evaporated to crystals, powdered, and smoked, snorted, or swallowed. Marijuana cigarettes can be soaked in ketamine solution.
  - ✓ Side effects are increased blood pressure and heart rate, respiratory depression, apnea, muscular hypertonus, and dystonic reactions. In overdose, seizures, polyneuropathy, increased intracranial pressure, and respiratory and cardiac arrest may occur.

LYSERGIC ACID DIETHYLAMIDE

- Physical signs and symptoms of **LSD** intoxication include mydriasis, tachycardia, diaphoresis, palpitations, blurred vision, tremor, incoordination, dizziness, weakness, and drowsiness; psychiatric signs and symptoms include perceptual intensification, depersonalization, derealization, illusions, psychosis, and synesthesia. There is no withdrawal syndrome after discontinuation.
- LSD and similar drugs stimulate presynaptic 5-HT_{1A} and 5-HT_{1B}, as well as postsynaptic 5-HT_2 receptors in the brain.
- Flashbacks may occur, especially in chronic users. It produces tolerance but is not addictive.
- LSD is sold as tablets, capsules, and a liquid. It is also added to absorbent paper and divided into small decorated squares, each square being one dose.

INHALANTS

- Organic solvents inhaled by abusers include **gasoline, glue, aerosols, amyl nitrite, butyl nitrite, typewriter correction fluid, lighter fluid, cleaning fluids, paint products, nail polish remover, waxes,** and **varnishes.** Chemicals in these products include **nitrous oxide, toluene, benzene, methanol, methylene chloride, acetone, methylethyl ketone, methylbutyl ketone, trichloroethylene,** and **trichloroethane.**
- Physiologic effects include CNS depression similar to the effects of alcohol, headache, nausea, anxiety, hallucinations, and delusions. With chronic

use, the drugs are toxic to virtually all organ systems. Death may occur from arrhythmias or suffocation by plastic bags.

DESIRED OUTCOME

- The goals of treatment are cessation of use of the drug, termination of associated drug-seeking behaviors, and return to normal functioning. The goals of treatment of the withdrawal syndrome are prevention of progression of withdrawal to life-threatening severity, thus enabling the patient to be sufficiently comfortable and functional in order to participate in a treatment program.

TREATMENT

INTOXICATION

- In treating acute intoxications, drug therapy should be avoided when possible, but it may be indicated if patients are agitated, combative, or psychotic (Table 74–3).
- When toxicology screens are desired, blood or urine should be collected immediately when the patient presents for treatment.
- **Flumazenil** is not indicated in all cases of suspected benzodiazepine overdose, and it is contraindicated when cyclic antidepressant involvement is known or suspected because of the risk of seizures. It should be used with caution when benzodiazepine physical dependence is suspected, as it may precipitate withdrawal.
- In opiate intoxication, **naloxone** may revive unconscious patients with respiratory depression. However, it may also precipitate physical withdrawal in dependent patients.
- **Cocaine** intoxication is treated pharmacologically only if the patient is agitated and psychotic. Injectable **lorazepam** can be used for agitation. Low-dose antipsychotics can be used short term if necessary for psychotic symptoms. Seizures are usually treated supportively, but IV lorazepam or **diazepam** can be used for status epilepticus.
- Many patients with **hallucinogen, marijuana**, or **inhalant** intoxication respond to reassurance, but short-term antianxiety and/or antipsychotic therapy can be used.

WITHDRAWAL

- Treatment of withdrawal from some common drugs of abuse is summarized in Table 74–4.

Alcohol

- Most clinicians agree that the **benzodiazepines** are the drugs of choice in the treatment of **alcohol** withdrawal.
- Lorazepam is preferred by many clinicians because it can be administered IV, intramuscularly, or orally with predictable results (Table 74–5).

TABLE 74–3	Pharmacologic Treatment of Substance Intoxication		
Drug Class	**Nonpharmacologic Therapy**	**Pharmacologic Therapy**	**Level of Evidence^{a,b}**
Benzodiazepines	Support vital functions	Flumazenil 0.2 mg/min IV initially, repeat up to 3 mg max.	Al
Alcohol, barbiturates, and sedative-hypnotics (nonbenzodiazepines)	Support vital functions	None	B3
Opiates	Support vital functions	Naloxone 0.4–2 mg IV every 3 min	A1
Cocaine and other CNS stimulants	Monitor cardiac function	Lorazepam 2–4 mg IM every 30 min to 6 hours as needed for agitation	B2
		Haloperidol 2–5 mg (or other antipsychotic agent) every 30 min to 6 hours as needed for psychotic behavior	B3
Hallucinogens, marijuana, and inhalants	Reassurance; "talk-down therapy"; support vital functions	Lorazepam and/or haloperidol as above	B3
Phencyclidine	Minimize sensory input	Lorazepam and/or haloperidol as above	B3

^{a}Strength of recommendations, evidence to support recommendation, A, good; B, moderate; C, poor.
^{b}Quality of evidence: 1, evidence from more than 1 properly randomized, controlled trial; 2, evidence from more than one well-designed clinical trial with randomization, from cohort or case-controlled analytic studies or multiple time series; or dramatic results from uncontrolled experiments; 3, evidence from opinions of respected authorities, based on clinical experience, descriptive studies, or reports of expert communities.
Data from O'Brien CP. Drug addiction and drug abuse. In: Brunton LL, Lazo JS, Parker KL, eds. Goodman and Gilman's The Pharmacological Basis of Therapeutics, 11th ed. New York: McGraw-Hill, 2006:614–615; Fudala PJ, Greenstein RA, O'Brien CP. Alternative pharmacotherapies for opiate addiction. In: Lowinson JH, Ruiz P, Millman RB, Langrod JG, eds. Substance Abuse: A Comprehensive Textbook, 4th ed. Baltimore, MD: Williams & Wilkins, 2005:641–653; Smith DE, Seymour RB. Benzodiazepines and other sedative-hypnotics. In: Galanter M, Kleber HD, eds. Textbook of Substance Abuse Treatment. Washington, DC: American Psychiatric Association, 1994:179–186; and Knapp CM, Ciraulo DA, Jaffe J. Opiates: Clinical aspects. In: Lowinson JH, Ruiz P, Millman RB, Langrod JG, eds. Substance Abuse: A Comprehensive Textbook, 4th ed. Baltimore, MD: Williams & Wilkins, 2005:180–195.

- With symptom-triggered therapy, medication is given only if symptoms emerge, resulting in shorter treatment duration and avoidance of over-sedation. A typical regimen would be lorazepam 2 mg administered every hour as needed when a structured assessment scale (e.g., Clinical Institute Withdrawal Assessment–Alcohol, Revised) indicates that symptoms are moderate to severe. Current guidelines recommend such individualized therapy over fixed-schedule therapy.
- Alcohol withdrawal seizures do not require anticonvulsant drug treatment unless they progress to status epilepticus. Patients with seizures should be

TABLE 74–4	Treatment of Withdrawal from Some Common Drugs of Abuse	
Drug or Drug Class	**Pharmacologic Therapy**	**Level of Evidence[a,b]**
Benzodiazepines		
Short to intermediate acting	Lorazepam 2 mg 3–4 times a day; taper over 5–7 days	A1
Long-acting	Lorazepam 2 mg 3–4 times a day; taper over additional 5–7 days	A1
Barbiturates	Pentobarbital tolerance test; initial detoxification at upper limit of tolerance test; decrease dosage by 100 mg every 2–3 days	B3
Opiates	Methadone 20–80 mg orally daily; taper by 5–10 mg daily or buprenorphine 4–32 mg orally daily, or clonidine 2 mcg/kg 3 times a day × 7 days; taper over additional 3 days	A1 (methadone and buprenorphine) B1 (clonidine)
Mixed-substance withdrawal		
Drugs are cross-tolerant	Detoxify according to treatment for longer-acting drug used	B3
Drugs are not cross-tolerant	Detoxify from one drug while maintaining second drug (cross-tolerant drugs), then detoxify from second drug	B3
CNS stimulants	Supportive treatment only; pharmacotherapy often not used; bromocriptine 2.5 mg 3 times a day or higher may be used for severe craving associated with cocaine withdrawal	B2

[a]Strength of recommendations, evidence to support recommendation, A, good; B, moderate; C, poor.
[b]Quality of evidence: 1, evidence from more than 1 properly randomized, controlled trial; 2, evidence from more than one well-designed clinical trial with randomization, from cohort or case-controlled analytic studies or multiple time series; or dramatic results from uncontrolled experiments; 3, evidence from opinions of respected authorities, based on clinical experience, descriptive studies, or reports of expert communities.
Data from O'Brien CP. Drug addiction and drug abuse. In: Brunton LL, Lazo JS, Parker KL, eds. Goodman and Gilman's The Pharmacological Basis of Therapeutics, 11th ed. New York: McGraw-Hill, 2006:614–615; TIP 40 Center for Substance Abuse Treatment. Clinical Guidelines for the Use of Buprenorphine in the Treatment of Opioid Addiction. Treatment Improvement Protocol (TIP) Series 40. DHHS Publication No. (SMA) 04-3939. Rockville, MD: Substance Abuse and Mental Health Services Administration, 2004. http://www.ncbi.nlm.nih.gov/bookshelf/br.fcgi?book=hssamhsatip&part=A72248; and Gorelick DA, Wilkins JN. Bromocriptine treatment for cocaine addiction: Association with plasma prolactin levels. Drug Alcohol Depend 2006;81:189–195.

treated supportively. An increase in the dosage and slowing of the tapering schedule of the **benzodiazepine** used for detoxification or a single injection of a benzodiazepine may be necessary to prevent further seizure activity.

Benzodiazepines

- For benzodiazepine withdrawal, the same drugs and dosages that are used for alcohol withdrawal are used (see **Table 74–5**).

TABLE 74–5 Pharmacologic Agents Used in the Treatment of Alcohol Withdrawal

Drug	Dose per Day (Unless Otherwise Stated)	Indication	Monitoring	Duration of Dosing	Level of Evidence[a]
Multivitamin	1 tablet	Malnutrition	Diet	At least until eating a balanced diet at caloric goal	B3
Thiamine	50–100 mg	Deficiency	CBC, WBC, nystagmus	Empiric × 5 days. More if evidence of deficiency	B2
Crystalloid fluids (typically D5-0.45 NS with 20 mEq of KCl per liter)	50–100 mL/hour	Dehydration	Weight, electrolytes, urine output, nystagmus if dextrose	Until intake and outputs stabilize and oral intake is adequate	A3
Clonidine oral	0.05–0.3 mg	Autonomic tone rebound and hyperactivity	Shaking, tremor, sweating, blood pressure	3 days or less	B2
Clonidine transdermal	TTS-1 to TTS-3	Autonomic tone rebound and hyperactivity	Shaking, tremor, sweating, blood pressure	1 week or less. One patch only	B3
Labetalol	20 mg IV every 2 hours as needed	Hypertensive urgencies and above	Blood pressure target	Individual doses as needed	B3
Antipsychotics, haloperidol	2.5 mg to 5 mg every four hours	Agitation unresponsive to benzodiazepines, hallucinations (tactile, visual, auditory, or otherwise) or delusions	Subjective response plus rating scale (CIWA-Ar or equivalent)	Individual doses as needed	B1

	Dose	Indication	Response	Comments	Strength[a]
Antipsychotics, atypical		Agitation unresponsive to benzodiazepines, hallucinations, or delusions in patients intolerant of conventional antipsychotics	Subjective response plus rating scale (CIWA-Ar or equivalent)	Individual doses as needed in addition to scheduled antipsychotic	C3
Quetiapine	25–200 mg				
Aripiprazole	5–15 mg				
Benzodiazepines		Tremor, anxiety, diaphoresis, tachypnea, dysphoria, seizures	Subjective response plus rating scale (CIWA-Ar or equivalent)	Individual doses as needed Underdosing is more common than overdosing	A2
Lorazepam	0.5–2 mg				
Chlordiazepoxide	5 mg–25 mg				
Clonazepam	0.5–2 mg				
Diazepam	2.5–10 mg				
Alcohol oral		Prevent withdrawal	Subjective signs of withdrawal	Wide variation	C3
Alcohol IV		Prevent withdrawal	Subjective signs of withdrawal	Wide variation	C3

CBC, complete blood count; CIWA-Ar, Clinical Institute Withdrawal Assessment for Alcohol, revised; D5, dextrose 5%; KCl, potassium chloride; NS, normal saline; WBC, white blood cell count.

[a]Strength of recommendations, evidence to support recommendation: A, good; B, moderate; C, poor.
Quality of evidence: 1, evidence from more than 1 properly randomized, controlled trial; 2, evidence from more than 1 well-designed clinical trial with randomization, from cohort or case-controlled analytic studies or multiple time series, or dramatic results from uncontrolled experiments; 3, evidence from opinions of respected authorities, based on clinical experience, descriptive studies, or reports of expert communities.

Data from Mayo-Smith MF. Pharmacological management of alcohol withdrawal. A meta-analysis and evidence-based practice guideline. American Society of Addiction Medicine Working Group on Pharmacological Management of Alcohol Withdrawal. JAMA 1997;278:144–151; and Mayo-Smith MF, Beecher LH, Fischer TL, et al. Working Group on the Management of Alcohol Withdrawal Delirium, Practice Guidelines Committee. American Society of Addiction Medicine. Management of alcohol withdrawal delirium. An evidence-based practice guideline [erratum Arch Intern Med 2004;164:2068]. Arch Intern Med 2004;164:1405–1412.

- The onset of withdrawal from long-acting benzodiazepines may be up to 7 days after discontinuation of the drug. Detoxification is approached by initiating treatment at usual doses and maintaining this dose for 5 days. The dose is then tapered over 5 days. Alprazolam withdrawal may require a more gradual taper of the benzodiazepine used for detoxification.

Opiates

- Unnecessary detoxification with drugs should be avoided if possible (e.g., if symptoms are tolerable). **Heroin** withdrawal reaches a peak within 36 to 72 hours, and the **methadone** withdrawal peak is reached at 72 hours.
- Conventional drug therapy for opiate withdrawal has been **methadone**, a synthetic opiate. Usual starting doses have been 20 to 40 mg/day. The dosage can be tapered in decrements of 5 to 10 mg/day until discontinued. Some clinicians use discontinuation schedules over 30 days or over 180 days.
- Other detoxification regimens (e.g., adrenergic agonists) also are effective. Regardless of detoxification strategy, most patients relapse to heroin use.
- **Buprenorphine** in two formulations (both assigned to schedule III) was recently made available for office-based management of opioid dependence by qualified physicians. Once-daily dosage is titrated to a target of 16 mg/day (range 4–24 mg/day).
- **Subutex** (**buprenorphine**) is typically used at the beginning of treatment for opiate abuse.
- **Suboxone** (**buprenorphine** and **naloxone**) is used in maintenance treatment of opiate addiction.
- **Clonidine** can attenuate the noradrenergic hyperactivity of opiate withdrawal without interfering significantly with activity at the opiate receptors. Monitoring should include blood pressure checks, supine and standing, at least daily.

SUBSTANCE DEPENDENCE

- The diagnosis of drug dependence requires at least three of the following during a 12-month period:
  - ✓ Tolerance
  - ✓ Withdrawal
  - ✓ Substance is taken in larger amounts over a longer period of time than intended.
  - ✓ Persistent desire or unsuccessful efforts to cut down or control substance use
  - ✓ Considerable time is spent in obtaining or using the substance or recovering from its effects.
  - ✓ Social, occupational, or recreational activities are reduced or given up because of substance use.
  - ✓ Substance use continues despite knowledge of having physical or psychological problems caused or exacerbated by the substance.

- The treatment of drug dependence or addiction is primarily behavioral. The goal of treatment is complete abstinence, and treatment is a lifelong process. Most drug-dependence treatment programs embrace treatment based on the Alcoholics Anonymous approach, that is, a 12-step model with peer-led self-help groups.

Alcohol

- **Disulfiram** deters a patient from drinking by producing an aversive reaction if the patient drinks. It inhibits aldehyde dehydrogenase in the pathway for alcohol metabolism, allowing acetaldehyde to accumulate, resulting in flushing, vomiting, headache, palpitations, tachycardia, fever, and hypotension. Severe reactions include respiratory depression, arrhythmias, MI, seizures, and death. Inhibition of the enzyme continues for as long as 2 weeks after stopping disulfiram. Disulfiram reactions have occurred with the use of alcohol-containing mouthwashes and aftershaves. The usual dosage is 250 to 500 mg/day.
- Prior to starting disulfiram, baseline liver function tests (LFTs) should be obtained, and patients should be monitored for hepatotoxicity. LFTs should be repeated at 2 weeks, 3 months, and 6 months, then twice yearly. The prescriber should wait at least 24 hours after the last drink before starting disulfiram, usually at a dose of 250 mg/day.
- **Naltrexone**, 50 to 100 mg/day, has been associated with reduced craving and fewer drinking days. It should not be given to patients currently dependent on opiates, as it can precipitate a severe withdrawal syndrome. A new depot formulation allows monthly administration in a usual dose of 380 mg intramuscularly.
- Naltrexone is hepatotoxic and contraindicated in patients with hepatitis or liver failure. LFTs should be monitored monthly for the first 3 months, then every 3 months. Side effects include nausea, headache, dizziness, nervousness, insomnia, and somnolence.
- Acamprosate-treated patients (999–1,998 mg/day and higher) have less craving and more success in maintaining abstinence than placebo-treated patients. The combination of acamprosate and naltrexone with psychosocial intervention may be more effective than acamprosate alone.
- The most common acamprosate side effects are GI related.

Nicotine

- The Agency for Healthcare Research and Quality released a new clinical guideline for smoking cessation in 2008. Every smoker should receive at least minimal treatment at every visit with the clinician.
- First-line pharmacotherapies for smoking cessation are **bupropion sustained release, nicotine gum, nicotine inhaler, nicotine lozenge, nicotine nasal spray, nicotine patch**, and **varenicline**. Combinations of these should be considered if a single agent has failed. Second-line pharmacotherapies include **clonidine** and **nortriptyline** and should be considered if first-line therapy fails.
- Interventions are more effective when they last >10 minutes, involve contact with multiple types of clinicians, involve at least four sessions, and provide **nicotine-replacement therapy** (NRT). Group and individual

counseling is effective, and interventions are more successful when they include social support and training in problem solving, stress management, and relapse prevention.

NICOTINE-REPLACEMENT THERAPY

- The role of pharmacotherapy in smoking cessation is summarized in **Table 74–6**. In general, use of NRT doubles the odds of successfully quitting compared to placebo.
- NRT should be used with caution in patients within 2 weeks post-MI, those with serious arrhythmias, and those with serious or worsening angina.
- The **2 mg gum** is recommended for those smoking fewer than 25 cigarettes a day, and the 4 mg gum for those smoking 25 or more cigarettes a day. Generally, the gum should be used for up to 12 weeks at doses of no more than 24 pieces per day. It should be chewed slowly until a peppery or minty taste emerges and then parked between the cheek and gums for about 30 minutes or until the taste dissipates. A fixed schedule may be more efficacious than as-needed use. Patients should be given specific dosing instruction, not just as needed.
- The **patch** is available as a prescription and nonprescription medication. Treatment of 8 weeks or less is as effective as longer treatments. The 16- and 24-hour patches have comparable efficacy. A new patch should be placed on a relatively hairless location each morning.
- **Nicotine nasal spray** requires a prescription. Recommended duration of therapy is 3 to 6 months at no more than 40 doses per day. A dose is one 0.5 mg delivery to each nostril (1 mg total). Initial doses are gradually increased as needed for symptom relief.
- NRT products have few side effects. Nausea and lightheadedness may indicate nicotine overdose. The patch site may be rotated to minimize skin irritation, and nonprescription **hydrocortisone** or **triamcinolone** cream may improve skin irritation. Sleep disturbances are reported in 23% of patients using the patch.

OTHER

- **Bupropion sustained release (SR)** is an effective smoking-cessation treatment. It is contraindicated in patients with a seizure disorder, a current or prior diagnosis of bulimia or anorexia nervosa, and concurrent use of a **monoamine oxidase inhibitor** or use within the previous 14 days. It can be used in combination with NRT.
- Insomnia and dry mouth are the most frequent side effects. Other side effects are tremor, rash, and anaphylactoid reactions.
- Bupropion SR should be dosed at 150 mg once daily for 3 days, then twice daily for 7 to 12 weeks or longer, with or without NRT. Patients should stop smoking during the second week of treatment. For maintenance treatment, bupropion SR 150 mg twice daily for up to 6 months can be given.
- **Varenicline** is a partial agonist that binds selectively to nicotinic acetylcholine receptors with a greater affinity than nicotine, thus producing an attenuated response compared with that of nicotine. It should be prescribed for 12 weeks, and a second 12-week treatment can be

TABLE 74–6 Pharmacologic Agents Used for Smoking Cessation

Drug	Place in Therapy	Dosage Range	Duration	Comments/Monitoring Parameters	LOE[d]
Buproprion SR[a,b]	First-line	Titrate up to 150 mg orally twice daily.	3 to 6 months	Patients receiving both bupropion and a nicotine patch should be monitored for hypertension.	A1
Clonidine[b,c]	Second-line	Titrate to response; 0.2 to 0.75 mg per day	6 to 12 months	Monitor baseline electrolyte and lipid profiles, renal function, uric acid, complete blood count, and blood pressure	B2
Nicotine polacrilex (gum)[a]	First-line	Initial dose depends on smoking history: 2 to 4 mg every 1 to 8 hours	12 weeks (taper down over time)	Heart rate and blood pressure should be monitored periodically during nicotine replacement therapy.	A1
Nicotine inhaler[a]	First-line	24 to 64 mg per day (total daily dose)	3 to 6 months (taper down over time)	Heart rate and blood pressure should be monitored periodically during nicotine replacement therapy.	A1
Nicotine nasal spray[a]	First-line	8 to 40 mg per day (total daily dose)	14 weeks (taper down over time)	Heart rate and blood pressure should be monitored periodically during nicotine replacement therapy.	A1
Nicotine patch[a]	First-line	Initial dose depends on smoking history: 7 to 21 mg topically once daily	6 weeks (taper down over time)	Heart rate and blood pressure should be monitored periodically during nicotine replacement therapy.	A1
Nortriptyline[b,c]	Second-line	Titrate up to 75 to 100 mg orally daily	6 to 12 months	Dry mouth, blurred vision, and constipation are dose-dependent adverse effects.	B2
Varenicline[b]	First-line	Titrate up to 1 mg orally twice daily	3 to 6 months	Monitor renal function, especially in elderly patients. Nausea, headache, insomnia are dose-dependent adverse effects.	A1

LOE, level of evidence.

[a]Nicotine replacement therapies can be combined with each other and/or bupropion to increase long-term abstinence rates.

[b]Do not abruptly discontinue. Taper up initially, and taper off once therapy is complete.

[c]Clonidine and nortriptyline are not FDA-approved for smoking cessation.

[d]Strength of recommendations, evidence to support recommendation: A, good; B, moderate; C, poor.
Quality of evidence: 1, evidence from more than 1 properly randomized, controlled trial; 2, evidence from more than 1 well-designed clinical trial with randomization, from cohort or case-controlled analytic studies or multiple time series; or dramatic results from uncontrolled experiments; 3, evidence from opinions of respected authorities, based on clinical experience, descriptive studies, or reports of expert communities.

Data from Fiore MC, Baily WC. Treating tobacco use and dependence. Clinical practice guidelines. Rockville, MD: U.S. Department of Health and Human Services, Public Health Service; 2000 (June), updated 2008 (May); and U.S. Department of Health and Human Services. The Health Consequences of Involuntary Exposure to Tobacco Smoke: A Report of the Surgeon General. Atlanta, GA: U.S. Department of Health and Human Services, Centers for Disease Control and Prevention, Coordinating Center for Health Promotion, National Center for Chronic Disease Prevention and Health Promotion, Office on Smoking and Health, 2006. http://www.surgeongeneral.gov/library/secondhandsmoke/report/citation.pdf.

prescribed if the patient is not abstinent. Its rate of cessation may be greater than that of bupropion.

- Side effects of varenicline include suicidal thoughts and erratic and aggressive behavior. A public health advisory stresses screening for psychiatric illness or behavior change after starting varenicline. The FDA required a boxed warning and updated medication guide.

SECOND-LINE MEDICATIONS

- **Clonidine**, delivered transdermally or orally, is an effective smoking-cessation treatment. It is given for 3 to 10 weeks and should not be discontinued abruptly. Abrupt discontinuation may cause nervousness, agitation, headache, tremor, and rapid rise in blood pressure.
- Dosing of clonidine initially is 0.1 mg orally twice daily or 0.1 mg/day transdermally, increasing by 0.1 mg/day each week if needed.
- The most common clonidine side effects are dry mouth, dizziness, sedation, and constipation. Blood pressure should be monitored.
- **Nortriptyline** is initiated 10 to 28 days before the quit date. The dose is initiated at 25 mg/day, gradually increasing to 75 to 100 mg/day. Treatment duration is commonly 12 weeks in trials, and common side effects are sedation, dry mouth, blurred vision, urinary retention, and lightheadedness.

See Chapter 74, Substance-Related Disorders: Overview and Depressants, Stimulants, and Hallucinogens, authored by Paul L. Doering, and Chapter 75, Substance-Related Disorders: Alcohol, Nicotine, and Caffeine, authored by Paul L. Doering and Robin Moorman Li, for a more detailed discussion of the topic.

CHAPTER 75

Acid–Base Disorders

DEFINITION

- Acid–base disorders are caused by disturbances in hydrogen ion (H^+) homeostasis, which is ordinarily maintained by extracellular buffering, renal regulation of hydrogen ion and bicarbonate, and ventilatory regulation of carbon dioxide (CO_2) elimination.

GENERAL PRINCIPLES

- General principles that are common to all types of acid–base disturbances are addressed first, followed by separate discussions of each type of acid–base disturbance.
- Buffering refers to the ability of a solution to resist change in pH after the addition of a strong acid or base. The body's principal extracellular buffer system is the carbonic acid/bicarbonate (H_2CO_3/HCO_3^-) system.
- Most of the body's acid production is in the form of CO_2 and is produced from catabolism of carbohydrates, proteins, and lipids.
- There are four primary types of acid–base disturbances, which can occur independently or together as a compensatory response.
- Metabolic acid–base disorders are caused by changes in plasma bicarbonate concentration (HCO_3^-). Metabolic acidosis is characterized by decreased HCO_3^-, and metabolic alkalosis is characterized by increased HCO_3^-.
- Respiratory acid–base disorders are caused by altered alveolar ventilation, producing changes in arterial carbon dioxide tension ($Paco_2$). Respiratory acidosis is characterized by increased $Paco_2$, whereas respiratory alkalosis is characterized by decreased $Paco_2$.

DIAGNOSIS

- Blood gases (**Table 75–1**), serum electrolytes, medical history, and clinical condition are the primary tools for determining the cause of acid–base disorders and for designing therapy.
- Arterial blood gases (ABG) are measured to determine oxygenation and acid–base status (**Fig. 75–1**). Low pH values (<7.35) indicate acidemia, whereas high values (>7.45) indicate alkalemia. The $Paco_2$ value helps to determine if there is a primary respiratory abnormality,

TABLE 75-1 Normal Blood Gas Values

	Arterial Blood	Mixed Venous Blood
pH	7.40 (7.35–7.45)	7.38 (7.33–7.43)
Pao_2	80–100 mm Hg (10.6–13.3 kPa)	35–40 mm Hg (4.7–5.3 kPa)
Sao_2	95%	70–75%
Pco_2	35–45 mm Hg (4.7–6 kPa)	45–51 mm Hg (4.7–6.8 kPa)
HCO_3^-	22–26 mEq/L (22–26 mmol/L)	24–28 mEq/L (24–28 mmol/L)

HCO_3^-, bicarbonate; $Paco_2$, partial pressure of carbon dioxide; Pao_2, partial pressure of oxygen; Sao_2, saturation of arterial oxygen

whereas the HCO_3^- concentration helps to determine if there is a primary metabolic abnormality. Steps in acid–base interpretation are described in **Table 75–2**.

DESIRED OUTCOME

- Initial treatment is aimed at stabilizing the acute condition, followed by identifying and correcting the underlying cause(s) of the acid–base disturbance. Additional treatment may be needed depending on the severity of symptoms and likelihood of recurrence, especially in patients with ongoing initiating events.

METABOLIC ACIDOSIS

PATHOPHYSIOLOGY

- Metabolic acidosis is characterized by decreased pH and serum HCO_3^- concentrations, which can result from adding organic acid to extracellular fluid (e.g., lactic acid and ketoacids), loss of HCO_3^- stores (e.g., diarrhea), or accumulation of endogenous acids due to impaired renal function (e.g., phosphates and sulfates).

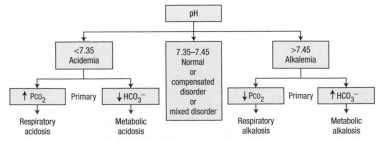

FIGURE 75–1. Analysis of arterial blood gases. (HCO_3^-, bicarbonate; $Paco_2$, partial pressure of carbon dioxide.)

TABLE 75–2 Steps in Acid–Base Diagnosis

1. Obtain arterial blood gases (ABGs) and electrolytes simultaneously.
2. Compare $[HCO_3^-]$ on ABG and electrolytes to verify accuracy.
3. Calculate anion gap.
4. Is acidemia (pH < 7.35) or alkalemia (pH > 7.45) present?
5. Is the primary abnormality respiratory (alteration in $Paco_2$) or metabolic (alteration in HCO_3^-)?
6. Estimate compensatory response (see Table 60–7 in *Pharmacotherapy: A Pathophysiologic Approach,* eighth edition).
7. Compare change in $[Cl^-]$ with change in $[Na^+]$.

$[Cl^-]$, chloride ion; $[HCO_3^-]$, bicarbonate; $[Na^+]$, sodium ion; $Paco_2$, partial pressure of carbon dioxide from arterial blood

- Serum anion gap (SAG) can be used to elucidate the cause of metabolic acidosis (**Table 75–3**). SAG is calculated as follows:

$$SAG = [Na^+] - [Cl^-] - [HCO_3^-]$$

The normal anion gap is ~9 mEq/L (9 mmol/L), with a range of 3 to 11 mEq/L (3–11 mmol/L). SAG is a relative rather than an absolute indication of the cause of metabolic acidosis.

- The primary compensatory mechanism is to decrease $Paco_2$ by increasing the respiratory rate.

CLINICAL PRESENTATION

- The major manifestation of chronic metabolic acidosis is bone demineralization with the development of rickets in children and osteomalacia and osteopenia in adults.
- The manifestations of acute severe metabolic acidemia (pH <7.15–7.2) involve the cardiovascular, respiratory, and central nervous systems. Hyperventilation is often the first sign of metabolic acidosis. Respiratory compensation may occur as Kussmaul respirations (i.e., deep, rapid respirations characteristic of diabetic ketoacidosis).

TREATMENT

- The primary treatment of metabolic acidosis is to correct the underlying disorder. Additional treatment depends on the severity and onset of acidosis.
- Asymptomatic patients with mild to moderate acidemia (HCO_3^- 12–20 mEq/L [12–20 mmol/L]; pH 7.2–7.4) can usually be managed with gradual correction of the acidemia over days to weeks using oral **sodium bicarbonate** or other alkali preparations (**Table 75–4**). The dose of bicarbonate can be calculated as follows:

$$\text{Loading dose (mEq or mmol/L)} = (Vd\ HCO_3^- \times \text{body weight}) \times (\text{desired } [HCO_3^-] - \text{current } [HCO_3^-]),$$

where $Vd\ HCO_3^-$ is the volume of distribution of HCO_3^- (0.5 L/kg).

| TABLE 75–3 | Common Causes of Metabolic Acidosis |

Increased Serum Anion Gap	Normal Serum Anion Gap/Hyperchloremic States
Lactic acidosis	**GI bicarbonate loss**
Diabetic ketoacidosis	Diarrhea
Renal failure (acute or chronic)	External pancreatic or small bowel drainage (fistula)
Methanol ingestion	Ureterosigmoidostomy, ileostomy
Ethylene glycol ingestion	**Drugs**
Salicylate overdosage	Cholestyramine (bile acid diarrhea)
Starvation	Magnesium sulfate (diarrhea)
	Calcium chloride (acidifying agent)
	Renal tubular acidosis
	Hypokalemia
	Proximal renal tubular acidosis (type II)
	Distal renal tubular acidosis (type I)
	Carbonic anhydrase inhibitors (e.g., acetazolamide)
	Hyperkalemia
	Generalized distal nephron dysfunction (type IV)
	Mineralocorticoid deficiency or resistance
	Tubulointerstitial disease
	Drug-induced hyperkalemia
	Potassium-sparing diuretics (amiloride, spironolactone, triamterene)
	Trimethoprim
	Pentamidine
	Heparin
	Angiotensin-converting enzyme inhibitors and receptor blockers
	Nonsteroidal antiinflammatory drugs
	Cyclosporin A
	Other
	Acid ingestion (ammonium chloride, hydrochloric acid, hyperalimentation)
	Expansion acidosis (rapid saline administration)

- Alkali therapy can be used to treat patients with acute severe metabolic acidosis due to hyperchloremic acidosis, but its role is controversial in patients with lactic acidosis. Therapeutic options include **sodium bicarbonate** and **tromethamine.**
  - ✓ Sodium bicarbonate has been recommended to raise arterial pH to 7.15 to 7.2. However, no controlled clinical studies have demonstrated reduced morbidity and mortality compared with general supportive care. If IV sodium bicarbonate is administered, the goal is to increase, not normalize, pH to 7.2 and HCO_3^- to 8 to 10 mEq/L (8–10 mmol/L).
  - ✓ Tromethamine, a highly alkaline solution, is a sodium-free organic amine that acts as a proton acceptor to prevent or correct acidosis. However, no evidence exists that tromethamine is beneficial or more efficacious than sodium bicarbonate. The usual empiric dosage for

TABLE 75–4 Therapeutic Alternatives for Oral Alkali Replacement

Generic Name	Trade Name(s)	Milliequivalents of Alkali	Dosage Form(s)	Comment
Shohl's solution, sodium citrate/citric acid	Bicitra (Willen)	1 mEq Na/mL; equivalent to 1 mEq bicarbonate	Solution (500 mg Na citrate, 334 mg citric acid/5 mL)	Citrate preparations increase absorption of aluminum
Sodium bicarbonate	Various (e.g., Sodamint)	3.9 mEq bicarbonate/tablet (325 mg)	325 mg tablet	Bicarbonate preparations can cause bloating because of carbon dioxide production
	Baking soda (various)	7.8 mEq bicarbonate/tablet (650 mg) 60 mEq bicarbonate/tsp (5 g/tsp)	650 mg tablet Powder	
Potassium citrate	Urocit-K (Mission)	5 mEq citrate/tablet	5 mEq tablet	See above
Potassium bicarbonate/potassium citrate	K-Lyte (Bristol)	25 mEq bicarbonate/tablet	25 mEq tablet (effervescent)	See above
	K-Lyte DS (Bristol)	50 mEq bicarbonate/tablet (double strength)	50 mEq tablet (effervescent)	
Potassium citrate/citric acid	Polycitra-K (Willen)	2 mEq K/mL; equivalent to 2 mEq bicarbonate	Solution (1,100 mg K citrate, 334 mg citric acid/5 mL)	See above
		30 mEq bicarbonate/unit dose packet	Crystals for reconstitution (3,300 mg K citrate, 1,002 mg citric acid/unit dose packet)	
Sodium citrate/potassium citrate/citric acid	Polycitra (Willen), Polycitra-LC (Willen)	1 mEq K, 1 mEq Na/mL; equivalent to 2 mEq bicarbonate	Syrup (Polycitra) solution (Polycitra-LC) (both contain 550 mg K citrate, 500 mg Na citrate, 334 mg citric acid/5 mL)	See above

tromethamine is 1 to 5 mmol/kg administered IV over 1 hour, and an individualized dose can be calculated as follows:

$$\text{Dose of tromethamine (in mL)} = 1.1 \times \text{body weight (in kg)}$$
$$\times (\text{normal [HCO}_3^-] - \text{current [HCO}_3^-])$$

METABOLIC ALKALOSIS

PATHOPHYSIOLOGY

- Metabolic alkalosis is *initiated* by increased pH and HCO_3^-, which can result from loss of H^+ via the GI tract (e.g., nasogastric suctioning, vomiting) or kidneys (e.g., diuretics, Cushing's syndrome) or from gain of bicarbonate (e.g., administration of bicarbonate, acetate, lactate, or citrate).
- Metabolic alkalosis is *maintained* by abnormal renal function that prevents the kidneys from excreting excess bicarbonate.
- The respiratory response to metabolic alkalosis is to increase $Paco_2$ by hypoventilation.

CLINICAL PRESENTATION

- No unique signs or symptoms are associated with mild to moderate metabolic alkalosis. Some patients complain of symptoms related to the underlying disorder (e.g., muscle weakness with hypokalemia or postural dizziness with volume depletion) or have a history of vomiting, gastric drainage, or diuretic use.
- Severe alkalemia (pH > 7.60) can be associated with cardiac arrhythmias and neuromuscular irritability.

TREATMENT

- Treatment of metabolic alkalosis should be aimed at correcting the factor(s) responsible for maintaining the alkalosis.
- Treatment depends on whether the disorder is sodium chloride responsive or resistant (**Fig. 75–2**).

RESPIRATORY ALKALOSIS

PATHOPHYSIOLOGY

- Respiratory alkalosis is characterized by a decrease in $Paco_2$ and an increase in pH.
- $Paco_2$ decreases when ventilatory CO_2 excretion exceeds metabolic CO_2 production, usually because of hyperventilation.
- Causes of respiratory alkalosis include increases in neurochemical stimulation via central or peripheral mechanisms, or physical increases in ventilation via voluntary or artificial means (e.g., mechanical ventilation).
- The earliest compensatory response is to chemically buffer excess bicarbonate by releasing hydrogen ions from intracellular proteins, phos-

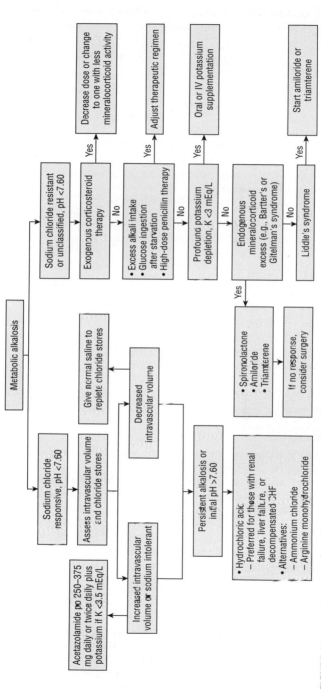

FIGURE 75–2. Treatment algorithm for patients with primary metabolic alkalosis. (CHF, chronic heart failure; K, potassium [serum potassium in mEq/L is numerically equal to mmol/L].)

phates, and hemoglobin. If respiratory alkalosis is prolonged (>6 hours), the kidneys attempt to further compensate by increasing bicarbonate elimination.

CLINICAL PRESENTATION

- Although usually asymptomatic, respiratory alkalosis can cause adverse neuromuscular, cardiovascular, and GI effects.
- Lightheadedness, confusion, decreased intellectual functioning, syncope, and seizures can be caused by decreased cerebral blood flow.
- Nausea and vomiting can occur, probably due to cerebral hypoxia.
- Serum electrolytes can be altered secondary to respiratory alkalosis. Serum chloride is usually increased; serum potassium, phosphorus, and ionized calcium are usually decreased.

TREATMENT

- Treatment is often unnecessary because most patients have few symptoms and only mild pH alterations (i.e., pH <7.50).
- Direct measures (e.g., treatment of pain, hypovolemia, fever, infection, or salicylate overdose) can be effective. A rebreathing device (e.g., paper bag) can help control hyperventilation in patients with anxiety/hyperventilation syndrome.
- Respiratory alkalosis associated with mechanical ventilation can often be corrected by decreasing the number of mechanical breaths per minute, using a capnograph and spirometer to adjust ventilator settings more precisely, or increasing dead space in the ventilator circuit.

RESPIRATORY ACIDOSIS

PATHOPHYSIOLOGY

- Respiratory acidosis is characterized by an increase in $Paco_2$ and a decrease in pH.
- Respiratory acidosis results from disorders that restrict ventilation or increase CO_2 production, airway and pulmonary abnormalities, neuromuscular abnormalities, or mechanical ventilator problems.
- The early compensatory response to acute respiratory acidosis is chemical buffering. If respiratory acidosis is prolonged (>12–24 hours), proximal tubular HCO_3^- reabsorption, ammoniagenesis, and distal tubular H^+ secretion are enhanced, resulting in an increase in serum HCO_3^- concentration that raises pH to normal.

CLINICAL PRESENTATION

- Neuromuscular symptoms include altered mental status, abnormal behavior, seizures, stupor, and coma. Hypercapnia can mimic a stroke or CNS tumor by producing headache, papilledema, focal paresis, and abnormal reflexes. CNS symptoms are caused by increased cerebral blood flow and are variable, depending in part on the acuity of onset.

TREATMENT

- Adequate ventilation should be provided if CO_2 excretion is acutely and severely impaired ($Paco_2$ >80 mm Hg [>10.6 kPa]) or if life-threatening hypoxia is present (arterial oxygen tension [Pao_2] <40 mm Hg [<5.3 kPa]). Ventilation can include maintaining a patent airway (e.g., emergency tracheostomy, bronchoscopy, or intubation), clearing excessive secretions, administering oxygen, and providing mechanical ventilation.
- The underlying cause of acute acidosis should be treated aggressively (e.g., administration of bronchodilators for bronchospasm or discontinuation of respiratory depressants such as narcotics and benzodiazepines). Bicarbonate administration is rarely necessary and is potentially harmful.
- In a patient with chronic respiratory acidosis (e.g., chronic obstructive pulmonary disease [COPD]), treatment is essentially similar to that for acute respiratory acidosis with a few important exceptions. Oxygen therapy should be initiated carefully and only if the Pao_2 is <50 mm Hg (<6.7 kPa) because the drive to breathe depends on hypoxemia rather than hypercarbia.
- For information on chronic respiratory acidosis, see Chap. 82.

MIXED ACID–BASE DISORDERS

PATHOPHYSIOLOGY

- Failure of compensation is responsible for mixed acid–base disorders such as respiratory acidosis and metabolic acidosis, or respiratory alkalosis and metabolic alkalosis. In contrast, excess compensation is responsible for metabolic acidosis and respiratory alkalosis, or metabolic alkalosis and respiratory acidosis.
- Respiratory and metabolic acidosis can develop in patients with cardiorespiratory arrest, with chronic lung disease and shock, and with metabolic acidosis and respiratory failure.
- The most common mixed acid–base disorder is respiratory and metabolic alkalosis, which occurs in critically ill surgical patients with respiratory alkalosis caused by mechanical ventilation, hypoxia, sepsis, hypotension, neurologic damage, pain, or drugs; and with metabolic alkalosis caused by vomiting or nasogastric suctioning and massive blood transfusions.
- Mixed metabolic acidosis and respiratory alkalosis occur in patients with advanced liver disease, salicylate intoxication, and pulmonary-renal syndromes.
- Metabolic alkalosis and respiratory acidosis can occur in patients with COPD and respiratory acidosis who are treated with salt restriction, diuretics, and possibly glucocorticoids.

TREATMENT

- Mixed respiratory and metabolic acidosis should be treated by responding to both the respiratory and metabolic acidosis. Improved oxygen delivery must be initiated to improve hypercarbia and hypoxia.

Mechanical ventilation can be needed to reduce $Paco_2$. During initial therapy, appropriate amounts of alkali should be given to reverse the metabolic acidosis.

- The metabolic component of mixed respiratory and metabolic alkalosis should be corrected by administering **sodium** and **potassium chloride solutions.** The respiratory component should be treated by readjusting the ventilator or by treating the underlying disorder causing hyperventilation.

- Treatment of mixed metabolic acidosis and respiratory alkalosis should be directed at the underlying cause.

- In metabolic alkalosis and respiratory acidosis, pH does not usually deviate significantly from normal, but treatment can be required to maintain Pao_2 and $Paco_2$ at acceptable levels. Treatment should be aimed at decreasing plasma bicarbonate with sodium and potassium chloride therapy, allowing renal excretion of retained bicarbonate from diuretic-induced metabolic alkalosis.

EVALUATION OF THERAPEUTIC OUTCOMES

- Patients should be monitored closely because acid–base disorders can be serious and even life threatening.

- ABG are the primary tools for evaluation of therapeutic outcome. They should be monitored closely to ensure resolution of simple acid–base disorders without deterioration to mixed disorders due to compensatory mechanisms.

See Chapter 61, Acid–Base Disorders, authored by John W. Devlin and Gary R. Matzke, for a more detailed discussion of this topic.

CHAPTER 76

Acute Kidney Injury

DEFINITIONS

- The term acute renal failure (ARF) describes an abrupt decrease in glomerular filtration rate (GFR) or creatinine clearance (CL_{cr}). ARF has been replaced by acute kidney injury (AKI) to emphasize that the disorder exists along a wide continuum, ranging from mild renal dysfunction to the need for renal replacement therapies (RRTs), such as hemodialysis and peritoneal dialysis.
- Risk, Injury, Failure, Loss of Kidney Function, and End-Stage Renal Disease (RIFLE) and Acute Kidney Injury Network (AKIN) criteria are two classification systems based on separate criteria for serum creatinine (S_{cr}) and urine output used to stage the severity of AKI (Table 76–1).
- Multiple studies have validated the ability of the RIFLE criteria to predict certain patient outcomes, particularly hospital mortality.

PATHOPHYSIOLOGY

- AKI can be categorized as prerenal (resulting from decreased renal perfusion in the setting of undamaged parenchymal tissue), intrinsic (resulting from structural damage to the kidney, most commonly the tubule from an ischemic or toxic insult), and postrenal (resulting from obstruction of urine flow downstream from the kidney) (Fig. 76–1).

CLINICAL PRESENTATION

- Patient presentation varies widely and depends on the underlying cause. Outpatients often are not in acute distress; hospitalized patients may develop AKI after a catastrophic event.
- Symptoms in the outpatient setting include acute change in urinary habits, weight gain, and flank pain. Signs include edema, colored or foamy urine, and, in volume-depleted patients, orthostatic hypotension.

DIAGNOSIS

- Thorough medical and medication histories, physical examination, assessment of laboratory values and, if needed, imaging studies are important in the diagnosis of AKI.
- S_{cr} cannot be used alone to diagnose AKI because it is insensitive to rapid changes in GFR and therefore may not reflect current renal function. The use of blood urea nitrogen (BUN) in AKI is very limited because urea's production and renal clearance are heavily influenced by extrarenal factors such as critical illness, volume status, protein intake, and medications.

TABLE 76–5	Common Causes of Diuretic Resistance in Patients with Severe Acute Kidney Injury

Causes of Diuretic Resistance	Potential Therapeutic Solutions
Excessive sodium intake (sources may be dietary, IV fluids, and drugs)	Remove sodium from nutritional sources and medications
Inadequate diuretic dose or inappropriate regimen	Increase dose, use continuous infusion or combination therapy
Reduced oral bioavailability (usually furosemide)	Use parenteral therapy; switch to oral torsemide or bumetanide
Nephrotic syndrome (loop diuretic protein binding in tubule lumen)	Increase dose, switch diuretics, use combination therapy
Reduced renal blood flow	
Drugs (NSAIDs ACEIs, vasodilators)	Discontinue these drugs if possible
Hypotension	Intravascular volume expansion and/or vasopressors
Intravascular depletion	Intravascular volume expansion
Increased sodium resorption	
Nephron adaptation to chronic diuretic therapy	Combination diuretic therapy, sodium restriction
NSAID use	Discontinue NSAID
Heart failure	Treat the heart failure, increase diuretic dose, switch to better-absorbed loop diuretic
Cirrhosis	High-volume paracentesis
Acute tubular necrosis	Higher dose of diuretic, diuretic combination therapy; add low-dose dopamine

ACEIs, angiotensin-converting enzyme inhibitors; IV, intravenous; NSAIDs, nonsteroidal antiinflammatory drugs.

- Nutritional management of critically ill patients with AKI is complex due to multiple mechanisms for metabolic derangements. Nutritional requirements are altered by stress, inflammation, and injury that lead to hypermetabolic and hypercatabolic states.

DRUG-DOSING CONSIDERATIONS

- Drug therapy optimization in AKI is a challenge. Confounding variables include residual drug clearance, fluid accumulation, and use of RRTs.
- Volume of distribution for water-soluble drugs is significantly increased due to edema. Use of dosing guidelines for CKD does not reflect the clearance and volume of distribution in critically ill patients with AKI.
- Patients with AKI may have a higher residual nonrenal clearance than those with CKD with similar creatinine clearances; this complicates drug therapy individualization, especially with RRTs.
- The mode of CRRT determines the rate of drug removal, further complicating individualization of drug therapy. The rates of ultrafiltration, blood flow, and dialysate flow influence drug clearance during CRRT.

TABLE 76–6	Key Monitoring Parameters for Patients with Established Acute Kidney Injury

Parameter	Frequency
Fluid ins/outs	Every shift
Patient weight	Daily
Hemodynamics (blood pressure, heart rate, mean arterial pressure, etc.)	Every shift
Blood chemistries	
Sodium, potassium, chloride, bicarbonate, calcium, phosphate, magnesium	Daily
Blood urea nitrogen/serum creatinine	Daily
Drugs and their dosing regimens	Daily
Nutritional regimen	Daily
Blood glucose	Daily (minimum)
Serum concentration data for drugs	After regimen changes and after renal replacement therapy has been instituted
Times of administered doses	Daily
Doses relative to administration of renal replacement therapy	Daily
Urinalysis	
Calculate measured creatinine clearance	Every time measured urine collection performed
Calculate fractional excretion of sodium	Every time measured urine collection performed
Plans for renal replacement	Daily

EVALUATION OF THERAPEUTIC OUTCOMES

- Vigilant monitoring of patient status is essential (**Table 76–6**).
- Drug concentrations should be monitored frequently because of changing volume status, changing renal function, and RRTs in patients with AKI.

See Chapter 51, Acute Kidney Injury, authored by William Dager and Jenana Halilovic, for a more detailed discussion of this topic.

CHAPTER 77

Chronic Kidney Disease

DEFINITION

- Chronic kidney disease (CKD), also called *chronic renal insufficiency* and *progressive kidney disease,* is a progressive loss of function over several months to years, characterized by gradual replacement of normal kidney architecture with parenchymal fibrosis.
- CKD is categorized by the level of kidney function, based on glomerular filtration rate (GFR), as stages 1 to 5, with each increasing number indicating a more advanced stage of the disease, as defined by a declining GFR. This classification system from the National Kidney Foundation's Kidney Dialysis Outcomes and Quality Initiative (K/DOQI) also accounts for structural evidence of kidney damage.
- CKD stage 5, previously referred to as end-stage renal disease (ESRD), occurs when the GFR falls below 15 mL/min/1.73m² (<0.14 mL/s/m²) or in patients receiving renal replacement therapy (RRT). In this chapter, *ESRD* refers specifically to patients who are receiving chronic dialysis.

PATHOPHYSIOLOGY

- *Susceptibility factors* increase the risk for kidney disease but do not directly cause kidney damage. They include advanced age, reduced kidney mass and low birth weight, racial or ethnic minority, family history, low income or education, systemic inflammation, and dyslipidemia.
- *Initiation factors* initiate kidney damage and can be modified by drug therapy. They include diabetes mellitus, hypertension, autoimmune diseases, polycystic kidney disease, systemic infections, urinary tract infections, urinary stones, and nephrotoxicity.
- *Progression factors* hasten the decline in kidney function after initiation of kidney damage. They include glycemia in diabetics, hypertension, proteinuria, hyperlipidemia, obesity, and smoking.
- Most progressive nephropathies share a final common pathway to irreversible renal parenchymal damage and ESRD (**Fig. 77–1**). Key pathway elements are loss of nephron mass, glomerular capillary hypertension, and proteinuria.

CLINICAL PRESENTATION

- CKD development and progression are insidious. Patients with stage 1 or 2 CKD usually do not have symptoms or metabolic derangements seen with stages 3 to 5, such as anemia, secondary hyperparathyroidism, cardiovascular disease, malnutrition, and fluid and electrolyte abnormalities that are more common as kidney function deteriorates.
- Uremic symptoms (fatigue, weakness, shortness of breath, mental confusion, nausea, vomiting, bleeding, and anorexia) are generally absent in stages 1 and 2, minimal during stages 3 and 4, and common in patients

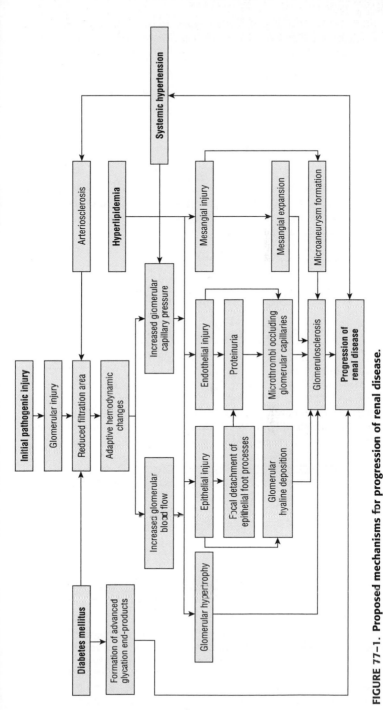

FIGURE 77-1. Proposed mechanisms for progression of renal disease.

with stage 5 CKD who may also experience itching, cold intolerance, weight gain, and peripheral neuropathies.

- Signs and symptoms of uremia are foundational to the decision to implement RRT.

DESIRED OUTCOME

- The goal is to delay the progression of CKD, minimizing the development or severity of complications.

TREATMENT: PROGRESSION-MODIFYING THERAPIES

- The treatment of CKD includes nonpharmacologic and pharmacologic strategies. Strategies differ depending on the presence (Fig. 77–2) or absence (Fig. 77–3) of diabetes.

NONPHARMACOLOGIC THERAPY

- A low-protein diet (0.6–0.75 g/kg/day) can delay progression of CKD in patients with or without diabetes, although the benefit is relatively small.

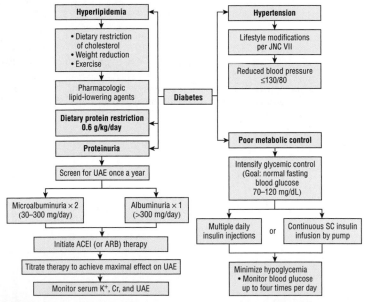

FIGURE 77–2. Therapeutic strategies to prevent progression of renal disease in diabetic individuals. (ACEI, angiotensin-converting enzyme inhibitor; ARB, angiotensin receptor blocker; Cr, creatinine; JNC VII, the seventh report of the Joint National Committee on Prevention, Detection, Evaluation, and Treatment of High Blood Pressure; K+, potassium; SC, subcutaneous; UAE, urinary albumin excretion.)

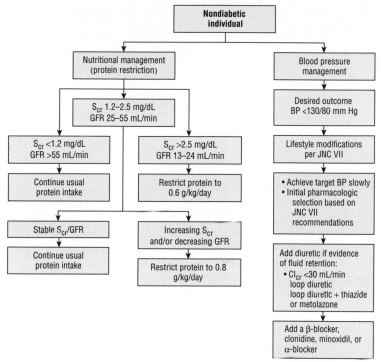

FIGURE 77–3. Therapeutic strategies to prevent progression of renal disease in nondiabetic individuals. (BP, blood pressure; CL_{cr}, creatinine clearance; GFR, glomerular filtration rate; JNC VII, the seventh report of the Joint National Committee on Prevention, Detection, Evaluation, and Treatment of High Blood Pressure; S_{cr}, serum creatinine.)

PHARMACOLOGIC THERAPY

Hyperglycemia

- Intensive therapy in patients with types 1 and 2 diabetes reduces microvascular complications, including nephropathy. This can include insulin or oral drugs and involves blood sugar testing at least three times daily.
- The progression of CKD can be limited by optimal control of hyperglycemia and hypertension.
- For more information on diabetes, see Chap. 19.

Hypertension

- Adequate blood pressure (BP) control (**Fig. 77–4**, see **Figs. 77–2** and **77–3**) can reduce the rate of decline in GFR and albuminuria in patients with or without diabetes.
- Antihypertensive therapy should be initiated in diabetic or nondiabetic CKD patients with an angiotensin-converting enzyme inhibitor (ACEI) or

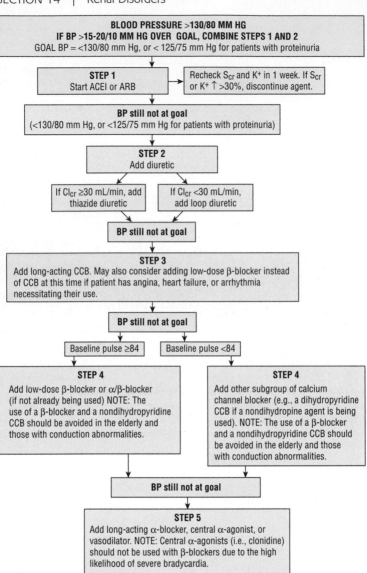

BLOOD PRESSURE >130/80 MM HG
IF BP >15-20/10 MM HG OVER GOAL, COMBINE STEPS 1 AND 2
GOAL BP = <130/80 mm Hg, or < 125/75 mm Hg for patients with proteinuria

STEP 1
Start ACEI or ARB

Recheck S_{cr} and K^+ in 1 week. If S_{cr} or K^+ ↑ >30%, discontinue agent.

BP still not at goal
(<130/80 mm Hg, or <125/75 mm Hg for patients with proteinuria)

STEP 2
Add diuretic

If Cl_{cr} ≥30 mL/min, add thiazide diuretic

If Cl_{cr} <30 mL/min, add loop diuretic

BP still not at goal

STEP 3
Add long-acting CCB. May also consider adding low-dose β-blocker instead of CCB at this time if patient has angina, heart failure, or arrhythmia necessitating their use.

BP still not at goal

Baseline pulse ≥84

Baseline pulse <84

STEP 4
Add low-dose β-blocker or α/β-blocker (if not already being used) NOTE: The use of a β-blocker and a nondihydropyridine CCB should be avoided in the elderly and those with conduction abnormalities.

STEP 4
Add other subgroup of calcium channel blocker (e.g., a dihydropyridine CCB if a nondihydropine agent is being used). NOTE: The use of a β-blocker and a nondihydropyridine CCB should be avoided in the elderly and those with conduction abnormalities.

BP still not at goal

STEP 5
Add long-acting α-blocker, central α-agonist, or vasodilator. NOTE: Central α-agonists (i.e., clonidine) should not be used with β-blockers due to the high likelihood of severe bradycardia.

FIGURE 77–4. Hypertension management algorithm for patients with chronic kidney disease. Dosage adjustments should be made every 2 to 4 weeks as needed. The dose of one agent should be maximized before another is added. (ACEI, angiotensin-converting enzyme inhibitor; ARB, angiotensin receptor blocker; BP, blood pressure; CCB, calcium channel blocker; Cl_{cr}, creatinine clearance; K^+, serum potassium; S_{cr}, serum creatinine.) *(Adapted from Bakris GL, Williams M, Dworkin L, et al. Preserving renal function in adults with hypertension and diabetes: A consensus approach. National Kidney Foundation Hypertension and Diabetes Executive Committees Working Group. Am J Kidney Dis 2000;36:646–661, with permission. Copyright Elsevier 2000.)*

an angiotensin II receptor blocker (ARB). Nondihydropyridine calcium channel blockers are generally used as second-line antiproteinuric drugs when ACEIs or ARBs are not tolerated.

- ACEI clearance is reduced in CKD; therefore, treatment should begin with the lowest possible dose followed by gradual titration to achieve target BP and, secondarily, to minimize proteinuria. No individual ACEI is superior to another.
- GFR typically decreases 25% to 30% within 3 to 7 days after starting ACEIs because this class reduces intraglomerular pressure. Sustained increases in the serum creatinine by >30% after starting ACEIs may be due to the ACEI, and discontinuation should be strongly considered. Serum potassium should also be monitored to detect development of hyperkalemia after initiating or increasing the dose of an ACEI.
- For more information on hypertension, see Chap. 10.

Supportive Therapies

- Dietary protein restriction (see Figs. 77–2 and 77–3), lipid-lowering medications, smoking cessation, and anemia management may help slow the rate of CKD progression.
- The primary goal of lipid-lowering therapies in CKD is to decrease the risk for progressive atherosclerotic cardiovascular disease (Table 77–1).

TABLE 77–1	Management of Dyslipidemia in Patients with Chronic Kidney Disease			
Dyslipidemia	**Goal**	**Initial Therapy**	**Modification in Therapy[a]**	**Alternative[a]**
TG ≥500 mg/dL (≥5.56 mmol/L)	TG <500 mg/dL (<5.56 mmol/L)	TLC	TLC + fibrate or niacin	Fibrate or niacin
LDL 100–129 mg/dL (2.56–3.34 mmol/L)	LDL <100 mg/dL (<2.56 mmol/L)	TLC	TLC + low-dose statin	Bile acid sequestrant or niacin
LDL ≥130 mg/dL (≥3.36 mmol/L)	LDL <100 mg/dL (<2.56 mmol/L)	TLC + low-dose statin	TLC + maximum-dose statin	Bile acid sequestrant or niacin
TG ≥200 mg/dL (≥2.26 mmol/L) and non-HDL ≥130mg/dL (≥3.36mmol/L)	Non-HDL <130 mg/dL (<3.36 mmol/L)	TLC + low-dose statin	TLC + maximum-dose statin	Fibrate or niacin

HDL, high-density lipoprotein; LDL, low-density lipoprotein; non-HDL, total cholesterol minus HDL cholesterol; TG, triglycerides; TLC, therapeutic lifestyle changes.

[a]Dosing of selected agents by class: fibrate (gemfibrozil 600 mg twice daily); niacin (1.5–3 g/day of immediate-release product); statin (simvastatin 10–40 mg/day if GFR <30 mL/min [<0.50 mL/s], 20–80 mg/day if GFR >30 mL/min [>0.50 mL/s]); bile acid sequestrant (cholestyramine 4–16 g/day).

See Chap. 28 in Pharmacotherapy: A Pathophysiologic Approach, eighth edition, for more complete dosing information. Reprinted from K/DOQI Clinical Practice Guidelines for managing dyslipidemias in patients with chronic kidney disease. Am J Kidney Dis 2003;41(4 suppl 3):S1–S91, Copyright 2003, with permission from Elsevier.

- A secondary goal is to reduce proteinuria and renal function decline seen with administration of statins (3-hydroxy-3-methylglutaryl coenzyme A reductase inhibitors).
- For more information on dyslipidemia, see Chap. 8.

TREATMENT: MANAGEMENT OF COMPLICATIONS

- Progression of CKD to ESRD can occur over years to decades, with the mechanism of kidney damage dependent on the etiology of the disease; however, the consequences and complications of marked reductions in kidney function are fairly uniform irrespective of the underlying etiology.
- No single toxin is responsible for all of the signs and symptoms of uremia observed in stage 4 or 5 CKD. Toxins accumulate as a result of increased secretion, decreased clearance secondary to reduced metabolism within the kidney, and/or decreased renal clearance of by-products of protein metabolism.
- The overall goal of therapy is to optimize the patient's duration and quality of life. Patients who reach CKD stage 4 almost inevitably progress to ESRD, requiring dialysis to sustain life.
- The most common complications associated with a decline in GFR are discussed below.

FLUID AND ELECTROLYTE ABNORMALITIES

- Serum sodium concentration is generally maintained by an increase in fractional excretion of sodium, resulting in a volume-expanded state. The most common manifestation of increased intravascular volume is systemic hypertension.
- The kidneys' ability to adjust to abrupt changes in sodium intake is diminished in patients with ESRD. Sodium restriction beyond a no-added-salt diet is not recommended unless hypertension or edema is present. A negative sodium balance can decrease renal perfusion and cause a further decline in GFR.
- Diuretic therapy or dialysis may be necessary to control edema or BP.
- Loop diuretics, particularly when administered by continuous infusion, increase urine volume and renal sodium excretion. Although thiazide diuretics are ineffective when creatinine clearance is <30 mL/min, adding them to loop diuretics can enhance excretion of sodium and water.

POTASSIUM HOMEOSTASIS

- Serum potassium concentration is usually maintained in the normal range until the GFR is <20 mL/min per 1.73 m^2, when mild hyperkalemia is likely to develop.
- The definitive treatment of severe hyperkalemia in ESRD is hemodialysis. Temporary measures include **calcium gluconate, insulin and glucose, nebulized albuterol,** and **sodium polystyrene sulfonate**.
- For more information on potassium homeostasis, see Chap. 79.

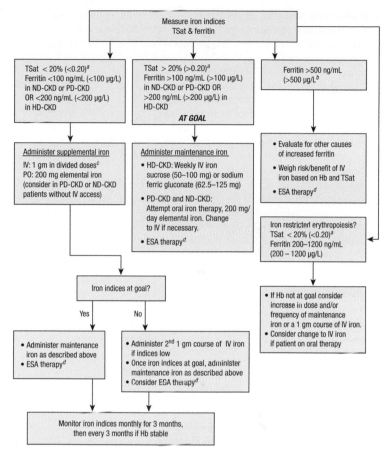

FIGURE 77-5. Algorithm for iron therapy in the management of the anemia of CKD. (ESA, erythropoiesis-stimulating agent; Hb, hemoglobin; TSat, transferrin saturation; ND-CKD, nondialysis CKD patients; PD-CKD, peritoneal dialysis patients; HD-CKD, hemodialysis patients.)

ANEMIA

- The primary cause of anemia in patients with CKD is erythropoietin deficiency. Other contributing factors are decreased life span of red blood cells, blood loss, deficiencies in vitamin B$_{12}$ or folate, and iron deficiency.
- The recommended target hemoglobin in all stage 5 CKD patients receiving erythropoietin-stimulating agents (ESAs) is 11 to 12 g/dL (110–120 g/L; 6.83–7.45 mmol/L).

- **Iron** supplementation is necessary to replete iron stores (**Fig. 77-5**). Parenteral iron therapy improves response to ESA therapy and reduces the dose required to achieve and maintain target indices. In contrast, oral therapy is limited by poor absorption and nonadherence with therapy primarily due to adverse effects.
- IV iron preparations have different pharmacokinetic profiles, which do not correlate with pharmacodynamic effect.
- Adverse effects of IV iron include allergic reactions, hypotension, dizziness, dyspnea, headaches, lower back pain, arthralgia, syncope, and arthritis. Some of these reactions can be minimized by decreasing the dose or rate of infusion. Sodium ferric gluconate and iron sucrose have better safety records than iron dextran.
- Subcutaneous (SC) administration of **epoetin alfa** is preferred because IV access is not required, and the SC dose that maintains target indices is 15% to 30% lower than the IV dose (**Fig. 77-6**).
- **Darbepoetin alfa** has a longer half-life than epoetin alfa and prolonged biologic activity. Doses are administered less frequently, starting at once a week when administered IV or SC.
- ESAs are well tolerated. Hypertension is the most common adverse event.

Evaluation of Therapeutic Outcomes

- Iron indices (transferrin saturation [TSat]; ferritin) should be evaluated before initiating an ESA (see **Fig. 77-5**). Iron status should be reassessed every month during initial ESA treatment and every 3 months for those on a stable ESA regimen.
- Hemoglobin should be monitored at least monthly, although more frequent monitoring (e.g., every 1–2 wk) is warranted after initiation of an ESA or after a dose change until hemoglobin is stable.
- Patients should be monitored for potential complications, such as hypertension, which should be treated before starting an ESA.
- For more information on anemia, see Chap. 33.

CHRONIC KIDNEY DISEASE–MINERAL AND BONE DISORDER AND RENAL OSTEODYSTROPHY

- Disorders of mineral and bone metabolism are common in the CKD population and include abnormalities in parathyroid hormone (PTH), calcium, phosphorus, the calcium–phosphorus product, vitamin D, and bone turnover, as well as soft tissue calcifications. Historically, these abnormalities have been described as classic characteristics of secondary hyperparathyroidism and renal osteodystrophy. The term CKD–mineral and bone disorder (CKD-MBD) has been advocated to encompass these abnormalities.

Pathophysiology and Clinical Presentation

- Calcium-phosphorus balance is mediated through a complex interplay of hormones and their effects on bone, the GI tract, kidneys, and the parathyroid gland. As kidney disease progresses, renal activation of vitamin D is impaired, which reduces gut absorption of calcium. Low blood calcium concentration stimulates secretion of PTH. As renal function declines,

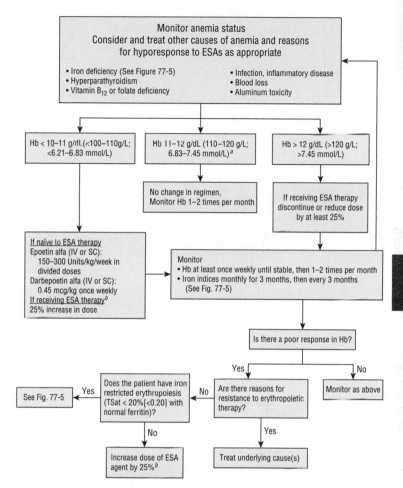

FIGURE 77-6. Algorithm for erythropoiesis-stimulating agent (ESA) therapy in the management of the anemia of CKD. (Hb, hemoglobin; SC, subcutaneous; TSat, transferrin saturation.)

serum calcium balance can be maintained only at the expense of increased bone resorption, ultimately resulting in renal osteodystrophy (ROD) (**Fig. 77-7**).

- Secondary hyperparathyroidism is associated with increased morbidity and mortality and sudden death in hemodialysis patients.
- ROD progresses insidiously for several years before the onset of symptoms such as bone pain and fractures. Skeletal complications include osteitis fibrosa cystica (high bone turnover), osteomalacia (low bone

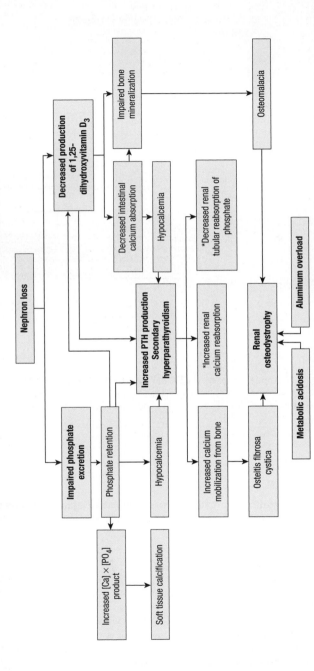

FIGURE 77–7. Pathogenesis of CKD–mineral and bone disorder (MBD) and renal osteodystrophy. *These adaptations are lost as renal failure progresses. (FGF-23, fibroblast growth factor-23.)

TABLE 77–2	Guidelines for Calcium, Phosphorus, Calcium–Phosphorus Product, and Intact Parathyroid Hormone		
	Chronic Kidney Disease		
Parameter	*Stage 3*	*Stage 4*	*Stage 5*
Corrected calcium	"Normal"	"Normal"	8.4–9.5 mg/dL[a] (2.10–2.38 mmol/L)
Phosphorus	2.7–4.6 mg/dL (0.87–1.49 mmol/L)	2.7–4.6 mg/dL (0.87–1.49 mmol/L)	3.5–5.5 mg/dL (1.13–1.78 mmol/L)
Ca × P	<55 mg^2/dL^2 [4.4 mmol^2/L^2]	<55 mg^2/dL^2 [4.4 mmol^2/L^2]	<55 mg^2/dL^2 [4.4 mmol^2/L^2]
Intact parathyroid hormone	35–70 pg/mL (35–70 ng/L)	70–110 pg/mL (70–110 ng/L)	150–300 pg/mL (150–300 mg/L)

[a]Recommend normal range for laboratory used, but keeping target at lower end of range.

From KFIGO clinical practice guideline for the diagnosis, evaluation, prevention, and treatment of chronic kidney disease-mineral and bone disorder (CKD-MBD). Kidney Int 2009;113(Supp):S1–130; and Eknoyan G, Levin A, Levin NW. Bone metabolism and disease in chronic kidney disease. Am J Kidney Dis 2003;42 (4 Suppl 3):1–201.

turnover) and adynamic bone disease. Prevention of ROD is key to minimizing long-term complications because once symptoms appear, the disease is not easily amenable to treatment.

Treatment

- Preventive measures should be initiated in patients in early stages of CKD to improve outcomes by the time they reach stage 5 CKD, or ESRD.
- The K/DOQI guidelines provide desired ranges of calcium, phosphorus, calcium-phosphorus product, and intact PTH based on the stage of CKD (Table 77–2). Measurements should be repeated every 12 months for stage 3, every 3 months for stage 4, and more frequently for stage 5.
- Dietary phosphorus restriction (800–1,000 mg/day) should be first-line intervention for stage 3 or higher CKD when the upper levels of serum phosphorus are reached.
- By the time ESRD develops, most patients require a combination of dietary intervention, phosphate-binding agents, vitamin D, and calcimimetic therapy to achieve K/DOQI goals.

PHOSPHATE-BINDING AGENTS

- Phosphate-binding agents decrease phosphorus absorption from the gut and are first-line agents for controlling both serum phosphorus and calcium concentrations (Table 77–3).
- K/DOQI guidelines recommend that elemental calcium from calcium-containing binders should not exceed 1,500 mg/day, and the total daily intake from all sources should not exceed 2,000 mg. This may necessitate a combination of calcium- and noncalcium-containing products (e.g., **sevelamer HCL** and **lanthanum carbonate**).

TABLE 77–3 Phosphate-binding Agents Used for the Treatment of Hyperphosphatemia in Patients with Chronic Kidney Disease

Compound	Trade Name	Compound Content (mg)	Dose Titration[a]	Starting Doses	Comments
Calcium carbonate[b] (40% elemental calcium)	Tums	500, 750, 1,000, 1,250	Increase or decrease by 500 mg per meal (200 mg elemental calcium)	0.5–1 g (elemental calcium) three times daily with meals	First-line agent; dissolution characteristics and phosphate binding may vary from product to product
	Oscal-500 Caltrate 600	1,250 1,500			Approximately 39 mg phosphorus bound per 1 g calcium carbonate
Calcium acetate (25% elemental calcium)	PhosLo	667	Increase or decrease by 667 mg per meal (168 mg elemental calcium)	0.5–1 g (elemental calcium) three times daily with meals	First-line agent; comparable efficacy to calcium carbonate with half the dose of elemental calcium
					Approximately 45 mg phosphorus bound per 1 g calcium acetate
					By prescription only
Sevelamer carbonate (available as tablet and powder for oral suspension)	Renvela	800	Increase or decrease by 800 mg per meal	800–1,600 mg three times daily with meals	First-line agent; lowers LDL cholesterol
					More expensive than calcium products; consider in patients at risk for extraskeletal calcification
					Associated with a lower risk of acidosis and GI adverse events than Renagel

Sevelamer hydrochloride	Renagel	400, 800	Increase or decrease by 800 mg per meal	Same as Renvela	Same as Renvela, plus acidosis
Lanthanum carbonate	Fosrenol	500, 750, 1,000	Increase or decrease by 750 mg/day	750–1,500 mg daily in divided doses with meals	First-line agent; available as chewable tablets
Aluminum hydroxide[b]	Alterna GEL	600 mg/5 mL	—	300–600 mg three times daily with meals	Not a first-line agent; do not use concurrently with citrate-containing products Reserve for short-term use (4 wk) in patients with hyperphosphatemia not responding to other binders

LDL, low-density lipoprotein.

[a]Based on phosphorus levels, titrate every 2 to 3 weeks until phosphorus goal is reached.

[b]Multiple preparations available that are not listed.

- Adverse effects of all phosphate binders are generally limited to GI effects, including constipation, diarrhea, nausea, vomiting, and abdominal pain. The risk of hypercalcemia may necessitate restriction of calcium-containing binder use and/or reduction in dietary intake. Aluminum binders have been associated with CNS toxicity and the worsening of anemia, whereas magnesium binder use may lead to hypermagnesemia and hyperkalemia.

VITAMIN D THERAPY

- Reasonable control of calcium and phosphorus must be achieved before initiation and during continued vitamin D therapy.
- **Calcitriol,** 1,25-dihydroxyvitamin D_3, directly suppresses PTH synthesis and secretion and upregulates vitamin D receptors, which ultimately may reduce parathyroid hyperplasia. The dose depends on the stage of CKD (**Table 77–4**).
- The newer vitamin D analogues **paricalcitol** and **doxercalciferol** may be associated with less hypercalcemia and, for paricalcitol, hyperphosphatemia. Vitamin D therapy, regardless of agent, is associated with decreased mortality.

CALCIMIMETICS

- **Cinacalcet** reduces PTH secretion by increasing the sensitivity of the calcium-sensing receptor. The most common adverse events are nausea and vomiting.
- The most effective way to use cinacalcet with other therapies has not been decided. The starting dose is 30 mg daily, which can be titrated to the desired PTH and calcium concentrations every 2 to 4 weeks and to a maximum of 180 mg daily.

METABOLIC ACIDOSIS

- A clinically significant metabolic acidosis is commonly seen when the GFR drops below 30 mL/min/1.73 m^2 (0.29 mL/s/m^2) (stage 4 CKD). The goals of therapy in CKD are to normalize the blood pH (7.35–7.45) and serum bicarbonate (22–26 mEq/L; 22–26 mmol/L).
- Consequences of metabolic acidosis include renal bone disease, reduced cardiac contractility, predisposition to arrhythmias, and protein catabolism.
- Oral alkalinizing salts (e.g., **sodium bicarbonate, Shohl solution,** and **Bicitra**) can be used in patients with stage 4 or 5 CKD. **Polycitra,** which contains potassium citrate, should not be used in patients with severe CKD because hyperkalemia may result.
- The replacement alkali dose can be approximated by multiplying bicarbonate's volume of distribution (0.5 L/kg) by the patient's weight (in kg) and by their deficit (24 mEq/L [24 mmol/L] minus the patient's serum bicarbonate value). The dose should be administered over several days. The daily maintenance dose is usually 12 to 20 mEq/mL (12–20 mmol/day) and should be titrated as needed.

TABLE 77–4 Available Vitamin D Agents

Generic Name	Trade Name	Form of Vitamin D	Dosage Range	Dosage Forms	Frequency of Administration
Vitamin D precursor					
Ergocalciferol[a]	Vitamin D₂	D₂	400–50,000 IU	PO	Daily (doses of 400–2000 IU)
Cholecalciferol[a]	Vitamin D₃	D₃			Weekly or monthly for higher doses (50,000 IU)
Active vitamin D					
Calcitriol	Calcijex		0.5–5 mcg	IV	Three times per week
	Rocaltrol		0.25–5 mcg	PO	Daily, every other day, or three times per week
Vitamin D analogs					
Paricalcitol	Zemplar		1–4 mcg	PO	Daily or three times per week
			2.5–15 mcg	IV	Three times per week
Doxercalciferol	Hectorol		5–20 mcg	PO	Daily or three times per week
			2–8 mcg	IV	Three times per week

[a]Multiple preparations are available that are not listed.

973

- Metabolic acidosis in patients undergoing dialysis can often be managed by using higher concentrations of bicarbonate or acetate in the dialysate.
- For more information on acid-base disorders, see Chap. 75.

HYPERTENSION

- The pathogenesis of hypertension in patients with CKD is multifactorial and includes fluid retention, increased sympathetic activity, decreased activity of vasodilators such as nitric oxide, elevated levels of endothelin-1, chronic erythropoietin use, hyperparathyroidism, and structural arterial changes.
- In early-stage CKD, the target BP for cardiovascular risk reduction is <130/80 mm Hg. The K/DOQI guidelines propose a predialysis BP <140/90 mm Hg and a postdialysis BP <130/80 mm Hg.
- Salt (2 g/day) and fluid intake should be restricted.
- Most patients with ESRD require three or more antihypertensive agents to achieve target BP. As with less advanced CKD (see Fig. 77–4), ACEIs, ARBs, and dihydropyridine calcium channel blockers are the preferred agents.
- BP should be monitored at each visit, and at home when feasible.
- For more information on hypertension, see Chap. 10.

HYPERLIPIDEMIA

- The prevalence of hyperlipidemia increases as renal function declines.
- Hyperlipidemia should be managed aggressively in patients with ESRD to a low-density lipoprotein cholesterol goal <100 mg/dL (2.59 mmol/L). **Statins** are the drugs of first choice. Although well tolerated by otherwise healthy patients, statins have the potential to cause myotoxic effects when administered in patients with hepatic disease or with interacting drugs such as azole antibiotics, cyclosporine, gemfibrozil, and niacin.
- In patients with ESRD, lipid profile should be reassessed at least annually and 2 to 3 months after changing treatment.
- For more information on dyslipidemias, see Table 77–1 and Chap. 8.

OTHER SECONDARY COMPLICATIONS

Nutritional Status

- Protein-energy malnutrition is common in patients with stage 4 or 5 CKD. Food intake is often inadequate because of anorexia, altered taste sensation, intercurrent illness, and unpalatability of prescribed diets.
- Daily protein intake should be 1.2 g/kg for patients undergoing hemodialysis and 1.2 to 1.3 g/kg for those undergoing peritoneal dialysis.
- Daily energy intake should be 35 kcal/kg (147 kJ/kg) for patients undergoing any type of dialysis. The intake should be lowered to 30 to 35 kcal/kg (126–147 kJ/kg) for patients older than 60 years.
- Vitamins A and E are elevated in ESRD, whereas water-soluble vitamins should be supplemented to replace dialysis-induced loss.
- For more information on nutrition requirements, see Chap. 58.

Uremic Bleeding

- The pathophysiology of uremic bleeding is multifactorial. The primary mechanisms are platelet biochemical abnormalities and alterations in platelet–vessel wall interactions.

See Chapter 52, Chronic Kidney Disease: Progression-Modifying Therapies, authored by Vimal K. Derebail, Abhijit V. Kshirsagar, and Melanie S. Joy, and Chapter 53, Chronic Kidney Disease: Management of Complications, authored by Joanna Q. Hudson, for a more detailed discussion of this topic.

Drug Therapy Individualization for Patients with Chronic Kidney Disease

GENERAL PRINCIPLES

- The pathophysiology, clinical manifestations, diagnosis, and treatment of acute renal failure and chronic kidney disease (CKD), or end-stage renal disease (ESRD), are discussed in Chaps. 76 and 77, respectively.
- Drug therapy individualization for patients with renal insufficiency sometimes requires only a simple proportional dose adjustment based on creatinine clearance (CL_{cr}) or the glomerular filtration rate (GFR). Alternatively, complex adjustments are required for drugs that are extensively metabolized or undergo dramatic changes in protein binding and distribution volume.
- Patients may respond differently to a given drug because of the physiologic and biochemical changes associated with CKD.

EFFECT ON DRUG ABSORPTION

- There is little quantitative information regarding the influence of impaired renal function on drug absorption and bioavailability.
- Factors that theoretically affect bioavailability include alterations in GI transit time, gastric pH, edema of the GI tract, vomiting and diarrhea, and concomitant drug therapy, especially antacid or H_2-antagonist administration.

EFFECT ON DRUG DISTRIBUTION

- The volume of distribution of many drugs is significantly increased or decreased in patients with CKD. Changes result from altered protein or tissue binding, or pathophysiologic alterations in body composition (e.g., fluid overload).
- Generally, plasma protein binding of acidic drugs (e.g., **warfarin** and **phenytoin**) is decreased in ESRD, whereas binding of basic drugs (e.g., **quinidine** and **lidocaine**) is usually normal or slightly decreased or increased.
- Ideally, unbound (vs total) drug concentrations should be monitored, especially for drugs that have a narrow therapeutic range, are highly protein bound (free fraction <20%), and have marked variability in the free fraction (e.g., **phenytoin** and **disopyramide**).
- Methods for calculating volume of distribution (V_D) can be influenced by renal disease. Of the commonly used terms (i.e., volumes of central compartment, terminal phase, and distribution at steady state [V_{SS}]), V_{SS} is the most appropriate for comparing patients with renal insufficiency to those with normal renal function because V_{SS} is independent of drug elimination.

EFFECT ON METABOLISM

- CKD may alter nonrenal clearance of drugs as the result of changes in cytochrome P450 (CYP)-mediated metabolism in the liver, predominantly drugs metabolized by CYP3A4, and other organs (Table 78–1). The

TABLE 78–1	Nonrenal Clearance of Many Drugs is Reduced in Patients with End-Stage Renal Disease	
Acyclovir	Didanosine	Nitrendipine
Aztreonam	Encainide	Nortriptyline
Bufuralol	Erythromycin	Procainamide
Bupropion	Guanadrel	Quinapril
Captopril	Imipenem	Reboxetine
Carvedilol	Isoniazid	Raloxifene
Cefipime	Ketoprofen	Repaglinide
Cefmetazole	Ketorolac	Rosuvastatin
Cefonicid	Lomefloxacin	Roxithromycin
Cefotaxime	Losartan	Simvastatin
Ceftriaxone	Lovastatin	Telithromycin
Ceftizoxime	Metoclopramide	Valsartan
Cervistatin	Minoxidil	Vancomycin
Cilastatin	Morphine	Verapamil
Cimetidine	Nicardipine	Zidovudine
Ciprofloxacin	Nimodipine	

degree of reduction in nonrenal clearance appears to be greater in patients with ESRD as compared with acute kidney injury (AKI).

- Patients with severe renal insufficiency can experience accumulation of metabolite(s), which can contribute to pharmacologic activity or toxicity.

EFFECT ON RENAL EXCRETION

- Altered renal filtration, secretion, and/or absorption can have dramatic effects on drug disposition. The impact depends on the fraction of drug normally eliminated unchanged by the kidneys and on the degree of renal insufficiency.
- Quantitative investigation of renal handling of drugs is needed to elucidate the relative contribution of tubular function to renal drug clearance. In the absence of clinically useful techniques to quantitate tubular function, clinical measurement or estimation of CL_{cr} or GFR remains the guiding factor for calculating drug dosage regimen design.

DRUG DOSAGE REGIMEN DESIGN FOR PATIENTS WITH CHRONIC KIDNEY DISEASE

- The optimal dosage regimen for patients with renal insufficiency requires an individualized assessment (Table 78–2). The optimal regimen depends on an accurate characterization of the relationship between the drug's pharmacokinetic parameters and renal function and on an accurate assessment of the patient's renal function (CL_{cr}).

TABLE 78–2	Stepwise Approach to Adjust Drug Dosage Regimens for Patients with Renal Insufficiency	
Step 1	Obtain history and relevant demographic/clinical information	Record demographic information, obtain past medical history, including history of renal disease, and record current laboratory information (e.g., serum creatinine)
Step 2	Estimate creatinine clearance	Use Cockcroft–Gault equation to estimate creatinine clearance, or calculate creatinine clearance from timed urine collection
Step 3	Review current medications	Identify drugs for which individualization of the treatment regimen will be necessary
Step 4	Calculate individualized treatment regimen	Determine treatment goals; calculate dosage regimen based on pharmacokinetic characteristics of the drug and the patient's renal function
Step 5	Monitor	Monitor parameters of drug response and toxicity; monitor drug levels if available/applicable
Step 6	Revise regimen	Adjust regimen based on drug response or change in patient status (including renal function) as warranted

- If the relationship between CL_{cr} and the kinetic parameters of a drug (i.e., total body clearance [CL] and elimination rate constant [k]) is known, these data should be used to individualize drug therapy (**Table 78–3**).
- If the relationship between CL_{cr} and the kinetic parameters is unknown, then the patient's kinetic parameters can be based on the fraction of drug eliminated renally unchanged (f_e) in subjects with normal renal function.
- This approach assumes that f_e is known, the change in CL and k are proportional to CL_{cr}, renal disease does not alter drug metabolism, any metabolites are inactive and nontoxic, the drug obeys first-order (linear) kinetic principles, and the drug is adequately described by a one-compartment model. The kinetic parameter/dosage adjustment factor (Q) can be calculated as

$$Q = 1 - [f_e(1 - KF)],$$

where KF is the ratio of the patient's CL_{cr} to the assumed normal value of 120 mL/min (equivalent to 2 mL/s). The estimated total body clearance of the patient (CL_{PT}) can then be calculated as:

$$CL_{PT} = CL_{norm} \times Q,$$

where CL_{norm} is the mean total body clearance in patients with normal renal function.
- The best method for adjusting the dosage regimen depends on whether the goal is maintaining a similar peak, trough, or average steady-state drug concentration. The principal choices are to decrease the dose, prolong the dosing interval, or both.

TABLE 78–3	Relationship Between Creatinine Clearance and Total Body Clearance and Terminal Elimination Rate Constant of Selected Drugs	
Drug	**Elimination Rate Constant**	**Total Body Clearance**[a]
Acyclovir		$CL = 3.37 (CL_{cr}) + 0.41$
Amikacin	$k = (0.0024 \times CL_{cr}) + 0.01$	$CL = 0.6 (CL_{cr}) + 9.6$
Aztreonam		$CL = 0.8 (CL_{cr}) + 26.6$
Cefazolin	$k = (0.0028 \times CL_{cr}) + 0.022$	$CL = 0.34 (CL_{cr}) + 6.6$
Ceftazidime	$k = (0.004 \times CL_{cr}) + 0.004$	$CL = 1.15 (CL_{cr}) + 10.6$
Ciprofloxacin		$CL = 2.83 (CL_{cr}) + 363$
Digoxin		$CL = 0.88 (CL_{cr}) + 23$
Gentamicin	$k = (0.0029 \times CL_{cr}) + 0.015$	$CL = 0.983 (Cl_{cr})$
Imipenem		$CL = 1.42 (CL_{cr}) + 54$
Lithium		$CL = 0.20 (CL_{cr})$
Ofloxacin		$CL = 1.04 (CL_{cr}) + 38.7$
Piperacillin	$k = (0.0049 \times CL_{cr}) + 0.21$	$CL = 1.36 (CL_{cr}) + 1.50$
Tobramycin	$k = (0.0029 \times CL_{cr}) + 0.01$	$CL = 0.801 (CL_{cr})$
Vancomycin	$k = (0.00083 \times CL_{cr}) + 0.0044$	$CL = 0.69 (CL_{cr}) + 3.7$

CL, total body clearance; CL_{cr}, creatinine clearance; k, elimination rate constant.
[a]Clearance in mL/min can be converted to mL/s through multiplication by 0.0167.

- Drug disposition parameters can be estimated if the relationship between the pharmacokinetic parameters of the drug and renal function are known.
- The ratio (Q) of the estimated elimination rate constant or total body clearance relative to normal renal function is used to determine the dose or dosing interval alterations needed (CL_{fail} is the clearance with impaired renal function).

$$Q = CL_{fail}/CL_{norm}$$

- The adjusted dosing interval (τ_f) or maintenance dose (D_f) is calculated from the following relationships, where τ_n is the normal dosing interval and D_n is the normal dose:

$$\tau_f = \tau_n/Q$$

$$D_f = D_n \times Q$$

- If V_D is significantly altered or a specific concentration is desired, estimation of a dosage regimen becomes more complex. The dosing interval (τ_f) is calculated as

$$\tau_f = \{(-1/k_f)[\ln (C_{min}/C_{max})]\} + t_{peak},$$

where C_{min} and C_{max} are minimum and maximum concentrations, respectively, and t_{peak} is time of peak concentration. The oral dose is calculated as

$$D = [FC^t_P V_D(k_a - k)]/\{k_a [e^{-kt}/(1 - e^{-kt})][e^{-k_a t}/(1 - e^{k_a t})]\},$$

where F equals the bioavailability, C_p^t equals the desired plasma concentration at time t, and k_a is the absorption rate constant. If the drug is absorbed extremely rapidly, τ_f is calculated as

$$\tau_f = (-1/k_f)[\ln (C_{min}/C_{max})]$$

and oral dose as

$$D = V_D \times (C_{max} - C_{min})$$

PATIENTS RECEIVING CONTINUOUS RENAL REPLACEMENT THERAPY

- Continuous renal replacement therapy (CRRT) is used for the management of fluid overload and removal of uremic toxins in patients with acute renal failure and other conditions. Drug therapy individualization for patients receiving CRRT is discussed in Chap. 76.

PATIENTS RECEIVING CHRONIC PERITONEAL DIALYSIS

- Peritoneal dialysis has the potential to affect drug disposition; however, drug therapy individualization is often less complicated because of the limited drug clearance achieved with this procedure.
- Factors that influence drug dialyzability by peritoneal dialysis include drug-specific characteristics (e.g., molecular weight, solubility, degree of ionization, protein binding, and V_D) and intrinsic properties of the peritoneal membrane (e.g., blood flow, pore size, and peritoneal membrane surface area).
- An inverse relationship exists between peritoneal drug clearance and molecular weight, protein binding, and V_D.
- In general, peritoneal dialysis is less effective in removing drugs than hemodialysis.

PATIENTS RECEIVING CHRONIC HEMODIALYSIS

- The impact of hemodialysis on drug therapy depends on drug characteristics (e.g., molecular weight, protein binding, and V_D), dialysis prescription (e.g., dialysis membrane composition, filter surface area, blood and dialysate flow rates, and reuse of the dialysis filter), and clinical indication for dialysis.
- High-flux dialysis allows free passage of most solutes with molecular weights up to 20,000. Therefore, high-flux dialysis is more likely to remove high-molecular-weight drugs (e.g., **vancomycin**) and drugs with low- to mid-molecular weights (i.e., 100–1,000) than conventional dialysis (**Table 78–4**).
- The dialysate recovery clearance approach has become the benchmark for determining dialyzer clearance. It can be calculated as

$$CL_D^r = R/AUC_{0-t}$$

where R is the total amount of drug recovered unchanged in dialysate and AUC_{0-t} is the area under the predialyzer plasma concentration–time curve

TABLE 78–4	**Drug Disposition during Dialysis Depends on Dialyzer Characteristics**			
	Hemodialysis Clearance (mL/min)[a]		**Half-Life during Dialysis (hours)**	
Drug	**Conventional**	**High Flux**	**Conventional**	**High Flux**
Cefazolin	15.1	30–38	NR	NR
Ceftazidime	60	155[b]	3.3	1.2[b]
Cefuroxime	NR	103[c]	3.8	1.6[c]
Foscarnet	183	253[c]	NR	NR
Gentamicin	58.2	116[c]	3	4.3[c]
Netilmicin	46	87–109	5–5.2	2.9–3.4
Ranitidine	43.1	67.2[c]	5.1	2.9[c]
Vancomycin	9–21	40–150[c]	35–38	4.5–11.8[c]
		72–116[d]		NR

NR, not reported.
[a]Clearance in mL/min can be converted to mL/s through multiplication by 0.0167.
[b]Polyamide filter.
[c]Polysulfone filter.
[d]Polymethylmethacrylate.
Data from Matzke GR. Status of hemodialysis of drugs in 2002. J Pharm Pract 2002;15:405–418.

during the time when the dialysate was collected. To determine AUC_{0-t}, at least two and preferably three or four plasma concentrations should be obtained during dialysis.

- Total clearance during dialysis can be calculated as the sum of the patient's residual renal and nonrenal clearance during the interdialytic period (CL_{RES}) and dialyzer clearance (CL_D):

$$CL_T = CL_{RES} + CL_D$$

- Half-life between hemodialysis (HD) treatments and during dialysis can then be calculated from the following relationships using a published estimate of the drug's V_D:

$$t_{1/2,\,offHD} = 0.693[V_D/CL_{RES}]$$

and

$$t_{1/2,\,onHD} = 0.693[V_D/CL_{RES} + CL_D)]$$

- Once key pharmacokinetic parameters are estimated (based on population data) or calculated, they can be used to simulate the plasma concentration–time profile of the drug for the patient and to ascertain how much drug to administer and when.

- Plasma concentrations of the drug over the interdialytic interval of 24 to 48 hours can be predicted. The concentration at the end of a 30-minute infusion (C_{max}) would be

$$C_{max} = [(D/t')(1 - e^{-kt'})]/CL_{RES}$$

- Plasma concentration before the next dialysis session (C_{bD}) can be calculated as

$$C_{bD} = C_{max} \times e^{-(CL_{RES}/V_D)} \times t$$

- Hemodialysis clearance of most drugs is dialysis-filter dependent, and a value can be extrapolated from the literature. The concentration after dialysis can be calculated as

$$C_{aD} = C_{bD} \times e^{-[(CL_{RES} + CL_D)/V_D] \times t}$$

- Postdialysis dose can be calculated as follows if the elimination half-life is prolonged relative to the infusion time and thus minimal drug is eliminated during the infusion period:

$$D = V_D \times (C_{max} - C_{min})$$

See Chapter 57, Drug Therapy Individualization for Patients with Chronic Kidney Disease, authored by Gary R. Matzke, for a more detailed discussion of this topic.

CHAPTER 79

Electrolyte Homeostasis

DEFINITION

- Fluid and electrolyte homeostasis is maintained by feedback mechanisms, hormones, and many organ systems and is necessary for the body's normal physiologic functions. Disorders of sodium and water, calcium, phosphorus, potassium, and magnesium homeostasis are addressed separately in this chapter.

DISORDERS OF SODIUM AND WATER HOMEOSTASIS

- Sixty percent of total body water is distributed intracellularly, and 40% is contained in the extracellular space.
- Addition of an isotonic solution to the extracellular fluid (ECF) does not change intracellular volume. Adding a hypertonic solution to the ECF decreases cell volume, whereas adding a hypotonic solution increases it (**Table 79–1**).
- Hypernatremia and hyponatremia can be associated with conditions of high, low, or normal ECF sodium and volume. Both conditions are most commonly the result of abnormalities of water metabolism.

HYPONATREMIA (SERUM SODIUM <135 mEq/L [<135 mmol/L])

Pathophysiology

- Hyponatremia predominantly results from an excess of extracellular water relative to sodium because of impaired water excretion.
- Causes of nonosmotic release of arginine vasopressin (AVP), commonly known as *antidiuretic hormone,* include hypovolemia; decreased effective circulating volume as seen in patients with congestive heart failure (CHF); nephrosis; cirrhosis; and syndrome of inappropriate antidiuretic hormone (SIADH).
- Depending on serum osmolality, hyponatremia is classified as isotonic, hypertonic, or hypotonic (**Fig. 79–1**).
- Hypotonic hyponatremia, the most common form of hyponatremia, can be further classified as hypovolemic, euvolemic, or hypervolemic.
- Hypovolemic hypotonic hyponatremia is associated with a loss of ECF volume and sodium, with the loss of more sodium than water. It is relatively common in patients taking **thiazide diuretics.**
- Euvolemic hyponatremia is associated with a normal or slightly decreased ECF sodium content and increased total body water and ECF volume. It is most commonly the result of SIADH release.
- Hypervolemic hyponatremia is associated with an increase in ECF volume in conditions with impaired renal sodium and water excretion, such as cirrhosis, CHF, and nephrotic syndrome.

TABLE 79-1 Composition of Intravenous Replacement Solutions

Solution	Dextrose	[Na⁺] (mEq/L or mmol/L)	[Cl⁻] (mEq/L or mmol/L)	Tonicity	Distribution		Free Water/L
					% ECF	% ICF	
D₅W	5 g/dL (50 g/L)	0	0	Hypotonic	40	60	1,000 mL
0.45% sodium chloride	0	77	77	Hypotonic	73	37	500 mL
0.9% sodium chloride	0	154	154	Isotonic	100	0	0 mL
3% sodium chloride[a]	0	513	513	Hypertonic	100	0	−2,331 mL

Cl⁻, chloride; D₅W, 5% dextrose in water; ECF, extracellular fluid; ICF, intracellular fluid; Na⁺, sodium.
[a]This solution will result in osmotic removal of water from the intracellular space.

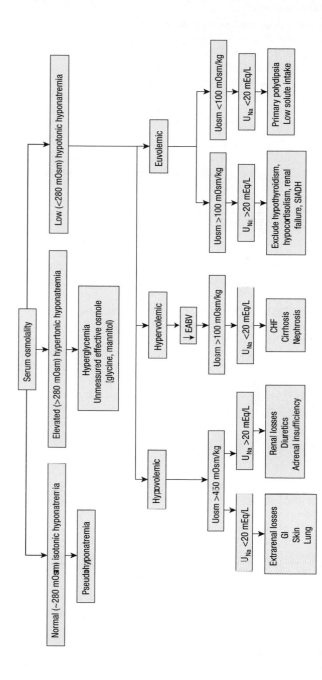

FIGURE 79–1. Diagnostic algorithm for the evaluation of hyponatremia. (CHF, congestive heart failure; EABV, effective arterial blood volume; SIADH, syndrome of inappropriate antidiuretic hormone; U_{Na}, urine sodium concentration [values in mEq/L are numerically equivalent to mmol/L]; Uosm, urine osmolality [values in mOsm/kg are numerically equivalent to mmol/kg].)

Clinical Presentation

- Most patients with hyponatremia are asymptomatic.
- The presence and severity of symptoms are related to the magnitude and rapidity of onset of hyponatremia. Symptoms progress from nausea and malaise to headache and lethargy and, eventually, to seizures, coma, and death if hyponatremia is severe or develops rapidly.
- Patients with hypovolemic hyponatremia present with decreased skin turgor, orthostatic hypotension, tachycardia, and dry mucous membranes.

Treatment

- Treatment of hyponatremia is associated with a risk of osmotic demyelination syndrome. The rate of administration of infusate should be adjusted to avoid exceeding a rise in serum sodium >12 mEq/L (12 mmol/L) per day.

ACUTE OR SEVERELY SYMPTOMATIC HYPOTONIC HYPONATREMIA

- Symptomatic patients, regardless of fluid status, should initially be treated with either a 0.9% or 3% concentrated saline solution until symptoms resolve. Resolution of severe symptoms may require only a 5% increase in serum sodium or an initial target serum sodium of 120 mEq/L (120 mmol/L).
- Patients with SIADH should be treated with 3% saline plus, if the urine osmolality exceeds 300 mOsm/kg (300 mmol/kg), a loop diuretic (**furosemide,** 40 mg IV every 6 hour).
- Patients with hypovolemic hypotonic hyponatremia should be treated with 0.9% saline, initially at infusion rates of 200 to 400 mL/hour until symptoms moderate.
- Patients with hypervolemic hypotonic hyponatremia should be treated with 3% saline and prompt initiation of fluid restriction. Loop diuretic therapy will also likely be required to facilitate urinary excretion of free water.

NONEMERGENT HYPOTONIC HYPONATREMIA

- Treatment of SIADH involves water restriction and correction of the underlying cause. Water should be restricted to ~1,000 to 1,200 mL/day. In some cases, administration of either sodium chloride or urea tablets and a loop diuretic or of **demeclocycline** can be required.
- AVP antagonists or "vaptans" (e.g., **conivaptan** and **tolvaptan**) can be used to treat SIADH as well as other causes of euvolemic and hypervolemic hypotonic hyponatremia that has been nonresponsive to other therapeutic interventions in patients with heart failure, cirrhosis, and SIADH. The vaptans have dramatic effects on water excretion and represent a breakthrough in the therapy of hyponatremia and disorders of fluid homeostasis.
- Treatment of asymptomatic hypervolemic hypotonic hyponatremia involves correction of the underlying cause and restriction of water intake to <1,000 to 1,200 mL/day. Dietary intake of sodium chloride should be restricted to 1,000 to 2,000 mg/day.

HYPERNATREMIA (SERUM SODIUM >145 mEq/L [>145 mmol/L])

Pathophysiology and Clinical Presentation

- Hypernatremia can result from either water loss (e.g., diabetes insipidus [DI]) or hypotonic fluids, or less commonly from hypertonic fluid administration or sodium ingestion.
- Symptoms of hypernatremia are primarily caused by decreased neuronal cell volume and can include weakness, restlessness, irritability, and confusion. Symptoms of a more rapidly developing hypernatremia include twitching, seizures, coma, and death.

Treatment

- Treatment of hypovolemic hypernatremia should begin with 0.9% saline. After hemodynamic stability is restored and intravascular volume is replaced, free-water deficit can be replaced with 5% dextrose or 0.45% saline solution.
- The correction rate should be ~1 mEq/L (1 mmol/L) per hour for hypernatremia that developed over a few hours and 0.5 mEq/L (0.5 mmol/L) per hour for hypernatremia that developed more slowly.
- Patients with central DI are usually treated with intranasal **desmopressin,** beginning with 10 mcg/day and titrating as needed, usually to 10 mcg twice daily.
- Patients with nephrogenic DI should decrease their ECF volume with a thiazide diuretic and dietary sodium restriction (2,000 mg/day), which often decreases urine volume by as much as 50%. Other treatment options include drugs with antidiuretic properties (Table 79–2).
- Patients with sodium overload should be treated with loop diuretics (**furosemide,** 20–40 mg IV every 6 hour) and 5% dextrose at a rate that decreases serum sodium by ~0.5 mEq/L (0.5 mmol/L per hour or, if hypernatremia developed rapidly, 1 mEq/L (1 mmol/L) per hour.

TABLE 79–2	Drugs Used to Manage Central and Nephrogenic Diabetes Insipidus	
Drug	**Indication**	**Dose**
Desmopressin acetate	Central and nephrogenic	5–20 mcg intranasally every 12 to 24 hours
Chlorpropamide	Central	125–250 mg orally daily
Carbamazepine	Central	100–300 mg orally twice daily
Clofibrate	Central	500 mg orally four times daily
Hydrochlorothiazide	Central and nephrogenic	25 mg orally every 12 to 24 hours
Amiloride	Lithium-related nephrogenic	5–10 mg orally daily
Indomethacin	Central and nephrogenic	50 mg orally every 8 to 12 hours

EDEMA

Pathophysiology and Clinical Presentation

- Edema, defined as a clinically detectable increase in interstitial fluid volume, develops when excess sodium is retained either as a primary defect in renal sodium excretion or as a response to a decrease in the effective circulating volume despite an already expanded or normal ECF volume.
- Edema can occur in patients with decreased myocardial contractility, nephrotic syndrome, or cirrhosis.
- Edema is usually first detected in the feet or pretibial area in ambulatory patients and in the presacral area in bed-bound individuals. Edema is defined as "pitting" when the depression caused by briefly exerting pressure over a bony prominence does not rapidly refill.

Treatment

- Diuretics are the primary pharmacologic therapy for edema. Loop diuretics are the most potent, followed by thiazide diuretics and then potassium-sparing diuretics.
- Pulmonary edema requires immediate pharmacologic treatment. Other forms of edema can be treated gradually with, in addition to diuretic therapy, sodium restriction and correction of underlying disease state.

DISORDERS OF CALCIUM HOMEOSTASIS

- ECF calcium is moderately bound to plasma proteins (46%), primarily albumin. Unbound or ionized calcium is the physiologically active form.
- Each 1 g/dL (10 g/L) drop in serum albumin concentration <4 g/dL (40 g/L) decreases total serum calcium concentration by 0.8 mg/dL (0.20 mmol/L).

HYPERCALCEMIA (TOTAL SERUM CALCIUM >10.5 mg/dL [>2.62 mmol/L])

Pathophysiology and Clinical Presentation

- Cancer and hyperparathyroidism are the most common causes of hypercalcemia. The primary mechanisms are increased bone resorption, increased GI absorption, and increased tubular reabsorption by the kidneys.
- Clinical presentation depends on the degree of hypercalcemia and rate of onset. Mild to moderate hypercalcemia (serum calcium concentration <13 mg/dL [<3.25 mmol/L] or ionized calcium concentration <6 mg/dL [<1.50 mmol/L]) can be asymptomatic.
- Hypercalcemia of malignancy develops quickly and is associated with anorexia, nausea and vomiting, constipation, polyuria, polydipsia, and nocturia. Hypercalcemic crisis is characterized by acute elevation of serum calcium to >15 mg/dL (>3.75 mmol/L), acute renal failure, and obtundation. Untreated hypercalcemic crisis can progress to oliguric renal failure, coma, and life-threatening ventricular arrhythmias.

- Chronic hypercalcemia (i.e., hyperparathyroidism) is associated with metastatic calcification, nephrolithiasis, and chronic renal insufficiency.
- Electrocardiogram (ECG) changes include shortening of the QT interval and coving of the ST-T wave.

Treatment

- The approach to hypercalcemia treatment depends on the degree of hypercalcemia, acuity of onset, and presence of symptoms requiring emergent treatment (**Fig. 79–2**).
- Management of patients with asymptomatic, mild to moderate hypercalcemia begins with attention to the underlying condition and correction of fluid and electrolyte abnormalities.
- Hypercalcemic crisis and symptomatic hypercalcemia are medical emergencies requiring immediate treatment. Rehydration with normal saline followed by loop diuretics can be used in patients with normal to moderately impaired renal function. Initiate treatment with **calcitonin** in patients in whom saline hydration is contraindicated (Table 79–3).
- Rehydration with saline and **furosemide** administration can decrease total serum calcium by 2 to 3 mg/dL (0.50–0.75 mmol/L) within 24 to 48 hours.
- Bisphosphonates are indicated for hypercalcemia of malignancy. Total serum calcium decline begins within 2 days and nadirs in 7 days. Duration of normocalcemia varies but usually doesn't exceed 2 to 3 weeks depending on treatment response of underlying malignancy.

HYPOCALCEMIA (TOTAL SERUM CALCIUM <8.5 mg/dL [<2.13 mmol/L])

Pathophysiology

- Hypocalcemia results from altered effects of parathyroid hormone and vitamin D on the bone, gut, and kidney. The primary causes are postoperative hypoparathyroidism and vitamin D deficiency.
- Symptomatic hypocalcemia commonly occurs because of parathyroid gland dysfunction secondary to surgical procedures involving the thyroid, parathyroid, and neck.
- Hypomagnesemia can be associated with severe symptomatic hypocalcemia that is unresponsive to calcium replacement therapy. Calcium normalization is dependent on magnesium replacement.

Clinical Presentation

- Clinical manifestations are variable and depend on the onset of hypocalcemia.
- Tetany is the hallmark sign of acute hypocalcemia, which manifests as paresthesias around the mouth and in the extremities; muscle spasms and cramps; carpopedal spasms; and, rarely, laryngospasm and bronchospasm.
- Cardiovascular manifestations result in ECG changes characterized by a prolonged QT interval and symptoms of decreased myocardial contractility often associated with CHF.

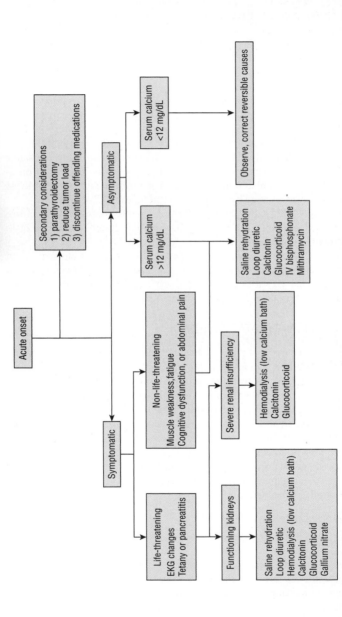

FIGURE 79–2. Pharmacotherapeutic options for the acutely hypercalcemic patient. Serum calcium of 12 mg/dL is equivalent to 3 mmol/L. (EKG, electrocardiogram.)

TABLE 79–3 Drug Therapy Used to Treat Acute Hypercalcemia

Drug	Starting Dosage	Time Frame to Initial Response	Contraindications	Adverse Effects
0.9% saline ± electrolytes	200–300 mL/hour	24–48 hours	Renal insufficiency; congestive heart failure	Electrolyte abnormalities; fluid overload
Loop diuretics	40–80 mg IV every 1 to 4 hours	N/A	Allergy to sulfas (use ethacrynic acid)	Electrolyte abnormalities
Calcitonin	4 units/kg every 12 hours SC/IM; 10–12 units/h IV	1–2 hours	Allergy to calcitonin	Facial flushing, nausea/vomiting, allergic reaction
Pamidronate	30–90 mg IV over 2 to 24 hours	2 days	Renal insufficiency	Fever
Etidronate	7.5 mg/kg per day IV over 2 hours	2 days	Renal insufficiency	Fever
Zoledronate	4–8 mg IV over 15 min	1–2 days	Renal insufficiency	Fever, fatigue, skeletal pain
Ibandronate	2–6 mg IV bolus	2 days	Renal insufficiency	Fever, musculoskeletal pain
Gallium nitrate	200 mg/m² per day	?	Severe renal insufficiency	Nephrotoxicity; hypophosphatemia; nausea/vomiting/diarrhea; metallic taste
Mithramycin	25 mcg/kg IV over 4 to 6 hours	12 hours	Decreased liver function; renal insufficiency; thrombocytopenia	Nausea/vomiting; stomatitis; thrombocytopenia; nephrotoxicity; hepatotoxicity
Glucocorticoids	40–60 mg oral prednisone equivalents daily	3–5 days	Serious infections; hypersensitivity	Diabetes; osteoporosis; infection

N/A, not available; SC, subcutaneous.

Treatment

- Acute, symptomatic hypocalcemia requires IV administration of soluble calcium salts (Fig. 79–3).
- Initially, 100 to 300 mg of elemental calcium (e.g., 1 g **calcium chloride,** 2 to 3 g **calcium gluconate**) should be given IV over 5 to 10 minutes (≤60 mg of elemental calcium per minute).
- The initial bolus dose is effective for only 1 to 2 hours and should be followed by a continuous infusion of elemental calcium (0.5–2 mg/kg/hour) usually for 2 to 4 hours and then by a maintenance dose (0.3–0.5 mg/kg/hour).
- **Calcium gluconate** is preferred over **calcium chloride** for peripheral administration because the latter is more irritating to veins.
- After acute hypocalcemia is corrected, the underlying cause and other electrolyte problems should be corrected.
- Magnesium supplementation is indicated for hypomagnesemia.
- Oral calcium supplementation (e.g., 1–3 g/day of elemental calcium initially, then 2–8 g/day in divided doses) is indicated for chronic hypocalcemia due to hypoparathyroidism and vitamin D deficiency. If serum calcium does not normalize, a vitamin D preparation should be added.

DISORDERS OF PHOSPHORUS HOMEOSTASIS

HYPERPHOSPHATEMIA (SERUM PHOSPHORUS >4.5 mg/dL [>1.45 mmol/L])

Pathophysiology

- The most common cause of hyperphosphatemia is decreased phosphorus excretion, secondary to decreased glomerular filtration rate (GFR).
- Large amounts of phosphorus can be released from intracellular stores in patients who have rhabdomyolysis and in patients who receive chemotherapy for acute leukemia and lymphoma (tumor lysis syndrome).

Clinical Presentation

- Acute symptoms include GI disturbances, lethargy, obstruction of the urinary tract, and, rarely, seizures. Calcium phosphate crystals are likely to form when the product of the serum calcium and phosphate concentrations exceeds 50 to 60 mg^2/dL^2 (4–4.8 $mmol^2/L^2$).
- The major effect of hyperphosphatemia is related to the development of hypocalcemia and damage resulting from calcium phosphate precipitation into soft tissues, intrarenal calcification, nephrolithiasis, or obstructive uropathy.
- For more information on hyperphosphatemia and renal failure, see Chap. 76.

Treatment

- The most effective way to treat nonemergent hyperphosphatemia is to decrease phosphate absorption from the GI tract with phosphate binders (see Chap. 77, Table 77–3).
- Severe symptomatic hyperphosphatemia manifesting as hypocalcemia and tetany is treated by the IV administration of calcium salts.

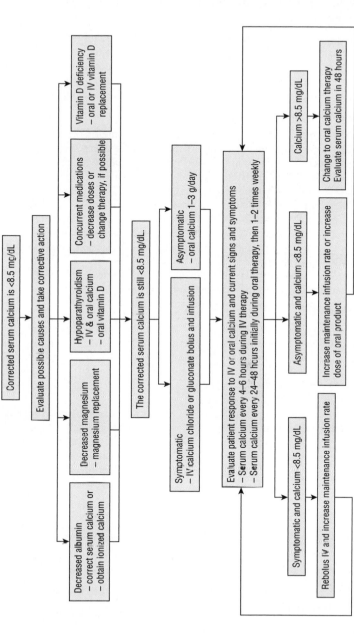

FIGURE 79–3. Hypocalcemia diagnostic and treatment algorithm. Serum calcium of 8.5 mg/dL is equivalent to 2.13 mmol/L.

HYPOPHOSPHATEMIA (SERUM PHOSPHORUS <2 mg/dL [<0.65 mmol/L])

Pathophysiology

- Hypophosphatemia can be the result of decreased GI absorption, reduced tubular reabsorption, or extracellular to intracellular redistribution.
- Hypophosphatemia is associated with chronic alcoholism, parenteral nutrition with inadequate phosphate supplementation, chronic ingestion of antacids, diabetic ketoacidosis, and prolonged hyperventilation.

Clinical Presentation

- Severe hypophosphatemia (serum phosphorus <1 mg/dL [<0.32 mmol/L]) has diverse clinical manifestations that affect many organ systems.
- Neurologic manifestations of severe hypophosphatemia include a progressive syndrome of irritability, apprehension, weakness, numbness, paresthesias, dysarthria, confusion, obtundation, seizures, and coma.
- Skeletal muscle dysfunction can cause myalgia, bone pain, weakness, and potentially fatal rhabdomyolysis. Respiratory muscle weakness and diaphragmatic contractile dysfunction can cause acute respiratory failure.
- Congestive cardiomyopathy, arrhythmias, hemolysis, and increased risk of infection can also occur.
- Chronic hypophosphatemia can cause osteopenia and osteomalacia because of enhanced osteoclastic resorption of bone.

Treatment

- Severe (<1 mg/dL; <0.32 mmol/L) or symptomatic hypophosphatemia should be treated with IV phosphorus replacement. The infusion of 15 mmol of phosphorus in 250 mL of IV fluid over 3 hours is a safe and effective treatment, but the recommended dosage of IV phosphorus (5–45 mmol or 0.08–0.64 mmol/kg) and infusion recommendations (over 4–12 hours) are highly variable.
- Asymptomatic patients or those who exhibit mild to moderate hypophosphatemia can be treated with oral phosphorus supplementation in doses of 1.5 to 2 g (50–60 mmol) daily in divided doses, with the goal of correcting serum phosphorus concentration in 7 to 10 days (Table 79–4).
- Patients should be closely monitored with frequent serum phosphorus and calcium determinations, especially if phosphorus is given IV or if renal dysfunction is present.
- Phosphorus, 12 to 15 mmol/L, should be routinely added to hyperalimentation solutions to prevent hypophosphatemia.

DISORDERS OF POTASSIUM HOMEOSTASIS

HYPOKALEMIA (SERUM POTASSIUM <3.5 mEq/L [<3.5 mmol/L])

Pathophysiology

- Hypokalemia results from a total body potassium deficit or shifting of serum potassium into the intracellular compartment.

TABLE 79–4	Phosphorus Replacement Therapy	
Product (Salt)	**Phosphate Content**	**Initial Dosing Based on Serum K**
Oral therapy (potassium phosphate + sodium phosphate)		
Neutra-Phos (7 mEq/ packet each of Na and K)	250 mg (8 mmol)/packet	1 packet three times daily[a]
Neutra-Phos-K (14.25 mEq/ packet of K)	250 mg (8 mmol)/packet	Serum K >5.5 mEq/L (>5.5 mmol/L); not recommended
K-Phos Neutral (13 mEq/ tablet Na and 1.1 mEq/ tablet K)	250 mg (8 mmol)/tablet	Serum K >5.5 mEq/L (>5.5 mmol/L) one tablet three times daily
Uro-KP-Neutral (10.9 mEq/ tablet Na and 1.27 mEq/ tablet K)	250 mg (8 mmol)/tablet	Serum K >5.5 mEq/L (>5.5 mmol/L) one tablet three times daily
Fleet Phospho-soda (sodium phosphate solution)	4 mmol/mL	Serum K >5.5 mEq/L (>5.5 mmol/L), 2 mL three times daily
IV therapy		
Sodium PO$_4$ (4 mEq/mL Na)	3 mmol/mL	Serum K >3.5 mEq/L (>3.5 mmol/L) 15–30 mmol IVPB
Potassium PO$_4$ (4.4 mEq/mL K)	3 mmol/mL	Serum K <3.5 mEq/L (<3.5 mmol/L) 15–30 mmol IVPB

IV, intravenous; IVPB, intravenous piggyback; K, potassium; Na, sodium; PO$_4$, phosphate.
[a]Monitor serum K closely.

- Many drugs can cause hypokalemia (**Table 79–5**), and it is most commonly seen with use of loop and thiazide diuretics. Other causes of hypokalemia are diarrhea, vomiting, and hypomagnesemia.

Clinical Presentation

- Signs and symptoms are nonspecific and variable and depend on the degree of hypokalemia and rapidity of onset. Mild hypokalemia is often asymptomatic.
- Cardiovascular manifestations include hypertension and cardiac arrhythmias (e.g., heart block, atrial flutter, paroxysmal atrial tachycardia, ventricular fibrillation, and digitalis-induced arrhythmias). In severe hypokalemia (serum concentration <2.5 mEq/L; <2.5 mmol/L), ECG effects include ST-segment depression or flattening, T-wave inversion, and U-wave elevation.
- Moderate hypokalemia is associated with muscle weakness, cramping, malaise, and myalgias.

TABLE 79–5 Mechanism of Drug-Induced Hypokalemia

Transcellular Shift	Enhanced Renal Excretion	Enhanced Fecal Elimination
β_2-Receptor agonists	Diuretics	Sodium polystyrene sulfonate
Epinephrine	Acetazolamide	Phenolphthalein
Albuterol	Thiazides	Sorbitol
Terbutaline	Indapamide	
Pirbuterol	Metolazone	
Salmeterol	Furosemide	
Isoproterenol	Torsemide	
Ephedrine	Bumetanide	
Pseudoephedrine	Ethacrynic acid	
Tocolytic agents	High-dose penicillins	
Ritodrine	Nafcillin	
Nylidrin	Ampicillin	
Theophylline	Penicillin	
Caffeine	Mineralocorticoids	
Insulin overdose	Miscellaneous	
	Aminoglycosides	
	Amphotericin B	
	Cisplatin	

Treatment

- In general, every 1 mEq/L (1 mmol/L) fall of potassium below 3.5 mEq/L (3.5 mmol/L) corresponds with a total body deficit of 100 to 400 mEq (100–400 mmol). To correct mild deficits, patients receiving chronic loop or thiazide diuretics generally need 40 to 100 mEq (40–100 mmol) of potassium.
- Whenever possible, potassium supplementation should be administered by mouth. Of the available salts, potassium chloride is most commonly used because it is the most effective for common causes of potassium depletion.
- IV use should be limited to patients who have severe hypokalemia, signs and symptoms of hypokalemia, or inability to tolerate oral therapy. IV supplementation is more dangerous than oral therapy due to the potential for hyperkalemia, phlebitis, and pain at the infusion site. Potassium should be administered in saline because dextrose can stimulate insulin secretion and worsen intracellular shifting of potassium. Generally, 10 to 20 mEq (10–20 mmol) of potassium is diluted in 100 mL of 0.9% saline and administered through a peripheral vein over 1 hour. If infusion rates exceed 10 mEq/h (10 mmol/hour), ECG should be monitored.
- Serum potassium concentration should be evaluated following infusion of each 30 to 40 mEq (30–40 mmol) to direct further potassium supplementation.

HYPERKALEMIA (SERUM POTASSIUM >5.5 mEq/L [>5 mmol/L])

Pathophysiology

- Hyperkalemia develops when potassium intake exceeds excretion or when the transcellular distribution of potassium is disturbed.
- Primary causes of true hyperkalemia are increased potassium intake, decreased potassium excretion, tubular unresponsiveness to aldosterone, and redistribution of potassium to the extracellular space.

Clinical Presentation

- Hyperkalemia is frequently asymptomatic. Patients might complain of heart palpitations or skipped heartbeats.
- The earliest ECG change (serum potassium 5.5–6 mEq/L; 5.5–6 mmol/L) is peaked T waves. The sequence of changes with further increases is widening of the PR interval, loss of the P wave, widening of the QRS complex, and merging of the QRS complex with the T wave resulting in a sine-wave pattern.

Treatment

- Treatment of hyperkalemia depends on the desired rapidity and degree of lowering (**Fig. 79–4, Table 79–6**). Dialysis is the most rapid way to lower serum potassium concentration.
- Calcium administration rapidly reverses ECG manifestations and arrhythmias, but it does not lower serum potassium concentrations. Calcium is short acting and therefore must be repeated if signs or symptoms recur.
- Rapid correction of hyperkalemia requires administration of drugs that shift potassium intracellularly (e.g., insulin and dextrose, sodium bicarbonate, or albuterol).
- **Sodium polystyrene sulfonate** is a cation-exchange resin suitable for asymptomatic patients with mild to moderate hyperkalemia. Each gram of resin exchanges 1 mEq (1 mmol) of sodium for 1 mEq (1 mmol) of potassium. The sorbitol component promotes excretion of exchanged potassium by inducing diarrhea. The oral route is better tolerated and more effective than the rectal route.

DISORDERS OF MAGNESIUM HOMEOSTASIS

HYPOMAGNESEMIA (SERUM MAGNESIUM <1.4 mEq/L [<0.70 mmol/L])

Pathophysiology

- Hypomagnesemia is usually associated with disorders of the intestinal tract or kidneys. Drugs (e.g., **aminoglycosides, amphotericin B, cyclosporine,** diuretics, **digitalis,** and **cisplatin**) or conditions that interfere with intestinal absorption or increase renal excretion of magnesium can cause hypomagnesemia.
- Hypomagnesemia is commonly associated with alcoholism.

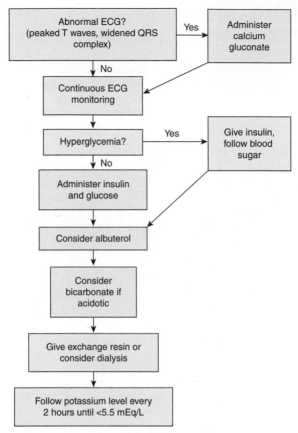

FIGURE 79–4. Treatment approach for hyperkalemia. Serum potassium of 5.5 mEq/L is equivalent to 5.5 mmol/L.

Clinical Presentation

- Although typically asymptomatic, the dominant organ systems involved are the neuromuscular and cardiovascular systems. Symptoms include heart palpitations, tetany, twitching, and generalized convulsions.
- Ventricular arrhythmias are the most important and potentially life-threatening cardiovascular effect.
- ECG changes include widened QRS complexes and peaked T waves in mild deficiency. Prolonged PR intervals, progressive widening of the QRS complexes, and flattening of T waves occur in moderate to severe deficiency.
- Many electrolyte disturbances occur with hypomagnesemia, including hypokalemia and hypocalcemia.

TABLE 79–6 Therapeutic Alternatives for the Management of Hyperkalemia

Medication	Dose	Route of Administration	Onset/Duration of Action	Acuity	Mechanism of Action	Expected Result
Calcium	1 g	IV over 5–10 min	1–2 min/10–30 min	Acute	Raises cardiac threshold potential	Reverses electrocardiographic effects
Furosemide	20–40 mg	IV	5–15 min/4–6 hours	Acute	Inhibits renal Na^+ reabsorption	Increased urinary K^+ loss
Regular insulin	5–10 units	IV or SC	30 min/2–6 hours	Acute	Stimulates intracellular K^+ uptake	Intracellular K^+ redistribution
Dextrose 10%	1,000 mL (100 g)	IV over 1–2 hours	30 min/2–6 hours	Acute	Stimulates insulin release	Intracellular K^+ redistribution
Dextrose 50%	50 mL (25 g)	IV over 5 min	30 min/2–6 hours	Acute	Stimulates insulin release	Intracellular K^+ redistribution
Sodium bicarbonate	50–100 mEq (50–100 mmol)	IV over 2–5 min	30 min/2–6 hours	Acute	Raises serum pH	Intracellular K^+ redistribution
Albuterol	10–20 mg	Nebulized over 10 min	30 min/1–2 hours	Acute	Stimulates intracellular K^+ uptake	Intracellular K^+ redistribution
Hemodialysis	4 hours	N/A	Immediate/variable	Acute	Removal from serum	Increased K^+ elimination
Sodium polystyrene sulfonate	15–60 g	Oral or rectal	1 hour/variable	Nonacute	Resin exchanges Na^+ for K^+	Increased K^+ elimination

K^+, potassium ion; Na^+, sodium ion; SC, subcutaneous.

TABLE 79–7	Guidelines for Treatment of Magnesium Deficiency in Adults

1. **Serum magnesium <1 mEq/L (<1.2 mg/dL [<0.5 mmol/L]) with life-threatening symptoms (seizure or arrhythmia)**

   Day 1

       2 g magnesium sulfate (1 g magnesium sulfate = 8.1 mEq Mg^{2+}) mixed with 6 mL 0.9% NaCl in 10 mL syringe and administer IV push over 1 min

       Follow with 1 mEq Mg^{2+}/kg lean body weight IV infusion over 24 hours

   Days 2–5

       0.5 mEq [0.25 mmol] Mg^{2+}/kg lean body weight per day divided in maintenance IV fluids

2. **Serum magnesium <1 mEq/L (<1.2 mg/dL [<0.5 mmol/L]) without life-threatening symptoms**

   Day 1

       Total of 1 mEq (0.5 mmol) Mg^{2+}/kg lean body weight per day as continuous IV infusion, or divided and given IM every 4 hours for five doses

   Days 2–5

       Total of 0.5 mEq (0.25 mmol) Mg^{2+}/kg lean body weight IV infusion per day as continuous IV infusion or divided and given IM every 6–8 hours

3. **Serum magnesium >1 mEq/L (>1.2 mg/dL [>0.5 mmol/L]) and <1.5 mEq/L (<1.8 mg/dL [<0.75 mmol/L]) without symptoms**

   As in no. 2 above, *or*

   Milk of magnesia 5 mL four times daily as tolerated, *or*

   Magnesium-containing antacid 15 mL three times daily as tolerated, *or*

   Magnesium oxide tablets 400 mg four times daily, increase to two tablets four times daily as tolerated

Mg^{2+}, magnesium ion; NaCl, sodium chloride.

Treatment

- The severity of magnesium depletion and the presence of symptoms dictate the route of magnesium supplementation (**Table 79–7**). Intramuscular magnesium is painful and should be reserved for patients with severe hypomagnesemia and limited venous access. IV bolus injection is associated with flushing, sweating, and a sensation of warmth.
- The optimal replacement regimen is unknown, but a common approach is to administer 8 to 12 g of magnesium sulfate in the first 24 hours, followed by 4 to 6 g/day for 3 to 5 days to adequately replace body stores. Approximately 50% of the administered dose is excreted in the urine.

HYPERMAGNESEMIA (SERUM MAGNESIUM >2 mEq/L [>1 mmol/L])

Pathophysiology

- Magnesium concentrations steadily increase as the GFR decreases below 30 mL/min/1.73m² (0.29 mL/s/m²).

- Other causes include magnesium-containing antacids in patients with renal insufficiency, enteral or parenteral nutrition in patients with multiorgan system failure, magnesium for treatment of eclampsia, lithium therapy, hypothyroidism, and Addison's disease.

Clinical Presentation

- Symptoms are rare when the serum magnesium concentration is <4 mEq/L (<2 mmol/L).
- The sequence of neuromuscular signs as serum magnesium increases from 5 mEq/L to 12 mEq/L (2.5–6 mmol/L) is sedation, hypotonia, hyporeflexia, somnolence, coma, muscular paralysis, and, ultimately, respiratory depression.
- The sequence of cardiovascular signs as serum magnesium increases from 3 mEq/L to 15 mEq/L (1.5–7.5 mmol/L) is hypotension, cutaneous vasodilation, QT-interval prolongation, bradycardia, primary heart block, nodal rhythms, bundle branch block, QRS- and then PR-interval prolongation, complete heart block, and asystole.

Treatment

- IV calcium (100–200 mg of elemental calcium; e.g., calcium gluconate 2 g IV) is indicated to antagonize the neuromuscular and cardiovascular effects of magnesium. Doses should be repeated as often as hourly in life-threatening situations.
- Forced diuresis with saline and loop diuretics (e.g., **furosemide,** 40 mg IV) can promote magnesium elimination in patients with normal renal function or stage 1, 2, or 3 CKD. In dialysis patients, their hemodialysis prescription should be changed to a magnesium-free dialysate.

EVALUATION OF THERAPEUTIC OUTCOMES

- The primary end point for monitoring treatment of fluid and electrolyte disorders is the correction of the abnormal serum electrolyte. In general, monitoring is initially performed at frequent intervals and, as homeostasis is restored, subsequently performed at less frequent intervals.
- All electrolytes should be monitored, as individual electrolyte abnormalities typically coexist with another abnormality (e.g., hypomagnesemia with hypokalemia and hypocalcemia, or hyperphosphatemia with hypocalcemia).
- Patients should be monitored for resolution of clinical manifestations of electrolyte disturbances and for treatment-related complications.

See Chapter 58, Disorders of Sodium and Water Homeostasis, authored by James D. Coyle and Gary R. Matzke; Chapter 59, Disorders of Calcium and Phosphorus Homeostasis, authored by Amy Barton Pai; and Chapter 60, Disorders of Potassium and Magnesium Homeostasis, authored by Donald F. Brophy and Jane Frumin, for a more detailed discussion of this topic.

CHAPTER 80

Allergic Rhinitis

DEFINITION

- Allergic rhinitis is inflammation of the nasal mucous membrane that occurs in sensitized individuals when inhaled allergenic materials contact mucous membranes and elicit a specific response mediated by immunoglobulin E (IgE). There are two types:
  - ✓ *Seasonal (hay fever):* occurs in response to specific allergens (pollen from trees, grasses, and weeds) present at predictable times of the year (spring and/or fall blooming seasons) and typically causes more acute symptoms.
  - ✓ *Perennial (intermittent or persistent):* occurs year-round in response to nonseasonal allergens (e.g., dust mites, animal dander, and molds) and usually causes more subtle, chronic symptoms.
- Many patients have a combination of both types, with symptoms year-round and seasonal exacerbations.

PATHOPHYSIOLOGY

- The initial reaction occurs when airborne allergens enter the nose during inhalation and are processed by lymphocytes, which produce antigen-specific IgE, thereby sensitizing genetically predisposed hosts to those agents. On nasal reexposure, IgE bound to mast cells interacts with airborne allergens, triggering release of inflammatory mediators.
- An immediate reaction occurs within seconds to minutes, resulting in the rapid release of preformed mediators and newly generated mediators from the arachidonic acid cascade. Mediators of immediate hypersensitivity include histamine, leukotrienes, prostaglandin, tryptase, and kinins. These mediators cause vasodilation, increased vascular permeability, and production of nasal secretions. Histamine produces rhinorrhea, itching, sneezing, and nasal obstruction.
- A late-phase reaction may occur 4 to 8 hours after the initial allergen exposure due to cytokine release from mast cells and thymus-derived helper lymphocytes. This inflammatory response is likely responsible for persistent, chronic symptoms, including nasal congestion.

CLINICAL PRESENTATION

- Symptoms include clear rhinorrhea, sneezing, nasal congestion, postnasal drip, allergic conjunctivitis, and pruritic eyes, ears, or nose.
- In children, physical examination may reveal dark circles under the eyes (allergic shiners), a transverse nasal crease caused by repeated rubbing of

the nose, adenoidal breathing, edematous nasal turbinates coated with clear secretions, tearing, and periorbital swelling.

- Patients may complain of loss of smell or taste, with sinusitis or polyps the underlying cause in many cases. Postnasal drip with cough or hoarseness can also be bothersome.
- Untreated rhinitis symptoms may lead to insomnia, malaise, fatigue, and poor work or school performance.
- Allergic rhinitis is a risk factor for asthma; the majority of asthma patients have nasal symptoms, and ~10% to 40% of allergic rhinitis patients have asthma.
- Recurrent and chronic sinusitis and epistaxis are complications of allergic rhinitis.

DIAGNOSIS

- To distinguish allergic rhinitis from other causes of rhinitis, the medical history includes a careful description of symptoms, environmental factors and exposures, results of previous therapy, use of medications, previous nasal injury or surgery, and family history.
- Microscopic examination of nasal scrapings typically reveals numerous eosinophils. The peripheral blood eosinophil count may be elevated, but it is nonspecific and has limited usefulness.
- Allergy testing can help determine whether rhinitis is caused by an immune response to allergens. Immediate-type hypersensitivity skin tests are commonly used. Percutaneous testing is safer and more generally accepted than intradermal testing, which is usually reserved for patients requiring confirmation. The radioallergosorbent test (RAST) can be used to detect IgE antibodies in the blood that are specific for a given antigen, but it is less sensitive than percutaneous tests.

DESIRED OUTCOME

- The goal of treatment is to minimize or prevent symptoms with minimal or no side effects and reasonable medication expense.
- Patients should be able to maintain a normal lifestyle, including participation in outdoor activities and playing with pets as desired.

TREATMENT

(Fig. 80–1)

ALLERGEN AVOIDANCE

- Avoidance of offending allergens is important but difficult to accomplish, especially for perennial allergens. Mold growth can be reduced by keeping household humidity <50% and removing obvious growth with bleach or disinfectant.

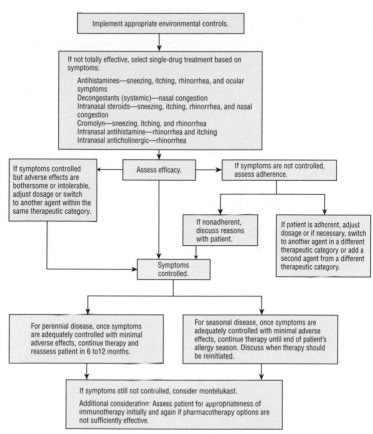

FIGURE 80–1. Treatment algorithm for allergic rhinitis.

- Patients sensitive to animals benefit most by removing pets from the home, if feasible. Reducing exposure to dust mites by encasing bedding with impermeable covers and washing bed linens in hot water has little clinical benefit, except perhaps in children.
- Patients with seasonal allergic rhinitis should keep windows closed and minimize time spent outdoors during pollen seasons. Filter masks can be worn while gardening or mowing the lawn.

PHARMACOLOGIC THERAPY

Antihistamines

- Histamine H_1-receptor antagonists bind to H_1 receptors without activating them, preventing histamine binding and action. They are more effective in preventing the histamine response than in reversing it.
- Oral antihistamines can be divided into two major categories: nonselective (first-generation or sedating antihistamines) and peripherally selective

TABLE 80–1	Relative Adverse Effect Profiles of Antihistamines	
Medication	**Relative Sedative Effect**	**Relative Anticholinergic Effect**
Alkylamine class, nonselective		
Brompheniramine maleate	Low	Moderate
Chlorpheniramine maleate	Low	Moderate
Dexchlorpheniramine maleate	Low	Moderate
Ethanolamine class, nonselective		
Carbinoxamine maleate	High	High
Clemastine fumarate	Moderate	High
Diphenhydramine hydrochloride	High	High
Ethylenediamine class, nonselective		
Pyrilamine maleate	Low	Low to none
Tripelennamine hydrochloride	Moderate	Low to none
Phenothiazine class, nonselective		
Promethazine hydrochloride	High	High
Piperidine class, nonselective		
Cyproheptadine hydrochloride	Low	Moderate
Phenindamine tartrate	Low to none	Moderate
Phthalazinone class, peripherally selective		
Azelastine (nasal only)	Low to none	Low to none
Piperazine class, peripherally selective		
Cetirizine	Low to moderate	Low to none
Levocetirizine	Low to moderate	Low to none
Piperidine class, peripherally selective		
Desloratadine	Low to none	Low to none
Fexofenadine	Low to none	Low to none
Loratadine	Low to none	Low to none

(second-generation or nonsedating antihistamines). However, individual agents should be judged on their specific sedating effects because variation exists among agents within these broad categories (**Table 80–1**). The central sedating effect may depend on the ability to cross the blood–brain barrier. Most older antihistamines are lipid soluble and cross this barrier easily. The peripherally selective agents have little or no central or autonomic nervous system effects.

- Symptom relief is caused in part by anticholinergic properties, which are responsible for the drying effect that reduces nasal, salivary, and lacrimal gland hypersecretion. Antihistamines antagonize increased capillary permeability, wheal-and-flare formation, and itching.
- Drowsiness is the most frequent side effect, and it can interfere with driving ability or adequate functioning at the workplace. Sedative effects

can be beneficial in patients who have difficulty sleeping because of rhinitis symptoms.

- Although anticholinergic (drying) effects contribute to efficacy, adverse effects such as dry mouth, difficulty in voiding urine, constipation, and potential cardiovascular effects may occur (see Table 80–1). Antihistamines should be used with caution in patients predisposed to urinary retention and in those with increased intraocular pressure, hyperthyroidism, and cardiovascular disease.
- Other side effects include loss of appetite, nausea, vomiting, and epigastric distress. Taking medication with meals or a full glass of water may prevent GI side effects.
- Antihistamines are more effective when taken ~1 to 2 hours before anticipated exposure to the offending allergen.
- Table 80–2 lists recommended doses of commonly used oral agents.
- **Azelastine** (Astelin) is an intranasal antihistamine that rapidly relieves symptoms of seasonal allergic rhinitis. However, patients should be cautioned about its potential for drowsiness because systemic availability is ~40%. Patients may also experience drying effects, headache, and diminished effectiveness over time.
- **Levocabastine** (Livostin) and **olopatadine** (Patanol) are ophthalmic antihistamines that can be used for allergic conjunctivitis that is often associated with allergic rhinitis. Systemic antihistamines are usually also effective for allergic conjunctivitis. Ophthalmic agents are a useful addition to nasal corticosteroids when ocular symptoms occur. They are also useful for patients whose only symptoms involve the eyes or for patients whose ocular symptoms persist on oral antihistamine treatment.

Decongestants

- Topical and systemic decongestants are sympathomimetic agents that act on adrenergic receptors in the nasal mucosa to produce vasoconstriction, shrink swollen mucosa, and improve ventilation. Decongestants work well in combination with antihistamines when nasal congestion is part of the clinical picture.
- Topical decongestants are applied directly to swollen nasal mucosa via drops or sprays (Table 80–3). They result in little or no systemic absorption.
- Prolonged use of topical agents (>3–5 days) can result in rhinitis medicamentosa, which is rebound vasodilation with congestion. Patients with this condition use more spray more often with less response. Abrupt cessation is an effective treatment, but rebound congestion may last for several days or weeks. Nasal steroids have been used successfully, but they take several days to work. Weaning the patient off the topical decongestant can be accomplished by decreasing the dosing frequency or concentration over several weeks. Combining the weaning process with nasal steroids may be helpful.
- Other adverse effects of topical decongestants are burning, stinging, sneezing, and dryness of the nasal mucosa.

TABLE 80–2	Oral Dosages of Commonly Used Antihistamines and Decongestants

	Dosage and Interval[a]	
Medication	*Adults*	*Children*
Nonselective (first-generation) antihistamines		
Chlorpheniramine maleate, plain[b]	4 mg daily every 6 hours	6–12 years: 2 mg daily every 6 hours 2–5 years: 1 mg every 6 hours
Chlorpheniramine maleate, sustained-release	8–12 mg daily at bedtime, 8 mg every 8–12 hours, or 12 mg every 12 hours	6–12 years: 8 mg at bedtime <6 years: Not recommended
Clemastine fumarate[b]	1.34 mg every 8 hours	6–12 years: 0.67 mg every 12 hours
Diphenhydramine hydrochloride[b]	25–50 mg every 8 hours	5 mg/kg/day divided every 8 hours (up to 25 mg per dose)
Peripherally selective (second-generation) antihistamines		
Loratadine[b]	10 mg once daily	6–12 years: 10 mg once daily 2–5 years: 5 mg once daily
Fexofenadine	60 mg twice daily or 180 mg once daily	6–11 years: 30 mg twice daily
Cetirizine[b]	5–10 mg once daily	>6 years: 5 mg once daily
Levocetirizine	5 mg in evening	6–11 years: 2.5 mg in evening
Oral decongestants		
Pseudoephedrine, plain	60 mg every 4–6 hours	6–12 years: 30 mg every 4–6 hours 2–5 years: 15 mg every 4–6 hours
Pseudoephedrine, sustained-release[c]	120 mg every 12 hours	Not recommended
Phenylephrine	10–20 mg every 4 hours	6–12 years: 10 mg every 4 hours 2–6 years: 0.25% drops, 1 mL every 4 hours

Note: Fexofenadine and levocetirizine are available by prescription only.
[a]Dosage adjustment may be needed in renal/hepatic dysfunction. Refer to manufacturers' prescribing information.
[b]Available in liquid form.
[c]Controlled-release product available: 240 mg once daily (60 mg immediate-release with 180 mg controlled-release).

TABLE 80–3	Duration of Action of Topical Decongestants
Medication	**Duration (Hours)**
Short-acting	
Phenylephrine hydrochloride	Up to 4
Intermediate-acting	
Naphazoline hydrochloride	4–6
Tetrahydrozoline hydrochloride	4–6
Long-acting	
Oxymetazoline hydrochloride	Up to 12
Xylometazoline hydrochloride	Up to 12

- These products should be used only when absolutely necessary (e.g., at bedtime) and in doses that are as small and infrequent as possible. Duration of therapy should always be limited to 3 to 5 days.
- **Pseudoephedrine** (see Table 80–2) is an oral decongestant that has a slower onset of action than topical agents but may last longer and cause less local irritation. Also, rhinitis medicamentosa does not occur with oral decongestants. Doses up to 180 mg produce no measurable change in blood pressure or heart rate. However, higher doses (210–240 mg) may raise both blood pressure and heart rate. Systemic decongestants should be avoided in hypertensive patients unless absolutely necessary. Severe hypertensive reactions can occur when pseudoephedrine is given concomitantly with monoamine oxidase inhibitors. Pseudoephedrine can cause mild CNS stimulation, even at therapeutic doses. Because of misuse as a component in the illegal manufacture of methamphetamine, legal requirements now restrict pseudoephedrine to behind-the-counter sale with a limit on monthly purchases.
- **Phenylephrine** has replaced pseudoephedrine in many nonprescription antihistamine–decongestant combination products because of the legal restriction on pseudoephedrine sales.
- Use of combination oral products containing a decongestant and antihistamine is rational because of the different mechanisms of action. Consumers should read product labels carefully to avoid therapeutic duplication.

Nasal Corticosteroids

- Intranasal corticosteroids effectively relieve sneezing, rhinorrhea, pruritus, and nasal congestion with minimal side effects (Table 80–4). They reduce inflammation by blocking mediator release, suppressing neutrophil chemotaxis, causing mild vasoconstriction, and inhibiting mast cell–mediated, late-phase reactions.
- These agents are an excellent choice for perennial rhinitis and can be useful in seasonal rhinitis, especially if begun in advance of symptoms. Some authorities recommend nasal steroids as initial therapy over antihistamines because of their high degree of efficacy when used properly along with allergen avoidance.

TABLE 80–4	Dosage of Nasal Corticosteroids
Medication	**Dosage and Interval**
Beclomethasone dipropionate, monohydrate	>12 years: 1–2 inhalations per nostril (42–84 mcg) twice daily 6–12 years: One inhalation per nostril twice daily to start
Budesonide	>6 years: Two sprays (64 mcg) per nostril in AM and PM or four sprays per nostril in AM (maximum 256 mcg)
Flunisolide	Adults: Two sprays (50 mcg) per nostril twice daily (maximum, 400 mcg) Children: One spray per nostril three times daily
Fluticasone	Adults: Two sprays (100 mcg) per nostril once daily; after a few days decrease to 1 spray per nostril Children >4 years and adolescents: One spray per nostril once daily (maximum 200 mcg/day)
Mometasone furoate	>12 years: Two sprays (100 mcg) per nostril once daily
Triamcinolone acetonide	>12 years: Two sprays (110 mcg) per nostril once daily (maximum 440 mcg/day)

- Side effects include sneezing, stinging, headache, epistaxis, and rare infections with *Candida albicans*.
- Some patients improve within a few days, but peak response may require 2 to 3 weeks. The dosage may be reduced once a response is achieved.
- Blocked nasal passages should be cleared with a decongestant or saline irrigation before administration to ensure adequate penetration of the spray.

Cromolyn Sodium

- **Cromolyn sodium** (Nasalcrom), a mast cell stabilizer, is available as a nonprescription nasal spray for symptomatic prevention and treatment of allergic rhinitis. It prevents antigen-triggered mast cell degranulation and release of mediators, including histamine. The most common side effect is local irritation (sneezing and nasal stinging).
- The dosage for persons at least 2 years of age is one spray in each nostril three or four times daily at regular intervals. Nasal passages should be cleared before administration, and inhaling through the nose during administration enhances distribution to the entire nasal lining.
- For seasonal rhinitis, treatment should be initiated just before the start of the offending allergen's season and continue throughout the season.
- In perennial rhinitis, the effects may not be seen for 2 to 4 weeks; antihistamines or decongestants may be needed during this initial phase of therapy.

Ipratropium Bromide

- **Ipratropium bromide** (Atrovent) nasal spray is an anticholinergic agent useful in perennial allergic rhinitis.

- It exhibits antisecretory properties when applied locally and provides symptomatic relief of rhinorrhea associated with allergic and other forms of chronic rhinitis.
- The 0.03% solution is given as two sprays (42 mcg) two or three times daily. Adverse effects are mild and include headache, epistaxis, and nasal dryness.

Montelukast

- **Montelukast** (Singulair) is a leukotriene receptor antagonist approved for treatment of perennial allergic rhinitis in children as young as 6 months and for seasonal allergic rhinitis in children as young as 2 years. It is effective alone or in combination with an antihistamine.
- The dosage for adults and adolescents older than 14 years is one 10-mg tablet daily. Children ages 6 to 14 years may receive one 5-mg chewable tablet daily. Children ages 6 months to 5 years may be given one 4-mg chewable tablet or oral granule packet daily.
- Leukotriene receptor antagonists are no more effective than peripherally selective antihistamines and less effective than intranasal corticosteroids. However, combined use with antihistamines is more effective than antihistamine treatment alone.

IMMUNOTHERAPY

- Immunotherapy is the slow, gradual process of injecting increasing doses of antigens responsible for eliciting allergic symptoms into a patient with the intent of inducing tolerance to the allergen when natural exposure occurs.
- Beneficial effects of immunotherapy may result from induction of IgG-blocking antibodies, reduction in specific IgE (long-term), reduced recruitment of effector cells, altered T-cell cytokine balance, T-cell anergy, and induction of regulatory T cells.
- Because immunotherapy is expensive, has potential risks, and requires a major time commitment from patients, it should only be considered in select patients. Good candidates include patients with a strong history of severe symptoms unsuccessfully controlled by avoidance and pharmacotherapy and patients who have been unable to tolerate the adverse effects of drug therapy. Poor candidates include patients with medical conditions that would compromise the ability to tolerate an anaphylactic-type reaction, patients with impaired immune systems, and patients with a history of nonadherence to therapy.
- In general, very dilute solutions are given initially once or twice weekly. The concentration is increased until the maximum tolerated dose or highest planned dose is achieved. This maintenance dose is continued in slowly increasing intervals over several years, depending on clinical response. Better results are obtained with year-round rather than seasonal injections.
- Common mild local adverse reactions include induration and swelling at the injection site. More severe reactions (generalized urticaria, bronchospasm, laryngospasm, vascular collapse, and death from anaphylaxis)

occur rarely. Severe reactions are treated with epinephrine, antihistamines, and systemic corticosteroids.

EVALUATION OF THERAPEUTIC OUTCOMES

- Patients should be monitored regularly for reduction in severity of identified target symptoms and the presence of side effects.
- Patients should be questioned about their satisfaction with the management of their allergic rhinitis. Management should result in minimal disruption to their life.
- The Medical Outcomes Study 36-Item Short Form Health Survey and the Rhinoconjunctivitis Quality of Life Questionnaire measure not only improvement in symptoms but also parameters such as sleep quality, nonallergic symptoms (e.g., fatigue and poor concentration), emotions, and participation in a variety of activities.

See Chapter 104, Allergic Rhinitis, authored by J. Russell May and Philip H. Smith, for a more detailed discussion of this topic.

Asthma

DEFINITION

- The National Asthma Education and Prevention Program (NAEPP) defines asthma as a chronic inflammatory disorder of the airways in which many cells and cellular elements play a role. In susceptible individuals, inflammation causes recurrent episodes of wheezing, breathlessness, chest tightness, and coughing. These episodes are usually associated with airflow obstruction that is often reversible either spontaneously or with treatment. The inflammation also causes an increase in bronchial hyperresponsiveness (BHR) to a variety of stimuli.

PATHOPHYSIOLOGY

- The major characteristics of asthma include a variable degree of airflow obstruction (related to bronchospasm, edema, and hypersecretion), BHR, and airway inflammation.
- Inhaled allergen challenge in allergic patients causes an early-phase allergic reaction characterized by activation of cells bearing allergen-specific immunoglobulin E (IgE) antibodies. There is rapid activation of airway mast cells and macrophages, which release proinflammatory mediators such as histamine and eicosanoids that induce contraction of airway smooth muscle, mucus secretion, vasodilation, and exudation of plasma in the airways. Plasma protein leakage induces a thickened, engorged, edematous airway wall and a narrowing of the airway lumen with reduced mucus clearance.
- The late-phase inflammatory reaction occurs 6 to 9 hours after allergen provocation and involves recruitment and activation of eosinophils, T lymphocytes, basophils, neutrophils, and macrophages. Eosinophils migrate to the airways and release inflammatory mediators (leukotrienes and granule proteins).
- T-lymphocyte activation leads to release of cytokines from type 2 T-helper (TH_2) cells that mediate allergic inflammation (interleukin [IL]-4, IL-5, and IL-13). Conversely, type 1 T-helper (TH_1) cells produce IL-2 and interferon-γ that are essential for cellular defense mechanisms. Allergic asthmatic inflammation may result from an imbalance between TH_1 and TH_2 cells.
- Mast cell degranulation in response to allergens results in release of mediators such as histamine; eosinophil and neutrophil chemotactic factors; leukotrienes C_4, D_4, and E_4; prostaglandins; and platelet-activating factor (PAF). Histamine is capable of inducing smooth muscle constriction and bronchospasm and may play a role in mucosal edema and mucus secretion.
- Alveolar macrophages release a number of inflammatory mediators, including PAF and leukotrienes B_4, C_4, and D_4. Production of neutrophil

chemotactic factor and eosinophil chemotactic factor furthers the inflammatory process.

- Neutrophils are also a source of mediators (PAFs, prostaglandins, thromboxanes, and leukotrienes) that contribute to BHR and airway inflammation.
- The 5-lipoxygenase pathway of arachidonic acid metabolism is responsible for production of cysteinyl leukotrienes. Leukotrienes C_4, D_4, and E_4 are released during inflammatory processes in the lung and produce bronchospasm, mucus secretion, microvascular permeability, and airway edema.
- Bronchial epithelial cells participate in inflammation by releasing eicosanoids, peptidases, matrix proteins, cytokines, and nitric oxide. Epithelial shedding results in heightened airway responsiveness, altered permeability of the airway mucosa, depletion of epithelial-derived relaxant factors, and loss of enzymes responsible for degrading inflammatory neuropeptides.
- The exudative inflammatory process and sloughing of epithelial cells into the airway lumen impair mucociliary transport. The bronchial glands are increased in size, and the goblet cells are increased in size and number. Expectorated mucus from patients with asthma tends to have high viscosity.
- The airway is innervated by parasympathetic, sympathetic, and nonadrenergic inhibitory nerves. The normal resting tone of airway smooth muscle is maintained by vagal efferent activity, and bronchoconstriction can be mediated by vagal stimulation in the small bronchi. Airway smooth muscle contains noninnervated β_2-adrenergic receptors that produce bronchodilation. The nonadrenergic, noncholinergic nervous system in the trachea and bronchi may amplify inflammation in asthma by releasing nitric oxide.

CLINICAL PRESENTATION

CHRONIC ASTHMA

- Classic asthma is characterized by episodic dyspnea associated with wheezing, but the clinical presentation of asthma is diverse. Patients may also complain of episodes of dyspnea, chest tightness, coughing (particularly at night), wheezing, or a whistling sound when breathing. These often occur with exercise but may occur spontaneously or in association with known allergens.
- Signs include expiratory wheezing on auscultation; a dry, hacking cough; and atopy (e.g., allergic rhinitis or eczema).
- Asthma can vary from chronic daily symptoms to only intermittent symptoms. The intervals between symptoms may be days, weeks, months, or years.
- The severity is determined by lung function, symptoms, nighttime awakenings, and interference with normal activity prior to therapy. Patients can present with mild intermittent symptoms that require no medications or only occasional use of short-acting inhaled β_2-agonists to severe chronic asthma symptoms despite receiving multiple medications.

ACUTE SEVERE ASTHMA

- Uncontrolled asthma can progress to an acute state in which inflammation, airway edema, excessive mucus accumulation, and severe bronchospasm result in profound airway narrowing that is poorly responsive to usual bronchodilator therapy.
- Patients may be anxious in acute distress and complain of severe dyspnea, shortness of breath, chest tightness, or burning. They may be able to say only a few words with each breath. Symptoms are unresponsive to usual measures (short-acting inhaled β-agonists).
- Signs include expiratory and inspiratory wheezing on auscultation; a dry, hacking cough; tachypnea; tachycardia; pallor or cyanosis; and hyperinflated chest with intercostal and supraclavicular retractions. Breath sounds may be diminished with very severe obstruction.

DIAGNOSIS

CHRONIC ASTHMA

- The diagnosis of asthma is made primarily by a history of recurrent episodes of coughing, wheezing, chest tightness, or shortness of breath and confirmatory spirometry.
- The patient may have a family history of allergy or asthma or have symptoms of allergic rhinitis. A history of exercise or cold air precipitating dyspnea or increased symptoms during specific allergen seasons also suggests asthma.
- Spirometry demonstrates obstruction (forced expiratory volume in 1 second [FEV_1]/forced vital capacity [FVC] <80%) with reversibility after inhaled β_2-agonist administration (at least a 12% improvement in FEV_1). Failure of pulmonary function to improve acutely does not necessarily rule out asthma. If baseline spirometry is normal, challenge testing with exercise, histamine, or methacholine can be used to elicit BHR.

ACUTE SEVERE ASTHMA

- Peak expiratory flow (PEF) and FEV_1 are <40% of normal predicted values. Pulse oximetry reveals decreased arterial oxygen and O_2 saturations. The best predictor of outcome is early response to treatment as measured by improvement in FEV_1 at 30 minutes after inhaled β_2-agonists.
- Arterial blood gases may reveal metabolic acidosis and a low partial pressure of oxygen (PaO_2).
- The history and physical examination should be obtained while initial therapy is being provided. A history of previous asthma exacerbations (e.g., hospitalizations and intubations) and complicating illnesses (e.g., cardiac disease and diabetes) should be obtained. The patient should be examined to assess hydration status; use of accessory muscles of respiration; and the presence of cyanosis, pneumonia, pneumothorax, pneumomediastinum, and upper airway

obstruction. A complete blood count may be appropriate for patients with fever or purulent sputum.

DESIRED OUTCOME

CHRONIC ASTHMA

- The NAEPP provides the following goals for chronic asthma management:
  - ✓ Reducing impairment: (1) prevent chronic and troublesome symptoms (e.g., coughing or breathlessness in the daytime, at night, or after exertion), (2) require infrequent use (≤2 days/wk) of inhaled short-acting β_2-agonist for quick relief of symptoms (not including prevention of exercise-induced bronchospasm [EIB]), (3) maintain (near-) normal pulmonary function, (4) maintain normal activity levels (including exercise and attendance at work or school), and (5) meet patients' and families' expectation of and satisfaction with care.
  - ✓ Reducing risk: (1) prevent recurrent exacerbations and minimize the need for emergency department visits or hospitalizations; (2) prevent loss of lung function; for children, prevent reduced lung growth; and (3) minimal or no adverse effects of therapy.

ACUTE SEVERE ASTHMA

- The goals of treatment are (1) correction of significant hypoxemia, (2) rapid reversal of airway obstruction (within minutes), (3) reduction of the likelihood of recurrence of severe airflow obstruction, and (4) development of a written action plan in case of a future exacerbation.

TREATMENT

- Fig. 81–1 depicts the NAEPP stepwise approach for managing chronic asthma. Fig. 81–2 illustrates the recommended therapies for home treatment of acute asthma exacerbations.

NONPHARMACOLOGIC THERAPY

- Patient education and the teaching of self-management skills should be the cornerstone of the treatment program. Self-management programs improve adherence to medication regimens, self-management skills, and use of healthcare services.
- Objective measurements of airflow obstruction with a home peak flow meter may not improve patient outcomes. The NAEPP advocates use of PEF monitoring only for patients with severe persistent asthma who have difficulty perceiving airway obstruction.
- Avoidance of known allergenic triggers can improve symptoms, reduce medication use, and decrease BHR. Environmental triggers (e.g., animals) should be avoided in sensitive patients, and those who smoke should be encouraged to stop.

- Patients with acute severe asthma should receive supplemental oxygen therapy to maintain arterial oxygen saturation >90% (>95% in pregnant women and patients with heart disease). Significant dehydration should be corrected; urine specific gravity may help guide therapy in young children, in whom assessment of hydration status may be difficult.

PHARMACOTHERAPY

β_2-Agonists

- The short-acting β_2-agonists (**Table 81–1**) are the most effective bronchodilators available. β_2-Adrenergic receptor stimulation activates adenyl cyclase, which produces an increase in intracellular cyclic adenosine monophosphate. This results in smooth muscle relaxation, mast cell membrane stabilization, and skeletal muscle stimulation.
- Aerosol administration enhances bronchoselectivity and provides a more rapid response and greater protection against provocations that induce bronchospasm (e.g., exercise and allergen challenges) than does systemic administration.
- **Albuterol** and other inhaled short-acting selective β_2-agonists are indicated for treatment of intermittent episodes of bronchospasm and are the first treatment of choice for acute severe asthma and EIB. Regular treatment (four times daily) does not improve symptom control over as-needed use.
- **Formoterol** and **salmeterol** are inhaled long-acting β_2-agonists indicated as adjunctive long-term control for patients with symptoms who are already on low to medium doses of inhaled corticosteroids prior to advancing to medium- or high-dose inhaled corticosteroids. Short-acting β_2-agonists should be continued for acute exacerbations. Long-acting agents are ineffective for acute severe asthma because it can take up to 20 minutes for onset and 1 to 4 hours for maximum bronchodilation after inhalation.
- In acute severe asthma, continuous nebulization of short-acting β_2-agonists (e.g., albuterol) is recommended for patients having an unsatisfactory response after three doses (every 20 min) of aerosolized β_2-agonists and potentially for patients presenting initially with PEF or FEV_1 values <30% of predicted normal. Dosing guidelines are presented in **Table 81–2**.
- Inhaled β_2-agonists agents are the treatment of choice for EIB. Short-acting agents provide complete protection for at least 2 hours after inhalation; long-acting agents provide significant protection for 8 to 12 hours initially, but the duration decreases with chronic regular use.
- In nocturnal asthma, long-acting inhaled β_2-agonists are preferred over oral sustained-release β_2-agonists or sustained-release theophylline. However, nocturnal asthma may be an indicator of inadequate antiinflammatory treatment.

Corticosteroids

- Corticosteroids increase the number of β_2-adrenergic receptors and improve receptor responsiveness to β_2-adrenergic stimulation, reduce mucus production and hypersecretion, reduce BHR, and reduce airway edema and exudation.

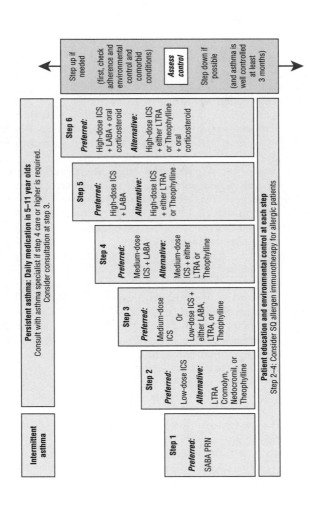

Persistent asthma: Daily medication in 5–11 year olds
Consult with asthma specialist if step 4 care or higher is required.
Consider consultation at step 3.

Intermittent asthma

Step 1
Preferred:
SABA PRN

Step 2
Preferred:
Low-dose ICS
Alternative:
LTRA,
Cromolyn,
Nedocromil, or
Theophylline

Step 3
Preferred:
Medium-dose
ICS
Or
Low-dose ICS +
either LABA,
LTRA, or
Theophylline

Step 4
Preferred:
Medium-dose
ICS + LABA
Alternative:
Medium-dose
ICS + either
LTRA or
Theophylline

Step 5
Preferred:
High-dose ICS
+ LABA
Alternative:
High-dose ICS
+ either LTRA
or Theophylline

Step 6
Preferred:
High-dose ICS
+ LABA + oral
corticosteroid
Alternative:
High-dose ICS
+ either LTRA
or Theophylline
+ oral
corticosteroid

Step up if
needed

(first, check
adherence and
environmental
control and
comorbid
conditions)

*Assess
control*

Step down if
possible

(and asthma is
well controlled
at least
3 months)

Patient education and environmental control at each step
Step 2–4: Consider SQ allergen immunotherapy for allergic patients

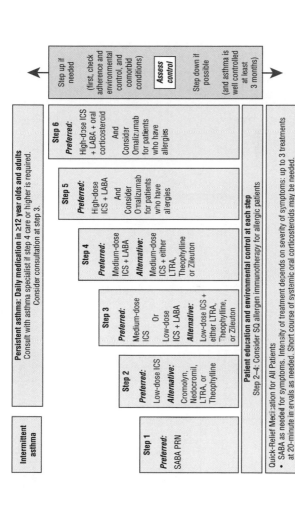

FIGURE 81–1. Stepwise approach for managing asthma in adults and children age 5 years and older. (EIB, exercise-induced bronchospasm; ICS, inhaled corticosteroid; LABA, long-acting β-agonist; LTRA, leukotriene receptor antagonist; SABA, short-acting β-agonist.) *(From NHLBI, National Asthma Education and Prevention Program. Full Report of the Expert Panel: Guidelines for the Diagnosis and Management of Asthma (EPR-3): July 2007. http://www.nhlbi.nih.gov/guidelines/asthma.)*

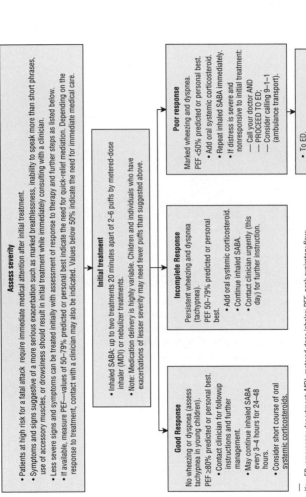

Assess severity

- Patients at high risk for a fatal attack require immediate medical attention after initial treatment.
- Symptoms and signs suggestive of a more serious exacerbation such as marked breathlessness, inability to speak more than short phrases, use of accessory muscles, or drowsiness should result in initial treatment while immediately consulting with a clinician.
- Less severe signs and symptoms can be treated initially with assessment of response to therapy and further steps as listed below.
- If available, measure PEF—values of 50–79% predicted or personal best indicate the need for quick-relief medication. Depending on the response to treatment, contact with a clinician may also be indicated. Values below 50% indicate the need for immediate medical care.

Initial treatment

- Inhaled SABA: up to two treatments 20 minutes apart of 2–6 puffs by metered-dose inhaler (MDI) or nebulizer treatments.
- Note: Medication delivery is highly variable. Children and individuals who have exacerbations of lesser severity may need fewer puffs than suggested above.

Good Response

No wheezing or dyspnea (assess tachypnea in young children).
PEF ≥80% predicted or personal best.
- Contact clinician for followup instructions and further management.
- May continue inhaled SABA every 3–4 hours for 24–48 hours.
- Consider short course of oral systemic corticosteroids.

Incomplete Response

Persistent wheezing and dyspnea (tachypnea).
PEF 50–79% predicted or personal best.
- Add oral systemic corticosteroid.
- Continue inhaled SABA.
- Contact clinician urgently (this day) for further instruction.

Poor response

Marked wheezing and dyspnea.
PEF <50% predicted or personal best.
- Add oral systemic corticosteroid.
- Repeat inhaled SABA immediately.
- If distress is severe and nonresponsive to initial treatment:
  — Call your doctor AND
  — PROCEED TO ED;
  — Consider calling 9-1-1 (ambulance transport).

- To ED.

Key: ED, emergency department; MDI, metered-dose inhaler; PEF, peak expiratory flow; SABA, short-acting beta₂-agonist (quick-relief inhaler)

FIGURE 81–2. Home management of acute asthma exacerbation. Patients at risk of asthma-related death should receive immediate clinical attention after initial treatment. Additional therapy may be required. *(From NHLBI, National Asthma Education and Prevention Program. Full Report of the Expert Panel: Guidelines for the Diagnosis and Management of Asthma (EPR-3); July 2007. http://www.nhlbi.nih.gov/guidelines/asthma.)*

TABLE 81-1	Relative Selectivity, Potency, and Duration of Action of the β-Adrenergic Agonists					
	Selectivity			**Duration of Action**[b]		
Agent	β_1	β_2	Potency, β_2[a]	*Bronchodilation (Hours)*	*Protection (Hours)*[c]	Oral Activity
Isoproterenol	+ + + +	+ + + +	1	0.5–2	0.5–1	No
Albuterol	+	+ + + +	2	4–8	2–4	Yes
Pirbuterol	+	+ + + +	5	4–8	2–4	Yes
Terbutaline	+	+ + + +	4	4–8	2–4	Yes
Formoterol	+	+ + + +	0.12	≥12	6–12	Yes
Salmeterol	+	+ + + +	0.5	≥12	6–12	No

[a]Relative molar potency to isoproterenol: 15, lowest potency.
[b]Median durations with the highest value after a single dose and lowest after chronic administration.
[c]*Protection* refers to the prevention of bronchoconstriction induced by exercise or nonspecific bronchial challenges.

- Inhaled corticosteroids are the preferred long-term control therapy for persistent asthma in all patients because of their potency and consistent effectiveness; they are also the only therapy shown to reduce the risk of dying from asthma. Comparative doses are included in Table 81–3. Most patients with moderate disease can be controlled with twice-daily dosing; some products have once-daily dosing indications. Patients with more severe disease require multiple daily dosing. Because the inflammatory response of asthma inhibits steroid receptor binding, patients should be started on higher and more frequent doses and then tapered down once control has been achieved. The response to inhaled corticosteroids is delayed; symptoms improve in most patients within the first 1 to 2 weeks and reach maximum improvement in 4 to 8 weeks. Maximum improvement in FEV₁ and PEF rates may require 3 to 6 weeks.
- Systemic toxicity of inhaled corticosteroids is minimal with low to moderate inhaled doses, but the risk of systemic effects increases with high doses. Local adverse effects include dose-dependent oropharyngeal candidiasis and dysphonia, which can be reduced by the use of a spacer device. The ability of spacer devices to enhance lung delivery is inconsistent and should not be relied on.
- Systemic corticosteroids (Table 81–4) are indicated in all patients with acute severe asthma not responding completely to initial inhaled β_2-agonist administration (every 20 min for three or four doses) Prednisone, 1 to 2 mg/kg/day (up to 40–60 mg/day), is administered orally in two divided doses for 3 to 10 days. Because short-term (1–2 wk), high-dose systemic steroids do not produce serious toxicities, the ideal method is to use a short burst and then maintain the patient on appropriate long-term control therapy with inhaled corticosteroids.
- In patients who require chronic systemic corticosteroids for asthma control, the lowest possible dose should be used. Toxicities may be decreased by alternate-day therapy or high-dose inhaled corticosteroids.

TABLE 81–2 Dosages of Drugs for Acute Severe Exacerbations of Asthma in the Emergency Department or Hospital

Medications	Dosages		Comments
	≥12 Years Old	<12 Years Old	
Inhaled β-agonists			
Albuterol nebulizer solution (5 mg/mL, 0.63 mg/3 mL, 1.25 mg/3 mL, 2.5 mg/3 mL)	2.5–5 mg every 20 min for three doses, then 2.5–10 mg every 1–4 hours as needed, or 10–15 mg/hour continuously	0.15 mg/kg (minimum dose 2.5 mg) every 20 min for three doses, then 0.15–0.3 mg/kg up to 10 mg every 1–4 hours as needed, or 0.5 mg/kg/hour by continuous nebulization	Only selective β₂-agonists are recommended; for optimal delivery, dilute aerosols to minimum of 4 mL at gas flow of 6–8 L/min
Albuterol MDI (90 mcg/puff)	4–8 puffs every 30 minutes up to 4 hours, then every 1–4 hours as needed	4–8 puffs every 20 min for three doses, then every 1–4 hours as needed	In patients in severe distress, nebulization is preferred
Levalbuterol nebulizer solution (0.31 mg/3 mL, 0.63 mg/3 mL, 2.5 mg/1 mL, 1.25 mg/3 mL)	Give at one-half the mg dose of albuterol above	Give at one-half the mg dose of albuterol above	The single isomer of albuterol is twice as potent on a mg basis
Levalbuterol MDI (45 mcg/puff)	See albuterol MDI dose	See albuterol MDI dose	
Pirbuterol MDI (200 mcg/puff)	See albuterol dose	See albuterol dose; one-half as potent as albuterol on a mcg basis	Has not been studied in acute severe asthma
Systemic β-agonists			
Epinephrine 1:1,000 (1 mg/mL)	0.3–0.5 mg every 20 min for three doses subcutaneously	0.01 mg/kg up to 0.5 mg every 20 min for three doses subcutaneously	No proven advantage of systemic therapy over aerosol
Terbutaline (1 mg/mL)	0.25 mg every 20 min for three doses subcutaneously	0.01 mg/kg every 20 min for three doses, then every 2–6 hours as needed subcutaneously	Not recommended

Anticholinergics

Ipratropium bromide nebulizer solution (0.25 mg/mL)	500 mcg every 30 min for three doses, then every 2–4 hours as needed	250 mcg every 20 min for 3 doses, then 250 mcg every 2–4 hours	May mix in same nebulizer with albuterol; do not use as first-line therapy; only add to β_2-agonist therapy
Ipratropium bromide MDI (18 mcg/puff)	8 puffs every 20 min as needed for up to 3 hours	4–8 puffs every 20 min as needed for up to 3 hours	

Corticosteroids

Prednisone, methylprednisolone, prednisolone	40–80 mg/day in one or two divided doses until FEF reaches 70% of predicted or personal best	1–2 mg/kg/day in two divided doses (max 60 mg/day) until PEF is 70% of predicted or personal best	For outpatient "burst," use 1–2 mg/kg/day (max 60 mg) for 3–10 days in children and 40–60 mg/day in one or two divided doses for 5–10 days in adults

FEV_1, forced expiratory volume in the first second of expiration; MDI, metered-dose inhaler; PEF, peak expiratory flow.

Note: No advantage has been found for very-high-dose corticosteroids in acute severe asthma, nor is there any advantage for IV administration over oral therapy. The usual regimen is to continue the oral corticosteroid for the duration of hospitalization. The final duration of therapy following a hospitalization or emergency department visit may be from 3 to 10 days. If the patient is then started on inhaled corticosteroids, there is no need to taper the systemic corticosteroid dose. The inhaled corticosteroids can be started at any time during the exacerbation.

| **TABLE 81–3** | Available Inhaled Corticosteroid Products, Lung Delivery, and Comparative Daily Dosages |

Inhaled Corticosteroids	Product	Lung Delivery[a]
Beclomethasone dipropionate (BDP)	40 and 80 mcg/actuation HFA MDI, 120 actuations	55–60%
Budesonide (BUD)	90 or 180 mcg/dose DPI, Flexhaler, 200 doses	32% (15–30%)
	200 and 500 mcg ampules, 2 mL each	5–8%
Ciclesonide (CIC)	80 or 160 mcg/actuation HFA MDI	50%
Flunisolide (FLU)	250 mcg/actuation CFC MDI, 100 actuations	20%
	80 mcg/actuation HFA MDI, 120 actuations	68%
Fluticasone propionate (FP)	44, 110, and 220 mcg/actuation HFA MDI, 120 actuations	20%
	50, 100, and 250 mcg/dose DPI, Diskus, 60 doses	15%
Mometasone furoate (MF)	110 and 220 mcg/dose DPI, Twisthaler, 14, 30, 60, and 120 doses	11%

	Comparative Daily Dosages (mcg) of Inhaled Corticosteroids		
	Low Daily Dose Child[a]/Adult	**Medium Daily Dose Child[a]/Adult**	**High Daily Dose Child[a]/Adult**
BDP			
HFA MDI	80–160/80–240	>160–320/>240–480	>320/>480
BUD			
DPI	180–360/180–540	>360–720/>540–1,080	>720/>1,080
Nebules	500/UK	1,000/UK	2,000/UK
CIC	80–160/160–320	>160–320/>320/640	>320/>640
FLU			
CFC MDI	500–750/500–1,000	1,000–1,250/1,000–2,000	>1,250/>2,000
HFA MDI	160/320	320/320–640	≥640/>640
FP			
HFA MDI	88–176/88–264	176–352/264–440	>352/>440
DPIs	100–200/100–300	200–400/300–500	>400/>500
MF, DPI	110/220	220–440/440	>440/>400

CFC, chlorofluorocarbon; DPI, dry-powder inhaler; HFA, hydrofluoroalkane; MDI, metered-dose inhaler.
[a]Five to 11 years of age, except for BUD Nebules, which is 2 to 11 years of age.

TABLE 81–4 Comparison of the Systemic Corticosteroids

Systemic	Antiinflammatory Potency	Mineralocorticoid Potency	Duration of Biologic Activity (Hours)	Elimination Half-Life (Hours)
Hydrocortisone	1	1	8–12	1.5–2
Prednisone	4	0.8	12–36	2.5–3.5
Methylprednisolone	5	0.5	12–36	3.3
Dexamethasone	25	0	36–54	3.4–4

Methylxanthines

- **Theophylline** appears to produce bronchodilation through nonselective phosphodiesterase inhibition. Methylxanthines are ineffective by aerosol and must be taken systemically (orally or IV). Sustained-release theophylline is the preferred oral preparation, whereas its complex with ethylenediamine (**aminophylline**) is the preferred parenteral product due to increased solubility. IV theophylline is also available.
- Theophylline is eliminated primarily by metabolism via hepatic cytochrome P450 mixed-function oxidase microsomal enzymes (primarily CYP1A2 and CYP3A4) with ≤10% excreted unchanged in the kidney. The hepatic cytochrome P450 enzymes are susceptible to induction and inhibition by various environmental factors and drugs. Clinically significant reductions in clearance can result from cotherapy with cimetidine, erythromycin, clarithromycin, allopurinol, propranolol, ciprofloxacin, interferon, ticlopidine, zileuton, and other drugs. Some substances that enhance clearance are rifampin, carbamazepine, phenobarbital, phenytoin, charcoal-broiled meat, and cigarette smoking.
- Because of large interpatient variability in theophylline clearance, routine monitoring of serum theophylline concentrations is essential for safe and effective use. A steady-state range of 5 to 15 mcg/mL is effective and safe for most patients.
- Fig. 81–3 gives recommended dosages, monitoring schedules, and dosage adjustments for theophylline.
- Sustained-release oral preparations are favored for outpatient therapy, but each product has different release characteristics, and some products are susceptible to altered absorption from food or gastric pH changes. Preparations unaffected by food that can be administered a minimum of every 12 hours in most patients are preferable.
- Adverse effects include nausea, vomiting, tachycardia, jitteriness, and difficulty sleeping; more severe toxicities include cardiac tachyarrhythmias and seizures.
- Sustained-release theophylline is less effective than inhaled corticosteroids and no more effective than oral sustained-release β_2-agonists, cromolyn, or leukotriene antagonists.

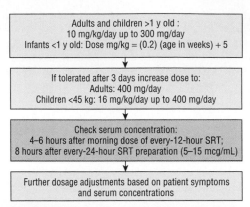

FIGURE 81–3. Algorithm for slow titration of theophylline dosage and guide for final dosage adjustment based on serum theophylline concentration measurement. For infants younger than 1 year of age, the initial daily dosage can be calculated by the following regression equation:

$$\text{Dose (mg/kg)} = (0.2)\,(\text{age in weeks}) + 5.$$

Whenever side effects occur, dosage should be reduced to a previously tolerated lower dose. (SRT, sustained-release theophylline.)

- The addition of theophylline to optimal inhaled corticosteroids is similar to doubling the dose of the inhaled corticosteroid and is less effective overall than the long-acting β_2-agonists as adjunctive therapy.

Anticholinergics

- **Ipratropium bromide** and **tiotropium bromide** are competitive inhibitors of muscarinic receptors; they produce bronchodilation only in cholinergic-mediated bronchoconstriction. Anticholinergics are effective bronchodilators but are not as effective as β_2-agonists. They attenuate but do not block allergen- or exercise-induced asthma in a dose-dependent fashion.
- The time to reach maximum bronchodilation from aerosolized ipratropium is longer than from aerosolized short-acting β_2-agonists (30–60 min vs 5–10 min). This is of little clinical consequence because some bronchodilation is seen within 30 seconds, and 50% of maximum response occurs within 3 minutes. Ipratropium bromide has a duration of action of 4 to 8 hours; tiotropium bromide has a duration of 24 hours.
- Inhaled ipratropium bromide is only indicated as adjunctive therapy in severe acute asthma not completely responsive to β_2-agonists alone because it does not improve outcomes in chronic asthma. Studies of tiotropium bromide in asthma are ongoing.

Mast Cell Stabilizers

- **Cromolyn sodium** has beneficial effects that are believed to result from stabilization of mast cell membranes. It inhibits the response to allergen challenge as well as EIB but does not cause bronchodilation.

- Cromolyn is effective only by inhalation and is available as a metered-dose inhaler and nebulizer solution. Cough and wheezing have been reported after inhalation.
- Cromolyn is indicated for the prophylaxis of mild persistent asthma in children and adults regardless of etiology. Its effectiveness is comparable to theophylline or leukotriene antagonists for persistent asthma. It is as effective as inhaled corticosteroids for controlling persistent asthma. It is not as effective as the inhaled β_2-agonists for preventing EIB, but it can be used in conjunction for patients not responding completely to inhaled β_2-agonists.
- Most patients experience improvement in 1 to 2 weeks, but it may take longer to achieve maximum benefit. Patients should initially receive cromolyn four times daily; after stabilization of symptoms, the frequency may be reduced to three times daily.

Leukotriene Modifiers

- **Zafirlukast** (Accolate) and **montelukast** (Singulair) are oral leukotriene receptor antagonists that reduce the proinflammatory (increased microvascular permeability and airway edema) and bronchoconstriction effects of leukotriene D_4. In adults and children with persistent asthma, they improve pulmonary function tests, decrease nocturnal awakenings and β_2-agonist use, and improve asthma symptoms. However, they are less effective in asthma than low-dose inhaled corticosteroids. They are not used to treat acute exacerbations and must be taken on a regular basis, even during symptom-free periods. The adult dose of zafirlukast is 20 mg twice daily, taken at least 1 hour before or 2 hours after meals; the dose for children ages 5 through 11 years is 10 mg twice daily. For montelukast, the adult dose is 10 mg once daily, taken in the evening without regard to food; the dose for children ages 6 to 14 years is one 5 mg chewable tablet daily in the evening.
- Zafirlukast and montelukast are generally well tolerated. Rare elevations in serum aminotransferase concentrations and clinical hepatitis have been reported. An idiosyncratic syndrome similar to the Churg–Strauss syndrome, with marked circulating eosinophilia, heart failure, and associated eosinophilic vasculitis, has been reported in a small number of patients; a direct causal association has not been established.
- **Zileuton** (Zyflo) is a 5-lipoxygenase inhibitor; its use is limited due to the potential for elevated hepatic enzymes, especially in the first 3 months of therapy, and inhibition of the metabolism of some drugs metabolized by CYP3A4 (e.g., theophylline and warfarin). The dose of zileuton tablets is 600 mg four times daily with meals and at bedtime. The recommended dose of zileuton extended-release tablets is two 600 mg tablets twice daily, within 1 hour after morning and evening meals (total daily dose 2,400 mg).

Combination Controller Therapy

- The addition of a second long-term control medication to inhaled corticosteroid therapy is one recommended treatment option in moderate to severe persistent asthma.

- Single-inhaler combination products containing fluticasone propionate and salmeterol (Advair) or budesonide and formoterol (Symbicort) are currently available. The inhalers contain varied doses of the inhaled corticosteroid with a fixed dose of the long-acting β_2-agonist. The addition of a long-acting β_2-agonist allows a 50% reduction in inhaled corticosteroid dosage in most patients with persistent asthma. Combination therapy is more effective than higher-dose inhaled corticosteroids alone in reducing asthma exacerbations in patients with persistent asthma.

Omalizumab

- **Omalizumab** (Xolair) is an anti-IgE antibody approved for the treatment of allergic asthma not well controlled by oral or inhaled corticosteroids. The dosage is determined by the patient's baseline total serum IgE (international units/mL) and body weight (kg). Doses range from 150 to 375 mg given subcutaneously at either 2- or 4-week intervals.
- Because of its high cost, it is only indicated as step 5 or 6 care for patients who have allergies and severe persistent asthma that is inadequately controlled with the combination of high-dose inhaled corticosteroids and long-acting β_2-agonists and at risk for severe exacerbations.
- Because it is associated with a 0.2% incidence of anaphylaxis, patients should remain in the physician's office for a reasonable period after the injection because 70% of reactions occur within 2 hours. Some reactions have occurred up to 24 hours after injection.

EVALUATION OF THERAPEUTIC OUTCOMES

CHRONIC ASTHMA

- Control of asthma is defined as reducing both impairment and risk domains. Regular follow-up is essential at 1- to 6-month intervals, depending on control.
- Components of the assessment of control include symptoms, nighttime awakenings, interference with normal activities, pulmonary function, quality of life, exacerbations, adherence, treatment-related adverse effects, and satisfaction with care. The categories of well controlled, not well controlled, and very poorly controlled are recommended. Validated questionnaires can be administered regularly, such as the Asthma Therapy Assessment Questionnaire, Asthma Control Questionnaire, and Asthma Control Test.
- Spirometric tests are recommended at initial assessment, after treatment is initiated, and then every 1 to 2 years. Peak flow monitoring is recommended in moderate to severe persistent asthma.
- Patients should also be asked about exercise tolerance.
- All patients on inhaled drugs should have their inhalation technique evaluated monthly initially and then every 3 to 6 months.
- After initiation of antiinflammatory therapy or an increase in dosage, most patients should begin experiencing a decrease in symptoms within 1 to 2 weeks and achieve maximum symptomatic improvement within

4 to 8 weeks. Improvement in baseline FEV_1 or PEF should follow a similar time frame, but a decrease in BHR as measured by morning PEF, PEF variability, and exercise tolerance may take longer and improve over 1 to 3 months.

ACUTE SEVERE ASTHMA

- Patients at risk for acute severe exacerbations should monitor morning peak flows at home.
- Lung function, either spirometry or peak flows, should be monitored 5 to 10 minutes after each treatment.
- Oxygen saturations can be easily monitored continuously with pulse oximetry. For young children and adults, pulse oximetry, lung auscultation, and observation for supraclavicular retractions are useful.
- Most patients respond within the first hour of initial inhaled β-agonists. Patients not achieving an initial response should be monitored every 0.5 to 1 hour.

See Chapter 33, Asthma, authored by H. William Kelly and Christine A. Sorkness, for a more detailed discussion of this topic.

Chronic Obstructive Pulmonary Disease

DEFINITIONS

- Chronic obstructive pulmonary disease (COPD) is a treatable and preventable disease characterized by airflow limitation that is not fully reversible. The airflow limitation is progressive and associated with abnormal inflammatory response of the lungs to noxious particles or gases. The two principal conditions comprising COPD are chronic bronchitis and emphysema.

- Chronic bronchitis is associated with chronic or recurrent excess mucus secretion into the bronchial tree with cough that occurs on most days for at least 3 months of the year for at least 2 consecutive years when other causes of cough have been excluded.

- Emphysema is defined as abnormal, permanent enlargement of the airspaces distal to the terminal bronchioles, accompanied by destruction of their walls, but without obvious fibrosis.

PATHOPHYSIOLOGY

- COPD is characterized by chronic inflammatory changes that lead to destructive changes and chronic airflow limitation. The most common etiology is exposure to environmental tobacco smoke, but other chronic inhalational exposures can also lead to COPD.

- Inhalation of noxious particles and gases stimulates the activation of neutrophils, macrophages, and CD8+ lymphocytes, which release a variety of chemical mediators, including tumor necrosis factor-α, interleukin-8, and leukotriene B_4. These inflammatory cells and mediators lead to widespread destructive changes in the airways, pulmonary vasculature, and lung parenchyma.

- Other pathophysiologic processes may include oxidative stress and an imbalance between aggressive and protective defense systems in the lungs (proteases and antiproteases). Increased oxidants generated by cigarette smoke react with and damage various proteins and lipids, leading to cell and tissue damage. Oxidants also promote inflammation directly and exacerbate the protease–antiprotease imbalance by inhibiting antiprotease activity.

- The protective antiprotease α_1-antitrypsin (AAT) inhibits several protease enzymes, including neutrophil elastase. In the presence of unopposed AAT activity, elastase attacks elastin, which is a major component of alveolar walls. A hereditary deficiency of AAT results in an increased risk for premature development of emphysema. In the inherited disease, there is an absolute deficiency of AAT. In emphysema resulting from cigarette smoking, the imbalance is associated with increased protease activity or reduced activity of antiproteases. Activated inflammatory cells release several other proteases, including cathepsins and metalloproteinases. In addition, oxidative stress reduces antiprotease (or protective) activity.

- An inflammatory exudate is often present in the airways that leads to an increased number and size of goblet cells and mucus glands. Mucus secretion increases, and ciliary motility is impaired. There is thickening of the smooth muscle and connective tissue in the airways. Chronic inflammation leads to scarring and fibrosis. Diffuse airway narrowing occurs and is more prominent in small peripheral airways.
- Parenchymal changes affect the gas-exchanging units of the lungs (alveoli and pulmonary capillaries). Smoking-related disease most commonly results in centrilobular emphysema that primarily affects respiratory bronchioles. Panlobular emphysema is seen in AAT deficiency and extends to the alveolar ducts and sacs.
- Vascular changes include thickening of pulmonary vessels that may lead to endothelial dysfunction of the pulmonary arteries. Later, structural changes increase pulmonary pressures, especially during exercise. In severe COPD, secondary pulmonary hypertension leads to right-sided heart failure (cor pulmonale).

CLINICAL PRESENTATION

- Initial symptoms of COPD include chronic cough and sputum production; patients may have these symptoms for several years before dyspnea develops.
- The physical examination is normal in most patients who present in the milder stages of COPD. When airflow limitation becomes severe, patients may have cyanosis of mucosal membranes, development of a "barrel chest" due to hyperinflation of the lungs, an increased resting respiratory rate, shallow breathing, pursing of the lips during expiration, and use of accessory respiratory muscles.
- Patients experiencing a COPD exacerbation may have worsening dyspnea, increase in sputum volume, or increase in sputum purulence. Other common features of an exacerbation include chest tightness, increased need for bronchodilators, malaise, fatigue, and decreased exercise tolerance.

DIAGNOSIS

- The diagnosis of COPD is based in part on the patient's symptoms and a history of exposure to risk factors such as tobacco smoke and occupational exposures.

SPIROMETRY

- Assessment of airflow limitation through spirometry is the standard for diagnosing and monitoring COPD. The forced expiratory volume after 1 second (FEV_1) is generally reduced except in very mild disease. The forced vital capacity (FVC) may also be decreased. The hallmark of COPD is a reduced FEV_1:FVC ratio to <70%. A postbronchodilator FEV_1 that is <80% of predicted confirms the presence of airflow limitation that is not fully reversible.

- An improvement in FEV_1 of less than 12% after inhalation of a rapid-acting bronchodilator is considered to be evidence of irreversible airflow obstruction.
- Peak expiratory flow measurements are not adequate for the diagnosis of COPD because of low specificity and a high degree of effort dependence. However, a low peak expiratory flow is consistent with COPD.

ARTERIAL BLOOD GASES

- Significant changes in arterial blood gases (ABG) are not usually present until the FEV_1 is <1 L. At this stage, hypoxemia and hypercapnia may become chronic problems. Hypoxemia usually occurs initially with exercise but develops at rest as the disease progresses.
- Patients with severe COPD can have a low arterial oxygen tension (partial pressure of O_2 [Pao_2] 45–60 mm Hg) and an elevated arterial carbon dioxide tension (partial pressure of CO_2 [$Paco_2$] 50–60 mm Hg). Hypoxemia results from hypoventilation (V) of lung tissue relative to perfusion (Q) of the area. The low V:Q ratio progresses over several years, resulting in a consistent decline in the Pao_2.
- Some patients lose the ability to increase the rate or depth of respiration in response to persistent hypoxemia. This decreased ventilatory drive may be due to abnormal peripheral or central respiratory receptor responses. This relative hypoventilation leads to hypercapnia; in this situation, the central respiratory response to a chronically increased $Paco_2$ can be blunted. Because these changes in Pao_2 and $Paco_2$ are subtle and progress over many years, the pH is usually near normal because the kidneys compensate by retaining bicarbonate.
- If acute respiratory distress develops (e.g., due to pneumonia or a COPD exacerbation), the $Paco_2$ may rise sharply, resulting in an uncompensated respiratory acidosis.

DIAGNOSIS OF ACUTE RESPIRATORY FAILURE IN CHRONIC OBSTRUCTIVE PULMONARY DISEASE

- The diagnosis of acute respiratory failure in COPD is made on the basis of an acute drop in Pao_2 of 10 to 15 mm Hg or any acute increase in $Paco_2$ that decreases the serum pH to ≤7.3.
- Additional acute clinical manifestations include restlessness, confusion, tachycardia, diaphoresis, cyanosis, hypotension, irregular breathing, miosis, and unconsciousness.
- The most common cause of acute respiratory failure in COPD is acute exacerbation of bronchitis with an increase in sputum volume and viscosity. This worsens obstruction and further impairs alveolar ventilation, thereby worsening hypoxemia and hypercapnia. Additional causes are pneumonia, pulmonary embolism, left ventricular failure, pneumothorax, and CNS depressants.

DESIRED OUTCOME

- The goals of therapy are to prevent or minimize disease progression, relieve symptoms, improve exercise tolerance, improve overall health status, prevent and treat exacerbations, prevent and treat complications, and reduce morbidity and mortality.

TREATMENT OF COPD

NONPHARMACOLOGIC THERAPY

- Smoking cessation is the most effective strategy to reduce the risk of developing COPD and the only intervention proven to affect the long-term decline in FEV_1 and slow the progression of COPD.
- Pulmonary rehabilitation programs include exercise training along with smoking cessation, breathing exercises, optimal medical treatment, psychosocial support, and health education.
- Annual vaccination with the inactivated intramuscular influenza vaccine is recommended.
- One dose of the polyvalent pneumococcal vaccine is indicated for patients at any age with COPD; revaccination is recommended for patients older than 65 years if the first vaccination was more than 5 years earlier and the patient was younger than age 65 years.
- Supplemental O_2 therapy increases survival in COPD patients with chronic hypoxemia. Once patients are stabilized as outpatients and pharmacotherapy is optimized, long-term O_2 therapy should be instituted if either the resting Pao_2 is <55 mm Hg or there is evidence of right-sided heart failure, polycythemia, or impaired neuropsychiatric function with a Pao_2<60 mm Hg. The most practical means of long-term O_2 delivery is via nasal cannula at 1 to 2 L/min, which provides 25% to 28% O_2. The goal is to raise the Pao_2 above 60 mm Hg.

PHARMACOLOGIC THERAPY

- Pharmacotherapy of COPD typically involves use of inhaled medications. A stepwise approach to managing stable COPD based on severity is shown in Fig. 82–1. Bronchodilators are used to control symptoms; no single pharmacologic class has been proven to provide superior benefit over others. Medication selection is based on likely patient adherence, individual response, and side effects. Medications can be used as needed or on a scheduled basis, and therapies should be added in a stepwise manner depending on response and disease severity. Bronchodilators relieve symptoms such as dyspnea, increase exercise capacity, and decrease air trapping. However, significant improvements in pulmonary function measurements such as FEV_1 may not be observed.
- Short-acting bronchodilators are the initial therapy for patients with COPD who experience intermittent symptoms. Short-acting β_2-agonists and anticholinergics are equally effective.
- Long-acting bronchodilators are recommended for patients with moderate to severe COPD who experience symptoms on a regular basis or in whom short-acting therapies do not provide adequate relief. These bronchodilators can be administered as either an inhaled long-acting β_2-agonist (LABA) or anticholinergic.

	I: Mild	II: Moderate	III: Severe	IV: Very severe
Characteristics	• FEV$_1$:FVC <70% • FEV$_1$ ≥80% • With or without symptoms	• FEV$_1$:FVC <70% • 50% > FEV$_1$ <80% • With or without symptoms	• FEV$_1$:FVC <70% • 30% > FEV$_1$ <50% • With or without symptoms	• FEV$_1$:FVC <70% • FEV$_1$ <30% or presence of chronic respiratory failure or right heart failure
	Avoidance of risk factor(s); influenza vaccination, pneumococcal vaccine			
	Add short-acting bronchodilator when needed			
		Add regular treatment with one or more long-acting bronchodilators *Add* rehabilitation		
			Add inhaled corticosteroids if repeated exacerbations	
				Add long-term oxygen if chronic respiratory failure *Consider* surgical treatments

FIGURE 82–1. Recommended therapy of stable chronic obstructive pulmonary disease (COPD). (FEV$_1$, forced expiratory volume in the first second of expiration; FVC, forced vital capacity.) *(From Global Initiative for Chronic Obstructive Lung Disease. Global Strategy for the Diagnosis, Management and Prevention of Chronic Obstructive Pulmonary Disease. NHLBI/WHO workshop report. Bethesda, MD: National Heart, Lung and Blood Institute, April 2001; updated November 2009. Available at http://www.goldcopd.com.)*

Sympathomimetics

- β_2-Selective sympathomimetics cause relaxation of bronchial smooth muscle and bronchodilation by stimulating the enzyme adenyl cyclase to increase the formation of cyclic adenosine monophosphate (cAMP). They may also improve mucociliary clearance.
- Administration via metered-dose inhaler (MDI) or dry-powder inhaler is at least as effective as nebulization therapy and is usually favored for reasons of cost and convenience. Refer to Table 81–1 in Chap. 81 for a comparison of the available agents.
- **Albuterol, levalbuterol, bitolterol, pirbuterol**, and **terbutaline** are the preferred short-acting agents because they have greater β_2 selectivity and longer durations of action than other short-acting agents (isoproterenol, metaproterenol, and isoetharine). The inhalation route is preferred to the oral and parenteral routes in terms of both efficacy and adverse effects.
- Short-acting agents can be used for acute relief of symptoms or on a scheduled basis to prevent or reduce symptoms. The duration of action of short-acting β_2-agonists is 4 to 6 hours.
- **Salmeterol, formoterol**, and **arformoterol** are LABAs that are dosed every 12 hours on a scheduled basis and provide bronchodilation throughout the dosing interval. In addition to providing greater convenience for patients with persistent symptoms, LABAs produce superior outcomes in terms of lung function, symptom relief, reductions in exacerbation frequency, and quality of life when compared with short-acting β_2-agonists. These agents are not recommended for acute relief of symptoms.

Anticholinergics

- When given by inhalation, anticholinergic agents produce bronchodilation by competitively inhibiting cholinergic receptors in bronchial smooth muscle. This activity blocks acetylcholine, with the net effect being a reduction in cyclic guanosine monophosphate, which normally acts to constrict bronchial smooth muscle.
- **Ipratropium bromide** is the primary short-acting anticholinergic agent used for COPD in the United States. It has a slower onset of action than short-acting β_2-agonists (15–20 min vs 5 min for albuterol). For this reason, it may be less suitable for as-needed use, but it is often prescribed in this manner. Ipratropium has a more prolonged bronchodilator effect than short-acting β_2-agonists. Its peak effect occurs in 1.5 to 2 hours, and its duration is 4 to 6 hours. The recommended dose via MDI is two puffs four times daily with upward titration often to 24 puffs/day. It is also available as a solution for nebulization. The most frequent patient complaints are dry mouth, nausea, and, occasionally, metallic taste. Because it is poorly absorbed systemically, anticholinergic side effects are uncommon (e.g., blurred vision, urinary retention, nausea, and tachycardia).
- **Tiotropium bromide** is a long-acting agent that protects against cholinergic bronchoconstriction for more than 24 hours. Its onset of effect is within 30 minutes, with a peak effect in 3 hours. It is delivered via the HandiHaler, a single-load, dry-powder, breath-actuated device. The recommended dose is inhalation of the contents of one capsule (18 mcg) once daily using the HandiHaler inhalation device. Because it acts locally, tiotropium is well tolerated; the most common complaint is dry mouth. Other anticholinergic effects have also been reported.

Combination Anticholinergics and Sympathomimetics

- The combination of an inhaled anticholinergic and β_2-agonist is often used, especially as the disease progresses and symptoms worsen over time. Combining bronchodilators with different mechanisms of action allows the lowest effective doses to be used and reduces adverse effects from individual agents. The combination of both short- and long-acting β_2-agonists with ipratropium has been shown to provide added symptomatic relief and improvements in pulmonary function.
- A combination product containing **albuterol** and **ipratropium** (**Combivent**) is available as an MDI for chronic maintenance therapy of COPD.

Methylxanthines

- **Theophylline** and **aminophylline** may produce bronchodilation by inhibition of phosphodiesterase (thereby increasing cAMP levels) and other mechanisms.
- Chronic theophylline use in COPD produces improvements in lung function, including vital capacity and FEV_1. Subjectively, theophylline reduces dyspnea, increases exercise tolerance, and improves respiratory drive. Nonpulmonary benefits may include improved cardiac function and decreased pulmonary artery pressure.

- Methylxanthines have a very limited role in COPD therapy. Inhaled bronchodilator therapy is preferred because of theophylline's risk for drug interactions and interpatient variability in dosage requirements. Theophylline may be considered in patients who are intolerant or unable to use an inhaled bronchodilator. A methylxanthine may also be added to the regimen of patients who have not achieved an optimal clinical response to an inhaled anticholinergic and β_2-agonist.
- As with other bronchodilators in COPD, parameters other than objective measurements such as FEV_1 should be monitored to assess efficacy. Subjective parameters, such as perceived improvements in dyspnea and exercise tolerance, are important in assessing the acceptability of methylxanthines for COPD patients.
- Sustained-release theophylline preparations improve patient compliance and achieve more consistent serum concentrations than rapid-release theophylline and aminophylline preparations. Caution should be used in switching from one sustained-release preparation to another because there are considerable variations in sustained-release characteristics.
- Theophylline maintenance therapy in nonacutely ill patients can be initiated at 200 mg twice daily and titrated upward every 3 to 5 days to the target dose; most patients require daily doses of 400 to 900 mg.
- Dose adjustments should be made based on trough serum concentrations. A therapeutic range of 8 to 15 mcg/mL is often targeted, especially in elderly patients, to minimize the likelihood of toxicity. Once a dose is established, concentrations should be monitored once or twice a year unless the disease worsens, medications that interfere with theophylline metabolism are added, or toxicity is suspected.
- The most common side effects of theophylline include dyspepsia, nausea, vomiting, diarrhea, headache, dizziness, and tachycardia. Arrhythmias and seizures may occur, especially at toxic concentrations.
- Factors that may decrease theophylline clearance and lead to reduced dosage requirements include advanced age, bacterial or viral pneumonia, heart failure, liver dysfunction, hypoxemia from acute decompensation, and use of drugs such as cimetidine, macrolides, and fluoroquinolone antibiotics.
- Factors that may enhance theophylline clearance and result in the need for higher doses include tobacco and marijuana smoking, hyperthyroidism, and use of drugs such as phenytoin, phenobarbital, and rifampin.

Corticosteroids

- The antiinflammatory mechanisms whereby corticosteroids exert their beneficial effect in COPD include reduction in capillary permeability to decrease mucus, inhibition of release of proteolytic enzymes from leukocytes, and inhibition of prostaglandins.
- The clinical benefits of systemic corticosteroid therapy in the chronic management of COPD are often not evident, and there is a high risk of toxicity. Consequently, chronic, systemic corticosteroids should be avoided if possible.
- Appropriate situations to consider corticosteroids in COPD include (1) short-term systemic use for acute exacerbations and (2) inhalation therapy for chronic stable COPD.

- The role of inhaled corticosteroids in COPD is controversial. Major clinical trials did not demonstrate any benefit from chronic treatment in modifying long-term decline in lung function. However, other important benefits in some patients may include a decrease in exacerbation frequency and improvements in overall health status.
- The current recommended role of inhaled corticosteroid therapy is for COPD patients with moderate to severe airflow obstruction (FEV_1<50% predicted) who experience frequent exacerbations despite bronchodilator therapy.
- Side effects of inhaled corticosteroids are relatively mild and include hoarseness, sore throat, oral candidiasis, and skin bruising. Severe side effects such as adrenal suppression, osteoporosis, and cataract formation are reported less frequently than with systemic corticosteroids, but clinicians should monitor patients receiving high-dose chronic inhaled therapy.
- Several studies have shown an additive effect with the combination of inhaled corticosteroids and long-acting bronchodilators. Combination therapy with salmeterol plus fluticasone or formoterol plus budesonide is associated with greater improvements in FEV_1, health status, and exacerbation frequency than either agent alone. The availability of combination inhalers makes administration of both drugs convenient and decreases the total number of inhalations needed daily.

TREATMENT OF EXACERBATION OF CHRONIC OBSTRUCTIVE PULMONARY DISEASE

DESIRED OUTCOMES

- The goals of therapy for patients experiencing COPD exacerbations are prevention of hospitalization or reduction in length of hospital stay, prevention of acute respiratory failure and death, resolution of symptoms, and a return to baseline clinical status and quality of life.

NONPHARMACOLOGIC THERAPY

- O_2 therapy should be considered for any patient with hypoxemia during an exacerbation. Caution must be used because many patients with COPD rely on mild hypoxemia to trigger their drive to breathe. Overly aggressive O_2 administration to patients with chronic hypercapnia may result in respiratory depression and respiratory failure. O_2 therapy should be used to achieve a $PaO_2 > 60$ mm Hg or O_2 saturation > 90%. ABG should be obtained after O_2 initiation to monitor CO_2 retention resulting from hypoventilation.
- Noninvasive positive-pressure ventilation (NPPV) provides ventilatory support with O_2 and pressurized airflow using a face or nasal mask with a tight seal but without endotracheal intubation. Use of NPPV reduces the complications that often arise with invasive mechanical ventilation. NPPV is not appropriate for patients with altered mental status, severe acidosis, respiratory arrest, or cardiovascular instability. Intubation and mechanical

ventilation may be considered in patients failing a trial of NPPV or those who are poor candidates for NPPV.

PHARMACOLOGIC THERAPY

Bronchodilators

- The dose and frequency of bronchodilators are increased during acute exacerbations to provide symptomatic relief. Short-acting β_2-agonists are preferred because of their rapid onset of action. Anticholinergic agents may be added if symptoms persist despite increased doses of β_2-agonists.
- Bronchodilators may be administered via MDIs or nebulization with equal efficacy. Nebulization may be considered for patients with severe dyspnea who are unable to hold their breath after actuation of an MDI.
- Clinical evidence supporting theophylline use during exacerbations is lacking; thus, theophylline should generally be avoided. It may be considered for patients not responding to other therapies.

Corticosteroids

- Results from clinical trials suggest that patients with acute COPD exacerbations should receive a short course of IV or oral corticosteroids. Although the optimal dose and duration of treatment are unknown, it appears that a regimen of prednisone 40 mg orally daily (or equivalent) for 10 to 14 days can be effective for most patients.
- If treatment is continued for longer than 2 weeks, a tapering oral schedule should be employed to avoid hypothalamic-pituitary-adrenal axis suppression.

Antimicrobial Therapy

- Although most exacerbations of COPD are thought to be caused by viral or bacterial infections, up to 30% of exacerbations are caused by unknown factors.
- Antibiotics are of most benefit and should be initiated if at least two of the following three symptoms are present: increased dyspnea, increased sputum volume, and increased sputum purulence. The utility of sputum Gram stain and culture is questionable because some patients have chronic bacterial colonization of the bronchial tree between exacerbations.
- Selection of empiric antimicrobial therapy should be based on the most likely organisms. The most common organisms for acute exacerbation of COPD are *Haemophilus influenzae*, *Moraxella catarrhalis*, *Streptococcus pneumoniae*, and *H. parainfluenzae*.
- Therapy should be initiated within 24 hours of symptoms to prevent unnecessary hospitalization and generally continued for at least 7 to 10 days. Five-day courses with some agents may produce comparable efficacy.
- In uncomplicated exacerbations, recommended therapy includes a **macrolide** (**azithromycin** or **clarithromycin**), **second- or third-generation cephalosporin**, or **doxycycline**. Trimethoprim–sulfamethoxazole should not be used because of increasing pneumococcal resistance. Amoxicillin and first-generation cephalosporins are not recommended because of

β-lactamase susceptibility. Erythromycin is not recommended because of insufficient activity against *H. influenzae*.

- In complicated exacerbations where drug-resistant pneumococci, β-lactamase-producing *H. influenzae* and *M. catarrhalis*, and some enteric gram-negative organisms may be present, recommended therapy includes **amoxicillin/clavulanate** or a fluoroquinolone with enhanced pneumococcal activity (**levofloxacin, gemifloxacin**, or **moxifloxacin**).
- In complicated exacerbations with risk of *Pseudomonas aeruginosa*, recommended therapy includes a fluoroquinolone with enhanced pneumococcal and *P. aeruginosa* activity (**levofloxacin**). If IV therapy is required, a β-lactamase-resistant penicillin with antipseudomonal activity or a third- or fourth-generation cephalosporin with antipseudomonal activity should be used.

EVALUATION OF THERAPEUTIC OUTCOMES

- In chronic stable COPD, pulmonary function tests should be assessed with any therapy addition, change in dose, or deletion of therapy. Other outcome measures are dyspnea score, quality-of-life assessments, and exacerbation rates (including emergency department visits and hospitalizations).
- In acute exacerbations of COPD, white blood cell count, vital signs, chest radiograph, and changes in frequency of dyspnea, sputum volume, and sputum purulence should be assessed at the onset and throughout the exacerbation. In more severe exacerbations, ABG and O_2 saturation should also be monitored.
- Patient adherence to therapeutic regimens, side effects, potential drug interactions, and subjective measures of quality of life must also be evaluated.

See Chapter 34, Chronic Obstructive Pulmonary Disease, authored by Dennis M. Williams and Sharya V. Bourdet, for a more detailed discussion of this topic.

CHAPTER 83

Benign Prostatic Hyperplasia

DEFINITION

- Benign prostatic hyperplasia (BPH), a nearly ubiquitous condition, is the most common benign neoplasm of American men.

PATHOPHYSIOLOGY

- The prostate gland comprises three types of tissue: epithelial or glandular, stromal or smooth muscle, and capsule. Both stromal tissue and capsule are embedded with α_1-adrenergic receptors.
- The precise pathophysiologic mechanisms that cause BPH are not clear. However, both intraprostatic dihydrotestosterone (DHT) and type II 5α-reductase are thought to be involved.
- BPH commonly results from both static (gradual enlargement of the prostate) and dynamic (agents or situations that increase α-adrenergic tone and constrict the gland's smooth muscle) factors. Examples of drugs that can exacerbate symptoms include testosterone, α-adrenergic agonists (e.g., decongestants), and those with significant anticholinergic effects (e.g., antihistamines, phenothiazines, tricyclic antidepressants, antispasmodics, and antiparkinsonian agents).

CLINICAL PRESENTATION

- Patients with BPH can present with a variety of signs and symptoms categorized as obstructive or irritative. Symptoms vary over time. Mild disease may stabilize, whereas other patients experience progressive disease over time.
- Obstructive signs and symptoms result when dynamic and/or static factors reduce bladder emptying. Patients experience urinary hesitancy, urine dribbles out of the penis, and the bladder feels full even after voiding.
- Irritative signs and symptoms are common and result from long-standing obstruction at the bladder neck. Patients experience frequency, urgency, and nocturia.
- Complications associated with BPH progression include chronic kidney disease, gross hematuria, urinary incontinence, recurrent urinary tract infection, bladder diverticula, and bladder stones.

DIAGNOSIS

- Diagnosis of BPH requires a careful medical history, physical examination, objective measures of bladder emptying (e.g., peak and average urinary

1041

flow rate and postvoid residual urine volume), and laboratory tests (e.g., urinalysis and prostate-specific antigen [PSA]).

- Medication history should include all prescription and nonprescription medications, as well as dietary supplements.
- On digital rectal examination, the prostate is usually but not always enlarged (>20 g), soft, smooth, and symmetric.

DESIRED OUTCOME

- BPH treatment is aimed primarily at relieving manifestations of the disease that are bothersome for the patient. A secondary aim is to prevent serious complications that can be life-threatening in this population.

TREATMENT

- Management options for BPH include watchful waiting, drug therapy, and surgical intervention. The choice depends on the severity of signs and symptoms (Table 83–1).
- Watchful waiting is appropriate for patients with mild disease and for those with moderate disease with only mildly bothersome symptoms and without complications (Fig. 83–1).
- Watchful waiting involves reassessment at yearly intervals. Patients should be educated about behavior modification, such as fluid restriction before bedtime, avoiding caffeine and alcohol, frequent emptying of the bladder, and avoiding drugs that exacerbate symptoms.

PHARMACOLOGIC THERAPY

- Pharmacologic therapy is appropriate for patients with moderately severe BPH and as an interim measure for patients with severe BPH.

TABLE 83–1	Categories of BPH Disease Severity Based on Symptoms and Signs	
Disease Severity	**AUA Symptom Score**	**Typical Symptoms and Signs**
Mild	≤7	Asymptomatic
		Peak urinary flow rate <10 mL/s
		Postvoid residual urine volume >25–50 mL
Moderate	8–19	All of the above signs plus obstructive voiding symptoms and irritative voiding symptoms (signs of detrusor instability)
Severe	≥20	All of the above plus one or more complications of BPH

AUA, American Urological Association; BPH, benign prostatic hyperplasia.

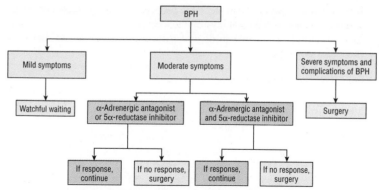

FIGURE 83–1. Management algorithm for benign prostatic hyperplasia (BPH).

- Pharmacologic therapy interferes with the stimulatory effect of testosterone on prostate gland enlargement (reduces the static factor) or relaxes prostatic smooth muscle (reduces the dynamic factor) (**Table 83–2**).
- Initial therapy with an α_1-adrenergic antagonist provides faster onset of symptom relief. A 5α-reductase inhibitor is preferred as initial therapy in patients with a prostate gland >40 g. Combination therapy should be considered for symptomatic patients with a prostate gland >40 g and PSA ≥1.4 ng/mL (1.4 mcg/L).
- Agents that interfere with androgen stimulation of the prostate are not popular in the United States because of adverse effects. The luteinizing

TABLE 83–2	Medical Treatment Options for Benign Prostatic Hyperplasia	
Category	**Mechanism**	**Drug (Brand Name)**
Reduces dynamic factor	Blocks α_1-adrenergic receptors in prostatic stromal tissue	Prazosin (Minipress)
		Alfuzosin (Uroxatral)
		Terazosin (Hytrin)
		Doxazosin (Cardura)
	Blocks α_{1A}-receptors in the prostate	Tamsulosin (Flomax)
		Silodosin (Rapaflo)
Reduces static factor	Blocks 5α-reductase enzyme	Finasteride (Proscar)
		Dutasteride (Avodart)
	Blocks DHT at its intracellular receptor	Bicalutamide (Casodex)[a]
		Flutamide (Eulexin)[a]
	Blocks pituitary release of luteinizing hormone	Leuprolide (Lupron)[a]
		Goserelin (Zoladex)[a]
	Blocks pituitary release of luteinizing hormone and blocks androgen receptor	Megestrol acetate (Megace)[a]

DHT, dihydrotestosterone.
[a]Not FDA approved for treatment of BPH.

hormone–releasing hormone agonists **leuprolide** and **goserelin** decrease libido and can cause erectile dysfunction, gynecomastia, and hot flashes. The antiandrogens **bicalutamide** and **flutamide** cause nausea, diarrhea, and hepatotoxicity.

α-Adrenergic Antagonists

- α-Adrenergic antagonists relax the smooth muscle in the prostate and bladder neck, thereby increasing urinary flow rates by 2 to 3 mL/sec in 60% to 70% of patients and reducing postvoid residual urine volumes.
- α_1-Adrenergic antagonists do not decrease prostate volume or PSA levels.
- **Prazosin, terazosin, doxazosin**, and **alfuzosin** are second-generation α_1-adrenergic antagonists. They antagonize peripheral vascular α_1-adrenergic receptors in addition to those in the prostate. Therefore, their adverse effects include first-dose syncope, orthostatic hypotension, and dizziness. Alfuzosin is less likely to cause cardiovascular adverse effects than other second-generation agents.
- Patients should be slowly titrated to a maintenance dose and should take these drugs at bedtime to minimize orthostatic hypotension and first-dose syncope with immediate-release formulations of terazosin and doxazosin. Sample titration schedules for terazosin include:

Titration Schedules	
Terazosin Slow	*Terazosin Quicker*
Days 1–3: 1 mg at bedtime	Days 1–3: 1 mg at bedtime
Days 4–14: 2 mg at bedtime	Days 4–14: 2 mg at bedtime
Weeks 2–6: 5 mg at bedtime	Weeks 2–3: 5 mg at bedtime
Weeks 7 and on: 10 mg at bedtime	Weeks 4 and on: 10 mg at bedtime

- **Tamsulosin** and **silodosin**, third-generation α_1-adrenergic antagonists, are selective for prostatic α_{1A}-receptors. Therefore, they do not cause peripheral vascular smooth muscle relaxation.
- Tamsulosin is a good choice for patients who cannot tolerate hypotension; have severe coronary artery disease, volume depletion, cardiac arrhythmias, severe orthostasis, or liver failure; or are taking multiple antihypertensives. Tamsulosin is also suitable for patients who want to avoid the delay of dose titration.
- Caution is needed to avoid potential drug interactions. Tamsulosin decreases metabolism of **cimetidine** and **diltiazem**. **Carbamazepine** and **phenytoin** increase catabolism of α_1-adrenergic antagonists. Large doses of phosphodiesterase inhibitors (e.g., sildenafil) in combination with α_1-adrenergic antagonists may result in systemic hypotension.
- A reduced daily dose of silodosin should be used in patients with moderate renal impairment or hepatic dysfunction.

5α-Reductase Inhibitors (Dutasteride and Finasteride)

- 5α-Reductase inhibitors interfere with the stimulatory effect of testosterone. These agents slow disease progression and decrease the risk of complications.

- Compared with α_1-adrenergic antagonists, 5α-reductase inhibitors have the disadvantages of requiring 6 months to maximally shrink an enlarged prostate, being less likely to induce objective improvement and causing more sexual dysfunction.
- Whether the pharmacodynamic advantages of **dutasteride** confer clinical advantages over **finasteride** is unknown. Dutasteride inhibits types I and II 5α-reductase, whereas finasteride inhibits only type II. Dutasteride more quickly and completely suppresses intraprostatic DHT (vs 80–90% for finasteride) and decreases serum DHT by 90% (vs 70%).
- 5α-Reductase inhibitors may be preferred in patients with uncontrolled arrhythmias, poorly controlled angina, use of multiple antihypertensives, or inability to tolerate hypotensive effects of α_1-adrenergic antagonists.
- 5α-Reductase inhibitors reduce serum PSA levels by 50%. PSA should be measured at baseline and repeated after 6 months. If PSA does not decrease by 50% after 6 months of therapy in a compliant patient, the patient should be evaluated for prostate cancer.
- 5α-Reductase inhibitors are in FDA pregnancy category X and are therefore contraindicated in pregnant women. Pregnant and potentially pregnant women should not handle the tablets or have contact with semen from men receiving 5α-reductase inhibitors.

SURGICAL INTERVENTION

- Prostatectomy, performed transurethrally or suprapubically, is the gold standard for treatment of patients with moderate or severe symptoms of BPH and for all patients with complications.
- Retrograde ejaculation is a complication of up to 75% of transurethral prostatectomy procedures. Other complications seen in 2% to 15% of patients are bleeding, urinary incontinence, and erectile dysfunction.

PHYTOTHERAPY

- Although widely used in Europe for BPH, phytotherapy with products such as saw palmetto berry (*Serenoa repens*), stinging nettle (*Urtica dioica*), and African plum (*Pygeum africanum*) should be avoided. Studies of these herbal medicines are inconclusive, and the purity of available products is questionable.

EVALUATION OF THERAPEUTIC OUTCOMES

- The primary therapeutic outcome of BPH therapy is restoring adequate urinary flow without causing adverse effects.
- Outcome depends on the patient's perception of effectiveness and acceptability of therapy. The American Urological Association Symptom Score is a validated standardized instrument that can be used to assess patient quality of life.
- Objective measures of bladder emptying (e.g., urinary flow rate and postvoid residual urine volumes) are useful measures in patients considering surgery.

- Laboratory tests (e.g., blood urea nitrogen, creatinine, and PSA) and urinalysis should be monitored regularly. In addition, patients should have an annual digital rectal examination.

See Chapter 93, Benign Prostatic Hyperplasia, authored by Mary Lee, for a more detailed discussion of this topic.

DEFINITION

- Erectile dysfunction (ED) is the failure to achieve a penile erection suitable for sexual intercourse. Patients often refer to it as impotence.

PATHOPHYSIOLOGY

- ED can result from an abnormality in one of the four systems necessary for a normal penile erection or from a combination of abnormalities. Vascular, nervous, or hormonal etiologies of ED are referred to as organic ED. Abnormality of the fourth system (i.e., patient's psychological receptivity to sexual stimuli) is referred to as psychogenic ED.
- The penis has two corpora cavernosa, which have many interconnected sinuses that fill with blood to produce an erection. The penis also has one corpus spongiosum, which surrounds the urethra and forms the glans penis.
- Acetylcholine works with other neurotransmitters (i.e., cyclic guanylate monophosphate, cyclic adenosine monophosphate, and vasoactive intestinal polypeptide) to produce penile arterial vasodilation and ultimately an erection.
- Causes of organic ED include diseases that compromise vascular flow to the corpora cavernosum (e.g., peripheral vascular disease, arteriosclerosis, and essential hypertension), impair nerve conduction to the brain (e.g., spinal cord injury and stroke), or impair peripheral nerve conduction (e.g., diabetes mellitus). Secondary ED is associated with hypogonadism.
- Causes of psychogenic ED include malaise, reactive depression or performance anxiety, sedation, Alzheimer's disease, hypothyroidism, and mental disorders. Patients with psychogenic ED generally have a higher response rate to interventions than patients with organic ED.
- Social habits (e.g., cigarette smoking and excessive ethanol intake) and medications (Table 84–1) can also cause ED.

CLINICAL PRESENTATION

- Signs and symptoms of ED can be difficult to detect. The patient's mate is often the first to report ED to the healthcare provider.
- Emotional manifestations include depression, performance anxiety, and embarrassment.
- Nonadherence to drugs thought to cause ED can be a sign of ED.

DIAGNOSIS

- The diagnostic workup should be designed to identify underlying causes of ED.

TABLE 84–1	Medication Classes That Can Cause Erectile Dysfunction	

Drug Class	Proposed Mechanism by Which Drug Causes Erectile Dysfunction	Special Notes
Anticholinergic agents (antihistamines, antiparkinsonian agents, tricyclic antidepressants, phenothiazines)	Anticholinergic activity	• Second-generation nonsedating antihistamines (e.g., loratadine, fexofenadine, or cetirizine) are associated with less erectile dysfunction than first-generation agents • Selective serotonin reuptake inhibitor (SSRI) antidepressants cause less erectile dysfunction than tricyclic antidepressants. Of the SSRIs, paroxetine, sertraline, and fluoxetine cause erectile dysfunction more commonly than venlafaxine, nefazodone, trazodone, or mirtazapine. • Phenothiazines with less anticholinergic effect (e.g., chlorpromazine) can be substituted in some patients if erectile dysfunction is a problem
Dopamine antagonists (e.g., metoclopramide, phenothiazines)	Inhibit prolactin inhibitory factor, thereby increasing prolactin levels	• Increased prolactin levels inhibit testicular testosterone production; depressed libido results
Estrogens, antiandrogens (e.g., luteinizing hormone–releasing hormone superagonists, digoxin, spironolactone, ketoconazole, cimetidine)	Suppress testosterone-mediated stimulation of libido	• In the face of a decreased libido, a secondary erectile dysfunction develops because of diminished sexual drive
Central nervous system depressants (e.g., barbiturates, narcotics, benzodiazepines, short-term use of large doses of alcohol, anticonvulsants)	Suppress perception of psychogenic stimuli	
Agents that decrease penile blood flow (e.g., diuretics, peripheral β-adrenergic antagonists, or central sympatholytics [methyldopa, clonidine, guanethidine])	Reduce arteriolar flow to corpora	• Any diuretic that produces a significant decrease in intravascular volume can decrease penile arteriolar flow • Safer antihypertensives include angiotensin-converting enzyme inhibitors, postsynaptic α_1-adrenergic antagonists (terazosin, doxazosin), calcium channel blockers, and angiotensin II receptor antagonists

(continued)

TABLE 84–1	Medication Classes That Can Cause Erectile Dysfunction (Continued)	
Drug Class	**Proposed Mechanism by Which Drug Causes Erectile Dysfunction**	**Special Notes**
Miscellaneous • Finasteride, dutasteride • Lithium carbonate • Gemfibrozil • Interferon • Clofibrate • Monoamine oxidase inhibitors	Unknown mechanism	

From Thomas A, Woodard C, Rovner ES, Wein AJ. Urologic complications of nonurologic medications. Urol Clin North Am 2003;30:123–131; and Lee M, Sharifi R. Sexual dysfunction in males. In Tisdale JE, Miller DA, eds. Drug-Induced Diseases: Prevention, Detection, and Management. Bethesda, MD: ASHP, 2005:455–467.

- Key diagnostic assessments include ED severity, medical and surgical history, concurrent medications, physical examination, and laboratory tests (i.e., serum blood glucose, lipid profile, and testosterone level).
- A standardized questionnaire can be used to assess the severity of ED.

DESIRED OUTCOME

- The goal of treatment is to improve the quantity and quality of penile erections suitable for intercourse.

TREATMENT

- The first step in management of ED is to identify and, if possible, reverse underlying causes. Psychotherapy can be used as monotherapy for psychogenic ED or as an adjunct to specific treatments.
- Treatment options include vacuum erection devices (VEDs), drugs (Table 84–2), and surgery. Although no option is ideal, the least invasive options are chosen first (Fig. 84–1).

VACUUM ERECTION DEVICE

- VEDs are first-line therapy for older patients. They should be limited to patients who have stable sexual relationships, because the onset of action is slow (i.e., ~30 minutes).
- To prolong the erection, the patient can also use constriction bands or tension rings, which are placed at the base of the penis to retain arteriolar blood and reduce venous outflow from the penis.

TABLE 84–2	Dosing Regimens for Selected Drug Treatments for Erectile Dysfunction		
Route of Administration	**Generic Name (Brand Name)**	**Dosage Form**	**Common Dosing Regimen**
Oral	Yohimbine (Aphrodyne, Yocon, Yohimex)	5.4 mg tablet or capsule	5.4 mg three times daily
	Sildenafil (Viagra)	25 mg, 50 mg, 100 mg tablet	25–100 mg 1 hour before intercourse
	Apomorphine (Uprima)[a]	10 mg sublingual tablet, 25 mg tablet and capsule	10–40 mg daily
	Fluoxymesterone (Halotestin)	2 mg, 5 mg, 10 mg, 50 mg tablet	5–20 mg daily
	Trazodone (Desyrel)	100 mg, 150 mg, 300 mg tablet	50–150 mg daily
	Vardenafil (Levitra)	2.5 mg, 5 mg, 10 mg, 20 mg tablet	5–10 mg 1 hour before intercourse
	Tadalafil (Cialis)	5 mg, 10 mg, 20 mg tablet	5–20 mg before intercourse or 2.5–5 mg daily
Topical	Testosterone patch (Testoderm)	4 mg/patch, 6 mg/patch	4–6 mg/day; apply to scrotum
	Testosterone patch (Testoderm TTS)	4 mg/patch, 6 mg/patch	4–6 mg/day; apply to arm, buttock, back
	Testosterone patch (Androderm)	2.5 mg/patch	2.5–5 mg/day; apply to arm, back, abdomen, thigh
	Testosterone gel (AndroGel 1%)	5 g/pkt, 10 g/pkt 5 g/activation	5–10 g/day; apply to shoulders, upper arms, abdomen
Intramuscular	Testosterone cypionate (Depo-Testosterone)	100 mg/mL, 200 mg/mL	200–400 mg every 2–4 weeks
	Testosterone enanthate (Delatestryl)	100 mg/mL, 200 mg/mL	200–400 mg every 2–4 weeks
Subcutaneous implant	Testosterone (Testopel)	75 mg pellet	150–450 mg every 3–4 months
Intraurethral	Alprostadil (MUSE)	125 mcg, 250 mcg, 500 mcg, 1,000 mcg pellet	125–1,000 mcg 5–10 min before intercourse
Intracavernosal	Alprostadil (Caverject)	5 mcg, 10 mcg, 20 mcg injection	2.5–60 mcg 5–10 min before intercourse
	Alprostadil (Edex)	5 mcg, 20 mcg, 40 mcg injection	2.5–60 mcg 5–10 min before intercourse

(continued)

TABLE 84–2	Dosing Regimens for Selected Drug Treatments for Erectile Dysfunction *(Continued)*		
Route of Administration	**Generic Name (Brand Name)**	**Dosage Form**	**Common Dosing Regimen**
	Papaverine[b]	30 mg/mL injection	Variable, usually used in combination with alprostadil and phentolamine
	Phentolamine[b]	2.5 mg/mL injection	Variable, usually used in combination with alprostadil and papaverine

[a]Not commercially available in the United States as a sublingual formulation; only available in the United States as a subcutaneous injection that is FDA approved for Parkinson's disease.
[b]Not FDA approved for this use.

- VEDs can be used as second-line therapy after failure of oral or injectable drugs. Adding **alprostadil** to a VED improves the response rate.
- VEDs are contraindicated in patients with sickle cell disease. They should be used cautiously in patients on warfarin because, through a poorly understood and idiosyncratic mechanism, it can cause priapism.

PHARMACOLOGIC TREATMENTS

Phosphodiesterase Inhibitors

- Phosphodiesterase mediates catabolism of cyclic guanylate monophosphate, a vasodilatory neurotransmitter in the corporal tissue.
- Unless otherwise stated, general information applies to the entire class of phosphodiesterase inhibitors. **Sildenafil** is highlighted because it was the first to be marketed and is the most thoroughly studied. The newer agents **tadalafil** and **vardenafil** have different pharmacokinetic profiles (Table 84–3), drug–food interactions, and adverse effects.
- Phosphodiesterase inhibitors are selective for isoenzyme type 5 in genital tissue. Inhibition of this isoenzyme in nongenital tissues (e.g., peripheral vascular tissue, tracheal smooth muscle, and platelets) can produce adverse effects.
- Phosphodiesterase inhibitors are first-line therapy for younger patients. Sildenafil, 25 to 100 mg, induces satisfactory erections in 56% to 82% of patients. Approximately half of nonresponders can have satisfactory responses after being instructed on the proper use of phosphodiesterase inhibitors. The effectiveness of these drugs appears to be dose related.
  - ✓ For the best response, patients must engage in sexual stimulation (foreplay).
  - ✓ For the fastest response, patients should take sildenafil on an empty stomach, at least 2 hours before meals. The other two agents can be taken without regard to meals.

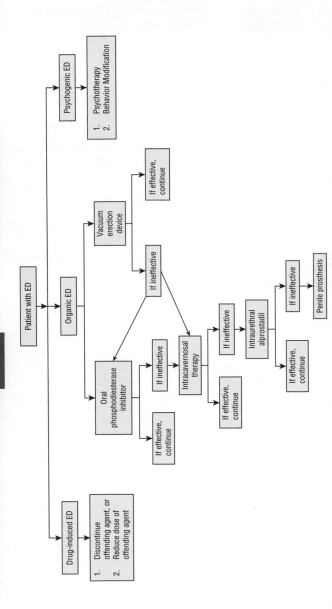

FIGURE 84–1. Algorithm for selecting treatment for erectile dysfunction (ED). For organic ED, oral agents are first-line therapy for younger patients, and vacuum erection devices are generally used first in older patients who are married or otherwise have a stable sexual relationship. These two approaches are sometimes used together in an effort to avoid surgical implantation of penile prostheses.

TABLE 84–3	Pharmacodynamics and Pharmacokinetics of Phosphodiesterase Inhibitors		
	Sildenafil[a]	**Vardenafil**[a]	**Tadalafil**[a]
Trade name	Viagra	Levitra	Cialis
Inhibits PDE-5	Yes	Yes	Yes
Inhibits PDE-6	Yes	Minimally	No
Inhibits PDE-11	No	No	Yes
Time to peak plasma level (hours)	0.5–1	0.7–0.9	2
Fatty meal decreases rate of oral absorption?	Yes	Yes	No
Mean plasma half-life (hours)	3.7	4.4–4.8	18
Percentage of dose excreted in feces	80	91–95	61
Percentage of dose excreted in urine	13	2–6	36
Duration (hours)	4	4	24–36
Usual dose (mg) before intercourse	25–100	5–20	5–20
Daily dose (mg)	Not applicable	Not applicable	2.5-5
Dose in patients ≥65 years (mg)	25	5	5–20
Dose in moderate renal impairment (mg)	25–100	5–20	5
Dose in severe renal impairment (mg)	25	5–20	5
Dose in mild hepatic impairment (mg)	25–100	5–20	10
Dose in moderate hepatic impairment (mg)	25–100	5–10	10
Dose in severe hepatic impairment (mg)	25	Not evaluated	Not recommended
Dose in patients taking cytochrome P450 3A4 inhibitors[a]	25 mg daily	2.5–5 mg every 24–72 hours	10 mg every 72 hours

PDE, phosphodiesterase

[a]Sildenafil doses should be decreased when any potent cytochrome P450 3A4 inhibitor is used (e.g., cimetidine, erythromycin, clarithromycin, ketoconazole, itraconazole, ritonavir, and saquinavir). Vardenafil doses vary according to the agent used (2.5 mg every 72 hours for ritonavir, 2.5 mg every 24 hours for indinavir, ketoconazole 400 mg daily, and itraconazole 400 mg daily; and 5 mg every 24 hours for ketoconazole 200 mg daily, itraconazole 200 mg daily, and erythromycin). Tadalafil doses are reduced only when the drug is used with the most potent cytochrome P450 3A4 inhibitors (e.g., ketoconazole and ritonavir).

✓ For maximal absorption, patients should avoid taking sildenafil or vardenafil with a fatty meal. A fatty meal does not affect absorption of tadalafil.
✓ If the first dose is not effective, patients should continue trying for five to eight doses. Some patients benefit from titration up to 100 mg of sildenafil, 20 mg of vardenafil, or 20 mg of tadalafil.
• Sildenafil and vardenafil have similar pharmacokinetic profiles with a rapid onset of action and short duration. Tadalafil has a delayed onset of action and prolonged duration of effect. All three drugs are metabolized

by cytochrome P450 enzymes, primarily 3A4. Patients should avoid exceeding prescribed doses because higher doses do not improve response. Depending on the phosphodiesterase inhibitor, the dose should be reduced if the patient is elderly, has renal or hepatic impairment, or receives an inhibitor of cytochrome P450 3A4 (see **Table 84–3**).

- In usual doses, the most common adverse effects are headache, facial flushing, dyspepsia, nasal congestion, and dizziness.
- Sildenafil and vardenafil decrease systolic/diastolic blood pressure by 8 to 10/5 to 6 mm Hg for 1 to 4 hours after a dose. Although most patients are asymptomatic, multiple antihypertensives, **nitrates**, and baseline hypotension increase the risk of developing adverse effects. Although tadalafil does not decrease blood pressure, it should be used with caution in patients with cardiovascular disease because of the inherent risk associated with sexual activity.
- Guidelines are available for stratifying patients on the basis of their cardiovascular risk (**Table 84–4**).

TABLE 84–4	Recommendations of the Second Princeton Consensus Conference for Cardiovascular Risk Stratification of Patients Being Considered for Phosphodiesterase Inhibitor Therapy	
Risk Category	**Description of Patient's Condition**	**Management Approach**
Low risk	Has asymptomatic cardiovascular disease with < 3 risk factors for cardiovascular disease Has well-controlled hypertension Has mild, stable angina Has mild CHF (NYHA class I) Has mild valvular heart disease Had MI >6 weeks ago	Patient can be started on phosphodiesterase inhibitor
Intermediate risk	Has ≥3 risk factors for cardiovascular disease Has moderate, stable angina Had recent MI or stroke within the past 6 weeks Has moderate CHF (NYHA class II)	Patient should undergo complete cardiovascular workup and treadmill stress test to determine tolerance to increased myocardial energy consumption associated with increased sexual activity
High risk	Has unstable or symptomatic angina, despite treatment Has uncontrolled hypertension Has severe CHF (NYHA class III or IV) Had recent MI or stroke within past 2 weeks Has moderate or severe valvular heart disease Has high-risk cardiac arrhythmias Has obstructive hypertrophic cardiomyopathy	Phosphodiesterase inhibitor is contraindicated; sexual intercourse should be deferred

CHF, congestive heart failure; MI, myocardial infarction; NYHA, New York Heart Association

From Kostis JB, Jackson G, Rosen R, et al. Sexual dysfunction and cardiac risk (the Second Princeton Consensus Conference). Am J Cardiol 2005;96:313–321.

- Phosphodiesterase inhibitors should be used cautiously in patients at risk for retinitis pigmentosa and by pilots who rely on blue and green lights to land airplanes. Patients who experience sudden vision loss should be evaluated before continuing treatment.
- Tadalafil inhibits type 11 phosphodiesterase, which is thought to account for the dose-related back and muscle pain seen in 7% to 30% of patients.
- Phosphodiesterase inhibitors are contraindicated in patients taking nitrates. They should be used cautiously in patients taking α-adrenergic antagonists.

Testosterone-Replacement Regimens

- **Testosterone**-replacement regimens restore serum testosterone levels to the normal range (300–1,100 ng/dL; 10.4–38.2 nmol/L). These regimens are indicated for symptomatic patients with hypogonadism as confirmed by both a decreased libido and low serum testosterone concentrations.
- Instead of directly correcting ED, testosterone-replacement regimens correct secondary ED by improving libido. Usually within days or weeks of starting therapy, they restore muscle strength and sexual drive and improve mood.
- Testosterone can be replaced orally, parenterally, or transdermally (see **Table 84–2**). Injectable regimens are preferred because they are effective, are inexpensive, and do not have the bioavailability problems or adverse hepatotoxic effects of oral regimens. Testosterone patches and gel are more expensive than other forms and should be reserved for patients who refuse injections.
- Before starting testosterone replacement, patients 40 years and older should be screened for benign prostatic hyperplasia (BPH) and prostate cancer. To ensure an adequate treatment trial, the patient should continue treatment for 2 to 3 months before a dosage increase is considered.
- Testosterone replacement can cause sodium retention, which can cause weight gain or exacerbate hypertension, congestive heart failure, and edema; gynecomastia; serum lipoprotein changes; and polycythemia. Exogenous testosterone can also exacerbate BPH and enhance prostate cancer growth.
- Oral testosterone replacement regimens can cause hepatotoxicity, ranging from mildly elevated hepatic transaminases to serious liver diseases (e.g., peliosis hepatitis, hepatocellular and intrahepatic cholestasis, and benign or malignant tumors).

Alprostadil

- **Alprostadil**, or prostaglandin E_1, stimulates adenyl cyclase to increase production of cyclic adenosine monophosphate, a neurotransmitter that ultimately enhances blood flow to and blood filling of the corpora.
- Alprostadil is approved as monotherapy for the management of ED. It is generally prescribed after failure of VEDs and phosphodiesterase inhibitors and for patients who cannot use these therapies. Of the available routes, the intracavernosal route is preferred over the intraurethral route because of better efficacy.

INTRACAVERNOSAL INJECTION

- Intracavernosal alprostadil is effective in 70% to 90% of patients. However, a high proportion of patients discontinue its use because of perceived ineffectiveness; inconvenience of administration; unnatural, nonspontaneous erection; needle phobia; loss of interest; and cost of therapy.
- Intracavernosal alprostadil has been used successfully in combination with VEDs or vasoactive agents (e.g., papaverine and phentolamine) that act by different mechanisms. Phosphodiesterase inhibitors should not be added to intracavernosal alprostadil because the combination can cause prolonged erections and priapism.
- Intracavernosal alprostadil acts rapidly, with an onset of 5 to 15 minutes. The duration of action is dose related and, within the usual dosage range, lasts <1 hour.
- The usual dose of intracavernosal alprostadil is 10 to 20 mcg up to a maximum of 60 mcg. Patients should start with 1.25 mcg, which should be increased by 1.25 to 2.5 mcg at 30-minute intervals to the lowest dose that produces a firm erection for 1 hour and does not produce adverse effects. In clinical practice, however, most patients start with 10 mcg and titrate quickly.
- To minimize the risk of complications, patients should use the lowest effective dose.
- Intracavernosal alprostadil should be injected 5 to 10 minutes before intercourse using a 0.5 in, 27- or 30-gauge needle or an autoinjector. The maximum number of injections is one daily and three weekly.
- Intracavernosal alprostadil is most commonly associated with local adverse effects, usually during the first year of therapy. Adverse events include cavernosal plaques or fibrosis at the injection site (2–12% of patients), penile pain (10–44%), and priapism (1–15%). Penile pain is usually mild and self-limiting, but priapism (i.e., painful, drug-induced erection lasting >1 hours) necessitates immediate medical attention.
- Intracavernosal injection therapy should be used cautiously in patients at risk of priapism (e.g., sickle cell disease or lymphoproliferative disorders) and bleeding complications secondary to injections.

INTRAURETHRAL ADMINISTRATION

- Intraurethral alprostadil, 125 to 1,000 mcg, should be administered 5 to 10 minutes before intercourse. Before administration, the patient should empty his bladder and void completely. No more than two doses daily are recommended.
- Intraurethral administration is associated with pain in 24% to 32% of patients, which is usually mild and does not require discontinuation of treatment. Prolonged painful erections are rare.
- Female partners may experience vaginal burning, itching, or pain, which is probably related to transfer of alprostadil from the man's urethra to the woman's vagina during intercourse.

Unapproved Agents

- A variety of commercially available and investigational agents have been used for management of ED. Examples include **trazodone** (50–200 mg/day),

yohimbine (5.4 mg three times daily), **papaverine** (7.5–60 mg [single-agent therapy] or 0.5–20 mg [combination therapy] intracavernosal injection), and **phentolamine** (1 mg [combination therapy] intracavernosal injection).

SURGERY

- Surgical insertion of a penile prosthesis, the most invasive treatment for ED, is used after failure of less invasive treatments and for patients who are not candidates for other treatments.
- Adverse effects of prosthesis insertion include early- and late-onset infection, mechanical failure, and erosion of the rods through the penis.

EVALUATION OF THERAPEUTIC OUTCOMES

- The primary therapeutic outcomes for ED are improving the quantity and quality of penile erections suitable for intercourse and avoiding adverse drug reactions and interactions.
- To assess improvement, the physician should conduct specific assessments at baseline and after a trial period of 1 to 3 weeks.
- To avoid adverse effects due to excessive use, patients with unrealistic expectations should be identified and should be counseled accordingly.

See Chapter 92, Erectile Dysfunction, authored by Mary Lee, for a more detailed discussion of this topic.

Urinary Incontinence

DEFINITION

- Urinary incontinence (UI) is the complaint of involuntary leakage of urine.

PATHOPHYSIOLOGY

- The urethral sphincter, a combination of smooth and striated muscles within and external to the urethra, maintains adequate resistance to the flow of urine from the bladder until voluntary voiding is initiated. Normal bladder emptying occurs with opening of the urethra concomitant with a volitional bladder contraction.
- Acetylcholine is the neurotransmitter that mediates both volitional and involuntary contractions of the bladder. Bladder smooth muscle cholinergic receptors are mainly of the M_2 variety; however, M_3 receptors are responsible for both emptying contraction of normal micturition and involuntary bladder contractions, which can result in UI. Therefore, most pharmacologic antimuscarinic therapy is anti-M_3 based.
- UI occurs as a result of overfunctioning or underfunctioning of the urethra, bladder, or both.
- Urethral underactivity is known as stress UI (SUI) and occurs during activities such as exercise, lifting, coughing, and sneezing. The urethral sphincter no longer resists the flow of urine from the bladder during periods of physical activity.
- Bladder overactivity is known as urge UI (UUI) and is associated with increased urinary frequency and urgency, with or without urge incontinence. The detrusor muscle is overactive and contracts inappropriately during the filling phase.
- Urethral overactivity and/or bladder underactivity is known as overflow incontinence. The bladder is filled to capacity but is unable to empty, causing urine to leak from a distended bladder past a normal outlet and sphincter. Common causes of urethral overactivity include benign prostatic hyperplasia (see Chap. 83); prostate cancer (see Chap. 66); and, in women, cystocele formation or surgical overcorrection after SUI surgery.
- Mixed incontinence includes the combination of bladder overactivity and urethral underactivity.
- Functional incontinence is not caused by bladder- or urethra-specific factors but rather occurs in patients with conditions such as cognitive or mobility deficits.
- Many medications can aggravate voiding dysfunction and UI (**Table 85–1**).

CLINICAL PRESENTATION

- Signs and symptoms of UI depend on the underlying pathophysiology (**Table 85–2**). Patients with SUI generally complain of urine leakage with

TABLE 85-1	Medications That Influence Lower Urinary Tract Function
Medication	**Effect**
Diuretics, acetylcholinesterase inhibitors	Polyuria, frequency, urgency
α-Receptor antagonists	Urethral relaxation and SUI in women
α-Receptor agonists	Urethral constriction and urinary retention in men
Calcium channel blockers	Urinary retention
Narcotic analgesics	Urinary retention from impaired contractility
Sedative hypnotics	Functional incontinence caused by delirium, immobility
Antipsychotics	Anticholinergic effects and urinary retention
Anticholinergics	Urinary retention
Antidepressants, tricyclic	Anticholinergic effects, α-antagonist effects
Alcohol	Polyuria, frequency, urgency, sedation, delirium
ACEIs	Cough as a result of ACEIs can aggravate SUI by increasing intraabdominal pressure

ACEIs, angiotensin-converting enzyme inhibitors; SUI, stress urinary incontinence

physical activity, whereas those with UUI complain of nocturia and nocturnal incontinence.

- Urethral overactivity and/or bladder underactivity is a rare but important cause of UI. Patients complain of lower abdominal fullness, hesitancy, straining to void, decreased force of stream, interrupted stream, and sense of incomplete bladder emptying. Patients can also have urinary frequency, urgency, and abdominal pain.

DIAGNOSIS

- Patients should undergo a complete medical history with assessment of symptoms, physical examination (i.e., abdominal examination to exclude

TABLE 85-2	Differentiating Bladder Overactivity from Urethral Underactivity	
Symptoms	**Bladder Overactivity**	**Urethral Underactivity**
Urgency (strong, sudden desire to void)	Yes	Sometimes
Frequency with urgency	Yes	Rarely
Leaking during physical activity (e.g., coughing, sneezing, lifting)	No	Yes
Amount of urinary leakage with each episode of incontinence	Large if present	Usually small
Ability to reach the toilet in time following an urge to void	No or just barely	Yes
Nocturnal incontinence (presence of wet pads or undergarments in bed)	Yes	Rare
Nocturia (waking to pass urine at night)	Usually	Seldom

distended bladder, pelvic examination in women looking for evidence of prolapse or hormonal deficiency, and genital and prostate examination in men), and brief neurologic assessment of the perineum and lower extremities.

- For SUI, the preferred diagnostic test is observation of urethral meatus while the patient coughs or strains.
- For UUI, the preferred diagnostic tests are urodynamic studies. Urinalysis and urine culture should be performed to rule out urinary tract infection.
- For urethral overactivity and/or bladder underactivity, digital rectal exam or transrectal ultrasound should be performed to rule out prostate enlargement. Renal function tests should be performed to rule out renal failure.

DESIRED OUTCOME

- The goal of therapy is to decrease the signs and symptoms of most distress to the patient.

TREATMENT

NONPHARMACOLOGIC TREATMENT

- Nonpharmacologic treatment (e.g., lifestyle modifications, toilet scheduling regimens, and pelvic floor muscle rehabilitation) is the chief form of UI management at the primary care level.
- Surgery rarely plays a role in the initial management of UI but can be required for secondary complications (e.g., skin breakdown or infection). Otherwise, the decision to surgically treat symptomatic UI requires that lifestyle compromise warrants an elective operation and that nonoperative therapy be proven undesirable or ineffective.

PHARMACOLOGIC TREATMENT

- The choice of pharmacologic therapy (Table 85–3) depends on the type of UI.
- Pharmacologic therapies should be combined with nonpharmacologic therapies.

Bladder Overactivity: Urge Urinary Incontinence

- The pharmacotherapy of first choice for UUI is anticholinergic/antispasmodic drugs, which antagonize muscarinic cholinergic receptors.

OXYBUTYNIN

- **Oxybutynin immediate-release** (IR) has been the drug of first choice for UUI and the "gold standard" against which other drugs are compared. Financial considerations favor generic oxybutynin IR.
- Many patients discontinue oxybutynin IR because of adverse effects due to antimuscarinic effects (e.g., dry mouth, constipation, vision impairment, confusion, cognitive dysfunction, and tachycardia), α-adrenergic

TABLE 85–3 Pharmacotherapeutic Options in Patients with Urinary Incontinence

Type	Drug Class	Drug Therapy (Usual Dose)	Comments
Overactive bladder	Anticholinergic agents/antispasmodics	Oxybutynin IR (2.5–5 mg two, three, or four times daily), oxybutynin XL (5–30 mg daily), oxybutynin TDS (3.9 mg/day; apply one patch twice weekly), oxybutynin gel (1 sachet [100 mg] topically daily), tolterodine IR (1–2 mg twice daily), tolterodine LA (2–4 mg daily), trospium chloride ER (60 mg daily), solifenacin (5–10 mg daily), darifenacin (7.5–15 mg daily), fesoterodine (4–8 mg daily)	Anticholinergics are first-line drug therapy (oxybutynin or tolterodine is preferred).
	Tricyclic antidepressants (TCAs)	Imipramine, doxepin, nortriptyline, or desipramine (25–100 mg at bedtime)	TCAs are generally reserved for patients with an additional indication (e.g., depression, neuropathic pain).
	Topical estrogen (only in women with urethritis or vaginitis)[a]	Conjugated estrogen vaginal cream (0.5 g) three times weekly for up to 8 months. Repeat course if symptom recurrence, or use estradiol vaginal insert/ring (2 mg [one ring]) and replace after 90 days if needed.	Marginally effective; few adverse effects with vaginal cream and insert.
Stress	Duloxetine[a]	40–80 mg/day (one or two doses)	Even though not FDA approved, duloxetine is first-line therapy; most adverse events diminish with time, so support patient during initial period of use.
	α-Adrenergic agonists	Pseudoephedrine (15–60 mg three times daily) with food, water, or milk Phenylephrine (10 mg four times daily)	Pseudoephedrine and phenylephrine are alternative first-line therapies for women with no contraindication (notably hypertension); phenylpropanolamine was the preferred agent in the class until its removal from the U.S. market in 2000.

(continued)

TABLE 85-3 Pharmacotherapeutic Options in Patients with Urinary Incontinence *(Continued)*

Type	Drug Class	Drug Therapy (Usual Dose)	Comments
	Estrogen	See estrogens (above). Works best if urethritis or vaginitis due to estrogen deficiency is present.	Considered a less-effective alternative to α-adrenergic agonists and duloxetine. Combined α-adrenergic agonist and estrogen may be somewhat more effective than α-adrenergic agonist alone in postmenopausal women.
	Imipramine	25–100 mg at bedtime	Imipramine is an optional therapy when first-line therapy is inadequate.
Overflow (atonic bladder)	Cholinomimetics	Bethanechol (25–50 mg three or four times daily) on an empty stomach	Avoid use if patient has asthma or heart disease. Short-term use only. Never give IV or IM because of life-threatening cardiovascular and severe gastrointestinal reactions.

ER, extended release; IR, immediate-release; IM, intramuscularly; IV, intravenously; LA, long-acting; TDS, transdermal system; XL, extended-release

^aNot FDA-approved for this use. Doses provided are those best supported by clinical trials to date.

inhibition (e.g., orthostatic hypotension), and histamine H_1 inhibition (e.g., sedation and weight gain).

- Oxybutynin IR is best tolerated when the dose is gradually escalated from no more than 2.5 mg twice daily to 2.5 mg three times daily after 1 month. Oxybutynin IR can be further increased in 2.5 mg/day increments every 1 to 2 months until the desired response, maximum recommended dose of 5 mg three times daily, or maximum tolerated dose is attained.

- **Oxybutynin extended-release** (ER) is better tolerated than oxybutynin IR and is as effective in reducing the number of UI episodes, restoring continence, decreasing the number of micturitions per day, and increasing urine volume voided per micturition.

- The maximum benefit of oxybutynin ER is not realized for up to 4 weeks after starting therapy or dose escalation.

- **Oxybutynin transdermal system** has similar efficacy but is better tolerated than oxybutynin IR presumably because this route avoids first-pass metabolism in the liver, which generates the metabolite thought to cause adverse events, especially dry mouth.

- **Oxybutynin gel** is also available for daily use. No data are available comparing it with an active control.

TOLTERODINE

- Tolterodine, a competitive muscarinic receptor antagonist, is considered first-line therapy in patients with urinary frequency, urgency, or urge incontinence.

- Controlled studies demonstrate that tolterodine is more effective than placebo and as effective as oxybutynin IR in decreasing the number of daily micturitions and increasing the volume voided per micturition. However, most studies have not shown a decrease in the number of daily UI episodes as compared with placebo.

- Tolterodine undergoes hepatic metabolism involving cytochrome (CYP) 2D6 and 3A4 isoenzymes. Therefore, elimination may be impaired by CYP 3A4 inhibitors, including **fluoxetine, sertraline, fluvoxamine**, macrolide antibiotics, azole antifungals, and grapefruit juice.

- Tolterodine's most common adverse effects are dry mouth, dyspepsia, headache, constipation, and dry eyes. The maximum benefit of tolterodine is not realized for up to 8 weeks after starting therapy or dose escalation.

- Fesoterodine fumarate is a prodrug for tolterodine and is considered an alternative first-line therapy for UI in patients with urinary frequency, urgency, or urge incontinence.

OTHER PHARMACOLOGIC THERAPIES
FOR URGE URINARY INCONTINENCE

- **Trospium chloride**, a quaternary ammonium anticholinergic, is superior to placebo and is equivalent to oxybutynin IR and tolterodine IR. However, clinical studies are limited by their focus on cystometric rather than clinical end points, small absolute benefits compared with placebo, and lack of comparisons with long-acting formulations.

- Trospium chloride causes the expected anticholinergic adverse effects with increased frequency in patients ≥75 years old.
- **Solifenacin succinate** and **darifenacin** are antagonists of M_1, M_2, and M_3 muscarinic cholinergic receptors. These antagonists do not offer significant advances over other anticholinergics despite being "uroselective" in preclinical studies. Both behave like nonselective anticholinergic in humans, causing dry mouth and other anticholinergic effects.
- Drug interactions are possible if CYP 3A4 inhibitors are given with solifenacin succinate or CYP 2D6 or 3A4 inhibitors with darifenacin.
- Other agents, including tricyclic antidepressants, **propantheline, flavoxate, hyoscyamine**, and **dicyclomine hydrochloride**, are less effective, not safer, or have not been adequately studied.
- Patients with UUI and elevated postvoid residual urine volume should be treated by intermittent self-catheterization along with frequent voiding between catheterizations.

Urethral Underactivity: Stress Urinary Incontinence

- The goal of treatment of SUI is to improve urethral closure by stimulating α-adrenergic receptors in the smooth muscle of the bladder neck and proximal urethra, enhancing supportive structures underlying the urethral epithelium, or enhancing serotonin and norepinephrine effects in the micturition reflex pathways.

ESTROGENS

- Historically, local and systemic **estrogens** have been the mainstays of pharmacologic management of SUI.
- In open trials, estrogens were administered orally, intramuscularly, vaginally, or transdermally. Regardless of the route, estrogens exerted variable effects on urodynamic parameters, such as maximum urethral closure pressure, functional urethral length, and pressure:transmission ratio.
- Results of four placebo-controlled comparative trials have not been as favorable, finding no significant clinical or urodynamic effect for oral estrogen compared with placebo.

α-ADRENERGIC RECEPTOR AGONISTS

- Many open trials support the use of a variety of α-adrenergic receptor agonists in SUI. Combining an α-adrenergic receptor agonist with an estrogen yields somewhat superior clinical and urodynamic responses compared with monotherapy.
- Contraindications to these agents include hypertension, tachyarrhythmias, coronary artery disease, myocardial infarction, cor pulmonale, hyperthyroidism, renal failure, and narrow-angle glaucoma.

DULOXETINE

- **Duloxetine**, a dual inhibitor of serotonin and norepinephrine reuptake indicated for depression and painful diabetic neuropathy, is approved in many countries for the treatment of SUI, but not in the United States. Duloxetine is thought to facilitate the bladder-to-sympathetic reflex pathway, increasing urethral and external urethral sphincter muscle tone during the storage phase.

- Six placebo-controlled studies showed that duloxetine reduces incontinent episode frequency and the number of daily micturitions, increases micturition interval, and improves quality-of-life scores. These benefits were statistically significant but clinically modest.
- To avoid drug interactions, clinicians should be careful when prescribing duloxetine concurrently with CYP 2D6 and 1A2 substrates or inhibitors.
- The adverse event profile might make adherence problematic. Adverse events include nausea, headache, insomnia, constipation, dry mouth, dizziness, fatigue, somnolence, vomiting, and diarrhea.

OVERFLOW INCONTINENCE

- Overflow incontinence secondary to benign or malignant prostatic hyperplasia may be amenable to pharmacotherapy (see Chaps. 66 and 83).

EVALUATION OF THERAPEUTIC OUTCOMES

- Total elimination of UI signs and symptoms may not be possible. Therefore, realistic goals should be established for therapy.
- In the long-term management of UI, the clinical symptoms of most distress to the individual patient need to be monitored.
- Survey instruments used in UI research along with quantitating the use of ancillary supplies (e.g., pads) can be used in clinical monitoring.
- Therapies for UI frequently have nuisance adverse effects, which need to be carefully elicited. Adverse effects can necessitate drug dosage adjustments, use of alternative strategies (e.g., chewing sugarless gum, sucking on hard sugarless candy, or use of saliva substitutes for xerostomia), or even drug discontinuation.

See Chapter 94, Urinary Incontinence, authored by Eric S. Rovner, Jean Wyman, Thomas Lackner, and David R.P. Guay, for a more detailed discussion of this topic.

APPENDIX

1

Allergic and Pseudoallergic Drug Reactions

TABLE A1–1 Classification of Allergic Drug Reactions

Type	Descriptor	Characteristics	Typical Onset	Drug Causes
I	Anaphylactic (IgE mediated)	Allergen binds to IgE on basophils or mast cells, resulting in release of inflammatory medicators.	Within 30 min to <2 hours	Penicillin immediate reaction Blood products Polypeptide hormones Vaccines Dextran
II	Cytotoxic	Cell destruction occurs because of cell-associated antigen that initiates cytolysis by antigen-specific antibody (IgG or IgM). Most often involves blood elements.	Typically >72 hours	Penicillin, quinidine, heparin, phenylbutazone, thiouracils, sulfonamides, methyldopa
III	Immune complex	Antigen–antibody complexes form and deposit on blood vessel walls and activate complement. Result is a serum sickness-like syndrome.	>72 hours	May be caused by penicillins, sulfonamides, minocycline, hydantoins
IV	Cell-mediated (delayed)	Antigens cause activation of T lymphocytes, which release cytokines and recruit effector cells (e.g., macrophages, eosinophils).	>72 hours	Tuberculin reaction Maculopapular rashes to a variety of drugs; Contact dermatitis Bullous exanthems Pustular exanthems

APPENDICES

TABLE A1–2	Top 10 Drugs or Agents Reported to Cause Skin Reactions

	Reactions per 1,000 Recipients
Amoxicillin	51.4
Trimethoprim–sulfamethoxazole	33.8
Ampicillin	33.2
Iopodate	27.8
Blood	21.6
Cephalosporins	21.1
Erythromycin	20.4
Dihydralazine hydrochloride	19.1
Penicillin G	18.5
Cyanocobalamin	17.9

Data from Roujeau JC, Stern RS. N Engl J Med 1994;331:1272–1285.

TABLE A1–3	Procedure for Performing Penicillin Skin Testing

A. Percutaneous (Prick) Skin Testing

Materials	Volume
Pre-Pen 6×10^6 M (currently not commercially available in the United States)	1 drop
Penicillin G 10,000 units/mL	1 drop
β-Lactam drug 3 mg/mL	1 drop
0.03% albumin-saline control	1 drop
Histamine control (1 mg/mL)	1 drop

1. Place a drop of each test material on the volar surface of the forearm.
2. Prick the skin with a sharp needle inserted through the drop at a 45° angle, gently tenting the skin in an upward motion.
3. Interpret skin responses after 15 minutes.
4. A wheal at least 2×2 mm with erythema is considered positive.
5. If the prick test is nonreactive, proceed to the intradermal test.
6. If the histamine control is nonreactive, the test is considered uninterpretable.

B. Intradermal Skin Testing

Materials	Volume
Pre-Pen 6×10^6 M (currently not commercially available in the United States)	0.02 mL
Penicillin G 10,000 units/mL	0.02 mL
β-Lactam drug 3 mg/mL	0.02 mL
0.03% albumin-saline control	0.02 mL
Histamine control (0.1 mg/mL)	0.02 mL

1. Inject 0.02–0.03 mL of each test material intradermally (amount sufficient to produce a small bleb).
2. Interpret skin responses after 15 minutes.
3. A wheal at least 6×6 mm with erythema and at least 3 mm greater than the negative control is considered positive.
4. If the histamine control is nonreactive, the test is considered uninterpretable.

Antihistamines may blunt the response and cause false-negative reactions.

From Sullivan TJ. Current Therapy in Allergy. St. Louis, MO: Mosby, 1985:57–61, with permission.

TABLE A1–4 Treatment of Anaphylaxis

1. Place patient in recumbent position and elevate lower extremities.
2. Monitor vital signs frequently (every 2–5 minutes) and stay with the patient.
3. Administer epinephrine 1:1,000 into nonoccluded site: (adults: 0.01 mL/kg up to a maximum of 0.2–0.5 mL every 5 minutes as needed, children: 0.01 mL/kg up to a maximum dose of 0.2–0.5 mL) subcutaneously or intramuscularly. If necessary, repeat every 5 minutes, up to 2 doses, then every 4 hours as needed.
4. Administer oxygen, usually 8–10 L/min; however, lower concentrations may be appropriate for patients with chronic obstructive pulmonary disease. Maintain airway with oropharyngeal airway device.
5. Administer the antihistamine diphenhydramine (Benadryl, adults 25–50 mg; children 1–2 mg/kg) usually given parenterally. Apply tourniquet proximal to site of antigen injection; remove every 10–15 minutes. Consider ranitidine 1 mg/kg diluted in D5W to a total volume of 20 mL given IV over 5 minutes.
6. If anaphylaxis is caused by an injection, administer aqueous epinephrine 1:1,000 into site of antigen injection; 0.15–0.3 mL into the injection site.
7. Treat hypotension with IV fluids or colloid replacement, and consider use of a vasopressor such as dopamine.
8. Treat bronchospasm resistant to epinephrine with nebulized albuterol 2.5–5 mg in 3 mL saline every 20 minutes for 3 doses; in children, 0.15 mg/kg via nebulizer every 20 minutes for 3 doses.
9. Give hydrocortisone, 5 mg/kg, or approximately 250 mg IV (prednisone 20 mg orally can be given in mild cases) to reduce the risk of recurring or protracted anaphylaxis. These doses can be repeated every six hours as required.
10. In refractory cases not responding to epinephrine because a β-adrenergic blocker is complicating management, glucagon 1 mg IV as a bolus may be useful. A continuous infusion of glucagon, 1–5 mg/hour, may be given if required.

Reprinted and adapted from J Allergy Clin Immunol 1998;101:S465–S528. Joint Task Force on Practice Parameters for Allergy and Immunology. The diagnosis and management of anaphylaxis: an updated practice parameter. J Allergy Clin Immunol 2005;115:S483–S523.

| TABLE A1–5 | Protocol for Oral Desensitization |

Phenoxymethyl Penicillin

Step[a]	Concentration (units/mL)	Volume (mL)	Dose (units)	Cumulative Dose (units)
1	1,000	0.1	100	100
2	1,000	0.2	200	300
3	1,000	0.4	400	700
4	1,000	0.8	800	1,500
5	1,000	1.6	1,600	3,100
6	1,000	3.2	3,200	6,300
7	1,000	6.4	6,400	12,700
8	10,000	1.2	12,000	24,700
9	10,000	2.4	24,000	48,700
10	10,000	4.8	48,000	96,700
11	80,000	1.0	80,000	176,700
12	80,000	2.0	160,000	336,700
13	80,000	4.0	320,000	656,700
14	80,000	8.0	640,000	1,296,700
		Observe for 30 min		
15	500,000	0.25	125,000	
16	500,000	0.5	250,000	
17	500,000	1.0	500,000	
18	500,000	2.25	1,125,000	

[a]The interval between steps is 15 min.

Reprinted from *Immunol Allerg Clin North*, Vol. 18, Weiss ME, Adkinson NF, Diagnostic Testing for Drug Hypersensivity, *Immunol Allerg Clin North*, 731–734, Copyright © 1998, with permission from Elsevier.

TABLE A1–6	Parenteral Desensitization Protocol		
Injection No.	Benzylpenicillin Concentration (units)	Volume (mL)	Route
1[a,b]	100	0.1	ID
2	100	0.2	SC
3	100	0.4	SC
4	100	0.8	SC
5[b]	1,000	0.1	ID
6	1,000	0.3	SC
7	1,000	0.6	SC
8[b]	10,000	0.1	ID
9	10,000	0.2	SC
10	10,000	0.4	SC
11	10,000	0.8	SC
12[b]	100,000	0.1	ID
13	100,000	0.3	SC
14	100,000	0.6	SC
15[b]	1,000,000	0.1	ID
16	1,000,000	0.2	SC
17	1,000,000	0.2	IM
18	1,000,000	0.4	IM
19	Continuous IV infusion at 1,000,000 units/hour		

[a]Administer doses at intervals of not less than 20 min.
[b]Observe and record skin wheal-and-flare response.
ID, intradermally; IM, intramuscularly; SC, subcutaneously.
Reprinted from Immunol Allerg Clin North, Vol. 18, Weiss ME, Adkinson NF, Diagnostic Testing for Drug Hypersensivity, Immunol Allerg Clin North, 731–734, Copyright © 1998, with permission from Elsevier.

See Chapter 97, Allergic and Pseudoallergic Drug Reactions, authored by Lynne M. Sylvia and Joseph T. DiPiro, for a more detailed discussion of this topic.

Geriatrics

TABLE A2-1	Physiologic Changes with Aging
Organ System	**Manifestation**
Body composition	↓ Total body water
	↓ Lean body mass
	↑ Body fat
	↔ or ↓ Serum albumin
	↑ α_1-Acid glycoprotein (↔ or ↑ by several disease states)
Cardiovascular	↓ Myocardial sensitivity to β-adrenergic stimulation
	↓ Baroreceptor activity
	↓ Cardiac output
	↑ Total peripheral resistance
Central nervous system	↓ Weight and volume of the brain
	Alterations in several aspects of cognition
Endocrine	Thyroid gland atrophies with age
	Increased incidence of diabetes mellitus, thyroid disease
	Menopause
Gastrointestinal	↑ Gastric pH
	↓ Gastrointestinal blood flow
	Delayed gastric emptying
	Slowed intestinal transit
Genitourinary	Atrophy of the vagina because of decreased estrogen
	Prostatic hypertrophy because of androgenic hormonal changes
	Age-related changes may predispose to incontinence
Immune	↓ Cell-mediated immunity
Liver	↓ Hepatic size
	↓ Hepatic blood flow
Oral	Altered dentition
	↓ Ability to taste sweetness, sourness, bitterness
Pulmonary	↓ Respiratory muscle strength
	↓ Chest wall compliance
	↓ Total alveolar surface
	↓ Vital capacity
	↓ Maximal breathing capacity
Renal	↓ Glomerular filtration rate
	↓ Renal blood flow
	↓ Filtration fraction
	↓ Tubular secretory function
	↓ Renal mass
Sensory	↓ Accommodation of the lens of the eye, causing farsightedness
	Presbycusis (loss of auditory acuity)
	↓ Conduction velocity

(continued)

TABLE A2–1	Physiologic Changes with Aging *(Continued)*
Organ System	**Manifestation**
Skeletal	Loss of skeletal bone mass (osteopenia)
Skin/hair	Skin dryness, wrinkling, changes in pigmentation, epithelial thinning, loss of dermal thickness
	↓ Number of hair follicles
	↓ Number of melanocytes in hair bulbs

Data from Kane RI, Ouslander JG, Abrass IB. Clinical implications of the aging process. In: essentials of Clinical Geriatrics, 5th ed. New York: McGraw-Hill, 2004:3–15; and Masoro EJ. Physiology of aging. In: Tallis R, Fillit H, eds. Brocklehurst's Textbook of Geriatric Medicine, 6th ed. London: Churchill-Livingstone, 2003:291–299.

TABLE A2–2	Age-Related Changes in Drug Pharmacokinetics
Pharmacokinetic Phase	**Pharmacokinetic Parameters**
Gastrointestinal absorption	Unchanged passive diffusion and no change in bioavailability for most drugs
	↓ Active transport and ↓ bioavailability for some drugs
	↓ First-pass extraction and ↑ bioavailability for some drugs
Distribution	↓ Volume of distribution and ↑ plasma concentration of water-soluble drugs
	↑ Volume of distribution and ↑ terminal disposition half-life ($t_{1/2}$) for fat-soluble drugs
	↑ or ↓ Free fraction of highly plasma protein-bound drugs
Hepatic metabolism	↓ Clearance and ↑ $t_{1/2}$ for some oxidatively metabolized drugs
	↓ Clearance and ↑ $t_{1/2}$ for drugs with high hepatic extraction ratios
Renal excretion	↓ Clearance and ↑ $t_{1/2}$ for renally eliminated drugs and active metabolites

Data from Cusack BJ. Pharmacokinetics in older persons. Am J Geriatr Pharm 2004;2:274–302; and Chapron DJ. Drug disposition and response. In: Delafuente JC, Stewart RB, eds. Therapeutics in the Elderly, 3rd ed. Cincinnati, OH: Harvey Whitney, 2000:257–288.

TABLE A2–3 Atypical Disease Presentation in Older Adults

Disease	Presentation
Acute myocardial infarction	Only ~50% present with chest pain. In general, older adults present with weakness, confusion, syncope, and abdominal pain; however, electrocardiographic findings are similar to those in younger patients.
Congestive heart failure	Instead of dyspnea, the older patient may present with hypoxic symptoms, lethargy, restlessness, and confusion.
Gastrointestinal bleed	Although the mortality rate is ~10%, presenting symptoms are nonspecific, ranging from altered mental status to syncope with hemodynamic collapse. Abdominal pain often is absent.
Upper respiratory infection	Older patients typically present with lethargy, confusion, anorexia, and decompensation of a preexisting medical condition. Fever, chills, and a productive cough may or may not be present.
Urinary tract infection	Dysuria, fever, and flank pain may be absent. More commonly, older adults present with incontinence, confusion, abdominal pain, nausea/vomiting, and azotemia.

Data from Fried LP, Storer DJ, King DE, et al. Diagnosis of illness presentation in the elderly. J Am Geriatr Soc 1991;39:117–123; and Jarrett PG, Rockwood K, Carver D, et al. Illness presentation in elderly patients. Arch Intern Med 1995;155:1060–1064.

TABLE A2–4 Inappropriate Medication Use in Nursing Homes Defined by CMS Criteria 2006

Antiinfective: Nitrofurantoin
Cardiovascular: Amiodarone (unless VT/Fib), disopyramide, methyldopa, nifedipine (SA), prazosin
Antiplatelets: Ticlopidine
Gastrointestinal: Antispasmodics (e.g., Donnatal), cimetidine, metoclopramide, trimethobenzamide (Tigan)

Analgesics: NSAIDs, propoxyphene, pentazocine, long-acting opioids (fentanyl patch, methadone, SR products)
Oral hypoglycemics: Chlorpropamide, glyburide
Psychotropics: Barbiturates, meprobamate, TCAs, MAOIs
Skeletal Muscle Relaxants Antihistamines: Chlorpheniramine, cyproheptadine, diphenhydramine, hydroxyzine, meclizine, promethazine

Data from Center for Medicaid & Medicare Services. Unnecessary Medication Use (Tag F329), 2007. http://www.cms.hhs.gov/transmittals/downloads/R22SOMA.pdf.

TABLE A2–5 Centers for Medicare and Medicaid Services Guidelines for Monitoring Medication Use

Drug	Monitoring	Monitoring Interval (in months)
Acetaminophen (>4 g/d)	Hepatic function tests	a
Amiodarone	Hepatic function tests, thyroid stimulating hormone level	6
Antiepileptic agents (carbamazepine, phenobarbital, phenytoin, primidone, valproate)	Drug levels	3–6
Angiotensin-converting enzyme inhibitors or Angiotensin I receptor blockers	Potassium levels	6
Antipsychotic agents	Extrapyramidal side effects, fasting serum glucose, serum lipid panel	6
Appetite stimulants	Weight, appetite	a
Digoxin	Serum blood urea nitrogen, creatinine, trough drug level	6
Diuretic	Serum sodium and potassium levels	3
Erythropoiesis stimulants	Blood pressure, iron and ferritin levels, complete blood count	1
Fibrates	Hepatic function test, complete blood count	6
Hypoglycemic agents	Fasting serum glucose level or glycated hemoglobin level	6
Iron	Iron and ferritin levels, complete blood count	a
Lithium	Trough serum drug levels	3
Metformin	Serum blood urea nitrogen, creatinine levels	
Niacin	Blood sugar levels, hepatic function tests	6
Statins	Hepatic function tests	6
Theophylline	Trough serum drug levels	3
Thyroid replacement	Thyroid stimulating hormone level on tests	6
Warfarin	Prothrombin time/international normalized ratio	1

aConsensus agreement about interval could not be reached.

Data from Center for Medicaid and Medicare Services. Unnecessary Medication Use (Tag F329), 2007. http://www.cms.hhs.gov/transmittals/downloads/R22SOMA.pdf; and Handler SM, Shirts BH, Perera S, et al. Frequency of laboratory monitoring of chronic medications administered to nursing facility residents: results of a national internet-based study. Consult Pharm 2008;23:387–395.

TABLE A2–6	Clinically Important Drug–Disease Interactions Determined by Expert Panel Consensus

Drug	Disease
Alpha-adrenergic blockers	Syncope
Anticholinergic agents	Benign prostatic hyperplasia, constipation, dementia, glaucoma (narrow-angle)
Aspirin	Peptic ulcer disease
Barbiturates	Dementia
Benzodiazepines	Dementia, falls
Bupropion	Seizures
Calcium channel blockers (first-generation)	Heart failure (systolic dysfunction)
Corticosteroids	Diabetes mellitus
Digoxin	Heart block
Metoclopramide	Parkinson disease
Nonaspirin nonsteroidal antiinflammatory drugs	Chronic renal failure, peptic ulcer disease
Opioid analgesics	Constipation
Sedative/hypnotics	Falls
Thioridazine	Postural hypotension
Tricyclic antidepressants	Benign prostatic hyperplasia, constipation dementia, falls, heart block, postural hypotension
Typical (first-generation) antipsychotics	Falls

Data from Lindblad CI, Hanlon JT, Gross CR, et al. Clinically important drug-disease interactions and their prevalence in older adults. Clin Ther 2006;28:1133–1143.

See Chapter 11, Geriatrics, authored by Emily R. Hajjar, Shelly L. Gray, David R.P. Guay, Catherine I. Starner, Steven M. Handler, and Joseph T. Hanlon, for a more detailed discussion of this topic.

APPENDIX 3

Drug-Induced Hematologic Disorders

TABLE A3-1 Drugs Associated with Aplastic Anemias

Observational Study Evidence	Case Report Evidence (*Probable* or *Definite* Causality Rating)
Carbamazepine	Acetazolamide
Furosemide	Aspirin
Gold salts	Captopril
Mebendazole	Chloramphenicol
Methimazole	Chloroquine
NSAIDs	Chlorothiazide
Oxyphenbutazone	Chlorpromazine
Penicillamine	Dapsone
Phenobarbital	Felbamate
Phenothiazines	Interferon alfa
Phenytoin	Lisinopril
Propylthiouracil	Lithium
Sulfonamides	Nizatidine
Thiazides	Pentoxifylline
Tocainide	Quinidine
	Sulindac
	Ticlopidine

NSAID, nonsteroidal antiinflammatory drug.

TABLE A3–2 Drugs Associated with Agranulocytosis

Observational Study Evidence	Case Report Evidence (*Probable* or *Definite* Causality Rating)	
β-Lactam antibiotics	Acetaminophen	Levodopa
Carbamazepine	Acetazolamide	Meprobamate
Carbimazole	Ampicillin	Methazolamide
Clomipramine	Captopril	Methyldopa
Digoxin	Carbenicillin	Metronidazole
Dipyridamole	Cefotaxime	Nafcillin
Ganciclovir	Cefuroxime	NSAIDs
Glyburide	Chloramphenicol	Olanzapine
Gold salts	Chlorpromazine	Oxacillin
Imipenem-cilastatin	Chlorpropamide	Penicillamine
Indomethacin	Chlorpheniramine	Penicillin G
Macrolide antibiotics	Clindamycin	Pentazocine
Methimazole	Clozapine	Phenytoin
Mirtazapine	Colchicine	Primidone
Phenobarbital	Doxepin	Procainamide
Phenothiazines	Dapsone	Propylthiouracil
Prednisone	Desipramine	Pyrimethamine
Propranolol	Ethacrynic acid	Quinidine
Spironolactone	Ethosuximide	Quinine
Sulfonamides	Flucytosine	Rifampin
Sulfonylureas	Gentamicin	Streptomycin
Ticlopidine	Griseofulvin	Terbinafine
Valproic acid	Hydralazine	Ticarcillin
Zidovudine	Hydroxychloroquine	Tocainide
	Imipenem-cilastatin	Tolbutamide
	Imipramine	Vancomycin
	Lamotrigine	

NSAID, nonsteroidal antiinflammatory drug.

TABLE A3–3 Drugs Associated with Hemolytic Anemia

Observational study evidence
Phenobarbital
Phenytoin
Ribavirin

Case report evidence *(probable* or *definite* causality rating)
Acetaminophen
Angiotensin-converting enzyme inhibitors
β-Lactam antibiotics
Cephalosporins
Ciprofloxacin
Clavulanate
Erythromycin
Hydrochlorothiazide
Indinavir
Interferon alfa
Ketoconazole
Lansoprazole
Levodopa
Levofloxacin
Methyldopa
Minocycline
NSAIDs
Omeprazole
p-Aminosalicylic acid
Phenazopyridine
Probenecid
Procainamide
Quinidine
Rifabutin
Rifampin
Streptomycin
Sulbactam
Sulfonamides
Sulfonylureas
Tacrolimus
Tazobactam
Teicoplanin
Tolbutamide
Tolmetin
Triamterene

NSAID, nonsteroidal antiinflammatory drug.

TABLE A3–4	Drugs Associated with Oxidative Hemolytic Anemia

Observational study evidence
Dapsone

Case report evidence (*probable* or *definite* causality rating)
Ascorbic acid
Metformin
Methylene blue
Nalidixic acid
Nitrofurantoin
Phenazopyridine
Primaquine
Sulfacetamide
Sulfamethoxazole
Sulfanilamide

TABLE A3–5	Drugs Associated with Megaloblastic Anemia

Case Report Evidence (*Probable* or *Definite* Causality Rating)

Azathioprine
Chloramphenicol
Colchicine
Cotrimoxazole
Cyclophosphamide
Cytarabine
5-Fluorodeoxyuridine
5-Fluorouracil
Hydroxyurea
6-Mercaptopurine
Methotrexate
Oral contraceptives
p-Aminosalicylate
Phenobarbital
Phenytoin
Primidone
Pyrimethamine
Sulfasalazine
Tetracycline
Vinblastine

TABLE A3–6 Drugs Associated with Thrombocytopenia

Observational study evidence	Diazoxide	Morphine
Carbamazepine	Diclofenac	Nalidixic acid
Phenobarbital	Diethylstilbestrol	Naphazoline
Phenytoin	Digoxin	Naproxen
Valproic acid	Ethambutol	Nitroglycerin
	Felbamate	Octreotide
Case report evidence	Fluconazole	Oxacillin
(*probable* or *definite*	Gold salts	p-Aminosalicylic acid
causality rating)	Haloperidol	Penicillamine
Abciximab	Heparin	Pentoxifylline
Acetaminophen	Hydrochlorothiazide	Piperacillin
Acyclovir	Ibuprofen	Primidone
Albendazole	Inamrinone	Procainamide
Aminoglutethimide	Indinavir	Pyrazinamide
Aminosalicylic acid	Indomethacin	Quinidine
Amiodarone	Interferonalfa	Quinine
Amphotericin B	Isoniazid	Ranitidine
Ampicillin	Isotretinoin	Recombinant hepatitis B
Aspirin	Itraconazole	vaccine
Atorvastatin	Levamisole	Rifampin
Captopril	Linezolid	Simvastatin
Chlorothiazide	Lithium	Sirolimus
Chlorpromazine	Low-molecular-weight	Sulfasalazine
Chlorpropamide	heparins	Sulfonamides
Cimetidine	Measles, mumps, and rubella	Sulindac
Ciprofloxacin	vaccine	Tamoxifen
Clarithromycin	Meclofenamate	Tolmetin
Clopidogrel	Mesalamine	Trimethoprim
Danazol	Methyldopa	Vancomycin
Deferoxamine	Minoxidil	
Diazepam		

See Chapter 112, Drug-Induced Hematologic Disorders, authored by Christine N. Hansen and Amy F. Rosenberg, for a more detailed discussion of this topic.

TABLE A4–1 An Approach to Evaluating a Suspected Hepatotoxic Reaction Using a Clinical Diagnostic Scale

Patient Presents with Elevated Liver Enzymes	Score	Component Subscore
Literature		
Literature supports this drug (drug combination) and pattern of liver enzyme elevation	+2	
No literature supports this, but the drug has been on the market less than 5 years	+0	–
No literature supports this and the drug has been on the market for 5 years or more	–3	
Alternative causes		
Alternative causes (e.g., viral, alcohol) are completely ruled out	+3	
Alternative causes are partially ruled out	+0	–
Alternative causes cannot be ruled out and are possible or even probable	–1	
Presentation		
The presentation includes 4 or more extrahepatic (fever, malaise, etc.) symptoms	+3	
The presentation includes 2–3 extrahepatic symptoms	+2	–
The presentation includes only 1 identifiable extrahepatic symptom	+1	
The presentation is essentially a laboratory abnormality, with no extrahepatic symptoms	+0	
Temporality		
Initiation of drug therapy to onset is 4–56 days	+3	
Initiation of drug therapy to onset is <4 or >56 days	+1	
Discontinuance of therapy to onset is 0–7 days	+3	–
Discontinuance of therapy to onset is 8–15 days	+0	
Discontinuance of therapy to onset is >15 days	–1	
Rechallenge		
Rechallenge was positive	+3	–
Rechallenge was negative or not attempted	+0	
Total Score		–

The likelihood that this presentation is an adverse reaction in the liver increases linearly with an increasing score. The maximum score is 14, and scores below 7 are associated with an ever decreasing likelihood that the drug or drug combination in question caused the problem. This approach is not designed for the assessment of hepatic cancers or cirrhotic conditions.

Reprinted from J Clin Epidemiol, Vol 46, Danan G, Benichou C. Causality assessment of adverse reactions to drugs–I. A novel method based on the conclusions of international consensus meetings: Application to drug-induced liver injuries: pages 1323–1330, Copyright © 1993, with permission from Elsevier.

TABLE A4–2	Environmental Hepatotoxins and Associated Occupations at Risk for Exposure
Hepatotoxin	**Associated Occupations at Risk for Exposure**
Arsenic	Chemical plant, agricultural workers
Carbon tetrachloride	Chemical plant workers, laboratory technicians
Copper	Plumbers, sculpture artists, foundry workers
Dimethylformamide	Chemical plant workers, laboratory technicians
2,4-Dichlorophenoxyacetic acid	Horticulturists
Fluorine	Chemical plant workers, laboratory technicians
Toluene	Chemical plant, agricultural workers, laboratory tech
Trichloroethylene	Printers, dye workers, cleaners, laboratory technicians
Vinyl chloride	Plastics plant workers; also found as a river pollutant

TABLE A4–3	Relative Patterns of Hepatic Enzyme Elevation versus Type of Hepatic Lesion			
Enzyme	**Abbreviations**	**Necrotic**	**Cholestatic**	**Chronic**
Alkaline phosphatase	Alk Phos, AP	↑	↑↑↑	↑
5′-Nucleotidase	5-NC, 5NC	↑	↑↑↑	↑
γ-Glutamyltransferase	GGT, GGTP	↑	↑↑↑	↑↑
Aspartate aminotransferase	AST, SGOT	↑↑↑	↑	↑↑
Alanine aminotransferase	ALT, SGPT	↑↑↑	↑	↑↑
Lactate dehydrogenase	LDH	↑↑↑	↑	↑

↑, <100% of normal; ↑↑, >100% of normal, ↑↑↑, >200% of normal.

TABLE A4–4	An Approach to Determining a Drug-Monitoring Plan to Detect Hepatotoxicity in Patients Initiated on Hepatotoxic Drugs

Draw a baseline set of blood samples for liver enzymes, bilirubin, and albumin before beginning the drug

↓

Is the patient pregnant?
Is the patient older than age 60 years?
Is the patient exposed to an environmental hepatotoxin at work or at home?
Is the patient drinking more than one alcoholic beverage per day or bingeing?
Is the patient using any injected recreational drug?
Is the patient using herbal remedies or tisanes that are associated with hepatic damage?
Is the patient's diet deficient in magnesium, vitamin E, vitamin C, or α- or β-carotenes?
Is the patient's diet excessive in vitamin A, iron, or selenium?
Does the patient have hypertriglyceridemia or type 2 diabetes mellitus?
Does the patient have juvenile arthritis or systemic lupus erythematosus?
Does the patient have chronic or chronic remitting viral hepatitis (hepatitis B or C)?

↓

Yes to one to two risk factors	No
↓	↓
Redraw liver enzymes every 180 days depending on the drug, for the first year	Redraw liver enzymes if other signs or symptoms manifest

Does the patient have more than two risk factors?
Is the drug identified as one that may cause a predictable hepatotoxic reaction?[a]

Yes	No	No
↓	↓	↓
Redraw liver enzymes every 60–90 days depending on the drug, for the first year	Redraw liver enzymes every 180 days as directed above for the first year	Redraw liver enzymes if other signs or symptoms manifest

If no toxicity is manifested during the first year of therapy, then redraw liver enzymes every 6–12 months; assess liver for cirrhosis every 1–2 years by ultrasound and every 4–6 years by CT or MRI scan; biopsy as directed by other findings

[a]A drug can become a predictable risk if it is administered concurrently with another drug or food that is known to induce or inhibit its metabolism.

See Chapter 45, Drug-Induced Liver Disease, authored by William R. Kirchain and Rondall E. Allen, for a more detailed discussion of this topic.

Drug-Induced Pulmonary Disease

TABLE A5–1 Drugs That Induce Apnea	
	Relative Frequency of Reactions
Central nervous system depression	
Narcotic analgesics	F
Barbiturates	F
Benzodiazepines	F
Other sedatives and hypnotics	I
Tricyclic antidepressants	R
Phenothiazines	R
Ketamine	R
Promazine	R
Anesthetics	R
Antihistamines	R
Alcohol	I
Fenfluramine	R
L-Dopa	R
Oxygen	R
Respiratory muscle dysfunction	
Aminoglycoside antibiotics	I
Polymyxin antibiotics	I
Neuromuscular blockers	I
Quinine	R
Digitalis	R
Myopathy	
Corticosteroids	F
Diuretics	I
Aminocaproic acid	R
Clofibrate	R

F, frequent; I, infrequent; R, rare.

TABLE A5–2 Drugs That Induce Bronchospasm

	Relative Frequency of Reactions
Anaphylaxis (IgE-mediated)	
Penicillins	F
Sulfonamides	F
Serum	F
Cephalosporins	F
Bromelin	R
Cimetidine	R
Papain	F
Pancreatic extract	I
Psyllium	I
Subtilase	I
Tetracyclines	I
Allergen extracts	I
L-Asparaginase	F
Pyrazolone analgesics	I
Direct airway irritation	
Acetate	R
Bisulfite	F
Cromolyn	R
Smoke	F
N-acetylcysteine	F
Inhaled steroids	I
Precipitating IgG antibodies	
β-Methyldopa	R
Carbamazepine	R
Spiramycin	R
Cyclooxygenase inhibition	
Aspirin/nonsteroidal antiinflammatory drugs	F
Phenylbutazone	I
Acetaminophen	R
Anaphylactoid mast-cell degranulation	
Narcotic analgesics	I
Ethylenediamine	R
Iodinated-radiocontrast media	F
Platinum	R
Local anesthetics	I
Steroidal anesthetics	I
Iron–dextran complex	I
Pancuronium bromide	R
Benzalkonium chloride	I
Pharmacologic effects	
α-Adrenergic receptor blockers	I–F
Cholinergic stimulants	I
Anticholinesterases	R
β-Adrenergic agonists	R
Ethylenediamine tetraacetic acid	R

(continued)

TABLE A5-2 Drugs That Induce Bronchospasm *(Continued)*	
	Relative Frequency of Reactions
Unknown mechanisms	
Angiotensin-converting enzyme inhibitors	I
Anticholinergics	R
Hydrocortisone	R
Isoproterenol	R
Monosodium glutamate	I
Piperazine	R
Tartrazine	R
Sulfinpyrazone	R
Zinostatin	R
Losartan	R

F, frequent; I, infrequent; R, rare.

TABLE A5-3 Tolerance of Antiinflammatory and Analgesic Drugs in Aspirin-Induced Asthma	
Cross-Reactive Drugs	**Drugs with No Cross-Reactivity**
Diclofenac	Acetaminophen[a]
Diflunisal	Benzydamine
Fenoprofen	Chloroquine
Flufenamic acid	Choline salicylate
Flurbiprofen	Corticosteroids
Hydrocortisone hemisuccinate	Dextropropoxyphene
Ibuprofen	Phenacetin[a]
Indomethacin	Salicylamide
Ketoprofen	Sodium salicylate
Mefenamic acid	
Naproxen	
Noramidopyrine	
Oxyphenbutazone	
Phenylbutazone	
Piroxicam	
Sulindac	
Sulfinpyrazone	
Tartrazine	
Tolmetin	

[a]A very small percentage (5%) of aspirin-sensitive patients react to acetaminophen and phenacetin.

TABLE A5–4	Drugs That Induce Pulmonary Edema	
	Relative Frequency of Reactions	
Cardiogenic pulmonary edema		
Excessive intravenous fluids	F	
Blood and plasma transfusions	F	
Corticosteroids	F	
Phenylbutazone	R	
Sodium diatrizoate	R	
Hypertonic intrathecal saline	R	
β_2-Adrenergic agonists	I	
Noncardiogenic pulmonary edema		
Heroin	F	
Methadone	I	
Morphine	I	
Oxygen	I	
Propoxyphene	R	
Ethchlorvynol	R	
Chlordiazepoxide	R	
Salicylate	R	
Hydrochlorothiazide	R	
Triamterene + hydrochlorothiazide	R	
Leukoagglutinin reactions	R	
Iron–dextran complex	R	
Methotrexate	R	
Cytosine arabinoside	R	
Nitrofurantoin	R	
Dextran 40	R	
Fluorescein	R	
Amitriptyline	R	
Colchicine	R	
Nitrogen mustard	R	
Epinephrine	R	
Metaraminol	R	
Bleomycin	R	
Iodide	R	
Cyclophosphamide	R	
VM-26	R	

F, frequent; I, infrequent; R, rare.

TABLE A5–5	Drugs That Induce Pulmonary Infiltrates with Eosinophilia (Löffler Syndrome)		
Drug	**Relative Frequency of Reactions**	**Drug**	**Relative Frequency of Reactions**
Nitrofurantoin	F	Imipramine	I
para-Aminosalicylic acid	F	Minocycline	I
		Nilutamide	I
Amiodarone	F	Propylthiouracil	I
Iodine	F	Sulfazalazine	I
Captopril	F	Tetracycline	R
Bleomycin	F	Procarbazine	R
L-tryptophan	F	Cromolyn	R
Methotrexate	F	Niridazole	R
Phenytoin	F	Chlorpromazine	R
Gold salts	F	Naproxen	R
Sulfonamides	I	Sulindac	R
Penicillins	I	Ibuprofen	R
Carbamazepine	I	Chlorpropamide	R
Granulocyte-macrophage colony stimulating factor	I	Mephenesin	R

F, frequent; I, infrequent; R, rare.

TABLE A5–6	Drugs That Induce Pneumonitis and Fibrosis		
Drug	**Relative Frequency of Reactions**	**Drug**	**Relative Frequency of Reactions**
Oxygen	F	Chlorambucil	R
Radiation	F	Melphalan	R
Bleomycin	F	Lomustine and semustine	R
Busulfan	F		
Carmustine	F	Zinostatin	R
Hexamethonium	F	Procarbazine	R
Paraquat	F	Teniposide	R
Amiodarone	F	Sulfasalazine	R
Mecamylamine	I	Phenytoin	R
Pentolinium	I	Gold salts	R
Cyclophosphamide	I	Pindolol	R
Practolol	I	Imipramine	R
Methotrexate	I	Penicillamine	R
Mitomycin	I	Phenylbutazone	R
Nitrofurantoin	I	Chlorphentermine	R
Methysergide	I	Fenfluramine	R
Sirolimus	I	Leflunomide	R
Azathioprine, 6-mercaptopurine	R	Mefloquine	R
		Pergolide	R

F, frequent; I, infrequent; R, rare.

TABLE A5–7 Possible Causes of Pulmonary Fibrosis

Idiopathic pulmonary fibrosis (fibrosing alveolitis)
Pneumoconiosis (asbestosis, silicosis, coal dust, talc berylliosis)
Hypersensitivity pneumonitis (molds, bacteria, animal proteins, toluene
   diisocyanate, epoxy resins)
Smoking
Sarcoidosis
Tuberculosis
Lipoid pneumonia
Systemic lupus erythematosus
Rheumatoid arthritis
Systemic sclerosis
Polymyositis/dermatomyositis
Sjägren syndrome
Polyarteritis nodosa
Wegener granuloma
Byssinosis (cotton workers)
Siderosis (arc welders' lung)
Radiation
Oxygen
Chemicals (thioureas, trialkylphosphorothioates, furans)
Drugs (see Tables A5–5, A5–6, and A5–8)

TABLE A5–8	Drugs That May Induce Pleural Effusions and Fibrosis	
	Relative Frequency of Reactions	
Idiopathic		
Methysergide	F	
Practolol	F	
Pindolol	R	
Methotrexate	R	
Nitrofurantoin	R	
Drug-induced lupus syndrome		
Procainamide	F	
Hydralazine	F	
Isoniazid	R	
Phenytoin	R	
Mephenytoin	R	
Griseofulvin	R	
Trimethadione	R	
Sulfonamides	R	
Phenylbutazone	R	
Streptomycin	R	
Ethosuximide	R	
Tetracycline	R	
Pseudolymphoma syndrome		
Cyclosporine	R	
Phenytoin	R	

F, frequent; I, infrequent; R, rare.

See Chapter 36, Drug-Induced Pulmonary Disease, authored by Hengameh H. Raissy, Michelle Harkins, and Patricia L. Marshik, for a more detailed discussion of this topic.

TABLE A6–1 Drug-Induced Renal Structural–Functional Alterations and Examples

Tubular epithelial cell damage

Acute tubular necrosis
- Aminoglycoside antibiotics
- Radiographic contrast media
- Cisplatin, carboplatin
- Amphotericin B
- Cyclosporine, tacrolimus
- Adefovir, cidofovir, tenofovir

- Pentamidine
- Foscarnet
- Zoledronate
Osmotic nephrosis
- Mannitol
- Dextran
- Intravenous immunoglobulin

Hemodynamically-mediated kidney injury

- Angiotensin-converting enzyme inhibitors
- Angiotensin II receptor blockers
- Nonsteroidal anti-inflammatory drugs

- Cyclosporine, tacrolimus
- OKT3

Obstructive nephropathy

Intratubular obstruction
- Acyclovir
- Sulfonamides
- Indinavir
- Foscarnet
- Methotrexate

Nephrolithiasis
- Sulfonamides
- Triamterene
- Indinavir
Nephrocalcinosis
- Oral sodium phosphate solution

Glomerular disease

- Gold
- Lithium

- Nonsteroidal antiinflammatory drugs, cyclooxygenase-2 inhibitors
- Pamidronate

Tubulointerstitial disease

Acute allergic interstitial nephritis
- Penicillins
- Ciprofloxacin
- Nonsteroidal anti-inflammatory drugs, cyclooxygenase-2 inhibitors
- Proton pump inhibitors
- Loop diuretics

Chronic interstitial nephritis
- Cyclosporine
- Lithium
- Aristolochic acid
Papillary necrosis
- NSAIDs, combined phenacetin, aspirin, and caffeine analgesics

Renal vasculitis, thrombosis, and cholesterol emboli

Vasculitis and thrombosis
- Hydralazine
- Propylthiouracil
- Allopurinol
- Penicillamine
- Gemcitabine
- Mitomycin C

- Methamphetamines
- Cyclosporine, tacrolimus
- Adalimumab
- Bevacizumab
Cholesterol emboli
- Warfarin
- Thrombolytic agents

TABLE A6–2	Potential Risk Factors for Aminoglycoside Nephrotoxicity

A. Related to aminoglycoside dosing:
   Large total cumulative dose
   Prolonged therapy
   Trough concentration exceeding 2 mg/L[a]
   Recent previous aminoglycoside therapy
B. Related to synergistic nephrotoxicity. Aminoglycosides in combination with
   Cyclosporine
   Amphotericin B
   Vancomycin
   Diuretics
   Iodinated radiographic contrast agents
   Cisplatin
   NSAIDs
C. Related to predisposing conditions in the patient:
   Preexisting kidney disease
   Diabetes
   Increased age
   Poor nutrition
   Shock
   Gram-negative bacteremia
   Liver disease
   Hypoalbuminemia
   Obstructive jaundice
   Dehydration
   Hypotension
   Potassium or magnesium deficiencies

[a]The equivalent concentration in SI molar units are 4.3 μmol/L for tobramycin, 4.2 μmol/L for gentamicin, and 1.4 μmol/L for vancomycin.

TABLE A6–3	Recommended Interventions for Prevention of Contrast Nephrotoxicity	
Intervention	**Recommendation**	**Recommendation Grade[a]**
Contrast	• Minimize contrast volume/dose	A-1
	• Use noniodinated contrast studies	A-2
	• Use low- or iso-osmolar contrast agents	A-2
Medications	• Avoid concurrent use of potentially nephrotoxic drugs, e.g., NSAIDs, aminoglycosides	A-2
Isotonic sodium chloride (0.9%)	• Initiate infusion 3–12 hours prior to contrast exposure and continue 6–24 hours postexposure	A-1
	• Infuse at 1–1.5 mL/kg/hour adjusting postexposure as needed to maintain urine flow rate of ≥150 mL/hour	
	• Alternatively, in urgent cases, initiate infusion at 3 mL/kg/hour, beginning 1 hour prior to contrast exposure, then continue at 1 mL/kg/hour for 6 hours postexposure	
Isotonic sodium bicarbonate [154 mEq/L (154 mmol/L)]	• Initiate and maintain infusion as per isotonic sodium chloride above	B-2
	• Alternatively, initiate infusion at 3 mL/kg/hour, beginning 1 hour prior to contrast exposure, then continue at 1 mL/kg/hour for 6 hours postexposure	
N-acetylcysteine	• Administer 600–1,200 mg by mouth (PO) every 12 hours, 4 doses beginning prior to contrast exposure (i.e., 1 dose prior to exposure and 3 doses postexposure)	B-1

[a]Strength of recommendations: A, B, and C are good, moderate, and poor evidence to support recommendation, respectively. Quality of evidence: 1, evidence from more than 1 properly randomized, controlled trial; 2, evidence from more than 1 well-designed clinical trial with randomization, from cohort or case-controlled analytic studies or multiple time series, or dramatic results from uncontrolled experiments; 3 evidence from opinions of respected authorities, based on clinical experience, descriptive studies, or reports of expert communities.

Data from Barrett BJ, Parfrey PS. Clinical practice. Preventing nephropathy induced by contrast medium. N Engl J Med 2006;354:379–386; McCullough PA. Contrast-induced acute kidney injury. J Am Coll Cardiol 2008;51:1419–1428; Fishbane S. N-acetylcysteine in the prevention of contrast-induced nephropathy. Clin J Am Soc Nephrol 2008;3:281–287; Weisbord SD, Palevsky PM. Prevention of contrast-induced nephropathy with volume expansion. Clin J Am Soc Nephrol 2008;3:273–280; Briguori C, Airoldi F, D'Andrea D, et al. Renal Insufficiency Following Contrast Media Administration Trial (REMEDIAL): A randomized comparison of 3 preventive strategies. Circulation 2007;115:1211–1217; and Schweiger MJ, Chambers CE, Davidson CJ, et al. Prevention of contrast induced nephropathy: Recommendations for the high risk patient undergoing cardiovascular procedures. Catheter Cardiovasc Interv 2006;69:135–140.

TABLE A6–4 Drugs Associated with Allergic Interstitial Nephritis

Antimicrobials

Acyclovir	Indinavir
Aminoglycosides	Rifampin
Amphotericin B	Sulfonamides
β-Lactams	Tetracyclines
Erythromycin	Trimethoprim-sulfamethoxazole
Ethambutol	Vancomycin

Diuretics

Acetazolamide	Loop diuretics
Amiloride	Triamterene
Chlorthalidone	Thiazide diuretics

Neuropsychiatric

Carbamazepine	Phenytoin
Lithium	Valproic acid
Phenobarbital	

Nonsteroidal antiinflammatory drugs

Aspirin	Ketoprofen
Indomethacin	Phenylbutazone
Naproxen	Diclofenac
Ibuprofen	Zomepirac
Diflunisal	Cyclooxygenase-2 inhibitors
Piroxicam	

Miscellaneous

Acetaminophen	Lansoprazole
Allopurinol	Methyldopa
Interferon-alfa	Omeprazole
Aspirin	P-aminosalicylic acid
Azathioprine	Phenylpropanolamine
Captopril	Propylthiouracil
Cimetidine	Radiographic contrast media
Clofibrate	Ranitidine
Cyclosporine	Sulfinpyrazone
Glyburide	Warfarin sodium
Gold	

See Chapter 55, Drug-Induced Kidney Disease, authored by Thomas D. Nolin and Jonathan Himmelfarb, for a more detailed discussion of this topic.

Index

Page numbers followed by *f* or *t* indicate figures or tables, respectively.

1097

Index

Index

Index

Index

Index

Index

Index

Index

Index

Index

Index

Index

Index

Nateglinide in diabetes mellitus, 224, 226*t*
National Asthma Education and
Prevention Program, 1013,
1019*f*, 1020*f*
National Cholesterol Education
Program, 60, 146*f*, 167
Adult Treatment Panel III, 88, 235
Nausea and vomiting
antiemetic use
in children, 319
during pregnancy, 318–319
chemotherapy-induced, 316
clinical presentation in, 308
desired outcome, 308
disorders of balance, 318
dosage recommendations for
chemotherapy-induced nausea
and vomiting (CINV) for adult
patients, 317*t*
drug class information for, 312–316
emetogenicity of chemotherapeutic
agents, 310*t*–311*t*
etiologies associated with, 308, 309*t*
nonchemotherapy etiologies of, 311*t*
pharmacologic management, 311
postoperative, 316, 318*t*
presentation of, 312
radiation-induced, 318
treatment of, general approach to 309
Necrolysis, toxic epidermal, 194
Necrotizing fasciitis, 525, 560*t*
Nefazodone
as antidepressant, 890*t*
in depression, 868, 877*t*, 890*t*
and cytochrome P450 activity, 890*t*
pharmacokinetics of, 885*t*
side effects of, 1048*t*
Neisseria gonorrhoeae infections. *See*
Gonorrhea
Neisseria meningitidis, 414
Infections, 411
Nelfinavir
in HIV infection, 476*t*, 478*t*
pharmacologic characteristics of, 478*t*
Neomycin
in colorectal surgery, 581
as poliovirus vaccine, 632
as rubella vaccine, 632
in surgical site infections, 577*t*
Nephritis, allergic interstitial, drugs
associated with, 1092*t*, 1095*t*

Nephrolithiasis in gout, 6
Nephropathy
in acute kidney injury, 952
in diabetes mellitus, 217, 234
in hyperglycemia, 961
renal structural–functional
alterations, 1092*t*
uric acid, 2
Nephrotoxin
in acute kidney injury, 954
interactions with other drugs, 406*t*
Nesiritide
in heart failure, 112–113
Netilmicin chronic kidney disease, 981*t*
dose adjustment in, 981*t*
Neurofibrillary tangles in Alzheimer's
disease, 635
Neurokinin₁ receptor antagonists in
nausea and vomiting, 315
Neuroleptic malignant syndrome,
906–909
Neurologic disorders, 635–714
Alzheimer's disease (AD), 635–643
from antipsychotic drugs, 875*t*
anxiety symptoms, 641*t*
in central nervous system infections,
410–411
coccidioidomycosis, 447–449
cryptococcal, 449–450
epilepsy, 644–669
and status epilepticus, 715–724
headache in, 670–685
Parkinson's disease, 706–714
Neuropathy
diabetic, 234, 686
optic, in glaucoma, 819
Neurosurgery, surgical site infections in,
580*t*, 583
Neurosyphilis, 405*t*, 546*t*, 547, 548*t*, 852*t*
Neutropenia, 6
Neutrophil count in infections, 399
Nevirapine in HIV infection, 474*t*, 478*t*
Niacin in hyperlipidemia, 92, 974
in cardiovascular disorders, 92–94
in combination therapy, 97
and coronary artery disease, 235
in dyslipidemia treatment, 93*t*, 97
in hypercholesterolemia, 96
myocardial infarction, secondary
prevention, 60
Nicardipine in hypertension, 119*t*, 134*t*

Index

Index

Index